SECOND EDITION

BREASTFEEDING ANSWERS

A Guide for Helping Families

SECOND EDITION

BREASTFEEDING ANSWERS

A Guide for Helping Families

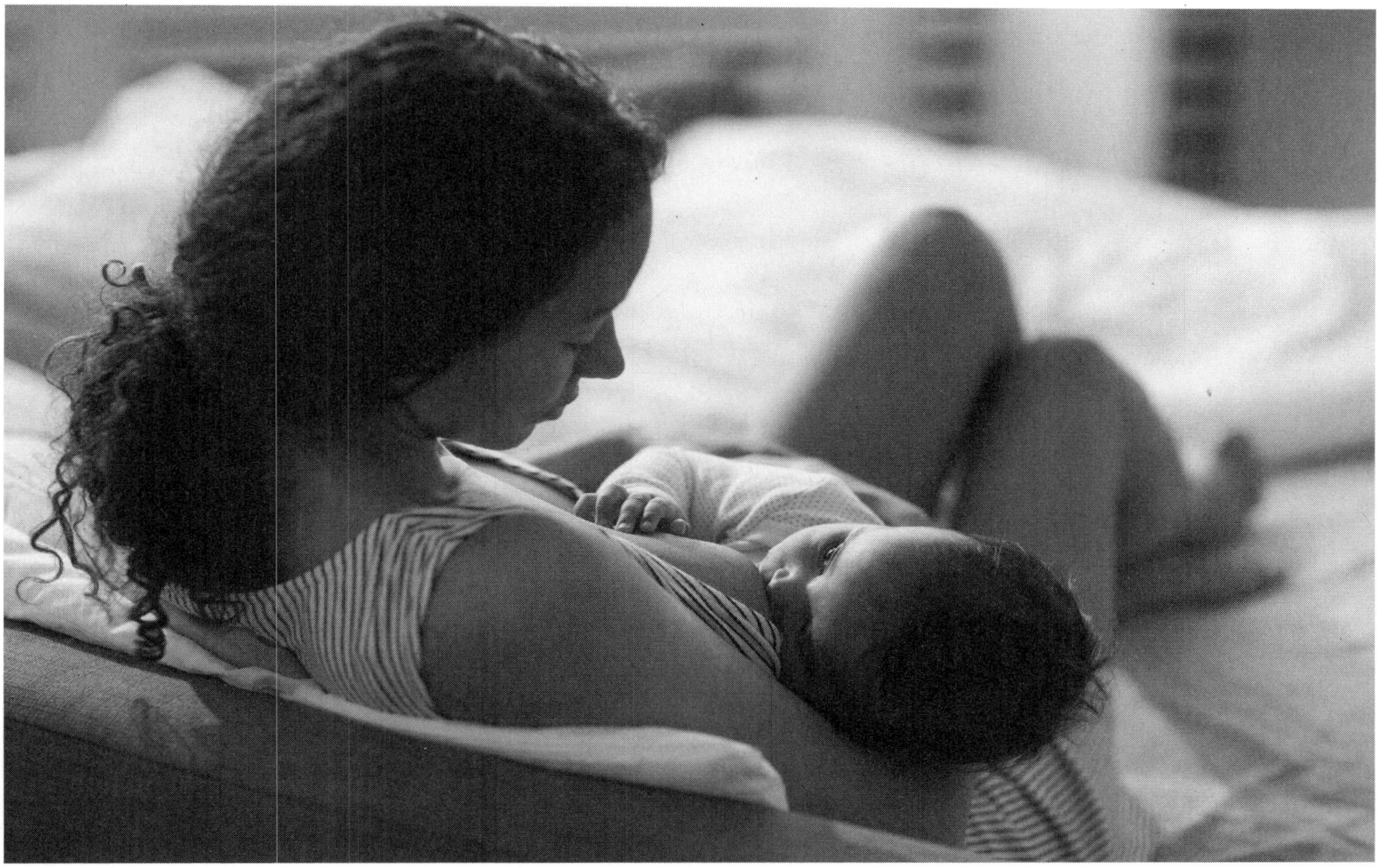

Nancy Mohrbacher, IBCLC, FILCA

NancyMohrbacher
SOLUTIONS, INC.
Arlington Heights, Illinois

Nancy Mohrbacher Solutions, Inc.
Arlington Heights, IL
630-336-9525
info@nancymohrbacher.com
www.NancyMohrbacher.com

Executive Editor: Nancy Mohrbacher
Project Editor: Kelly Sijapati
Proofreader: Heather Behles
Indexer: Gina Guilinger, Weight of the Word LLC
Cover and Text Designer: Julie Anderson

Cover photo credit: Fotolia

BREASTFEEDING ANSWERS: A Guide for Helping Families, Second Edition

ISBN: 978-1-7345239-0-4

Library of Congress Control Number: 2020905538

Printed in the United States of America.

10 9 8 7 6 5 4 3 2 1

This second edition is dedicated to the memory of

Jill Dye

(November 13, 1949 — September 26, 2019)

A dear friend and respected colleague who devoted much of her life to supporting new families as an LLL leader, an IBCLC in private practice, and a guiding light to several U.K. breastfeeding organizations. Like so many of my sisters and brothers in lactation, Jill's tireless efforts as a breastfeeding advocate made our world a better, more loving place. My thanks for a job well done!

Brief Contents

Contents

4 • Solid Foods

5 • Weaning from Nursing

PART II • BABY

6 • Weight Gain and Growth

7 • Newborn Hypoglycemia and Jaundice

8 • Baby's Anantomy and Health Issues

9 • The Preterm Baby

PART III • THE NURSING PARENT

10 • Making Milk

11 • Milk Expression and Storage

12 • Sex, Fertility, and Contraception

13 • Nutrition, Exercise, and Lifestyle Issues

A • Techniques

B • Tools and Products

Foreword

Over many decades of practicing pediatrics, my greatest privilege has been sharing the first moments of new parenthood. I realize that what's most important about promoting a positive breastfeeding experience is rarely mentioned. As each mother masters the initial challenges, breastfeeding becomes the steppingstone between the wishful expectations for motherhood and the foundation of confidence in oneself as a provider, nurturer, and protector.

Parents know breastmilk is best for babies. But when nursing challenges become defeating, their stories paint a picture of silenced dreams, information gaps, and too little help too late. Lack of motivation or personal choice does not accurately account for the high percentage of parents who decide to stop. A strong determinant rests with the infrastructure of support for newly delivered parents. What happens (or doesn't happen) in the earliest hours matters the most. Indeed, the first hours after delivery hold the greatest opportunity to prevent problems, which otherwise become less remedial with time.

There is good news. Nancy Mohrbacher's comprehensive review of the science, her focus on practical management, cultural considerations, and in-depth exploration of the key issues suggest numerous opportunities to leverage for change, once we recognize that establishing breastfeeding is exquisitely time sensitive. And so, in Chapter 2 Nancy highlights "The First 2 Hours," when first milk matters most. This understanding potentiates a shift from the paradigm of ***problem-oriented*** lactation management to ***problem-prevention***.

The goal of prevention is deceptively simple, but the challenges are significant. Nancy pieces together the research that each of her readers can use to identify the weaknesses of the status quo and create pathways for consistent, timely and accurate assistance.

Equipped with this excellent resource, informed readers who interact with new parents can share in these confidence-building hours, escorting parents over these steppingstones of parenthood. And in the weeks, months, and years ahead, they will find in these pages the strategies and evidence needed to smooth their paths every step of the way.

Jane Morton, MD
Adj. Cl. Professor of Pediatrics, Emerita
Stanford Medical Center, California

www.firstdroplets.com — A website designed to safeguard breastfeeding by placing timely and simple education and guidance in the hands of parents before delivery.

Acknowledgements

My sincere thanks goes first to all the families who allowed me to be a part of their lactation journey. It was a true privilege to learn from you and to share your joys and sorrows.

I am also grateful to the many generous people whose contributions were vital to this second edition. Tom Hale graciously granted me the rights to this book when he closed Hale Publishing in 2016. Many creators aspire to own their own work, but without Tom's kindness, this ideal would never have become a reality for me.

My thanks goes, too, to the world-class experts who took the time to review these pages and provide invaluable feedback, which made this a better book. They include otolaryngologist Margo McKenna Benoit, MD, Catherine Watson Genna, BS, IBCLC, Karleen Gribble, BRurSC, PhD, Lisa Marasco, MA, IBCLC, FILCA, Christina Smillie, MD, FAAP, IBCLC, FABM, Alice Farrow, BSc, IBCLC, Cert PPH, Hilary Flower, PhD, Sarah Shapiro, IBCLC, Alyssa Schnell, MS, IBCLC, and Jill Dye, MA, IBCLC. In addition, I'd like to thank my colleague Trevor MacDonald, who provided me with key help at the beginning of this project in crafting this edition's more inclusive, gender-neutral language. Special thanks to Dr. Jane Morton—whose work is featured prominently in this second edition—for taking time out of her incredibly hectic schedule to write the Foreword.

I also extend my sincere gratitude to those who provided the images. Special thanks to Dr. Gina Weissman, who shared many clinical tongue-tie photos, and my talented daughter-in-law Anna Mohrbacher, who created line drawings especially for these pages. Thanks, too, to Catherine Watson Genna, BS, IBCLC, a gifted lactation consultant and kind friend who generously allowed me to reprint 11 of her clinical photos, most from her indispensable books, *Supporting Sucking Skills in Breastfeeding Infants* and *Selecting and Using Breastfeeding Tools*. Thanks also to Barbara Wilson-Clay, BS, IBCLC, FILCA and Kay Hoover, MEd, IBCLC, FILCA, who kindly gave me permission to reprint two photos from their excellent *Breastfeeding Atlas*. Thanks also to the many families who contributed a vast array of nursing photos. I'm grateful to you all!

I couldn't have completed this project without the help of my publishing support team. Many thanks to Julie Anderson, my talented book designer, who worked tirelessly with me through nights and weekends for the entire 2 years of this project. Thanks also to Gina Guilinger, professional indexer extraordinaire, Eric Platou and his team at Sheridan Books, and my colleague and friend Kelly Sijapati, IBCLC for her many hours spent pouring over these pages and for her insights, and words of wisdom. Thanks, too, to Heather Behles, who not only provided proofreading help and this book's short links, but also shared lovely nursing photos of her and her daughter Jovie.

And last but never least, I thank my family. My three sons, Carl, Peter, and Ben, each played a vital role in this edition. I appreciate every day that you grew into such wonderful men. Sincere thanks, also, to my husband of 43 years, Michael, who made sure I was well fed and was (mostly) patient and understanding as I kept my eye on the prize and nose to the grindstone to complete this work.

Introduction

During the 2 years I labored over this revision, my hope was to create a comprehensive resource that accurately reflects our current understanding of lactation science and techniques. I know from my 10 years in private practice how difficult it can be to keep up with the latest evidence while working with families. For this reason, I often think of my job as "I read the research so you don't have to." At this writing, it has been a decade since the debut of the last edition of this book, and much has changed.

The Evolution of This Book

Just last week, I came to a startling realization: I've been working on this book in one form or another for most of my adult life. While watching a video of myself in 1989 (the only video recorded when our three boys were young), I laughed when my much younger self announced that I was working on a book whose working title was *The Breastfeeding Management Handbook*. Later retitled *The Breastfeeding Answer Book* (more widely known as the *BAB*), this was the first book published by La Leche League International (LLLI) for lactation helpers rather than for nursing families. It was a worldwide success, and for many years, the sales of its three editions (debuting in 1991, 1996, and 2003) played a significant role in supporting the work of that nonprofit organization.

In 2008, I knew the *BAB* was in serious need of revision, and I pondered my options. LLLI's reference library had closed, so I had no access from that source to the research I needed to complete the revision. LLLI's publications department also closed, so they could no longer support my work in-house. That's when Dr. Thomas Hale offered to provide me with access to the research and the support of his staff if I agreed to sign over the rights to Hale Publishing. After signing on the dotted line, we retitled the book *Breastfeeding Answers Made Simple (BAMS)*, but there were still questions. Was this 2010 book really the book's first edition or the fourth edition of the *BAB*? Although I wrote the *BAB* (along with my coauthor Julie Stock) and its unique two-column format remained the same, I did not own the rights to the *BAB*. It belonged to LLLI, so this next version of the book became *BAMS'* first edition.

In June 2016, Hale Publishing closed its doors, which profoundly affected our plans for this second edition. Having discovered that my local public library could provide me with access to the research, I requested ownership of my work, and Tom Hale generously agreed. For the first time (just like Taylor Swift!) I owned my own work. As a result, with this second edition, I've personally overseen all aspects of this book's development, design, and printing, which was a fascinating and gratifying learning experience. Its title was also tweaked. A complication we didn't consider when we chose *Breastfeeding Answers Made Simple* was the confusion created by its similarity to my book for parents: *Breastfeeding Made Simple*. For clarity's sake, I shortened the title of this edition to simply *Breastfeeding Answers* (*BAB* for short?), which also hearkens back to its roots.

What Drew Me to Lactation

How did I get so invested in lactation? My story begins even before I nursed my own babies. My initial encounter with breastfeeding support occurred in June of 1980, when I attended my first La Leche League meeting. I was 5 months pregnant with my first child, and I arrived feeling curious about motherhood and wondering if I could make nursing work.

That was also the night I fell in love with nursing. It happened as I watched a mother and her 3-week-old baby interact at the breast. In my mind's eye, I can still see her stroking, smiling, and talking to her newborn girl while they stared into each other's eyes. I was stunned by how alive that tiny baby was to her mother's overtures! Others told me that newborns were incapable of real interaction, but that mother and baby proved them wrong. Although I didn't know it then, what I witnessed that night was the mother-baby synchrony described in Chapter 1, and after that experience, I would never be the same. I don't remember a word that mother said to the larger group that night, but the impression she left on me was indelible. I knew immediately this was the kind of intimacy I wanted with my own baby. When I left that meeting, I was confident that with this group's help I could nurse, and I felt even more excited about becoming a mother.

After that meeting and many more, I went on to nurse my three sons and threw my heart and soul into helping other nursing families. In 1982, before lactation was a career choice, I became a La Leche League leader. In 1984, I began reading lactation research and reporting on lactation trends in the articles I wrote for La Leche League publications (in those days I wrote with pen on yellow pad and typed final drafts on a typewriter). In 1991, with my coauthor Julie Stock, I finished the first version of this book (my first work on a computer) and joined a new profession as a board-certified lactation consultant. In 1993, I founded and ran what became a large Chicago-area private lactation practice that over the next 10 years helped thousands of families. Next, I worked in a variety of roles. I organized professional seminars for an international breast pump company, which put me in contact with some of the most creative and inspiring minds in lactation. I helped families by phone for a U.S. corporate lactation program. I developed a smartphone app and other digital lactation tools for parents and professionals. I wrote three books for nursing parents. More recently, I created and taught a 90-hour course for aspiring lactation consultants in China, and I contracted with U.S. hospitals to improve their breastfeeding practices, helping several to become Baby Friendly.

What's New in This Edition

As part of this book's revision, I reviewed more than 4,000 studies, some of which advance our knowledge and may potentially improve practice. Every chapter and appendix was fully updated with new information and approaches, as well as the latest digital, online, and print resources. Many more images were added, and nearly every page was substantially rewritten. Some of the countless updates include:

- Simple post-delivery strategies that prevent excess weight loss and exaggerated newborn jaundice (p. 189, 249, and 474)
- New research on rapid weight gain in nursing babies and the effect of early formula supplementation on allergy risk (p. 63 and 563)

- Guidelines for nursing parents with COVID-19 (p. 813)
- New high- and low-tech biilirubin measuring tools for newborns (p. 247) and new low-tech jaundice treatment options (p. 256-257)
- How to use newborns' inborn feeding behaviors to make early latching easier in any feeding position (p. 29)
- Nursing the baby with Type 1 diabetes (p. 315)
- How nursing outcomes differ in early term babies (p. 389)
- Complementary therapies found to boost milk production and milk yields during pumping (p. 448-449 and 493-494)
- LGBTQ nursing and the effects of chest masculinization (top) surgery on milk production (p. 432 and 797)
- Factors affecting nursing outcomes in obese parents (p. 574-580)
- Updated recommendations on when to start highly allergenic solid foods in nursing babies (p. 137-138)
- The effects of parental diabetes and insulin resistance on milk production (p. 843)
- The use of breast massage and Chinese manual therapy techniques to treat lactation challenges (p. 879-884)
- New treatments for nipple pain and mastitis (p. 721 and 764)

Language and Gender

In addition to the changes in knowledge and skills, this book reflects the changes in language that occurred over the last decade. Why does language change? The short answer is to better reflect the current reality. For example, in the early 1980s, when I was new to lactation, adoptive nursing was synonymous with induced lactation. Then came new reproductive technologies, and now parents induce lactation for their biological children, who are carried and birthed by surrogates.

For this edition, the most significant change in language was necessary because mothers are no longer the only ones who nurse their babies. Transgender men give birth and nurse (aka chestfeed), too (p. 433 and 797). Transgender men, such as my colleague Trevor MacDonald, not only nurse their babies, they also change the world by persuading LLLI to update its policies so that transgender men can now become accredited as La Leche League leaders.

Because the families who come to us for lactation help—and indeed also some of our colleagues—include those who are not heterosexual and cisgender, it's important to widen our worldview and for the language in this book to be appropriately inclusive. I don't think the words "mother" or "mother's milk" will ever go out of style, so you'll continue to find them in these pages. (After all, many transgender women happily embrace these words, along with many cisgender women.) But I also use other, more inclusive terms throughout, such as "birthing parent" and "nursing parent." My hope is that by using these broader terms, it will help us all remember that our work has expanded to include a wider range of loving and nurturing families, which—for me at least—is a cause for celebration.

Regarding the use of pronouns, in the first edition, the nursing parent was always presumed to be "she" and baby was referred to as "he." In this edition, you'll see the word "parents" used more often with the pronoun "they" and baby's gender will alternate by chapter, with odd chapters using "he" and even chapters using "she."

Using This Book

In the years since my first La Leche League meeting, approaches to lactation help have undergone radical shifts. When I began helping families in 1982, we shared basic information, offered encouragement, and conveyed our faith that given patience and persistence, nursing problems would resolve. As we learned more—often through trial and error—many in our fledging profession began teaching all families—not just those with problems—latching and positioning techniques that in hindsight made nursing feel complicated. Today, a deeper understanding of basic lactation dynamics (or "natural laws"), make it possible for us to simplify our approach (see Chapter 1).

My personal philosophy of lactation help has long been: "Do what works, and don't do what doesn't work." But as simple as this sounds, many parents and clinicians continue using the same strategies even after it is clear they are not working. When using this book, please remember this "do what works" philosophy. After a fair trial, if one of the many strategies in these pages isn't working, move on to the next. Differences in personal preferences, cultural beliefs, anatomy, and circumstances make each nursing couple unique. A "one-size-fits-all" or "cookbook" approach to lactation help is often counter-productive and does not do families justice.

Another important point to keep in mind is that what initially drew many of us to lactation was not the wonders of human milk (which are considerable) but the miraculous way nursing deepens the parent-child bond. The real power of nursing lies in the profound intimacy I witnessed between that mother and her newborn at my first La Leche League meeting. Experiencing that—even second-hand—created a hunger in me for that intimacy with my own newborn. Experiencing it myself was my main motivation for wanting to help other families feel that same amazing magic.

Let us keep our eye on that prize. Approaching lactation help with intimacy and attachment as a focus (p. 12) enables us to better reinforce parents' instincts and leave them feeling empowered rather than incompetent. My hope is that this second edition will provide you with the knowledge and tools you need to both help families nurse and enhance their bond with their baby. Many of the new insights in these pages take us back to our roots but this time with a firmer grasp of the underlying forces at work. We are entering an exciting time in lactation. The best is definitely yet to come, both for us and for the families we help.

PART I

The Nursing Relationship

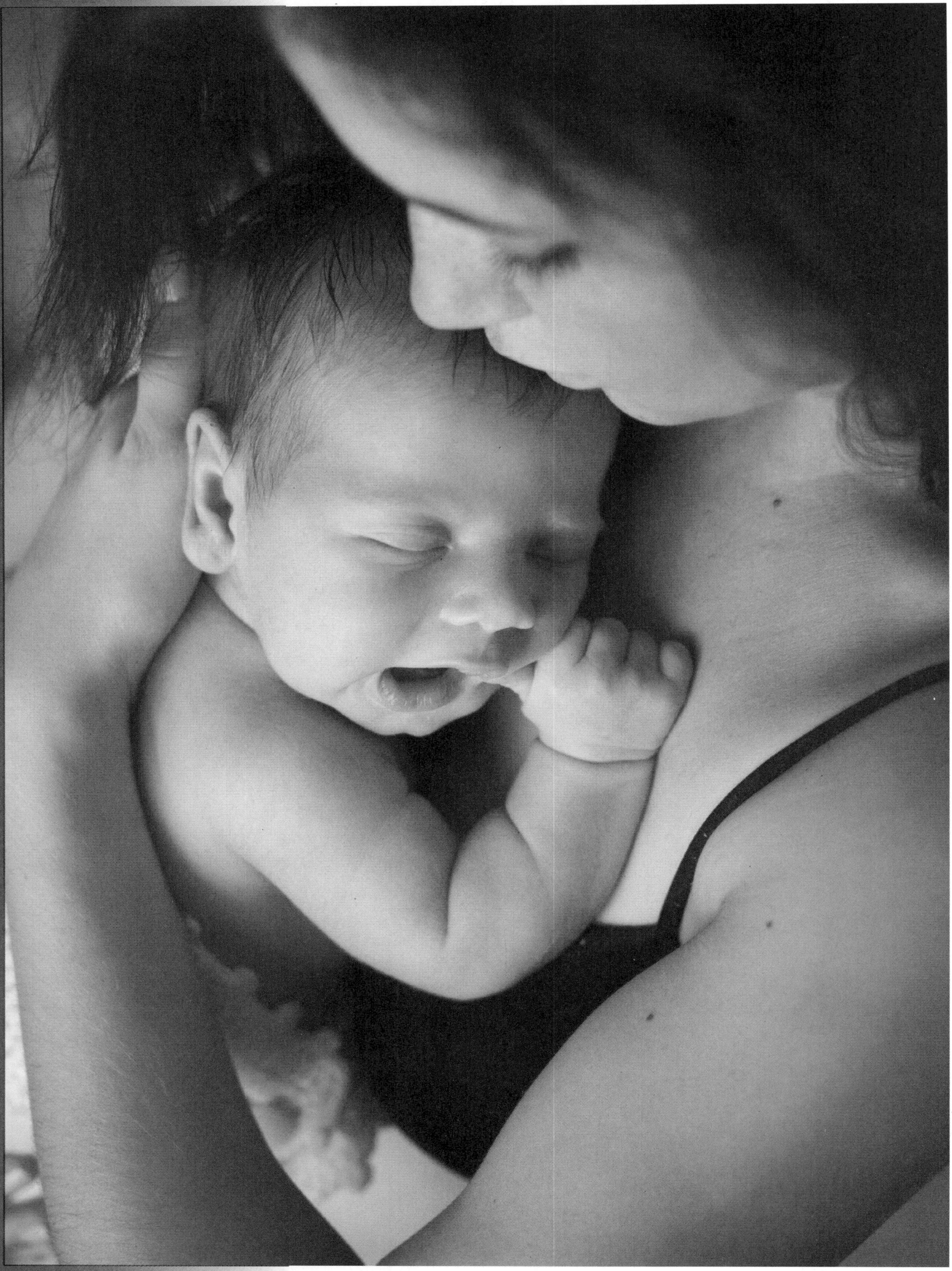

Basic Nursing Dynamics

1

Think of nursing as part of an intimate relationship rather than a skill to be taught.

This chapter describes the hardwiring nature builds into humans to make early nursing easier and how helpers can best support families as they learn. During the first weeks after birth, the milk is just one part of why nursing matters. Perhaps even more important is the role this intimate interaction plays in enhancing their emotional connection, which is just as crucial for human survival as food. At first, many new parents feel pressure to "get nursing right." Some even consider it their first parenting "test." Most families find it reassuring to know that their job is not to "make baby nurse," but to calm and comfort their baby (p. 19). Calming baby with eye contact, talking, and touch builds their bond while helping baby settle and feed. But there is more to it. By sensitively responding to baby's cues, families can "get in sync" with their newborn (p. 12). This synchrony—or lack of it—is the first of a baby's essential life lessons on what it means to be human. Better parent-child synchrony is linked to better mental and physical health (Baker & McGrath, 2011). One 2018 review (Krol & Grossmann, 2018) found that nursing improves this synchrony and families' social and emotional lives.

KEY CONCEPT

To give effective lactation support, we need a basic grasp of the emotional side of nursing and how our approach affects the families we help.

According to the Australian research summarized on p. 16-18, different approaches to lactation help can enhance or undermine both early nursing and the parent-child relationship. For this reason, knowing about the emotional side of nursing and the power of words are vital for effective support.

With each new baby, families must learn what works and tailor their responses accordingly. A good first step is a basic understanding of what nature builds into babies and using this to make early nursing easier.

BABY'S INBORN FEEDING BEHAVIORS

Under the right conditions, like all mammal newborns, healthy term human babies emerge from the womb with the innate behaviors needed to get to their food source and feed.

We take for granted that all other mammal newborns are born with what's needed to get to their food source and feed. After all, their very survival depends on it. But for much of modern history, the human newborn was considered completely helpless, dependent on adults for feeding. Then in 1987, Swedish researchers discovered that after birth if laid tummy down on the mother's chest in skin-to-skin contact, newborns could make their own way to the nipple and nurse without help (Widstrom et al., 1987). Science has documented the innate feeding behaviors humans possess at birth, known as the ***breast crawl***, and we are beginning to understand more fully how these inborn behaviors can make early nursing easier at the first feed and for weeks and months afterward.

The Breast Crawl

After decades of study, we have a better understanding of the breast crawl.

In a 2011 Swedish study (Widstrom et al., 2011), researchers videotaped 28 full-term newborns during the first hours after birth to understand more clearly, the sequence of behaviors that unfolds from birth to the first nursing. The researchers grouped these behaviors into nine instinctive stages (see p. 47). According to several studies, when newborns did the breast crawl, the time it took from birth to the first feed averaged less than 60 minutes, but some babies took as long as 75 minutes (Girish et al., 2013; Matthiesen, Ransjo-Arvidson, Nissen, & Uvnas-Moberg, 2001; Widstrom et al., 2011).

• • •

Nursing outcomes during the hospital stay appear to be better when babies do the breast crawl at the first feed. An Indian prospective, single-blinded, randomized controlled clinical trial of 100 healthy term newborns (Girish et al., 2013) divided these babies into two groups. In the first group, the babies were placed on their mother's abdomen immediately after birth and allowed to do the breast crawl for the first feed. The second group was removed from the mother's body after birth, weighed, measured, and given vitamin K injections then returned to the mother within 30 to 60 minutes for feeding. The researchers found significant differences in breastfeeding outcomes between the two groups. Nipple pain occurred in 44% of the mothers whose babies did not do the breast crawl compared with 24% of those who did. Delay in milk increase occurred in 60% of the mothers whose babies did not do the breast crawl compared with only 24% of the mothers whose babies did. Mean weight loss on Day 3 was significantly higher among babies who did not do the breast crawl compared with those who did.

Newborns had better breastfeeding outcomes when they were allowed to do the breast crawl at the first feed.

• • •

In a classic Swedish study (Righard & Alade, 1990), two birth interventions derailed the breast crawl in some babies: a short separation of mother and baby and the use of the pain medication pethidine (Demerol) during labor. This study convinced many that these feeding behaviors were fragile and short-lived.

It is now common knowledge that inborn feeding behaviors—once thought to be fragile and short-lived—can be triggered for months and even years.

One of the first to describe these behaviors as long-lasting was U.S. pediatrician Christina Smillie (Smillie, 2017). When she began helping families with feeding problems in her clinic, she noticed that when babies were held with their torso in contact with their nursing parent's chest they all exhibited similar feeding behaviors. This occurred with term and preterm babies, young babies and older babies.

Being new to lactation, Smillie had few preconceived notions, and her fresh eyes led to new insights. Smillie observed that these feeding behaviors persisted long after the newborn period (Smillie, 2017, p. 107):

> "Although we know of anecdotal instances of infants as old as 10 and even 20 months who, with no prior experience at the breast, have surprised their mothers by independently initiating feeding for the first time in this manner, such instances are rare. It is much easier for infants in the first 3 months of life. After infants reach 4 or 5 months of age, when developmentally they are more and more distractible, their curiosity and high activity can interfere with the behavioral state that allows them to follow through on their instincts for the breast."

In Australia, these breast-seeking behaviors have been observed in adopted children between 8 months to 12 years old (Gribble, 2005).

• • •

When the nursing couple both take an active role during feeding, this simplifies the process and enhances their relationship. Positive nursing experiences reinforce effective feeding, which can prevent problems. Supporting rather than suppressing these feeding behaviors can also help overcome feeding problems, such as latching struggles or distress during feeding attempts. which may arise from negative experiences at previous feeds (Smillie, 2017). For details, see Chapter 3, "Latching and Nursing Struggles."

Supporting the baby's feeding behaviors can help avoid and overcome nursing problems.

Primitive Neonatal Reflexes

Researchers identified 20 inborn reflexes—components of the breast crawl—that help babies make their way to the nipple and feed.

Until 2008, only a small number of reflexes—rooting, sucking, and swallowing—were formally identified by neurologists as being crucial to newborn feeding. To learn more, U.K. research midwife Suzanne Colson videotaped 40 British and French mothers and babies during the first month after birth (S. D. Colson, Meek, & Hawdon, 2008). Twenty-four hours of videotaped breastfeeding footage from 93 separate feeding episodes was analyzed to identify the underlying reflexes responsible for these inborn feeding behaviors and to better understand their contribution to nursing. The authors referred to them as ***primitive neonatal reflexes***, or PNRs.

> **KEY CONCEPT**
>
> *Knowing something about the reflexes human babies are born with can make early nursing easier.*

These 20 reflexes (Table 1.1) appeared to have two primary purposes: 1) to find the nipple and latch, and 2) to transfer milk. One of their new insights: a strong "foot to mouth connection," with the mother's stroking of the baby's feet triggering reflexive movements of the baby's toes and feet and active sucking. The baby's gestational age, age when videotaped, ethnicity, and state of alertness had no effect on the triggering of these reflexes.

• • •

The feeding reflexes the babies used varied from feed to feed and from position to position.

The U.K. researchers described in the previous point found that not all babies used all 20 of these reflexes at all feeds (S. D. Colson et al., 2008). And the number of reflexes observed varied by the mother's body position. When the mothers used semi-reclined, or starter positions (see p. 23-29) the researchers observed more feeding reflexes.

• • •

These same reflexes are seen in preterm babies as young as 29 weeks.

Inborn feeding behaviors are a part of a newborn's survival skills. As such, they are present in all babies, not just those born healthy and full-term. Studies from Sweden (Nyqvist, 2008; Nyqvist, Sjoden, & Ewald, 1999) confirm that preterm babies born as early as 29 weeks gestation made their own way to the nipple and sucked. For details see Chapter 9, "The Preterm Baby."

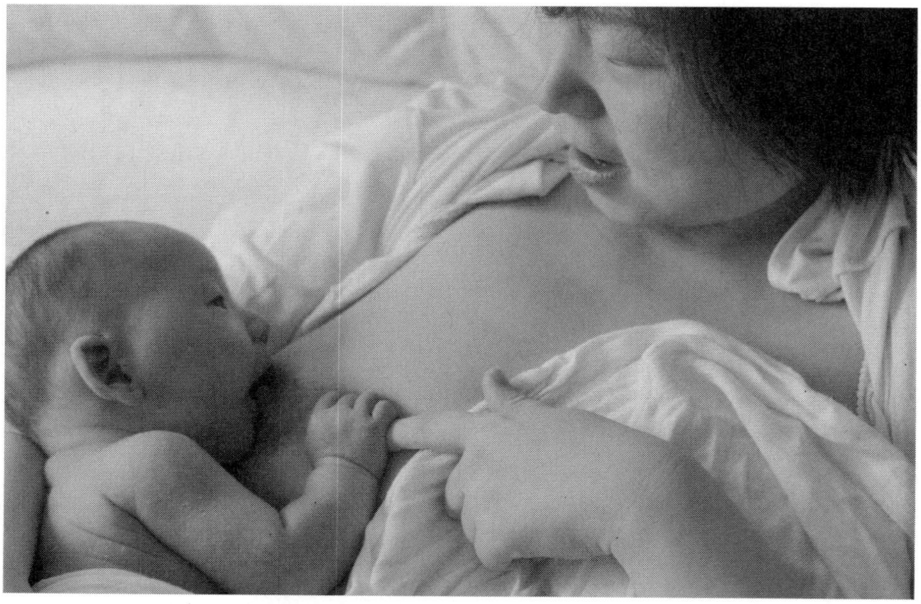

©2020 Melanie Ham, used with permission

TABLE 1.1 Primitive Neonatal Reflexes by Function

Function	Reflex
Finding/latching	Hand to mouth Finger flex/extend Mouth gape Tongue dart, tick Arm cycle Leg cycle Foot/hand flex Head lift Head right Head bob/nod Root Placing
Finding/latching, milk transfer	Palmar grasp Plantar grasp Babinski toe fan Step (withdrawal) Crawl
Milk transfer	Suck Jaw jerk Swallow

Adapted from (S. D. Colson et al., 2008)

• • •

Several Swedish studies found that even when the mothers who participated were specifically instructed not to interact with their babies after birth (an unnatural intervention), their hormonal levels changed with their babies' actions (Matthiesen et al., 2001; Righard & Alade, 1990; Widstrom et al., 1987). In one Swedish study (Matthiesen et al., 2001), researchers videotaped the movements 10 babies made between an unmedicated birth and the first nursing. At the same time, the researchers measured the mothers' blood oxytocin levels. Oxytocin has wide-ranging physical effects, including milk ejection and uterine contractions. Oxytocin also has a calming and relationship-enhancing effect. The babies' actions during the breast crawl increased the mothers' blood oxytocin levels and the researchers concluded (Matthiesen et al., 2001, p. 13):

Newborns' movements affect nursing parents' hormonal levels, strengthening their bond and making milk more accessible to the baby.

> "Newborns use their hands as well as their mouths to stimulate maternal oxytocin release after birth, which may have significance for uterine contraction, milk ejection, and mother-infant interaction."

• • •

The U.K. researcher team that identified the 20 primitive neonatal reflexes (S. D. Colson et al., 2008) noted that these specific reflexes are similar to reflexes innate in other mammal species (like dogs and cats) whose newborns feed on their tummies. The researchers concluded that human newborns—like many other mammal newborns—are hardwired to be ***abdominal feeders*** (feeding best when on their abdomens) rather than ***dorsal feeders*** (pressure applied to their backs during nursing). In the years since this study was published, practitioners in other parts of the world (Douglas & Keogh, 2017) found this approach to early positioning an effective way to prevent nursing problems and to overcome them when they occur. (For an overview of this approach to early positioning, see the free video at: **NaturalBreastfeeding.com**.)

The specific reflexes identified led researchers to conclude that human newborns are hardwired to feed most easily resting on their abdomens rather than with pressure applied to their backs.

Normal Rooting, Sucking, and Swallowing

The touch of baby's chin on the mammary tissue helps baby locate the nipple, open wide, attach, and begin sucking.

Latching on and sucking occurs in a predictable sequence of actions (Genna, 2017):

- Baby finds the nipple, usually by rooting (moving his head from side to side with an open mouth),
- The touch of the baby's chin on the mammary tissue stimulates his natural response: to open his mouth wide (gape),
- He then drops his tongue and extends its tip over his lower lip as he attaches and begins to suck.

When babies take an active role in seeking the nipple, they make their way there using different strategies (Smillie, 2017). Some babies drop slowly to the mammary gland with their cheek lightly touching. Some lunge quickly, turning their head only when their cheek touches the nipple. Others crawl slowly, using their whole body. Some make their way by touching each cheek alternately to the mammary tissue.

• • •

Swallowing is easier for the baby if his head is tilted back slightly, also known as the instinctive feeding position.

After latching, swallowing milk is easier if the baby can tilt his head back slightly. Both adults and babies find drinking easier with this slight head extension, because this opens the throat for easier swallowing. For this reason, Australian midwife and lactation consultant Rebecca Glover refers to this head tilt as the ***instinctive feeding position*** (Glover & Wiessinger, 2017).

• • •

The baby draws milk from the mammary gland through a combination of tongue and jaw movements.

Research from the 1980s suggested that babies remove milk from the mammary gland almost entirely through a wavelike movement of their tongue (peristalsis) to compress the breast and press milk into their mouth (Woolridge, 1986). Later research found that vacuum generated by the dropping of the back of the tongue also plays a major role (Geddes, Kent, Mitoulas, & Hartmann, 2008). In 2014, an Israeli research team used ultrasonic movie clips (Elad et al., 2014) to determine that during milk transfer, the front (anterior) of baby's tongue moves as a rigid body with the cycling movement of baby's lower jaw, while the back (posterior) section of baby's tongue moves in a wavelike motion essential for swallowing. A small amount of suction, or negative pressure (about -20 mmHg) is needed for baby to keep the mammary tissue in his mouth. While the baby sucks, the movement of baby's lower jaw causes the pressure inside his mouth to vary. A 2016 Australian ultrasound study (Geddes & Sakalidis, 2016) found these pressures varied in part by baby's age, with the mean pressure in babies younger than 1 month measuring -98 mmHg, while the mean pressure in babies older than 1 month was lower, about -50 mmHg.

• • •

How deeply the nipple extends into the baby's mouth during nursing may affect the nursing parent's comfort, the rate of milk flow, and whether baby stays active or falls asleep quickly.

The depth of latch is also called by some the ***intraoral breast tissue volume*** (Douglas & Keogh, 2017). If the baby takes the nipple shallowly into his mouth with the nipple pressed against his hard palate, this can contribute to nipple pain or trauma and slow milk flow. If the milk flow is slow enough, the baby may not gain weight well, suck less actively, or fall asleep quickly.

According to ultrasound studies of healthy, thriving babies during normal nursing, when baby is latched comfortably, the nipple extends on average to within about 4 to 5 mm of the junction of the baby's hard and soft palates (Elad et al., 2014; Geddes et al., 2008; Geddes & Sakalidis, 2016; Jacobs, Dickinson, Hart, Doherty, & Faulkner, 2007). A deep latch has several advantages: nursing is less likely to cause nipple pain or trauma (Kent et al., 2015), baby transfers more milk with every suck, and it stimulates in the baby longer, more active sucking. Some call this area in the baby's mouth, where there is no friction or pressure on the nipple during feeds the ***comfort zone*** (Mohrbacher & Kendall-Tackett, 2010).

WHAT SUPPORTS AND UNDERMINES BABY

Triggers of Inborn Feeding Behaviors

The way parents naturally hold their babies for cuddling triggers babies' feeding behaviors. U.K. research midwife Suzanne Colson suggested that nursing parents lean back and put their baby on top with unrestricted access to the nipple so that "every part of the baby's body is facing, touching, and closely applied to one of the mother's curves or to part of the surrounding environment" (S. Colson, 2012, p. 9). This full frontal contact of the baby triggers his "internal navigation system," so he can orient himself and focus on feeding.

A newborn's innate feeding behaviors are primarily triggered and maintained by touch, specifically the full-frontal contact of the baby against the adult's body.

A 2014 Australian observational study of 78 newborns during the first hour after birth (Cantrill, Creedy, Cooke, & Dykes, 2014) found that effective sucking during the first hour after birth was predicted by positioning babies so they could instinctively nudge their chin into the underside of the mammary gland as they neared the nipple and latched.

U.S. pediatrician Christina Smillie suggested parents hold their baby with his torso against their chest (Smillie, 2017). From there, the baby begins making his way to the nipple. Smillie has observed that if a parent sits upright and part of the baby's torso loses contact with the parent's body—such as when the baby curls up or moves away—these behaviors stop. If this happens, upright parents can bring the baby's torso, hips, and legs in close contact with their body again to stimulate these behaviors again.

• • •

A newborn's reflexes can be triggered even when he is not hungry, but if enough time goes by since the last feed, the biochemistry of hunger begins to play a role. When a baby's blood sugar drops, the first sign of hunger may be to put his hands to his mouth, perhaps chewing or sucking on his hand. If he cannot get to the nipple, eventually he will start to cry.

Hunger and thirst may also play a role in triggering a baby's feeding behaviors.

• • •

The stimulation of the baby's feet, either by the parent or by contact with something else in the environment, appears to help stimulate a baby's movement toward the nipple (S. D. Colson et al., 2008). When the parent is in a semi-reclined, starter position (see later section on p. 23) and the top of the baby's feet brush against the parent's body, this releases the stepping reflex, which

The baby can move to the nipple more easily if his legs and feet have contact with the nursing parent's thigh or another nearby object.

can help a baby make his way to the nipple. U.K. research midwife Suzanne Colson noted that when semi-reclined mothers had their hands free, they often "spontaneously stroked their baby's feet, triggering toe fanning and toe grasping, which appeared at the same time to release their baby's lip and tongue reflexes" (S. D. Colson et al., 2008). This same behavior was not seen when mothers sat upright (possibly in part because the mothers didn't have a free hand in these positions). If a baby's body is tummy down with legs draped over the nursing parent's side, pillows or other objects could also stimulate this response.

• • •

When a baby's cheek is touched, he turns his head in that direction, which can either help or hinder nursing.

The rooting response is a part of a baby's inborn feeding behaviors that helps a baby locate the nipple and take it into his mouth. This response can help a baby locate the nipple, but it can also be a barrier if nursing parents accidentally trigger this response by touching baby's cheek with their fingers, causing him to turn away from the nipple.

• • •

Hearing, smell, and sight also play a role in orienting the baby to the nipple.

In their book, *Your Amazing Newborn* (Klaus & Klaus, 2000), Marshall and Phyllis Klaus noted that shortly after birth, healthy term newborns make eye contact, turn toward their birthing parents' voice, and can recognize their smell.

Many studies found that babies use smell to orient themselves to their birthing parent and to the mammary gland. One overview of the literature described several studies (Porter & Winberg, 1999). In one, breast pads were suspended over a baby's face, one clean and one with the smell of the mother's breast (Macfarlane, 1975). Babies consistently turned toward the pad with the mother's smell. Another study found that even 2-week-old exclusively formula-fed babies turned first to smell a pad with an unfamiliar mother's milk on it over a pad with the more familiar smell of formula (Porter, Makin, Davis, & Christensen, 1991). In another study of 30 newborns and their mothers, one breast was washed with an odorless soap just before the newborn was placed between the mother's breasts after birth and allowed to choose which breast to go to (Varendi, Porter, & Winberg, 1994). Twenty-two babies (73%) preferred the unwashed breast. The authors noted that the infants' attraction to breast odors clearly influenced their behaviors and was "analogous to the role of 'nipple search pheromone' in guiding young rabbits and piglets to the nipple" (Porter & Winberg, 1999). In another study in which the mother wasn't present, babies 36 to 72 hours old were placed tummy down in a warming bed, and a breast pad was placed 17 cm away from the babies' nose (Varendi & Porter, 2001). Within 3 minutes, 18 of the 22 babies (85%) made their way to the breast pad with the mother's scent on it as compared with only three of 22 babies (15%) with the control pad. Being on their abdomens made it possible for these babies to get to the pads. In addition to helping a baby find the nipple, the smell of the mother's breast is another sensory stimulus that increases sucking during breastfeeding (Russell, 1976).

KEY CONCEPT

Touch is the primary trigger for a newborn's feeding behaviors.

Pediatrician T. Berry Brazelton found that newborn babies will turn toward the sound of their mother's voice, and even preferred that voice to others talking at the same time (Brazelton & Nugent, 2011). Newborns were also found to have a more intense change in heart rate and breathing in response to their mother's face than to other faces (Fifer & Moon, 1994).

The Importance of Positional Stability

If a baby feels physically unstable, before he can focus on feeding, he first attempts to stabilize his body. Australian lactation consultant and midwife Rebecca Glover once said: "A baby without positional stability is like a ballerina on a moving stage." As Glover and her co-author U.S. lactation consultant Diane Wiessinger (Glover & Wiessinger, 2017, p. 125) wrote:

> "Picture a mammal, any mammal, as a newborn. Imagine it on its back. What does it do? It thrashes and tries to get onto its stomach, where it feels stable and in control. Human newborns are no different. A baby needs to hug its mother's body, front to front, in order to feel truly secure."

This type of insecurity is obvious when a newborn is laid on his back on a scale when being weighed. The distress it causes is one reason newborns are routinely weighed on the sides or tummies in some parts of the world (see p. 919).

Babies need to feel physically stable before they can focus on feeding.

• • •

With more mature nervous systems, adults, children, and older babies feel stable in many different body positions. Not so with newborns. Young babies need a stable midsection or "core" and equal use of both sides of their body, known, as ***midline stability*** (Glover & Wiessinger, 2017). That's why babies born with muscle asymmetry (such as torticollis, see p. 107) often struggle with feeding (Genna, 2015). Feeding is more difficult if baby's body is twisted or turned.

For positional stability, a newborn needs a stable core and midline stability.

U.K. research midwife Suzanne Colson noted that after birth, a baby's position in the womb may influence his comfort while nursing. For example, if a baby was in a posterior position or had his arms or legs extended in the womb, during the early weeks he may not feel comfortable nursing with his body well aligned. This is one reason to encourage families to find their own best feeding position. What's most important is that both parent and baby are comfortable.

With a stable core, a newborn can more easily coordinate his head-and-neck movements. This is known as ***proximal stability***, which explains why it is easier for adults to control their wrist and hand movements when their elbow rests on a firm surface. Both midline stability and a stable core make it easier for newborns to coordinate their movements and feed effectively. Resting tummy down on the nursing parent's body provides a newborn the most stable place for feeding.

Factors That May Undermine Baby

Without full frontal contact, frustration and feeding struggles can occur. See the later section, "Positioning Basics" for ways to maximize full frontal contact and other strategies that make early nursing easier.

When gaps form between a hungry newborn and the nursing parent, baby may become disoriented and frustrated.

• • •

When a nursing parent tries to help baby latch deeply (or help maintain a deep latch), it can be tempting in upright feeding positions to push on the back of a baby's head. However, this often causes more feeding problems than it solves.

When the back of a baby's head is touched, a reflex may be triggered that causes baby to push back, which may lead to feeding struggles.

As previously described, babies find swallowing easier when their heads are slightly tilted back (extended) during feeds. Applying pressure (even gentle pressure) to the back of baby's head may tilt baby's head forward, chin to chest, making swallowing more difficult (Glover & Wiessinger, 2017). Pushing baby's nose into the mammary tissue may obstruct baby's breathing. Babies are also born with a reflex (which helps them exit the birth canal) that causes them to push back when pressure is applied to the back of their head. If a baby reacts to this head pressure by pushing back, this can contribute to feeding struggles.

• • •

An upset baby needs to be calmed before he can settle and feed.

Babies who are fussing and crying may have a difficult time settling to feed. That's one reason the American Academy of Pediatrics recommended feeds begin when baby is showing early feeding cues, such as rooting and hand-to-mouth (AAP, 2012). When a baby is very upset, the first step is to calm him. Skin-to-skin contact is one excellent strategy in this situation. For more details, see the section on the next page, "Baby's State, Readiness, and Engagement."

HELPING NURSING COUPLES GET IN SYNC

Responsive parenting is key to getting in sync with baby.

Most lactation supporters know that nursing a baby on cue (rather than on a schedule) is the best way to ensure both healthy growth for baby and healthy milk production. But being responsive to a baby has other long-term positive effects. According to infant neuroscience, the best physical and emotional outcomes for both children and parents occur in families that use responsive parenting styles that promote parent-child ***synchrony*** (Evans & Porter, 2009; Leclere et al., 2014; Swain, Konrath, Dayton, Finegood, & Ho, 2013).

What is synchrony? It's defined as "a dynamic process by which hormonal, physiological, and behavioral cues are exchanged between parent and young during social contact" (Feldman, 2012, p. 42). Others describe it as harmonious, rhythmical interactions that involve mutual and reciprocal behaviors (Leclere et al., 2014).

Getting in sync with a newborn involves experimenting to find what helps lower baby's stress levels and helps baby stay calm (Ball, Douglas, Kulasinghe, Whittingham, & Hill, 2018). Scientists use the word ***co-regulation*** to describe how adults help settle babies. As the next chapter describes in more detail, through close body contact after delivery, nursing parents co-regulate their newborns' physiology (body temperature, blood sugar, heart rate, and breathing), as well as enhance growth. This crucial physical and hormonal part of getting in sync with a newborn helps babies make a safer, smoother transition from womb to world (Winberg, 2005).

Not surprisingly, the behaviors that help calm babies include holding, talking, eye contact, and of course, nursing. This is how adults naturally respond when babies fuss. In the long term, responsive care is how parents teach babies how to handle stress and strong emotions and how to relate to others (Parsons, Young, Murray, Stein, & Kringelbach, 2010). One U.S. study of 101 6-month-old babies and their mothers (Evans & Porter, 2009) found that strong mother-baby synchrony was associated with better mental and psychomotor development at 9 months. Some research indicates that responsive parenting may enhance emotional resilience in children and even prevent the development of mood and anxiety disorders, as well as serious psychiatric problems (Swain, 2011).

A 2011 review of the literature on mother-baby synchrony (Baker & McGrath, 2011) concluded that babies in sync with their mothers had a closer emotional bond, which helped the babies learn to better manage their emotions and state. This review also concluded that getting in sync helps a child learn language and develop healthy relationships with others. It concluded that responsive parenting is good for parents, too, because it helps them adjust more easily to the new baby's arrival. In addition to enjoying a closer relationship, parents who get in sync with their babies feel a greater sense of competence and are at reduced risk of depression and anxiety. They are also less likely to adopt a negative-control parenting style that puts them at odds with their child.

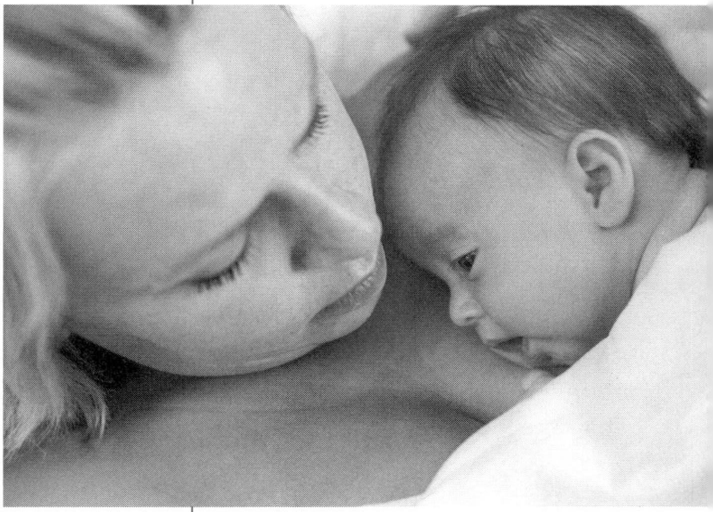

Nursing makes it easier for families to get in sync with their baby. With the use of MRI brain scans, U.S. researchers viewed brain changes in two groups of mothers—one group breastfed, the other formula-fed—during the first month after birth (Kim et al., 2011). They found that when their babies cried, breastfeeding mothers showed greater activation of the brain regions associated with nurturing behavior and empathy, as compared with formula-feeding mothers. A 2018 Japanese study of 25 first-time breastfeeding mothers (Matsunaga, Tanaka, & Myowa, 2018) found that the act of nurturing their babies increased mothers' sensitivity to perceiving and interpreting facial expressions in both babies and adults. Longer breastfeeding duration was associated with a longer period of sensitivity. They concluded that the experience in nurturing that mothers gain enhances their sensitivity to others. A Dutch study (Tharner et al., 2012) found an association between duration of breastfeeding and sensitive responsiveness and a more secure attachment.

Baby's State, Readiness, and Engagement

A baby's state of alertness affects his feeding behaviors and his ability to nurse.

One infant assessment guide, the Neonatal Behavior Assessment Scale (Brazelton & Nugent, 2011), describes six infant states:

- Deep sleep
- Light sleep
- Drowsy
- Quiet alert
- Fussy
- Crying

Babies nurse best in quiet alert, drowsy, and light sleep states. Before nursing, most fussy or crying babies first need to be calmed. Nursing is usually easiest and most effective when babies are in the quiet alert state, when they are drowsy, and even in light sleep (eyes moving under eyelids or other body movement). There may even be advantages to nursing some babies when drowsy or in light sleep. One U.K. study followed 12 late preterm babies born between 35 to 37 weeks gestation during their hospital stay after birth (S. Colson, DeRooy, & Hawdon, 2003). Their mothers were asked to keep their babies on their bodies as much of each day as they were comfortable to help ease their transition from womb to world. As these late preterm babies slept tummy down on their mothers' semi-reclined bodies, they showed feeding cues. When they rooted or head-bobbed with their eyes closed, their mothers helped them latch. On average, these late preterm babies—a group at serious risk for underfeeding because of their excessive sleepiness—nursed actively on average 2.5 hours of every 24-hour day, including those active feeds that occurred during light sleep.

Innate feeding behaviors continue to be triggered when babies are in a light sleep (S. Colson, 2019). If when awake a baby appears distressed during attempts to nurse, it may help for nursing parents to get into a semi-reclined position with baby resting on their body during sleep. U.K. research midwife Suzanne Colson suggested that sleep may "blunt" negative reactions to nursing that can interfere with feeding reflexes. Attempting nursing while baby is in a light sleep may help baby attach with less resistance. For more details, see Chapter 3, "Latching and Nursing Struggles."

• • •

Whenever possible, suggest nursing before baby starts crying.

One of the most common questions new parents ask is when to feed their baby. Although many parenting books describe how a new parent learns over time to tell the difference between a "hungry cry" and a "tired cry," babies should ideally be fed before they are crying at all. In its policy statement on breastfeeding (AAP, 2012), the American Academy of Pediatrics describes crying as "a late indicator of hunger" and suggests nursing before a baby gets to this point. It recommends nursing whenever babies show any of these early feeding cues:

- Increased alertness
- Physical activity
- Mouthing (including putting hand to mouth)
- Rooting (turning head from side to side with an open mouth as cheeks are touched)

Especially during the early weeks, suggest nursing whenever the baby will suck, whether he's hungry or not. Because a newborn's feeding reflexes can be triggered at any time, encourage nursing to relieve any mammary fullness (to prevent engorgement) or just as a way to enjoy greater closeness with the baby. The more opportunities babies have to nurse, the more quickly it becomes comfortable and automatic. Frequent feeds in the early weeks are also associated with better health outcomes and a healthy milk production (see next chapter).

• • •

When adults and babies interact, this active engagement can improve the baby's coordination during feeding attempts.

When U.S. pediatrician Christina Smillie studied the neurobehavioral literature, she discovered that eye contact, talking to baby, and touch (aspects of getting in sync) can improve baby's feeding coordination (Smillie, 2017). French neurologists looked for ways to simplify infant neurological exams and noticed that when babies were engaged through eye contact, talking, and touch that their coordination markedly improved and they could do motor tasks far beyond their age expectations (Amiel-Tison & Grenier, 1983). These researchers suggested that when babies appeared "charmed" by others, this "communicative state" was different from states previously identified. In this state, infants appeared to be "liberated" from many distracting reflexive behaviors, which made it possible for them to better control their actions. One remarkable photo from this study showed a 17-day-old "charmed" infant (with just a little head support provided by two of the researcher's fingers) sitting upright and reaching for a toy.

Similarly, in an overview article, U.S. neuropsychoanalyst Allan Schore (Schore, 2001) described that when caregivers and babies talk, look into each other's eyes, and touch, this interaction can create a direct intimate connection that allows the adult to help regulate baby's state. Schore called the resonance between a parent and baby ***affective synchrony***, which he said allows—as described at the beginning of this section—the newborn's immature systems to be "co-regulated by the caregiver's more mature and differentiated nervous system."

This information helped Smillie better understand the role of the parent-baby relationship to mastering nursing. By encouraging nursing parents to focus on their babies rather than learning specific feeding positions and techniques, the babies became more coordinated while latching, and as a result, they fed better with fewer problems (Smillie, 2017).

The Nursing Parent: Instincts and Learning

For parents, nursing appears to be partly learned and partly innate.

Some research suggests that mothers–like newborns–have biological triggers and innate responses. For example, without even thinking, a mother's body helps regulate her baby's body temperature (Chiu, Anderson, & Burkhammer, 2005).

The hormone oxytocin, released during nursing and skin-to-skin contact, makes most mothers feel like touching and stroking their baby (Uvnas-Moberg, 2014). Some of these behaviors may have an innate component. U.S. pediatrician Christina Smillie noted strong similarities in the way the mothers in her practice touch and stroke their babies (Smillie, 2017).

In one U.K. study (S. D. Colson et al., 2008), the researchers noted that during the first month after birth many of the mothers who were videotaped during breastfeeding made the same movements to trigger their babies' reflexes. For example, when the mothers were in a semi-reclined position with their hands free, they often helped their baby get into the same type of vertical position used in neurological exams and used their fingers to stroke their baby's feet, triggering toe fanning and toe grasping, which released lip and tongue reflexes and helped the baby latch and suck. The researchers wrote that the mothers "appeared to trigger instinctively the right reflex at the right time" and suggested that some aspects of breastfeeding may be innate for mothers as well.

KEY CONCEPT

For newborns, feeding is reflex-driven, but parents can overthink it, and their intellect can override their instincts.

But while newborns' behaviors are reflex-driven, adults can overthink nursing. Unlike other mammals, human mothers can use their intellect to overrule innate behaviors and emotions. In fact, U.K. research midwife Suzanne Colson suggested that engaging nursing mothers' intellect unnecessarily can even alter their hormonal state, making it more difficult for them to know what their body is telling them (S. Colson, 2019). This is why when nursing is going well, it is important for those supporting nursing parents after birth to engage their intellect only when families ask for input.

The Role of the Helper

Sensitive lactation help can boost families' "breastfeeding self-efficacy," a key influencer of nursing initiation, exclusivity, and duration.

Scientists refer to ***breastfeeding self-efficacy*** (BSE) to describe the level of confidence parents have in their ability to meet their nursing goals. BSE is measured with its short form (Dennis, 2003), which was validated worldwide. Whenever research examines the factors that influence nursing initiation, exclusivity, and duration, BSE is nearly always mentioned. A high or low BSE explains why some families nurse or don't nurse and why some persevere in spite of serious challenges while others give up at the slightest obstacle. BSE appears to be more important to nursing duration than the use of supplements or perceived support (Dunn, Davies, McCleary, Edwards, & Gaboury, 2006).

Lactation helpers can boost BSE through encouragement and by helping families overcome early feeding problems (Kilci & Coban, 2016). A 2017 systematic review and meta-analysis (Brockway, Benzies, Carr, & Aziz, 2018) concluded that BSE can be modified and that by using strategies that boost BSE, helpers can lengthen nursing duration. But the approach used to provide lactation help can make all the difference. If a family feels like the helper is taking over without permission or "talking at them" rather than involving them in decision-making, BSE can be lowered. The next section provides more details.

Approaches to Lactation Help

When helping nursing families, our underlying assumptions about our own role and the role of the nursing parent influence the quality of our interactions.

Providing families with effective lactation help is about more than just knowledge and clinical skills. Attitude and approach also play a key role in how families feel about the help they receive. Several studies from Australia provide insights into how lactation help is perceived and raise questions about the short- and long-term consequences of helping approaches on parenting style.

One of these qualitative studies (Burns, Fenwick, Sheehan, & Schmied, 2013) was conducted in publicly funded hospitals in two different areas of Australia. Its researchers made audio recordings of conversations between healthcare providers (midwives and lactation consultants) and breastfeeding mothers. They also observed the participants, interviewed them, and held focus groups. The researchers used a technique called "discourse analysis" to slow down recorded conversations to more clearly understand the assumptions underlying the interactions. They found that the healthcare providers primarily focused on lactation help used two basic approaches. One of these approaches was perceived by families as supportive. The other was perceived by many to be undermining.

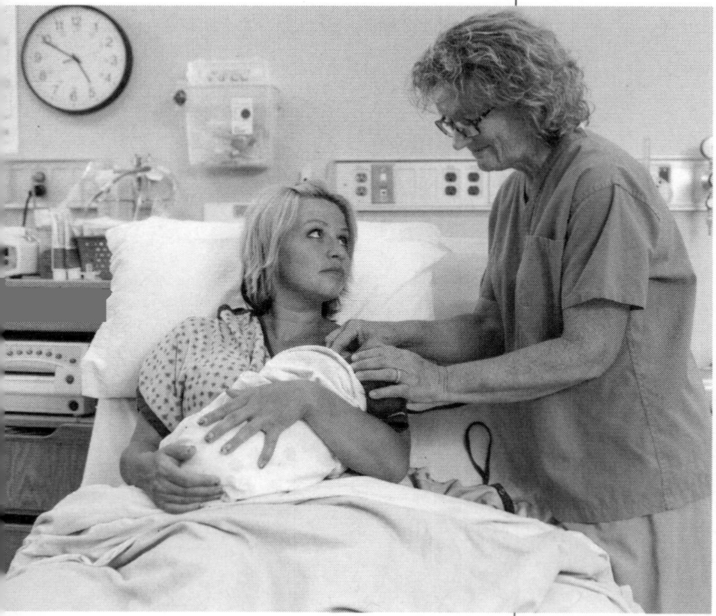

Approach 1: Helper as Expert. Table 1.2 describes these two basic approaches. Approach 1, which 80% of the study health professionals used, represents what the researchers called a medicalized approach to lactation help. This approach reflected the Cartesian view of medicine, in which the body is thought to be like a machine, with the focus on whatever body part is malfunctioning: the heart, the lungs, the kidneys, etc. This Cartesian view of medicine—also known as a "technocratic" approach—can work well when dealing with physical disease or dysfunction, but not so well with healthy processes like birth and nursing.

TABLE 1.2 Approaches to Lactation Help

	Approach 1: Helper as Expert	Approach 2: Mother as Expert
Top Priority	Nutrition: getting milk from breast into baby	Relationship: mother-baby, helper-family (equal partnership)
Perception of Mother	Novice in need of training in mechanical process, "milk machine"	Expert on baby and own needs, in need of support
Perception of Baby	Baby as independent decision-maker, personality traits (stubborn, lazy) can undermine nursing	Baby behaviors are normal, any struggles are part of the early learning process
Helper's Role	Make sure mother is "doing it right," helper provides information thought to be important	Reframe any negative interpretations, support family to "do it their way"
Helper's Communication Style	Closed-ended questions (yes or no answers), one-way "information dumps"	Open-ended questions, two-way conversations, customized suggestions via careful listening

Adapted from (Burns et al., 2013; Burns, Fenwick, Sheehan, & Schmied, 2016)

The midwives and lactation consultants who used Approach 1 considered themselves the lactation experts and their top priority a physical one: getting the milk from the breast into the baby. They emphasized the value of the "liquid gold." They saw the mother as a novice they needed to train in the mechanical process of breastfeeding. When nursing challenges arose, those using Approach 1 often attributed the problems to the baby's personality (referring to babies, for example, as "stubborn" or "lazy") and suggested baby made a conscious decision to cooperate with nursing or not (Burns et al., 2016). These lactation helpers often took over the latching process, sometimes without consent, and spoke critically of the mothers' latching techniques. Communications were often one-sided, with the lactation helpers doing what the researchers called an "information dump," giving long spiels of information they thought the mothers needed to know. These helpers often quickly turned to lactation tools, such as breast pumps and nipple shields, if nursing wasn't immediately successful. Many mothers felt these helpers were intrusive and their interactions undermining rather than supportive. With the focus on the breast and the milk, some mothers described feeling "invisible."

Approach 2: Mother as Expert. The second approach, which was used by only 9% of the study professionals, was based on an entirely different set of underlying assumptions. These midwives and lactation consultants viewed mothers as the experts on their baby and their own needs. Both through language and non-verbal cues, they expressed confidence in mothers' ability to breastfeed. These lactation helpers saw their top priority as helping the family establish a close relationship with their new baby and considered nursing a central part of that. They used open-ended questions (questions without a "yes" or "no" answer) to get needed information and built in ample time for the family to ask questions. To facilitate the mother-baby relationship, they often asked mothers to describe what they had learned about their baby. They viewed their relationship with the family as more of an equal partnership. Rather than seeing new mothers as novices, they considered both mother and baby to be in the "learning phase," which requires the support they were there to provide.

If the mothers described their baby in negative terms, these helpers reframed their comments to better reflect reality. For example, rather than "My baby is being stubborn," the helper might say, "Many newborns react this way. It may help to be patient and see if there is an adjustment that can help him calm and nurse." Rather than focusing on helping mothers "do it right," these helpers encouraged mothers to find their own way to make breastfeeding work. Helpers using Approach 2 primarily used "hands-off" lactation help but did help position the baby if asked. Rather than giving long "information dumps" of general facts, these helpers tailored any strategies to the mother's individual situation. The mothers considered these lactation helpers truly supportive, valued their assistance, and felt empowered and more confident with their help. These strategies boosted rather than lowered breastfeeding self-efficacy.

• • •

The kind of support that empowers nursing families does not usually involve teaching or taking over.

An Australia metasynthesis of both peer and professional support of breastfeeding mothers drew from both qualitative studies and large-scale surveys that included qualitative data (Schmied, Beake, Sheehan, McCourt, & Dykes, 2011). The researchers found that families perceived lactation help on a continuum from most supportive to undermining.

Authentic presence and a facilitative style were at the "most-supportive" end of the continuum. The authors called these lactation helpers an "authentic presence." These interactions with the mothers reflected trust and connectedness, and the helpers were perceived as empathetic. Helpers at this end of the spectrum used what the researchers called a "facilitative style." This meant that during their two-way discussions with families they provided realistic information. They didn't sugar-coat how challenging early nursing could be. They were proactive with practical help and the mothers described their approach as encouraging and the accurate information they provided sufficiently detailed to be of genuine help.

Disconnected encounters and a reductionist approach fell at the "undermining" end of the spectrum. Families viewed these helpers as dogmatic. These interactions often included conflicting advice and standard information that was not appropriate to their situation. Families felt these helpers were critical of them and blamed them for whatever issues that caused their struggles. This type of lactation help felt rushed and was based on telling rather than listening, and the families reported feeling pressured by the helpers to do things their way rather than feeling empowered. Helpers who had disconnected encounters with families also gave "hands-on" help in a way that the mothers spoke pointedly about. As the authors (Schmied et al., 2011, p. 57) noted:

> **KEY CONCEPT**
>
> *Families want realistic lactation help that acknowledges how challenging early nursing can be and tailors suggestions to their situation.*

> "...attempts by professionals to help in this way were often experienced as intrusive and rough. This insensitive and invasive touch meant some women felt as though they were being treated in a disembodied way—as though the breast was just a 'feeding implement.' In contrast, practical help, such as with latching on the baby, was appreciated if performed sensitively and within the context of a relationship with rapport and empathy."

It may help to keep in mind that learning to nurse is not an intellectual process. It is a part of parents' intimate relationship with their baby.

Early Helping Strategies: Keep It Simple

Due to the brain changes that occur during pregnancy and after birth, keep explanations simple.

During pregnancy and the early weeks after delivery, birthing parents undergo brain changes that make it more difficult to follow instructions and remember facts. A 2018 Chinese study used a resting-state MRI to record brain changes in 22 women during pregnancy and after birth and 23 controls. The researchers found significant decreases in the functions of the posterior cingulate cortex and the prefrontal cortex (Zheng et al., 2018). These changes may affect memory, planning, and reasoning. Some families call this change the "mommy brain," and some researchers referred to it as a "cognitive deficiency" (Eidelman, Hoffmann, & Kaitz, 1993) or "cognitive impairment" (Zheng et al., 2018). However, other scientists offer a more positive take on these changes, which they describe as an increase in brain plasticity that makes the adjustment to parenthood easier (Kim, 2016).

Due to these brain changes, a simplified approach to lactation help is more consistent with a birthing parent's physiology. One way this can be done is described by U.S. physician Christina Smillie. When Smillie began encouraging active engagement between mother and baby (holding, eye contact, talking), she noticed the babies who were engaged (in a "charmed" state) became more coordinated and proficient at feeding and the mothers became more confident. She also noticed that this engagement helped solve their feeding problems, and she became more effective at helping families meet their feeding goals.

• • •

Using a simplified approach with nursing families makes it easier for them to be responsive to their baby and to focus on their relationship.

Think of the more complicated approaches to lactation help as "head" knowledge and simplified approaches as "heart" or "body" knowledge. Some learning is best done with books and classes. Other learning is best done in other ways. Learning to ride a bicycle, for example, is best learned by feel.

In some ways, nursing is similar. The "feel" that guides parents as they learn to nurse comes from the physiological responses that draw parent and baby to one another. It's why they love to look at each other, touch each other, and interact. Much of this behavior is guided by the emotions that spring from our natural hormonal responses. Nursing is a natural outcome of this "heart" interaction between nursing parent and baby. A 2013 Spanish questionnaire study completed by 311 mothers (Diaz Meneses, 2013) found that nursing was more strongly rooted in the emotions rather than cognitive decision-making.

U.S. physician Dr. Christina Smillie emphasizes to families that "there is no one right way" to nurse (Smillie, 2017) and focuses instead on:

- Displaying confidence that nursing will work
- Encouraging parents to talk to their baby and maintain eye contact
- Reassuring them that their baby's actions are normal

Her main message to parents is that their job is not to learn to nurse (a "head" action) or to make their baby learn to nurse. Their job is to get comfortable, make sure the baby is well supported, and help the baby stay calm, relaxed, and comfortable.

In their overview of what families need to get breastfeeding off to the best start, U.S. midwife Robyn Schafer and U.S. lactation consultant Catherine Watson Genna (Schafer & Genna, 2015, p. 551), wrote:

"If she does not do so spontaneously, the woman can be encouraged to calm and encourage her newborn through voice and touch. Providers should offer reassuring communication, interpreting newborn behavior as normal and positive, praising how the woman responds to her newborn's physical cues, and reinforcing how the newborn reacts to the mother's efforts. Through the use of verbal and nonverbal communication that conveys self-efficacy in the dyad's ability to breastfeed independently, providers can facilitate maternal-newborn interaction and strengthen maternal confidence to build a successful breastfeeding relationship."

• • •

Teaching families specific feeding positions has drawbacks.

Naming and teaching feeding positions can make nursing seem unnecessarily complicated. U.S. physician Christina Smillie noted that we don't teach bottle-feeding positions (e.g., "the highchair hold," "the car-seat hold"). We trust that when families feed their babies by bottle, they will find their own comfortable feeding positions. She suggests the same should be true when supporting nursing.

Another drawback to teaching specific nursing positions is that it may put the focus on the wrong things. Parents expressing concern about whether they are doing specific positions "right" or trying to exactly duplicate a position they see in a photo or class takes their focus off their baby's response. There are no "right" or "wrong," "proper" or "improper" feeding positions. But some aspects of body positions can work for or against nursing. For details, see the next section.

Nursing parents and babies come in different shapes and sizes, and there are hundreds of possible feeding positions. This is a much more helpful message than implying that nursing parents are limited to just a few positions or being too directive about how they should hold their babies. It boosts new parents' confidence in their own abilities when they find comfortable positions on their own and when nursing parent and baby work this out without outside help.

KEY CONCEPT

Being too specific about feeding positions can make nursing feel difficult and complicated.

In one randomized trial of 160 first-time mothers in Australia, the mothers were assigned to one of two groups (Henderson, Stamp, & Pincombe, 2001). During the first 24 hours after birth, one group received one-on-one positioning-and-attachment teaching (the experimental group). The other group didn't. Although the mothers who received the training reported less nipple pain on the second day in the hospital, these mothers also had a trend toward lower breastfeeding rates and less satisfaction with breastfeeding at 3 and 6 months. The researchers noted that it wasn't possible to rule out the training as the cause (Henderson et al., 2001, p. 41):

"...[A] possible unintended consequence of the emphasis on instruction and assessment of positioning and attachment may have been to raise anxiety in first-time mothers....The physical and psychological events of childbirth may also influence the amount of information a new mother can process. Therefore this intervention may have contributed to a feeling that breastfeeding was too difficult for women in the experimental group."

• • •

Early nursing ideally occurs in an environment that enhances nursing parents' hormonal response to their baby, which is linked to increased duration of nursing (Nissen et al., 1996). Creating a relaxing and supportive environment includes:

- Ensuring privacy, warmth, and comfort
- Respecting nursing parents' choices and reinforcing what they do right
- Enhancing their feelings of competence as they learn to care for their newborn by minimizing information/teaching unless requested or when necessary

When supporting normal nursing, keep the focus on creating a conducive environment, getting comfortable, and giving encouragement rather than instructions.

Instruction can disrupt nursing parents' ability to tap into and trust their natural responses, which may ultimately undermine nursing. Instructions trigger thinking, which also takes the focus off the baby and may even cause nursing parents to question their competence. Too much information at the wrong time can also be overwhelming. Finding a comfortable, private place to interact freely with the baby allows the inborn hardwiring described in this chapter to unfold and allows each family to find their own best approach to nursing. This approach also enhances both self-confidence and their relationship with their new baby. As two U.S. authors wrote in their overview article describing an evidence-based, physiologic approach to breastfeeding initiation (Schafer & Genna, 2015, p. 548):

> "...contemporary theories of breastfeeding initiation have shifted away from mechanical positioning-and-attachment models toward a focus on supporting a relationship-centered breastfeeding experience incorporating innate breastfeeding abilities."

POSITIONING BASICS

Every family brings a different blend of anatomy and temperament to nursing. For this reason, it's wise to approach positioning with an attitude of flexibility, along with a basic understanding of what nature builds into babies and parents. Australian physician Pamela Douglas and nurse-lactation consultant Renee Keogh describe many of the anatomical factors that can affect positioning for women and infants (Douglas & Keogh, 2017, p. 510):

Every nursing couple is unique, so encourage an open mind about feeding positions, using comfort as a guide.

> "A woman's unique anatomy, including breast size and elasticity, abdominal shape; lap length; nipple shape, size and direction; and upper and forearm length and shape, and her infant's unique anatomy, including palate contour; oral connective tissue length, attachments and elasticities; tongue length, oral cavity size; and chin recession or shape need to fit together in a way that supports positional stability, nipple protection or healing, and optimal milk transfer. This is particularly important in mother-infant pairs facing anatomic challenges, including (but not limited to) inelastic breast tissue, pendulous breasts, recessed infant mandible, high infant palate, and obesity."

When considering feeding positions, the baby's age also makes a difference. During the first 4 to 6 weeks, for example, newborns have very little head-and-neck control, which means that until baby matures, some positions may be easier for a newborn than others. (See the next section "Starter Positions: The Early Weeks.)

• • •

There is no advantage to varying positions at every nursing session, unless there is a special need.

In the past, some nursing parents were told to routinely vary their positions at each feed. This idea became popular at a time when nipple pain and trauma were erroneously thought to be a normal part of nursing and was based on the premise that using different positions would more evenly spread the pain and damage, making nursing more tolerable.

With a better understanding of the causes of nipple trauma, this recommendation no longer makes sense, except in special situations, such as babies with untreated tongue-tie, an unusually shaped palate, or another anatomic variation that makes nursing painful despite a deep latch.

• • •

Feeding positions fall into two general categories: primarily baby-driven and primarily parent-driven.

The earlier section, "Baby's Inborn Feeding Behaviors," described how—like all other mammal newborns—healthy human newborns come into the world with behaviors built in by nature that allow them to get to their food source and feed. But these behaviors only lead to successful feeding if the conditions are right. In some positions, these same inborn feeding behaviors can act as barriers to successful feeding.

All feeding positions can be put into one of two basic categories. The first of these two approaches (which is described in more detail in the next section) is especially well suited to newborns.

Primarily baby-driven approach to positioning. As a U.K. research team (S. D. Colson et al., 2008) found, newborns' primitive neonatal reflexes are more likely to lead to successful feeding when the nursing parent leans back into a semi-reclined position and baby rests tummy down on the parent's body. These ***starter positions*** (see next section) include many variations, allowing families to tailor them to their unique anatomies and temperaments. Although this approach has often mistakenly been referred to as one (the "laid-back") position, this is far from true, as the next section describes. This approach has as many variations as its alternative approach.

Primarily parent-driven approach to positioning. This second approach includes the sitting-up-straight feeding positions that in decades past lactation supporters traditionally taught: the cradle hold, the cross-cradle hold, and the football/rugby or clutch hold. While these positions may be helpful in some cases, drawbacks to using these feeding positions during the newborn period include:

- **Full frontal contact (which orients baby) is easily lost.** The pull of gravity often causes gaps to form between them, which can lead to latching struggles.
- **Positional stability (which baby needs to keep his focus on feeding) is more difficult to achieve and maintain** against the pull of gravity.

- **Baby's primitive neonatal reflexes may become barriers to nursing.** In the sitting-up-straight positions, the same reflexes nature builds in (such as arm and leg cycling) can become barriers to feeding (batting at the nipple and kicking) (S. D. Colson et al., 2008).
- **Managing milk flow is more difficult for some newborns,** leading to coughing and sputtering during feeds.
- **Nursing parents have the primary responsibility for achieving a deep latch.** If they are unskilled, the result may be a shallow latch, one cause of feeding struggles, ineffective milk transfer, and nipple pain. One 2016 retrospective cross-sectional Australian analysis (Thompson et al., 2016) found a 4-fold increase in the incidence of nipple trauma among women using the cross-cradle hold compared with those using other holds.
- **Requires detailed instructions to achieve a deep latch** by inexperienced nursing parents, which may be difficult for them to master and remember due to brain changes during the early weeks after birth. In these upright positions, without head-and-neck control, the newborn cannot take an active role in latching.
- **Pressure is put on the tender perineum** in sitting-up-straight positions, which can cause discomfort after a vaginal delivery.
- **Muscle strain and fatigue are common** from supporting baby's weight in arms, making nursing tiring. This motivates some to keep feeds short, which may contribute to milk production issues.
- **Muscle relaxation can cause a deep latch to become shallow.** The hormones of nursing naturally relax muscles during feeds, which may turn a deep latch shallow for painful feeds.

Starter Positions: The Early Weeks

As described in the section, "Baby's Inborn Feeding Behaviors," healthy term babies are born with an internal navigation system triggered by full frontal contact that guides them to the nipple and helps them latch and feed. If families know how to activate and use this internal navigation system, they can avoid many early feeding struggles (S. D. Colson et al., 2008; Douglas & Keogh, 2017).

During the first 4 to 6 weeks after birth, starter positions—which involve a primarily baby-driven approach to positioning—are easier for many new families than sitting-up-straight nursing holds.

In starter feeding positions (Figure 1.1), newborns can take an active role in getting to the nipple and latching. When using this approach, the nursing parent relaxes into a semi-reclined position with a body slope between about 15 and 65 degrees (Figure 1.2). In these positions, parents need enough arm and body support so they can relax all their muscles. Baby rests tummy down, hands free on the parent's body with easy access to the nipple. The nursing parents' arms act as guardrails to keep baby safely on their body and, as needed, as head support for the newborn.

Some advantages of starter positions during the newborn period include:

- **Full frontal contact (which orients baby) is guaranteed,** reducing latching struggles.
- **Positional stability (which keeps baby focused on feeding) is nearly automatic.**

Figure 1.1 Starter positions.

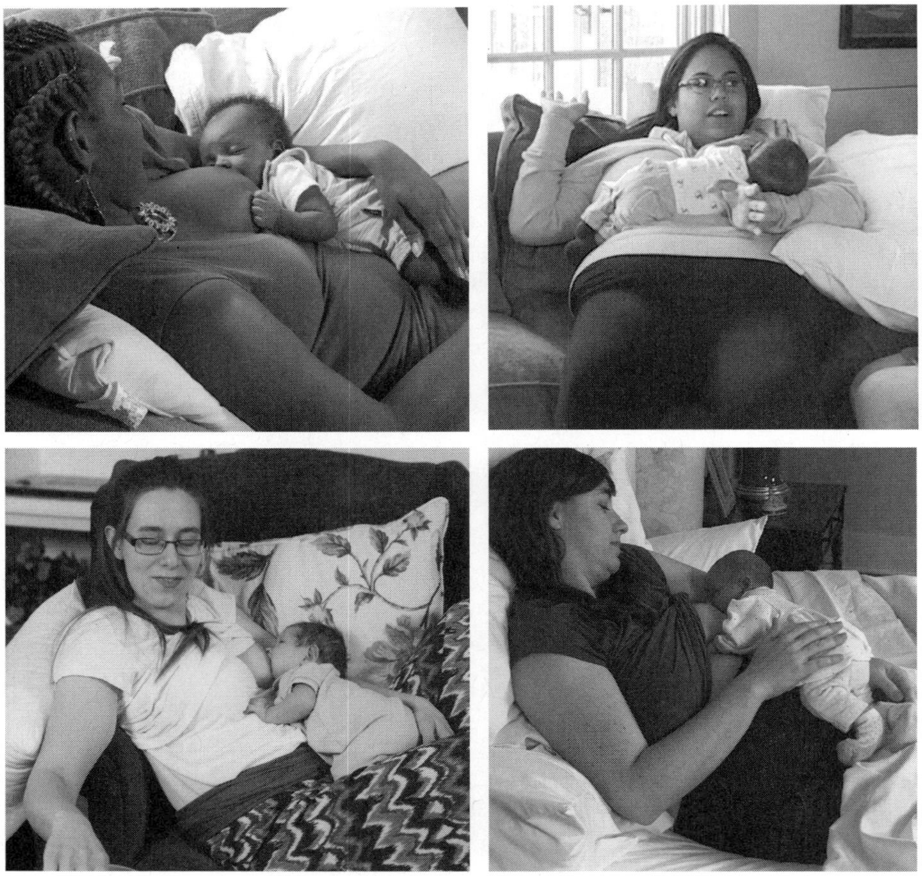

- **Gravity works in harmony with baby's primitive neonatal reflexes,** leading to more successful feeding (S. D. Colson et al., 2008; Douglas & Keogh, 2017).
- **Babies manage milk flow more easily** (Marmet & Shell, 2017) due either to the effects of gravity, a more stable feeding position, or both (Douglas & Keogh, 2017).
- **The baby has primary responsibility for latching.** Babies are hardwired at birth to self-attach. In these positions, newborns can adjust the latch as needed until it feels optimal.
- **Avoids the need for complicated positioning and latch instructions,** so the nursing parent can focus on the baby and on providing the baby with any needed help or support.
- **Avoids pressure on the tender perineum,** eliminating one common source of discomfort after a vaginal birth.
- **Eliminates muscle strain and fatigue,** as baby's weight is supported by the nursing parent's body rather than in arms. In these positions, parents can rest and recover during feeds. When nursing is relaxed and comfortable, parents are more likely to nurse longer, enhancing early milk production.
- **Muscle relaxation from the hormones of nursing causes baby's latch to deepen during feeds** due to the effects of gravity, making nursing more comfortable and effective.

These positions can also be helpful with young babies who have nursing challenges related to tongue-tie or a small or receding lower jaw, because gravity pulls the tongue and chin forward (Marmet & Shell, 2017).

In many parts of the world, after birth, parents are in these positions while baby does the breast crawl (Girish et al., 2013). Yet at the next feed, many are told to sit up straight to nurse. Because of their many advantages during the first 4 to 6 weeks, all parents deserve to know that these positions are an option. When babies can take an active role in finding the nipple and latching, this often prevents or alleviates early feeding problems (Smillie, 2017).

Australian physician Pamela Douglas describes starter positions in her approach to early nursing (Douglas & Keogh, 2017), which she calls ***gestalt breastfeeding***, meaning the whole is greater than the sum of its parts.

• • •

Starter positions have advantages for lactation helpers, such as saving time and eliminating the need for detailed latching instructions (S. Colson, 2012). This approach can also reduce job-related back, neck, and shoulder pain from bending over while assisting with nursing.

Starter positions have advantages for lactation helpers, too, but those who are more familiar with sitting-up-straight nursing holds may need new skills and new ways of thinking about positioning.

Many lactation specialists originally learned to help families with the traditional sitting-up-straight holds. But different skills and a different vocabulary are needed when families customize starter positions to their anatomy and comfort. This author, along with U.S. obstetrician Theresa Nesbitt, developed a simplified vocabulary for helping families with starter positions. These terms are not copyrighted or trademarked, so they can be used without the need for permission. The descriptions of the three basic adjustments are: "adjust your body," "adjust your baby," and "adjust your breast." The following points provide the details. They are also featured in a free video at **NaturalBreastfeeding.com**.

• • •

"Adjust your body" refers to the following possible adjustments of the nursing parent's body.

"Adjust your body" refers to adjustments used to get comfortable and support the baby.

Parent's body slope. U.K. research midwife Suzanne Colson and her team concluded from their study that the most effective body slope for triggering feeding reflexes is between 15 and 65 degrees. Fortunately, a helper does not need a protractor to determine body slope. An easy way to think about it is that nursing parents need to be reclined enough so that if they raise their hands, the baby stays in place. In other words, baby's weight is fully resting on the parent's body rather than being held in position by their hands or arms. Their torso also needs to be elevated enough to make baby's face easily visible without neck strain. Colson recommended against nursing while lying flat on their back (supine) to prevent the newborn's breathing from becoming unknowingly obstructed (S. Colson, 2014). Although parents can use these semi-reclined positions anywhere, hospital beds can easily be adjusted to many angles, making it simple to try different body slopes.

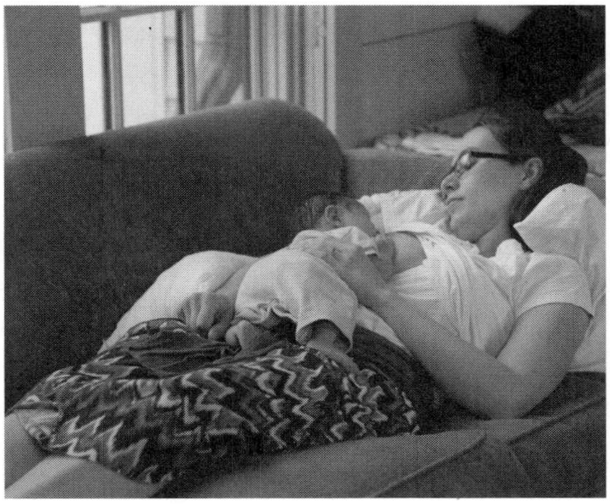

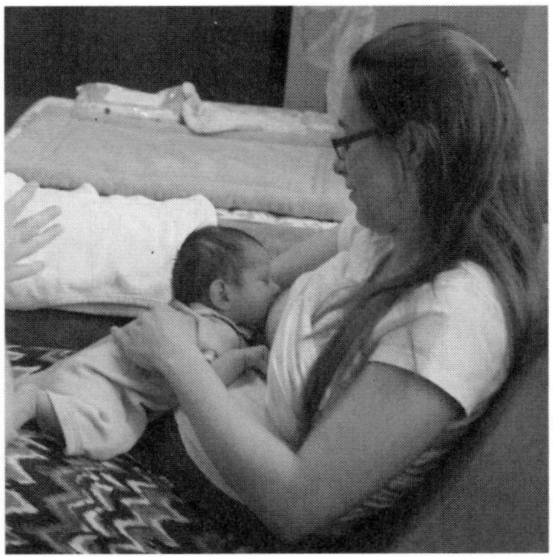

Figure 1.2 Starter positions include all body slopes between 15° and 65°.

Parent's body support. Ideally in starter positions, nursing parents can relax all

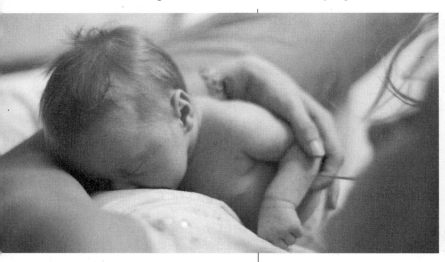

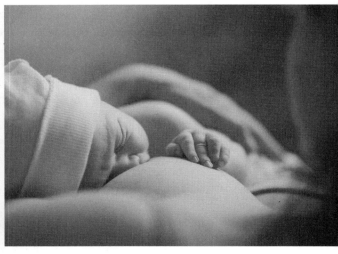

Figure 1.3 Left: Face plant. Right: Mother's left arm lowered slightly for breathing space.

their muscles. To do this, it may help to position pillows or cushions behind their back, under their arms, and/or behind their head. To determine whether more support is needed, stand back and check to see if a shoulder is raised or if any muscles seem tense. If so, offer rolled cloths or pillows. In the similar "gestalt breastfeeding" approach, Australian physician Douglas described how after receiving permission, helpers sometimes put their hands or arms on the parent's body to help them relax (Douglas & Keogh, 2017).

Parents' arms and hands are used differently in starter positions than in sitting-up-straight holds. With baby's weight resting fully on the parent's body, their arms are not needed to support baby's weight. Since baby self-attaches when using this approach, there's no need to push or guide baby on deeply during latch. Instead their arms are used as guardrails to help keep the baby safely on their body and as head support during feeds. Depending on the length of the parent's arms and mammary size, baby may rest his head on their upper or lower arm during nursing. In starter positions, often parents' hands are completely free.

Arm adjustments to safeguard baby's breathing. If baby does a face plant into the mammary tissue and has trouble breathing, suggest slightly lowering the arm that's supporting baby's head to provide breathing space (Figure 1.3), or try positioning baby's body differently (see next point). Usually all that's needed to ensure unrestricted breathing is a small adjustment.

Support the mammary gland? Nursing is usually easier when the mammary gland lays at its natural level. Lifting it can cause feeding problems. Australian authors described some of the drawbacks of routine breast lifting, as are exceptions to this recommendation (Douglas & Keogh, 2017, p. 517):

> "Teaching women to lift and shape her breast increases the risk of nipple pain 4-fold (Thompson et al., 2016). This is because when she lets go of the breast, a vector of force is generated by the downward pull of gravity on the breast, which conflicts with the direction of the intraoral vacuum [inside the baby's mouth]. Sometimes, the breast requires the support of a folded cloth underneath to expose an adequate landing pad [for the baby to latch]. Occasionally, women with very generous breasts or downward pointing nipples need to lift the breast a little with the hand to expose an adequate landing pad."

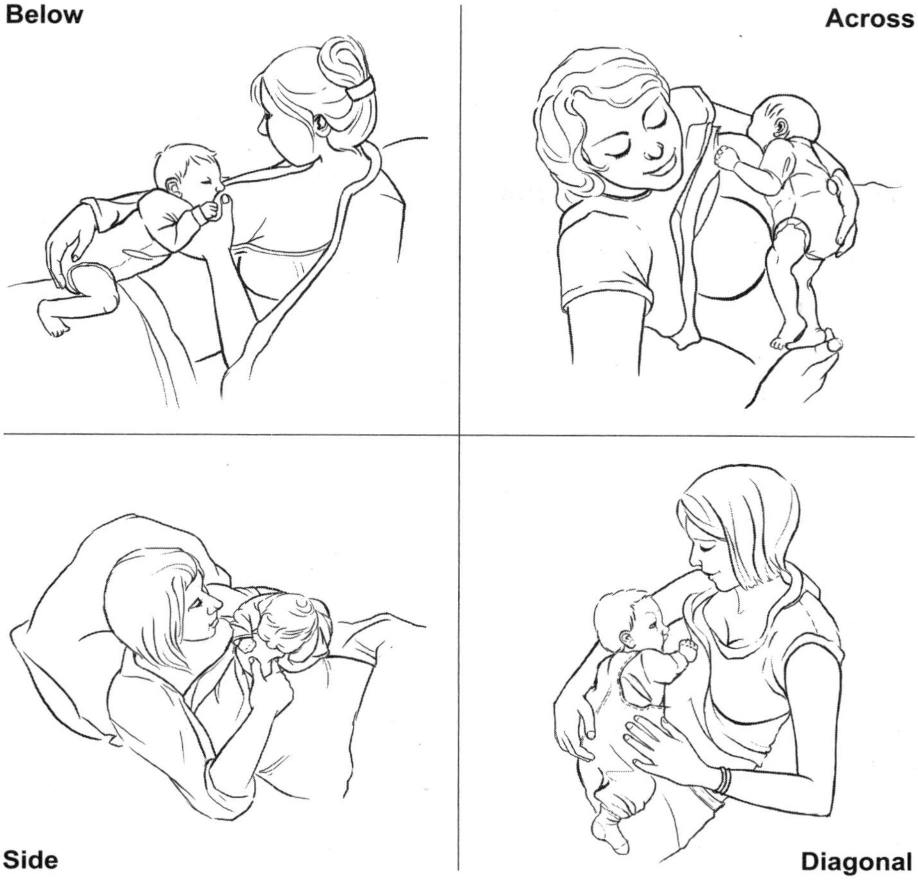

Figure 1.4 Some of baby's many lie options ©2020 Nancy Mohrbacher Solutions, Inc.

• • •

"Adjust your baby" refers to several adjustments parents can make for greater comfort and feeding effectiveness.

The baby's body can be adjusted in several ways that may make nursing easier.

Baby's body direction. Because the nipple is a circle, a baby can approach it in a tummy-down position from many different angles. Think of the nipple like a clock face. In most cases, babies will approach the nipple somewhere between 3 o'clock and 9 o'clock. That means baby will likely lie on the parent's body vertically, horizontally, or diagonally. After a cesarean birth, avoid a vertical lie to prevent baby's weight from resting on the surgical incision. But there are many other choices. The baby may be supported at the parent's side (see the lower left section of Figure 1.4) or even over the parent's shoulder.

Baby's hands are free and uncovered. Babies' hands serve many purposes before and during nursing. Having control of their hands helps babies locate the nipple, stimulate the release of oxytocin, and stabilize and calm themselves (Genna & Barak, 2010). Babies' hands are also a part of their internal navigation system.

Frog legs. To help baby orient himself and more easily find the nipple, he needs to be fully tummy down on the parent's body. To check that his hips are not twisted, put a hand under the baby's groin area and lift slightly. If baby's legs are splayed apart (look like frog legs), this ensures full frontal contact.

Baby's head higher than bottom. Most babies feel unstable when held in a head-down position, and rather than focusing on feeding, devote their energy to trying to get stable. If baby's head is lower than his bottom, suggest the nursing parent rotate their hips or readjust their body position until baby's head is higher than his bottom so he can focus on feeding.

Foot contact. Another part of baby's internal navigation system involves foot contact. Baby orients more easily if either the tops or soles of baby's feet are touching the nursing parent's body or something else. If baby's feet are out in thin air, try rolling up a towel or baby blanket and wedging it under baby's feet or shift baby's body position until his feet touch the parent's body.

• • •

"Adjust your breast" is not always needed, but if baby still struggles to latch after the other adjustments are made, some gentle shaping can sometimes help.

Even though the nursing couple is well positioned, in some cases, the baby may still struggle to latch. This can happen with engorged or naturally taut mammary tissue. Some newborns need a little help getting their mouth around the mammary tissue. In this case, gentle shaping may be just enough for the baby to get a deep latch.

Shaping the mammary tissue means placing the fingers far enough back from the areola so that they don't get in baby's way during latch (Figure 1.5) and then squeezing gently. The goal is to change the circle into an oval that runs parallel to baby's lips (wider at the corners and narrower between the upper and lower jaws). If the oval runs perpendicular to baby's lips, this makes latching more challenging, like trying to take a bite out of a sandwich held vertically rather than horizontally in front of our mouth. Another quick, easy way to describe this dynamic is to suggest shaping the tissue "like a hamburger, not a taco" (using hand motions to illustrate). Although we usually turn our heads to the side to eat a taco so that the filling doesn't fall out, this analogy usually gets the idea across.

TABLE 1.3 Starter Positions Checklist

Adjustments To Try	YES	NO
Is the baby upset and needs to be calmed first?		
Is the nursing parent semi-reclined (body slope between 15° and 65°) and fully supported and relaxed?		
When the nursing parent's hands are raised, does baby stay in place?		
Is baby fully tummy down in a frog-legs position?		
Is baby's head higher than his bottom?		
Have they tried varying the direction of baby's lie?		
Are baby's feet in contact with the parent or something else?		
Have they tried shaping the mammary tissue (hamburger not taco)?		
If baby's breathing is blocked, have they tried slightly lowering the arm that supports baby's head or varying the direction of baby's lie?		

Adapted from **NaturalBreastfeeding.com**

• • •

To help understand some of the basic differences between traditional upright holds and starter positions, it's helpful to know which strategies commonly used with upright holds are best avoided with the starter positions.

Some strategies are best avoided when using starter positions.

- **Nursing pillows** make sense in traditional holds as an alternative to supporting baby's weight in arms. In starter positions, though, they simply get in the way. Any pillows are best used to support the nursing parent rather than the baby.
- **Pressure to baby's back or shoulders during latch.** This action is necessary for a deep latch when the nursing couple is fighting gravity in upright positions. It is not necessary in starter positions. Some babies respond negatively to being pushed onto the nipple during latch by tensing their jaw. Swedish researchers suggested that pushing baby on during latch may contribute to nursing aversion in some babies (Svensson, Velandia, Matthiesen, Welles-Nystrom, & Widstrom, 2013).
- **Asymmetrical latch** makes achieving a deep latch easier in upright positions. In starter positions, though, it is not necessary. Baby can make whatever adjustments are needed to ensure the nipple extends into the comfort zone, where there is no friction or pressure.
- **After latch, checking baby's lips.** An Australian physician notes that this action often inadvertently pulls mammary tissue out of the back of baby's mouth (Douglas & Keogh, 2017). It's not necessary to see baby's lips. What is most important to know is whether nursing is comfortable and baby is feeding actively. If both are true, leave baby's lips and the mammary tissue alone.

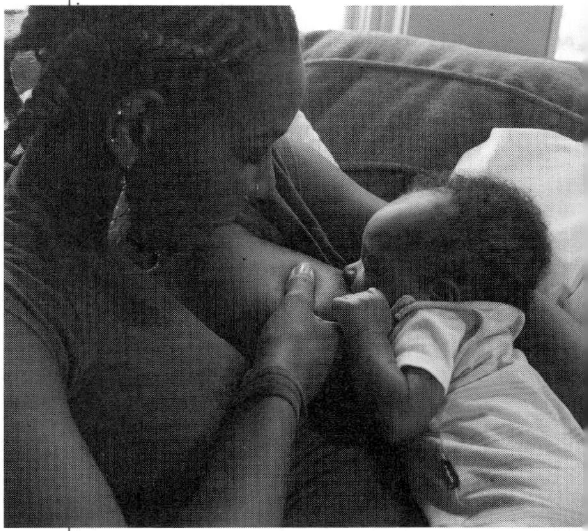

Figure 1.5 If baby struggles to latch, gentle shaping of the mammary tissue can sometimes help.

- **Covering or restraining baby's hands.** Restraining baby's hands by swaddling baby during feeds or pinning baby's arms behind the nursing parent's body is sometimes recommended in upright positions. But when gravity works in harmony with baby's reflexes in starter positions, it is not only unnecessary, it can cause feeding struggles (Schafer & Genna, 2015).
- **Touching the back of baby's head.** This action can complicate nursing in upright and starter positions, as one of baby's reflexes (which is used to exit the birth canal) causes babies to push back, which can lead to latching struggles.

Basic Body Dynamics in Any Position

Due to individual differences, no single positioning strategy works with all nursing families all the time, so be prepared with alternatives.

For the vast majority of nursing families, starter positions work well during the newborn period because they make the most of a young baby's inborn feeding behaviors and allow him to take an active role in latching, but there are always exceptions. Also, babies don't stay newborns for very long. For these reasons, lactation helpers need to be ready when families want or need alternatives. In the following situations, it makes sense to try upright or side-lying positions.

- **The nursing parent does not want to use starter positions.** Some prefer to nurse upright or side-lying. Affirming what feels right to the nursing parent is one critical aspect of supportive lactation help.

- **After trying all the adjustments, the baby still struggles to latch or feed.** Some babies become upset when they get near the nipple due to previous negative nursing attempts. Some babies struggle to nurse due to anatomical variations, minimal mammary tissue from chest masculinization or other surgeries, an undiagnosed infant health problem, or other factors. For strategies, see Chapter 3, "Latching and Nursing Struggles."

Also, as babies grow, most nursing parents want to expand their repertoire with other holds, such as side-lying for night feeds or upright positions for nursing in public, and they may ask for help in making them work.

• • •

Knowing something about inborn infant feeding behaviors can help avoid struggles and make nursing easier in any position.

The same dynamics that make starter positions work can be used in many other positions as well. For example:

- **Positional stability** involves making sure baby feels physically stable, with his head higher than bottom.
- **Full frontal contact** is key to baby feeling oriented in any position. For full frontal contact, baby's body needs to fully face the parent's body. If gaps form between them, suggest pulling baby in closer.
- **Foot and eye contact.** Foot contact helps orient baby. Ensure that either the tops or soles of baby's feet touch the parent's body or something else, such as a rolled-up towel or baby blanket. Eye contact is important, especially when the nursing parent has primary responsibility for the latch. A 2017 Japanese study used special eye-tracking equipment to evaluate the gaze of 74 nursing mothers of 1-month-old babies during the latching process (Kikuchi et al., 2017). The mothers gazed primarily at the breast, the lower half of baby's face, the space between the breast and baby's face, and the area where the baby's face made contact with the breast.
- **Nose to nipple with baby's head slightly tilted back** for easier swallowing. If needed, baby's body position can be adjusted.
- **Chin touching the mammary tissue, then wait for the gape.** The contact of the chin and the parent's body triggers the wide-open mouth (gape) needed for a deep latch.
- **Asymmetrical latch** (Figure 1.6), which means during latching baby's lower jaw is as far from the nipple as possible to allow the nipple to extend deeper into baby's mouth. This isn't necessary in starter positions but can be important for comfortable, effective nursing in other positions. For more details, see p. 878.
- **Gentle pressure behind baby's shoulders during latch, avoiding the back of baby's head,** as this can cause arching and feeding struggles. If head support is needed, position palm on baby's back and thumb and index finger behind baby's ears (Figure 1.6).
- **Continued gentle pressure behind baby's shoulders during the feed.** This prevents gaps from forming and provides the baby with more core stability and coordination. In a side-lying position, this gentle pressure can be provided with a rolled-up towel or baby blanket wedged behind baby's back (Figure 1.9).

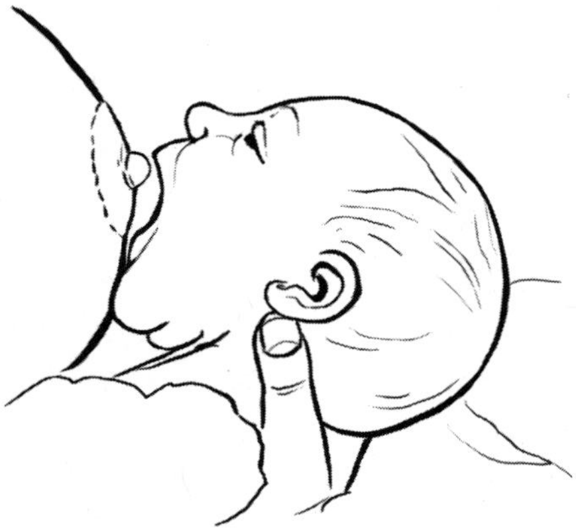

Figure 1.6 Asymmetrical latch. ©2020 Nancy Mohrbacher Solutions, Inc.

Side-Lying

In side-lying positions, parent and baby lie on their sides facing one another. As described previously, to focus on feeding, babies must feel physically stable. In side-lying positions—assuming the surface doesn't shift—the surface provides automatic positional stability. This may be one reason a randomized controlled trial of 152 women in Thailand after cesarean births (Puapornpong, Raungrongmorakot, Laosooksathit, Hanprasertpong, & Ketsuwan, 2017) found that during the hospital stay nursing outcomes were the same in its two groups: those who used starter positions and those who used side-lying positions.

Side-lying, which is often used for night nursing, is a good second choice during the newborn period, because the surface provides positional stability.

• • •

Side-lying positions allow nursing parents to rest while baby feeds, so they are ideal for night nursing. In all versions of side-lying, parents and babies face one another on their sides with the nipple directly in front of baby's mouth. When used with a newborn, the parent needs to help baby latch with a hand on baby's upper back. Babies older than 6 weeks or so have usually developed enough head-and-neck control so they can latch by themselves. Try the following variations until the nursing couple finds its own best fit:

To help nursing couples make side-lying work, experiment with its variations.

- Baby's head lies flat on the surface with parent's lower arm out of the way or cradling baby (Figure 1.7).

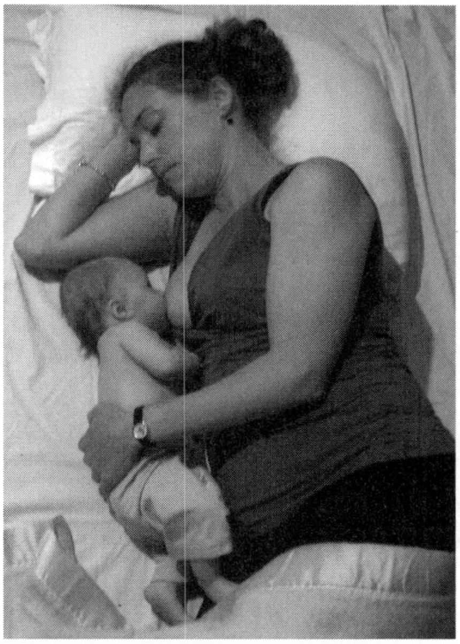

Figure 1.7 This baby's head rests on the bed, feet against mother's thigh. ©2020 Mary Jane Chase, used with permission.

- Baby's head is supported by the parent's lower arm. (Figure 1.8).

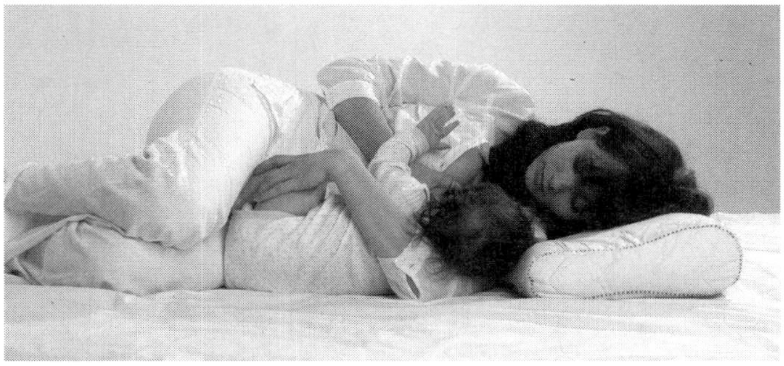

Figure 1.8 Mother's lower arm supports baby's head.

- To keep a newborn on his side and pulled in close, the parent can either place the hand of their upper arm on baby's back or wedge a rolled-up towel or baby blanket behind baby's back. Note: Baby's head needs to be free to tilt back slightly for easier swallowing (Figure 1.9).

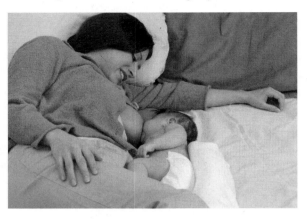

Figure 1.9 Newborn has a rolled cloth wedged behind his back to keep him on his side.

- When switching sides, either hold baby to chest and roll over or lean over so baby can latch to the upper breast in the same position (Figure 1.10).

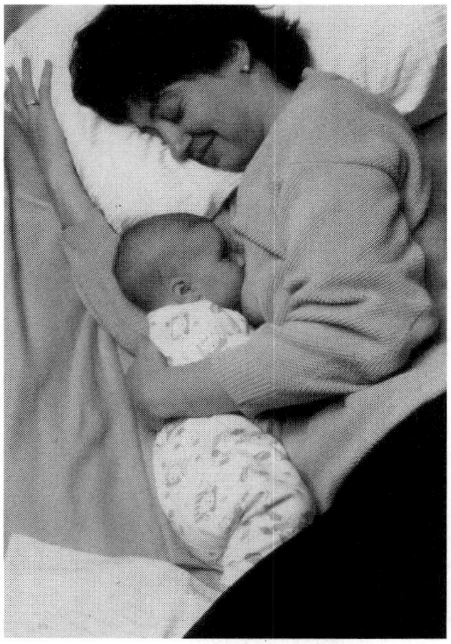

Figure 1.10 Switching sides by leaning over. ©2020 Barbara Hardin, used with permission.

It may also help to add pillows for support under parents' head and their upper knee. Depending on the size and shape of the mammary tissue and the location of the nipples, some find it helpful to lean back slightly into a pillow for support (Figure 1.9).

Upright Holds

Nursing goes more smoothly in upright holds when baby is in full frontal contact with the nursing parent.

The most commonly taught upright holds are the cradle hold (Figure 1.11), the cross-cradle hold (Figure 1.12), and the football/rugby or clutch hold (Figure 1.13). The football/rugby hold is sometimes recommended after a cesarean birth to keep baby's weight away from the incision. The best way to achieve positional stability in these holds is for nursing parents to make sure the baby's entire front (torso, hips, legs, and feet) are gently pressed against their body.

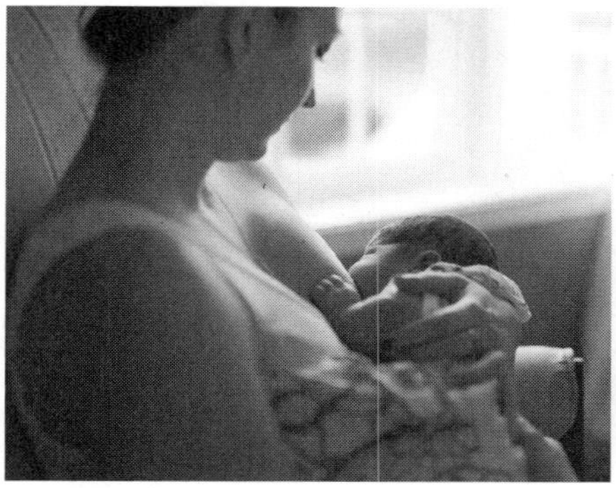

Figure 1.11 Cradle hold.

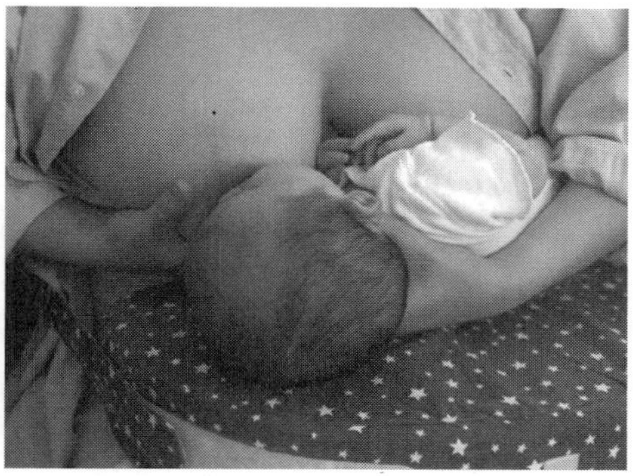

Figure 1.12 Cross-cradle hold. This mother pulls baby's body in close with her left elbow. ©2020 Catherine Watson Genna, used with permission.

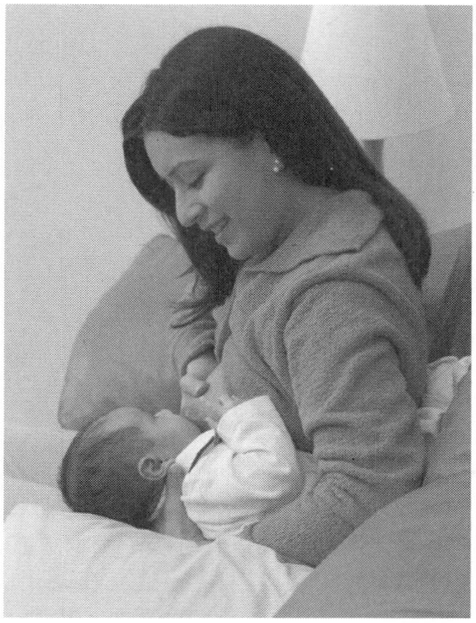

Figure 1.13 Football/rugby hold. The soles of this baby's feet rest on the sofa behind mother.

In upright positions, keeping baby at nipple height and his body close can feel awkward, tiring, and lead to muscle strain. The use of pillows or cushions to support baby's weight may help, provided they support the baby at the right height: not too high, which makes getting a deep latch challenging, and not too low, which may lead to back or neck pain from bending over during feeds. Without support during nursing, a deep latch may become shallower as the feed progresses. One Australian retrospective cross-sectional analysis of 653 mother-infant records of home visits (Thompson et al., 2016) concluded that mothers who used the cross-cradle hold were 4 times more likely to experience nipple pain and trauma compared with those who used other feeding positions. The authors wrote in the study's abstract that the use of the cross-cradle hold "…appeared to limit the baby's instinctive ability to activate neuro-sensory mammalian behaviours to freely locate and effectively draw the nipple and breast tissue without causing trauma." The cross-cradle hold does give parents a clear view of the baby's face, which may make a deep latch easier. If a nursing parent finds the cross-cradle hold helpful during latch, one option to increase comfort is to latch baby in the cross-cradle hold and then relax back into a semi-reclined position, with baby's weight resting on the parent's body.

As with other positions, upright holds need to be tailored to the nursing parents' body type and the baby's response. For details on how to help nursing parents whose anatomy is challenging, see p. 114.

Supporting or Shaping Mammary Tissue

Depending on body shape, feeding position, and nipple location in relation to the baby, a nursing parent may or may not support their mammary tissue during feeds. This is best left to the parent's discretion. See the earlier point "Adjust your breast," on p. 28.

Some nursing parents use their hands to support their mammary tissue during feeds; others do not; and some vary this from feed to feed.

• • •

When supporting mammary tissue in an upright position, suggest keeping it at or near its natural level.

The closer the mammary tissue is to its natural height, the less work is involved in maintaining it during feeds. If nursing is easier with support, suggest focusing primarily on the section near the nipple and areola, as this is the area the baby needs to manage during nursing. For more strategies, see p. 114.

Positions for Special Situations

Straddle Hold

A straddle hold may be helpful for babies with a cleft palate, hip dysplasia, airway abnormalities, low muscle tone, and for some neurologically impaired babies.

In a straddle hold—either upright (Figure 1.14) or semi-reclined (Figure 1.15)—parent and baby face each other with baby supported on the parent's lap and baby's legs straddling the parent's leg. This provides full frontal contact but its upright version can be tiring, as nursing parents must use their hands and arms to latch deeply and keep baby close. This may be helpful to babies who do better with more body flexion (such as those with hip dysplasia) or more head extension during feeds (Marmet & Shell, 2017).

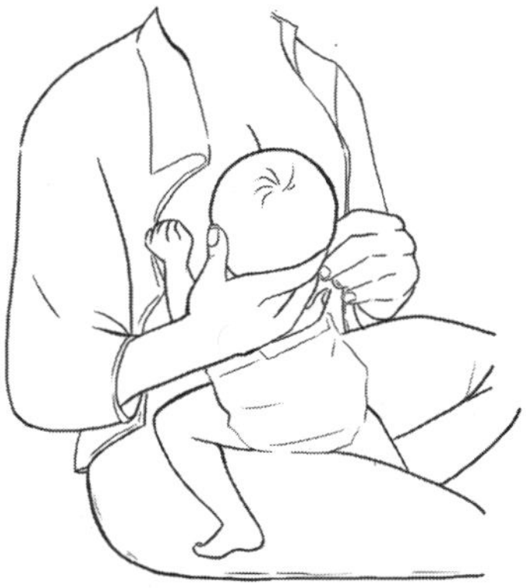

Figure 1.14 Straddle or koala hold upright. ©2020 Nancy Mohrbacher Solutions, Inc.

In some variations of the straddle hold, the nursing parent may lean forward or back. According to one Australian midwife-lactation consultant, this position is sometimes referred to as the ***koala hold***, and Australian midwives are routinely trained in this technique (Thomson, 2013, p. 148):

> "…this can be particularly useful for mothers with large breasts who have difficulty aligning the nipple to the baby's mouth. Some mothers may find increased comfort by positioning the baby away from the suture line following a cesarean section."

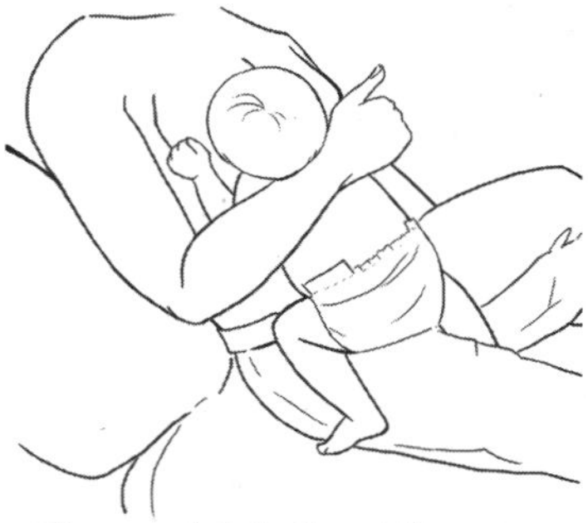

Figure 1.15 Straddle or koala hold semi-reclined. ©2020 Nancy Mohrbacher Solutions, Inc.

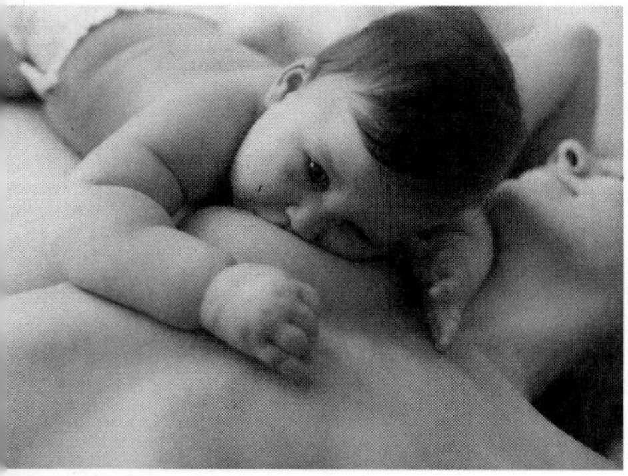

Figure 1.16 The over-the-shoulder hold.

Over-the-Shoulder Hold

The over-the-shoulder hold is not used often, because it is awkward and makes eye contact impossible, but it may work well after a cesarean birth, to help relieve a plugged duct, or when unresolved nipple pain creates a need to vary positions.

Most nursing parents prefer having both eye and body contact with their baby during nursing. The over-the-shoulder hold provides neither, but it can be helpful at times, such as after a cesarean birth, when due to pain from surgery or injury the nursing parent wants to avoid body contact. When nipple pain occurs after birth, getting a deeper latch is usually enough to alleviate it. But when the cause of the nipple pain cannot be quickly corrected, such as an unreleased tongue-tie and/or an unusually shaped palate, being able to use positions that rotate the nipple damage can sometimes make it possible to continue nursing without interruption. Also, when a nursing parent develops a plugged or blocked duct, nursing with baby's nose pointing toward the plug can sometimes help to relieve it more quickly (see next point for more on this). Depending on its location, that can lead to unusual nursing positions.

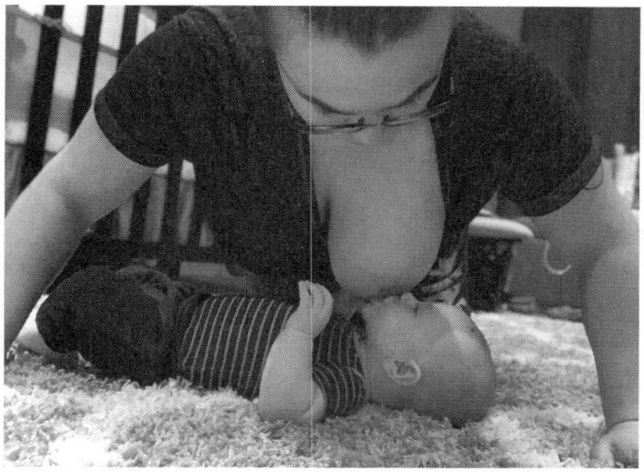

Figure 1.17 The all-fours dangle position.

All-Fours Dangle (Hands-and-Knees) Positions

Some relieve a plugged duct faster when they get up on their hands and knees and dangle the mammary tissue into baby's mouth.

One of the recommended strategies to more quickly relieve a plugged or blocked duct is to position the nursing baby so his nose points toward the plug (Wambach, 2021, p. 284). While amusing and often awkward, some report that the all-fours dangle positions can make it easier to accomplish this, especially if the plug is in an area where this is difficult in the usual holds. Although the effectiveness of these positions in resolving plugged ducts faster has not yet been studied, if a family asks for ways to relieve a plugged duct, these positions are one option.

Nursing Two Babies at the Same Time

There are many positioning options when simultaneously nursing two babies.

Parents of twins, triplets, or higher-order multiples often prefer to nurse two babies together at some feeds and separately at others. Nursing two babies together can be a big time-saver and it may be more effective at increasing blood prolactin levels, which can contribute to increased milk production, especially in the early weeks. Nursing two babies at once can also be helpful when one baby nurses more effectively than the other baby. When they nurse together, the more-effective sibling can get the milk flow started and maintained for the less-effective sibling.

Figure 1.18 illustrates some of the many ways two babies can be positioned for nursing. Encourage families to use the positions that feel most natural and comfortable for them and their babies.

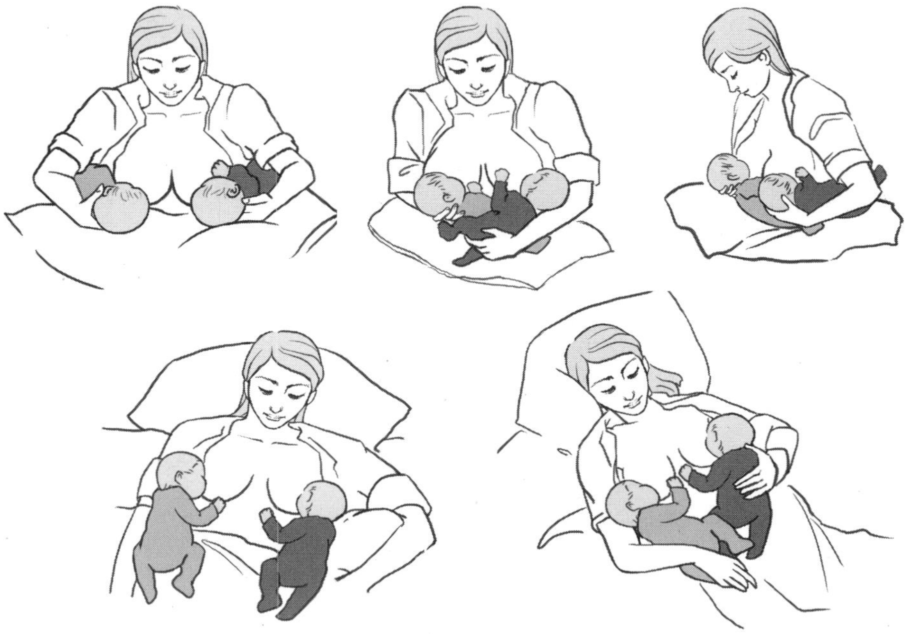

Figure 1.18 Some different ways to nurse two babies simultaneously. ©2020 Nancy Mohrbacher Solutions, Inc.

HOW FEEDS END

When taking baby off before he's finished, be sure to suggest first breaking the suction.

To avoid nipple pain or trauma, when ending the feed, suggest inserting a clean finger quickly into the corner of baby's mouth between his gums so that he can't bear down on the nipple as he comes off.

• • •

When nursing is going well, suggest nursing on one side until the baby comes off on his own and then offer the other side.

Some babies are fast feeders and some are slow feeders. Although there may be average feeding lengths for babies of different ages, not all babies are average. If a baby is thriving, there is no advantage to timing feeds or switching sides after a specific number of minutes. Encourage letting the baby finish the first side before offering the other side. How to know when baby is "finished?" Not all babies drop off, but they will usually eventually release the nipple. If unsure if baby is done, suggest wriggling or gently moving the mammary tissue. If baby has had enough milk, he will come off. If the baby falls asleep while nursing on the first side and comes off, suggest offering the other side when he awakens. For more details on feeding frequency and length, see the next chapter.

RESOURCES

Colson, S. (2019). *Biological Nurturing: Instinctual Breastfeeding,* 2nd edition. Amarillo, TX: Praeclarus Press.

GlobalHealthMedia.org/videos—A website with a large selection of free and downloadable nursing videos. "Attaching Your Baby at the Breast" at **bit.ly/BA2-Attaching** is particularly good.

Mohrbacher, N. & Kendall-Tackett, K. (2010). *Breastfeeding Made Simple: Seven Natural Laws for Nursing Mothers.* Oakland, CA: New Harbinger Publications.

NaturalBreastfeeding.com—A free 38-minute video with narration that demonstrates why the starter positions can make early breastfeeding easier and the three basic adjustments.

NaturalBreastfeeding.com/professional—Annual subscription to Professional Package offers licensing rights for educational use of video clips, images, staff-training videos, and a digital lactation course that can be shared with an unlimited number of families.

YouTube.com/NancyMohrbacher—A channel featuring a variety of free short videos (none longer than 5 minutes) showing diverse women of different races, shapes, and sizes using the starter positions with their newborns.

REFERENCES

AAP (2012). Breastfeeding and the use of human milk. *Pediatrics, 129*(3), e827-e841.

Amiel-Tison, C., & Grenier, A. (1983). Expression of liberated motor activity (LMA) following manual immobilization of the head (J. Steichen, steichen-Asch, P., Braun, C.P., Trans.). In C. Amiel-Tison, Grenier, A. (Ed.), *Neurologic Evaluation of the Newborn and the Infant* (pp. 87-109). New York, NY: Masson Publishing.

Baker, B., & McGrath, J. M. (2011). Maternal-infant synchrony: An integrated review of the literature. *Neonatal Paediatric and Child Health Nursing, 14*(3), 2-13.

Ball, H. L., Douglas, P. S., Kulasinghe, K., et al. (2018). The Possums Infant Sleep Program: Parents' perspectives on a novel parent-infant sleep intervention in Australia. *Sleep Health, 4*(6), 519-526.

Brazelton, T. B., & Nugent, J. K. (2011). *The Neonatal Behavioral Assessment Tool.* London, UK: Mac Keith Press.

Brockway, M., Benzies, K. M., Carr, E., et al. (2018). Breastfeeding self-efficacy and breastmilk feeding for moderate and late preterm infants in the Family Integrated Care trial: A mixed methods protocol. *International Breastfeeding Journal, 13,* 29.

Burns, E., Fenwick, J., Sheehan, A., et al. (2013). Mining for liquid gold: Midwifery language and practices associated with early breastfeeding support. *Maternal and Child Nutrition, 9*(1), 57-73.

Burns, E., Fenwick, J., Sheehan, A., et al. (2016). 'This little piranha': A qualitative analysis of the language used by health professionals and mothers to describe infant behaviour during breastfeeding. *Maternal and Child Nutrition, 12*(1), 111-124.

Cantrill, R. M., Creedy, D. K., Cooke, M., et al. (2014). Effective suckling in relation to naked maternal-infant body contact in the first hour of life: An observation study. *BMC Pregnancy and Childbirth, 14,* 20.

Chiu, S. H., Anderson, G. C., & Burkhammer, M. D. (2005). Newborn temperature during skin-to-skin breastfeeding in couples having breastfeeding difficulties. *Birth, 32*(2), 115-121.

Colson, S. (2012). Biological nurturing: The laid-back breastfeeding revolution. *Midwifery Today International Midwife*(101), 9-11, 66.

Colson, S. (2014). Does the mother's posture have a protective role to play during skin-to-skin contact? *Clinical Lactation, 5*(2), 41-50.

Colson, S. (2019). *Biological Nurturing: Instinctual Breastfeeding* (2nd ed.). Amarillo, TX: Praeclarus Press.

Colson, S., DeRooy, L., & Hawdon, J. (2003). Biological nurturing increases duration of breastfeeding for a vulnerable cohort. *MIDIRS Midwifery Digest, 13*(1), 92-97.

Colson, S. D., Meek, J. H., & Hawdon, J. M. (2008). Optimal positions for the release of primitive neonatal reflexes stimulating breastfeeding. *Early Human Development, 84*(7), 441-449.

Dennis, C. L. (2003). The breastfeeding self-efficacy scale: Psychometric assessment of the short form. *Journal of Obstetric, Gynecologic & Neonatal Nursing, 32*(6), 734-744.

Diaz Meneses, G. (2013). Breastfeeding: An emotional instinct. *Breastfeeding Medicine, 8,* 191-197.

Douglas, P., & Keogh, R. (2017). Gestalt breastfeeding: Helping mothers and infants optimize positional stability and intraoral breast tissue volume for effective, pain-free milk transfer. *Journal of Human Lactation, 33*(3), 509-518.

Dunn, S., Davies, B., McCleary, L., et al. (2006). The relationship between vulnerability factors and breastfeeding outcome. *Journal of Obstetric, Gynecologic & Neonatal Nursing, 35*(1), 87-97.

Eidelman, A. I., Hoffmann, N. W., & Kaitz, M. (1993). Cognitive deficits in women after childbirth. *Obstetrics & Gynecology, 81*(5 (Pt 1)), 764-767.

Elad, D., Kozlovsky, P., Blum, O., et al. (2014). Biomechanics of milk extraction during breast-feeding. *Proceedings of the National Academy of Sciences U.S.A., 111*(14), 5230-5235.

Evans, C. A., & Porter, C. L. (2009). The emergence of mother-infant co-regulation during the first year: Links to infants' developmental status and attachment. *Infant Behavior and Development, 32*(2), 147-158.

Feldman, R. (2012). Parent-infant synchrony: A biobehavioural model of mutual influences in the formation of affiliative bonds. *Monographs of the Society for Research in Child Development, 77*(2), 42-51.

Fifer, W. P., & Moon, C. M. (1994). The role of mother's voice in the organization of brain function in the newborn. *Acta Paediatrica Supplement, 397,* 86-93.

Geddes, D. T., Kent, J. C., Mitoulas, L. R., et al. (2008). Tongue movement and intra-oral vacuum in breastfeeding infants. *Early Human Development, 84*(7), 471-477.

Geddes, D. T., & Sakalidis, V. S. (2016). Ultrasound imaging of breastfeeding--A window to the inside: Methodology, normal appearances, and application. *Journal of Human Lactation, 32*(2), 340-349.

Genna, C. W. (2015). Breastfeeding infants with congenital torticollis. *Journal of Human Lactation, 31*(2), 216-220.

Genna, C. W. (2017). Breastfeeding: Normal sucking and swallowing. In C. W. Genna (Ed.), *Supporting Sucking Skills in Breastfeeding Infants* (3rd ed., pp. 1-48). Burlington, MA: Jones & Bartlett Learning.

Genna, C. W., & Barak, D. (2010). Facilitating autonomous infant hand use during breastfeeding. *Clinical Lactation, 1*(1), 15-20.

Girish, M., Mujawar, N., Gotmare, P., et al. (2013). Impact and feasibility of breast crawl in a tertiary care hospital. *Journal of Perinatology, 33*(4), 288-291.

Glover, R., & Wiessinger, D. (2017). They can do it, you can help: Building breastfeeding skill and confidence in mother and helper. In C. W. Genna (Ed.), *Supporting Sucking Skills in Breastfeeding Infants* (3rd ed., pp. 113-155). Burlington, MA: Jones & Bartlett Learning.

Gribble, K. D. (2005). Post-institutionalized adopted children who seek breastfeeding from their new mothers. *Journal of Prenatal & Perinatal Psychology & Health, 19*(3), 217-235.

Henderson, A., Stamp, G., & Pincombe, J. (2001). Postpartum positioning and attachment education for increasing breastfeeding: A randomized trial. *Birth, 28*(4), 236-242.

Jacobs, L. A., Dickinson, J. E., Hart, P. D., et al. (2007). Normal nipple position in term infants measured on breastfeeding ultrasound. *Journal of Human Lactation, 23*(1), 52-59.

Kent, J. C., Ashton, E., Hardwick, C. M., et al. (2015). Nipple pain in breastfeeding mothers: Incidence, causes and treatments. *International Journal of Environmental Research and Public Health, 12*(10), 12247-12263.

Kikuchi, K., Toyota, M., Endo, K., et al. (2017). Maternal gaze behaviors during latching-on for breastfeeding. *Breastfeeding Medicine, 12*(6), 359-364.

Kilci, H., & Coban, A. (2016). The correlation between breastfeeding success in the early postpartum period and the perception of self-efficacy in breastfeeding and breast problems in the late postpartum. *Breastfeeding Medicine, 11,* 188-195.

Kim, P. (2016). Human maternal brain plasticity: Adaptation to parenting. *New Directions for Child and Adloscent Development*(153), 47-58.

Kim, P., Feldman, R., Mayes, L. C., et al. (2011). Breastfeeding, brain activation to own infant cry, and maternal sensitivity. *Journal of Child Psychology and Psychiatry, 52*(8), 907-915.

Klaus, M., & Klaus, P. (2000). *Your Amazing Newborn.* Boston, MA: De Capo Lifelong Books.

Krol, K. M., & Grossmann, T. (2018). Psychological effects of breastfeeding on children and mothers. *Bundesgesundheitsblatt Gesundheitsforschung Gesundheitsschutz, 61*(8), 977-985.

Leclere, C., Viaux, S., Avril, M., et al. (2014). Why synchrony matters during mother-child interactions: A systematic review. *PLoS One, 9*(12), e113571.

Macfarlane, A. (1975). Olfaction in the development of social preferences in the human neonate. In R. Porter & M. O'Connor (Eds.), *Parent-Infant Interactions* (pp. 103-113). New York, New York: Elsevier.

Marmet, C., & Shell, E. (2017). Therapeutic positioning for breastfeeding. In C. W. Genna (Ed.), *Supporting Sucking Skills in Breastfeeding Infants* (3rd ed., pp. 399-416). Burlington, MA: Jones & Bartlett Learning.

Matsunaga, M., Tanaka, Y., & Myowa, M. (2018). Maternal nurturing experience affects the perception and recognition of adult and infant facial expressions. *PLoS One, 13*(10), e0205738.

Matthiesen, A. S., Ransjo-Arvidson, A. B., Nissen, E., et al. (2001). Postpartum maternal oxytocin release by newborns: Effects of infant hand massage and sucking. *Birth, 28*(1), 13-19.

Mohrbacher, N., & Kendall-Tackett, K. (2010). *Breastfeeding Made Simple: Seven Natural Laws for Nursing Mothers* (2nd ed.). Oakland, CA: New Harbinger Publications.

Nissen, E., Uvnas-Moberg, K., Svensson, K., et al. (1996). Different patterns of oxytocin, prolactin but not cortisol release during breastfeeding in women delivered by caesarean section or by the vaginal route. *Early Human Development, 45*(1-2), 103-118.

Nyqvist, K. H. (2008). Early attainment of breastfeeding competence in very preterm infants. *Acta Paediatrica, 97*(6), 776-781.

Nyqvist, K. H., Sjoden, P. O., & Ewald, U. (1999). The development of preterm infants' breastfeeding behavior. *Early Human Development, 55*(3), 247-264.

Parsons, C. E., Young, K. S., Murray, L., et al. (2010). The functional neuroanatomy of the evolving parent-infant relationship. *Progress in Neurobiology, 91*(3), 220-241.

Porter, R. H., Makin, J. W., Davis, L. B., et al. (1991). An assessment of the salient olfactory environment of formula-fed infants. *Physiology & Behavior, 50*(5), 907-911.

Porter, R. H., & Winberg, J. (1999). Unique salience of maternal breast odors for newborn infants. *Neuroscience & Biobehavioral Reviews, 23*(3), 439-449.

Puapornpong, P., Raungrongmorakot, K., Laosooksathit, W., et al. (2017). Comparison of breast-feeding outcomes between breastfeeding positions in mothers delivering by cesarean section: A randomized controlled trial. *Breastfeeding Medicine, 12,* 233-237.

Righard, L., & Alade, M. O. (1990). Effect of delivery room routines on success of first breast-feed. *Lancet, 336*(8723), 1105-1107.

Russell, M. J. (1976). Human olfactory communication. *Nature, 260*(5551), 520-522.

Schafer, R., & Genna, C. W. (2015). Physiologic breastfeeding: A contemporary approach to breastfeeding initiation. *Journal of Midwifery&Women's Health, 60*(5), 546-553.

Schmied, V., Beake, S., Sheehan, A., et al. (2011). Women's perceptions and experiences of breastfeeding support: A metasynthesis. *Birth, 38*(1), 49-60.

Schore, A. N. (2001). The effects of a secure attachment relationship on right brain development, affect regulation, and infant mental health. *Infant Mental Health Journal, 22,* 7-66.

Smillie, C. M. (2017). How infants learn to feed: A neurobehavioral model. In C. W. Genna (Ed.), *Supporting Sucking Skills in Breastfeeding Infants* (3rd ed., pp. 89-111). Burlington, MA: Jones & Bartlett Learning.

Svensson, K. E., Velandia, M. I., Matthiesen, A. S., et al. (2013). Effects of mother-infant skin-to-skin contact on severe latch-on problems in older infants: A randomized trial. *International Breastfeeding Journal, 8*(1), 1.

Swain, J. E. (2011). Becoming a parent: Biobehavioral and brain science perspectives. *Current Problems in Pediatric and Adolescent Health Care, 41*(7), 192-196.

Swain, J. E., Konrath, S., Dayton, C. J., et al. (2013). Toward a neuroscience of interactive parent-infant dyad empathy. *Behavioral and Brain Sciences, 36*(4), 438-439.

Tharner, A., Luijk, M. P., Raat, H., et al. (2012). Breastfeeding and its relation to maternal sensitivity and infant attachment. *Journal of Developmental & Behavioral Pediatrics, 33*(5), 396-404.

Thompson, R., Kruske, S., Barclay, L., et al. (2016). Potential predictors of nipple trauma from an in-home breastfeeding programme: A cross-sectional study. *Women and Birth, 29*(4), 336-344.

Thomson, S. C. (2013). The koala hold from down under: Another choice in breastfeeding position. *Journal of Human Lactation, 29*(2), 147-149.

Uvnas-Moberg, K. (2014). *Oxytocin: The Biological Guide to Motherhood.* Amarillo, TX: Praeclarus Press.

Varendi, H., & Porter, R. H. (2001). Breast odour as the only maternal stimulus elicits crawling towards the odour source. *Acta Paediatrica, 90*(4), 372-375.

Varendi, H., Porter, R. H., & Winberg, J. (1994). Does the newborn baby find the nipple by smell? *Lancet, 344*(8928), 989-990.

Wambach, K. (2021). Breast-related problems. In K. Wambach & B. Spencer (Eds.), *Breastfeeding and Human Lactation* (6th ed., pp. 281-312). Burlington, MA: Jones & Bartlett Learning.

Widstrom, A. M., Lilja, G., Aaltomaa-Michalias, P., et al. (2011). Newborn behaviour to locate the breast when skin-to-skin: A possible method for enabling early self-regulation. *Acta Paediatrica, 100*(1), 79-85.

Widstrom, A. M., Ransjo-Arvidson, A. B., Christensson, K., et al. (1987). Gastric suction in healthy newborn infants. Effects on circulation and developing feeding behaviour. *Acta Paediatrica Scandanavica, 76*(4), 566-572.

Winberg, J. (2005). Mother and newborn baby: Mutual regulation of physiology and behavior--a selective review. *Developmental Psychobiology, 47*(3), 217-229.

Woolridge, M. W. (1986). The 'anatomy' of infant sucking. *Midwifery, 2*(4), 164-171.

Zheng, J. X., Chen, Y. C., Chen, H., et al. (2018). Disrupted spontaneous neural activity related to cognitive impairment in postpartum women. *Frontiers in Psychology, 9,* 624.

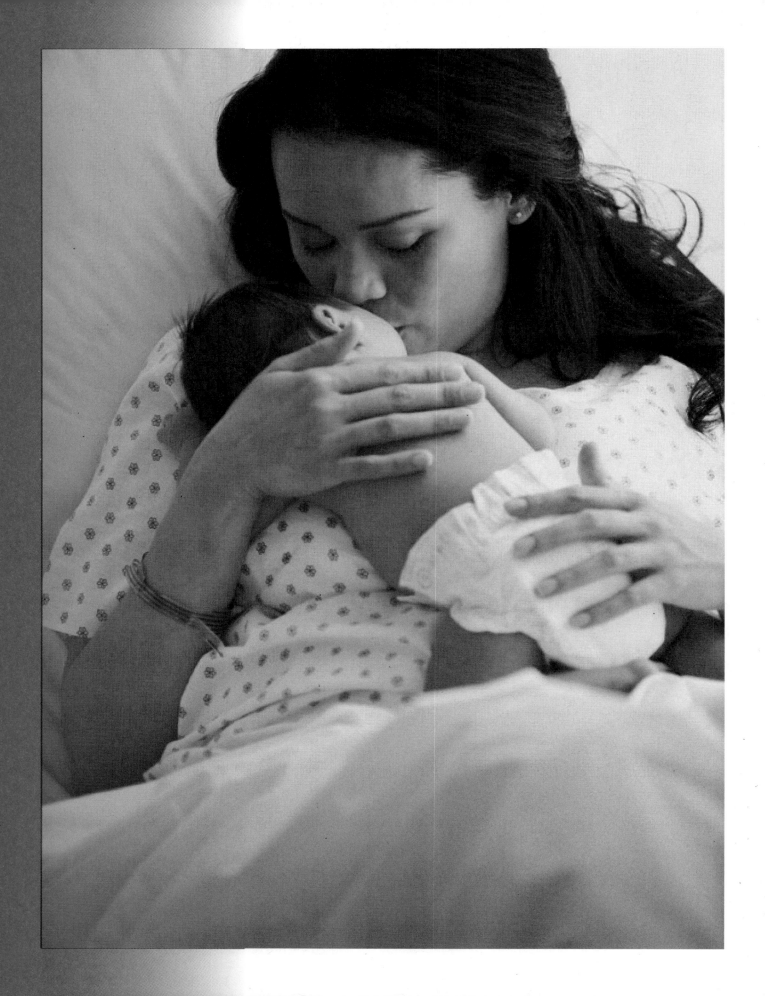

Nursing Rhythms

2

"Nursing rhythm" is the natural fluctuation in feeding patterns over time.

Nursing rhythms encompass many aspects of feeding: how often and how long baby nurses at a session, whether baby takes one side or more, the day and night changes in feeding frequency, and how these variables change over time as baby matures. Both biology and culture affect nursing rhythms.

BIRTH PRACTICES AND EARLY NURSING

Practices that prolong labor or make birth more stressful or traumatic can undermine early nursing and delay milk increase.

Whether a birth is easy or difficult, ecstatic or traumatic, it is a life-changing event that profoundly influences the rhythms of early nursing. Practices that prolong labor include keeping laboring parents immobile and on their back, leaving them alone to labor, withholding food and drink, induction of labor by drugs, using forceps and/or vacuum extractors, and performing cesarean deliveries (L. J. Smith, 2017).

Research found an association between stressful birth—either physically or psychologically stressful—and a delay in increased milk production (secretory activation, also known as lactogenesis II) (Beck & Watson, 2008; Chen, Nommsen-Rivers, Dewey, & Lonnerdal, 1998; Dewey, Nommsen-Rivers, Heinig, & Cohen, 2003; Dimitraki et al., 2016). This may be due to elevated blood cortisol levels after a long, stressful, or difficult birth (Grajeda & Perez-Escamilla, 2002). One U.S. study found more than 1 hour spent pushing during stage II labor was associated with delayed milk increase (Dewey et al., 2003). An association was also found between mild to moderate postpartum hemorrhage during birth and decreased milk production (Willis & Livingstone, 1995).

KEY CONCEPT

Birth practices may profoundly affect early nursing.

When parents perceive a birth as traumatic, some develop posttraumatic stress disorder (PTSD), which may affect their intention to nurse. A 2017 systematic review (Dekel, Stuebe, & Dishy, 2017) examined 36 quality international studies and estimated the incidence of acute PTSD among women who successfully delivered full-term babies was 5% to 6%. Up to 17% of the study women experienced clinically significant PTSD symptoms.

How do PTSD and its symptoms affect nursing? A national survey conducted in England of 5,332 mothers (Beck, Gable, Sakala, & Declercq, 2011) found that flashbacks associated with a traumatic birth convinced some women to stop breastfeeding, as they believed that weaning brought them closer to their "normal," pre-birth selves again. Others found that the act of breastfeeding triggered flashbacks of their traumatic birth, which convinced them to wean. Conversely, in other interview studies (Beck & Watson, 2008; Elmir, Schmied, Wilkes, & Jackson, 2010), some women with a history of birth trauma reported that breastfeeding gave them a welcome respite from their trauma symptoms and that nursing comforted them and aided in their healing. For recommended trauma-informed treatment options, see p. 841.

• • •

Emotional support received during labor is associated with earlier nursing.

The desire to nurse and care for a baby may be enhanced by emotional support during labor. One study of 209 first-time mothers in Nigeria (Morhason-Bello, Adedokun, & Ojengbede, 2009) found that the time to the first breastfeed was significantly shorter among the mothers who had a companion with them during labor. A shorter interval between birth and the first breastfeed was associated with longer duration of breastfeeding and greater infant survival (see next section).

• • •

Establishing a definitive cause-and-effect relationship between labor medications and nursing problems is challenging, in part because most families are unlikely to agree to participate in research that randomly assigns them to a "medicated-labor" or "non-medicated-labor" group. Another confounding factor that may affect the results of non-randomized studies is that motivation to nurse may significantly differ between those who decide to use pain medications during labor and those who don't. In other words, many families who feel strongly about nursing also feel strongly about avoiding pain medications during childbirth. Not surprisingly, research on the effects of pain medications on early nursing is conflicting.

Extra lactation support is needed when labor medications are used, because they may affect baby's alertness, inborn feeding behaviors, and feeding effectiveness.

Epidurals and early nursing. A 2016 systematic review examined the effects of epidural anesthesia on early nursing (French, Cong, & Chung, 2016) by examining 23 studies. Twelve of these studies found a negative association between epidurals and nursing success, 10 studies found no effect, and 1 study showed a positive association.

Research on the effects of fentanyl—a drug often used with epidurals—is also conflicting and inconclusive. In a U.S. prospective comparative study (Brimdyr et al., 2015), mothers self-selected into the epidural or no-epidural groups. An inverse association was found between exposure to fentanyl and the babies' ability to do the breast crawl and feed while in skin-to-skin contact during the first hour after birth. A U.S. randomized controlled trial of women who had previously breastfed compared nursing outcomes among 60 women who received no fentanyl in their epidural, 59 who received an intermediate dose of fentanyl in their epidural, and 58 who received a high dose of fentanyl in their epidural (Beilin et al., 2005). The researchers found that the mothers who received the high dose of fentanyl were more likely to stop breastfeeding by 6 weeks compared with the mothers who received no fentanyl or an intermediate dose of fentanyl. A third 2017 U.S. randomized double-blind controlled trial of 345 women who had fully breastfed previous children also considered the effects of fentanyl on nursing outcomes and measured levels of the labor medications in the mothers' blood and the umbilical cord after delivery (Lee et al., 2017). The women were randomized into three groups, all of whom received epidurals. One group received no fentanyl, one received a lower dose of fentanyl, and the third received a higher dose. They found no differences in nursing outcomes among the three groups.

What is the takeaway message? The Academy of Breastfeeding Medicine (ABM) noted in its 2018 Clinical Protocol #28, "Peripartum Analgesia and Anesthesia for the Breastfeeding Mother" (Martin, Vickers, Landau, & Reece-Stremtan, 2018, p. 165):

> "Like many other aspects of breastfeeding, [epidural] analgesia likely has minimal effects on women who strongly intend to breastfeed and have good support, but may present one more subtle challenge to women whose intention to breastfeed is more vulnerable."

For this reason, the authors of the ABM protocol suggested that when epidural anesthesia is used, nursing parents receive good lactation support and closer follow-up. As an example of how hospital practices that support nursing can affect this dynamic, one Italian retrospective cohort study of 2,480 women (Zuppa et al., 2014) found that among those with partial rooming-in, more mothers who did not receive epidurals either exclusively or predominantly breastfed. This difference did not exist, however, among the women who had full rooming-in. Among those rooming-in around the clock, breastfeeding exclusivity was the same in both groups.

Longer-acting opioid pain medications. The timing of using drugs, such as meperidine/pethidine (Demerol) or morphine, during labor is crucial. If they are given between 1 and 4 hours before delivery, this increases baby's risk of depressed breathing and heart rate and negatively affects a newborn's ability to latch (Martin et al., 2018). Several Swedish studies noted that meperidine/pethidine (Demerol) given during labor was negatively associated with newborns' ability to complete the breast crawl at the first feed (Nissen et al., 1997; Ransjo-Arvidson et al., 2001; Righard & Alade, 1990; Widstrom et al., 2011). An Australian ultrasound study of 35 babies born vaginally and by cesarean (Sakalidis et al., 2013) found that after cesarean delivery, babies whose mothers received meperidine/pethidine for pain relief after birth were more likely to suck abnormally during nursing than the babies born vaginally whose mothers did not use this drug. Two Australian randomized controlled trials (J. Fleet, Belan, Jones, Ullah, & Cyna, 2015; J. A. Fleet, Jones, & Belan, 2017) found that even at 6 weeks, more of the babies whose mothers received pethidine via intramuscular shots during labor had trouble establishing breastfeeding compared with those whose mothers received epidurals during labor.

For more details on the effects of labor medications on nursing, download the free the ABM Clinical Protocol #28 at: **bfmed.org/protocols**.

• • •

Use of synthetic oxytocin during the third stage of labor may negatively affect nursing and baby's feeding reflexes and increase depression and anxiety among exposed parents.

Synthetic oxytocin (Pitocin) is often given during the third stage of labor (delivery of the placenta) to prevent hemorrhage. Several studies raised concerns about the effects of synthetic oxytocin on nursing and mood.

One concerning study was a large 2009 U.K. retrospective cohort study of 48,366 women (Jordan et al., 2009), which found a 6% to 8% reduction in breastfeeding at 48 hours among mothers given synthetic oxytocin after their baby's birth. This effect was strongest in women whose labor was induced or augmented or who also received epidural or spinal anesthesia. A smaller 2014 retrospective self-questionnaire completed by 288 mothers who had a vaginal birth (Brown & Jordan, 2014) found that those who received the synthetic oxytocin after delivery were significantly more likely to stop breastfeeding by 3 and 6 months compared with those who did not. A Spanish prospective cohort study followed 98 mothers for 6 months who gave birth in a Baby Friendly hospital (Fernandez-Canadas Morillo et al., 2017). Of these women, 53 were given synthetic oxytocin after delivery and 45 were not. The researchers found no statistically significant differences in exclusive breastfeeding between the two groups at 3 and 6 months. The authors of a 2018 Portuguese retrospective cohort study (Gomes, Trocado, Carlos-Alves, Arteiro, & Pinheiro, 2018) suggested that previous research had failed to control for differences among mothers. This study looked more closely at maternal factors and concluded that use of synthetic oxytocin was a predictor of impaired breastfeeding during the first hour after birth and that a high body mass index before pregnancy predicted impaired breastfeeding at 3 months. The impact of synthetic oxytocin on the first feed was explained in part in a 2015 Spanish cohort prospective study (Marin Gabriel et al., 2015), which found that synthetic oxytocin given at birth reduced infant feeding behaviors (primitive neonatal reflexes) during the first hour. The researchers suggested that the synthetic oxytocin might "alter the neurohormonal status of the newborn brain."

The nursing parent's brain may also be affected by synthetic oxytocin, according to a 2017 U.S. population-based retrospective study (Kroll-Desrosiers et al., 2017). The study found that of the 9,684 mothers who received the synthetic oxytocin after delivery, both those with a history of depression and those without this history were at a substantially increased risk of depression and anxiety (36% increased risk versus 32% increased risk).

A 2017 integrated review of the evidence to date (Erickson & Emeis, 2017) found that 17 of 34 studies demonstrated an association between the use of synthetic oxytocin and less optimal breastfeeding outcomes, while 8 of 34 found no association. In 9 of the 34, findings were mixed.

• • •

Cesarean delivery puts exclusive nursing at risk for several reasons.

A cesarean birth puts exclusive nursing at risk. For earlier milk increase and more comfortable feeds after a surgical delivery, families need help and support.

Effects on exclusive nursing. Research worldwide found cesarean birth to be a risk factor for lower rates of exclusive nursing (Cohen et al., 2018).

- A 2018 systematic review and meta-analysis of nursing in China over 15 years (Zhao, Zhao, Du, Binns, & Lee, 2017) concluded that mothers who gave birth by cesarean were 47% less likely to exclusively breastfeed than those who gave birth vaginally.
- In Latin America and the Caribbean, about one third of newborns received other foods (called "pre-lacteal feeds") during the first few days after birth, which was more likely after a cesarean (Boccolini, Perez-Escamilla, Giugliani, & Boccolini Pde, 2015).
- In Sweden (where nursing is the cultural norm), a longitudinal, population-based study of 679 women (Cato, Sylven, Lindback, Skalkidou, & Rubertsson, 2017) linked cesarean birth with increased likelihood of discontinuing exclusive nursing by 2 months.

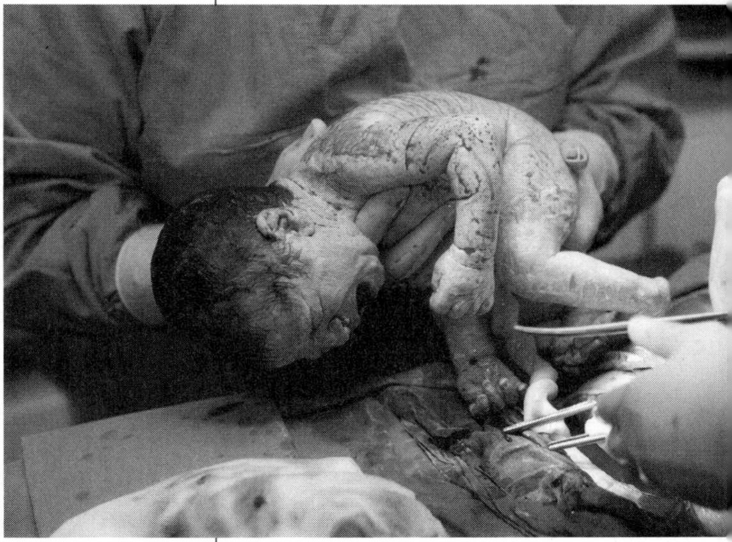

Three U.S. studies (Regan, Thompson, & DeFranco, 2013; Wallenborn, Graves, & Masho, 2017; Wallenborn & Masho, 2016) found that women undergoing repeat cesarean deliveries were significantly more likely to never breastfeed than those who attempted a vaginal birth after a cesarean.

Cesarean delivery and milk increase after birth. Post-birth patterns of normal weight loss and weight gain differ significantly between babies born via cesarean versus those delivered vaginally (Flaherman et al., 2015). Weight loss charts (nomograms) of exclusively breastfed newborns show that babies born by cesarean lose more weight and lose weight for a longer time than babies born vaginally. These differences in weight loss and weight gain may convince parents and healthcare providers to supplement. What factors account for these differences?

- ***IV fluids given during surgery,*** which if excessive (more than 1500 mL), inflate baby's birth weight and act as a diuretic after birth to stimulate more urination, leading to greater weight loss (Noel-Weiss, Woodend, & Groll, 2011)

- ***Differences in hormonal responses.*** A Swedish study (Nissen et al., 1996) found that on the second day of life mothers who had a cesarean delivery had lower levels of oxytocin pulsatility and lower levels of blood prolactin than those delivering vaginally.
- ***Longer time to the first feed and fewer feeds per day.*** One common side effect of a surgical delivery is a later start to nursing and fewer feeds per day due to discomfort and difficulty accessing the baby (Tully & Ball, 2014). Later and fewer nursing sessions could account for difference patterns of early weight loss. One small Turkish study of 40 mothers (Sozmen, 1992) found that women who delivered by cesarean and nursed sooner experienced an earlier increase in milk production than women whose first nursing was later.

One Turkish study of 288 women who delivered by cesarean (Ilhan et al., 2018) found an association between delayed milk increase (secretory activation or lactogenesis II) and surgical deliveries performed between sunset and dawn. The researchers recommend that families whose cesareans are performed at night receive extra nursing support.

Interventions to support nursing after a cesarean delivery. Families whose babies are born by cesarean can do several things to help nursing go more smoothly.

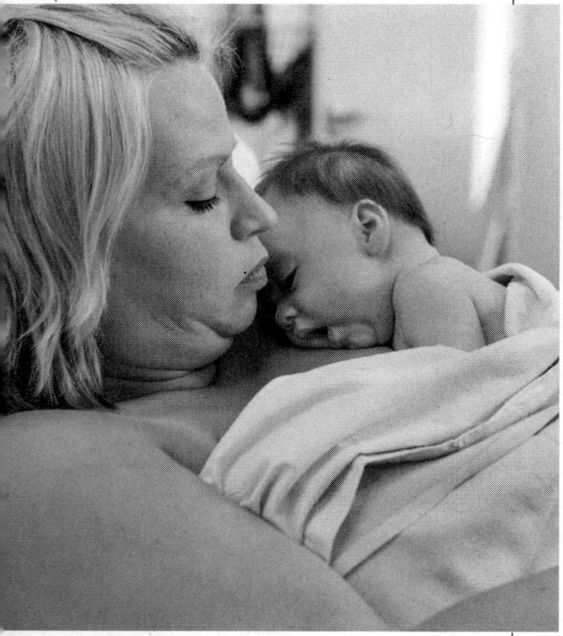

- ***Immediate skin-to-skin contact and early nursing.*** Many birthing facilities support these practices after a cesarean (Dudeja, Sikka, Jain, Suri, & Kumar, 2018; Stevens, Schmied, Burns, & Dahlen, 2014). An Italian prospective cohort study (Guala et al., 2017) found that after a cesarean birth, more of the mothers who had early skin-to-skin contact exclusively breastfed at hospital discharge, as well as at 3 and 6 months compared with those who did not have early skin-to-skin contact.
- ***Hand expression after nursing,*** spoon-feeding baby this extra colostrum as "dessert" to prevent excess weight loss and stimulate earlier milk increase. For more, see p. 474 and U.S. pediatrician Jane Morton's videos for parents at **firstdroplets.com** (Morton, 2019).
- ***Help with nursing, especially at night.*** Some of the challenges expressed in one U.K. study based on interviews with 115 mothers after a cesarean birth (Tully & Ball, 2014) were the need for help with positioning, mobility limitations, and the frustration of needing assistance, including being able to get the newborn out of the bassinet to nurse. The mothers surveyed in another U.K. study overwhelmingly preferred a side-car bassinet (which attached to the hospital bed and made the baby more accessible for night feeds) over a separate bassinet (Tully & Ball, 2012).
- ***Guidance about normal nursing patterns and infant condition.*** In one U.K. study (Tully & Ball, 2014), after a cesarean birth, many mothers expressed concern about their newborn's condition, not realizing that after a cesarean delivery issues like less responsiveness and expelling mucus before the first feed are normal. They were also unfamiliar with normal nursing patterns during the first few days. Providing families with realistic expectations may make these early days less worrisome and promote best nursing practices. This study also found that the mothers who expressed their desire to breastfeed for both maternal and infant reasons were more likely to exclusively breastfeed than those who said they breastfed for baby reasons alone.

- ***Practical suggestions and answers to common questions.*** Simple adjustments, like inserting an IV into the nursing parent's forearm rather than hand, may make early nursing easier after a cesarean. Reassurance about the compatibility of any drugs (anesthesia, pain medications, antibiotics) may also encourage more early nursing. See the first chapter for practical nursing positions after a surgical delivery.

For more on cesarean delivery and milk production, see p. 439.

ESTABLISHING NURSING

The early weeks after birth are a vulnerable time for nursing and for the family's relationship with their new baby.

For most mammals, the time after birth is a sensitive period that has long-term effects on the mother-baby relationship. As one example, separation of mother and baby after birth causes many mammalian mothers, such as ewes, to reject their newborns (Levy et al., 1991). To care for their babies, many animal mothers must feel the sensations of birth and experience the touch, taste, and smell of their newborn. When any of these are missing, their attachment to the newborn can be disrupted. Human parents can override these innate responses, but during this vulnerable time, post-delivery practices should be tailored to support—rather than undermine—the natural forces at work. This sensitive period requires particular care.

The First 2 Hours

After birth, nursing goes more smoothly when the birthing parent and baby stay together in skin-to-skin contact in a relaxed, warm, private place.

Nursing is a physical part of the intimate relationship between nursing parent and baby, so the ideal environment after birth is one that keeps them together and enhances their feelings of intimacy. Early nursing works best when parents can attend to their baby without distraction. In their overview article (Schafer & Genna, 2015), American midwife Robyn Schafer and lactation consultant Catherine Watson Genna described the most physiologic way to begin nursing after birth. They emphasized the importance of an environment free from disruptions and interventions so the nursing couple can relax. Being relaxed enhances the release of hormones, such as oxytocin, prolactin and others, which play several important roles after delivery to:

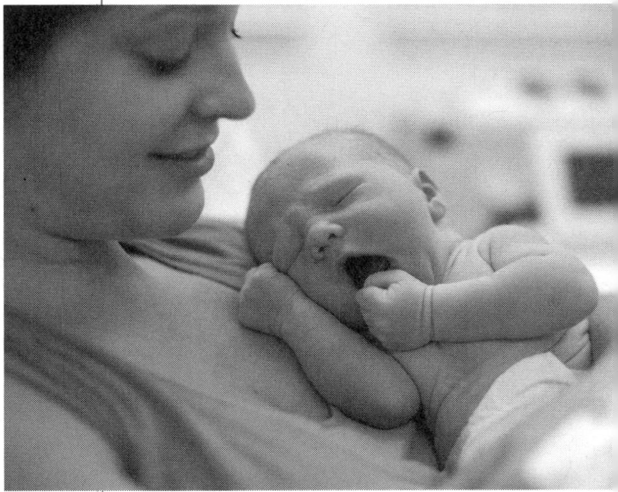

- Regulate baby's body temperature and blood glucose levels (Christensson et al., 1992; Takahashi & Tamakoshi, 2018; Walters, Boggs, Ludington-Hoe, Price, & Morrison, 2007)
- Increase baby's nursing effectiveness (Aghdas, Talat, & Sepideh, 2014)
- Reduce risk of uterine hemorrhage (Abedi, Jahanfar, Namvar, & Lee, 2016; Marin Gabriel et al., 2015)

Schafer and Genna (Schafer & Genna, 2015, p. 549) wrote:

> "Physiologic breastfeeding support is based on a fundamental trust in women's bodies and innate newborn breastfeeding abilities. In the model of physiologic breastfeeding initiation, the role of the

clinician is to allow the woman and her newborn to follow their natural instincts to establish breastfeeding and maintain an environment in which they both feel calm, comfortable, and supported."

U.K. research midwife Suzanne Colson took this one step further by suggesting that it is not just the first hour after birth that is critical, but the first weeks of life, and that the primary role of the nursing supporter is to promote a hormone-enhancing environment (Colson, 2019). A relaxing and comfortable environment is key to the release of the nursing parent's and baby's reciprocal behaviors, one way they get to know one another. Nursing provides a biological intimacy that helps mothers and babies establish their relationship (Colson, 2019).

In one Australian study, researchers created a special private room designed to enhance comfort and relaxation (called a ***Snoezelen room***), where families could take their babies to be alone or receive one-on-one help. The mothers reported that in this private setting, their anxiety decreased and they were better able to focus on their baby. One mother (Y. L. Hauck, Summers, White, & Jones, 2008, p. 20) wrote:

> "I wanted to experiment and explore it on my own because I'm not a complete idiot, sometimes you just need a chance to try it for yourself. You want some time out to yourself to see if you can do it yourself and I knew that in that space I was just going to have some time to find out for myself and not have any interruptions."

The next section describes in more detail how skin-to-skin contact during the first hours after birth improves infant stability and provides the natural triggers for early nursing. The American Academy of Pediatrics recommends: "Direct skin-to-skin contact with mothers immediately after delivery until the first feeding is accomplished" (AAP, 2012, p. e835). The AAP also encourages skin-to-skin contact throughout the early days and weeks after birth.

• • •

Even a short separation after birth can inhibit baby's inborn feeding behaviors.

When the birthing parent and newborn are healthy, best practice is routine skin-to-skin contact (see next section). Even a short time apart before the first feed can inhibit baby's inborn feeding behaviors and short-circuit the first nursing. In a classic 1990 Swedish study (Righard & Alade, 1990), some of the study babies were taken from their mothers for 20 minutes for a bath and measurements before their first nursing. When mothers and babies were reunited, half of the babies did not nurse successfully, which was significantly different from the babies who remained in skin-to-skin contact from birth, nearly all of whom had a successful first feed. A 2016 French study of 30 mothers and babies after birth (Robiquet et al., 2016) found an association between interruption of skin-to-skin contact before the first feed (done to perform routine infant care) and failure to breastfeed within the first 2 hours.

• • •

Suctioning of the newborn after delivery can interfere with the first feed and is no longer recommended.

Oronasopharyngeal suctioning after birth was regularly performed in many hospitals around the world. However, it is no longer recommended. A review of the research (M. B. Evans & Po, 2016) noted that while this procedure was once thought to help promote better lung aeration after birth by removing fluids, studies found that suctioning can cause vagal stimulation, induced bradycardia (slowed heart rate), and apnea. It can also cause injuries that lead to infection. Suctioning after birth was also linked to oral aversion, which can lead to inability to latch (L. J. Smith, 2017).

• • •

After decades of study, in 2011 the Swedish research team that first identified the breast crawl categorized babies' inborn feeding behaviors into nine instinctive stages (Table 2.1), which occur after birth when newborns are left undisturbed on their birthing parent's body in skin-to-skin contact (Widstrom et al., 2011). In this 2011 study, researchers videotaped 28 healthy term newborns during the first hours after birth to understand more clearly the sequence of behaviors that unfolds from birth to the sleep that follows the first nursing. (See Chapter 1 for more details about babies' inborn feeding behaviors.) Since the publication of this study, many maternity facilities train birth attendants in these nine instinctive stages (Crenshaw et al., 2012). Knowing what to expect from newborns after birth helps task-oriented healthcare professionals be patient and allow these behaviors to happen without interference. According to several studies (Girish et al., 2013; Matthiesen, Ransjo-Arvidson, Nissen, & Uvnas-Moberg, 2001; Widstrom et al., 2011), when doing the breast crawl, most newborns go from birth to the first feed within 60 minutes, but some take as long as 75 minutes.

For the first feed after birth, research found that letting newborns experience the 9 instinctive stages of the breast crawl was associated with fewer early feeding problems.

An Indian prospective, single-blinded, randomized controlled clinical trial of 100 healthy term newborns (Girish et al., 2013) divided these babies into two groups. In the first group, the babies were placed on the mothers' abdomen immediately after birth and allowed to do the breast crawl to initiate the first feed. The second group was removed from the mothers' body after birth and weighed, measured, and given vitamin K injections, then returned to the mother within 30 to 60 minutes for feeding. The researchers found significant differences in nursing outcomes between the two groups. Nipple pain occurred in 44% of the mothers whose babies did not do the breast crawl compared with 24% of those who did. Delay in milk increase occurred in 60% of the mothers whose babies did not do the breast crawl compared with only 24% of those who did. Mean weight loss on Day 3 was significantly higher among babies who did not

TABLE 2.1 Nine Instinctive Stages after Birth

Stages of the Breast Crawl	Description
Stage 1 Birth cry	The intense crying after birth
Stage 2 Relaxation phase	A period of recovery where there is no movement of baby's mouth, head, arms, legs, or body
Stage 3 Awakening phase	Signs of activity, such as head movements, small movements of limbs and shoulders
Stage 4 Active phase	More determined movements of head and limbs, pushing and rooting with no shifting of body
Stage 5 Crawling phase	Pushing, which shifts body position
Stage 6 Resting phase	More resting, this time with some movements of mouth or sucking on hand
Stage 7 Familiarization phase	After reaching areola/nipple, brushing and licking activities
Stage 8 Sucking phase	Taking nipple in mouth and sucking
Stage 9 Sleeping phase	Closed eyes

Adapted from (Widstrom et al., 2011). See these 9 stages in action at **bit.ly/BA2-BF1stHours**

do the breast crawl compared with those who did. Why would the breast crawl affect milk production? The researchers (Girish et al., 2013, p. 290) wrote:

> "We believe that by allowing breast crawl, a cycle is established in which early and effective feeds result in a strong oxytocin and prolactin response, causing better lactation and exclusive breastfeeding, thereby ensuring prolonged lactation."

An earlier Swedish study (Matthiesen et al., 2001) videotaped 10 babies doing the breast crawl after birth and measured the mothers' oxytocin blood levels. They found that babies' body and hand movements during the breast crawl increased the mothers' blood oxytocin levels, one way of preparing her body for milk release. The researchers concluded that "newborns use their hands as well as their mouths to stimulate maternal oxytocin release after birth, which may have significance for uterine contraction, milk ejection, and mother-infant interaction" (Matthiesen et al., 2001, p. 13).

• • •

Some studies found that newborns are more likely to complete the breast crawl after birth when born vaginally rather than by cesarean.

According to some studies, babies are more likely to complete the breast crawl after a vaginal birth than after a cesarean delivery. A 2016 Iranian study of 399 women who delivered at a large teaching hospital (Heidarzadeh, Hakimi, Habibelahi, Mohammadi, & Shahrak, 2016) found differences in breast-crawl outcomes among those who delivered by unmedicated vaginal delivery when compared with those who delivered by elective cesarean section. In this study, 88% of those born vaginally successfully completed the breast crawl within 60 minutes compared with only 11% of those born by elective cesarean. Oddly, on average the babies born by cesarean delivery took less time to complete the breast crawl (an average of 28 versus 45 minutes). Other studies have also found that fewer babies born by cesarean successfully completed the breast crawl (K. C. Evans, Evans, Royal, Esterman, & James, 2003; Patel, Liebling, & Murphy, 2003; Zanardo et al., 2010).

• • •

Nursing within the first hour or two after birth is associated with greater infant survival, earlier increase in milk production, and fewer feeding problems.

Creating an environment that promotes early nursing (within the first hour or two) benefits families in many ways.

Greater infant survival. In some parts of the world, delaying the first nursing longer than an hour or two increases the risk of illness and death. A 2013 study examined secondary data from 67 countries and concluded that nursing within the first hour of life was negatively correlated with newborn death (Boccolini, Carvalho, Oliveira, & Perez-Escamilla, 2013). This correlation was strongest among countries with more than 29 neonatal deaths per 1,000 births. Countries with the lowest rates of nursing had 24% higher neonatal mortality rates, even when adjusted for potential confounders. A 2013 systematic review of 18 studies (Debes, Kohli, Walker, Edmond, & Mullany, 2013) found a direct negative association between early initiation of nursing and newborn illness and death. Initiating nursing within 1 hour of birth was estimated to avert up to 22% to 29% of all newborn deaths (Debes et al., 2013; Edmond et al., 2006; Group, 2016). A 2014 overview article on neonatal mortality in *The Lancet's* Every Newborn series (Bhutta et al., 2014) estimated that nursing within the first hour could reduce neonatal mortality in some parts of the world by as much as 44%. One possible reason early nursing has such a profound effect on infant survival is the positive association some research found between early nursing and exclusive nursing for the first 6 months (Mawaddah, 2018).

Earlier increase in milk production. A study done in Russia with a team of Swedish, Russian, and Canadian researchers examined the effects of post-birth practices on 176 mothers and their newborns (Bystrova et al., 2007). This study found a positive association between the timing of the first feed and milk intake on Day 4. Newborns who breastfed for the first time within 2 hours of birth took on average 55% more milk on Day 4 (284 mL), as compared with the babies whose first feed occurred more than 2 hours after birth (184 mL). The researchers noted that the babies who fed within the first 2 hours weighed more on average and were born closer to term than those babies who did not.

Fewer feeding problems. A 2019 systematic review (Karimi, Sadeghi, Maleki-Saghooni, & Khadivzadeh, 2019) found that skin-to-skin contact increases the success and duration of the first breastfeed. A 2016 French study of 30 mothers and babies after birth (Robiquet et al., 2016) found an association between interruption of skin-to-skin contact before the first feed (due to routine infant care) and failure to breastfeed within the first 2 hours after birth. A 2013 Australian cross-sectional study of 581 healthy term newborns (Carberry, Raynes-Greenow, Turner, & Jeffery, 2013) found that for each hour the first nursing was delayed after birth the greater the risks of nursing problems. This effect was still evident even after controlling for factors such as number of children, type of birth, maternal body mass index, age, ethnicity and health problems in mother or baby.

Promoting nursing soon after birth is one of the Ten Steps to Successful Breastfeeding developed as part of the Baby Friendly Hospital Initiative (BFHI), which was launched in 1991 by the World Health Organization and UNICEF. These Ten Steps were expanded in 2018 (Box 2.1). A 2016 systematic review of the research on the impact of BFHI on nursing (Perez-Escamilla, Martinez, & Segura-Perez, 2016) found a dose-response relationship between how many of the Ten Steps the study families were exposed to and the likelihood of improved nursing outcomes, such as early initiation of nursing, exclusive nursing at hospital discharge, and duration of exclusive nursing.

The First Few Days

The first few days after birth are a critical period for infant stability, as well as for establishing both nursing and strong relationships.

Togetherness, Separation, and Newborn Stability

The first hours after birth may be a sensitive period during which skin-to-skin contact is important to infant stability and early nursing.

Many factors affect infant feeding rhythm on the first day of life. In addition to the birth, another major influencer is how much time baby spends on the nursing parent's body, which is key to infant stability and is the stimulus for inborn feeding behaviors. During this time of rapid adjustment from womb to world, the newborn needs help staying warm. For the first time, baby begins to breathe air and to feed intermittently, rather than receiving oxygen and food continuously through the umbilical cord. Research suggests that at this vulnerable time, skin-to-skin contact—with the naked baby lying prone on the parent's bare chest—often covered by a warm blanket—eases baby's transition. Separation appears to be a major stressor, which among other things, contributes to feeding problems (Righard & Alade, 1990).

BOX 2.1 Ten Steps to Successful Breastfeeding Expanded

Critical Management Procedures

1a. Comply fully with the International Code of Marketing of Breast-milk Substitutes and relevant World Health Assembly resolutions.

1b. Have a written infant-feeding policy that is routinely communicated to staff and parents.

1c. Establish ongoing monitoring and data management systems.

2. Ensure that staff have sufficient knowledge, competence, and skills to support breastfeeding.

Key Clinical Practices

3. Discuss the importance and management of breastfeeding with pregnant women and their families.

4. Facilitate immediate and uninterrupted skin-to-skin contact and support mothers to initiate breastfeeding as soon as possible after birth.

5. Support mothers to initiate and maintain breastfeeding and manage common difficulties.

6. Do not provide breastfed newborns any food or fluids other than breast milk, unless medically indicated.

7. Enable mothers and their infants to remain together and to practice rooming-in 24 hours a day.

8. Support mothers to recognize and respond to their infants' cues for feeding.

9. Counsel mothers on the use and risks of feeding bottles, teats and pacifiers.

10. Coordinate discharge so that parents and their infants have timely access to ongoing support and care.

Adapted from **bit.ly/BA2-BFHI** *(World Health Organization and UNICEF, revised 2018)*

The authors of a Cochrane Review examined 46 trials involving 3,850 mothers and babies in 21 countries (Moore, Bergman, Anderson, & Medley, 2016) and concluded that healthy newborns in early skin-to-skin contact after birth:

- Had greater cardio-respiratory stability
- Had higher blood glucose levels
- Were more likely to breastfeed successfully during their first feed and breastfeed longer.

These authors wrote: "This time frame immediately post birth may represent a 'sensitive period' for programming future physiology and behavior." Also, no evidence of harm in any of the included studies was found for early skin-to-skin contact.

• • •

When separated, newborn mammals—including humans—display predictable stress responses that can cause instability.

When a newborn mammal is separated from her mother, she emits a distinctive distress cry and experiences predictable physiological changes. South African researcher and public health physician Nils Bergman decided to investigate these changes after he conducted a study of preterm babies in Zimbabwe (N. J. Bergman & Jurisoo, 1994) that found an increase in survival rates from 10%

to 50% in very low birth weight preemies when they were kept in skin-to-skin contact with their mothers after birth. Bergman found part of the explanation in animal studies. Human newborns—like other mammals—have inborn physiological programming that is key to survival and growth (N. Bergman, 2017). Using biologists' terminology, he referred to the newborn's changing environments (womb, mother's body, family, the larger world) as "habitats," with the mother's body being baby's natural "habitat" after birth. The feel of the birthing parent's body acts as a trigger for the behaviors and responses necessary for physiological regulation and optimal growth.

If a newborn is removed from her normal habitat—her parent's body—this triggers different responses. Bergman explains that in all mammal babies there are three basic physiological programs governed by the hindbrain that are key to survival: nutrition, reproduction, and defense. They regulate hormones, nerves, and muscles that affect the entire body. However, at any given time only one of these programs can run. If the defense program is running, the body shuts off the nutrition program and with it, growth.

When a newborn is removed from her parent's body, she goes into defense mode, beginning with a distinctive cry known as the "separation distress call" (Christensson, Cabrera, Christensson, Uvnas-Moberg, & Winberg, 1995). Biologists refer to the set of behaviors during parent-baby separation as the ***protest-despair response***. If the baby's cries are unanswered, she goes into the despair mode, where to increase the odds of survival, her body uses less energy by changing her heart rate, breathing rate, and body temperature (Alberts, 1994). In this mode, her stress hormones increase as the baby physically prepares to fight for survival, shutting down gut function, digestion, and growth.

• • •

Early separation increases infant instability in several ways.

Because of the physical changes described in the previous point, research linked early newborn separation to a number of concerning issues:

- Agitated state, more crying, and less sleep (Christensson et al., 1995; Ferber & Makhoul, 2004; Michelsson, Christensson, Rothganger, & Winberg, 1996)
- More feeding problems (Armbrust, Hinkson, von Weizsacker, & Henrich, 2016; Christensson et al., 1992)
- Lower blood glucose levels independent of feeding (Christensson et al., 1995; Mazurek et al., 1999; Takahashi & Tamakoshi, 2018)

Some of the conditions that put newborns at risk, such as hypoglycemia, may be triggered or worsened by early separation. A 2019 Danish quasi-experimental study (Dalsgaard, Rodrigo-Domingo, Kronborg, & Haslund, 2019) found that 2 hours of immediate skin-to-skin contact after birth along with frequent nursing were effective strategies for preventing hypoglycemia among babies born to mothers with gestational diabetes.

In a 2014 summary of the effects of separation on infant physiology (N. J. Bergman, 2014), Bergman made the case for ***zero separation*** during the first few days of life for term and preterm babies. He cited one South African study in which healthy term newborns acted as their own controls (Morgan, Horn, & Bergman, 2011). It found that in comparison to when

KEY CONCEPT

The more time newborns spend on their parents' body during the first few days, the easier the physical transition from womb to world.

the 2-day-olds slept in skin-to-skin contact, when they slept in a bassinet, they had:

- Higher cortisol levels
- Greater heart-rate variability
- 176% higher autonomic nervous system activation
- 86% decrease in time spent in quiet sleep

Bergman explained that when cortisol regulates a baby's system, it creates metabolic ***set-points*** that do a poor job of maintaining a healthy balance (homeostasis). According to a Swedish study (Hochberg et al., 2011), once established, these metabolic set-points may remain for life.

Bergman suggested that lifelong metabolic set-points created during early separation may lead to higher rates of many of the health problems plaguing the developed world, such as obesity, cardiovascular disease, and Type 2 diabetes. He also suggested that although the separated babies in the Morgan study appeared to be asleep, their physiological readings showed them to be in a state of "near-terror" or "freeze state" (a survival strategy used by newborns of other species to avoid attracting predators in the wild). If this "freeze state" is prolonged, it, too, could lead to long-term problems (Misslin, 2003).

KEY CONCEPT

Skin-to-skin contact reduces physical stress in newborns, stimulates earlier and more exclusive nursing, and elicits nurturing behaviors in parents.

In contrast, keeping newborns in skin-to-skin contact during this critical period may have lifelong positive health effects. When a parent holds a newborn in skin-to-skin contact, the nutrition program is activated. Research found (Modi & Glover, 1996; Mooncey, 1997) that skin-to-skin contact decreased blood levels of stress hormones by 74%. The amazing increase in preterm survival rates that Bergman found is the direct result of the baby remaining in the right habitat (in skin-to-skin contact), which turned on the program that enhanced baby's physiological regulation. In the nutrition program, babies had a lower level of stress hormones, their gut more easily processed food, and their heart rate and breathing were not elevated or slowed. Skin-to-skin contact also leads to a more successful beginning for nursing, because this parent-baby body contact elicits parents' nurturing behaviors, enhances their bond, and triggers the baby's inborn feeding reflexes.

• • •

Immediate skin-to-skin contact after a cesarean birth reduced admissions to special care.

As awareness spreads about the benefits of immediate skin-to-skin contact after birth, more and more birthing facilities are finding ways to implement this practice after cesarean deliveries (de Alba-Romero et al., 2014; Guala et al., 2017; Stevens, Schmied, Burns, & Dahlen, 2018). An overview article about U.S. maternity care trends from 2007 to 2015 (Boundy, Perrine, Barrera, Li, & Hamner, 2018) found that skin-to-skin contact after a vaginal birth increased from 40% to 83% and after a cesarean birth from 29% to 70%. A U.S. study of 2,841 babies born by planned cesarean section (Schneider, Crenshaw, & Gilder, 2017) found that one benefit of immediate skin-to-skin contact among babies born by cesarean was a significant reduction in the number of newborns admitted to the neonatal intensive care unit (NICU) for observation. Before beginning immediate skin-to-skin contact during cesarean delivery, the rate of NICU admission after cesarean delivery was 5.6%. After immediate skin-to-skin contact was implemented, the admission rate dropped to 1.75%.

• • •

In many busy birthing hospitals, it can be tempting to focus on completing assigned tasks rather than recommended practices (Sobel, Silvestre, Mantaring, Oliveros, & Nyunt, 2011). Recommendations vary on the best timing for a newborn's first bath. The World Health Organization recommended delaying the first bath for 24 hours after birth, and if that is not culturally appropriate, to delay the bath for a minimum of 6 hours (WHO, 2017). The American Academy of Pediatrics (AAP) and American College of Obstetricians and Gynecologists (ACOG) recommended delaying the first bath until after the first feed (AAP & ACOG, 2017). In its 2018 guidelines, the Association of Women's Health, Obstetric and Neonatal Nurses (AWHONN) recommended the first bath be delayed for 6 to 24 hours (AWHONN, 2018). Delaying baby's first bath makes sense for several reasons.

Delaying baby's first bath for 12 to 24 hours may promote better infant stability and improve early feeding.

Maintain a healthy body temperature. Some studies found that bathing baby within the first hour after birth can lead to low body temperature (hypothermia) (Bergstrom, Byaruhanga, & Okong, 2005; Takayama, Teng, Uyemoto, Newman, & Pantell, 2000). A U.S. 2018 study examined the effects on newborn body temperature when the first bath occurred at 3, 6, and 9 hours (Kelly et al., 2018) and found no clinically significant differences in body temperature or in breastfeeding rates at these different time periods.

More exclusive nursing. Bathing baby within the first hour interferes with both early skin-to-skin contact and nursing. One U.S. retrospective chart review (Preer, Pisegna, Cook, Henri, & Philipp, 2013) found that delaying the first bath from a mean time of 2 hours to 13 hours increased exclusive breastfeeding rates during the hospital stay by 39%. After the bath was routinely delayed for at least 12 hours, nursing initiation also increased 166%. A 2019 U.S. study of 996 mothers and babies (DiCioccio, Ady, Bena, & Albert, 2019) found that delaying the first bath for at least 12 hours (before this intervention average time was 1.7 hours) was associated with a 60% increase in exclusive breastfeeding rates during the hospital stay.

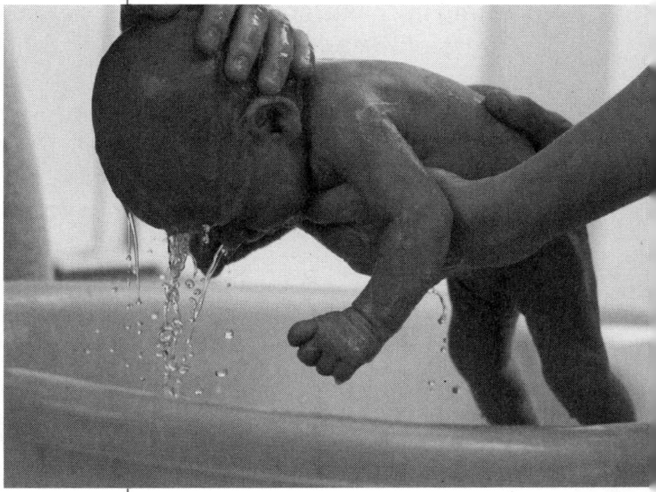

More parent participation. Delaying the first bath also makes it possible for the parents to participate, which one U.S. study found parents preferred (Brogan & Rapkin, 2017).

Better use of baby's vernix. Newborns emerge from the womb coated with *vernix caseosa*, a white, creamy substance that acts as a waterproof barrier and skin moisturizer. Vernix also has anti-microbial properties and is considered part of a newborn's defense system (Jha, Baliga, Kumar, Rangnekar, & Baliga, 2015; Tollin et al., 2005). Leaving the vernix on baby's skin after birth—rather than washing it off right away—may be beneficial. Although many health professionals worry that parents will react negatively to "birth dirt," a U.K. multicultural study (Finigan & Long, 2014) found most parents prefer immediate skin-to-skin contact rather than an early bath.

• • •

The 2016 Cochrane Review on early skin-to-skin contact in healthy term newborns (Moore et al., 2016) found that skin-to-skin contact was associated with more exclusive breastfeeding in the hospital and a longer duration of breastfeeding.

Early skin-to-skin contact is associated with longer exclusive nursing and can help overcome feeding problems.

Several studies found skin-to-skin contact can be an effective intervention to overcome early feeding problems, including severe latching struggles (Chiu, Anderson, & Burkhammer, 2008; Meyer & Anderson, 1999; K. E. Svensson, Velandia, Matthiesen, Welles-Nystrom, & Widstrom, 2013). A 2013 Swedish study (K. E. Svensson et al., 2013) randomized 103 mother-baby pairs having severe latching problems into two groups. In one group, attempts to feed were made in skin-to-skin contact, and in the other group, during feeding attempts the babies were clothed. The same percentage of mother-baby pairs in both groups overcame their nursing struggles, but the resolution of their feeding problems happened twice as fast in the skin-to-skin contact group.

In a U.S. prospective exploratory study of healthy, ethnically diverse mothers who reported feeding problems (Chiu et al., 2008), four sessions of skin-to-skin contact before nursing during the first 2 days successfully helped these mothers and babies overcome their feeding problems. Despite the initial feeding problems, 81% of these mothers were still breastfeeding at a 1-month follow-up call. Other research found that time spent before nursing in skin-to-skin contact acted as a stress-reliever and lowered blood pressure in mothers (Jonas et al., 2008).

• • •

Encourage families to follow safety recommendations concerning early nursing and skin-to-skin contact to ensure newborns' unobstructed breathing.

The term Sudden Unexpected Postnatal Collapse, or SUPC, is used in the medical literature to describe the death and near-death event of apparently healthy newborns during the first week or so of life (Herlenius & Kuhn, 2013). The incidence of SUPC is estimated as 40 per 100,000 in Scotland, 2.6 per 100,000 in Germany, 0.5 per 100,000 in Australia, and the risk of SUPC is highest during the first 2 hours after birth (Piumelli et al., 2017).

During the early days of life, any obstruction of newborns' breathing puts them at risk of SUPC. Some reported cases of SUPC occurred while mothers were on their smartphone and didn't notice their baby's breathing issues (Rodriguez, Hageman, & Pellerite, 2018). According to one review (Becher, Bhushan, & Lyon, 2012), among those cases where a physical cause (such as metabolic disease, congenital malformation, infection, etc.) could not be found, 80% involved a baby whose breathing was blocked. In 2019, researchers examined a large volume of data over nearly a decade from the U.S. Centers for Disease Control and Prevention WONDER and statistics from births in Massachusetts (Bartick, 2019) and found that during the period when more and more U.S. babies were born in Baby Friendly hospitals and skin-to-skin care was implemented more broadly, the incidence of SUPC in the U.S. decreased. Although these events are rare--accounting for only 0.72% of U.S. newborn deaths--parents can take the following simple steps to reduce risk during nursing and skin-to-skin contact in the early days of life (see Figure 2.1):

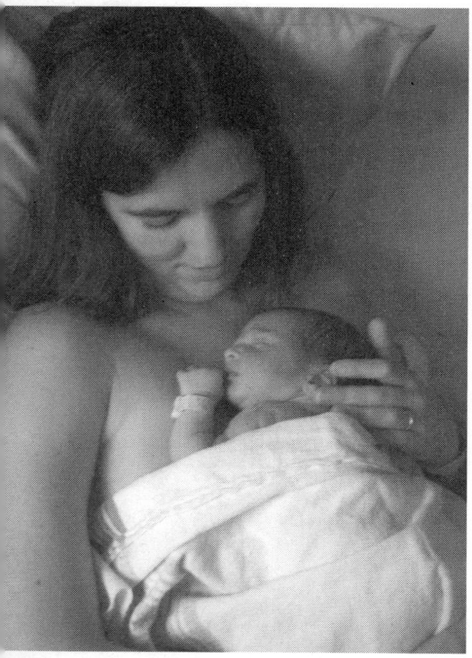

Figure 2.1 Safe skin-to-skin contact.

- The nursing parent leans back into a semi-reclined position (not flat or supine) and is either awake and undistracted (set aside electronic devices until later) or a nearby adult will monitor them.
- Baby rests tummy down on the nursing parent's body with her face visible and nose and mouth uncovered.
- Baby's neck is straight (not bent forward) and her chin is slightly raised in "sniff position."

Two articles (Davanzo et al., 2015; Ludington-Hoe, Morrison-Wilford, DiMarco, & Lotas, 2018) provide checklists for hospital use.

Early Nursing Patterns

On their first day, newborns may want to nurse often or may seem disinterested in feeding.

What happens in the first day of life will not "make or break" long-term milk production, but the number of feeds in the first 24 hours can have a significant effect on health outcomes, such as weight loss and bilirubin levels during the baby's first week.

The birth experience and routine practices after birth can profoundly influence nursing rhythms during the first 24 hours. In the introduction to her 2001 article on breastfeeding patterns during the first 60 hours, Australian researcher Stephanie Benson described her granddaughter's nursing pattern after an unmedicated home birth. It began with an early first feed at which she nursed for 2 to 3 minutes (Benson, 2001, p. 27).

> "An hour later she had a second breastfeed which lasted much longer and after about 60 minutes we decided to detach her. This was the beginning of a very long night. The baby roused and demanded a feed every 30-40 minutes and continued this whether we left her in bed with her mother or wrapped her and put her in the cot or whether I took her and cuddled her! Early the next morning she shared a warm bath with her mum, where she again fed and then slipped into deep sleep that lasted four-and-a-half hours. Then began a new pattern of feeding where she fed every 2 to 4 hours."

In her work as a hospital midwife, Benson noted that after medicated labors and routine separation after birth, many babies were very difficult to awaken and did not feed well during the first days. Where labor medication and separation are routine, sleepy and disinterested babies may seem to be the norm. In this setting, babies with a strong desire to nurse may be viewed as problematic. Benson wrote that some members of her hospital staff considered the babies who wanted to nurse like her home-birthed granddaughter "overly demanding, particularly at night."

Defining 'a Feed'

Especially at first, the sensory experience of nursing may be as important as the milk the newborn receives.

There are many ways to define a feed. At its essence, nursing is an intimate act that enhances the relationship of the nursing couple and provides the baby with food and other ingredients needed for normal growth and development. Many families depend as much on the calming, comforting aspects of nursing as they do on the milk it provides.

The sensory stimulation of nursing is also important. Some researchers consider the smell and touch a baby experiences as key to stability and neurodevelopment. The neurological effects of skin-to-skin contact and nursing are the focus of South African public health physician and researcher Nils Bergman. According to Bergman, during a baby's journey to the nipple after birth, the birthing parent's smell, taste, and touch activate nerve pathways that lead to a baby's amygdala, the seat of emotional memory in the brain, and stimulate the baby's limbic system, which helps regulate her autonomic nervous system, improving stability. Based on a large body of research, Bergman suggested that nursing and uninterrupted skin-to-skin contact after birth are vital for optimal newborn brain wiring (N. Bergman, 2017).

• • •

A more "milk-oriented" definition of a nursing is when baby takes milk from one side.

When focusing on the milk aspect of nursing, any definition of a feed will be based at least in part on the needs of the definer. One group of Swedish researchers, whose study's focus was time (Aarts, Hornell, Kylberg, Hofvander, & Gebre-Medhin, 1999; Hornell, Aarts, Kylberg, Hofvander, & Gebre-Medhin, 1999), defined a feed as at least 2 minutes spent nursing, with at least 30 minutes in between.

An Australian research team used another definition better suited to its goals, defining a feed as whenever a baby took milk from one side (Kent et al., 2006). This group examined feeding patterns among 71 exclusively nursed 1- to 6-month-old babies and needed to distinguish whether babies took one side or more and measured milk intake from left and right sides. In this study, if a baby went longer than 30 minutes before wanting to feed again, this was considered an "unpaired" feed. If baby took both sides within 30 minutes, this was considered a "paired" feed. If after taking both sides baby took the first side again within 30 minutes, this was considered a "clustered" feed. They defined a "meal" as a one-sided unpaired feed, a two-sided paired feed, or a three-or-more-sided clustered feed.

• • •

Cultural beliefs affect what nursing parents consider "a feed."

Nursing rhythms vary among families and may also vary considerably from place to place. A "feed" means something very different in different cultures. Western families, for example, may consider a "feed" a lengthy, ritualized activity that involves changing the baby's diaper, making the nursing parent a drink, turning off the phone, settling into a certain chair, and then nursing baby for an extended time. Many Western attitudes about feeding, such as the belief that babies should feed at set time intervals, such as every few hours, are influenced by bottle-feeding norms. In contrast, in many developing countries, a nursing baby may be kept on the parent's body, nursing at the slightest cue for just a few minutes 15 to 20 times each day (Hartmann, 2007). Babies in the West and babies in the developing world average about the same daily milk intake, but the immense cultural differences in their feeding rhythms affect early nursing.

Health Outcomes and Early Nursing

When a baby nurses effectively, more feeds in the first 24 hours are associated with more milk intake and less weight loss days later.

The number of times a baby nurses on the first day of life affects how quickly the nursing parent's milk production increases. A classic prospective Japanese study of 140 mothers and babies after vaginal births (Yamauchi & Yamanouchi, 1990) found that the babies who nursed 7 to 11 times on their first day consumed 86% more milk on Day 3 than the babies who nursed fewer than 7 times. The babies who nursed more on the first day also lost less weight initially and began regaining their birth weight more quickly. The difference in milk intake between these two groups continued to be significant through the fifth day of life.

• • •

More feeds on the first day were associated with fewer cases of exaggerated newborn jaundice on Day 6.

Exaggerated newborn jaundice can affect feeding rhythm because elevated bilirubin levels can make a baby sleepy and less responsive. But frequent feeds on the first day can help prevent exaggerated newborn jaundice later. The prospective Japanese study described in the previous point (Yamauchi & Yamanouchi, 1990) found an association between more feeds on the first day of life and lower bilirubin levels on Day 6. This study found a significant correlation between number of nursing sessions during a baby's first 24 hours with both frequency of meconium passage and bilirubin levels on Day 6. The fewer times the babies fed during their first 24 hours, the more likely they were to have bilirubin levels higher than 14 mg/dL (238 μmol/L) on Day 6:

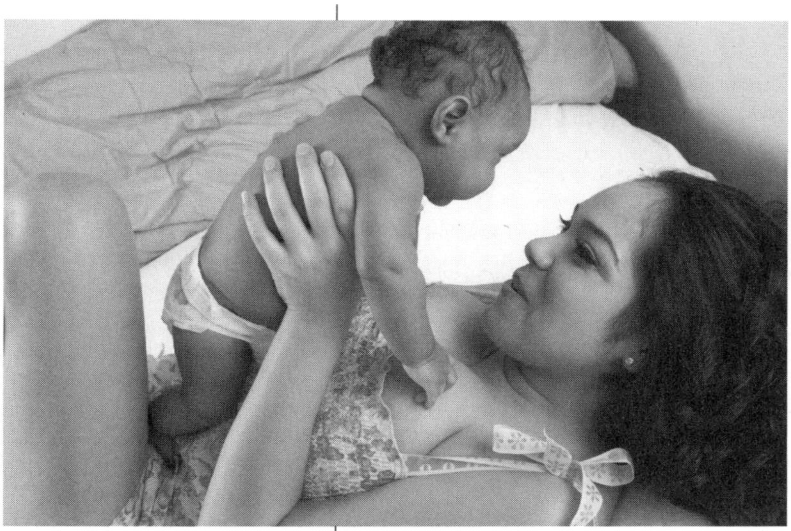

- 28.1% who fed two or fewer times
- 24.5% who fed three to four times
- 15.2% who fed five to six times
- 11.8% who fed seven to eight times
- 0% of those who fed nine or more times

A 2017 Iranian study (Boskabadi & Zakerihamidi, 2017) also found an association between more nursing sessions during the first 4 days and lower bilirubin levels (for more details, see p. 243-244).

• • •

Feeding often is crucial, but so is feeding effectively.

In the classic Japanese study described in the previous points, its babies clearly nursed effectively, but in other studies, some babies did not. In one U.S. study of 73 mothers and babies, the researchers noted that the baby who had the most feeds per day (12) lost the most weight and was 30% below birth weight on Day 11. The authors wrote that frequent nursing "...particularly when associated with low bowel output strongly suggests the need for evaluation of baby's weight, the mother milk's supply, and the baby's ability to remove milk from the breasts (Shrago, Reifsnider, & Insel, 2006, p. 200). See p. 201-205 in Chapter 6, "Weight Gain and Growth" for ways to evaluate a baby's milk intake during nursing.

Rooming-In

Rooming-in is associated with better nursing outcomes

As described in the previous section, the more times each day baby nurses during the first few days after birth, the better the health outcomes and the faster milk production increases. To encourage frequent nursing, it makes sense for nursing parents and newborns to stay together day and night and spend as much time as possible with baby resting on the nursing parent's body. Full frontal contact, whether in skin-to-skin contact or not, triggers baby's inborn feeding behaviors. Both the Baby Friendly Hospital Initiative and Academy of Breastfeeding Medicine Clinical Protocol #7: "Model Maternity Policy Supportive of Breastfeeding" recommends 24-hour rooming in (Hernandez-Aguilar, Bartick, Schreck, Harrel, & Academy of Breastfeeding, 2018). Any needed infant assessments can be performed in the parent's room.

• • •

Keeping baby on the nursing parent's body as much as possible during the early days helps baby make a smoother transition from womb to world.

Zero separation of nursing parent and baby in the early days is promoted by infant neuroscience (N. Bergman, 2017; N. J. Bergman, 2014) as the healthiest way to transition newborns from life in utero to life on the outside in terms of both infant stability in the short term and healthier physiological programming in the longer term. For more details, see p. 49-52 in the earlier section "Togetherness, Separation, and Newborn Stability."

• • •

Rooming in during the first 48 hours is associated with significantly more total sleep.

A 2018 Irish study of 30 first-time mothers with no history of sleep disorders (Hughes, Mohamad, Doyle, & Burke, 2018) used a sleep questionnaire to examine the mothers' sleep patterns during the first 48 hours after giving birth at term. Type of birth fell evenly into three categories. One third (10) had spontaneous vaginal births, one third (10) had instrument-assisted vaginal births, and one third (10) had cesarean births. All mothers roomed-in with their babies except during the times some of the babies were taken to the neonatal intensive care unit. Eighteen (60%) planned to breastfeed, and all of these women nursed through Day 2, when the study ended. Twelve (40%) planned to bottle-feed from birth, and these mothers had no help with night feeds from hospital staff or relatives.

Reasons the study mothers reported being awake at night included:

- Feeding (90%)
- Overwhelming emotions, anxiety, watching baby sleep (33%)
- Hospital background noise (27%)

All mothers slept more during the second 24 hours than the first, and these differences were statistically significant. Demographic factors (age, marital status, employment status, educational level) did not affect sleep duration, nor did post-birth analgesia. Total sleep time also did not vary among women whose babies were admitted for a time to the special-care nursery and those who kept their babies with them in their room. The researchers (Hughes et al., 2018, p. 3) wrote:

> "Interestingly, environmental factors including background noise, shared room, type of delivery, need for neonatal intensive care unit bed, pain and worrying about the neonate did not influence the total time slept. Perhaps contrary to popular belief, in our study, breastfeeding was the only factor to significantly influence sleep, increasing it."

The women who breastfed reported on average 2.6 hours more sleep during the first 48 hours than those who bottle-fed, and this difference was statistically significant.

Overcoming Barriers to Early Nursing

Sleepy newborns feed more—even in light sleep—when resting on the nursing parent's body.

About 2 hours after birth, most newborns fall into a long sleep stretch. To reach a goal of 8 to 12 feeds during the first day, it helps to let go of the assumption that newborns must nurse at regular time intervals (such as every 2 hours). To encourage frequent feeds, take advantage of newborns' natural inclination to "cluster" their feeds together during some parts of the day. Suggest nursing parents keep their baby on their body in semi-reclined positions (see Chapter 1) and attempt nursing often whenever the baby is awake and alert. Full frontal contact with the nursing parent also triggers feeding behaviors, which may not happen if baby is swaddled in a bassinet (Figure 2.2).

Also keep in mind that the baby doesn't have to be awake and alert to feed. Babies can feed actively while drowsy or in a light sleep. One small U.K. study found that when kept on their mothers' bodies in semi-reclined positions, late preterm babies breastfed effectively during sleep, averaging 2.5 hours of active nursing every 24 hours (Colson, 2003). Helping a baby latch in light sleep (eyes

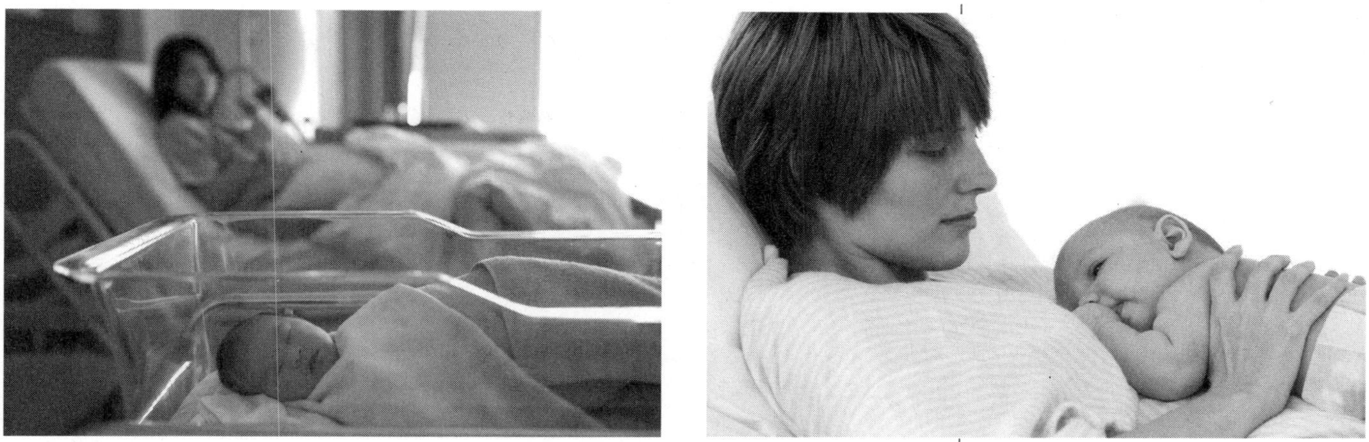

Figure 2.2 For more feeds in the early days, spend less time with baby swaddled in a box and more time with baby on the nursing parent's body.

moving under eyelids, any body movement) can also be an effective strategy for babies having feeding struggles (Smillie, 2017).

• • •

Step 7 of the Baby-Friendly Hospital Initiative requires that Baby Friendly hospitals provide 24-hour rooming-in. In one Swedish study of 132 mothers (K. Svensson, Matthiesen, & Widstrom, 2005), more of the mothers who chose to send their newborns to the hospital nursery at night thought the staff believed their babies should stay in the nursery. Of the mothers who chose to keep their babies with them at night, 93% felt positively about the experience, which was counter to how the hospital staff thought the mothers felt. Of those mothers who didn't keep their babies with them, 73% thought night rooming-in was a good idea. The researchers suggested that hospital staff may mistakenly believe that when babies are with mothers at night, they will cry as much as they do while in the hospital nursery. Research found that mothers and babies actually get more sleep at night when together than when separated (Keefe, 1988; Waldenstrom & Swenson, 1991).

The attitude hospital staff conveys about night rooming-in can influence families' choices.

• • •

Many hospitals are concerned about safety issues, such as preventing falls. One U.K. study (Ball, Ward-Platt, Heslop, Leech, & Brown, 2006) randomly assigned 64 mothers and babies after vaginal births with no opiate analgesia to one of three different sleep locations during their first 2 days. When the study mothers were ready to sleep, they placed their newborns:

1. In a separate stand-alone crib/cot in their room
2. In bed with them
3. In a side-car bed closed on three sides and attached to the mother's bed for easy access.

Hospital sleeping arrangements that give easy access to the baby—such as side-cars—result in more nursing and reduce safety risks.

Researchers videotaped the sleep episodes to evaluate the effects of the different sleep locations on infant safety, breastfeeding frequency, and mothers' sleep.

The researchers found that the babies placed in their mother's bed or in the side-car attempted to breastfeed and actually breastfed significantly more times than the babies in the stand-alone crib/cot. The median frequency per hour of attempted feeds was 1.3 in the mother's bed, 2.1 in the side-car, and 0.7 in the stand-alone crib, and of actual feeds was 1.2 in the mother's bed, 1.3 in the side-car, and 0.5 in the stand-alone crib. This study found no difference in sleep duration among the three groups, even when mother and baby shared a bed.

KEY CONCEPT

Share insights and strategies with nursing families that can help even sleepy newborns feed at least 8 or more times each day.

The researchers evaluated "potential infant safety risk exposures" as breathing risk, overheating, falling, entrapment, and overlaying. None of the newborns in the study experienced any adverse events, but researchers identified more potential risks among those who slept in their mothers' beds than in the other two groups. However, each sleep setting had some potential risk exposures. For example, the one infant found to have the most potential safety risk exposures included: "...observed bouts of airway covering occurred while sleeping in the stand-alone cots and were all related to swaddling" (Ball et al., 2006, p. 1008). The researchers concluded that the side-car crib appeared to be the best of the three sleep options, increasing breastfeeding frequency while providing a safe-sleep setting.

Another smaller U.K. randomized controlled trial compared the experiences of 35 mothers and babies after a cesarean birth (Tully & Ball, 2012). In this study, 20 of the babies were randomized to sleep at night in a side-car attached to their mother's bed, while the other 15 babies were randomized to sleep at night in a stand-alone bassinet. Although the use of the side-car did not result in more nursing in this study, the women much preferred the side-car. The researchers noted that stand-alone bassinets introduced an unnecessary obstacle to nursing after surgery and posed a hazard for newborns due to their mothers' compromised mobility after a cesarean delivery.

• • •

Unnecessary newborn supplementation—which is common worldwide—can interfere with frequent nursing. Nursing outcomes can be improved with simple strategies.

Supplementing healthy term newborns with formula without a medical indication is common practice worldwide (Biggs et al., 2018; Boban & Zakarija-Grkovic, 2016; Parry, Ip, Chau, Wu, & Tarrant, 2013). A 2016 U.S. review examined the statistics from all U.S. birthing facilities in responses to the Maternity and Infant Nutrition and Care (mPINC) surveys from 2009 to 2013 (J. M. Nelson, Perrine, Scanlon, & Li, 2016). Its authors found that nearly one quarter of U.S. hospitals supplement more than half of healthy term nursing newborns with formula. More than 65% of the formula use was attributed to "mother's choice," the most common reason given.

Why families request formula. One U.S. study of 97 low-income mothers (DaMota, Banuelos, Goldbronn, Vera-Beccera, & Heinig, 2012) shed new light on why so many parents supplement their newborns in the hospital. During discussion groups with these mothers, the underlying cause of most supplementation was unfamiliarity with normal newborn behaviors and nursing patterns. In other words, their newborns' behavior ran counter to their expectations of how their newborns "should" behave. These new mothers considered formula the "solution" to nonexistent problems, such as infant waking and frequent feeding cues. The researchers reported that the first request for formula in the hospital was most often triggered by typical newborn behaviors and unmet expectations about how long their baby would sleep or how often the baby wanted to nurse. Clearly, knowing more about typical newborn feeding and sleeping patterns before giving birth could help prevent supplementation for these reasons.

Risk factors for supplementation. An Australian retrospective study of more than 1,500 babies found that 15% were supplemented during their hospital stay (Kalmakoff, Gray, & Baddock, 2018). Supplements were independently associated with maternal overweight, first baby, early-term birth (at 37 or 38 weeks), birth weight below 2500 g (5.5 lb.), and use of synthetic oxytocin at birth. The researchers concluded that in families with these risk factors, longer time in skin-to-skin contact may be beneficial as well as extra education and support.

> **KEY CONCEPT**
>
> *Most unnecessary formula supplementation—which can undermine early nursing—is rooted in families' misconceptions about newborn norms.*

Supplement options. The healthiest first choice, whether a supplement is medically indicated or not, is expressed mother's milk. U.S. pediatrician Jane Morton suggests that parents learn and practice regular hand expression during the last month of an uncomplicated pregnancy (see p. 474), and after birth routinely express extra colostrum after nursing and spoon-feed it to their newborn. This practice prevents excess weight loss and stimulates earlier milk increase, as well as giving parents confidence in their ability to provide the milk their baby needs (Morton, 2019). See Dr. Morton's free videos for parents at **firstdroplets.com**. When expressed milk is unavailable, another option in a growing number of facilities is donor milk from a milk bank. Once used almost exclusively for preterm or sick babies, many facilities now offer the option of donor milk to supplement healthy term babies (Belfort et al., 2018; Sen et al., 2018). One U.S. study consisting of semi-structured interviews of 24 mothers (Rabinowitz, Kair, Sipsma, Phillipi, & Larson, 2018) asked them if they would prefer to supplement with donor milk or formula. About 56% chose donor milk. The 44% who chose the formula did so because they were unfamiliar with donor milk and had questions about its cost and safety.

Volume of supplement. Whatever supplement is chosen, the volume is key to better nursing outcomes, as overfeeding can lead to less interest in nursing. The Academy of Breastfeeding Medicine's Clinical Protocol #5 on supplementation (Kellams, Harrel, Omage, Gregory, & Rosen-Carole, 2017) is free and downloadable at **bfmed.org/protocols**. The authors of this ABM protocol recommend supplemental volumes based on baby's age. These are comparable to the average volume of milk baby receives while nursing (Table 2.2).

Swaddling/Bundling

Swaddling, also known as bundling, was practiced historically in many parts of the world (Blatt, 2015). From about 2 to 3 weeks of age until about 12 weeks, many babies have daily fussy periods, when they are inconsolable. At that time, swaddling may be a useful tool for calming an unhappy baby who is unwilling to nurse.

Although swaddling can help calm some fussy babies, during the first few days, skin-to-skin contact is a better calming strategy.

TABLE 2.2 Recommended Volume of Supplment Per Feed By Baby's Age

Baby's Age in Hours	Volume of Milk Per Feed in mL (oz.)
First 24	2-10 mL (0.1-0.3 oz.)
24-48	5-15 mL (0.2-0.5 oz.)
48-72	15-30 mL (0.5-1 oz.)
72-96	30-60 mL (1-2 oz.)

Adapted from (Kellams et al., 2017)

However, some parenting authors recommend that from birth all families should swaddle their newborns from 12 to 20 hours per day (Karp, 2002). There is no evidence to support this practice, and it could potentially undermine early nursing. As described in the previous sections, frequent feeds after birth are crucial to faster milk increase. Swaddled babies who are laid in a bassinet arouse less, show fewer feeding cues, and sleep for longer stretches (Franco et al., 2005). To increase baby's interest in frequent feeds, as much as parents are comfortable, encourage them to keep baby on their bodies in full frontal contact (Figure 2.2). Skin-to-skin contact is ideal, but body contact when lightly dressed stimulates feeding behaviors, too. Resting on the nursing parent's (or partner's) body will stimulate infant feeding behaviors, even in light sleep (Colson, 2003, 2019).

A 2017 integrative review of the literature on swaddling (A. M. Nelson, 2017) noted that early skin-to-skin contact is important to establishing nursing and suggested that if newborns are swaddled between episodes of skin-to-skin contact, they may need to be awakened to feed often enough. It concluded that according to the limited evidence available, swaddling probably has no long-term negative effect on breastfeeding. This integrative review also found a strong association between tight swaddling around baby's hips and hip dysplasia and noted that while swaddling can calm babies, it may slightly increase the risk of Sudden Infant Death Syndrome (SIDS).

Feeding Volumes and Newborn Stomach Size

During their first 24 hours, newborns consume on average about 7 mL of colostrum per nursing session, with feeds increasing significantly in volume over the next few days.

Before birth, a baby never feels hunger. After birth, intermittent feeding is a new experience. To make this transition easier, the mammary glands provide small, gradually increasing volumes of milk. The volume of colostrum a newborn receives per feed on the first day varies greatly from one nursing couple to another. An Australian study of nine babies (Saint, Smith, & Hartmann, 1984) found that milk intake on the first day ranged from 7 to 123 mL, with an average daily intake of 37 mL and average feed volume of 7 mL By the second day, a Dutch study of 18 mothers and babies (Houston, Howie, & McNeilly, 1983) estimated the average milk intake per feed was 14 mL, with a range of daily intake of 44 to 335 mL. When nursing is going normally, each day during the first week of life, the baby takes more milk as the milk production increases. For more details, see p. 421 in the section "Making Milk during the First Year and Beyond" in Chapter 10.

• • •

For the newborn, small feeds have advantages over larger feeds.

Some worry that the small volume of colostrum available during the early days is insufficient. But small feeds have advantages for the newborn.

Newborns have small stomachs. Stomach capacity varies by birth weight, with larger babies having larger stomachs. A 2013 review of the literature (N. J. Bergman, 2013) concluded that average stomach capacity of a newborn is about 20 mL (two thirds of an ounce). When both stomach capacity and gastric emptying time of human milk are considered, according to Bergman, this translates to biologically appropriate feeding intervals of about 1 hour.

On the first day, newborn stomachs don't stretch. In one U.S. study that measured newborns' stomach elasticity with a balloon at the end of a nasogastric tube (Zangen et al., 2001), researchers found that during the first day of life, the walls of a newborn's stomach stay firm and don't yet stretch as they will later. By 3 days of age, as the baby takes more small, frequent feeds, her stomach begins to expand more easily to hold more milk.

• • •

Although new parents are sometimes encouraged to "top up" babies after nursing to fill them as full as possible as a way to help them stay satisfied or sleep longer, there are several disadvantages to this approach.

Supplementing a newborn with too much milk has short- and long-term drawbacks.

Early exposure to non-human milks puts newborns at greater risk of allergy sensitization and a longer period of intestinal permeability. In the early weeks, feeding non-human milks is not recommended unless there is a medical indication (Kellams et al., 2017), in part because a newborn's gut junctions are more open and permeable than they will be later. Introducing foreign proteins such as those in cow's-milk-based formulas during this vulnerable time increases the risk of allergy sensitization (Gil et al., 2017; Host, Husby, & Osterballe, 1988). A 2019 Irish study (E. Kelly, et al., 2019) found formula supplementation of nursing babies during the first 24 hours increased their risk of cow's milk allergy 7-fold. For details, see p. 563. Some research (Le Huerou-Luron, Blat, & Boudry, 2010) suggested that feeding formula during the early weeks may extend the period of intestinal permeability by several more weeks, which makes a newborn vulnerable to sensitization and illness for a longer time. As a baby's gut matures, her gut junctions become tighter and these risks decrease. Giving non-human milks also changes a newborn's gut flora to more closely resemble that of an adult, which puts her at greater risk of gut inflammation and infection (Moodley-Govender, Mulol, Stauber, Manary, & Coutsoudis, 2015).

If formula is fed to nursing newborns during the first 3 days, the type of formula may affect allergy sensitization. A 2019 Japanese randomized controlled trial followed 312 nursing newborns for 2 years (Urashima et al., 2019). During their first 3 days, the babies supplemented with an amino-acid-based elemental formula (like Nutramigen AA or Neocate) were much less likely to develop cow-milk-protein allergy than those fed regular formula. At 2 years, 17% of the group supplemented with elemental formula developed cow-milk-protein allergy as compared with 32% of the group supplemented with regular formula.

Large milk volumes raise baby's expectations. Even when expressed mother's milk is used as a supplement, be sure not to overfeed. Use the feeding volumes listed in Table 2.2, which are consistent with nursing norms. Feeding a baby too much milk after the first day can stretch a newborn's stomach, leaving her feeling dissatisfied later by the smaller volumes she receives while nursing, which can lead to feeding problems.

A 2018 U.S. randomized controlled trial (Flaherman et al., 2018) is a good example of how small volumes of supplement can meet the needs of at-risk babies without negatively affecting nursing patterns. This study included 164 exclusively breastfed newborns 24 to 48 hours old who had lost ≥5% of birth weight. They were randomized into two groups: one group continued to exclusively breastfeed, and after each nursing the other group received a supplement of 10 mL of formula until the mother's milk increased. At that time, the supplements were discontinued. At 1 week, 96% of the babies in the supplemented group and 94% of those who did not receive early supplements were still nursing. At 1 month, 55% of the babies who received early supplements were exclusively nursing compared with 66% of the babies who did not receive the

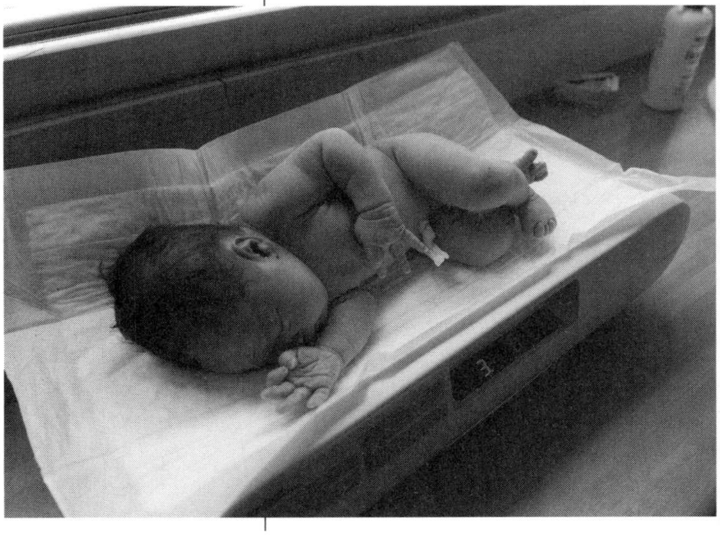

early supplements. Hospital readmission occurred in 5% of the unsupplemented babies and none of the supplemented babies. Examination of the supplemented babies' microbiome found that the 10 mL formula supplements did not decrease the abundance of the types of bacteria, *Lactobacillus* and *Bifidobacterium*, which are usually abundant in exclusively nursing babies. And there was no expansion of bacteria such as *Clostridium*, which is more common in formula-fed infants and adults.

However, this study has at least two major issues. First, a better choice of supplement—to reduce the risk of allergy sensitization—is expressed mother's milk or donor milk. Second, as other studies found, the excess IV fluids many receive during labor can artificially inflate baby's birth weight and increase weight loss during the first 24 hours of life (Noel-Weiss et al., 2011). That's why many now recommend against using baby's birth weight as a gauge of feeding adequacy. Instead, research (DiTomasso & Paiva, 2018) found that babies' 24-hour weight can safely be used as a basis for evaluating the need for supplements. On the plus side, the biologically appropriately 10 mL supplements appeared to be enough to prevent hospital readmission in the supplemented group.

Overfeeding during the first week is associated with obesity later in life. A U.S. prospective longitudinal study followed 653 formula-fed babies from birth to age 20 to 32 years and found that greater weight gain in the first week of life was associated with adult overweight. The researchers suggested that birth to 8 days may be a "critical period" during which human physiology is programmed. They concluded that: "In formula fed infants, weight gain during the first week of life may be a critical determinant for the development of obesity several decades later" (Stettler et al., 2005, p. 1897). For more research on this dynamic and details about normal newborn weight loss and gain after birth, see p. 184.

Day and Night Early Feeding Patterns

Most babies are born with their days and nights mixed up and feed more often at night.

Nursing patterns in the first 60 hours of life were documented in an Australian study of 37 mothers and babies after an unmedicated vaginal birth (Benson, 2001). The researchers found that the newborns nursed the fewest times from 3 a.m. to 9 a.m. Feeding frequency increased throughout the day with the most feeds occurring between 9 p.m. to 3 a.m.

> **KEY CONCEPT**
>
> *The more familiar families are with normal newborn behaviors, the less likely they are to give unnecessary supplements.*

Realistic expectations about feeding frequency at night are helpful during the early weeks. This is even more vital when families are discharged from the birthing facility on the second day. If new parents are unaware that frequent night feeds are common during this time, they may mistakenly assume that their baby's' desire to feed so often at night is a sign of inadequate milk or another nursing problem, which can lead to unnecessary supplementation.

An excellent one-page handout for parents is "Baby's Second Night," written by Jan Barger, RN, MA, IBCLC, which describes nursing as the "closest thing to home" the newborn knows in a scary new world and is available from: **bit.ly/BA2-Babys2ndNight**.

• • •

Suggest safe sleep locations that make nursing easier.

For details, see the last section "Night Feed" at the end of this chapter.

• • •

Babies' nursing rhythm and stool color change as milk production increases.

With increasing milk production around the third or fourth day, nursing patterns often change, with feeds becoming shorter and babies being satisfied for longer stretches. Stool color should change from black meconium to green transitional stools and by Day 4 or 5 to yellow. An earlier-than-usual transition to yellow stools is a reliable sign that nursing is going especially well, which usually means less weight loss and earlier weight gain (Nommsen-Rivers, Heinig, Cohen, & Dewey, 2008). For more details about how parents can gauge healthy milk intake, see p. 201-205.

The First 40 Days

Feeding Intensity and Milk Production

During the first 40 days, suggest families expect their newborn to nurse intensely as they establish full milk production.

Feeding rhythms change over the weeks, months, and years as baby grows. As with early feeding rhythms, some changes are rooted in biology and some in culture. The first 40 days after birth is a time when the birthing parent's body is primed and ready to make milk. Although hormones play a role in initiating milk production, the major driver is the rhythm and effectiveness of milk removal from the mammary glands, either by nursing or expressing milk. This dynamic is also known as ***autocrine control*** (or local control) of milk production (for details, see p. 410). When a baby is nursing effectively, the baby's feeding rhythm is the main driver of the rate of milk production. When nursing is going normally, by the end of the first 40 days, a nursing parent will produce just about as much milk as the baby will ever need. During this time, expect the baby to nurse at irregular intervals, "clustering" or bunching her feeds close together during some parts of the day.

The first week. With frequent nursing, by the end of the first week, milk production increases more than 10-fold—from an average of a little more than 1 ounce (37 mL) per day total on the first day to about 10 to 19 ounces (280 to 576 mL) per day by Day 7 (Kent, Gardner, & Geddes, 2016). During this same time, the baby's stomach expands and can comfortably hold about 1 to 2 ounces (30 to 59 mL) of milk at a feed. With rapid growth, baby's stomach grows along with milk production.

The second and third weeks. With frequent feeds, milk production continues to build. Now baby consumes about 2 to 3 ounces (59 to 89 mL) per feed and takes about 20 to 25 ounces (591 to 750 mL) of milk per day. At this stage, babies often increase the number and length of feeds to increase milk production to meet her growing needs. These periods of longer, more frequent feedings are sometimes called ***growth spurts*** or ***frequency days***.

The fourth and fifth weeks. Babies now take an average of about 3 to 4 ounces (89 to 118 mL) per feed, and daily milk intake increases to an average of about 25 to 30 ounces (750 to 887 mL) per day (Kent et al., 2013). At 1 month, most nursing parents produce nearly as much milk per day as their nursing baby will ever need. Because babies' growth and metabolic rate slow as they age, they continue to need about the same daily volume of milk from 1 month to 6 months of age. For more details, see p. 426 in Chapter 6, "Weight Gain and Growth."

But not every baby is average. One Australian prospective study of 71 exclusively breastfed babies from 1 to 6 months old (Kent et al., 2006) found a large range of daily milk intake among these healthy, thriving babies, from 15.5 to 43 ounces (440 to 1220 g).

• • •

Encourage the family to arrange for extra help during this hectic time, so they can focus on the baby and on nursing.

When parents expect nursing to be intense during the first 40 days, they can plan ahead to get help with meals, household chores, and any older children. Perhaps equally important, with a good understanding of normal nursing patterns during this time, they will be less likely to assume something is wrong because the baby wants to nurse so often. Emphasize that after this "adjustment period," typically babies begin to take more milk in less time and number of feeds per day decreases slightly, which will make nursing easier to fit into the family's other activities.

Care of the Nursing Parent

Nurturing practices used by some traditional societies after birth may help prevent the "baby blues" and other mood disorders.

Many cultures consider the first 40 days a time to provide special care for the birthing parent. Many Hispanics refer to it as "la cuarentina" (the quarantine), and in China it is called "doing the month." In years past in the U.S., it was called the "lying-in" period. In contrast, many Western parents today are encouraged to "get back to normal" quickly, which can compromise both nursing and feelings of well-being.

After studying postpartum practices in many cultures, anthropologists Gwen Stern and Larry Kruckman noted in their 1983 cross-cultural review (Stern & Kruckman, 1983) that postpartum/postnatal depression, including the "baby blues," were almost unheard of in some traditional societies. In contrast, in developed countries like the U.S., 50% to 85% of new mothers experience the "baby blues," and 15% to 25% or more experience the more severe postpartum depression (K. A. Kendall-Tackett, 2017). Stern and Kruckman found that all the cultures with a low incidence of baby blues and postpartum depressive symptoms had several supportive practices in common.

The period after birth is seen as different and distinct. In almost all the societies studied, the postpartum/postnatal period is considered a time distinct from normal life. During this time, experienced mothers help new mothers learn to care for their babies.

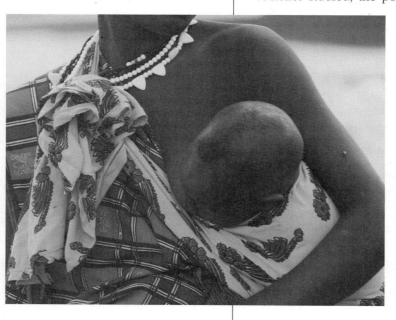

New mothers rest and are cared for in seclusion. During this time, new mothers are seen as especially vulnerable, so social seclusion is widely practiced. While they rest, they are expected to restrict their normal activities separate from others, which promotes frequent nursing. This is a time to rest, regain strength, and learn baby care.

Mothers are relieved of household duties. In order for seclusion and mandated rest to be practical, mothers' normal workload must be taken on by someone else. In these cultures, someone else takes care of older children and household duties. Some women stay in their parents' homes during this time, where help is more available.

A woman's new status is publicly recognized. In these cultures, much personal attention is given to the mother, often described as "mothering the mother." In some places, the new status of the mother is recognized through social rituals, such as bathing, washing of hair, massage, binding of the abdomen, and other types of personal care.

• • •

In many Western cultures, greater concern and support are expressed during the pregnancy than after the baby is born. After birth, the focus on the birthing parent vanishes. Hospital discharge in the U.S. is usually 24 to 48 hours after a vaginal birth and 2 to 4 days after a cesarean birth. Many nursing parents have no help or support at home--chances are no one at the hospital even asked. The partner (if there is one) will probably return to work within the week, leaving the nursing parent home alone to prepare meals, learn to nurse, and recover from birth. Those who provided attention during pregnancy are no longer there, and the people who visit are often more interested in the baby. There is the unspoken understanding not to "bother" medical caregivers unless there is a medical reason.

Encourage families to adopt as many of these practices as they can during the first 40 days.

Caring for a newborn—especially a first baby—takes far more time and work than most parents expect. The combination of hormonal shifts, physical discomfort, lack of sleep, body changes, and the intensity of being on duty day and night are some of the reasons many Western parents find nursing overwhelming and the first 40 days stressful. If help is not provided through a national health-care system, encourage families to seek help from family and friends or to seek professional services available to families, such as doulas. Another valuable source of support is peer-support groups—both in person and online—which can alleviate the isolation many Western families feel after birth.

FEEDING RHYTHMS AS BABY GROWS

Biology and Culture

Although many consider humans in a different category from other mammals, our biology profoundly influences us. When it comes to feeding rhythms, in general, the more mature the newborn mammal is at birth and the more protein and fat in its mother's milk, the less often that species' newborn feeds. Each of the more than 4,000 species of mammals falls into one of these two general categories: mammals whose mothers are in intermittent contact with their newborns (cache, follow, and nest mammals) and mammals whose mothers and newborns are in continuous contact (N. Bergman, 2017; Lozoff, Brittenham, Trause, Kennell, & Klaus, 1977).

The natural feeding pattern of each mammal species varies by its maturity at birth and the composition of its milk.

Cache mammals. These include the deer, the rabbit, and the seal. Seal mothers may leave their babies on shore for up to several days at a time as they hunt for fish in the sea. Land mammals in this category stash their newborns in a safe place (the "cache") and may leave them for 12 hours at a time. Their milk is very high in fat and protein to sustain the newborns for the long periods their mother is away.

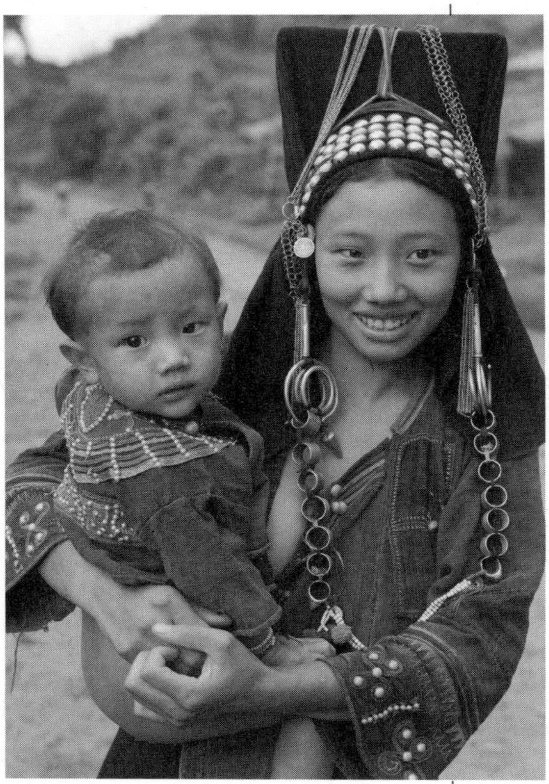

Follow mammals. These include the giraffe and cow. Their newborns are mature enough at birth to follow their mothers around and feed. They feed more often than the cache mammals and their milk is lower in fat and protein.

Nest mammals. These include the dog and cat. These mothers leave their litter of newborns together in a "nest" and return every few hours to feed. Their milk is correspondingly lower in fat and protein.

Carry mammals. Also referred to as continuous contact mammals, this group includes the apes and marsupials, like the kangaroo. These mammals are the most immature at birth, need to be held against their mother's body to stay warm, and are carried constantly. Their milk has the lowest levels of fat and protein, and as a result, they need to be fed often around the clock.

Humans are in this last group. With our larger brains and smaller pelvises, we are born very early. At birth our brains are less mature than most other mammals, some scientists believe so that our heads do not become too big to fit through our mothers' narrow pelvis. Most other mammals are born at about 80% of adult brain growth, but humans are born at less than 50%, with most brain growth occurring after birth. We also know that humans are carry mammals, because human milk is among the lowest in fat and protein content of all mammalian milks (Lawrence & Lawrence, 2016, p. 92). From the composition of our milk and our immaturity at birth, it is clear that from a biological standpoint, human newborns are meant to be carried constantly and fed often around the clock.

• • •

During most of history, frequent nursing and constant carrying have been the human norm.

Nursing and baby-care practices of hunter-gatherer societies provide a good idea of "natural human feeding rhythms" independent of cultural influences. These practices reflect how human babies were fed for more than 99% of human history. In an article comparing baby-care practices worldwide, U.S. pediatricians Betsy Lozoff and Gary Brittenham wrote: "If all human history were represented by an hour, the last one/one-hundredth of a second would represent the 200 years of industrialization"(Lozoff & Brittenham, 1979, p. 479). Hunter-gatherer societies like the !Kung tribe in Botswana and Namibia and the people living in North Fore in the Highlands of New Guinea still live this ancient way. Among hunter-gatherers, similar nursing patterns are reported, whether babies are born in Botswana, New Guinea, Tanzania, or to the Aboriginal tribes in Australia (Crittenden et al., 2018; Hartmann, 2007; Konner & Worthman, 1980). Babies born to hunter-gatherer cultures typically are carried on their mothers' bodies and nursed for a few minutes several times each hour for the first 2 years of life and continue nursing less intensely for months or years longer (Stuart-Macadam, 1995).

• • •

Many nursing babies do not conform to Western feeding and sleep expectations.

Western parenting recommendations about infant feeding and sleep are often based on bottle-feeding norms (McKenna, Ball, & Gettler, 2007), with babies expected to stay full for hours after feeds and to sleep alone for long stretches at night (Ezzo & Bucknam, 2019; Weissbluth, 2015). While some nursing babies follow these feeding and sleep patterns, many do not easily conform to these expectations. In an Australian study of 71 exclusively breastfed 1- to 6-month-old babies, 11 feeds per day was average (Kent et al., 2006). Number of daily feeds among these babies ranged from 6 to 18. In a prospective U.S. study (Thomas & Foreman, 2005), nearly 30% of the babies 4 to 10 weeks old fed 13 or more times in 24 hours. For differences in sleep patterns among nursing and formula-fed babies, see the later section "Sleep and Night Feeds" on p. 78.

Rhythm versus Schedule

Feeding schedules are recommended to nursing families in some Western societies.

As described in the previous section, human babies are born expecting constant carrying and frequent feeds. Human babies' hardwiring hasn't changed since the stone age, so there is often a disconnect between modern expectations and babies' needs. Feeding schedules and "sleep training" are recent developments that are an outgrowth of bottle-feeding norms and are part of an approach to child-rearing sometimes referred to as "scientific mothering." This approach became popular in the early 20th century and was based on the beliefs of behaviorist psychologists, such as John Watson (Mohrbacher & Kendall-Tackett, 2010). Although many of these underlying beliefs have been proven wrong by science, when the natural feeding patterns of a nursing baby are in conflict with cultural beliefs, this creates anxiety among new parents and can lead to feeding problems and premature weaning.

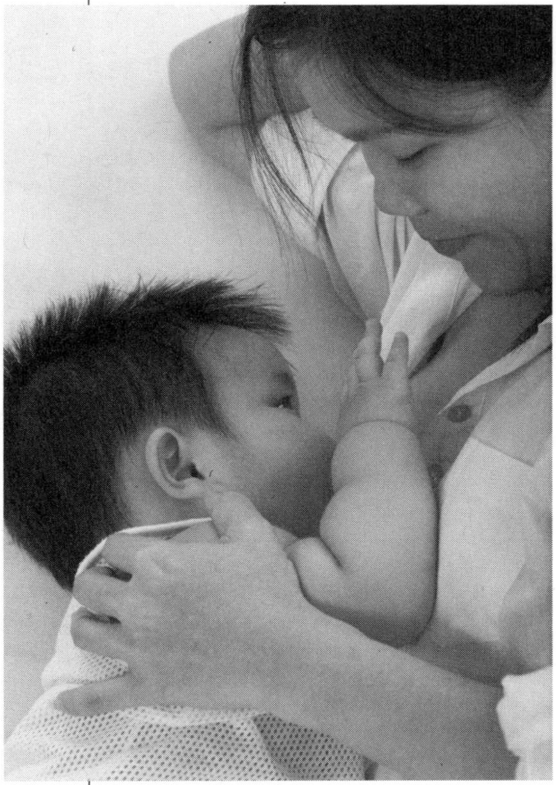

Despite being disproved by science, some of scientific mothering's basic tenets have become a part of Western cultural beliefs and actively undermine nursing. Ideas like "babies cry to manipulate adults" and "responding to a baby's cries encourages crying" are believed by many. However, the opposite was proven true in studies around the world. In the U.S., longitudinal studies compared mothers responsive to their babies during infancy with mothers who were less responsive and found that babies who were responded to promptly cried less (Bates, Maslin, & Frankel, 1985; Crockenberg, 1986). More recent research done in the U.K. and Denmark found the same (St James-Roberts et al., 2006).

Parenting beliefs can also be tested by observing cultures untouched by industrialization and scientific mothering, such as the !Kung, a hunter-gatherer tribe in which babies sleep with their mothers and are held most of the time. Their mothers often wear them in a carrier on their bodies, where the babies have near constant access to their mothers' breasts and breastfeed at will. !Kung babies rarely cry, and as toddlers, they were found to be more independent than their U.S. counterparts (Konner, 1976).

• • •

Feeding schedules are more compatible with bottle-feeding than nursing and may increase risk of overweight and obesity.

Due to the bottle's faster, more consistent flow, on average babies fed by bottle consume more milk per feed and feed fewer times per day as compared with nursing babies (Sievers, Oldigs, Santer, & Schaub, 2002). These faster feeds establish an overfeeding pattern early in life, increasing the risk of childhood obesity (R. Li, Magadia, Fein, & Grummer-Strawn, 2012). In Western cultures where bottle-feeding was common for several generations, new parents and their families may be more familiar with bottle-feeding norms and may attempt to apply those norms to nursing. Bottle-feeding a baby "by the clock" works for some babies because a reluctant feeder can sometimes be coaxed to feed by pushing the firm bottle nipple into the back of a young baby's mouth, which triggers active sucking. But during nursing, a baby must actively draw the nipple into her mouth, so these same strategies will not work. Also, some research found an association between feeding babies on a schedule and more rapid weight gain (Mihrshahi, Battistutta, Magarey, & Daniels, 2011).

Flexibility in the frequency and length of feeding is important when nursing because it allows a baby to regulate milk production as needed. If the mammary gland gave the same amount of milk day and night, and if all nursing parents produced milk at the exactly the same rate and had the same storage capacity, a prescribed feeding schedule could work. But that's not the reality (see next section), which is why when nursing flexibility in feeding is important.

Storage capacity (see p. 416), which varies considerably among nursing parents, significantly affects how often the baby needs to feed in order to thrive, as well as to keep the rate of milk production steady. This individual variation can have a profound effect on a baby's feeding rhythm (see the later section "Rhythm and Storage Capacity" on p. 71).

Daily Milk Ebb and Flow

Many nursing babies feed more often in the evening and less often in the morning.

In Western cultures, nursing parents report that with young babies, time of day influences feeding rhythm. Milk production may have a natural ebb and flow during the day.

Morning abundance. As newborns turn their days and night around to be more in tune with the rest of the family, they nurse less often at night (Kent et al., 2013), which means more milk accumulates by morning. Also, when researchers measure the hormonal levels of breastfeeding women, they find that prolactin, one hormone long thought to be related to milk production, is at its highest level in the middle of the night (Neville, 1999).

Evening low ebb. In the evening, many Western babies nurse more often to get the milk they need. Experienced nursing parents know that the young baby who was happily full for hours between feeds in the morning is often the same baby who wants to feed every hour, every half hour, or even continuously during the evening. Called "the witching hour" in the U.S. and "hell hour" in Australia, this feeding frenzy often happens just about the time the family's thoughts turn to getting the evening meal on the table. In some cases, these frequent feeds may continue all evening. One Israeli study that analyzed the milk expressed for 22 preterm babies for 7 weeks (Lubetzky, Mimouni, Dollberg, Salomon, & Mandel, 2007) found a consistent "circadian variation" in the fat content of the milk, with milk fat levels being higher during the evening (when the mammary glands were less full) as compared to the morning (when they were fuller), which reflected this difference in milk volumes by time of day. Other studies (Khan et al., 2013) also found these same variations in fat content over the course of a 24-hour day.

• • •

No matter what the time intervals between feeds, overall babies consume about the same amount of fat over the course of a day.

Some families worry that if their baby nurses often she won't get the fatty hindmilk she needs. However, U.S. and Australian researchers found that as long as a baby nurses effectively, no matter what her feeding rhythm, she will receive about the same amount of fat over the course of a day (Casey, Neifert,

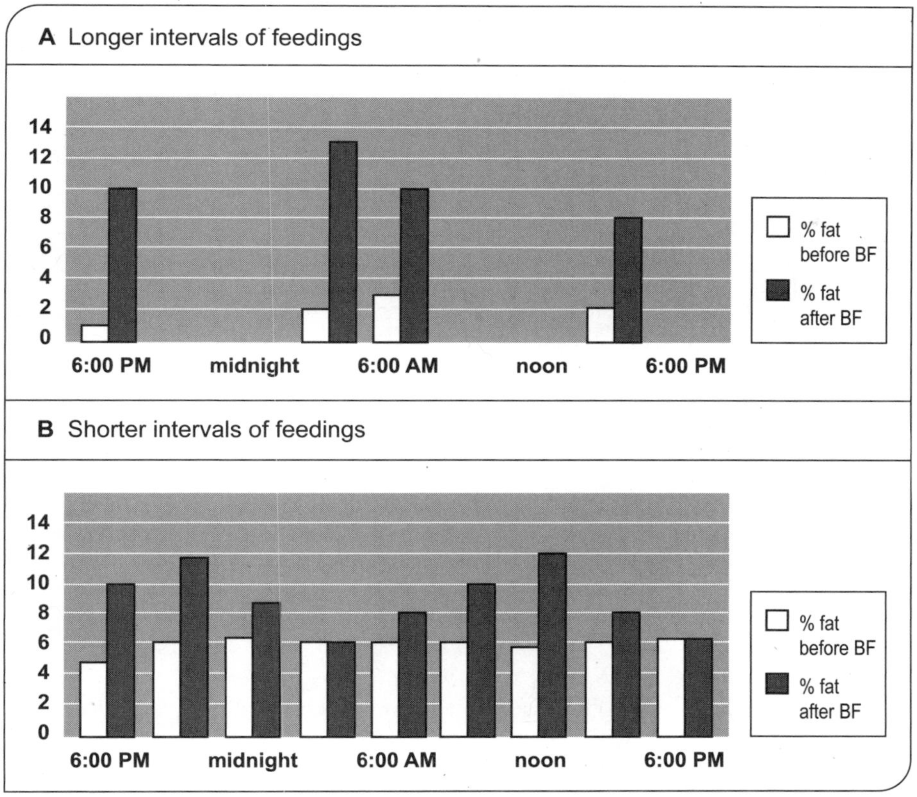

Figure 2.3 Percentage of fat in the milk before and after breastfeeding with longer (A) and shorter (B) feeding intervals. Adapted from (Kent, 2007).

Seacat, & Neville, 1986; Kent, 2007). This is because the baby who nurses more often gets foremilk higher in fat and hindmilk lower in fat than the baby who nurses less often (Figure 2.3).

• • •

Whatever the feeding rhythm, daily milk intake is what's most important to a baby's growth.

Exclusively nursing babies are usually happy to nurse in spite of the ebb and flow of daily milk production. What's most important to a baby's weight gain and growth is the total volume of milk consumed every 24 hours. On average, babies between 1 and 6 months of age consume about 25 to 30 ounces (750 to 900 mL) per day (Kent et al., 2013). As far as growth is concerned, it doesn't matter if a baby takes 1 ounce (30 mL) every hour or 3 ounces (89 mL) every 3 hours, as long as she receives enough milk overall. In fact, researchers found that whether babies practice the frequent feeds of the hunter-gatherers or the longer intervals between feeds of Western societies, babies take about the same amount of milk each day (Hartmann, 2007).

Rhythm and Storage Capacity

Two physical dynamics that affect feeding rhythm are baby's stomach size and the nursing parent's storage capacity.

A baby's feeding rhythm will be determined in part by how much milk her stomach can hold and how much milk is available from the mammary gland. Baby's stomach size is determined in part by age, with a newborn's stomach capable of holding on average about 20 mL (two thirds of an ounce) of milk at birth (N. J. Bergman, 2013) (see p. 62 in this chapter.) Stomach size increases with age and growth.

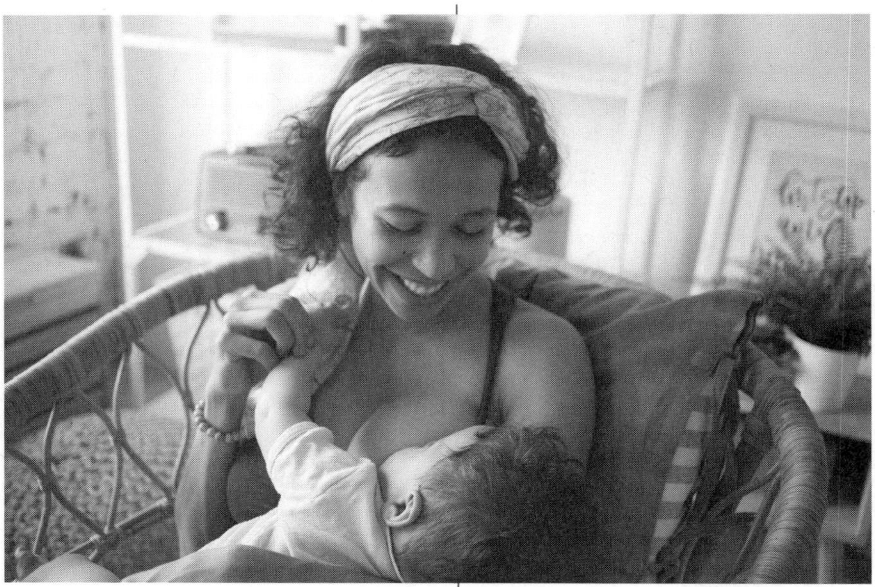

The other part of the equation is how much milk is available from the mammary gland during feeding. Since humans are "carry" mammals and intended to feed often, large feeds and long intervals between feeds were not part of nature's design for our babies. We were not designed with large milk storage areas, like the cistern in a cow's udder. So when babies feed often, which seems to be our natural pattern, there is no need for much milk storage.

Western cultural beliefs, however, sometimes test these boundaries. When nursing parents follow nursing "rules" and encourage their babies to feed as infrequently as possible, this tests milk-storage limits, which as milk accumulates can lead to discomfort and mastitis. As more milk fills the glands, internal pressure increases. According to lactation theory, when this pressure is combined with the accumulation of a substance in the milk some refer to as feedback inhibitor of lactation (FIL) (Prentice, 1989). this slows the rate of milk production. As described in detail on p. 415 in Chapter 10, "Making Milk," drained glands make milk faster and full glands make milk slower.

The term ***storage capacity*** refers to the maximum volume of milk available to the baby when the mammary gland is at its fullest time of the day. Because this volume of milk varies—sometimes greatly—from nursing parent to nursing parent, this concept helps explain why feeding rhythms can vary so much from one nursing couple to another. One Australian study of 71 mothers and babies found a storage-capacity range among its mothers of 74 to 382 mL (2.6 to 12.9 oz.) per breast (Kent et al., 2006), while another Australian study (Daly, Owens, & Hartmann, 1993) found an even broader range among its mothers, from 81 to 606 mL (2.7 to 20.5 oz.).

Storage capacity is not related to the size of the mammary gland, which is usually determined by the amount of fatty tissue present. This means that nursing parents with smaller mammary glands could have a large storage capacity and nursing parents with large mammary glands could have a small storage capacity.

• • •

With a large storage capacity, Western babies may thrive on one side per feed and fewer feeds per day.

One side or two. One side per feed may be plenty for a 3-month-old baby whose nursing parent can comfortably hold 4 ounces (118 mL) of milk or more in each side. Even if many hours pass before the baby takes that side again, with a large storage capacity, milk production may not slow as a result. In fact, spacing out larger feeds may help prevent the opposite problem—overabundant milk. (For details, see p. 457 in Chapter 10, "Making Milk.")

Number of feeds per day may also be affected by storage capacity. Between 1 and 6 months of age, the Western baby typically takes on average about 3 to 4 ounces (76 to 118 mL) of milk per feed (Kent et al., 2013; Kent et al., 2006), so for baby to get enough milk over 24 hours, she needs to nurse on average about eight times. But as baby's stomach grows and stretches, she can take more milk at a feed. If a nursing parent also has a large storage capacity, this may lead to the need for fewer feeds. Since the volume of milk a baby needs in a day stays about the same from months 1 to 6 (see next section), if she increases her milk intake at feeds, her number of feeds per day will drop. If the nursing parent has a large storage capacity, the baby may have previously needed to nurse eight times per day to get 25 ounces (750 mL) per day, but as she grows, she may only need to feed six times per day to get the same volume of milk. One Australian study of 71 mothers and babies between 1 and 6 months found an inverse relationship between milk consumed at each feed and the number of feeds per day (Kent et al., 2006).

• • •

When a nursing parent has a small storage capacity, for the baby to grow well and thrive, she may need both sides per feed and more feeds per day.

Nursing parents with a small storage capacity can produce plenty of milk for their babies. In one study, Australian researchers found that all of the study babies with mothers who had a small storage capacity gained weight well (Kent et al., 2006). There were no issues with low milk production or slow weight gain, but these babies had different feeding rhythms compared with other babies.

One difference in feeding rhythm was that more often these babies took both sides at a feed and removed more of the available milk (Kent, 2007). On average, babies took one side at some feeds and both sides at some feeds (Kent et al., 2006), but mothers with a small storage capacity are not average.

Small storage capacity may also influence the number of feeds needed per day. Doing the math explains why. After 1 month of age, a baby needs on average 25 ounces (750 mL) of milk per day. If the most a baby can consume at a feed is a little more than 2 ounces (74 mL) of milk per feed, she will need to feed at least 12 times to get this needed daily volume. If she can take 3 ounces (89 mL) of milk per feed, she will need at least eight feeds in a day. As one researcher wrote: "There is a significant tendency for babies of mothers with smaller storage capacities to feed more frequently than babies of mothers with larger storage capacities" (Kent, 2007, p. 568).

• • •

On average, babies take one side at some feeds and both sides at some feeds.

In general, it is best to let each nursing couple work out their own best feeding rhythm without too many "rules" imposed. For example, babies whose nursing parents have a very large storage capacity may do best with one side per feed, whereas babies whose nursing parents are on the other end of the storage-capacity spectrum may do better when they take both sides. In an Australian study of 71 exclusively nursing 1- to 6-month-old babies in which 775 feeds were monitored, 53% of the feeds were "unpaired," meaning babies were happy with one side for at least 1 hour, 44% of the feeds were "paired," meaning both sides were taken within a 30-minute period, and 3% of the feeds were "clustered," meaning the baby took both sides plus the first side a second time during the "meal."

Milk Intake as Baby Grows

Despite rapid growth, the volume of milk a nursing baby consumes per day between 1 and 6 months of age remains remarkably stable.

At around 5 weeks of age, a nursing baby reaches her peak daily milk intake of about 25 to 30 ounces (750 to 887 mL) of milk per day, and this stays roughly the same until she begins solid foods at 6 months and her need for milk begins to decrease. Because babies' growth and metabolic rate slow as they age, they continue to need about the same volume of milk from 1 month to 6 months of age. (For more details, see p. 426.)

• • •

There is a significant difference in the volume of milk a nursing baby consumes per feed and per day compared with a baby who is bottle-fed formula.

On average, formula-fed babies consume much more milk per feed and per day compared with nursing babies: 15% more milk at 3 months, 23% more at 6 months, 20% more at 9 months, and 18% more at 12 months (Heinig, Nommsen, Peerson, Lonnerdal, & Dewey, 1993). Researchers noted that breastfed babies continued to gain less weight even after solid foods were started, and if availability of food was the reason, they could have consumed more solids to make up for the difference, but they didn't (Dewey, Heinig, Nommsen, & Lonnerdal, 1991). It is helpful for nursing parents to know about this difference in milk intake because sometimes they assume they need to pump as much milk for a feed as their formula-feeding friends' babies take from the bottle.

The reasons for these differences are explained in detail on p. 192-194. One reason is the differences in the milk itself, as formula is missing hormones, such as leptin, ghrelin, and adiponectin, which help babies regulate appetite and energy metabolism (R. Li, Fein, & Grummer-Strawn, 2008). Also, the overfeeding associated with the fast flow of the bottle increases the risk of obesity later in life (Appleton et al., 2018; R. Li et al., 2012).

• • •

The Western expectation that number of feeds per day will decrease significantly as babies grow is based on bottle-feeding norms.

The Western familiarity with bottle-feeding norms is most likely the reason many parents are advised to eliminate feeds as their babies get older and heavier. It is common for formula-fed babies to take larger and fewer feeds as they get older, but this is not a nursing norm. One 2013 Australian study (Kent et al., 2013) found that the number of feeds per day among exclusively nursing babies was remarkably similar at 4 and 13 weeks (8 versus 7). Following this advice without taking into account storage capacity can lead to decreased milk production and slowed weight gain in some families.

Doing the math explains why. As previously explained, a nursing baby continues to need about the same daily volume of milk from 1 to 6 months, on average 25 ounces (750 mL) per day. If her nursing parent has a small storage capacity and the most the baby can take at a feed is 3 ounces (89 mL) and she needs a daily average of 25 ounces (750 mL), she will need at least eight feeds per day. What will happen if her nursing parent attempts to drop some feeds as she grows? The baby's daily milk intake will decrease because it is impossible for her to take more milk at each feed to make up for the dropped feed(s). And as a result, her nursing parent's milk production would likely slow. In this case, with fewer feeds the baby's weight gain may slow or stop. Depending on the number of feeds dropped, she may even lose weight.

• • •

After 1 year, feeding rhythm varies from child to child and from place to place.

By the time the nursing baby is 15 months old and is eating many other foods, the baby will need less mother's milk but may still nurse often for comfort and closeness. In Australia and the U.S., mothers' daily milk production at 15 months was measured at between 95 and 315 mL per day (Kent, Mitoulas, Cox, Owens, & Hartmann, 1999; Neville et al., 1991). However, in Zaire, where nursing older babies is the norm, research found that at 30 months mothers produced on average of 300 mL per day (Hennart, Delogne-Desnoeck, Vis, & Robyn, 1981). For more details on nursing expectations for older babies, see p. 162-163 and 168 Chapter 5, "Weaning from the Breast."

PACIFIERS/DUMMIES

Pacifiers/dummies are not recommended for healthy term infants during the first month of nursing.

Pacifiers are used to help settle fussy babies and prolong the intervals between feeds. However, during the intense first 40 days of nursing, fussy newborns should ideally be settled by nursing, which also helps establish healthy milk production. If used often enough, regular use of a pacifier during this critical time can decrease the number of feeds per day, potentially undermining milk production. Even health organizations that recommend pacifier use to prevent SIDS (see later point) recommend that families who intend to use pacifiers delay their introduction in healthy term babies until after milk production is firmly established, usually after the first 3 to 4 weeks or so (AAP, 2012, 2016).

• • •

In some places, nursing parents are cautioned not to let their baby "use them as a pacifier."

In some areas where bottle-feeding is common, a pacifier is considered by many to be a baby's preferred source of comfort, and parents are cautioned to limit their baby's time nursing, so their baby doesn't "use them as a pacifier." Because nursing is a newborn's natural source of comfort and pre-dates the pacifier, this way of thinking is clearly misguided. It is more accurate to consider the pacifier a nursing substitute rather than the reverse.

• • •

Pacifiers can be an appropriate tool in some situations.

Like any tool, a pacifier can be used appropriately or inappropriately. In the following situations, pacifier use may actually promote nursing.

Pacifier use speeds the transition of preterm babies from tube feeding to oral feeds. A 2018 Turkish prospective randomized controlled trial with 90 preterm babies born at less than 1500 g (3.3 lb.) and at less than 32 weeks gestation (Say, Simsek, Canpolat, & Oguz, 2018) found the use of a pacifier during gavage feeding significantly decreased both the length of their hospital stay and the transition time from gavage to full oral feeds. A 2016 Cochrane review and meta-analysis (Foster, Psaila, & Patterson, 2016) also concluded that use of a pacifier with hospitalized preterm babies decreased the transition time from tube feeding to full oral feeds and decreased the length of hospital stay. Although some studies found a positive effect of pacifier use during tube feeding on weight gain, this systematic review and meta-analysis found no significant effect.

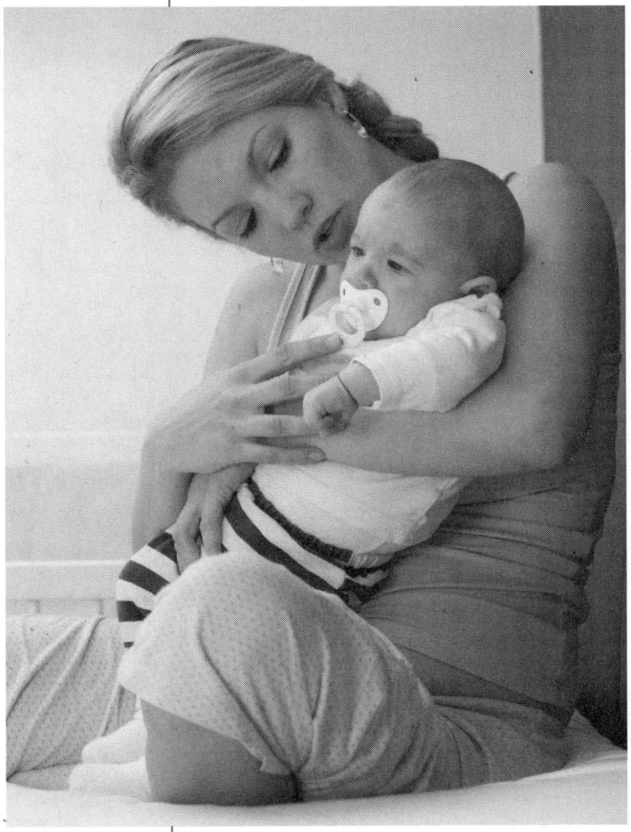

Pacifier use helps some low-tone babies overcome feeding problems. U.S. lactation consultants Barbara Wilson-Clay and Kay Hoover described another potential therapeutic use of a pacifier in babies with low lip tone who struggle to form a seal during nursing: "Use a finger, bottle teat, or pacifier with a round-shaped nipple to play 'tug of war' as a way to exercise and strengthen lip tone" (Wilson-Clay & Hoover, 2017, p. 18).

Pacifier use can soothe babies during painful procedures when parents are not available. Another appropriate use of a pacifier is for comfort during painful procedures where the nursing parent cannot be present to comfort the baby with skin-to-skin contact or nursing.

A 2017 review article (Lubbe & Ten Ham-Baloyi, 2017) summarized the situations in which pacifier use can be justified in a Baby Friendly hospital. According to its authors, pacifier use may be beneficial to babies who:

- Are low birth-weight or preterm
- Are separated from their nursing parent or for whom breastfeeding is contraindicated
- Need extra stimulation to develop and maintain a mature sucking reflex
- Need help with neurobehavioral organization (calming)

This article mentioned the recommendation of the American Academy of Pediatrics and the American Association of Family Physicians to wean babies from pacifier use by the second 6 months of life to minimize interference with speech and to prevent dental issues such as malocclusions, which was associated with long-term pacifier use (Costa et al., 2018).

• • •

Research on the effects of pacifier use on nursing outcomes is mixed. Parents' motivation to nurse may be a major factor.

The previous edition of this book described many observational studies that found a negative association between pacifier use and nursing, both exclusivity and duration (DiGirolamo, Grummer-Strawn, & Fein, 2008; Ullah & Griffiths, 2003). However, nursing is a complex social behavior, and association is not the same as causation. Sometimes the relationship between variables is not easily explained. For example, in many Western cultures, lower socioeconomic status is associated with less exclusivity and shorter duration of nursing. One small 2018 U.S. prospective observational study of 51 mothers and babies (Pineda, Luong, Ryckman, & Smith, 2018) found that lower socioeconomic status predicted both less breastfeeding and more pacifier use. If researchers did not control for socioeconomic status, this could significantly affect a study's conclusion.

Motivation to nurse appears to affect whether pacifier use decreases nursing exclusivity and duration. When motivation to nurse is considered, researchers found no statistically significant association between pacifier use and nursing outcomes, at least for the first 4 months. A 2016 Cochrane Review, which included two randomized controlled trials involving 1,306 healthy babies (Jaafar, Ho, Jahanfar, & Angolkar, 2016), concluded that there was moderate-quality evidence that in motivated mothers pacifier use with healthy term babies during the first 4 months of life does not affect the exclusivity or duration of nursing. One problem with randomized controlled trials evaluating the effects of pacifier use is that compliance in both groups tends to be low (Chapman, 2009). In other words, many in the "no-pacifier" group actually do use pacifiers, and many in the "pacifier" group have babies who do not accept pacifiers or don't use them as directed. But these issues aside, what is the effect of pacifier use on nursing in families who are not as motivated to nurse? This question has yet to be answered, and it's an important question from a public-health standpoint.

The Brazilian perspective. Articles from Brazil about pacifiers and nursing, however, tell a different story. One 2017 systematic review and meta-analysis examined 46 studies (G. D. S. Buccini, Perez-Escamilla, Paulino, Araujo, & Venancio, 2017) and found a consistent association between pacifier use and risk of interruption of exclusive nursing. A 2016 Brazilian study conducted secondary cross-sectional analyses of two waves of infant-feeding surveys that included data from more than 42,000 children less than 6 months old (Buccini Gdos, Perez-Escamilla, & Venancio, 2016). Multivariate logistic regression was used to test associations in a pooled sample within each survey wave, and they were adjusted for socioeconomic, demographic, and biomedical confounders. Pacifier use was strongly associated with interruption of exclusive nursing. Another 2018 Brazilian article analyzed these same datasets (G. Buccini, Perez-Escamilla, D'Aquino Benicio, Justo Giugliani, & Isoyama Venancio, 2018) and found that in Brazil from 1999 to 2008 there was a 15% increase in exclusive breastfeeding and a corresponding 17% decrease in pacifier use. The researchers concluded that the reduction in pacifier use explained a 5.5% increase in exclusive breastfeeding. Comparing both rates of nursing and pacifier use with the rates in New Zealand, the Brazilian researchers predicted that if pacifier use decreased from 42% (the 2008 statistic) to 14%, they would expect an additional increase in exclusive breastfeeding of about 12%.

Pacifier use lowers progesterone levels, contributing to an earlier return to fertility. Motivation to nurse may play a role in nursing outcomes when pacifiers are used, but there is also a hormonal impact of pacifier use that may matter to some families. Usually, time spent sucking on a pacifier means less time nursing. Less time spent nursing has a direct effect on nursing parents' hormonal levels and therefore their return to fertility. One U.K. prospective cohort study of 85 breastfeeding mothers (Ingram, Hunt, Woolridge, & Greenwood, 2004) found that both formula use and pacifier use were associated with lower progesterone levels, which significantly contributed to earlier resumption of menstruation. The researchers concluded: "Higher postnatal progesterone levels are associated with delayed menstruation, while the use of pacifiers and infant formula milk are associated with earlier return to menstruation" (Ingram et al., 2004, p. 197).

KEY CONCEPT

Many factors influence the effect of pacifier use on nursing, but families should know that regular use may lead to an earlier return to fertility.

• • •

In a large U.S. university teaching hospital, researchers discovered in a retrospective comparison (Kair, Kenron, Etheredge, Jaffe, & Phillipi, 2013) that eliminating routine distribution of pacifiers to parents of healthy term babies without also restricting access to formula significantly reduced rates of exclusive nursing from 79% to 68%. After making this change, the researchers found an increase in both supplementation of nursing babies with formula and the decision to switch to exclusive formula feeding.

In some cultures, restricting hospital pacifier distribution to families without restricting access to formula may negatively affect nursing outcomes.

• • •

The question of whether pacifier use negatively affects nursing outcomes is an important one when considering the recommendation of the American Academy of Pediatrics (AAP) that once nursing is fully established (within about 3 to 4 weeks), all nursing babies should be given a pacifier while going to sleep (AAP, 2016). This recommendation is based on a meta-analysis and a case-controlled study (F. R. Hauck, Omojokun, & Siadaty, 2005; D. K. Li et al., 2006) that found a strong association between pacifier use at sleep time and decreased risk of Sudden Infant Death Syndrome (SIDS). The mechanism responsible for this effect is unknown.

To prevent SIDS, one U.S. health organization recommended all nursing babies older than 1 month be given a pacifier while going to sleep.

It is also not yet clear whether nursing a baby to sleep provides the same protective effect as giving a pacifier at sleep time. After conducting their own research on SIDS in the Netherlands, Dutch researchers recommended pacifier use at sleep time only for bottle-fed babies (L'Hoir et al., 1999). Dr. M. Jane Heinig, editor of the *Journal of Human Lactation* when the first recommendations were published by the AAP in 2006 (Heinig & Banuelos, 2006, p. 8) wrote:

> "If sucking was associated with the arousal effect, it follows that the breastfed child who feeds during the night would be afforded the same protection. However, at this time, this mechanism has not been established, and fewer than half the studies included in the meta-analysis collected data on breastfeeding practices."

For more on nursing and SIDS, see the next section.

SLEEP AND NIGHT FEEDS

Sleep Patterns

To help newborns move their longest sleep stretch from day to night, keep stimulation at night to a minimum.

Most babies are born with their days and nights mixed up (Benson, 2001), and many have one long 4- to 5-hour sleep stretch, which may happen at any time. Unless the parents want to try to encourage the baby to sleep longer at night, there is no need to wake a baby during this longer sleep stretch. The exception is the baby who feeds fewer than 8 times in 24 hours.

To gently shift a baby's longest sleep period from day to night, suggest parents start by reducing all sensory stimulation at night:

- Keep lights low—for just enough light to see, leave on a closet light with door partly closed or use a nightlight
- Keep sound and movements to a minimum
- Change diapers only when necessary—when baby is soaked or passed a stool

Over time this will help baby sleep more at night and be more alert during the day. In one U.S. study of 37 mothers and babies 4 to 10 weeks old, 78% of the babies took their longest sleep stretch at night (Thomas & Foreman, 2005).

• • •

To get more rest, encourage nursing parents to sleep when their baby sleeps and find a feeding position, such as side-lying, that allows them to safely doze during feeds.

Learning to nurse in a side-lying or semi-reclined starter position (see p. 23-29 in Chapter 1) makes it possible to catch up on rest during feeds. In one U.S. repeated-measure study of 20 breastfeeding mothers, after nursing in a side-lying position the study mothers reported less fatigue than after nursing in an upright cradle or clutch position (Milligan, Flenniken, & Pugh, 1996). In a semi-reclined position, nursing parents can support their baby's weight on their body, which offers a similar benefit (Colson, 2019).

Parents are often encouraged to "sleep when the baby sleeps" in order to reduce fatigue, but one U.S. intensive within-subject study found that many mothers used this time to do other things, rather than catching up on their rest (Thomas & Foreman, 2005). Encourage any tired nursing parent to take advantage of the baby's sleep time to get some extra rest.

• • •

Fatigue is a fact of life for new parents no matter how a baby is fed. Some families think weaning will help them get more rest, but according to one U.S. prospective longitudinal study, weaning does not necessarily change fatigue levels (Wambach, 1998). Contrary to popular belief, feeding method doesn't seem to affect the total time babies sleep, but it may affect how much sleep parents get. Some studies found no difference in the amount of sleep exclusively nursing families got at night compared to mixed-fed and formula-feeding families (Montgomery-Downs, Clawges, & Santy, 2010). But in the following studies, nursing mothers got more sleep and better-quality sleep than those who mixed-fed and exclusively formula fed.

Research found that exclusively breastfeeding mothers slept more deeply and got either the same amount or more sleep per night than those who mixed-fed or formula fed.

Exclusively nursing mothers (and their partners) got more sleep. Some parents think that giving their baby formula at night will mean longer sleep stretches. However, one U.S. study that used data from a randomized clinical trial of 133 new mothers and fathers during the first 3 months after birth found that mothers who exclusively breastfed averaged 40 to 45 minutes more sleep at night than those who also gave their babies infant formula (Doan, Gardiner, Gay, & Lee, 2007). These same researchers conducted another longitudinal study of mostly low-income ethnically diverse first-time mothers (Doan, Gay, Kennedy, Newman, & Lee, 2014) and found again that the exclusively breastfeeding mothers got more sleep. In this case, they averaged 30 more minutes of sleep per night than those who gave formula at night.

Why didn't giving babies formula mean more sleep for parents? In the two Doan studies described above, exclusively breastfeeding mothers averaged between 30 and 40 to 45 minutes more sleep per night during the first 3 months. The authors wrote (Doan et al., 2007, p. 204):

> "...formula feeding not only failed to improve parent sleep, but actually resulted in parents getting less sleep, even when fathers helped during the night with supplementation feedings."

The researchers thought this was due to time spent preparing bottles and the disruption of sleep mothers experienced even when their partners fed the baby. They found that when mothers handled all night feeds they (and their partners) slept more than when night feeds were shared. Another U.S. study that compared 72 breastfeeding and non-breastfeeding families during the first month found that both the mothers and fathers in exclusively breastfeeding families got slightly more sleep overall than in families not breastfeeding, with mothers sleeping 384 minutes versus 364 minutes and fathers sleeping 407 minutes versus 386 minutes (Gay, Lee, & Lee, 2004).

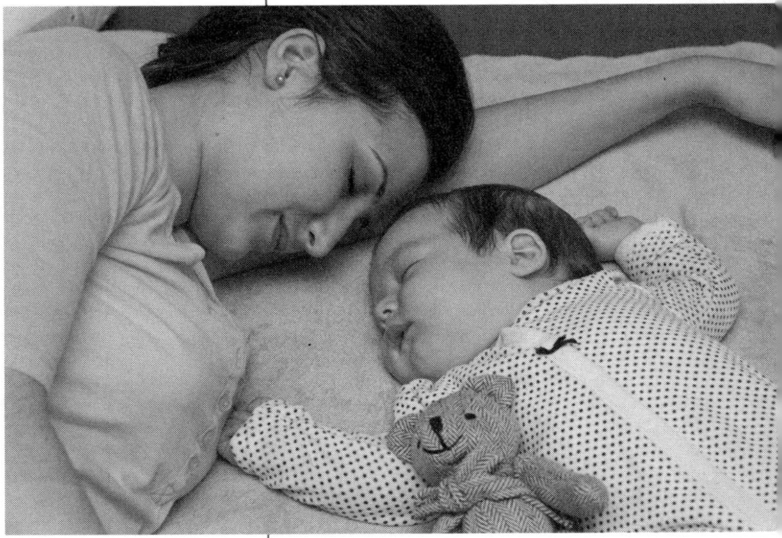

Nursing mothers spend more time in deep sleep. An Australian sleep study of 31 women, 12 who were breastfeeding, 12 age-matched women without infants, and seven bottle-feeding mothers found that mothers who exclusively breastfed had "a marked alteration in their sleep architecture," giving them longer periods of a type of deep sleep known as slow-wave sleep (SWS) than bottle-fed mothers with babies the same age (Blyton, Sullivan, & Edwards, 2002). These researchers concluded that "enhanced SWS may be another important factor to support breastfeeding in the postnatal period."

• • •

Giving nursing babies formula or early solids so they will sleep longer may undermine milk production and increase other risks.

Some parents decide to give their baby formula before bed or start solids early to increase the length of their baby's longest sleep stretch. But these decisions may not produce the desired results and may have unintended consequences.

Formula-fed babies are harder to arouse from sleep, increasing risk of SIDS. More difficult to arouse may sound like a positive to some tired families, but easier arousal from sleep is an important mechanism that protects babies from Sudden Infant Death Syndrome (SIDS) (Horne et al., 2010). In an Australian study that compared sleep in formula-fed and breastfed babies, the researchers found the formula-fed babies were more difficult to arouse from sleep (Horne, Parslow, Ferens, Watts, & Adamson, 2004). Any amount of nursing is protective against SIDS, with exclusive nursing providing the strongest protection (Y. L. Hauck, Hall, Dhaliwal, Bennett, & Wells, 2012; Vennemann et al., 2009). If giving formula does extend the time of baby's longest sleep stretch, this may lower milk production by reducing the number of night feeds, but it may also increase the risk of SIDS in a baby that has arousal issues.

Feeding solids early may not help babies "sleep through the night." Feeding babies early solid foods is commonly believed to help babies sleep longer, but the evidence of this is mixed (Brown & Harries, 2015; Perkin et al., 2018). For details see p. 141-142.

Sleeping longer at night is something babies do when they're developmentally ready, and manipulating a baby's diet will not necessarily change this.

• • •

The nursing parent's storage capacity may affect the baby's need to nurse at night.

Nearly all young babies wake at night to feed, no matter how they're fed. But as they mature, sleeping patterns still vary from one baby to another. As described in the previous section "Rhythm and Storage Capacity," a nursing parent's storage capacity is one variable that can affect how often a baby needs to nurse to grow and gain weight normally. Storage capacity can also affect the longest interval between feeds and, therefore, number of night feeds.

Nursing parents with a large storage capacity. This baby may take more milk per feed and need fewer feeds per day. When developmentally ready, she is more likely to "sleep through the night" at an earlier age than other babies. Yet even with longer stretches between feeds at night, this nursing parent may not feel uncomfortably full by morning, since their mammary glands can hold more milk. A large storage capacity makes it possible to maintain milk production in spite of longer stretches between night feeds.

Nursing parents with a small storage capacity. For this baby, night feeds may need to continue longer. Because this baby has access to less milk per feed, she may need night feeds to get her required daily milk intake. Because fullness causes milk production to slow, for continued adequate milk production, night feeds may need to continue. In an Australian study of 71 mothers and babies, all the babies of the mothers with the smallest storage capacity breastfed during the night (Kent et al., 2006). If a nursing parent with a small storage capacity tries to "sleep train" the baby, this may slow both milk production and the baby's weight gain.

• • •

Sleep patterns vary by baby's feeding method.

According to research, there may be some significant differences between the sleep/wake patterns of nursing babies versus babies fed cow's-milk-based formulas. These effects, however, are complex.

Formula-fed babies slept longer and deeper. The differences may be in part because the cow's milk formula is more difficult to digest. Babies fed formula—at least the formulas that were available when the research was done—slept longer and deeper earlier in life than nursing babies, who fed more often day and night (Anuntaseree et al., 2008).

But the total 24-hour sleep duration was the same. One study (Quillin, 1997) compared the sleeping patterns of formula-fed and nursing babies. Although the total number of times the babies awakened differed between the two groups, the 24-hour sleep duration was the same. The nursing babies in this study had more awakenings, but even so, the research cited in the previous points suggested that breastfeeding mothers got the same amount of sleep or even more sleep overall compared with formula-feeding mothers.

Nursing babies woke more often but had an easier time falling asleep. An Australian study (Galbally, Lewis, McEgan, Scalzo, & Islam, 2013) found that breastfeeding babies at 6 months woke more frequently at night and found it more difficult to sleep alone compared with formula-fed babies. But nursing was not associated with problems falling asleep or having restless sleep. This ease of falling sleep may be due in part to the presence of the hormone melatonin in mother's milk (Katzer et al., 2016). This hormone is secreted during the night in adults but not in babies and has a hypnotic effect as well as a relaxing effect on the smooth muscle of the gastrointestinal tract. One German study (Cohen Engler, Hadash, Shehadeh, & Pillar, 2012) compared formula-fed and breastfed 2- to 4-month-old babies and found that exclusive breastfeeding was associated with improved sleep and a reduction in irritability and colic.

• • •

When families know about normal sleep patterns in nursing babies and receive support for meeting their baby's needs at night, they report feeling less stressed

Western expectations of infant sleep are based on research conducted on non-nursing babies put to sleep in a separate room (Bartick, Tomori, & Ball, 2018; McKenna et al., 2007). Based on this outdated research and the cultural expectations about infant sleep that arose from it, many parents believe that at night their nursing babies should sleep alone for long stretches by 3 to 4 months of age.

As described in the previous section "Biology and Culture," human babies are born expecting continuous contact and frequent feeds around the clock for well past their first few months. This disconnect between cultural expectations and biology creates stress for many families, whose nursing babies do not follow bottle-feeding sleep norms.

Current research on attachment and infant neuroscience found that parenting strategies that enhance parent-infant synchrony produce the best physical, developmental, and emotional outcomes (Leclere et al., 2014; Swain, Konrath, Dayton, Finegood, & Ho, 2013). (For more details, see p. 12-13 in Chapter 1.) Getting in sync with a baby essentially means learning to interpret baby's cues and to respond to them appropriately. One essential parenting task during baby's first year is to help her learn to regulate her emotions. This involves the help parents give in keeping baby calm by holding, nursing, and soothing. Or as one study put it: "learning what responses keep their baby's stress circuitry dialed down" (Ball, Douglas, Kulasinghe, Whittingham, & Hill, 2018, p. 520). Of course, this task doesn't end at sunset.

There are many reasons other than hunger that babies wake at night to nurse, even into the toddler years: teething, restlessness from rapid development, individual differences in normal sleep patterns, and loneliness. Unfortunately, in many Western countries, parents have unrealistic expectations of infant sleep. Techniques intended to teach nursing babies to sleep for longer stretches at night (see next point) are often recommended to new parents who are convinced their baby has a "sleep problem." Rather than encouraging synchrony, this approach to infant sleep discourages parental responsiveness.

An entirely different approach was taken in one 2018 Australian mixed-methods study (Ball et al., 2018) that examined the results of a sleep program conducted at a clinic for new parents. This program taught parents about the wide variation in normal infant sleep in nursing babies and encouraged them to use a "cue-based" approach, which involved responding to their baby's cues at night until they were developmentally ready to sleep longer. This study was conducted by an independent U.K. sleep expert who was not affiliated with this program. Rather than using an approach that involved reducing parents' responses to their baby at night, which most behavioral sleep interventions do, the philosophy of this program was to encourage synchrony between parents and children, in line with current understanding of infant neuroscience and healthy family dynamics. The upper-income parents who took part in this study reported that this approach was acceptable to them and they considered it "highly valued." After participating in the program, the parents reported a better quality of life with less stress, and less concern about frequent night-waking.

• • •

Sleep-training strategies disrupt parent-baby synchrony, have the potential to undermine nursing, and may encourage a more unresponsive parenting style long term.

As more and more families nurse their babies, the Western idea that babies should sleep undisturbed for long stretches early in life became more and more problematic. As a result, a whole industry arose to help parents solve infant "sleep problems." Those who participated in this industry (Ezzo & Bucknam, 2019; Weissbluth, 2015) promoted new concepts:

- Babies should learn early to fall asleep alone
- Babies should learn to soothe themselves back to sleep without parents' help when they wake at night

Some parenting authors warn parents that if their babies don't learn these skills, sleep problems will develop or continue (Ezzo & Bucknam, 2019; Weissbluth, 2015).

While some strategies to encourage infant sleep have a positive or neutral effect on parent-baby synchrony, such as adopting a regular bedtime routine, one of the common strategies suggested to achieve these sleep goals involves ***extinction*** (not responding to baby's cues) in an attempt to discourage babies from "signaling" (crying) at night. These methods include "crying it out," "controlled crying," and variations ("gradual extinction" methods), in which parents spend some time with their baby while she goes to sleep but without picking her up. Although some research reviews suggested that these methods can "work" to reduce night waking (Crichton & Symon, 2016), others strongly disagree (Douglas & Hill, 2013).

Many parents reported that using extinction methods was stressful, especially using them at home as opposed to in a study lab (Loutzenhiser, Hoffman, & Beatch, 2014; Sadeh et al., 2016). That's because responding to baby's cries is essential for human survival and is built into our biology. Extinction methods run directly counter to parents' natural physical and emotional reactions and undermine parent-baby synchrony. (For details on why parent-infant synchrony is important, see p. 12-13 in Chapter 1.

Some research results are genuinely concerning. A New Zealand study (Middlemiss, Granger, Goldberg, & Nathans, 2012) found that parents' stress levels (measured by the stress hormone cortisol in their saliva) eventually decreased after several days of letting their babies cry. In other words, these parents stopped responding physically to their baby's cries. However, the babies in this study continued to experience high cortisol levels, even though they stopped crying as often at night. According to a research review by the U.K. sleep researchers at the University of Durham at **bit.ly/BA2-SleepTrain**:

> "The response of the babies in this study lends support to the theory that babies who undergo sleep training via extinction may be learning to 'give up' rather than to 'settle'—outwardly the two behaviors appear the same, but inwardly the babies' physiology is very different. As well as being physically separated from their mothers, the sleep-trained babies were no longer in physical synchrony with their mothers as their mutual stress response link (maintaining by infant crying) had been broken."

According to research, these extinction sleep-training methods are much less successful at home as compared with as part of a clinical trial (Loutzenhiser et al., 2014). Many families are also unaware that they are not a permanent solution to night-waking. In other words, their effects are temporary. They may reduce night-waking for a time, but with developmental changes, baby begins waking regularly at night again. According to one Australian researcher (Douglas & Hill, 2013, p. 497):

> "...these strategies have not been shown to decrease infant crying, prevent sleep and behavioral problems in later childhood, or protect against postnatal depression....[but they have] unintended outcomes, including increased amount of crying, premature cessation of breastfeeding, worsened maternal anxiety, and if the infant is required to sleep either day or night in a room separate from the caregiver, an increased risk of [SIDS]."

An excellent overview of the research on sleep training is freely available on the website created by U.K. sleep researchers at the University of Durham: **basisonline.org.uk** (Babies Sleep Info Source). This website features the latest evidence-based information on all aspects of infant sleep and nursing, along with a free app and free downloadable handouts for families. At this writing, these researchers express concern that encouraging babies to sleep longer and deeper than is normal may have negative consequences, especially in babies younger than 6 months. These possible consequences include increased risk of SIDS and fewer night feeds, which may negatively affect milk production. They also note that most studies define "sleep problems" primarily as a disconnect between parental expectations and baby's sleep patterns, rather than using objective definitions. They suggest that the best approach may be to help reframe normal infant sleep for parents and develop programs, such as one developed in an Australian clinic (Ball et al., 2018), that encourage parental flexibility and responsiveness to babies' cues. Rather than trying to maximize infant sleep duration, an alternative approach is to respond to babies in a way that meets the baby's underlying need, which also preserves parent-child synchrony.

Where Should Babies Sleep?

If a nursing parent is exhausted, explore sleep options that make nursing easier and are less disruptive of sleep.

When a baby's sleep patterns do not conform to cultural expectations, parents may become frustrated and upset. They may wonder what they're doing "wrong" to cause the baby's night-waking and be concerned that unless something is done to "correct" this, they may not be caring for the baby properly.

If a nursing family is worried that the baby's frequent waking is not normal, acknowledge their frustrations and concerns. Assure them that night waking is normal in nursing babies during the first year of life and beyond and discuss ways to make night feeds easier that help the parents get more sleep while meeting their baby's needs. For example, if the baby sleeps in a crib in another room, share with them the recommendations to keep the baby in their room at night for ideally the first 12 months, but 6 months minimum (AAP, 2016), which will make it easier to hear the baby stir before she is fully awake and starts to cry. Most parents and babies fall back to sleep faster if they have not been fully awakened.

Many different sleeping arrangements can make night feeds easier:

- A bassinet or cradle next to the parents' bed
- Baby's crib attached to the parents' bed in a "side-car" arrangement
- A co-sleeper bed that attaches to the parents' bed
- Baby put to sleep on a pallet or mattress on the floor away from the walls and furniture in the parents' room, so nursing parents can lie down and sleep while feeding the baby and return to their bed if desired after the baby goes back to sleep.
- Baby sleeps in the parents' bed, either for part of the night—after baby awakens the first time—or for the whole night

When considering sleep arrangements, suggest families use the free Infant Sleep Info app (available in the App Store and Google Play), which was created by the U.K. sleep researchers at the University of Durham.

Encourage the family to do what works best for them while following safe sleeping practices. The Infant Sleep Info app listed in the Resources section at the end of this chapter includes guidance on safe sleeping practices.

• • •

To prevent Sudden Infant Death Syndrome (SIDS), most health organizations recommend that babies sleep on their backs and in their parents' room at night.

"Back to sleep" and room-sharing have become generally accepted around the world as effective SIDS-prevention strategies, and parents everywhere are encouraged to follow them. As a result, during the late 1990s and early 2000s, SIDS rates worldwide dropped dramatically. For a review of the literature that supports both "back to sleep" and sleeping in the parents' room, see the 2016 American Academy of Pediatrics' Task Force on Sudden Infant Death Syndrome

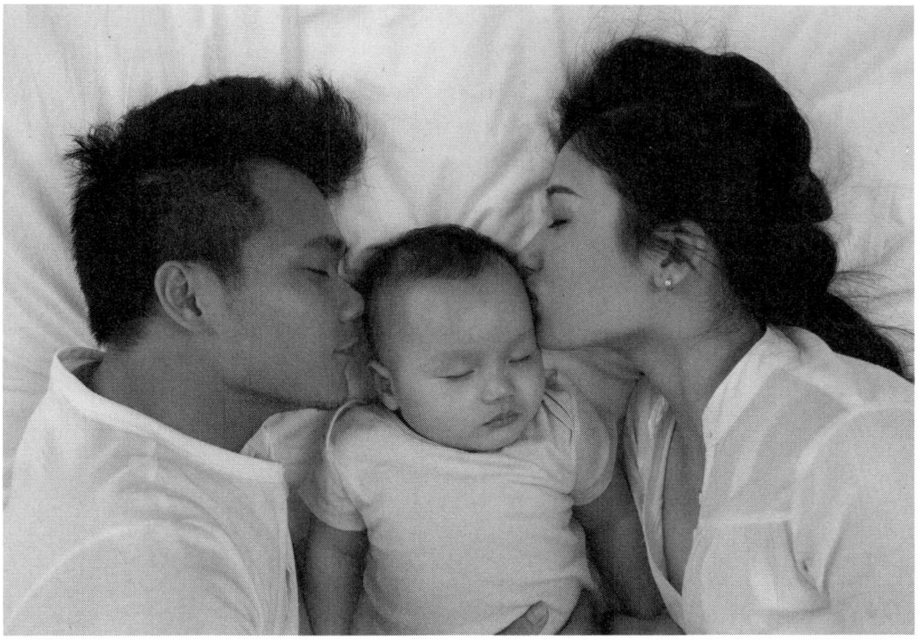

(AAP, 2016) at **bit.ly/BA2-SafeSleep**. According to this policy statement, room-sharing is recommended for ideally the first 12 months, but at least the first 6 months, because it is associated with a decrease in SIDS rates by as much as 50%.

• • •

Bed-sharing among nursing families is common worldwide and is associated with more sleep and longer and more exclusive nursing.

Babies' needs are the same everywhere, but cultural beliefs on where babies should sleep vary. Western health organizations promote close but separate sleep surfaces for babies (AAP, 2016), but many nursing families bed-share at night so that the baby can nurse with the least disruption of sleep (Volpe & Ball, 2015). In cultures where nursing is the norm, parents expect babies to wake frequently to feed at night until they have matured enough to outgrow this behavior, which may take many months or years. In some parts of the world, a wakeful baby—even a wakeful older baby or toddler—is considered neither unusual nor a problem to be solved. As researchers studying infant sleep in Thailand wrote: "All infants normally arouse briefly on average 4 to 6 times throughout the night" (Anuntaseree et al., 2008, p. 565).

U.S. research indicated that mothers got more sleep when they shared a bed with their baby than when they slept alone (Quillin & Glenn, 2004). Research conducted internationally found a positive association between bed-sharing and more frequent, longer, and more exclusive nursing (Ball et al., 2016; Bovbjerg, Hill, Uphoff, & Rosenberg, 2018; Gettler & McKenna, 2011). U.S. anthropologist Dr. James McKenna suggested that sharing sleep at night is so biologically normal for nursing families that we should change our terminology from bed-sharing to "breastsleeping" (McKenna & Gettler, 2016).

• • •

In Western cultures, some recommend against bed-sharing, but it is still common among Western families.

Bed-sharing is considered by some in the West to be potentially dangerous. The 2016 policy statement of American Academy of Pediatrics' Task Force on Sudden Infant Death Syndrome (AAP, 2016) recommended that new parents put their babies to sleep "in the parent's room but on a separate surface," ideally a separate crib or bassinet made for babies.

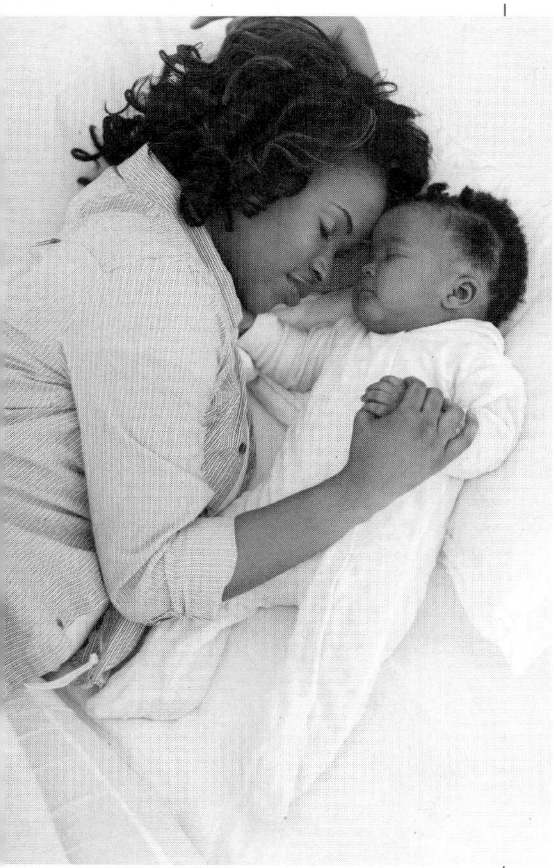

Yet even with U.S. health organizations recommending against bed-sharing, research indicates that large numbers of U.S. parents still bed-share. One 2016 study used a nationally representative sample of 3,218 mothers who spoke English or Spanish and were enrolled at 32 birth hospitals (L. A. Smith et al., 2016). The researchers found that nearly 21% of those surveyed bed-shared, while 65% room-shared. They found that mothers who bed-shared were more than twice as likely to report exclusive breastfeeding. A U.S. survey of 4,789 mothers of babies 0 to 12 months old (K. Kendall-Tackett, Cong, & Hale, 2010) found that almost 60% bed-shared and this occurred throughout the first year. A U.S. open-ended semi-structured interview study (Tully, Holditch-Davis, & Brandon, 2015) found that 12% of the 52 mothers of both late-preterm (22) and term (30) babies planned during pregnancy to bed-share to make infant care at night more convenient. Other reasons were to help baby sleep and for reassurance of the baby's well-being. One mother of a preterm baby said that because her baby was born early, she bed-shared because she did not yet have a bassinet at home. However, although only 12% planned to bed-share during pregnancy, 47% of the mothers in this study bed-shared after birth.

U.K. sleep researcher Dr. Helen Ball suggested that—unlike a change in sleep position—bed-sharing is not an infant-care behavior that is easily changed by simple recommendations. She wrote (Ball & Volpe, 2013, p. 84): "Failure to recognize the importance of infant sleep location to ethnic and sub-culture identity has led to inappropriate and ineffective risk-reduction messages that are rejected by their target populations."

• • •

Attempts to avoid bed-sharing can inadvertently lead to dangerous sleeping practices.

When new parents are encouraged to exclusively nurse and also to avoid bed-sharing, they may ask themselves the next logical question: "What is the alternative?" In an article written for U.S. pediatricians, Laura Wilwerding, MD, FAAP wrote that if a new mother is advised not to sleep with her baby (Wilwerding, 2008):

> "...she may get out of bed at night and nurse or bottle-feed her baby in another location with no intention of sleeping. The result in the sleep-deprived mother is often inadvertently sleeping on a couch or recliner. This is far more dangerous to the infant than a firm adult mattress" (Wilwerding, 2008, p. 3).

Parents can easily become exhausted from spending their nights nursing in upright positions while trying to avoid falling asleep in bed, on a sofa, or in a chair. Some find themselves nodding off after several night feeds and nearly (or actually) dropping their baby or falling asleep somewhere much more hazardous than an adult bed. In the 2015 U.S. open-ended semi-structured interview study described in the previous point (Tully et al., 2015), many of the study mothers who chose not to bed-share did so because they were afraid for their baby's safety. One study mother instead slept with her baby in a reclining chair, which is much riskier from a safety perspective than bed-sharing in an adult bed. (AAP, 2016). In the U.S. survey of 4,789 mothers of babies 0 to 12 months old (K. Kendall-Tackett et al., 2010), of the 55% of mothers whose night feeds happened in another location rather than an adult bed, 44% admitted to falling asleep while feeding their baby in a chair, recliner, or sofa. After experiences like these, many parents begin to see bed-sharing as a safer alternative.

BOX 2.2 Bed-sharing Practices for Nursing Families

Elements of Safe Bed-sharing in Order of Importance

1. Never sleep with the baby on a sofa, armchair, or pillow.
2. Keep the sleeping baby away from anyone impaired by alcohol or drugs.
3. Position baby for sleep on her back.
4. Keep the sleeping baby away from secondhand smoke, any routine smoker, and clothing that smells of smoke.
5. Position the bed away from walls and furniture so baby cannot become wedged.
6. Choose a bed with a firm surface and without thick covers or objects that could block baby's breathing.
7. Do not leave the baby alone in an adult bed.
8. The best sleeping position for the nursing couple is the "cuddle curl," with baby's head across from the nipple, adult's arms and legs curled around baby, and baby on her back away from pillows.
9. Follow cultural norms about where to position the baby in relation to both parents.

Adapted from (Blair, et al., 2020)

Putting parents in this quandary may also put nursing at risk. As one British researcher explained, parents may view their choices as (Ball, 2003, pp. 185-186):

> "(1) feeding the baby formula (or formula plus some 'heavy' indigestible substance, such as cereal or baby rice) so that he or she does not require frequent (or any) night feeding; (2) undertake an 'infant-training' program…to encourage them to lengthen their sleep bouts until they 'sleep through the night' (midnight to 5:00 AM); or (3) sleep next to the baby, allowing easy access to breasts, and eliminating the need for either mother or baby to wake fully for breastfeeds."

Since the release of the first edition of its policy statement in 2005, which cautioned against any bed-sharing, the AAP Task Force on SIDS made one addition that acknowledges the research showing that when parents attempt to strictly follow the recommendation to avoid bed-sharing, this sometimes leads to falling asleep somewhere far worse. In its 2016 policy statement, the AAP suggested a course of action for exhausted parents if they think they may fall asleep while feeding the baby (AAP, 2016, p. e13):

> "…the AAP acknowledges that parents frequently fall asleep while feeding the infant. Evidence suggests that it is less hazardous to fall asleep with the infant in the adult bed than on a sofa or armchair, should the parent fall asleep."

An alternative to issuing a blanket recommendation against bed-sharing is to recommend parents adopt safer bed-sharing practices. In its 2020 clinical protocol on bed-sharing and breastfeeding (Blair et al., 2020), the Academy of Breastfeeding Medicine makes the scientific case that the best way to decrease infant deaths during sleep is to openly discuss the specific ways parents who bed-share (intentionally or unintentionally) can reduce risk (summarized in Box 2.2). Download the ABM's Clinical Protocol #6 on bed-sharing and breastfeeding in multiple languages at **bfmed.org/protocols**.

RESOURCES

basisonline.org.uk—Website of Baby Sleep Info Source from the University of Durham in the U.K., which features information and free downloadable handouts for parents on normal infant sleep and research on sleep strategies, as well as resources for professionals.

bit.ly/BA2-BF1stHours—Free 10-minute video on GlobalHealthMedia.org showing the 9 instinctive stages of the breast crawl in action.

firstdroplets.com—Free videos for parents by U.S. pediatrician Jane Morton show how to avoid excess newborn weight loss, maximize milk production, and increase self-confidence by learning hand expression before birth and using it in the first days after birth to provide newborns with "dessert" by spoon after nursing.

Infant Sleep Info app available free from the App Store and Google Play. Created for parents by the U.K. sleep researchers at the University of Durham. Includes a sleep log that tracks and displays baby's sleep patterns on a chart depicting the range of normal sleep at different ages, a bed-sharing decision guide, and a guide to safe sleep.

Nagle, M. (2015). *Boobin' All Day—Boobin' All Night: A Gentle Approach to Sleep for Breastfeeding Families.* Sunshine Coast, Australia: The Milk Meg.

Wiessinger, D., West, D., Smith, L., and Pitman, T. (2014). *Sweet Sleep: Nighttime and Naptime Strategies for the Breastfeeding Family.* New York: Ballantine Books.

REFERENCES

AAP. (2012). Breastfeeding and the use of human milk. *Pediatrics, 129*(3), e827-e841.

AAP. (2016). SIDS and other sleep-related infant deaths: Updated 2016 recommendations for a safe infant sleeping environment. *Pediatrics, 138*(5).

AAP, & ACOG. (2017). Care of the newborn. In S. J. Kilpatrick, L.-A. Papile, & G. A. Macones (Eds.), *Guidelines for Perinatal Care* (8th ed., pp. 347-408). Elk Grove Village, IL: American Academy of Pediatrics.

Aarts, C., Hornell, A., Kylberg, E., et al. (1999). Breastfeeding patterns in relation to thumb sucking and pacifier use. *Pediatrics, 104*(4), e50.

Abedi, P., Jahanfar, S., Namvar, F., et al. (2016). Breastfeeding or nipple stimulation for reducing postpartum haemorrhage in the third stage of labour. *Cochrane Database of Systematic Reviews(*1), CD010845.

Aghdas, K., Talat, K., & Sepideh, B. (2014). Effect of immediate and continuous mother-infant skin-to-skin contact on breastfeeding self-efficacy of primiparous women: A randomised control trial. *Women and Birth, 27*(1), 37-40.

Alberts, J. R. (1994). Learning as adaptation of the infant. *Acta Paediatrica Supplement, 397,* 77-85.

Anuntaseree, W., Mo-Suwan, L., Vasiknanonte, P., et al. (2008). Night waking in Thai infants at 3 months of age: Association between parental practices and infant sleep. *Sleep Medicine, 9*(5), 564-571.

Appleton, J., Russell, C. G., Laws, R., et al. (2018). Infant formula feeding practices associated with rapid weight gain: A systematic review. *Maternal and Child Nutrition, 14*(3), e12602.

Armbrust, R., Hinkson, L., von Weizsacker, K., et al. (2016). The Charite cesarean birth: A family orientated approach of cesarean section. *Journal of Maternal-Fetal & Neonatal Medicine, 29*(1), 163-168.

AWHONN. (2018). *Neonatal Skin Care: Evidence-based Clinical Practice Guidelines.* Washington, DC: Association of Women's Health, Obstetric and Neonatal Nurses.

Ball, H. L. (2003). Breastfeeding, bed-sharing, and infant sleep. *Birth, 30*(3), 181-188.

Ball, H. L., Douglas, P. S., Kulasinghe, K., et al. (2018). The Possums Infant Sleep Program: Parents' perspectives on a novel parent-infant sleep intervention in Australia. *Sleep Health, 4*(6), 519-526.

Ball, H. L., Howel, D., Bryant, A., et al. (2016). Bed-sharing by breastfeeding mothers: Who bed-shares and what is the relationship with breastfeeding duration? *Acta Paediatrica, 105*(6), 628-634.

Ball, H. L., & Volpe, L. E. (2013). Sudden Infant Death Syndrome (SIDS) risk reduction and infant sleep location — Moving the discussion forward. *Social Science & Medicine, 79,* 84-91.

Ball, H. L., Ward-Platt, M. P., Heslop, E., et al. (2006). Randomised trial of infant sleep location on the postnatal ward. *Archives of Disease in Childhood, 91*(12), 1005-1010.

Bartick, M., Tomori, C., & Ball, H. L. (2018). Babies in boxes and the missing links on safe sleep: Human evolution and cultural revolution. *Maternal and Child Nutrition, 14*(2), e12544.

Bartick, M., Boisvert, M.E., Philipp, B.L., et al. (2019). Trends in breastfeeding interventions, skin-to-skin care, and sudden infant deat in the first 6 days after birth. *Journal of Pediatrics,* doi: 1016/jpeds.2019.09.069.

Bates, J. E., Maslin, C. A., & Frankel, K. A. (1985). Attachment security, mother-child interaction, and temperament as predictors of behavior-problem ratings at age three years. *Monographs of the Society for Research in Child Development, 50*(1-2), 167-193.

Becher, J. C., Bhushan, S. S., & Lyon, A. J. (2012). Unexpected collapse in apparently healthy newborns--A prospective national study of a missing cohort of neonatal deaths and near-death events. *Archives of Disease in Childhood. Fetal and Neonatal Edition, 97*(1), F30-34.

Beck, C. T., Gable, R. K., Sakala, C., et al. (2011). Posttraumatic stress disorder in new mothers: Results from a two-stage U.S. national survey. *Birth, 38*(3), 216-227.

Beck, C. T., & Watson, S. (2008). Impact of birth trauma on breast-feeding: A tale of two pathways. *Nursing Research, 57*(4), 228-236.

Beilin, Y., Bodian, C. A., Weiser, J., et al. (2005). Effect of labor epidural analgesia with and without fentanyl on infant breast-feeding: A prospective, randomized, double-blind study. *Anesthesiology, 103*(6), 1211-1217.

Belfort, M. B., Drouin, K., Riley, J. F., et al. (2018). Prevalence and trends in donor milk use in the well-baby nursery: A survey of northeast United States birth hospitals. *Breastfeeding Medicine, 13*(1), 34-41.

Benson, S. (2001). What is normal? A study of normal breastfeeding dyads during the first sixty hours of life. *Breastfeeding Review, 9*(1), 27-32.

Bergman, N. (2017). Breastfeeding and perinatal neuroscience. In C. W. Genna (Ed.), *Supporting Sucking Skills in Breastfeeding Infants* (3rd ed., pp. 49-63). Burlington, MA: Jones & Bartlett Learning.

Bergman, N. J. (2013). Neonatal stomach volume and physiology suggest feeding at 1-h intervals. *Acta Paediatrica, 102*(8), 773-777.

Bergman, N. J. (2014). The neuroscience of birth--and the case for zero separation. *Curationis, 37*(2), e1-e4.

Bergman, N. J., & Jurisoo, L. A. (1994). The 'kangaroo-method' for treating low birth weight babies in a developing country. *Tropical Doctor, 24*(2), 57-60.

Bergstrom, A., Byaruhanga, R., & Okong, P. (2005). The impact of newborn bathing on the prevalence of neonatal hypothermia in Uganda: A randomized, controlled trial. *Acta Paediatrica, 94*(10), 1462-1467.

Bhutta, Z. A., Das, J. K., Bahl, R., et al. (2014). Can available interventions end preventable deaths in mothers, newborn babies, and stillbirths, and at what cost? *Lancet, 384*(9940), 347-370.

Biggs, K. V., Hurrell, K., Matthews, E., et al. (2018). Formula milk supplementation on the postnatal ward: A cross-sectional analytical study. *Nutrients, 10*(5).

Blair, P. S., Ball, H. L., McKenna, J. J., et al. (2020). Bedsharing and breastfeeding: The Academy of Breastfeeding Medicine Protocol #6, Revision 2019. *Breastfeeding Medicine.* doi:10.1089/bfm.2019.29144.psb

Blatt, S. H. (2015). To swaddle, or not to swaddle? Paleoepidemiology of developmental dysplasia of the hip and the swaddling dilemma among the indigenous populations of North America. *American Journal of Human Biology, 27*(1), 116-128.

Blyton, D. M., Sullivan, C. E., & Edwards, N. (2002). Lactation is associated with an increase in slow-wave sleep in women. *Journal of Sleep Research, 11*(4), 297-303.

Boban, M., & Zakarija-Grkovic, I. (2016). In-hospital formula supplementation of healthy newborns: Practices, reasons, and their medical justification. *Breastfeeding Medicine, 11,* 448-454.

Boccolini, C. S., Carvalho, M. L., Oliveira, M. I., et al. (2013). Breastfeeding during the first hour of life and neonatal mortality. *Jornal de Pediatria (Rio J), 89*(2), 131-136.

Boccolini, C. S., Perez-Escamilla, R., Giugliani, E. R., et al. (2015). Inequities in milk-based prelacteal feedings in Latin America and the Caribbean: The role of cesarean section delivery. *Journal of Human Lactation, 31*(1), 89-98.

Boskabadi, H., & Zakerihamidi, M. (2017). The correlation between frequency and duration of breastfeeding and the severity of neonatal hyperbilirubinemia. *Journal of Maternal-Fetal & Neonatal Medicine, 31*(4), 457-463.

Boundy, E. O., Perrine, C. G., Barrera, C. M., et al. (2018). Trends in maternity care practice skin-to-skin contact indicators: United States, 2007-2015. *Breastfeeding Medicine, 13*(5), 381-387.

Bovbjerg, M. L., Hill, J. A., Uphoff, A. E., et al. (2018). Women who bedshare more frequently at 14 weeks postpartum subsequently report longer durations of breastfeeding. *Journal of Midwifery & Women's Health, 63*(4), 418-424.

Brimdyr, K., Cadwell, K., Widstrom, A. M., et al. (2015). The association between common labor drugs and suckling when skin-to-skin during the first hour after birth. *Birth, 42*(4), 319-328.

Brogan, J., & Rapkin, G. (2017). Implementing evidence-based neonatal skin care with parent-performed, delayed immersion baths. *Nursing for Women's Health, 21*(6), 442-450.

Brown, A., & Harries, V. (2015). Infant sleep and night feeding patterns during later infancy: Association with breastfeeding frequency, daytime complementary food intake, and infant weight. *Breastfeeding Medicine, 10*(5), 246-252.

Brown, A., & Jordan, S. (2014). Active management of the third stage of labor may reduce breastfeeding duration due to pain and physical complications. *Breastfeeding Medicine, 9*(10), 494-502.

Buccini, G., Perez-Escamilla, R., D'Aquino Benicio, M. H., et al. (2018). Exclusive breastfeeding changes in Brazil attributable to pacifier use. *PLoS One, 13*(12), e0208261.

Buccini Gdos, S., Perez-Escamilla, R., & Venancio, S. I. (2016). Pacifier use and exclusive breastfeeding in Brazil. *Journal of Human Lactation, 32*(3), NP52-60.

Buccini, G. D. S., Perez-Escamilla, R., Paulino, L. M., et al. (2017). Pacifier use and interruption of exclusive breastfeeding: Systematic review and meta-analysis. *Maternal and Child Nutrition, 13*(3).

Bystrova, K., Widstrom, A. M., Matthiesen, A. S., et al. (2007). Early lactation performance in primiparous and multiparous women in relation to different maternity home practices. A randomised trial in St. Petersburg. *International Breastfeeding Journal, 2,* 9.

Carberry, A. E., Raynes-Greenow, C. H., Turner, R. M., et al. (2013). Breastfeeding within the first hour compared to more than one hour reduces risk of early-onset feeding problems in term neonates: A cross-sectional study. *Breastfeeding Medicine, 8*(6), 513-514.

Casey, C. E., Neifert, M. R., Seacat, J. M., et al. (1986). Nutrient intake by breast-fed infants during the first five days after birth. *American Journal of Diseases of Children, 140*(9), 933-936.

Cato, K., Sylven, S. M., Lindback, J., et al. (2017). Risk factors for exclusive breastfeeding lasting less than two months-Identifying women in need of targeted breastfeeding support. *PLoS One, 12*(6), e0179402.

Chapman, D. J. (2009). Does pacifier introduction at 15 days disrupt well-established breastfeeding? *Journal of Human Lactation, 25*(4), 466-467.

Chen, D. C., Nommsen-Rivers, L., Dewey, K. G., et al. (1998). Stress during labor and delivery and early lactation performance. *American Journal of Clinical Nutrition, 68*(2), 335-344.

Chiu, S. H., Anderson, G. C., & Burkhammer, M. D. (2008). Skin-to-skin contact for culturally diverse women having breastfeeding difficulties during early postpartum. *Breastfeeding Medicine, 3*(4), 231-237.

Christensson, K., Cabrera, T., Christensson, E., et al. (1995). Separation distress call in the human neonate in the absence of maternal body contact. *Acta Paediatrica, 84*(5), 468-473.

Christensson, K., Siles, C., Moreno, L., et al. (1992). Temperature, metabolic adaptation and crying in healthy full-term newborns cared for skin-to-skin or in a cot. *Acta Paediatrica, 81*(6-7), 488-493.

Cohen Engler, A., Hadash, A., Shehadeh, N., et al. (2012). Breastfeeding may improve nocturnal sleep and reduce infantile colic: Potential role of breast milk melatonin. *European Journal of Pediatrics, 171*(4), 729-732.

Cohen, S. S., Alexander, D. D., Krebs, N. F., et al. (2018). Factors associated with breastfeeding initiation and continuation: A meta-analysis. *Journal of Pediatrics, 203,* 190-196 e121.

Colson, S. (2003). Biological nurturing increases duration of breastfeeding for a vulnerable cohort. *MIDRIS Midwifery Digest, 13*(1), 92-97.

Colson, S. (2019). *Biological Nurturing: Instinctual Breastfeeding* (2nd ed.). Amarillo, TX: Praeclarus Press.

Costa, C. T. D., Shqair, A. Q., Azevedo, M. S., et al. (2018). Pacifier use modifies the association between breastfeeding and malocclusion: A cross-sectional study. *Brazilian Oral Research, 32,* e101.

Crenshaw, J. T., Cadwell, K., Brimdyr, K., et al. (2012). Use of a video-ethnographic intervention (PRECESS Immersion Method) to improve skin-to-skin care and breastfeeding rates. *Breastfeeding Medicine, 7*(2), 69-78.

Crichton, G. E., & Symon, B. (2016). Behavioral management of sleep problems in infants under 6 months--What works? *Journal of Developmental & Behavioral Pediatrics, 37*(2), 164-171.

Crittenden, A. N., Samson, D. R., Herlosky, K. N., et al. (2018). Infant co-sleeping patterns and maternal sleep quality among Hadza hunter-gatherers. *Sleep Health, 4*(6), 527-534.

Crockenberg, S., McCluskey, K. (1986). Change in maternal behavior during the baby's first year of life. *Child Development, 57,* 746-753.

Dalsgaard, B. T., Rodrigo-Domingo, M., Kronborg, H., et al. (2019). Breastfeeding and skin-to-skin contact as non-pharmacological prevention of neonatal hypoglycemia in infants born to women with gestational diabetes; A Danish quasi-experimental study. *Sexual & Reproductive Healthcare, 19,* 1-8.

Daly, S. E., Owens, R. A., & Hartmann, P. E. (1993). The short-term synthesis and infant-regulated removal of milk in lactating women. *Experimental Physiology, 78*(2), 209-220.

DaMota, K., Banuelos, J., Goldbronn, J., et al. (2012). Maternal request for in-hospital supplementation of healthy breastfed infants among low-income women. *Journal of Human Lactation, 28*(4), 476-482.

Davanzo, R., De Cunto, A., Paviotti, G., et al. (2015). Making the first days of life safer: Preventing sudden unexpected postnatal collapse while promoting breastfeeding. *Journal of Human Lactation, 31*(1), 47-52.

de Alba-Romero, C., Camano-Gutierrez, I., Lopez-Hernandez, P., et al. (2014). Postcesarean section skin-to-skin contact of mother and child. *Journal of Human Lactation, 30*(3), 283-286.

Debes, A. K., Kohli, A., Walker, N., et al. (2013). Time to initiation of breastfeeding and neonatal mortality and morbidity: A systematic review. *BMC Public Health, 13* Suppl 3, S19.

Dekel, S., Stuebe, C., & Dishy, G. (2017). Childbirth induced posttraumatic stress syndrome: A systematic review of prevalence and risk factors. *Frontiers in Psychology, 8,* 560.

Dewey, K. G., Heinig, M. J., Nommsen, L. A., et al. (1991). Adequacy of energy intake among breast-fed infants in the DARLING study: Relationships to growth velocity, morbidity, and activity levels. *Davis Area Research on Lactation, Infant Nutrition and Growth. Journal of Pediatrics, 119*(4), 538-547.

Dewey, K. G., Nommsen-Rivers, L. A., Heinig, M. J., et al. (2003). Risk factors for suboptimal infant breastfeeding behavior, delayed onset of lactation, and excess neonatal weight loss. *Pediatrics, 112*(3 Pt 1), 607-619.

DiCioccio, H. C., Ady, C., Bena, J. F., et al. (2019). Initiative to improve exclusive breastfeeding by delaying the newborn bath. *Journal of Obstetric, Gynecologic & Neonatal Nursing.* doi:10.1016/j.jogn.2018.12.008

DiGirolamo, A. M., Grummer-Strawn, L. M., & Fein, S. B. (2008). Effect of maternity-care practices on breastfeeding. *Pediatrics, 122 Suppl 2,* S43-49.

Dimitraki, M., Tsikouras, P., Manav, B., et al. (2016). Evaluation of the effect of natural and emotional stress of labor on lactation and breast-feeding. *Archives of Gynecology and Obstetrics, 293*(2), 317-328.

DiTomasso, D., & Paiva, A. L. (2018). Neonatal weight matters: An examination of weight changes in full-term breastfeeding newborns during the first 2 weeks of life. *Journal of Human Lactation, 34*(1), 86-92.

Doan, T., Gardiner, A., Gay, C. L., et al. (2007). Breast-feeding increases sleep duration of new parents. *Journal of Perinatal & Neonatal Nursing, 21*(3), 200-206.

Doan, T., Gay, C. L., Kennedy, H. P., et al. (2014). Nighttime breastfeeding behavior is associated with more nocturnal sleep among first-time mothers at one month postpartum. *Journal of Clinical Sleep Medicine, 10*(3), 313-319.

Douglas, P. S., & Hill, P. S. (2013). Behavioral sleep interventions in the first six months of life do not improve outcomes for mothers or infants: A systematic review. *Journal of Developmental & Behavioral Pediatrics, 34*(7), 497-507.

Dudeja, S., Sikka, P., Jain, K., et al. (2018). Improving first-hour breastfeeding initiation rate after cesarean deliveries: A quality improvement study. *Indian Pediatrics, 55*(9), 761-764.

Edmond, K. M., Zandoh, C., Quigley, M. A., et al. (2006). Delayed breastfeeding initiation increases risk of neonatal mortality. *Pediatrics, 117*(3), e380-386.

Elmir, R., Schmied, V., Wilkes, L., et al. (2010). Women's perceptions and experiences of a traumatic birth: A meta-ethnography. *Journal of Advanced Nursing, 66*(10), 2142-2153.

Erickson, E. N., & Emeis, C. L. (2017). Breastfeeding outcomes after oxytocin use during childbirth: An integrative review. *Journal of Midwifery & Women's Health, 62*(4), 397-417.

Evans, K. C., Evans, R. G., Royal, R., et al. (2003). Effect of caesarean section on breast milk transfer to the normal term newborn over the first week of life. *Archives of Disease in Childhood. Fetal and Neonatal Edition, 88*(5), F380-382.

Evans, M. B., & Po, W. D. (2016). Clinical question: Does medical evidence support routine oronasopharyngeal suction at delivery? *Journal of the Oklahoma State Medical Association, 109*(4-5), 140-142.

Ezzo, G., & Bucknam, R. (2019). *On Becoming Babywise.* Sisters, OR: Hawksflight & Associates.

Ferber, S. G., & Makhoul, I. R. (2004). The effect of skin-to-skin contact (kangaroo care) shortly after birth on the neurobehavioral responses of the term newborn: A randomized, controlled trial. *Pediatrics, 113*(4), 858-865.

Fernandez-Canadas Morillo, A., Marin Gabriel, M. A., Olza Fernandez, I., et al. (2017). The relationship of the administration of intrapartum synthetic oxytocin and breastfeeding initiation and duration rates. *Breastfeeding Medicine, 12,* 98-102.

Finigan, V., & Long, T. (2014). Skin-to-skin contact: Multicultural perspectives on birth fluids and birth 'dirt'. *International Nursing Review, 61*(2), 270-277.

Flaherman, V. J., Narayan, N. R., Hartigan-O'Connor, D., et al. (2018). The effect of early limited formula on breastfeeding, readmission, and intestinal microbiota: A randomized clinical trial. *Journal of Pediatrics, 196,* 84-90 e81.

Flaherman, V. J., Schaefer, E. W., Kuzniewicz, M. W., et al. (2015). Early weight loss nomograms for exclusively breastfed newborns. *Pediatrics, 135*(1), e16-23.

Fleet, J., Belan, I., Jones, M. J., et al. (2015). A comparison of fentanyl with pethidine for pain relief during childbirth: A randomised controlled trial. *British Journal of Obstetrics and Gynaecology, 122*(7), 983-992.

Fleet, J. A., Jones, M., & Belan, I. (2017). The influence of intrapartum opioid use on breastfeeding experience at 6 weeks post partum: A secondary analysis. *Midwifery, 50,* 106-109.

Foster, J. P., Psaila, K., & Patterson, T. (2016). Non-nutritive sucking for increasing physiologic stability and nutrition in preterm infants. *Cochrane Database of Systematic Reviews, 10,* CD001071.

Franco, P., Seret, N., Van Hees, J. N., et al. (2005). Influence of swaddling on sleep and arousal characteristics of healthy infants. *Pediatrics, 115*(5), 1307-1311.

French, C. A., Cong, X., & Chung, K. S. (2016). Labor epidural analgesia and breastfeeding: A systematic review. *Journal of Human Lactation, 32*(3), 507-520.

Galbally, M., Lewis, A. J., McEgan, K., et al. (2013). Breastfeeding and infant sleep patterns: An Australian population study. *Journal of Paediatrics and Child Health, 49*(2), E147-152.

Gay, C. L., Lee, K. A., & Lee, S. Y. (2004). Sleep patterns and fatigue in new mothers and fathers. *Biological Research for Nursing, 5*(4), 311-318.

Gettler, L. T., & McKenna, J. J. (2011). Evolutionary perspectives on mother-infant sleep proximity and breastfeeding in a laboratory setting. *American Journal of Physical Anthropology, 144*(3), 454-462.

Gil, F., Amezqueta, A., Martinez, D., et al. (2017). Association between caesarean delivery and isolated doses of formula feeding in cow milk allergy. *International Archives of Allergy and Immunology, 173*(3), 147-152.

Girish, M., Mujawar, N., Gotmare, P., et al. (2013). Impact and feasibility of breast crawl in a tertiary care hospital. *Journal of Perinatology, 33*(4), 288-291.

Gomes, M., Trocado, V., Carlos-Alves, M., et al. (2018). Intrapartum synthetic oxytocin and breastfeeding: A retrospective cohort study. *Journal of Obstetrics and Gynaecology, 38*(6), 745-749.

Grajeda, R., & Perez-Escamilla, R. (2002). Stress during labor and delivery is associated with delayed onset of lactation among urban Guatemalan women. *Journal of Nutrition, 132*(10), 3055-3060.

Group, N. S. (2016). Timing of initiation, patterns of breastfeeding, and infant survival: Prospective analysis of pooled data from three randomised trials. *Lancet Global Health, 4*(4), e266-275.

Guala, A., Boscardini, L., Visentin, R., et al. (2017). Skin-to-skin contact in cesarean birth and duration of breastfeeding: A cohort study. *Scientific World Journal,* 2017, 1940756.

Hartmann, P. E. (2007). Mammary gland: Past, present, and future. In T. W. Hale & P. E. Hartmann (Eds.), *Hale & Hartmann's Textbook of Human Lactation.* Amarillo, TX: Hale Publishing.

Hauck, F. R., Omojokun, O. O., & Siadaty, M. S. (2005). Do pacifiers reduce the risk of sudden infant death syndrome? A meta-analysis. *Pediatrics, 116*(5), e716-723.

Hauck, Y. L., Hall, W. A., Dhaliwal, S. S., et al. (2012). The effectiveness of an early parenting intervention for mothers with infants with sleep and settling concerns: A prospective non-equivalent before-after design. *Journal of Clinical Nursing, 21*(1-2), 52-62.

Hauck, Y. L., Summers, L., White, E., et al. (2008). A qualitative study of Western Australian women's perceptions of using a Snoezelen room for breastfeeding during their postpartum hospital stay. *International Breastfeeding Journal, 3,* 20.

Heidarzadeh, M., Hakimi, S., Habibelahi, A., et al. (2016). Comparison of breast crawl between infants delivered by vaginal delivery and cesarean section. *Breastfeeding Medicine, 11*(6), 305-308.

Heinig, M. J., & Banuelos, J. (2006). American Academy of Pediatrics task force on sudden infant death syndrome (SIDS) statement on SIDS reduction: Friend or foe of breastfeeding? *Journal of Human Lactation, 22*(1), 7-10.

Heinig, M. J., Nommsen, L. A., Peerson, J. M., et al. (1993). Energy and protein intakes of breast-fed and formula-fed infants during the first year of life and their association with growth velocity: the DARLING Study. *American Journal of Clinical Nutrition, 58*(2), 152-161.

Hennart, P., Delogne-Desnoeck, J., Vis, H., et al. (1981). Serum levels of prolactin and milk production in women during a lactation period of thirty months. *Clinical Endocrinology, 14*(4), 349-353.

Herlenius, E., & Kuhn, P. (2013). Sudden unexpected postnatal collapse of newborn infants: A review of cases, definitions, risks, and preventive measures. *Translational Stroke Research, 4*(2), 236-247.

Hernandez-Aguilar, M. T., Bartick, M., Schreck, P., et al. (2018). ABM Clinical Protocol #7: Model maternity policy supportive of breastfeeding. *Breastfeeding Medicine, 13*(9), 559-574.

Hochberg, Z., Feil, R., Constancia, M., et al. (2011). Child health, developmental plasticity, and epigenetic programming. *Endocrine Reviews, 32*(2), 159-224.

Horne, R. S., Parslow, P. M., Ferens, D., et al. (2004). Comparison of evoked arousability in breast and formula fed infants. *Archives of Disease in Childhood, 89*(1), 22-25.

Horne, R. S., Witcombe, N. B., Yiallourou, S. R., et al. (2010). Cardiovascular control during sleep in infants: Implications for Sudden Infant Death Syndrome. *Sleep Medicine, 11*(7), 615-621.

Hornell, A., Aarts, C., Kylberg, E., et al. (1999). Breastfeeding patterns in exclusively breastfed infants: A longitudinal prospective study in Uppsala, Sweden. *Acta Paediatrica, 88*(2), 203-211.

Host, A., Husby, S., & Osterballe, O. (1988). A prospective study of cow's milk allergy in exclusively breast-fed infants. Incidence, pathogenetic role of early inadvertent exposure to cow's milk formula, and characterization of bovine milk protein in human milk. *Acta Paediatrica Scandavica, 77*(5), 663-670.

Houston, M. J., Howie, P. W., & McNeilly, A. S. (1983). Factors affecting the duration of breast feeding: 1. Measurement of breast milk intake in the first week of life. *Early Human Development, 8*(1), 49-54.

Hughes, O., Mohamad, M. M., Doyle, P., et al. (2018). The significance of breastfeeding on sleep patterns during the first 48 hours postpartum for first time mothers. *Journal of Obstetrics and Gynaecology, 38*(3), 316-320.

Ilhan, G., Atmaca, F. V., Cumen, A., et al. (2018). Effects of daytime versus night-time cesarean deliveries on Stage II lactogenesis. *Journal of Obstetrics and Gynaecology Research, 44*(4), 717-722.

Ingram, J., Hunt, L., Woolridge, M., et al. (2004). The association of progesterone, infant formula use and pacifier use with the return of menstruation in breastfeeding women: A prospective cohort study. *European Journal of Obstetrics, Gynecology, and Reproductive Biology, 114*(2), 197-202.

Jaafar, S. H., Ho, J. J., Jahanfar, S., et al. (2016). Effect of restricted pacifier use in breastfeeding term infants for increasing duration of breastfeeding. *Cochrane Database of Systematic Reviews*(8), CD007202.

Jha, A. K., Baliga, S., Kumar, H. H., et al. (2015). Is there a preventive role for vernix caseosa?: An invitro study. *Journal of Clinical and Diagnostic Research, 9*(11), SC13-16.

Jonas, W., Nissen, E., Ransjo-Arvidson, A. B., et al. (2008). Short- and long-term decrease of blood pressure in women during breastfeeding. *Breastfeeding Medicine, 3*(2), 103-109.

Jordan, S., Emery, S., Watkins, A., et al. (2009). Associations of drugs routinely given in labour with breastfeeding at 48 hours: Analysis of the Cardiff Births Survey. *British Journal of Obstetrics and Gynaecology, 116*(12), 1622-1629; discussion 1630-1622.

Kair, L. R., Kenron, D., Etheredge, K., et al. (2013). Pacifier restriction and exclusive breastfeeding. *Pediatrics, 131*(4), e1101-1107.

Kalmakoff, S., Gray, A., & Baddock, S. (2018). Predictors of supplementation for breastfed babies in a Baby-Friendly hospital. *Women and Birth, 31*(3), 202-209.

Karimi, F. Z., Sadeghi, R., Maleki-Saghooni, N., et al. (2019). The effect of mother-infant skin to skin contact on success and duration of first breastfeeding: A systematic review and meta-analysis. *Taiwanese Journal of Obstetrics & Gynecology, 58*(1), 1-9.

Karp, H. (2002). *The Happiest Baby on the Block: The New Way to Calm Crying and Help Your Newborn Baby Sleep Longer.* New York, NY: Bantam Books.

Katzer, D., Pauli, L., Mueller, A., et al. (2016). Melatonin concentrations and antioxidative capacity of human breast milk according to gestational age and the time of day. *Journal of Human Lactation, 32*(4), NP105-NP110.

Keefe, M. R. (1988). The impact of infant rooming-in on maternal sleep at night. *Journal of Obstetric, Gynecologic & Neonatal Nursing, 17*(2), 122-126.

Kellams, A., Harrel, C., Omage, S., et al. (2017). ABM Clinical Protocol #3: Supplementary feedings in the healthy term breastfed neonate, revised 2017. *Breastfeeding Medicine, 12,* 188-198.

Kelly, E., DunnGalvin, G., Murphy, B.P., et al. (2019). Formula supplementation remains a risk for cow's milk allergy in breast-fed infants. *Pediatric Allergy and Immunology.* doi: 10.1111/pai.13108

Kelly, P. A., Classen, K. A., Crandall, C. G., et al. (2018). Effect of timing of the first bath on a healthy newborn's temperature. *Journal of Obstetric, Gynecologic & Neonatal Nursing, 47*(5), 608-619.

Kendall-Tackett, K., Cong, Z., & Hale, T. W. (2010). Mother-infant sleep location and nighttime feeding behavior: U.S. data from the Survey of Mothers' Sleep and Fatigue. *Clinical Lactation, 1*(1), 27-31.

Kendall-Tackett, K. A. (2017). *Depression in New Mothers: Causes, Consequences and Treatment Alternatives.* London and New York: Routledge.

Kent, J. C. (2007). How breastfeeding works. *Journal of Midwifery & Women's Health, 52*(6), 564-570.

Kent, J. C., Gardner, H., & Geddes, D. T. (2016). Breastmilk production in the first 4 weeks after birth of term infants. *Nutrients, 8*(12).

Kent, J. C., Hepworth, A. R., Sherriff, J. L., et al. (2013). Longitudinal changes in breastfeeding patterns from 1 to 6 months of lactation. *Breastfeeding Medicine, 8,* 401-407.

Kent, J. C., Mitoulas, L., Cox, D. B., et al. (1999). Breast volume and milk production during extended lactation in women. *Experimental Physiology, 84*(2), 435-447.

Kent, J. C., Mitoulas, L. R., Cregan, M. D., et al. (2006). Volume and frequency of breastfeedings and fat content of breast milk throughout the day. *Pediatrics, 117*(3), e387-395.

Khan, S., Hepworth, A. R., Prime, D. K., et al. (2013). Variation in fat, lactose, and protein composition in breast milk over 24 hours: Associations with infant feeding patterns. *Journal of Human Lactation, 29*(1), 81-89.

Konner, M. (1976). Maternal care, infant behavior and development among the !Kung. In R. B. Lee & I. DeVore (Eds.), *Kalahari Hunter-Gatherers: Studies of the !Kung San and Their Neighbors.* Cambridge, MA: Harvard University Press.

Konner, M., & Worthman, C. (1980). Nursing frequency, gonadal function, and birth spacing among !Kung hunter-gatherers. *Science, 207*(4432), 788-791.

Kroll-Desrosiers, A. R., Nephew, B. C., Babb, J. A., et al. (2017). Association of peripartum synthetic oxytocin administration and depressive and anxiety disorders within the first postpartum year. *Depression and Anxiety, 34*(2), 137-146.

L'Hoir, M. P., Engelberts, A. C., van Well, G. T., et al. (1999). Dummy use, thumb sucking, mouth breathing and cot death. *European Journal of Pediatrics, 158*(11), 896-901.

Lawrence, R. A., & Lawrence, R. M. (2016). *Breastfeeding: A Guide for the Medical Profession* (8th ed.). Philadelphia, PA: Elsevier.

Le Huerou-Luron, I., Blat, S., & Boudry, G. (2010). Breast- v. formula-feeding: Impacts on the digestive tract and immediate and long-term health effects. *Nutrition Research Reviews, 23*(1), 23-36.

Leclere, C., Viaux, S., Avril, M., et al. (2014). Why synchrony matters during mother-child interactions: A systematic review. *PLoS One, 9*(12), e113571.

Lee, A. I., McCarthy, R. J., Toledo, P., et al. (2017). Epidural labor analgesia-fentanyl dose and breastfeeding success: A randomized clinical trial. *Anesthesiology, 127*(4), 614-624.

Levy, F., Gervaise, R., Kindermann, U., et al. (1991). Effects of early post-partum separation on maintenance of maternal responsiveness and selectivity in parturient ewes. *Applied Animal Behaviour Science, 31*(1-2), 101-110.

Li, D. K., Willinger, M., Petitti, D. B., et al. (2006). Use of a dummy (pacifier) during sleep and risk of sudden infant death syndrome (SIDS): Population based case-control study. *British Medical Journal, 332*(7532), 18-22.

Li, R., Fein, S. B., & Grummer-Strawn, L. M. (2008). Association of breastfeeding intensity and bottle-emptying behaviors at early infancy with infants' risk for excess weight at late infancy. *Pediatrics, 122* Suppl 2, S77-84.

Li, R., Magadia, J., Fein, S. B., et al. (2012). Risk of bottle-feeding for rapid weight gain during the first year of life. *Archives of Pediatric & Adolescent Medicine, 166*(5), 431-436.

Loutzenhiser, L., Hoffman, J., & Beatch, J. (2014). Parental perceptions of the effectiveness of graduated extinction in reducing infant night-waking. *Journal of Reproductive and Infant Psychology, 32*(3).

Lozoff, B., & Brittenham, G. (1979). Infant care: Cache or carry. *Journal of Pediatrics, 95*(3), 478-483.

Lozoff, B., Brittenham, G. M., Trause, M. A., et al. (1977). The mother-newborn relationship: Limits of adaptability. *Journal of Pediatrics, 91*(1), 1-12.

Lubbe, W., & Ten Ham-Baloyi, W. (2017). When is the use of pacifiers justifiable in the Baby-Friendly Hospital Initiative context? A clinician's guide. *BMC Pregnancy and Childbirth, 17*(1), 130.

Lubetzky, R., Mimouni, F. B., Dollberg, S., et al. (2007). Consistent circadian variations in creamatocrit over the first 7 weeks of lactation: A longitudinal study. *Breastfeeding Medicine, 2*(1), 15-18.

Ludington-Hoe, S. M., Morrison-Wilford, B. L., DiMarco, M., et al. (2018). Promoting newborn safety using the RAPPT assessment and considering Apgar criteria: A quality improvement project. *Neonatal Network, 37*(2), 85-95.

Marin Gabriel, M. A., Olza Fernandez, I., Malalana Martinez, A. M., et al. (2015). Intrapartum synthetic oxytocin reduce the expression of primitive reflexes associated with breastfeeding. *Breastfeeding Medicine, 10*(4), 209-213.

Martin, E., Vickers, B., Landau, R., et al. (2018). ABM Clinical Protocol #28, Peripartum analgesia and anesthesia for the breastfeeding mother. *Breastfeeding Medicine, 13*(3), 164-171.

Matthiesen, A. S., Ransjo-Arvidson, A. B., Nissen, E., et al. (2001). Postpartum maternal oxytocin release by newborns: Effects of infant hand massage and sucking. *Birth, 28*(1), 13-19.

Mawaddah, S. (2018). The relationship of early breastfeeding initiation with exclusive breastfeeding for babies. *Jurnal Info Kesehatan, 15*(2).

Mazurek, T., Mikiel-Kostyra, K., Mazur, J., et al. (1999). [Influence of immediate newborn care on infant adaptation to the environment]. *Medycyna Wieku Rozwojowego, 3*(2), 215-224.

McKenna, J. J., Ball, H. L., & Gettler, L. T. (2007). Mother-infant cosleeping, breastfeeding and sudden infant death syndrome: What biological anthropology has discovered about normal infant sleep and pediatric sleep medicine. *American Journal of Physical Anthropology, Suppl 45,* 133-161.

McKenna, J. J., & Gettler, L. T. (2016). There is no such thing as infant sleep, there is no such thing as breastfeeding, there is only breastsleeping. *Acta Paediatrica, 105*(1), 17-21.

Meyer, K., & Anderson, G. C. (1999). Using kangaroo care in a clinical setting with fullterm infants having breastfeeding difficulties. *MCN American Journal of Maternal and Child Nursing, 24*(4), 190-192.

Michelsson, K., Christensson, K., Rothganger, H., et al. (1996). Crying in separated and non-separated newborns: Sound spectrographic analysis. *Acta Paediatrica, 85*(4), 471-475.

Middlemiss, W., Granger, D. A., Goldberg, W. A., et al. (2012). Asynchrony of mother-infant hypothalamic-pituitary-adrenal axis activity following extinction of infant crying responses induced during the transition to sleep. *Early Human Development, 88*(4), 227-232.

Mihrshahi, S., Battistutta, D., Magarey, A., et al. (2011). Determinants of rapid weight gain during infancy: Baseline results from the NOURISH randomised controlled trial. *BMC Pediatrics, 11,* 99.

Milligan, R. A., Flenniken, P. M., & Pugh, L. C. (1996). Positioning intervention to minimize fatigue in breastfeeding women. *Applied Nursing Research, 9*(2), 67-70.

Misslin, R. (2003). The defense system of fear: Behavior and neurocircuitry. *Neurophysiologie Clinique, 33*(2), 55-66.

Modi, N., & Glover, V. (1996). Non-pharmacological reduction of hypercortisolaemia in preterm infants. *Infant Behavior and Development, 21,* 86.

Mohrbacher, N., & Kendall-Tackett, K. (2010). *Breastfeeding Made Simple: Seven Natural Laws for Nursing Mothers* (2nd ed.). Oakland, CA: New Harbinger Publications.

Montgomery-Downs, H. E., Clawges, H. M., & Santy, E. E. (2010). Infant feeding methods and maternal sleep and daytime functioning. *Pediatrics, 126*(6), e1562-1568.

Moodley-Govender, E., Mulol, H., Stauber, J., et al. (2015). Increased exclusivity of breastfeeding associated with reduced gut inflammation in infants. *Breastfeeding Medicine, 10*(10), 488-492.

Mooncey, S. (1997). The effect of mother-infant skin-to-skin contact on plasma cortisol and beta-endorphin concentrations in preterm newborns. *Infant Behavior and Development, 20,* 553.

Moore, E. R., Bergman, N., Anderson, G. C., et al. (2016). Early skin-to-skin contact for mothers and their healthy newborn infants. *Cochrane Database of Systematic Reviews, 11,* CD003519.

Morgan, B. E., Horn, A. R., & Bergman, N. J. (2011). Should neonates sleep alone? *Biological Psychiatry, 70*(9), 817-825.

Morhason-Bello, I. O., Adedokun, B. O., & Ojengbede, O. A. (2009). Social support during childbirth as a catalyst for early breastfeeding initiation for first-time Nigerian mothers. *International Breastfeeding Journal, 4,* 16.

Morton, J. (2019). Hands-on or hands-off when first milk matters most? *Breastfeeding Medicine, 14*(5), 295-297.

Nelson, A. M. (2017). Risks and benefits of swaddling healthy infants: An integrative review. *MCN American Journal of Maternal and Child Nursing, 42*(4), 216-225.

Nelson, J. M., Perrine, C. G., Scanlon, K. S., et al. (2016). Provision of non-breast milk supplements to healthy breastfed newborns in U.S. hospitals, 2009 to 2013. *Maternal and Child Health Journal, 20*(11), 2228-2232.

Neville, M. C. (1999). Physiology of lactation. *Clinics in Perinatology, 26*(2), 251-279.

Neville, M. C., Allen, J. C., Archer, P. C., et al. (1991). Studies in human lactation: Milk volume and nutrient composition during weaning and lactogenesis. *American Journal of Clinical Nutrition, 54*(1), 81-92.

Nissen, E., Uvnas-Moberg, K., Svensson, K., et al. (1996). Different patterns of oxytocin, prolactin but not cortisol release during breastfeeding in women delivered by caesarean section or by the vaginal route. *Early Human Development, 45*(1-2), 103-118.

Nissen, E., Widstrom, A. M., Lilja, G., et al. (1997). Effects of routinely given pethidine during labour on infants' developing breastfeeding behaviour. Effects of dose-delivery time interval and various concentrations of pethidine/norpethidine in cord plasma. *Acta Paediatrica, 86*(2), 201-208.

Noel-Weiss, J., Woodend, A. K., & Groll, D. L. (2011). Iatrogenic newborn weight loss: Knowledge translation using a study protocol for your maternity setting. *International Breastfeeding Journal, 6*(1), 10.

Nommsen-Rivers, L. A., Heinig, M. J., Cohen, R. J., et al. (2008). Newborn wet and soiled diaper counts and timing of onset of lactation as indicators of breastfeeding inadequacy. *Journal of Human Lactation, 24*(1), 27-33.

Parry, J. E., Ip, D. K., Chau, P. Y., et al. (2013). Predictors and consequences of in-hospital formula supplementation for healthy breastfeeding newborns. *Journal of Human Lactation, 29*(4), 527-536.

Patel, R. R., Liebling, R. E., & Murphy, D. J. (2003). Effect of operative delivery in the second stage of labor on breastfeeding success. *Birth, 30*(4), 255-260.

Perez-Escamilla, R., Martinez, J. L., & Segura-Perez, S. (2016). Impact of the Baby-friendly Hospital Initiative on breastfeeding and child health outcomes: A systematic review. *Maternal and Child Nutrition, 12*(3), 402-417.

Perkin, M. R., Bahnson, H. T., Logan, K., et al. (2018). Association of early introduction of solids with infant sleep: A secondary analysis of a randomized clinical trial. *JAMA Pediatrics,* e180739.

Pineda, R., Luong, A., Ryckman, J., et al. (2018). Pacifier use in newborns: Related to socioeconomic status but not to early feeding performance. *Acta Paediatrica, 107*(5), 806-810.

Piumelli, R., Davanzo, R., Nassi, N., et al. (2017). Apparent life-threatening events (ALTE): Italian guidelines. *Italian Journal of Pediatrics, 43*(1), 111.

Preer, G., Pisegna, J. M., Cook, J. T., et al. (2013). Delaying the bath and in-hospital breastfeeding rates. *Breastfeeding Medicine, 8*(6), 485-490.

Prentice, A. (1989). Evidence for local feedback control of human milk secretion. *Biochemical Society Transactions, 17,* 489-492.

Quillin, S. I. (1997). Infant and mother sleep patterns during 4th postpartum week. *Issues in Comprehensive Pediatric Nursing, 20*(2), 115-123.

Quillin, S. I., & Glenn, L. L. (2004). Interaction between feeding method and co-sleeping on maternal-newborn sleep. *Journal of Obstetric, Gynecologic, and Neonatal Nursing, 33*(5), 580-588.

Rabinowitz, M. R., Kair, L. R., Sipsma, H. L., et al. (2018). Human donor milk or formula: A qualitative study of maternal perspectives on supplementation. *Breastfeeding Medicine, 13*(3), 195-203.

Ransjo-Arvidson, A. B., Matthiesen, A. S., Lilja, G., et al. (2001). Maternal analgesia during labor disturbs newborn behavior: Effects on breastfeeding, temperature, and crying. *Birth, 28*(1), 5-12.

Regan, J., Thompson, A., & DeFranco, E. (2013). The influence of mode of delivery on breastfeeding initiation in women with a prior cesarean delivery: A population-based study. *Breastfeeding Medicine, 8,* 181-186.

Righard, L., & Alade, M. O. (1990). Effect of delivery room routines on success of first breast-feed. *Lancet, 336*(8723), 1105-1107.

Robiquet, P., Zamiara, P. E., Rakza, T., et al. (2016). Observation of skin-to-skin contact and analysis of factors linked to failure to breastfeed within 2 hours after birth. *Breastfeeding Medicine, 11,* 126-132.

Rodriguez, N. A., Hageman, J. R., & Pellerite, M. (2018). Maternal distraction from smartphone use: A potential risk factor for sudden unexpected postnatal collapse of the newborn. *Journal of Pediatrics, 200,* 298-299.

Sadeh, A., Juda-Hanael, M., Livne-Karp, E., et al. (2016). Low parental tolerance for infant crying: An underlying factor in infant sleep problems? *Journal of Sleep Research, 25*(5), 501-507.

Saint, L., Smith, M., & Hartmann, P. E. (1984). The yield and nutrient content of colostrum and milk of women from giving birth to 1 month post-partum. *British Journal of Nutrition, 52*(1), 87-95.

Sakalidis, V. S., Williams, T. M., Hepworth, A. R., et al. (2013). A comparison of early sucking dynamics during breastfeeding after cesarean section and vaginal birth. *Breastfeeding Medicine, 8*(1), 79-85.

Say, B., Simsek, G. K., Canpolat, F. E., et al. (2018). Effects of pacifier use on transition time from gavage to breastfeeding in preterm infants: A randomized controlled trial. *Breastfeeding Medicine, 13*(6), 433-437.

Schafer, R., & Genna, C. W. (2015). Physiologic breastfeeding: A contemporary approach to breastfeeding initiation. *Journal of Midwifery & Women's Health, 60*(5), 546-553.

Schneider, L. W., Crenshaw, J. T., & Gilder, R. E. (2017). Influence of immediate skin-to-skin contact during cesarean surgery on rate of transfer of newborns to NICU for observation. *Nursing for Women's Health, 21*(1), 28-33.

Sen, S., Benjamin, C., Riley, J., et al. (2018). Donor milk utilization for healthy infants: Experience at a single academic center. *Breastfeeding Medicine, 13*(1), 28-33.

Shrago, L. C., Reifsnider, E., & Insel, K. (2006). The Neonatal Bowel Output Study: Indicators of adequate breast milk intake in neonates. *Pediatric Nursing, 32*(3), 195-201.

Sievers, E., Oldigs, H. D., Santer, R., et al. (2002). Feeding patterns in breast-fed and formula-fed infants. *Annals of Nutrition and Metabolism, 46*(6), 243-248.

Smillie, C. M. (2017). How infants learn to feed: A neurobehavioral model. In C. W. Genna (Ed.), *Supporting Sucking Skills in Breastfeeding Infants* (3rd ed., pp. 89-111). Burlington, MA: Jones & Bartlett Learning.

Smith, L. A., Geller, N. L., Kellams, A. L., et al. (2016). Infant sleep location and breastfeeding practices in the United States, 2011-2014. *Academic Pediatrics, 16*(6), 540-549.

Smith, L. J. (2017). Impact of birth practices on infant suck. In C. W. Genna (Ed.), *Supporting Sucking Skills in Breastfeeding Infants* (3rd ed., pp. 65-88). Burlington, MA: Jones & Bartlett Learning.

Sobel, H. L., Silvestre, M. A., Mantaring, J. B., 3rd, et al. (2011). Immediate newborn care practices delay thermoregulation and breastfeeding initiation. *Acta Paediatrica, 100*(8), 1127-1133.

Sozmen, M. (1992). Effects of early suckling of cesarean-born babies on lactation. *Biology of the Neonate, 62,* 67-68.

St James-Roberts, I., Alvarez, M., Csipke, E., et al. (2006). Infant crying and sleeping in London, Copenhagen and when parents adopt a "proximal" form of care. *Pediatrics, 117*(6), e1146-1155.

Stern, G., & Kruckman, L. (1983). Multi-disciplinary perspectives on post-partum depression: An anthropological critique. *Social Science & Medicine, 17*(15), 1027-1041.

Stettler, N., Stallings, V. A., Troxel, A. B., et al. (2005). Weight gain in the first week of life and overweight in adulthood: A cohort study of European American subjects fed infant formula. *Circulation, 111*(15), 1897-1903.

Stevens, J., Schmied, V., Burns, E., et al. (2014). Immediate or early skin-to-skin contact after a caesarean section: A review of the literature. *Maternal and Child Nutrition, 10*(4), 456-473.

Stevens, J., Schmied, V., Burns, E., et al. (2018). Who owns the baby? A video ethnography of skin-to-skin contact after a caesarean section. *Women and Birth, 31*(6), 453-462.

Stuart-Macadam, P. (1995). Breastfeeding in prehistory. In P. Stuart-Macadam & K. A. Dettwyler (Eds.), *Breastfeeding: Biocultural Perspectives* (pp. 75-99). New York, NY: Aldine de Gruyter.

Svensson, K., Matthiesen, A. S., & Widstrom, A. M. (2005). Night rooming-in: Who decides? An example of staff influence on mother's attitude. *Birth, 32*(2), 99-106.

Svensson, K. E., Velandia, M. I., Matthiesen, A. S., et al. (2013). Effects of mother-infant skin-to-skin contact on severe latch-on problems in older infants: A randomized trial. *International Breastfeeding Journal, 8*(1), 1.

Swain, J. E., Konrath, S., Dayton, C. J., et al. (2013). Toward a neuroscience of interactive parent-infant dyad empathy. *Behavioral and Brain Sciences, 36*(4), 438-439.

Takahashi, Y., & Tamakoshi, K. (2018). The positive association between duration of skin-to-skin contact and blood glucose level in full-term infants. *Journal of Perinatal & Neonatal Nursing, 32*(4), 351-357.

Takayama, J. I., Teng, W., Uyemoto, J., et al. (2000). Body temperature of newborns: What is normal? *Clinical Pediatrics (Philadelphia), 39*(9), 503-510.

Thomas, K. A., & Foreman, S. W. (2005). Infant sleep and feeding pattern: Effects on maternal sleep. *Journal of Midwifery & Women's Health, 50*(5), 399-404.

Tollin, M., Bergsson, G., Kai-Larsen, Y., et al. (2005). Vernix caseosa as a multi-component defence system based on polypeptides, lipids and their interactions. *Cellular and Molecular Life Sciences, 62*(19-20), 2390-2399.

Tully, K. P., & Ball, H. L. (2012). Postnatal unit bassinet types when rooming-in after cesarean birth: Implications for breastfeeding and infant safety. *Journal of Human Lactation, 28*(4), 495-505.

Tully, K. P., & Ball, H. L. (2014). Maternal accounts of their breast-feeding intent and early challenges after caesarean childbirth. *Midwifery, 30*(6), 712-719.

Tully, K. P., Holditch-Davis, D., & Brandon, D. (2015). The relationship between planned and reported home infant sleep locations among mothers of late preterm and term infants. *Maternal and Child Health Journal, 19*(7), 1616-1623.

Ullah, S., & Griffiths, P. (2003). Does the use of pacifiers shorten breastfeeding duration in infants? *British Journal of Community Nursing, 8*(10), 458-463.

Urashima, M., Mezawa, H., Okuyama, M., et al. (2019). Primary prevention of cow's milk sensitization and food allergy by avoiding supplementation with cow's milk formula at birth: A randomized clinical trial. *JAMA Pediatrics.* doi:10.1001/jamapediatrics.2019.3544

Vennemann, M. M., Bajanowski, T., Brinkmann, B., et al. (2009). Sleep environment risk factors for sudden infant death syndrome: The German Sudden Infant Death Syndrome Study. *Pediatrics, 123*(4), 1162-1170.

Volpe, L. E., & Ball, H. L. (2015). Infant sleep-related deaths: Why do parents take risks? *Archives of Disease in Childhood, 100*(7), 603-604.

Waldenstrom, U., & Swenson, A. (1991). Rooming-in at night in the postpartum ward. *Midwifery, 7*(2), 82-89.

Wallenborn, J. T., Graves, W. C., & Masho, S. W. (2017). Breastfeeding initiation in mothers with repeat cesarean section: The impact of marital status. *Breastfeeding Medicine, 12,* 227-232.

Wallenborn, J. T., & Masho, S. W. (2016). The interrelationship between repeat cesarean section, smoking status, and breastfeeding duration. *Breastfeeding Medicine, 11,* 440-447.

Walters, M. W., Boggs, K. M., Ludington-Hoe, S., et al. (2007). Kangaroo care at birth for full term infants: A pilot study. *MCN American Journal of Maternal and Child Nursing, 32*(6), 375-381.

Wambach, K. A. (1998). Maternal fatigue in breastfeeding primiparae during the first nine weeks postpartum. *Journal of Human Lactation, 14*(3), 219-229.

Weissbluth, M. (2015). *Healthy Sleep Habits, Happy Child, 4th Edition: A Step-by-Step Program for a Good Night's Sleep.* New York, NY: Ballantine Books.

WHO. (2017). *WHO Recommendations on Newborn Health: Guidelines Approved by the WHO Guidelines Review Committee.* Geneva, Switzerland: World Health Organization.

Widstrom, A. M., Lilja, G., Aaltomaa-Michalias, P., et al. (2011). Newborn behaviour to locate the breast when skin-to-skin: A possible method for enabling early self-regulation. *Acta Paediatrica, 100*(1), 79-85.

Willis, C. E., & Livingstone, V. (1995). Infant insufficient milk syndrome associated with maternal postpartum hemorrhage. *Journal of Human Lactation, 11*(2), 123-126.

Wilson-Clay, B., & Hoover, K. (2017). *The Breastfeeding Atlas* (6th ed.). Manchaca, TX: LactNews Press.

Wilwerding, L. (2008). Minimize bed-sharing risks for mom and baby. *American Academy of Pediatrics' Section on Breastfeeding Newsletter* (Summer), 3.

Yamauchi, Y., & Yamanouchi, I. (1990). Breast-feeding frequency during the first 24 hours after birth in full-term neonates. *Pediatrics, 86*(2), 171-175.

Zanardo, V., Svegliado, G., Cavallin, F., et al. (2010). Elective cesarean delivery: Does it have a negative effect on breastfeeding? *Birth, 37*(4), 275-279.

Zangen, S., Di Lorenzo, C., Zangen, T., et al. (2001). Rapid maturation of gastric relaxation in newborn infants. *Pediatric Research, 50*(5), 629-632.

Zhao, J., Zhao, Y., Du, M., et al. (2017). Does caesarean section affect breastfeeding practices in China? A systematic review and meta-analysis. *Maternal and Child Health Journal, 21*(11), 2008-2024.

Zuppa, A. A., Alighieri, G., Riccardi, R., et al. (2014). Epidural analgesia, neonatal care and breastfeeding. *Italian Journal of Pediatrics, 40,* 82.

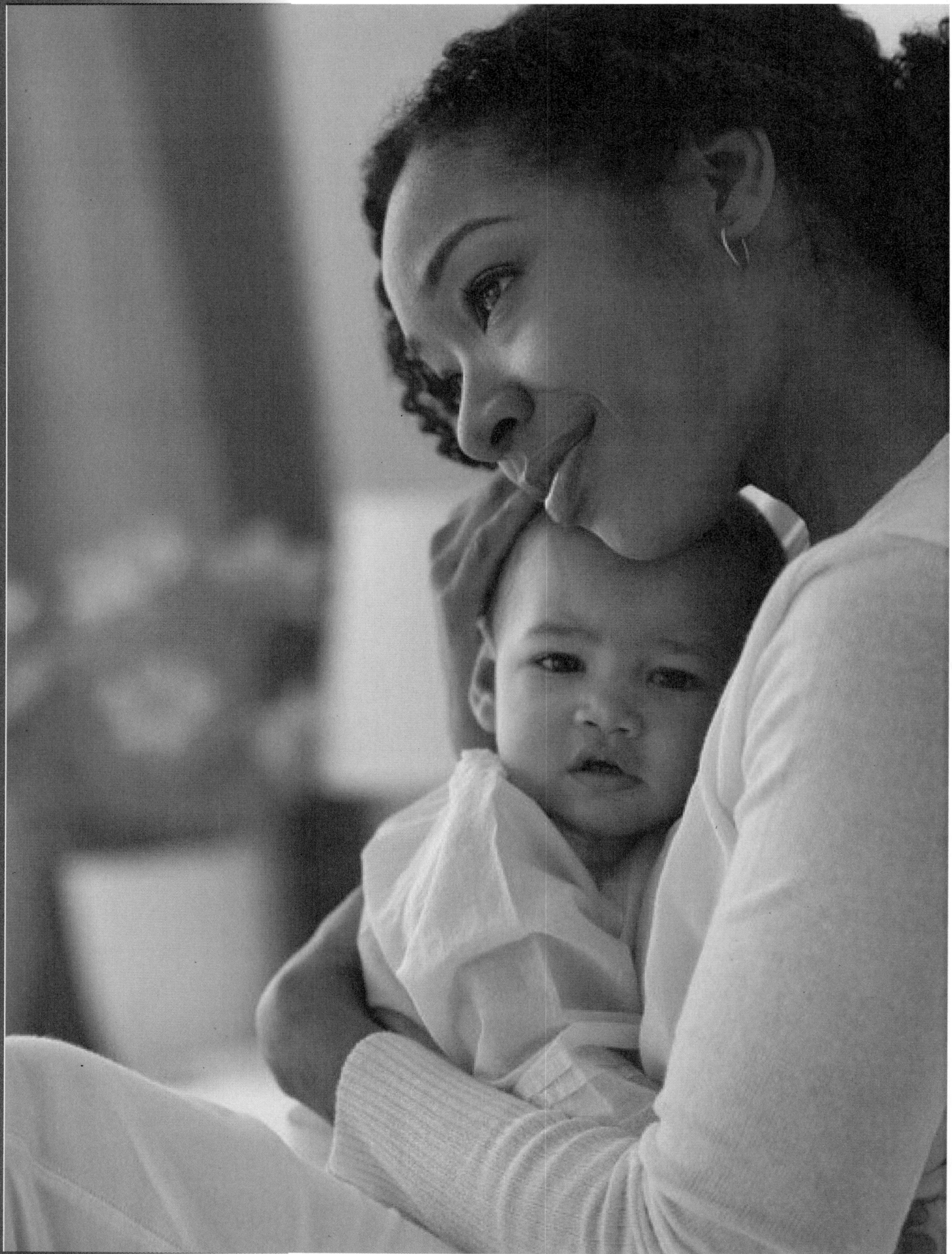

Latching and Nursing Struggles

3

Latching and nursing struggles are common and include different types of problems.

The focus of this chapter is problems associated with the act of nursing: difficulty latching, ineffective nursing or inconsistent feeding effectiveness, and not latching at all to one or both sides. One prospective U.S. survey of 532 first-time mothers (Wagner, Chantry, Dewey, & Nommsen-Rivers, 2013) found that by the third day of life, 92% of its mothers reported one or more breastfeeding problems. More than half—52%--of these mothers reported their baby was struggling at the breast. In a 2018 Danish cross-sectional, mixed-methods study of 1,437 mothers with full-term singleton babies (Feenstra, Jorgine Kirkeby, Thygesen, Danbjorg, & Kronborg, 2018), 40% of the mothers with breastfeeding problems reported latching struggles.

One of the most challenging problems is the baby who seems distressed during latch attempts and unable to nurse. These and other nursing struggles can usually be overcome, but to safeguard nursing, it's important to first feed the baby, second protect the milk production, and third use careful detective work to find the cause of the problem so appropriate strategies can be used to help the baby transition most easily to direct nursing.

SAFEGUARDING NURSING

Nursing struggles are stressful and demoralizing and often lead to premature weaning.

When parents easily soothe and satisfy their nursing baby, their self-confidence is enhanced. The opposite is also true. Feeding struggles undermine their feelings of competence and self-worth, as well as their desire to continue nursing. When nursing is going well, it has a positive effect on mood (Hatton et al., 2005; McCoy, Beal, Shipman, Payton, & Watson, 2006), but nursing struggles can contribute to depressive symptoms. A 2017 Australian prospective observational study followed 229 mothers (Cooklin et al., 2018) and found an association between two or more breastfeeding problems lasting 2 weeks or longer and poorer maternal mood. One Canadian study (Rempel, 2004) found that no matter what the baby's age, the less control the study mothers felt they had over breastfeeding, the weaker their intentions to continue and the earlier they weaned.

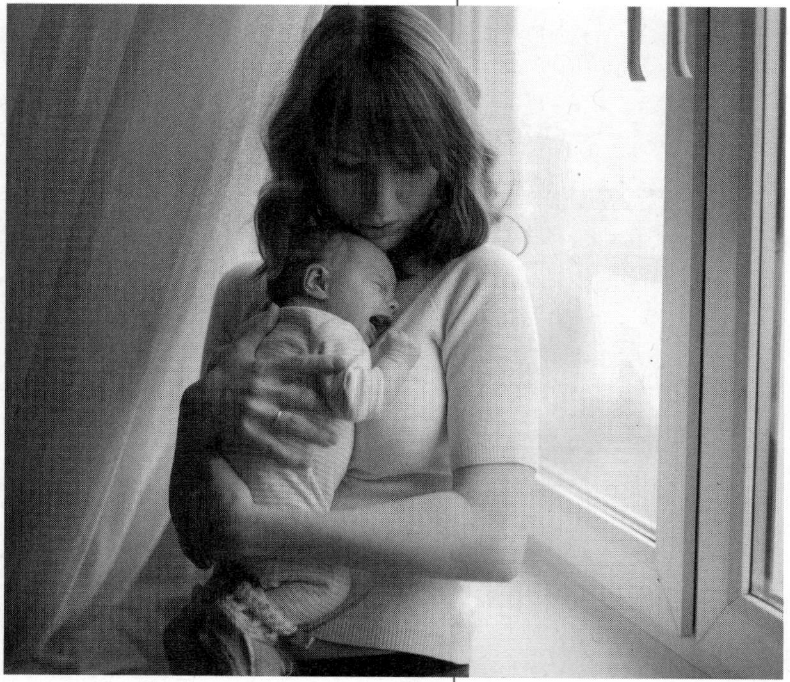

Strong feelings often arise with nursing struggles (Feenstra, Nilsson, & Danbjorg, 2018). The nursing parent may feel upset and frustrated and worry that the baby's behavior is a sign of poor parenting, or—even worse—personal rejection. Some parents are plagued by anxiety about their ability to care for the baby or by worry about baby's health. Many feel guilty and wonder if their baby's behavior is somehow their fault. Many who struggle with nursing feel like a failure.

It's important for parents to have an outlet where they can express their worries, fears, and doubts. Sharing and acknowledging these feelings makes it possible for them to consider their situation more objectively. Assure them that their baby needs them now more than ever, that there are reasons for the baby's behavior, and that with effective strategies, most often nursing struggles can be overcome.

Feed the Baby

Gather some basic information to determine whether supplements are needed.

Ask the baby's age, weight, diaper output, and how many times each day nursing goes well and at which feeds. One of the first concerns is likely to be how to make sure the baby gets the milk he needs. This and the nursing parent's comfort should be the top priorities. The specifics will determine how this is done. For example, the needs of a 10-month-old baby on a nursing strike may be met with expressed milk in a cup along with solid foods, while the nursing parent expresses milk to stay comfortable and works to get him back to nursing.

Because being underfed can compromise a baby's nursing effectiveness, in some situations part of getting nursing going smoothly may involve feeding the baby expressed milk, donor milk, or a substitute. The strategy of withholding milk until the baby "gets hungry enough" is ineffective for many and will put some young babies at risk for dehydration.

KEY CONCEPT

While formulating a plan, the baby's weight gain is the most reliable gauge of whether or not he needs a supplement.

Baby's weight gain. There are several ways to gauge whether the baby needs a supplement. The most reliable is the baby's weight gain. For healthy weight gain by age, see p. 191, Table 6.1 and see also p. 227-228 in Chapter 6, "Weight Gain and Growth."

Stool color and output during the early weeks. A less reliable gauge of milk intake—but one that can be helpful during the early weeks in combination with weight checks—is stool color and output. In the first week of life, some aspects of diaper output can provide good clues about whether the baby is receiving the milk he needs. In one U.S. prospective descriptive study of 131 newborns during the first 14 days of life (Shrago, Reifsnider, & Insel, 2006), a transition to yellow stools by Day 6 or earlier was associated with acceptable levels of weight loss and earlier weight gain. In another U.S. prospective study of 242 exclusively breastfed newborns (Nommsen-Rivers, Heinig, Cohen, & Dewey, 2008), breastfeeding inadequacy was predicted by less than three stools per day along with the mother's perception that her milk had not yet increased within 72 hours post-delivery. However, nursing was actually going well with 41% of the mothers with these two indicators.

KEY CONCEPT

Stool output is at best only a rough indicator of milk intake, but tracking it may be reassuring between weight checks.

Although stool color and output are not as accurate as weight gain in determining whether a baby is getting enough milk, they can be used during the early weeks as a rough gauge between weight checks. During the first 4 to 6 weeks or so (Courdent, Beghin, Akre, & Turck, 2014), daily stool output is even less reliable than it was during the first week, but between weight checks it can be another rough indicator of whether milk intake is adequate. An average is at least four stools the diameter of a U.S. quarter (2.5 cm) or larger (Shrago et al., 2006). If the baby has fewer stools but is gaining weight well, this is a normal variation and not a problem. After 4 to 6 weeks of age, stool count is no longer a helpful sign because many nursing babies have fewer stools, even when getting plenty of milk. For more details, see p. 202-204 in Chapter 6.

• • •

If the baby needs to be supplemented, offer to discuss possible supplements and feeding methods.

A variety of feeding methods are available for young babies, including spoon, cup, bowl, eyedropper, nursing supplementer, feeding bottle, and others. Ask if the family wants to discuss them. If so, see p. 894-904, "Alternative Feeding Methods," in Appendix B, "Tools and Products," and support their choice. If the baby is older than 6 to 8 months, baby can drink expressed milk from a cup. The best supplement is nearly always mother's milk. If that is not available and donor milk is a local option, that is an excellent second choice. Otherwise, suggest consulting with the baby's healthcare provider for a recommended supplement. See also on p. 222-228, the section "When and How to Supplement" in Chapter 6, "Weight Gain and Growth."

Protect Milk Production

If a newborn is not nursing or is nursing ineffectively, encourage effective milk expression at least eight times per day.

If a baby is not nursing at all or is nursing ineffectively, milk expression can help keep the nursing parent comfortable and establish or maintain milk production. How often to express and what expression method to use depends on the situation. For a young baby who is not removing the milk effectively, suggest expressing milk at least eight times per day—as often as a newborn would nurse. Especially during the first 2 weeks after birth, encourage frequent expression, because the nursing parent's body is more responsive to stimulation during that time. In the first 2 weeks post-delivery, mammary stimulation produces a much greater hormonal response. See p. 425 in Chapter 10, "Making Milk," to learn how to take maximum advantage of this extra, time-limited responsiveness to boost the "lactation curve" and ensure healthy long-term milk production and p. 497-504, the section "Establishing Full Milk Production with Pumping" in Chapter 11, "Milk Expression and Storage."

• • •

If the baby is nursing well at some feeds, tailor the expression plan to the need.

Each situation is different and requires a different milk-expression plan. How often to express milk depends on the baby's age, the number of times per day he feeds well, any other food or drink he receives, the level of milk production, and the baby's weight. Table 3.1 describes average milk intake by age per day and per feed. Discuss the specifics of the situation and calculate how much expressed milk the baby needs. Assure the family that when nursing is going well, the baby will likely be able to maintain milk production without the need for milk expression.

• • •

If the nursing struggles started after milk production was well established, maintaining milk production may require less milk expression.

The number of milk expressions per day needed to maintain milk production depends in part on baby's age, how much other foods baby consumes, and the nursing parent's storage capacity. For details, see p. 504-506 in the section "Maintaining Full Milk Production" in Chapter 11, "Milk Expression and Storage."

TABLE 3.1 Milk Intake by Age

Baby's Age	Average Milk Per Feeding	Average Milk Per Day
First week (after Day 4)	1-2 oz. (30-59 mL)	10-20 oz. (296-591 mL)
Weeks 2 and 3	2-3 oz. (59-89 mL)	15-25 oz. (443-750 mL)
Months 1-6	3-4 oz. (89-118 mL)	25-30 oz. (750-887 mL)

Adapted from (Kent, Gardner, & Geddes, 2016; Kent et al., 2013)

STRUGGLES DURING THE EARLY WEEKS

Gathering Basic Information

Before suggesting strategies, first try to determine the cause(s) of the nursing struggle.

Determining the cause(s) of a nursing struggle will help determine the most effective strategies. Babies with a medical problem—such as an ear infection or thrush—may need diagnosis and treatment. If distractibility is the primary cause, minimizing distractions may be the best approach. For the baby who's teething, comfort measures may help. If engorgement is one of the issues, using reverse pressure softening (p. 885) before nursing and feeding more often may help. The baby who struggles with a fast milk flow may find a change in feeding position (see the ***starter positions*** on p. 23-29 in Chapter 1) makes it easier for him to manage the milk flow.

Some situations require time, patience, and specialized information, such as a poor fit between the nipple size and baby's mouth. Other examples include nursing struggles caused by prematurity, variations in baby's oral anatomy, pain from birth injuries, reflux disease, an airway abnormality, neurological impairment, or other health issue.

In some cases, such as emotional upset due to family stresses, tincture of time and some common-sense suggestions may be all that are needed. Occasionally, an allergy, hypersensitivity, or intolerance to a food, drug, perfume, or other product may be the trigger. In this case, experimenting with dietary or product elimination may bring improvement. Sometimes, the cause of the nursing struggle is never found.

When an obvious issue is identified, it can be tempting to assume that addressing it will lead to settled nursing. But sometimes more than one factor is at work. In one Australian study (Kent et al., 2015), researchers examined the clinical records from 708 consults over a one-year period at a lactation clinic. They found that of the nursing mothers suffering from nipple pain, in 89% of the cases, the pain was due to more than one cause. When a strategy is tried and improvement is seen, be sure the problem is completely resolved. More detective work may be needed.

• • •

Ask questions in a calm, relaxed manner, and affirm nursing families for what they are doing right.

Asking questions in a calm, relaxed manner rather than in quick succession will help put the family at ease. Try to word sensitive questions as tactfully as possible. Make sure they know that not all of the factors discussed will cause nursing struggles. Individual differences in parents and babies create a wide range of reactions to the same factor. For example, a baby who easily coordinates sucking, swallowing, and breathing may be able to cope well with an overabundant milk production, while another baby who is not as well-coordinated may find the same milk flow overwhelming and stop latching altogether. One baby may nurse well no matter what his nursing parent's diet, while another baby may be sensitive to some foods. One baby is easygoing and resilient, while another baby fusses or stops nursing whenever household stress runs high.

The intensity of a baby's response may also vary with the same factor, causing one baby to fuss while latching and another to go on a "nursing strike." To make nursing parents less likely to blame themselves for the feeding struggle, emphasize these individual differences, which also explains why many families notice nursing differences from one child to the next. There are general dynamics at work, but there are no hard-and-fast nursing rules.

When nursing struggles happen, many parents feel vulnerable, so be sure to affirm them for what they are doing right and for their efforts to overcome the problem.

• • •

Ask the baby's age now, his age when the nursing struggles started, and at what point during the feed the problem starts.

Knowing at what age the feeding problem began provides a good starting point and valuable clues to the causes(s) of the problem. See Box 3.1 for an overview of nursing struggles starting at birth and Box 3.2 for an overview of feeding problems that start from Day 2 to 5. Knowing when during the feed the problem starts may also help in determining the cause.

Problem starts before milk ejection. Consider:

- Positioning issues causing discomfort or shallow latch
- Shallow latch caused by positioning issues or taut mammary tissue
- Pain from a birth injury, medical procedure, or other cause
- Oral anatomical variations in the baby
- Health problems, such as prematurity, airway abnormality, or neurological impairment

Problem starts with milk ejection. If the baby coughs or gasps when the milk ejection occurs, he may have problems coping with milk flow. In this case, suggest trying a semi-reclined starter position with baby tummy down on the parent's body (see p. 23-29 in Chapter 1). Other contributing factors could be abundant milk production, variations in baby's oral anatomy, airway abnormality, or neurological impairment.

Problem starts later in the feed. If the baby gets fussier and fussier as the feed goes on, the baby may simply need to burp or pass a stool. Consider the need to burp when the baby gulps loudly as he nurses, which may indicate he's swallowing a lot of air. Another possible cause is low milk production.

Interactive Factors

Positioning

Ask what feeding positions they are using.

Nursing can be more challenging in the early weeks if upright feeding positions are used, because the newborn has little head-and-neck control, which limits his ability to take an active role during latching. This is not an issue for the baby older than about 6 weeks, who has more head-and-neck control. A newborn, however, needs much more help in upright positions. Nursing parents must support baby's weight in arms, keep baby's body pressed against theirs, and keep baby well-aligned to the nipple. A parent nursing for the first time may be unaware of how much support a newborn needs in upright positions, and this can lead to common problems: a shallow latch, latching struggles, and other challenges. Both U.K. and Australian research (S. D. Colson, Meek, & Hawdon, 2008; Douglas & Keogh, 2017) found that semi-reclined feeding positions (using a 15° to 65° parental body slope) with baby resting tummy down on the nursing parent's body, make early nursing easier for most families. When the conditions are right, babies are hardwired to find the nipple and latch with very little help.

When positioning seems to be contributing to nursing struggles, suggest trying these starter positions and experiment by using the three basic adjustments described in Chapter 1 (adjust your body, adjust your baby, adjust your breast) until they find their own best fit. (Families can watch a demonstration video of these adjustments at **NaturalBreastfeeding.com**.) Nursing goes more smoothly for some babies if they are first allowed to lie for a few minutes on their parent's body in a position similar to the one they assumed in the womb (S. Colson, 2005). Ideally, in any position, the nursing parent should have enough body support to nurse with relaxed neck and shoulder muscles and can maintain the position comfortably for at least 30 to 60 minutes. For more details, see the section "Positioning Basics," starting on p. 21 in Chapter 1, "Basic Nursing Dynamics."

> **KEY CONCEPT**
>
> *Semi-reclined starter positions can reduce nursing struggles for many families, especially during the newborn period.*

• • •

Ask about nipple pain or trauma.

Nipple pain and trauma can indicate:

- **A shallow latch,** which may be due to positioning issues or baby's inability to draw taut mammary tissue deeply into his mouth.
- **Abnormal tongue movements** during nursing, due to oral restrictions, such as tongue-tie or "superficial nipple sucking" from early exposure to bottles or pacifiers (Praborini et al., 2016; Righard, 1998).

BOX 3.1 Factors Contributing to Nursing Struggles That Start at Birth

Interactive Factors

- Post-delivery practices that interfere with inborn feeding behaviors (see Chapter 2), such as labor medications, routine suctioning, unnecessary formula supplements, and separation
- Positioning issues and/or shallow latch (attachment)
- Poor fit (large nipple/small mouth)

Baby Factors

- Pain from birth injury
- Feeding aversion from rough suctioning or rough handling during latch
- Oral anatomical variations (tongue-tie, lip tie, unusual palate, etc.)
- Health problems (i.e., cardiac defect, illness, etc.)
- Airway abnormality (laryngomalacia, tracheomalacia, vocal cord paralysis)
- Neurological impairment (Down syndrome, etc.)

Parent Factors

- Birth-related pain or trauma
- Naturally taut mammary tissue
- Anatomical variations (size or shape of nipples, mammary tissue)

Post-Delivery Practices

For early nursing struggles, ask about the birth and their early nursing experiences.

Interventions, such as medications during labor and delivery, aggressive suctioning after birth, the use of bottles and pacifiers, and separation after birth can contribute to nursing struggles in some babies. For details, see p. 45-64 on the effects of birth and post-delivery practices on nursing in Chapter 2, "Nursing Rhythms."

• • •

Ask if the baby nursed well during the first 2 hours after birth.

Was the baby allowed to do the breast crawl after birth (see p. 47 in Chapter 2)? Research (Girish et al., 2013) found fewer feeding problems among babies who did the breast crawl at the first feed compared with those who didn't. One French study (Robiquet et al., 2016) found an association between interrupted skin-to-skin contact before the first feed and feeding problems. Suctioning after birth is another possible contributor to early feeding problems, and if done roughly, can sometimes lead to oral aversion. Some question the health benefits of routine suctioning in newborns and recommend against it (Evans & Po, 2016).

• • •

Ask if the baby used a pacifier or was fed by bottle.

Although the existence of ***nipple confusion*** is controversial, in some cases—but not all—early use of artificial nipples/teats may affect nursing. A 2015 review of the literature examined 14 articles (Zimmerman & Thompson, 2015) and found emerging evidence to suggest the presence of nipple confusion with early bottle use but not pacifiers. A 2016 Indian study of 58 non-latching babies (Praborini et al., 2016) attributed their latching issues to bottle-feeding during the first week of life. However, nearly 80% of these babies were also tongue-tied, which led to the use of bottles. After mothers and babies were hospitalized together to provide 24-hour breastfeeding help and frenotomies were performed on the tongue-tied babies, within 5 days 92% went on to nurse successfully. In one Swedish study (Righard, 1998), early use of bottles and pacifiers was associated with a type of ineffective feeding the researchers called "superficial nipple sucking." In this study, 73% of the babies given artificial nipples used this less-effective type of sucking, as compared with only 30% of those babies who were not.

In *The Breastfeeding Atlas,* U.S. lactation consultants Barbara Wilson-Clay and Kay Hoover suggested that nipple anatomy may also play a role in a baby's response to a bottle teat or pacifier. These authors wrote: "If women have erectile nipples with good elasticity, their babies may not be vulnerable to early exposure to bottle teats" (Wilson-Clay & Hoover, 2017, p. 47). In other words, bottles or pacifiers may pose a greater risk of feeding problems in babies whose nursing parents have flat or inverted nipples. Wilson-Clay and Hoover suggest the fast flow of the bottle and the firm teat provide a "supernormal stimulus" in the baby's mouth, which may lead to feeding problems, especially for mothers with non-protruding nipples.

KEY CONCEPT

In some babies, the use of bottles and pacifiers during the first weeks may contribute to nursing struggles.

The way a baby is bottle-fed may also be a factor in his response. One U.S. lactation consultant reported that if a baby is given a bottle in a similar way that he is latched during nursing (lips touched first, nipple inserted only after baby opens wide, etc.), bottle-feeding may not be as likely to cause feeding problems, and in some cases may even be used as a "tool to reinforce breastfeeding" (Kassing, 2002).

BOX 3.2 Factors Contributing to Nursing Struggles Starting on Days 2-5

Baby Factors
• Inability to cope with increased milk flow due to anatomical variations, such as tongue-tie, airway abnormality, or other health issues • Pain from circumcision or any other painful medical procedure
Parent Factors
• Newly taut mammary tissue from edema (due to excess IV fluids), fullness from increased milk production, and/or engorgement • Delay in milk production, baby underfed (weight loss ≥10%) • Fast milk flow from overabundant milk production, overwhelming baby

Poor Fit

Do very wide or long nipples prevent the baby from nursing effectively or comfortably?

The term ***poor fit*** is used to describe the combination of a nursing parent with very large nipples (wide and/or long) and a baby with a very small mouth. No matter how ideal their nursing dynamics, in some cases, due to a poor nipple-baby fit, the baby may only be able to fit the nipple, rather than the nipple and some of the areola, in his mouth, which can lead to nipple pain and/or slow milk flow. This is considered an "interactive factor" because if this same nursing parent had a larger baby with a larger mouth, nursing might go smoothly. For more details, see the last point on p. 113 in the section, "Nipple Size and Shape."

Baby Factors

If one of the following baby factors is affecting milk intake, keep the basic priorities in mind throughout the process.

This section includes strategies to try when the following baby factors contribute to nursing struggles. While helping families achieve settled nursing, keep in mind the basic priorities:

1. Feed the baby
2. Safeguard the milk production

This means ensuring that the baby receives the milk he needs throughout the process. This may involve finding strategies right away that allow the baby to nurse effectively and often. Or, if that's not possible, discuss with the family which supplemental feeding method they prefer and discuss supplement options (expressed milk, donor milk, formula, and depending on baby's age, solid foods and other fluids). If the baby is not nursing at all or is not latching and feeding often enough, make sure the family has the information they need to establish or maintain adequate milk production, with hand expression and/or pumping (for details, see Chapter 11, "Milk Expression and Storage").

Sleepy Baby

Ask about the baby's wake and sleep patterns.

During the first few weeks after birth, some babies spend so much time sleeping that it is difficult to nurse at least eight times each day. If so, suggest the following strategies:

- **Make sure the baby is not too warm.** Unwrap the baby or dress in lighter clothes; an overheated baby is a sleepy baby.

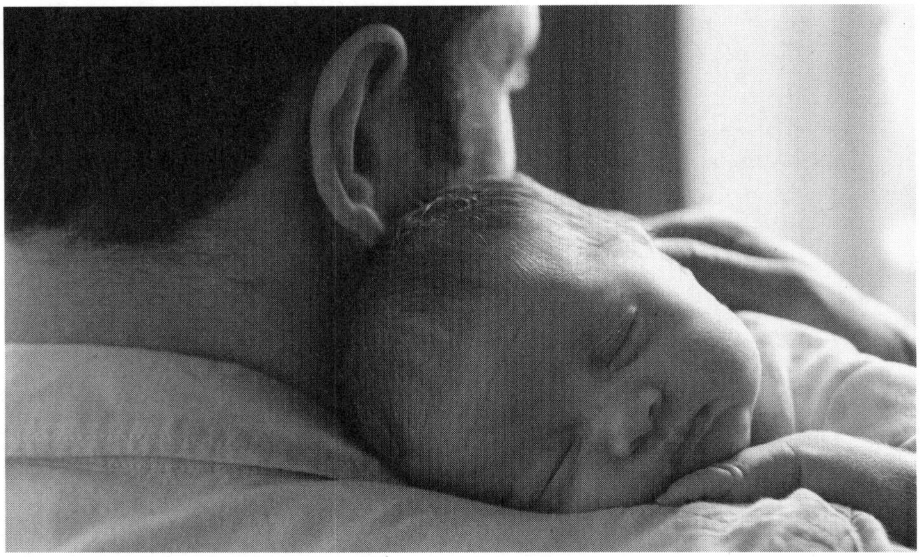

- **Keep the baby tummy down on the parent's semi-reclined body** as much as possible, either in skin-to-skin contact or lightly dressed, to trigger baby's inborn feeding behaviors. Being swaddled and laid in a crib or bassinet can cause some babies to miss feeds (Nelson, 2017).
- **Cluster or bunch feeds together** during baby's naturally occurring alert times.
- **Guide baby to latch when he is in a light sleep.** Don't wait until baby is wide awake to feed; help him latch when there are any movements (eyes moving under eyelids, mouth or hand movements, etc.), which are signs baby is in a light sleep.

U.K. research midwife Suzanne Colson (S. Colson, DeRooy, & Hawdon, 2003) found that newborns—even late preterm newborns—can nurse effectively while in a light sleep. Some babies even latch more easily and feed more effectively in this state.

KEY CONCEPT

Babies can nurse effectively while in light sleep.

Newborns move in and out of sleep often. A long stretch of up to 4 to 5 hours of sleep is not a cause for concern, as long as the baby nurses at least 8 times in 24 hours. Make sure the parents know that nursing babies do not typically feed at regular time intervals (Benson, 2001) and that there is no advantage to doing so. Suggest counting the number of feeds over a 24-hour period without worrying about the time intervals between feeds.

• • •

Ask about the baby's weight gain and stool output.

Baby's weight gain indicates whether or not low milk intake is a factor in baby's sleepiness (see next section). If a newborn is consistently underfed, eventually the baby will start sleeping more and more and become difficult to rouse. This kind of extreme sleepiness may mistakenly convince parents that their baby is satisfied or just a "good sleeper." Be sure to rule out underfeeding as the cause of sleepiness by asking about baby's weight gain and stool output. Between the fourth or fifth day of life until about 3 months (when weight gain slows), expect babies to gain about 1 ounce (28 g) per day. Although diaper output is not a reliable gauge of milk intake (DiTomasso & Paiva, 2018; Nommsen-Rivers et al., 2008), the color and number of stools can provide a clue to milk intake. By Day 6, expect each day at least four yellow stools the size of a U.S. quarter (2.5 cm) or larger (Shrago et al., 2006).

A newborn who is well fed may also be sleepy, but his weight gain will be average or above. For more details about diaper output and weight gain, see the last point on p. 202 in Chapter 6, Weight Gain and Growth."

• • •

Ask if the baby's sleepiness began when the mammary tissue felt fuller.

Taut mammary tissue may occur naturally and be ongoing, or it may be temporary. When feelings of fullness are due to increased milk production, fullness or firmness usually occurs around Day 4 or 5 after birth. Mammary firmness from excess IV fluids may occur within a day or two after delivery and in some rare cases may prolong engorgement for as long as 10 to 14 days (Cotterman, 2004; Gonik & Cotton, 1984).

If the baby's sleepiness started after mammary fullness occurred, it may be because the baby is unable to draw the firmer tissue deeply into his mouth (which triggers active sucking), and he may need help in the form of tissue shaping or reverse pressure softening. For details, see the later section "Taut Mammary Tissue" and p. 884-888 in Appendix A, "Techniques."

• • •

Ask if the baby quickly falls asleep after latching.

The most common cause of babies falling asleep quickly during feeds is a shallow latch. Active sucking is triggered by the stimulation of the tissue deep within the baby's mouth. When a baby latches shallowly, this trigger may be missing. Helping the baby latch deeper is often all that's needed to turn a sleepy feeder into an actively sucking baby. Strategies to achieve a deeper latch include using starter positions so baby self-attaches (p. 23-29) or an asymmetrical latch (p. 878) in other positions.

Combining breast compression with a deeper latch can help speed milk flow and stimulate a longer period of active sucking in the baby. For details on breast compression, see p. 889 in Appendix A, "Techniques."

• • •

Ask about the labor and birth and whether the baby is jaundiced or ill.

A difficult labor and delivery can leave baby exhausted. Some labor medications can sedate baby, decreasing alertness, and make the baby appear less interested in nursing (Martin, Vickers, Landau, & Reece-Stremtan, 2018). For details on the link between some labor medications and a baby's feeding effectiveness, see p. 40-43 in the section "Birth Practices and Early Nursing" in Chapter 2, "Nursing Rhythms."

A baby who is severely jaundiced or ill may be less alert. For details, see p. 250 in Chapter 7, "Newborn Hypoglycemia and Jaundice." Ask when the baby was last seen by his healthcare provider and whether he has any health issues. If the baby appears to have no health issues affecting his sleepiness, suggest the strategies listed in the first point in this section.

Underfed Baby

Ask how many times each day the baby nurses, how much time he spends on each side, and baby's birth weight and weight now.

As described in the previous section, baby's weight gain can rule in or out nursing struggles caused by low milk intake. If a baby is not getting enough milk, this can lead to fussiness during feeds or even inability to latch. But low milk intake can also cause a loss of energy and alertness, and over time, babies begin to shut down. When underfed, some babies start sleeping more and more and become difficult to rouse. They may also fall asleep quickly during feeds.

KEY CONCEPT

The first priority is to feed the underfed baby with mother's milk, donor milk, and/or infant formula..

If low milk intake is an issue, the first priority is to feed the baby, with expressed mother's milk, donor milk, or if neither is available, a substitute recommended by the baby's healthcare provider. Next, it is important to get to the root cause of the baby's low milk intake, which may be due to one or more of the following:

- **Baby is not nursing often or long enough** (see p. 205-208, the section "Basic Nursing Dynamics" in Chapter 6, "Weight Gain and Growth.")
- **Low milk production** (see p. 433-457, the section "Low Milk Production" in Chapter 10, "Making Milk.")
- **Baby nurses ineffectively** (see p. 211-212, the section "Ineffective Nursing" in Chapter 6, "Weight Gain and Growth.")

If the baby's weight gain is average or high, consider other causes for the nursing struggles.

• • •

Ask if the parent or the baby was diagnosed with any health problems and if either is taking any medications.

A variety of health problems in the nursing parent can affect early milk production, such as Type 1 diabetes (which can delay milk increase after birth by a day or so), gestational ovarian theca lutein cysts, and hypothyroidism (which can cause low milk production at any stage of lactation), as can some medications (see Table 10.2 on p. 419 in Chapter 10, "Making Milk"). A baby's feeding effectiveness can also be affected by health problems, such as cardiac disease, cleft palate, Down syndrome, and other conditions and illnesses (see Chapter 8, "Baby's Anatomy and Health Issues").

Discomfort or Pain During Nursing

Birth Injury

Ask about the length of labor, if the baby was born in an unusual position (i.e., breech, posterior, etc.), or if he suffered any birth injuries.

A long and difficult labor is stressful for both birthing parent and baby and may leave baby sore or uncomfortable in some or all feeding positions. If forceps were used, the baby may be bruised or have a headache or hematoma. The pain of a dislocated hip or a broken clavicle may decrease a baby's interest in feeding. If the baby seems fussy much of the time, ask if he was carefully examined by a healthcare professional to rule out pain or injury.

If the baby has a painful physical condition that makes feeding difficult, suggest experimenting with different positions (see Chapter 1) and using those that are most comfortable. Also suggest the family ask the baby's healthcare provider about pain medication for the baby. If a comfortable feeding position cannot be found and the baby is not latching, suggest expressing milk for the baby until the injuries have healed enough to nurse comfortably. To establish full milk production with milk expression, see p. 498-504 in Chapter 11, "Milk Expression and Storage."

Circumcision

If the baby is a boy, ask if he has been circumcised.

In some babies, the pain of circumcision causes nursing struggles. After this procedure, a baby may have trouble settling to nurse or may shut down and be unresponsive. Although a 2016 U.S. retrospective study of 797 newborns (Mondzelewski, Gahagan, Johnson, Madanat, & Rhee, 2016) found no association between timing of circumcision during the hospital stay and exclusive breastfeeding rates at hospital discharge, babies' responses to circumcision vary. If circumcision appears to be the cause of nursing struggles, suggest asking the baby's healthcare provider to recommend pain medication for the baby while he recovers.

KEY CONCEPT

Babies in pain may have difficulty nursing.

Torticollis

U.S. research estimated that 10% of babies younger than 8 weeks old prefer to hold their heads to one side (Boere-Boonekamp & van der Linden-Kuiper, 2001). In some cases, this may be a sign of torticollis, from the Latin words meaning "twisted neck," which can be caused by a confined position in the womb. When a baby's neck muscles are pulled to one side, this pulls the baby's lower jaw and affects jaw development in utero, which may give the baby's jaw an asymmetrical look. In some cases, the baby also may be in pain (Mojab, 2007).

Ask if the baby keeps his head turned to one side and if the baby's lower jaw looks tilted.

One review of the literature (Wall & Glass, 2006) described 11 babies with asymmetrical lower jaws (mandibles), whose lower gumlines looked tilted to one side rather than parallel. Ten of the 11 mothers had labor and birth complications. All had breastfeeding problems, including nipple pain, latching difficulties, and ineffective feeding. Nine of the 11 babies needed supplementation. The authors suggested that nursing struggles may be the first symptoms in babies with undiagnosed torticollis.

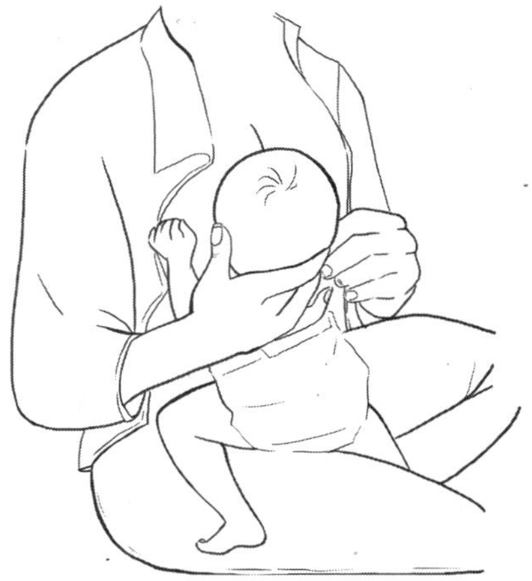

Figure 3.1 Upright type of straddle feeding position.

For babies with this condition, encourage experimenting with different feeding positions until they find the positions most comfortable for them both. If one position is clearly best, encourage the family to use that one for now. U.S. lactation consultant Catherine Watson Genna wrote in an article describing approaches to nursing the baby with torticollis (Genna, 2015, p. 217):

> "The mechanistic approach to positioning and latch (place tab A into slot B) can exacerbate breastfeeding difficulties. Infants are more likely to achieve comfortable stable positions if placed prone on their reclining mother. Postpartum women respond to support for their intuition and language that paints a picture rather than 'left-brained' lists of instruction."

Very different positions may work best on each side. Sometimes the baby may need to be positioned in the same way on both sides (LeVan, 2011). This can often be done by simply sliding baby's body to the other side. An occupational or physical therapist can recommend therapeutic exercises to help improve the baby's range of motion.

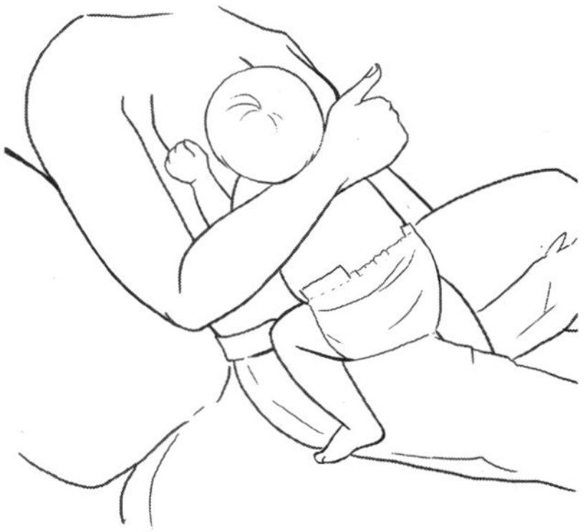

Figure 3.2 Semi-reclined type of straddle feeding position.

Hip Dysplasia

Hip dysplasia occurs when a baby's hip socket did not form correctly, requiring a brace or cast to keep the thigh bone pressed into the hip socket. Unusual stress on the baby's hip should be avoided, which makes positioning for feeding more challenging, because a brace or cast may make it impossible for the baby to completely relax his body against his parent. For this reason, an upright (Figure 3.1) or semi-reclined (Figure 3.2) straddle position may make nursing more comfortable. The nursing parent may also find it helpful to use a pillow for support between the baby's legs (Marmet & Shell, 2017).

If the baby has hip dysplasia and wears a brace or cast, finding a comfortable feeding position can be challenging.

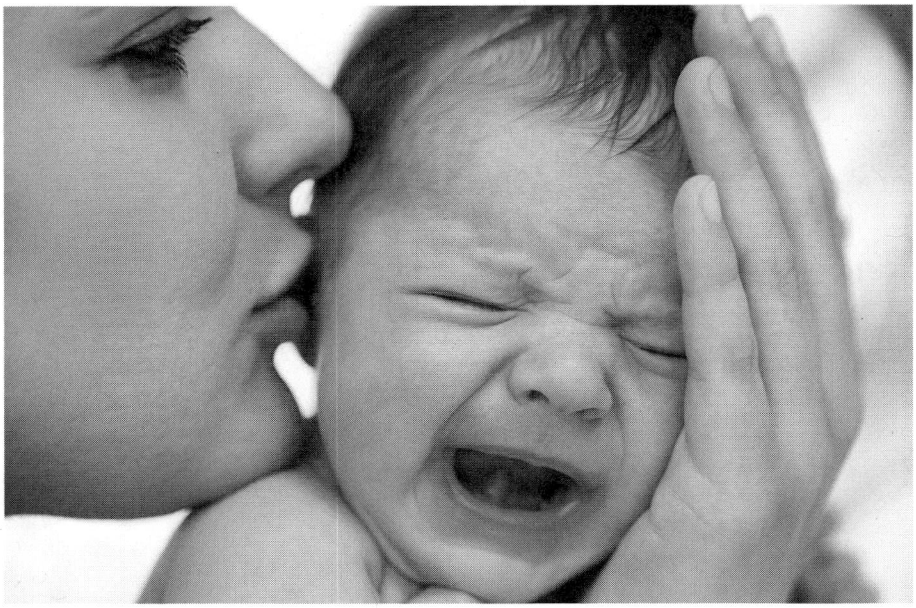

Baby Causes of Ineffective Nursing

Ask if the baby's swallowing is audible during feeds and ask about other signs of feeding effectiveness.

If a baby is not gaining adequate weight (or losing weight) and it is clear that he is only feeding effectively at some feeds, discuss some of the signs that indicate effective nursing. One is wide jaw movements and ear wiggling during nursing. Others are swallowing sounds, increasing relaxation, and baby coming off satisfied. Some pauses during nursing are normal. If needed, share the following signs of possible ineffective nursing:

- **No swallowing heard.** At milk ejection, most babies swallow after every one or two sucks, swallowing less and less often as feeds progress. Some babies feed effectively but swallow too quietly to be heard. In this case, the baby will be gaining weight well and have profuse diaper output.
- **Baby never seems satisfied.** Families often say the ineffective baby nurses "all the time."
- **Shallow latch.** When the baby nurses shallowly, with the nipple in the front of his mouth (instead of farther back in the "comfort zone"), the angle of baby's jaws will appear narrow. A shallow latch may cause one or more of the following: slow milk flow, less milk intake, nipple pain, and/or difficulty staying latched.
- **Coughing or sputtering during feeds.** This can occur with very fast milk flow and also with uncoordinated sucking and swallowing or an airway abnormality.
- **Low or high muscle tone.** "Floppy" babies with low tone include those with Down syndrome and other neurological impairments. Babies with high tone may be in the high-normal range or be neurologically impaired. High-tone babies may appear tense and arch away when nursing, especially in upright feeding positions. For nursing strategies for high- and low-tone babies, see p. 227-229 in the section "Other Strategies for Babies with High/Low Tone" in Chapter 8, "Baby's Anatomy and Health Issues."

- **A clicking sound** during nursing usually indicates suction is being broken. If baby is gaining weight well, this is not a problem.
- **Cheek dimpling** during feeds indicates the baby's mouth is empty and can occur with or without loss of suction. Again, if the baby is gaining weight well, this is not a problem.
- **Nipple pain or trauma** can be due to a shallow latch, unusual tongue movements, or anatomical variations, such as tongue-tie.
- **Unrelieved mammary fullness or recurring mastitis** can be a sign of ineffective milk removal.

If baby's swallowing cannot be heard, audible swallowing stops early in the feeds, or the baby falls asleep quickly, suggest increasing the time spent actively nursing by getting a deeper latch and using breast compression (for details, see p. 889 and p. 878).) for a faster milk flow. If these strategies do not improve feeding effectiveness, try to determine possible underlying causes (see Box 3.2).

Variations in Baby's Oral Anatomy

Some—but not all—babies with tongue-tie and other oral variations nurse ineffectively. Ask if anyone in the family is tongue-tied.

The frenulum is the string-like membrane that attaches the tongue to the floor of the mouth. When the frenulum restricts normal tongue movement, this is called tongue-tie or ankyloglossia. Tongue-tie may run in families. A 2017 Spanish study of 302 babies with feeding problems (Ferres-Amat et al., 2017) found that 25% of those identified as tongue-tied (171 or 60%) had a family history of this oral variation. One U.S. study of 88 tongue-tied babies with breastfeeding problems (Ballard, Auer, & Khoury, 2002) noted a positive family history for tongue-tie in 21% of the babies identified. Also ask about a family history of speech therapy, orthodontia, and sleep apnea, which can occur with undiagnosed tongue-tie.

For more details on tongue-tie and other oral variations that may affect nursing, such as lip-tie, an unusually shaped palate, small or recessed lower jaw, and others, see the section "Oral Anatomy of the Nursing Baby" starting on p. 262.

Keep in mind that like the poor fit described on p. 103 (the mismatch between nipple size and baby's mouth), whether a baby's oral variation affects nursing depends not just on the baby, but also the fit between the baby and the nursing parent. A tongue-tied baby, for example, may have a much more difficult time feeding effectively when mammary tissue is taut and an easier time when mammary tissue is looser (Genna, 2017).

Airway Abnormality

If the baby often coughs or sputters during nursing and/or makes a high-pitched "squeaky" sound, consider the possibility of an airway abnormality.

A young baby who struggles to keep up with a fast milk flow may cough or sputter during nursing (see next point). If a high-pitched squeaky sound known as ***stridor*** occurs during feeds or at other times, this may be a sign that the baby has a narrowed airway and is one sign of an airway abnormality, such as laryngomalacia (narrowing of the upper airway), tracheomalacia (narrowing of the lower airway), vocal-cord paralysis, or other respiratory issues.

For effective nursing, a baby needs to coordinate sucking, swallowing, and breathing. A baby with an airway malformation or instability usually breathes faster (more breaths per minute) to get the oxygen he needs. Faster breathing means less time to swallow, and when a baby has to choose between breathing and feeding, breathing always wins.

• • •

Baby's weight gain can help distinguish milk-flow issues from breathing issues.

When a respiratory issue compromises a baby's ability to nurse, this can lead to ineffective feeding, coughing and gasping while nursing, and even a nursing aversion or "strike." When babies struggle with milk flow, some assume this is a sign of overabundant milk production, also known as ***hyperlactation*** or ***hypergalactia*** (Eglash, 2014). But babies with an airway abnormality often gain weight slowly. When overabundant milk production is an issue, however, babies usually gain weight faster than average, well above 2 pounds (900 grams) per month. See p. 292-293, "Airway Abnormality" in Chapter 8, "Baby's Anatomy and Health Issues."

Neurological Impairment

Babies with a neurological impairment often have either high or low muscle tone, which may cause nursing struggles.

A baby may be neurologically impaired due to immaturity or obvious physical problems, such as a brain bleed, seizures, or one of many syndromes, such as Prader-Willi and Williams. When a baby's brain or nervous system is affected, it can compromise his ability to organize his movements and feed effectively, leading to feeding problems (Genna, LeVan Fram, & Sandora, 2017). However, with practice, patience, and maturity, many of these babies can learn to nurse.

Typically, neurological impairment leads to either high or low muscle tone. Babies with high tone may arch their bodies, over-respond to stimulation, and bite or clench during nursing. Babies with low muscle tone tend to under-respond to feeding triggers. Both high- and low-tone babies may have trouble coordinating sucking, swallowing, and breathing. For details and strategies, see p. 323-329, the section "Neurological Impairment" in Chapter 8, Baby's Anatomy and Health Issues."

Parent Factors

Birth-Related Pain or Trauma

A traumatic delivery can affect how birthing parents experience nursing.

Families react differently to birth trauma. A national survey conducted in England of 5,332 mothers (Beck, Gable, Sakala, & Declercq, 2011) found that flashbacks associated with a traumatic birth convinced some women to stop breastfeeding, because they believed that weaning brought them closer to their "normal," pre-birth selves again. Others found that the act of breastfeeding triggered flashbacks of their traumatic birth, which convinced them to wean. Conversely, in other interview studies (Beck & Watson, 2008; Elmir, Schmied, Wilkes, & Jackson, 2010), some women with a history of birth trauma reported that breastfeeding gave them a welcome respite from their trauma symptoms and that nursing comforted them and aided in their healing.

KEY CONCEPT

A traumatic birth may contribute to nursing struggles, or nursing may be perceived as comforting and healing.

Research found an association between stressful birth and a delay in increased milk production (secretory activation, also known as lactogenesis II) (Beck & Watson, 2008; Chen, Nommsen-Rivers, Dewey, & Lonnerdal, 1998; Dewey, Nommsen-Rivers, Heinig, & Cohen, 2003; Dimitraki et al., 2016). For more details, see the section "Inhibited Milk Increase after Birth," starting on p. 435 of Chapter 10, "Making Milk."

• • •

Mothers described the challenges of breastfeeding after a caesarean birth in one U.K. study based on interviews with 115 women (Tully & Ball, 2014). These challenges included the need for help with positioning, mobility limitations, and the frustration of needing assistance, including being able to get the newborn out of the bassinet to nurse. See Chapter 1, "Basic Nursing Dynamics" for details and illustrations of comfortable semi-reclined starter positions that do not put pressure on the surgical incision. U.K. research midwife Suzanne Colson described how these positions can be used after a cesarean birth (S. Colson, 2005, pp. 29-30):

After a cesarean section, suggest comfortable feeding positions that do not put pressure on the surgical incision.

> "In the first postnatal hours, many mothers are afraid that any body contact with the baby near the recent surgical site will be painful.... [M]others in comfortable semi-reclined...postures can either use an over-the-shoulder position with baby...or...the baby's body draped across her upper torso. Trying different lies often helps a worried mother to breastfeed almost immediately, thus avoiding any direct friction with her fresh wound."

To get a sense of the positioning possibilities, Colson suggests thinking of the mammary gland as a 360-degree circle and the baby being positioned anywhere around the circle, like the hands of a clock.

If upright feeding positions are used, to avoid any contact with the incision, the football/rugby or clutch hold can be used with baby along the parent's side. In a side-lying position, a rolled-up towel or baby blanket can be put between parent and baby to protect the incision during nursing. One drawback is that this barrier will also prevent the close body contact that triggers baby's inborn feeding behaviors.

Mammary Gland and Nipple Challenges

Taut Mammary Tissue

Within the first day or two after birth—even before the milk increases—IV fluids received during labor can cause tissue swelling that can make feedings difficult. Some lactation specialists report seeing an increase over time in the incidence of mammary swelling or edema (Cotterman, 2004, p. 227):

Ask if the ankles or mammary glands are swollen.

> "Over the years, I have observed a rising incidence of severe edema in the postpartum breast, sometimes making it nearly impossible to soften the areola by hand expression, causing unnecessary postpartum and neonatal problems, despite optimal management of early breastfeeding."

Edema increases the tautness of the mammary tissue, which can flatten the nipple and make it more difficult for the baby to draw it deeply into his mouth. To understand this dynamic, imagine trying to use suction to draw a firm beach ball or soccer ball deeply into the back of the mouth. When mammary tissue is taut, it can lead to frustration and latching struggles.

KEY CONCEPT

Excess IV fluids during labor can lead to swollen mammary tissue, making early nursing challenging.

In some cases, more IV fluids are given than were ordered by the doctor (Gonik & Cotton, 1984). Also, one type of commonly used IV fluid (crystalloid) both adds to the body's fluid load and reduces the ability to process excess fluid, extending the amount of time it takes for swelling to resolve. See the next point for strategies.

• • •

When taut mammary tissue makes nursing challenging, suggest starting with reverse pressure softening and mammary shaping.

If the areola is taut, swollen, or engorged, suggest first trying reverse pressure softening (RPS), a technique that moves swelling further back into the mammary tissue to soften the areola and make it easier for the baby to draw the nipple deeper into his mouth. This technique, along with mammary shaping, is often enough to make feedings easier. For details on these techniques, see p. 884 and 885 in Appendix A, "Techniques."

If RPS is not enough to soften the area around the areola and the milk has increased (usually sometime between Day 2 and 5), another approach is to express enough milk to soften the areola. Hand expression is the first choice because its use of positive pressure on the areola is less likely than the negative pressure (suction) of a pump to cause more areolar swelling (Cotterman, 2004). Removing milk will not make fullness or engorgement worse. Removing milk will help decrease engorgement faster. For details, see p. 751 in Chapter 18, "Breast or Chest Issues."

Another strategy to help the baby draw the nipple farther back in his mouth is mammary shaping. For details, see p. 884-885 in Appendix A, "Techniques." Also, suggest trying to nurse in one of the many starter positions (semi-reclined). In these positions, gravity may help draw the swelling away from the areola.

• • •

Ask if the mammary tissue feels full or engorged and how often the baby is nursing.

Between the second and fifth day after birth, normal mammary fullness may become engorgement. This is more likely if the baby has not nursed often or long. Engorgement can cause feeding problems if fullness makes the area around the areola taut. When this happens, some babies are unable to latch. Others try to nurse shallowly. If the tautness of the areola causes the baby to take only the nipple, it can make nursing painful and reduce the milk flow, further aggravating the engorgement.

If severe engorgement occurs despite frequent nursing, this may be a sign the baby is not nursing effectively. If so, suggest the baby be checked for oral variations and other health problems. Also, suggest milk expression to relieve engorgement, safeguard milk production, and provide milk to feed the baby.

• • •

If mammary tissue is naturally taut, suggest shaping techniques.

Some nursing parents have naturally taut mammary tissue. In this case, mammary shaping may be helpful in achieving effective nursing during the early learning period. Usually, as babies get older, stronger, and more coordinated, taut mammary tissue is less of a challenge for them. For details on mammary shaping strategies, see p. 884-885 in Appendix A, "Techniques."

Nipple Shape and Size

Ask if one or both nipples are flat or inverted.

After birth, learning to nurse takes time and patience. If the baby has difficulty latching to flat or inverted nipples, review the suggestions in the checklist at the bottom of p. 28 in Chapter 1, "Basic Nursing Dynamics" and those in the last section of this chapter. See also p. 738-739 in the section "Flat and Inverted

Nipples" in Chapter 17, "Nipple Issues." Most important is patience and persistence. Assure the family that with gentle persuasion and time the baby will likely master nursing.

KEY CONCEPT

With flat or inverted nipples, the main focus should be on getting a deep latch.

Research found an association between flat and inverted nipples and early nursing struggles, but in these studies (Dewey et al., 2003; Kent et al., 2015), the breastfeeding mothers used upright feeding positions rather than the semi-reclined starter positions described on p. 23-29 in Chapter 1. An Iranian study of first-time mothers (Vazirinejad, Darakhshan, Esmaeili, & Hadadian, 2009) examined the effect of "breast variations" (including flat and inverted nipples and "abnormally large breasts") on weight gain during the first 7 days. At 7 days of life, the mean weight of the babies whose mothers had one or more of these "breast variations" was below birth weight, whereas the mean weight among the babies whose mothers did not have a variation was above birth weight.

Although flat and inverted nipples can make the early learning period more challenging for some nursing couples, protruding (everted) nipples are not a requirement for effective nursing. Most babies are happy to suck on anything they can get into their mouth, including caregivers' arms, shoulders, and necks. In *The Breastfeeding Atlas* (2017), authors Wilson-Clay and Hoover suggest that the babies whose mothers have flat or inverted nipples may be more at risk for nursing struggles after experiencing the "supernormal stimulus" of bottles and pacifiers/dummies. Ultimately, what is most important is the baby feeling the stimulation of the mammary tissue deeply in his mouth (protruding nipple or not) to trigger active sucking. So the primary focus should be on getting a deep latch.

Research from India (Kesaree, Banapurmath, Banapurmath, & Shamanur, 1993) found that using a suction device to draw out the flat or inverted nipple before feeding may help resolve the struggle. In this study, a makeshift suction device was used, which consisted of a syringe with one end cut off and the plunger inserted backwards for a smooth surface against the mammary tissue. Several manufactured products made for this purpose are described on p. 740 and 908-910.

• • •

Ask if the nipples were flat before birth.

In some cases, flat nipples may not be what they seem. IV fluids given during labor can cause mammary tissue swelling (edema) that causes nipples that once protruded to appear flat within a day or so after birth (Cotterman, 2004). In this case, the nursing struggle is not due to "flat nipples," but taut mammary tissue (see the previous section).

• • •

Does either nipple seem too large for the baby, or does the nipple texture seem to make nursing more challenging?

Called a poor nipple-baby fit (see earlier section on p. 103), this can happen when very large nipples (wide and/or long) are paired with a baby with a very small mouth. No matter how ideal their nursing dynamics, in some cases, the baby may fit only the nipple in his mouth, which can lead to nipple pain and/or slow milk flow. If long nipples extend far enough back to trigger the baby's gag reflex, nursing struggles and even aversion may occur. With a poor fit, the most reliable solution is tincture of time. Fortunately, newborns grow quickly, and it may take only a few weeks of growth before a baby can nurse well. Since the baby's "oral reach" (the distance from the lips to the area near his hard and soft palate junction) increases as he grows, babies will outgrow poor fit. If the nursing parent establishes full milk production with milk expression, the baby can begin nursing as soon as their fit issues are outgrown.

In *The Breastfeeding Atlas* (2017), Wilson-Clay and Hoover suggested nipple texture may also play a role in a baby's ability to nurse, with "pliable" large nipples easier to manage than "meaty" large nipples.

Mammary Gland Size and Nipple Placement

Do large mammary glands make it difficult to find a comfortable nursing position?

Many assume that large mammary glands make early nursing more challenging, but research on this is mixed. A 2019 Israeli prospective observational study of 109 mothers of term babies (Mangel, Mimouni, Mandel, Mordechaev, & Marom, 2019) divided them into four groups by prepregnancy body mass index (BMI). They found that the higher the BMI, the larger the breasts. Nipple diameter, nipple length and areola diameter correlated significantly with breast size, too. Surprisingly, the percentage of mothers who had latching difficulties during the newborn period was about the same in all four groups: 15.5%. Large mammary glands and/or unusual nipple placement, however, may require creative positioning. Assure the family that it's common to feel awkward during early nursing attempts and that with practice it will get easier. One common challenge in this situation is difficulty seeing baby's face during latch. Suggest avoiding positioning baby on his back so that heavy mammary tissue does not rest on his chest during feeds (Brown & Hoover, 2013).

Figure 3.3 illustrates one nursing couple's solution. (Although it's not visible, the mother's left arm supports the baby's head.) Begin with a comfortable, well-supported semi-reclined position and place the baby tummy down on the parent's body, allowing his inborn feeding behaviors to be triggered before latching. Tissue support or shaping may also be helpful for some babies, but encourage starting with the mammary gland at its natural height to see if the baby can latch well. The less lifting and support that is done, the easier nursing will be.

Milk Flow

Depending on the baby, either fast or slow milk flow may contribute to nursing struggles.

Milk flow that is either fast or slow can contribute to nursing struggles. At one end of the spectrum, a very fast milk flow, often linked to overabundant milk production, can be difficult for a baby to manage. He may gulp, cough, and sputter at milk ejection, and latch on and off many times during each feed to catch his breath. At the other end of the spectrum, slow milk flow may cause the underfed baby to become frustrated.

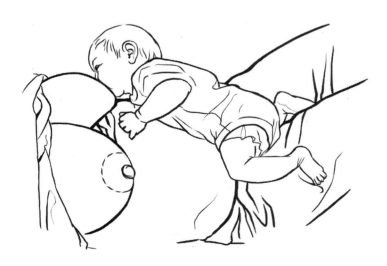

Figure 3.3 One possible starter position for those with large mammary glands and nipples pointing down. ©2020 Nancy Mohrbacher Solutions, Inc.

Overabundant Milk Production

If fast milk flow might be the problem, ask about the baby's weight gain.

If the baby is coughing, gasping, and pulling off at feeds, determine first if this is due to an overabundance of milk or other reasons. If he is gaining significantly more than 2 pounds (900 g) per month, it is likely that overabundant milk production may be a factor. See p. 459. In this case, the nursing parent may also experience discomfort from fullness between feeds or have a history of recurring mastitis. If overabundant milk production is a contributing factor, suggest taking steps to slow milk production. For details, see p. 461-464, the section "Strategies for Making Less Milk" in Chapter 10, "Making Milk." If the baby's weight gain is not above average, see the next point.

• • •

When a baby struggles with milk flow and is not gaining quickly, consider physical causes.

If a baby has difficulty coping with the milk flow and it is clear from baby's weight gain that milk production is at best average, suggest experimenting with feeding positions (see next point), and if that doesn't help, have the baby's healthcare provider rule out any physical problems. The following factors, which are covered in more detail in previous sections, are some that could contribute to a baby's inability to cope with average milk production:

- Upright feeding positions in which the milk is flowing "downhill" into baby's mouth
- Tongue-tie, an unusually shaped palate, or other oral variations
- Pain or discomfort during feeds
- Airway abnormality
- Neurological impairment (these babies would have obvious physical problems) or other health issues

• • •

To give the baby more control over milk flow, suggest trying semi-reclined positions with baby's head tilted slightly back, with baby free to pull off the nipple as needed.

One common recommendation for babies having problems coping with milk flow is to use a feeding position such as Figure 3.3 in which the baby nurses "uphill," with his head and throat higher than the nipple. In these positions, gravity gives the baby more control over flow, plus his inborn feeding behaviors are more effectively triggered (S. D. Colson et al., 2008). When the baby latches, suggest making sure baby's head is tilted back (extended) slightly, rather than chin down or head turned to the side. A slight head extension makes swallowing easier (Glover & Wiessinger, 2017).

Because the baby may need to latch on and off several times during feeds to catch his breath, suggest positioning baby in a way that makes this possible. In other words, avoid holding baby's head to the nipple, which could contribute to a feeding aversion.

> **KEY CONCEPT**
>
> *Semi-reclined starter positions give babies more control over milk flow.*

• • •

For babies struggling with milk flow, nursing more often may make the flow more manageable.

Rather than postponing nursing, which may be a parent's first impulse when the baby is struggling, more frequent nursing often reduces the amount of available milk, making milk flow more manageable.

• • •

Some babies handle milk flow more easily when a nipple shield is used.

If the other suggestions didn't lead to settled nursing, suggest trying a thin, silicone nipple shield. The shield slows the milk flow, which may help the baby better cope with feeds while trying other strategies, such as slowing milk production. For details on nipple shield fit, application, and use, see p. 912-917, the section "Nipple Shields" in Appendix B, "Tools and Products."

Low Milk Production

Slow milk flow can frustrate a hungry baby, which sometimes causes nursing struggles.

If milk production is low, see p. 442 in Chapter 10, "Making Milk" for strategies to increase it, and if it is very low, see also Chapter 16, "Relactation, Induced Lactation, and Emergencies." When there is little milk, this can create frustration and feeding problems in some babies.

STRUGGLES AFTER THE EARLY WEEKS

When feeding struggles start after several weeks of uneventful nursing, anatomical variations and other conditions present at birth are less likely to be the cause.

If the baby is more than a couple of weeks old and nursing was going well—parent was comfortable and baby was gaining weight as expected—it is less likely that many of the physical causes described in the previous section (birth injury, neurological impairment, mammary gland and nipple challenges, etc.) would cause problems now. However, it is not impossible, so definitely keep them in mind. For example, a nursing parent with an abundant milk production may have a baby whose nursing effectiveness is marginal due to a tongue-tie or an airway abnormality. After the first few weeks, as the hormones of childbirth settle down, milk production may decrease drastically because the baby is unable to remove the milk effectively. Some babies do well in the early weeks when the milk production is ample, but as milk production adjusts downward and the baby's feeding effectiveness is poor, problems may develop. This section describes causes of nursing struggles that start later.

• • •

Ask how old the baby was when the nursing struggles started.

The baby's age can provide clues to the cause of the problem. If a baby begins having feeding issues after the first couple of weeks, consider the causes listed in Box 3.3, which provides an overview of many possible causes and the ages at which they are most likely to appear.

• • •

Ask when during the feed the difficulty usually starts and what it is.

The baby's behaviors may provide clues to the cause. Is the problem on one side or both? The timing of the nursing struggle during a feed can also provide clues.

Nursing struggle starts before milk ejection. When an issue begins at the start of a feed, consider:

- **Positioning issues** causing discomfort or frustration. Has the baby recently been immunized or could he be sore from an injury?

BOX 3.3 Factors Contributing to Nursing Struggles after the Early Weeks

Baby Issues

- Change in baby's sucking patterns from use of artificial nipples. Can occur when bottles or pacifiers are used. More likely in the baby younger than 1 month.
- Temperament. Some previously easygoing babies "wake up" at 2 to 3 weeks of age and become colicky.
- Illness, such as ear infection, cold, or others. Can happen at any age.
- Gastroesophageal reflux disease (GERD). Symptoms usually first appear after about 4 weeks or so.
- Hypersensitivity, intolerance, or allergy, causing discomfort, congestion, skin rash. Symptoms usually appear after about 3 or 4 weeks of age.
- Pain when held. May be caused by immunization, medical procedure, or injury. Can occur at any age.
- Candida (thrush). Can occur at any age.
- Teething. Usually occurs after about 3 to 4 months of age.
- Distractibility. Usually starts at around 3 months and increases over time.
- Reaction to a new product the nursing parent uses, such as deodorant, detergents, etc.
- Nursing strike. Usually occurs after 2 months or so.

Parent Issues

- Overabundant or low milk production, causing fast or slow milk flow.
- Mastitis or other issues related to mammary health.
- Stress, overstimulation, or upset, such as household move, holidays, anything that delays or decreases nursing, reducing milk production.

- **Use of pacifiers/dummies or bottles.** This can contribute to nursing struggles in some babies (Zimmerman & Thompson, 2015).
- **Mammary gland or milk-flow issues.** Is the mammary tissue taut from missed feeds? Is the baby sleeping longer at night, causing milk production to slow? Has excess milk expression created an oversupply? Could the nursing parent have mastitis?

Nursing struggle starts at milk ejection. If the baby coughs or gasps, this may be a sign the baby has problems coping with milk flow. If so, suggest adjusting positioning, so baby's head is higher than the nipple. Discuss possible overabundant milk production or health problems in the baby.

Nursing struggle starts later in the feed. When baby starts fussing later, consider:

- **The need to burp or pass a stool.** Loud gulping indicates air being swallowed, and regular burping may help. Babies often fuss before passing a stool.
- **Low milk production.** Is the baby's weight gain borderline or low?

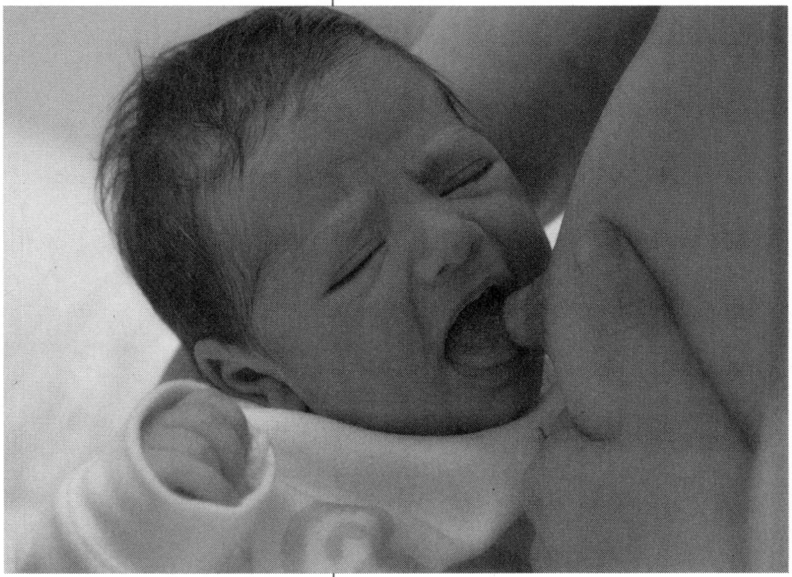

- **Overabundant milk production.** Is the baby gaining much more than the average of 2 pounds (900 grams) per month?
- **Gastroesophageal reflux disease (GERD).** Babies with GERD fuss because feeds are painful. These symptoms usually begin after about 4 weeks of age.
- **Hypersensitivity, intolerance, or allergy.** Expect other symptoms, like rash or wheezing/congestion.

If the baby's weight gain has slowed and the fussiness increases over the course of the feed, suggest the family ask the baby's healthcare provider to rule out allergy and/or reflux disease.

• • •

Ask about their usual nursing pattern—feeds per day, time on each side—and the baby's weight at birth and now.

If baby's weight gain is borderline or low and baby is nursed by the clock, the nursing parent puts limits on number of feeds or feeding length, the baby may not be getting enough milk.

Also ask if baby is fed by bottle and if he takes a pacifier. If yes, ask how often. Ask, too, if the baby is eating solid foods. Overuse of bottles, pacifiers, and solid foods can cause a rapid decrease in the number of times each day baby nurses. When number of feeds decreases, this reduces milk production, causing slow milk flow. Some babies react to slow milk flow by fussing during feeds. If the exclusively nursing baby's weight gain is normal or high, consider other causes. Very fast weight gain may indicate overabundant milk production.

• • •

Ask about any nipple pain or mastitis.

Nipple pain after a period of comfortable nursing can be caused by a shallow latch, candida (thrush), or teething (usually in a baby older than 3 or 4 months. Ask if there is a history of nipple cracks or bleeding. If so, this increases the risk for a bacterial infection and/or an overgrowth of candida.

If there was a recent bout of mastitis, the baby may be reacting to the slower milk flow on the affected side or the salty taste of the milk that is associated with mastitis. If so, assure the family that milk production will rebound after about a week of frequent nursing or milk expression.

Baby Factors

Physical Causes

Ask if the baby has nasal congestion.

When a baby with a stuffy nose closes his mouth around the nipple, he may struggle to breathe. Although a sick baby almost always copes more easily with nursing than with bottle-feeding, neither will be easy when his nose is blocked. Congestion can be caused by the common cold or other viruses and can lead to an ear infection. Persistent congestion may be a symptom of allergy or illness. For nursing strategies and more details, see the section "Colds, Flu, Congestion, and Ear Infections," starting on p. 298 in Chapter 8, "Baby's Anatomy and Health Issues."

> **KEY CONCEPT**
>
> *Knowing when the struggle starts during nursing can help determine the cause.*

• • •

Colic is defined as crying at least 3 hours per day at least 3 days a week for at least 3 weeks (Wessel, Cobb, Jackson, Harris, & Detwiler, 1954). It often starts when a baby is about 2 to 3 weeks old and is estimated to affect between 8% to 40% of babies (Howard, Lanphear, Lanphear, Eberly, & Lawrence, 2006). Sometimes called "high-need," colicky babies may spend much of their first 3 months crying, both during and between feeds. Parents may describe the baby as demanding or intense and find it difficult to help him settle and nurse. Living with a colicky baby is stressful. A 2016 Irish study that included almost 6,000 mothers and babies (Taut, Kelly, & Zgaga, 2016) found that the more difficult the baby's temperament, the shorter time the families were likely to nurse. The parents who participated in a U.S. prospective cohort study of 700 babies (Howard et al., 2006) reported the strategies that worked best to comfort their crying babies (in order of effectiveness) were holding, nursing, walking, and rocking. If the baby has trouble settling to feed, also suggest the following strategies:

Ask how much of the day the baby cries and at what age this started.

KEY CONCEPT

Colic symptoms may be caused by hypersensitivity, intolerance, allergy, or an overabundant milk supply.

Before nursing

- Be sure baby is not too warm or too cold and that his clothing is not binding.
- To help calm baby, if needed, offer a clean, trimmed finger to suck on, pad side up.

During nursing

- Keep sound and lights low.
- Begin nursing while baby is in a light sleep and not yet fully awake.
- Use a semi-reclined starter feeding position (see p. 23-29 in Chapter 1) with the baby tummy down on the parent's body, so gravity works in harmony with baby's inborn feeding behaviors. Allow the baby to self-attach.
- Let the baby finish feeding on one side before offering the other.

At other times

- Devote as much time as possible to holding baby either in skin-to-skin contact, lightly dressed, or in a soft baby carrier or sling.

A 2018 meta-analysis (Sung et al., 2018) concluded that giving exclusively nursing colicky babies a probiotic containing *Lactobacillus reuteri* DSM17938 significantly reduced colic symptoms and improved quality of life. This intervention was not effective in babies receiving infant formula.

• • •

What appears to be colic may be caused by health issues, such as allergy or overabundant milk production.

The regular, inconsolable crying of colic may be a symptom of hypersensitivity, intolerance, or allergy (Hill et al., 2005), which may also be associated with gastroesophageal reflux disease GERD (Gupta, 2007; Sicherer, 2003). For details and strategies, see p. 309-313, the section "Allergy" in Chapter 8, "Baby's Anatomy and Health Issues." One symptom of allergy or sensitivity is crying during or after feeds. Others include skin rashes, congestion or wheezing, gastrointestinal symptoms, and sleep problems. These types of reactions are more common when there is a family history of allergy. If one parent has allergies, the baby has a 20% to 40% risk of being allergic, and if both parents have allergies, the baby's risk increases to 50-80% (Ferreira & Seidman, 2007).

Colic-like symptoms can also occur with overabundant milk production (Eglash, 2014). If the baby has gained significantly more than 2 pounds (900 grams) per month, discuss this possibility and consider taking steps to slow the milk production. For more details, see p. 461-464, the section "Strategies for Making Less Milk" in Chapter 10, "Making Milk."

• • •

Ask if the baby could be teething.

Sore gums from teething can make a baby unsettled during nursing. While teething, which usually occurs after about 3 to 4 months of age, a baby may nurse differently, bearing down on the mammary tissue, or even making chewing movements because pressure helps ease gum discomfort. He may even go "on strike" when the pain is at its peak. For strategies, see p. 712-715, the section "Teething and Biting" in Chapter 17, "Nipple Issues."

• • •

Ask if the baby has white patches on the inside of his cheeks and if there is nipple pain.

The organism that most commonly causes oral thrush, *Candida albicans,* is a fungus that thrives in dark, moist places, such as the nipple and the baby's mouth and diaper area. An overgrowth of candida in a baby's mouth, also known as thrush, can be painful. He may latch eagerly, but pull away repeatedly from the pain.

To determine whether or not this may be a factor in baby's feeding issues, ask if the baby has white patches inside his cheeks that when wiped off look red or bleed. (A white tongue is normal in a nursing baby.) Another possible sign is a red diaper rash, with or without raised dots. Nipple pain may become an issue after a time of comfortable nursing. For more details and treatment options, see p. 727-731, the section "Candida/Thrush" in Chapter 17, "Nipple Issues."

• • •

Ask the nursing parent to check inside the baby's mouth for anything unusual.

If the baby bumped his mouth and has a sore area inside, this could affect his feeding comfort. Also, any sores in the mouth, such as cold sores, could affect feeding.

• • •

Ask if the baby recently had an injection, a medical procedure, or was injured.

Babies sometimes resist nursing if a sensitive area is touched. This could be an injection site or a bruise. If so, suggest trying a different feeding position until the sore area heals.

• • •

Ask if the baby's been distractible and if that might be contributing to his nursing struggles.

Each stage of development brings new skills that can distract a baby from nursing and change his feeding behaviors. For nursing strategies at different ages and stages, see p. 217 in the section "Other Nursing Dynamics" in Chapter 6, "Weight Gain and Growth."

Distractibility is part of baby's normal development and is not a sign he's ready to wean. For more details, see p. 168-169 in Chapter 5, "Weaning from Nursing." If the nursing parent is concerned because the baby is nursing for such a short time, explain that older babies can get a lot of milk quickly and that the baby may only need to nurse for 5 to 10 minutes. His weight gain will indicate whether or not the shorter nursing is a cause for concern.

Environmental Causes

Ask if the family has been under unusual stress lately or if there have been any major changes in the baby's routine.

Moving a household, family tensions, or the nursing parent's return to work all have the potential to affect nursing, especially in a sensitive baby. Even a positive stress, like holiday preparations, can sometimes affect a baby's willingness to feed.

• • •

Ask if any new body-care products are being used.

Use of some nipple creams or ointments may change the taste, causing the baby to become unsettled during feeds or go "on strike." A sensitive baby may register his dislike for a new product, like a new deodorant, body lotion, or even laundry detergent, by becoming unsettled while nursing or refusing to nurse altogether. If this might be the cause, suggest rinsing the area with clear water before the next feed. If deodorant is the cause, changing from a spray to a stick may be all that's needed.

Parent Factors

Milk Flow

With overabundant milk production, a baby may have trouble coping with milk flow and gain weight faster than average.

An overabundant milk production means making much more milk than the baby needs (see p. 457). As a result, the milk flow may be very fast and hard to manage. The baby struggling with milk flow may:

- Swallow a lot of air from gulping during feeds
- Spit up regularly
- Pass a lot of gas
- Wake soon after falling asleep and act hungry, even if he just nursed
- Have symptoms of colic
- Fuss during feeds, gasping, sputtering, or arching away when the milk ejects
- Have regular or occasional explosive green or watery stools

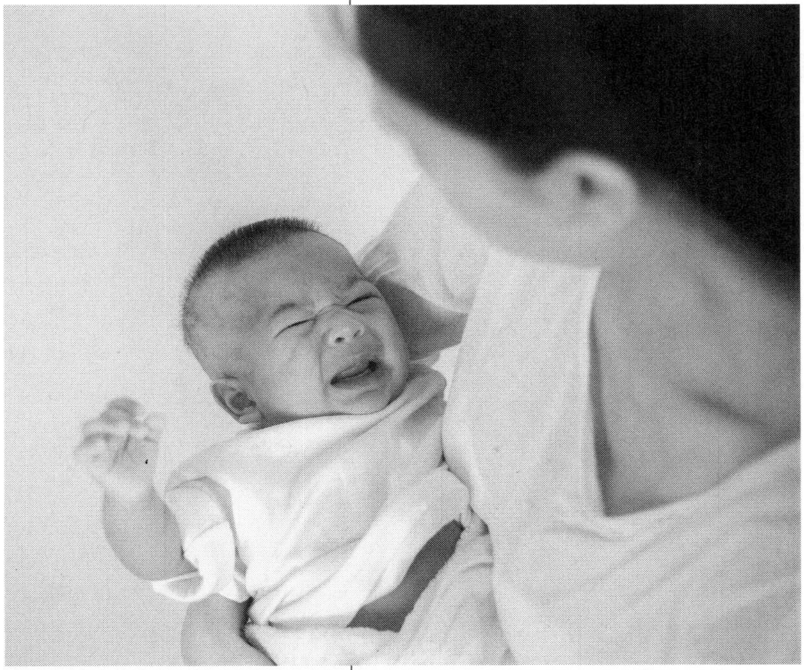

Similar symptoms may also occur in the baby with colic, reflux disease, and allergy.

The baby may have a strong suck, strong muscle tone, and want to nurse often. Or he may refuse some feeds. Some parents report that their baby's fussiness continues as the baby gets older. The nursing parent may leak milk profusely during and between feeds, and the milk ejection may feel painful.

• • •

Over time, a baby who struggles with fast milk flow may develop other feeding problems.

As baby gets older, if fast milk flow continues to be an issue, some babies:

- Become reluctant to nurse at all, even when obviously hungry
- Will not nurse to sleep, preferring instead to suck their fingers or thumb
- Use chewing or "biting" motions to avoid triggering fast milk flow
- Go on a nursing strike

• • •

Ask about the baby's weight gain, which may help find the underlying cause.

When a baby has trouble with milk flow, before considering slowing milk production, be sure that the baby is gaining much more than the average 2 pounds (900 grams) per month. For strategies for coping with fast milk flow and slowing overabundant milk production, see p. 459-461 of Chapter 10, "Making Milk."

If the baby is sputtering and coughing when the milk ejection occurs but weight gain is not above average, see the earlier section on airway abnormalities.

If a baby's weight gain is borderline or low, a baby's nursing struggles could be related to low milk production and slow milk flow. The baby may be frustrated during nursing or underfed. If the baby's weight is average or below, consider other causes. To boost milk production, see the section, "Strategies for Making More Milk," starting on p. 442 of Chapter 10, "Making Milk."

• • •

Ask if the nursing struggles happen during menstruation.

Although it is unusual, some babies become unsettled while nursing or will not nurse when their parent's menstrual cycle begins. According to two U.S. physicians (Lawrence & Lawrence, 2016), some families report that their baby rejects nursing for a day or so with each menstruation.

Mammary Health

Ask if there is a lump, swelling, or any discomfort in one or both mammary glands.

One cause of nursing struggles is mastitis, which includes plugged ducts, infection, and abscess. Although mastitis usually occurs in one side, in some cases, both sides are affected. Some babies nurse reluctantly on the affected side; others refuse that side altogether.

KEY CONCEPT

During a bout of mastitis, milk flow on the affected side is slowed, and the taste of the milk changes.

During a bout of mastitis, milk flow from the affected mammary gland is slowed (Fetherston, Lai, & Hartmann, 2006; Matheson, Aursnes, Horgen, Aabo, & Melby, 1988; Wambach, 2003). Also, sodium and chloride levels increase, giving the milk a saltier taste, and sugar levels (lactose and glucose) decrease, making the milk less sweet (Fetherston et al., 2006).

Assure the family that by following the treatment recommendations for mastitis (see the section "Mastitis Treatments," starting on p. 760 of Chapter 18, "Breast or Chest Issues"), as the mastitis clears, the milk production will rebound and its original taste will return, usually within a week or so. To help the baby accept the affected side again, suggest following the strategies in the last section of this chapter and continue nursing on the other side. Also suggest expressing milk from the affected side as often or more often than the baby was nursing, so the mastitis clears more quickly and the milk production in the affected side returns to normal faster.

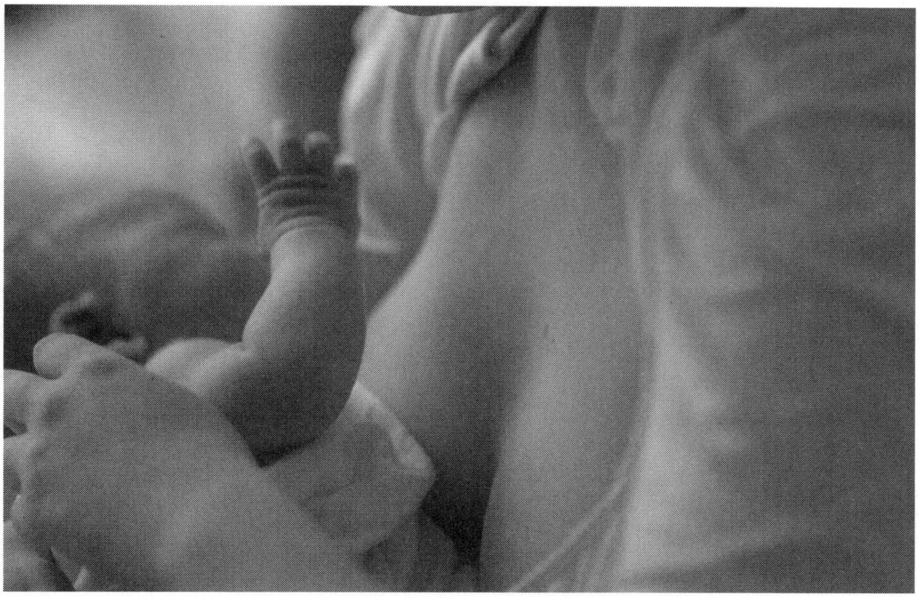

NOT LATCHING TO ONE OR BOTH SIDES

If beginning at birth a baby does not latch to one or both sides, suggest seeing the baby's healthcare provider to rule out medical reasons, such as torticollis, birth injury, oral anatomical variations, airway abnormalities, and illness.

When a baby seems unable or unwilling to latch to one or both sides, the first step is to rule out medical issues in the baby.

When a baby begins struggling to latch to one or both sides after a time of uneventful nursing, ruling out a medical issue is also important. Nasal congestion, ear infection, allergy, reflux disease, mouth injury, and other health problems can lead to nursing struggles. See Box 3.3 on p. 117 for a summary of possible causes after the newborn period.

Not Latching to One Side

One-sided latching is not unusual.

Although often unexplained, many young babies latch and feed well on one side and not on the other. Two Saudi studies reported on this behavior. One retrospective chart review found that of the 2,091 patients whose medical records they examined (Baslaim, Al-Amoudi, & Ashoor, 2011), in 54 (nearly 3%) their babies nursed on one side only. This study also found, not surprisingly, that the mothers who nursed on one breast only were more likely to have complaints (symptoms of mastitis, heaviness) on the unused breast as compared with the used breast.

The second Saudi study, a population-based, cross-sectional survey of 478 mothers (Al-Abdi, Al Omran, Al-Aamri, Al Nasser, & Al Omran, 2015), found that 1 in 4 of the study babies (25%) nursed on one breast only. More than half of the study mothers whose babies latched to only one breast (54%) did not know why their babies did not latch to the other breast. (There was no obvious difference in the nipple shape, breast health, or milk flow.) The researchers called this "infant unexplained preference." In other words, there was no specific reason others could determine for why these babies did not latch to the other side. This one-sided nursing most often began at around 1 month of age.

• • •

If a newborn does not latch to one side, ask if the nipples differ in size or shape or if the tissue on one side feels firmer.

Nipple differences. In the Al-Abdi study described in the previous point, 19% of the mothers whose babies latched to just one breast attributed their babies' one-sided nursing to the small or inverted nipple of the unused breast. If one nipple is more everted (protruding) or less inverted than the other, the baby may latch to only one side. The same can happen if the baby responds better to the size or texture of one nipple over the other. To help the baby latch to both sides, suggest using a semi-reclined starter position and first trigger the baby's inborn feeding behaviors so that he has an active role in latching (see p. 23-29 in Chapter 1). Another strategy is to use mammary support and shaping to make it easier for the baby to latch deeper. Helping the baby get a more asymmetrical latch may also help, especially in upright feeding positions. For details, see p. 878-879 in Appendix A, "Techniques." If one nipple is too large for the baby to easily manage, see the earlier section on p. 112.

Mammary firmness. If one side is consistently firmer than the other, the baby may find it more difficult to latch deeply or latch at all. Suggest starting with the reverse pressure softening technique to first soften the area around the areola before offering that side (see p. 885 in Appendix A, "Techniques"). Expressing just enough milk to soften the area around the areola may also help. Suggest also trying mammary support and shaping techniques described on p. 884-885. Softening the areola and helping the baby get on deeper may solve this problem.

• • •

Ask if there may be differences in milk production or milk flow between the sides.

In the Al-Abdi study mentioned in the first point in this section, 17% of the mothers whose babies nursed from one breast only attributed their babies' one-sided nursing to less milk production in the unused breast. But babies may

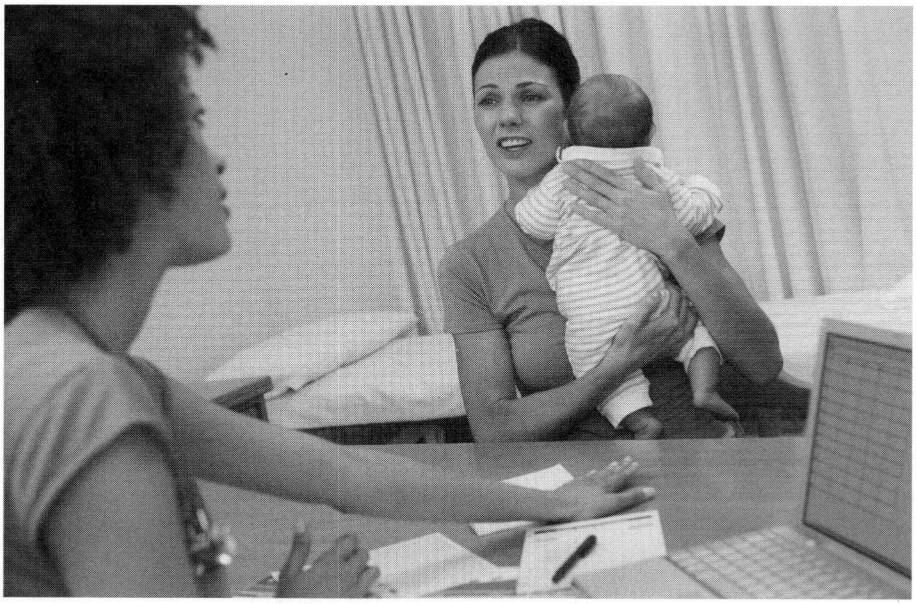

respond this way to either high or low milk production in the unused side. At any stage, it is common for rates of milk production to vary significantly between the mammary glands (Engstrom, Meier, Jegier, Motykowski, & Zuleger, 2007). Also, over time, rate of milk production may change. If a baby nurses more often on one side, for example, that will stimulate faster production there. Also, a case of mastitis may cause milk production in one side to drastically decrease (see later point).

Baby nurses better with faster flow. In this case, suggest stimulating milk ejection before offering the unused side, so the baby won't have to wait.

Baby nurses better with slower flow. In this case, suggest trying a semi-reclined starter position on the difficult side, with baby tummy down on the parent's body. These positions ensure full frontal contact and gravity gives him more control over milk flow, which may make that side easier to manage. For more strategies, see p. 459-461, the section "Coping with Too Much Milk" in Chapter 10, "Making Milk."

• • •

If the baby is a newborn, ask what feeding positions they use.

Some newborns feel discomfort when held in certain positions and may latch to the difficult side if a more comfortable position is used. In upright positions with the baby in front (cradle or cross-cradle holds), typically the baby's head points in one direction when on the right side and points in the opposite direction on the left side. In these upright positions, during latch attempts on the challenging side, suggest sliding the baby over in exactly the same body position (called the "slide-over position") that worked on the easy side, so baby's head points in the same direction on both sides. Babies who struggle to latch when their position changes include those with:

> **KEY CONCEPT**
>
> *Babies may take the more difficult side if a more comfortable position is used.*

- Torticollis (see p. 107), who may find it difficult or painful to turn their head
- A birth injury, who feel pain when pressure is applied in some positions
- Recent immunization or injury

In some cases, a nursing parent may be more coordinated on one side and nursing may go more smoothly when using the dominant hand to help the baby.

• • •

Ask if the mammary tissue on the difficult side is very firm or if there is a noticeable lump or a painful or swollen area.

Mammary fullness and mastitis may cause nursing struggles in a baby of any age. Tissue fullness can make a deep latch difficult. Mastitis can change the taste of the milk, making it saltier and slowing milk flow (see next point). If mastitis is a possibility (sore area or lump in one side), see the "Mastitis" section starting on p. 754 of Chapter 19, "Breast or Chest Issues."

• • •

Although exclusive nursing is possible with one-sided feeding, a good first step is to see if it's possible to nurse on both sides.

Families have exclusively nursed twins, triplets, and even higher-order multiples (Berlin, 2007), so it is safe to say that it's possible in most cases to produce enough milk on one side to satisfy one baby. However, depending on their storage capacity (see p. 416 in Chapter 10, "Making Milk"), the baby doing one-sided nursing may feed more often than a baby taking both sides.

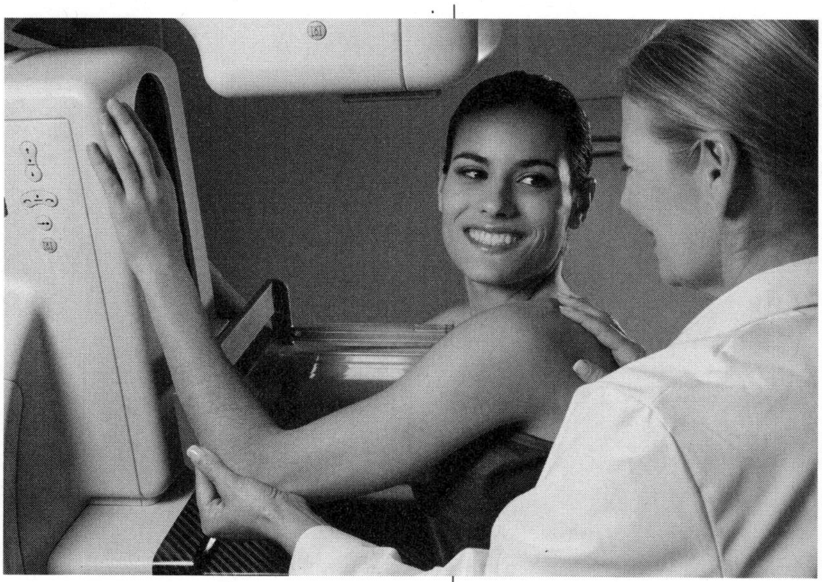

A common worry about one-sided nursing is whether the mammary glands will ever be the same size again, as the used side may become noticeably larger than the unused side. If this is a concern, assure the family that after weaning the mammary glands should return to the same size they were before pregnancy. If they were the same size before pregnancy, they will most likely be the same size again after nursing ends.

If nursing parents want to help baby nurse on the challenging side, suggest during their normal waking hours they express milk from the unused side to establish or maintain good milk flow on that side. Strategies to make it easier for baby to latch and feed on the unused side include:

- **Start nursing on the easier side,** and after milk ejection, slide the baby over to the other side without changing his body position.
- **Offer the unused side after first stimulating milk ejection.**
- **Experiment with different positions,** starting with semi-reclined starter positions (see p. 23-29).
- **Give the baby more help with mammary shaping and support** during latch attempts on the unused side (for details, see p. 884-885 in Appendix A, "Techniques").
- **Offer the unused side when baby is in a light sleep** and less aware.
- **Try nursing in a darkened room.**
- **Try the unused side while walking or rocking** to distract baby.

• • •

If baby's milk intake is a concern, suggest monitoring baby's weight.

See Table 6.1 on p. 191, which lists adequate weight gains for different ages. If the baby's weight gain is too low while nursing on one side alone and there is not enough expressed or donor milk available to use as a supplement, suggest consulting with the baby's healthcare provider for advice on choosing an appropriate supplement. See also the section "When and How to Supplement," starting on page 222 of Chapter 6, "Weight Gain and Growth."

• • •

If a baby suddenly stops latching to one side without obvious cause, suggest parents see their healthcare provider to rule out mammary-related medical causes.

Several articles suggested that when a baby who was nursing well from both sides suddenly becomes unwilling to latch to one side for no apparent reason, this is a possible indicator of mammary disease. One Saudi journal article reported that of eight mothers whose babies suddenly stopped nursing from one breast, two had a breast abscess, two had an infected galactocele, and four had malignant breast cancer (Makanjuola, 1998). (For more details on these conditions, see Chapter 18, "Breast or Chest Issues." Two U.S. articles described cases of mothers whose babies switched suddenly to one-sided nursing who after weeks or months were eventually diagnosed with malignant breast cancer (Goldsmith, 1974; Saber, Dardik, Ibrahim, & Wolodiger, 1996). Encourage nursing parents in this situation to see their healthcare provider as soon as possible to rule out mammary disease as the cause of the one-sided nursing.

The Non-Latching Baby in the Early Weeks

Ask the baby's age and how long it has been since he stopped nursing.

If the baby has never nursed, suggest having the baby's healthcare provider rule out physical causes (see Box 3.1). If the nursing struggles started between the second and fifth day, consider engorgement or a delay in milk increase (see Box 3.2). If nursing struggles started within the first month and the baby received artificial nipples, consider that as a possible contributing factor (Praborini et al., 2016; Righard, 1998; Zimmerman & Thompson, 2015).

• • •

Ask if the baby was suctioned roughly at birth or if there were many stressful nursing attempts.

Some babies are roughly aspirated at birth or shoved roughly during latch attempts without regard to their inborn feeding behaviors (see Chapter 1). In some cases, parents are so motivated to nurse that they spend time at every feed trying to get their baby to latch while he is clearly upset. Some babies will go on to nurse after such experiences, but some may develop negative associations or aversions (Svensson, Velandia, Matthiesen, Welles-Nystrom, & Widstrom, 2013). If this appears to be the case, suggest devoting some time to developing positive associations by making sure all the time spent on the nursing parent's body is time that the baby is happy (for details, see the last section).

• • •

Try to determine what the baby is looking for during latch attempts that he is not finding.

Non-latching babies often struggle to nurse because they are looking for something they cannot find, such as:

- The feel of the nursing parent's body against the front of their body to trigger their inborn feeding behaviors
- The chance to make their own way to the nipple in their own time
- The feeling of a deep latch, which stimulates active sucking
- A faster milk flow or a slower, more manageable milk flow
- A firm, protruding nipple (in babies who have been fed by bottle or given pacifiers)

In some cases, all that is needed to help the non-latching baby latch is to allow them to take an active role in latching. At a time when the baby is not too hungry, suggest nursing parents get into a comfortable, semi-reclined position with the nipple accessible to the baby and put the baby tummy down on their body near the nipple, triggering his inborn feeding behaviors, and letting the baby go to the nipple in his own time.

If a baby latches shallowly, he may not feel the sensation in the back of his mouth that triggers active sucking, and he may become frustrated. In this case, the nursing parent may need to help the baby latch deeply by using mammary support or shaping. If they are using an upright position, it may also help to use an asymmetrical latch (see p. 884-885 in Appendix A, "Techniques"). If the baby's inability to feel the nipple in the back of his mouth is related to engorgement, see the earlier section "Taut Mammary Tissue." For more strategies, see the last section in this chapter.

If a baby received artificial nipples and is becoming frustrated with the soft nipple, suggest trying mammary shaping and support to help the baby feel the nipple deeper in his mouth. Sometimes dripping milk on the nipple during latch attempts can help as well. In some cases, a thin, silicone nipple shield may be needed to help the baby transition to direct nursing. For using a nipple shield (style, fit, application, and weaning from the shield), see that section on p. 912-917 in Appendix B, "Tools and Products."

Nursing Strike

A nursing strike is most common after about 2 months of age, and sometimes, but not always, the cause can be determined.

The term ***nursing strike*** describes the baby who has been nursing well and suddenly completely stops. When babies go "on strike," some nursing parents wonder if this is their baby's way of weaning. However, if the baby is younger than 1 year, this is unlikely, since babies this age have a physical need for mother's milk. Something else that distinguishes a nursing strike from a natural weaning is that the baby is usually unhappy about it. Typically, a nursing strike lasts 2 to 4 days, but it may last as long as 10 days and may require some ingenuity and careful analysis to find the cause and help the baby transition back to nursing. Sometimes the cause is never determined.

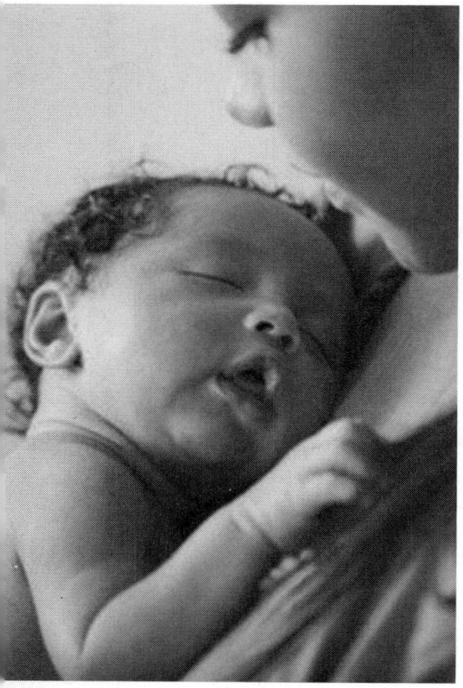

It is helpful to at least try to determine the cause. All previous possible causes of nursing struggles should be considered. Individual babies respond to these factors differently, with some fussing at latch attempts, while others reject nursing completely. The causes of a nursing strike fall into two general categories:

Physical causes:

- Ear infection, cold, or other illness
- Gastroesophageal reflux (GERD), which can make feedings painful
- Overabundant milk production, as a very fast milk flow can upset baby
- Hypersensitivity, intolerance, or allergy
- Pain when held resulting from injury, medical procedure, or injection
- Mouth pain due to teething, thrush, or mouth injury
- Reaction to a new product, such as deodorant, lotion, laundry detergent, etc.

Environmental causes:

- Stress, upset, overstimulation, or a chaotic home environment
- Feeding on a strict schedule, timed feeds, or frequent interruptions
- Baby left to cry for long periods
- Major changes in baby's routine, like traveling, a household move, or parent's return to work
- Arguments with others or yelling while nursing
- A strong reaction when the baby bites
- An unusually long separation of nursing parent and baby.

Finding a cause is reassuring and may influence which strategies to try. Even if the cause is unknown, suggest the strategies described in the last section, "Strategies to Achieve Settled Nursing."

• • •

Safeguard nursing by making sure the baby is well fed and milk production is protected.

Suggest expressing milk as often as the baby was nursing to avoid uncomfortable fullness and to maintain milk production. Feed baby the expressed milk using any method the family chooses, which will depend in part on the baby's age. If a baby is at least 6 to 8 months old, feeding expressed milk in a cup has advantages, as it does not satisfy a baby's sucking urge like a bottle nipple/teat. Without a sucking outlet, the baby may be more motivated to go back to nursing more quickly. A younger baby can be supplemented with a cup, spoon, eyedropper, or bowl. For details, see the section "Alternative Feeding Methods" starting on p. 894 in Appendix B, "Tools and Products." If it's possible to avoid giving the baby artificial nipples, this may shorten the strike. If the baby uses a pacifier, suggest discontinuing it for now.

STRATEGIES TO ACHIEVE SETTLED NURSING

Knowing the cause of the baby's nursing struggles will affect the strategies used.

Knowing the cause of latching issues can help determine the best approach. For example, the baby with a medical problem, such as an ear infection or other illness, will need diagnosis and treatment. For environmental causes, minimizing distractions and creating a calmer setting may help. For the baby in pain, comfort measures and a tincture of time may be most important. But no matter what the cause, the basic strategies described in this section may be helpful.

• • •

Before suggesting strategies, review basic nursing dynamics.

Ask about what happens during nursing attempts and compare that with the dynamics described in Chapter 1.

- Is baby calm?
- Are they looking into each other's eyes, touching, and talking?
- Is the baby in full frontal contact with the nursing parent and baby's body stable and well supported? Does the baby have foot contact?
- Is gravity working for or against nursing?
- Is the baby relaxed with no muscle tension on either side of his body?
- Is baby's chin or cheek touching the parent's body?
- Can the baby's head tilt back slightly for easier swallowing?

Discuss the baby's alignment with the nipple. Is there pressure on the back of baby's head? Must baby tuck his chin to latch? If so, suggest adjusting their body positions, so he can tilt his head slightly back during latch.

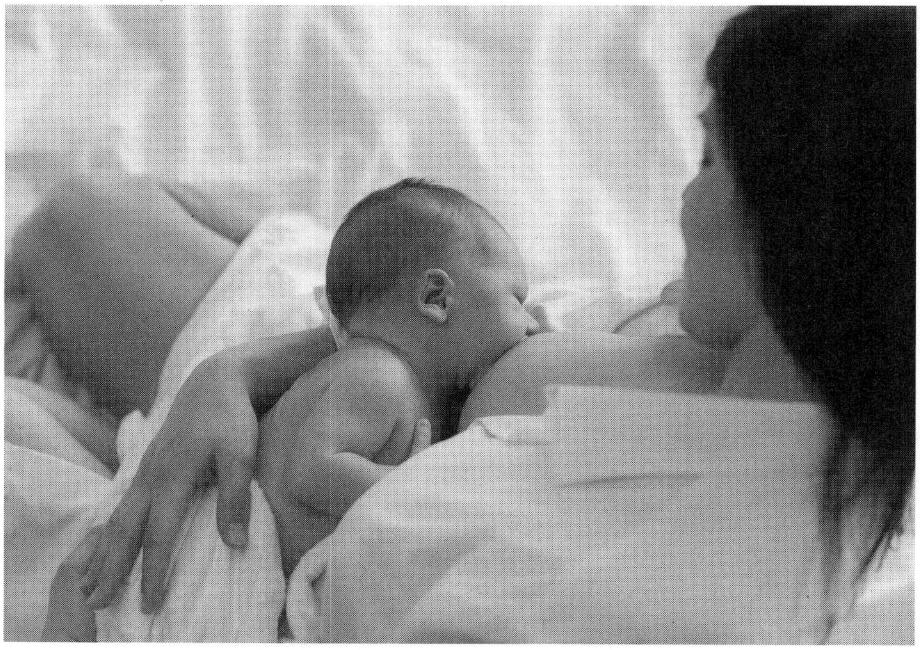

• • •

Time-tested approaches to reduce stress at feeds can help nursing go more smoothly and help the baby who's "on strike" nurse again.

Approaches to decrease stress at feeds include:

- **Make sure the nursing parent's body is a pleasant place to be,** not a battleground. If nursing feels stressful, feed another way and instead give baby lots of cuddle time, including allowing baby to nap with his head resting near the nipple (Smillie, 2017).
- **Spend time touching and in skin-to-skin contact.** Between feeds, suggest holding the baby as much as possible in skin-to-skin contact, with baby's bare torso resting against the nursing parent's bare chest. This is soothing to them both and the oxytocin released makes them more open to one another (Uvnas-Moberg, 2014). In one U.S. group, prospective exploratory study of 48 healthy, ethnically diverse mothers, four sessions of skin-to-skin contact before breastfeeding during the first 2 days successfully helped overcome early nursing problems (Chiu, Anderson, & Burkhammer, 2008). At 1 month, 81% of these mothers were still nursing, more than the local average. A Swedish prospective randomized trial of 103 nursing couples with severe latching problems divided them into two groups (Svensson et al., 2013). In one group, mother and baby were in skin-to-skin contact during latch attempts, and in the other group, they were not. The same percentage of couples in both groups eventually resolved their latching struggles, but those in the skin-to-skin contact group did so in half the time.
- **Attempt nursing while baby is in a light sleep or drowsy.** Some babies latch more easily when in a relaxed, sleepy state.
- **Use feeding positions baby likes best** and experiment, beginning first with semi-reclined starter positions (see p. 23-29 in Chapter 1).
- **Trigger a milk ejection before latch attempts** to give an instant reward, or try first expressing a little milk onto baby's lips.

- **Try mammary shaping or support.** These techniques may help the baby latch deeper to trigger active sucking. For details, see p. 884-885 in Appendix A, "Techniques."
- **Try nursing in motion**—walking or rocking.
- **Spend as much time as possible nursing** at those times the baby nurses well.
- **Supplement if baby's weight gain slows or stops** to make sure the baby gets the milk he needs to feel calm and open to nursing. For a choice of feeding methods, see the section "Alternative Feeding Methods," starting on p. 894 in Appendix B, "Tools and Products."

• • •

Tools and other strategies can help in some situations.

Drip expressed milk on the nipple. If the baby attempts latching but won't stay there, ask a helper to use a spoon or eyedropper to drip expressed milk on the nipple or in the corner of baby's mouth. Swallowing triggers sucking, which can get baby started nursing. Give more milk if baby comes off.

Feed a little milk first. Some babies are more willing to try nursing if they are not very hungry. Suggest giving the baby one-third to half a feeding, and then offer to nurse. Another variation of this is called ***bait and switch*** (Wilson-Clay & Hoover, 2017), which begins by bottle-feeding in a nursing position (see p. 683 in Chapter 16 for photos). After baby actively sucks and swallows for a minute or two, pull out the bottle teat and insert the nipple. Some babies just keep sucking.

If using an upright feeding position, try a pillow for support. For a nursing parent with a disability or one who prefers an upright feeding position, a pillow for support may make nursing easier. Rarely, a baby may find close body contact too stimulating. In these rare cases, a baby may be more willing to latch and feed if a firm pillow is used to provide good body support while he nurses.

If flat or inverted nipples are an issue, draw them out with a suction device before nursing. Research from India found this an effective strategy for overcoming feeding problems in mothers with inverted nipples (Kesaree et al., 1993). For details on these devices, see p. 908-910.

Try a thin, silicone nipple shield. In some situations, nipple shields can be a useful tool to preserve nursing. Consider it for the non-latching baby, the baby whose feeding problems may be caused in part by bottle-feeding and pacifier use, the baby with oral anatomical variations, like tongue- or lip-ties or an unusual palate, the nursing parent with inverted nipples, preterm babies who are not yet feeding effectively or able to stay latched throughout the feed. For details on use, fit, and application, see the section "Nipple Shields," starting on p. 912 of Appendix B, "Tools and Products."

Try a nursing supplementer. If slow milk flow is an issue, this type of device will provide an immediate and steady milk flow and may help the baby latch and keep nursing. If slow flow is not the cause, this may not be a good choice, as for some, the addition of the tubing can make latching more challenging (Borucki, 2005). For details, see the section "Nursing Supplementers," starting on p. 897 in Appendix B, "Tools and Products."

REFERENCES

Al-Abdi, S. Y., Al Omran, S. A., Al-Aamri, M. A., et al. (2015). Prevalence and characteristics of infant's unexplained breast preference for nursing one breast: A self-administered survey. *Breastfeeding Medicine, 10*(10), 474-480. doi:5.0116

Ballard, J. L., Auer, C. E., & Khoury, J. C. (2002). Ankyloglossia: Assessment, incidence, and effect of frenuloplasty on the breastfeeding dyad. *Pediatrics, 110*(5), e63.

Baslaim, M. M., Al-Amoudi, S. A., & Ashoor, A. A. (2011). Unilateral breastfeeding: An unusual practice that might be the reason for future development of contralateral breast disease. *Breastfeeding Medicine, 6*(3), 131-135.

Beck, C. T., Gable, R. K., Sakala, C., et al. (2011). Posttraumatic stress disorder in new mothers: Results from a two-stage U.S. national survey. *Birth, 38*(3), 216-227.

Beck, C. T., & Watson, S. (2008). Impact of birth trauma on breast-feeding: A tale of two pathways. *Nursing Research, 57*(4), 228-236.

Benson, S. (2001). What is normal? A study of normal breastfeeding dyads during the first sixty hours of life. *Breastfeeding Review, 9*(1), 27-32.

Berlin, C. M. (2007). "Exclusive" breastfeeding of quadruplets. *Breastfeeding Medicine, 2*(2), 125-126.

Boere-Boonekamp, M. M., & van der Linden-Kuiper, L. L. (2001). Positional preference: prevalence in infants and follow-up after two years. *Pediatrics, 107*(2), 339-343.

Borucki, L. C. (2005). Breastfeeding mothers' experiences using a supplemental feeding tube device: Finding an alternative. *Journal of Human Lactation, 21*(4), 429-438.

Brown, D., & Hoover, K. (2013). Breastfeeding tips for women with large breasts. *Journal of Human Lactation, 29*(2), 261-262.

Chen, D. C., Nommsen-Rivers, L., Dewey, K. G., et al. (1998). Stress during labor and delivery and early lactation performance. *American Journal of Clinical Nutrition, 68*(2), 335-344.

Chiu, S. H., Anderson, G. C., & Burkhammer, M. D. (2008). Skin-to-skin contact for culturally diverse women having breastfeeding difficulties during early postpartum. *Breastfeeding Medicine, 3*(4), 231-237.

Colson, S. (2005). Maternal breastfeeding positions: Have we got it right? (2). *Practical Midwife, 8*(11), 29-32.

Colson, S., DeRooy, L., & Hawdon, J. (2003). Biological nurturing increases duration of breastfeeding for a vulnerable cohort. *MIDIRS Midwifery Digest, 13*(1), 92-97.

Colson, S. D., Meek, J. H., & Hawdon, J. M. (2008). Optimal positions for the release of primitive neonatal reflexes stimulating breastfeeding. *Early Human Development, 84*(7), 441-449.

Cooklin, A. R., Amir, L. H., Nguyen, C. D., et al. (2018). Physical health, breastfeeding problems and maternal mood in the early postpartum: A prospective cohort study. *Archives of Women's Mental Health, 21*(3), 365-374.

Cotterman, K. J. (2004). Reverse pressure softening: A simple tool to prepare areola for easier latching during engorgement. *Journal of Human Lactation, 20*(2), 227-237.

Courdent, M., Beghin, L., Akre, J., et al. (2014). Infrequent stools in exclusively breastfed infants. *Breastfeeding Medicine, 9*(9), 442-445.

Dewey, K. G., Nommsen-Rivers, L. A., Heinig, M. J., et al. (2003). Risk factors for suboptimal infant breastfeeding behavior, delayed onset of lactation, and excess neonatal weight loss. *Pediatrics, 112*(3 Pt 1), 607-619.

Dimitraki, M., Tsikouras, P., Manav, B., et al. (2016). Evaluation of the effect of natural and emotional stress of labor on lactation and breast-feeding. *Archives of Gynecology and Obstetrics, 293*(2), 317-328.

DiTomasso, D., & Paiva, A. L. (2018). Neonatal weight matters: An examination of weight changes in full-term breastfeeding newborns during the first 2 weeks of life. *Journal of Human Lactation, 34*(1), 86-92.

Douglas, P., & Keogh, R. (2017). Gestalt breastfeeding: Helping mothers and infants optimize positional stability and intraoral breast tissue volume for effective, pain-free milk transfer. *Journal of Human Lactation, 33*(3), 509-518.

Eglash, A. (2014). Treatment of maternal hypergalactia. *Breastfeeding Medicine, 9*(9), 423-425.

Elmir, R., Schmied, V., Wilkes, L., et al. (2010). Women's perceptions and experiences of a traumatic birth: A meta-ethnography. *Journal of Advanced Nursing, 66*(10), 2142-2153.

Engstrom, J. L., Meier, P. P., Jegier, B., et al. (2007). Comparison of milk output from the right and left breasts during simultaneous pumping in mothers of very low birth weight infants. *Breastfeeding Medicine, 2*(2), 83-91.

Evans, M. B., & Po, W. D. (2016). Clinical question: Does medical evidence support routine oronasopharyngeal suction at delivery? *Journal of the Oklahoma State Medical Association, 109*(4-5), 140-142.

Feenstra, M. M., Jorgine Kirkeby, M., Thygesen, M., et al. (2018). Early breastfeeding problems: A mixed method study of mothers' experiences. *Sexual & Reproductive Healthcare, 16,* 167-174.

Feenstra, M. M., Nilsson, I., & Danbjorg, D. B. (2018). Broken expectations of early motherhood: Mothers' experiences of early discharge after birth and readmission of their infants. *Journal of Clinical Nursing.* doi:10.1111/jocn.14687

Ferreira, C. T., & Seidman, E. (2007). Food allergy: A practical update from the gastroenterological viewpoint. *Jornal de Pediatria (Rio J), 83*(1), 7-20.

Ferres-Amat, E., Pastor-Vera, T., Rodriguez-Alessi, P., et al. (2017). The prevalence of ankyloglossia in 302 newborns with breastfeeding problems and sucking difficulties in Barcelona: A descriptive study. *European Journal of Paediatric Dentistry, 18*(4), 319-325.

Fetherston, C. M., Lai, C. T., & Hartmann, P. E. (2006). Relationships between symptoms and changes in breast physiology during lactation mastitis. *Breastfeeding Medicine, 1*(3), 136-145.

Genna, C. W. (2015). Breastfeeding infants with congenital torticollis. *Journal of Human Lactation, 31*(2), 216-220.

Genna, C. W. (2017). The influence of anatomic and structural issues on sucking skills. In C. W. Genna (Ed.), *Supporting Sucking Skills in Breastfeeding Infants* (3rd ed., pp. 209-267). Burlington, MA: Jones & Bartlett Learning.

Genna, C. W., LeVan Fram, J., & Sandora, L. (2017). Neurological issues and breastfeeding. In C. W. Genna (Ed.), *Supporting Sucking Skills in Breastfeeding Infants* (3rd ed., pp. 335-397). Burlington, MA: Jones & Bartlett Learning.

Girish, M., Mujawar, N., Gotmare, P., et al. (2013). Impact and feasibility of breast crawl in a tertiary care hospital. *Journal of Perinatology, 33*(4), 288-291.

Glover, R., & Wiessinger, D. (2017). They can do it, you can help: Building breastfeeding skill and confidence in mother and helper. In C. W. Genna (Ed.), *Supporting Sucking Skills in Breastfeeding Infants* (3rd ed., pp. 113-155). Burlington, MA: Jones & Bartlett Learning.

Goldsmith, H. S. (1974). Milk-rejection sign of breast cancer. *American Journal of Surgery, 127*(3), 280-281.

Gonik, G., & Cotton, D. B. (1984). Peripartum colloid osmotic pressure changes influence of intravenous hydration. *American Journal of Obstetrics and Gynecology, 150,* 174-177.

Gupta, S. K. (2007). Update on infantile colic and management options. *Current Opinion in Investigational Drugs, 8*(11), 921-926.

Hatton, D. C., Harrison-Hohner, J., Coste, S., et al. (2005). Symptoms of postpartum depression and breastfeeding. *Journal of Human Lactation, 21*(4), 444-449; quiz 450-444.

Hill, D. J., Roy, N., Heine, R. G., et al. (2005). Effect of a low-allergen maternal diet on colic among breastfed infants: A randomized, controlled trial. *Pediatrics, 116*(5), e709-715.

Howard, C. R., Lanphear, N., Lanphear, B. P., et al. (2006). Parental responses to infant crying and colic: The effect on breastfeeding duration. *Breastfeeding Medicine, 1*(3), 146-155.

Kassing, D. (2002). Bottle-feeding as a tool to reinforce breastfeeding. *Journal of Human Lactation, 18*(1), 56-60.

Kent, J. C., Ashton, E., Hardwick, C. M., et al. (2015). Nipple pain in breastfeeding mothers: Incidence, causes and treatments. *International Journal of Environmental Research and Public Health, 12*(10), 12247-12263.

Kent, J. C., Gardner, H., & Geddes, D. T. (2016). Breastmilk production in the first 4 weeks after birth of term infants. *Nutrients, 8*(12).

Kent, J. C., Hepworth, A. R., Sherriff, J. L., et al. (2013). Longitudinal changes in breastfeeding patterns from 1 to 6 months of lactation. *Breastfeeding Medicine, 8,* 401-407.

Kesaree, N., Banapurmath, C. R., Banapurmath, S., et al. (1993). Treatment of inverted nipples using a disposable syringe. *Journal of Human Lactation, 9*(1), 27-29.

Lawrence, R. A., & Lawrence, R. M. (2016). *Breastfeeding: A Guide for the Medical Profession* (8th ed.). Philadelphia, PA: Elsevier.

LeVan, J. (2011). Helping your baby with torticollis. *Journal of Humam Lactation, 27*(4), 399-400.

Makanjuola, D. (1998). A clinico-radiological correlation of breast diseases during lactation and the significance of unilateral failure of lactation. *West African Journal of Medicine, 17*(4), 217-223.

Mangel, L., Mimouni, F. B., Mandel, D., et al. (2019). Breastfeeding difficulties, breastfeeding duration, maternal body mass index, and breast anatomy: Are they related? *Breastfeeding Medicine, 14*(5), 342-346.

Marmet, C., & Shell, E. (2017). Therapeutic positioning for breastfeeding. In C. W. Genna (Ed.), *Supporting Sucking Skills in Breastfeeding Infants* (3rd ed., pp. 399-416). Burlington, MA: Jones & Bartlett Learning.

Martin, E., Vickers, B., Landau, R., et al. (2018). ABM Clinical Protocol #28, Peripartum analgesia and anesthesia for the breastfeeding mother. *Breastfeeding Medicine, 13*(3), 164-171.

Matheson, I., Aursnes, I., Horgen, M., et al. (1988). Bacteriological findings and clinical symptoms in relation to clinical outcome in puerperal mastitis. *Acta Obstetricia et Gynecologica Scandinavica, 67*(8), 723-726.

McCoy, S. J., Beal, J. M., Shipman, S. B., et al. (2006). Risk factors for postpartum depression: A retrospective investigation at 4-weeks postnatal and a review of the literature. *Journal of the American Osteopathic Association, 106(*4), 193-198.

Mojab, C. G. (2007). Congenital torticollis in the nursling. *Journal of Human Lactation, 23*(1), 12.

Mondzelewski, L., Gahagan, S., Johnson, C., et al. (2016). Timing of circumcision and breastfeeding initiation among newborn boys. *Hospital Pediatrics, 6*(11), 653-658.

Nelson, A. M. (2017). Risks and benefits of swaddling healthy infants: An integrative review. *MCN American Journal of Maternal and Child Nursing, 42*(4), 216-225.

Nommsen-Rivers, L. A., Heinig, M. J., Cohen, R. J., et al. (2008). Newborn wet and soiled diaper counts and timing of onset of lactation as indicators of breastfeeding inadequacy. *Journal of Human Lactation, 24*(1), 27-33.

Praborini, A., Purnamasari, H., Munandar, A., et al. (2016). Hospitalization for nipple confusion: A method to restore healthy breastfeeding. *Clinical Lactation, 7*(2), 69-76.

Rempel, L. A. (2004). Factors influencing the breastfeeding decisions of long-term breastfeeders. *Journal of Human Lactation, 20*(3), 306-318.

Righard, L. (1998). Are breastfeeding problems related to incorrect breastfeeding technique and the use of pacifiers and bottles? *Birth, 25*(1), 40-44.

Robiquet, P., Zamiara, P. E., Rakza, T., et al. (2016). Observation of skin-to-skin contact and analysis of factors linked to failure to breastfeed within 2 hours after birth. *Breastfeeding Medicine, 11,* 126-132.

Saber, A., Dardik, H., Ibrahim, I. M., et al. (1996). The milk rejection sign: A natural tumor marker. *American Surgeon, 62*(12), 998-999.

Shrago, L. C., Reifsnider, E., & Insel, K. (2006). The Neonatal Bowel Output Study: Indicators of adequate breast milk intake in neonates. *Pediatric Nursing, 32*(3), 195-201.

Sicherer, S. H. (2003). Clinical aspects of gastrointestinal food allergy in childhood. *Pediatrics, 111*(6 Pt 3), 1609-1616.

Smillie, C. M. (2017). How infants learn to feed: A neurobehavioral model. In C. W. Genna (Ed.), *Supporting Sucking Skills in Breastfeeding Infants* (3rd ed., pp. 89-111). Burlington, MA: Jones & Bartlett Learning.

Sung, V., D'Amico, F., Cabana, M. D., et al. (2018). Lactobacillus reuteri to treat infant colic: A meta-analysis. *Pediatrics, 141*(1).

Svensson, K. E., Velandia, M. I., Matthiesen, A. S., et al. (2013). Effects of mother-infant skin-to-skin contact on severe latch-on problems in older infants: A randomized trial. *International Breastfeeding Journal, 8*(1), 1.

Taut, C., Kelly, A., & Zgaga, L. (2016). The association between infant temperament and breastfeeding duration: A cross-sectional study. *Breastfeeding Medicine, 11,* 111-118.

Tully, K. P., & Ball, H. L. (2014). Maternal accounts of their breast-feeding intent and early challenges after caesarean childbirth. *Midwifery, 30*(6), 712-719.

Uvnas-Moberg, K. (2014). *Oxytocin: The Biological Guide to Motherhood.* Amarillo, TX: Praeclarus Press.

Vazirinejad, R., Darakhshan, S., Esmaeili, A., et al. (2009). The effect of maternal breast variations on neonatal weight gain in the first seven days of life. *International Breastfeeding Journal, 4,* 13.

Wagner, E. A., Chantry, C. J., Dewey, K. G., et al. (2013). Breastfeeding concerns at 3 and 7 days postpartum and feeding status at 2 months. *Pediatrics, 132*(4), e865-875.

Wall, V., & Glass, R. (2006). Mandibular asymmetry and breastfeeding problems: Experience from 11 cases. *Journal of Human Lactation, 22*(3), 328-334.

Wambach, K. A. (2003). Lactation mastitis: a descriptive study of the experience. *Journal of Human Lactation, 19*(1), 24-34.

Wessel, M. A., Cobb, J. C., Jackson, E. B., et al. (1954). Paroxysmal fussing in infancy, sometimes called colic. *Pediatrics, 14*(5), 421-435.

Wilson-Clay, B., & Hoover, K. (2017). *The Breastfeeding Atlas* (6th ed.). Manchaca, TX: LactNews Press.

Zimmerman, E., & Thompson, K. (2015). Clarifying nipple confusion. *Journal of Perinatology, 35*(11), 895-899.

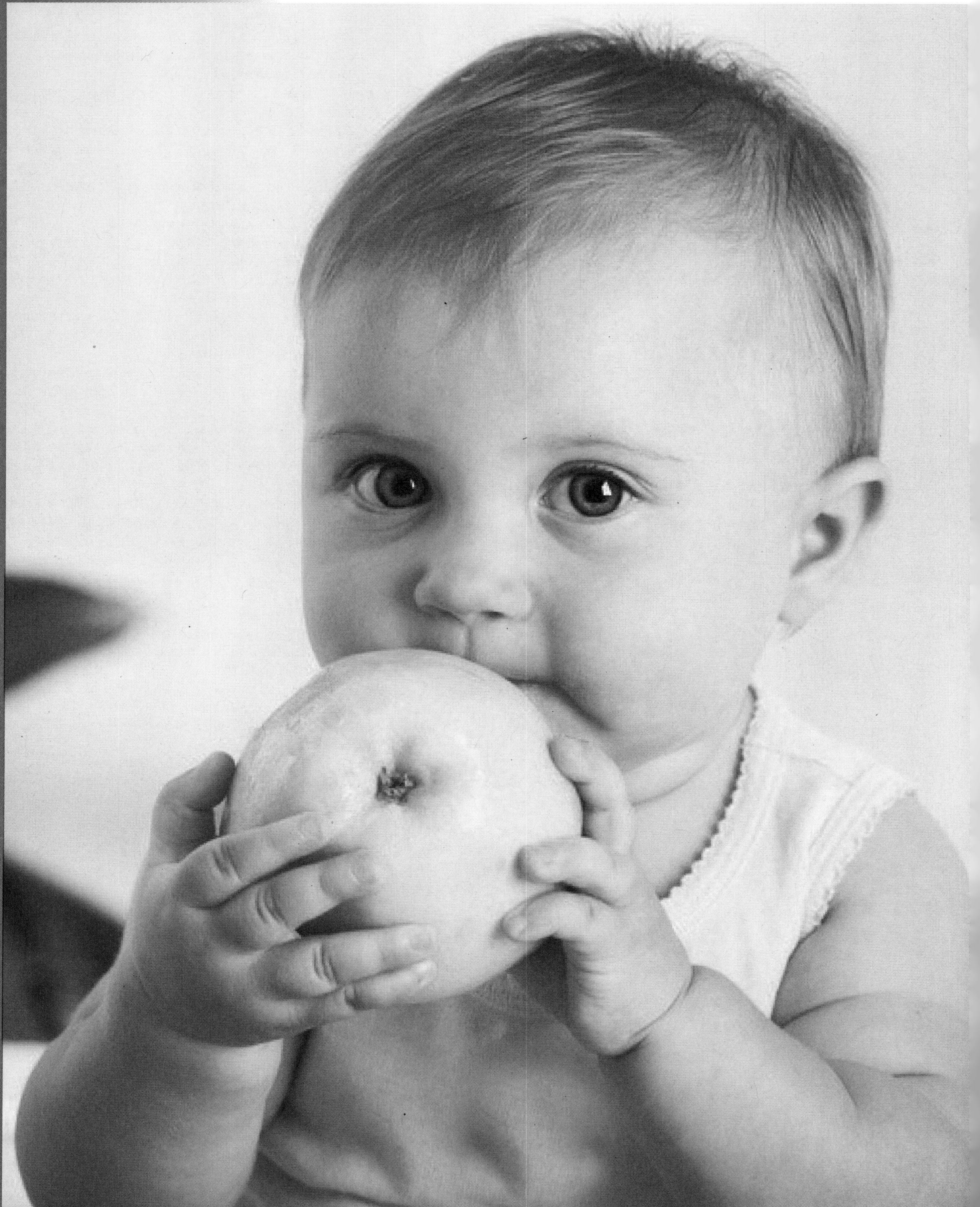

Solid Foods

4

Starting solid foods is a part of the weaning process, which begins when a baby takes any food other than milk and ends with the last nursing. In the U.K., "weaning" refers to starting solid foods, which are referred to as "weaning foods."

WHEN TO BEGIN SOLIDS

Many health organizations recommend exclusive breastfeeding for the first 6 months, with solid foods introduced at about 6 months with continued nursing.

Not Too Early

Health Outcomes

Starting solid foods before 6 months is associated with more negative health outcomes in nursing parents and babies.

For most of human history, babies began eating solid foods only when they were mature enough to begin feeding themselves. In many times and places, 9 months to 1 year was a common time to introduce solids (Brown, 2017b). But in the 1920s, male baby-care experts began to recommend significant changes in practice. These doctors and scientists, whose goal was to make baby care more "scientific," recommended parents feed babies on strict schedules and start solid foods at younger ages. As a result of their efforts and the growing influence of the prospering baby-food industry (Bentley, 2014), by the mid-20th century, it became accepted in developed countries to start feeding babies solid foods during the early months of life (Truby King, 1941). In the 1950s, some health providers recommended starting newborns on solid foods as early as 2 to 3 days of age (Sackett, 1953). During the 1970s, the health community began to question these practices (Wilkinson & Davies, 1978).

After much debate, in 1997, the American Academy of Pediatrics (AAP) published its recommendation that babies begin eating solid foods no earlier than 4 to 6 months of age (AAP, 1997). Another change in recommendations occurred again in 2001, when the World Health Organization published a report by its expert panel (WHO, 2001), which reviewed over 3,000 studies and concluded that starting solids before 6 months of age had health drawbacks for both mothers and babies:

- Babies who start solid foods before 6 months are at greater risk of gastrointestinal infections and diarrhea in both developed and developing countries (M.S. Kramer & Kakuma, 2002).
- Mothers lose less weight and become fertile sooner.

The WHO expert panel agreed that most babies who are exclusively nursed for 6 months grow normally and that the benefits of waiting until 6 months to start solid foods outweigh any risks (WHO, 2001).

After reviewing research from around the world, others agreed (Black & Victora, 2002):

> "A reanalysis of studies in Brazil and Bangladesh has found that breastfed infants in the first 6 months of life who were given additional foods had a two-fold to three-fold higher mortality from diarrhea and pneumonia in comparison with infants who were exclusively breastfed."

Although updated several times since 2003, when the first Cochrane Review recommended 6 months as the optimal duration of exclusive breastfeeding, the conclusions of its authors have not changed since then (M. S. Kramer & Kakuma, 2012):

> "Infants breastfed exclusively for 6 months have a reduced risk of gastrointestinal infection and no observed deficits in growth.…No benefits of introducing complementary foods between 4 and 6 months have been demonstrated….."

In its regularly updated online articles for families and professionals, the World Health Organization continues to recommend starting solid foods at 6 months of age (WHO, 2018).

Some studies in the 2000s found an association between too-early solids and increased risk of Type 1 diabetes (Rosenbauer, Herzig, Kaiser, & Giani, 2007) and celiac disease (Norris et al., 2005), a serious and hereditary autoimmune disorder in which the small intestine is hypersensitive to gluten, a protein found in wheat, rye, and barley. Since then, however, the research on these associations has been mixed. A 2017 systematic review of infant feeding and Type 1 diabetes concluded that the evidence on the association between early exposure to both cow's milk and early solids and increased risk of Type 1 diabetes is inconclusive (Piescik-Lech, Chmielewska, Shamir, & Szajewska, 2017). A 2016 systematic review of the introduction of gluten, and celiac disease found that in light of conflicting evidence, no conclusions are possible (Silano, Agostoni, Sanz, & Guandalini, 2016).

• • •

As a 2018 Cochrane Review on parent education about solid foods (Arikpo, Edet, Chibuzor, Odey, & Caldwell, 2018) noted:

Starting solid foods too early and unsafe feeding practices can cause serious and widespread health problems. In the developing world, which makes this a major public-health issue.

> "Inappropriate complementary feeding practices, with their associated adverse health consequences, remain a significant global public health problem. This is because inappropriate complementary feeding practices, such as introduction of semi-solid foods too early (before 6 months of age), poor hygiene, or giving foods that do not contain adequate nutrients, are all major causes of…malnutrition, diarrhoea, poor growth, infections and poor mental development of children."

In some parts of the world, mixing unsafe water with solid foods leads to serious illness and death in many small children. But no matter where a family lives, using clean feeding utensils and following safe hygiene practices when starting solid foods is important.

• • •

The incidence of peanut allergy has increased significantly worldwide in Westernized countries. In the United States, peanut allergy is estimated to have tripled over one 10- to 15-year period, with about 1% of the population now allergic to peanut (Sicherer, Munoz-Furlong, Godbold, & Sampson, 2010). Because peanut allergy is severe and life-threatening, this is a major public-health concern.

To prevent peanut allergy in babies with severe allergic symptoms, introducing tiny, nearly medicinal amounts of peanut regularly under medical supervision is recommended between 4 and 11 months of age by several health organizations.

Until about 2015, the prevailing wisdom on the best strategy to prevent allergy was to delay the introduction of any solid foods until 6 months and then delay the introduction of highly allergenic foods like peanuts and egg whites until 1 year (Greer, Sicherer, & Burks, 2008). But this recommendation has changed. Based in part on the findings of the U.K. LEAP study (Du Toit et al., 2015), the American Academy of Pediatrics published revised recommendations (Fleischer et al., 2015) that take a different approach. In 2017, the European Society for Paediatric Gastroenterology, Hepatology, and Nutrition (ESPGHAN) published similar recommendations (Fewtrell et al., 2017).

These revised recommendations involve introducing peanut earlier than 1 year with the intent of preventing peanut allergy. These recommendations apply to all babies: babies with no signs of allergy, and babies already showing signs of allergy, such as eczema, even before other solids are started.

The LEAP study, a randomized controlled trial on which these revised guidelines are based, followed 640 babies with severe eczema or egg allergy during their first 5 years. One group avoided exposure to peanut for the 5-year period of the study. The other group consumed tiny, nearly medicinal amounts of peanut 3 times per week (about 6 g in total per week) for their first 5 years. The peanut was intended simply to expose the babies, not to provide nutrition. According to the researchers, regular exposure to peanut resulted in a 10% to 25% reduction in the risk of peanut allergy. Table 4.1 describes the revised recommendations, which provide different strategies, depending into which of its three categories a baby falls.

The most significant change involves introducing peanut earlier than the previously suggested 1 year. The revised guidelines recommend that all babies start peanut at around 6 months, about the same time as other foods. The highly allergenic babies, on the other hand, may be exposed to peanut (rather than eating peanut in nutritional quantities) between 4 and 6 months.

A 2016 systematic review and meta-analysis (Lerodiakonou et al., 2016) found that exposing babies to eggs between 4 and 6 months appears to reduce egg allergies in at-risk babies, however, at this writing, the recommendations have not yet been expanded to include early egg exposure.

TABLE 4.1 New Recommendations for Peanut Exposure During Infancy

Guideline	Infant Criteria	Recommendations	Earliest Age of Peanut Introduction
Group 1	Severe eczema, egg allergy, or both	Provider first evaluates with peanut-specific IgE, skin-prick test, or both	4 to 5 months—based on test result(s), introduce peanut under medical supervision
Group 2	Mild-to-moderate eczema	Introduce peanut-containing foods	Around 6 months
Group 3	No eczema or food allergy	Introduce peanut-containing foods	Age-appropriate by family preference

Adapted from (Togias et al., 2017)

• • •

What does science tell us about the timing of solid foods and the development of allergy? It's complicated, as prolific researcher Dr. Amy Brown from Swansea University in Wales explains in her 2017 book *Why Starting Solids Matters* (Brown, 2017b, pp. 33-34):

> "I looked at more than 100 papers on timing of solids and allergies, and I'm still at 'no one quite knows'....One problem in allergy research is that different studies look at different things—some look at introducing any food, while others look at the most allergenic foods. Some look at introducing to children with a family history of allergy, others look at all children. Some consider only food allergies, while others look at any allergy. The wording can be misleading; some studies talk about early introduction, but actually mean the introduction of allergenic foods at around 9 months! These studies have looked at earlier introduction compared to when many parents introduce allergenic foods. This is totally different from looking at the timing of introduction of any solids."

The association between the timing of solid foods and allergies is complicated.

Another reason so many conflicting studies exist is due to the many confounding variables that influence this equation. Genetics, environment, diet during pregnancy and lactation, timing of the introduction of solid foods, all of these factors affect an individual's likelihood of becoming allergic. For a deeper understanding of these dynamics, see the 2017 comprehensive review article (Munblit et al., 2017) compiled by a large group of international experts that describes many of these factors and their currently understood influence on how asthma, eczema, and food allergies develop in infants.

• • •

From a practical standpoint, the following developmental changes that occur between 4 and 6 months of age—which also indicate readiness for solid foods—are good reasons to wait until 6 months.

In addition to better health outcomes, starting solid foods at around 6 months has practical advantages that makes this process easier for the whole family.

- **Tongue-thrust reflex fades** between 4 and 6 months of age. Until this happens, babies push out their tongue when their mouth is touched, so little food is swallowed, making feedings frustrating and messy.
- **Baby can sit up and reach for foods.** At 6 months, most babies can take a more active role in feeding themselves, because they can sit up alone, reach for foods, and put them in their mouth.
- **Eruption of teeth.** Teething encourages chewing and makes it easier for babies to break down their food for easier swallowing.

• • •

Some suggest—based on the results of a study published in the 1960s of children with learning and physical disabilities (Illingworth & Lister, 1964)—that there is a narrow time window during which children learn to chew and if that window is missed, there may be feeding difficulties. Although the researchers of this older study suggested that this "critical period" was around 6 months, some have suggested that waiting until 6 months might mean missing this "window of opportunity." However, a 2016 U.K. study (Hollis et al., 2016) examined the incidence of feeding problems at age three and found that the children who waited until 6 months to start solid foods had fewer feeding difficulties than those who started earlier.

Waiting until 6 months to introduce solid foods was associated with fewer feeding difficulties at 3 years.

Talking with Parents

Many parents are eager to give their baby solid foods.

Many parents—especially first-time parents—look forward to giving their baby solid foods. When their baby starts solids, many parents feel "proud" and consider it a "big achievement" (Anderson et al., 2001; Danowski & Gargiula, 2002). For the exclusively nursing baby, solid foods may be the first time others become involved in baby's feeding, which can be an exciting time for the whole family. Parents' eagerness to start solids can sometimes lead them to start earlier than is recommended (Clayton, Li, Perrine, & Scanlon, 2013).

• • •

Parents' willingness to delay solid foods until 6 months varies by geography, cultural beliefs, and education.

A study that examined the average age of starting solid foods in five European countries (Belgium, Germany, Italy, Poland, and Spain) found that overall about 25% of children started solids before 4 months of age, and at 6 months at least 90% had eaten solid food (Schiess et al., 2010). In Sweden and Norway, it is common practice for babies to receive small "tastes" of pureed foods between 4 and 6 months of age and to start solids in earnest at around 6 months (Fewtrell et al., 2017). In other parts of the world, public-health workers have spent decades promoting the delay of solid foods until around 6 months. These dedicated efforts have resulted in improved practices in the United States (Barrera, Hamner, Perrine, & Scanlon, 2018), Kuwait (Scott, Dashti, Al-Sughayer, & Edwards, 2015) and Australia (Brodribb & Miller, 2013), where the vast majority of parents start solids closer to the recommended age than in years past. In these countries, starting solids earlier than 4 months is often associated with lower parental educational levels and lower socioeconomic status. In these areas, waiting to start solids until at least 4 months is more common among nursing families than in families where babies are formula-fed or mixed-fed (Armstrong, Abraham, Squair, Brogan, & Merewood, 2014; Barrera et al., 2018).

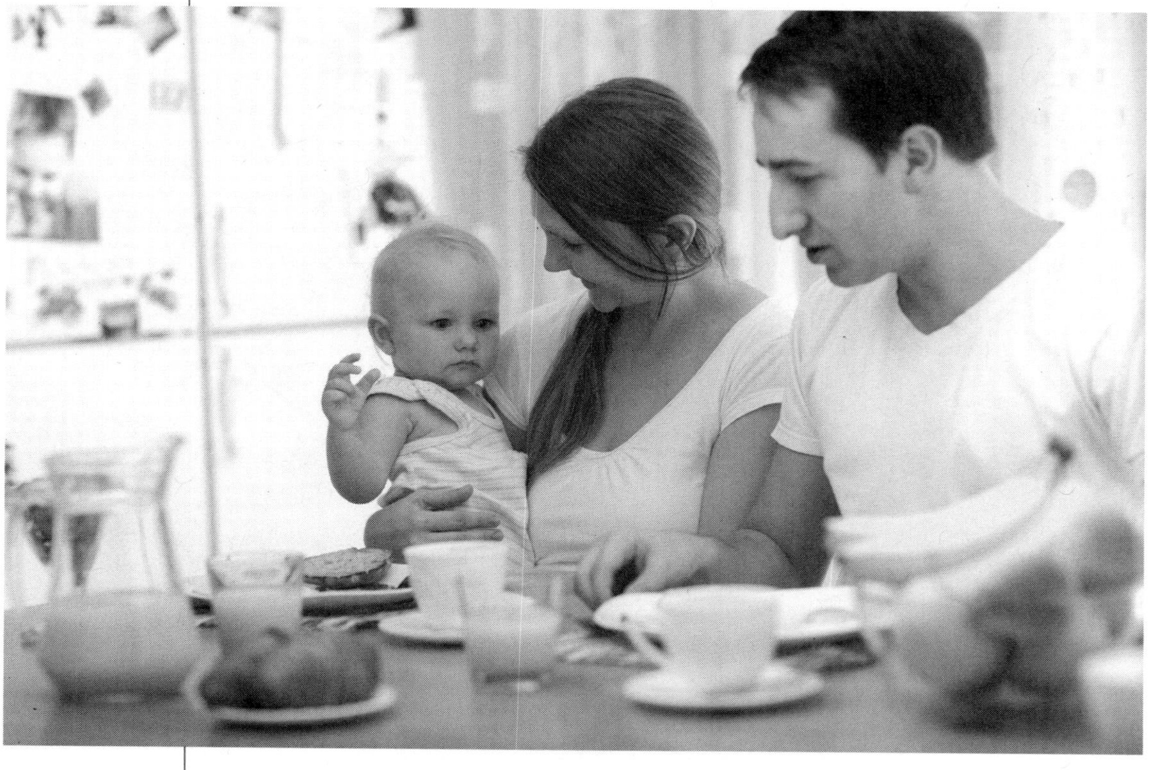

In other parts of the world, despite World Health Organization recommendations, starting solid foods younger than 4 months is much more common. Examples include Pakistan (Manikam et al., 2018) and some developing countries (Marriott, Campbell, Hirsch, & Wilson, 2007).

• • •

Family and friends are major influencers of new parents on what foods to give and when to give them (Alder et al., 2004; Crocetti, Dudas, & Krugman, 2004; Gijsbers, Mesters, Andre Knottnerus, Legtenberg, & van Schayck, 2005). Research also found that many parents start solids early because they believe infant crying is a sign of hunger and that giving solids will help "settle" their baby (Wasser et al., 2011).

Many parents are influenced by cultural beliefs and advice from others to start solids early, thinking their babies will cry less and sleep more.

The belief that solids will help their babies "sleep better" is another reason parents give for early introduction of solids, which is often reinforced by family and friends. As one mother in a 2012 Scottish qualitative serial interview study said about starting her baby on solids early (Hoddinott, Craig, Britten, & McInnes, 2012, p. 9):

> "He was waking every kind of hour and half/two hours wanting to feed, so I tried him on the solids after speaking to the health visitor. I just would like to sleep and I just don't know why he's not sleeping at night time, so I just have to see if food will help."

In this same study, researchers concluded that many parents give early solids and may also give up on nursing when they feel like something significant needs to change as a result of their baby's (usually normal) sleeping or feeding patterns.

As prolific U.K. researcher Dr. Amy Brown wrote (Brown, 2017b, p. 134):

> "A common belief is that if a baby is not sleeping through the night, introducing solids, or giving more of them just before bed, will help them to sleep. Around a quarter of mothers in the U.K. Infant Feeding Survey gave this reason for introducing solids with around a third giving this reason if they introduced solids at 3 to 4 months. Unfortunately, this is a persistent myth. My own research shows that the amount of solids given does not affect sleep (and while we're on the subject, milk type does not affect sleep once the baby is past a few weeks old either—stopping breastfeeding will not help your baby to sleep)."

Popular beliefs to the contrary, research is mixed on the association between solid foods and babies sleeping longer at night (Keane, 1988; Macknin, Medendorp, & Maier, 1989). One 2015 study, in which 715 U.K. mothers completed questionnaires about their 6- to 12-month-old babies, found that nearly 75% of the babies woke at least once during the night, with more than 50% receiving at least one feeding, making this normal behavior. The researchers found that breastfeeding, solid foods, and infant weight were not associated with frequency of night waking. However, a 2018 U.K. study that included more than 1,300 exclusively breastfed babies (Perkin et al., 2018) reported an association between early introduction of solid foods (at 3 months) and slightly more sleep at night, as compared with the group of babies who exclusively breastfed until solids were started at 6 months. Beginning at about 5 months, the babies in this study who started solid foods at around 3 months slept on average nearly 17 more minutes each night and woke fewer times at night (1.7 night wakings versus 2.0 night wakings). These differences were statistically significant. The parents in the early solids group also reported fewer "sleep problems" than the group who started solid foods at 6 months. It's important to note, though, that at study enrollment, the babies in the early introduction group were already sleeping significantly longer than the babies in the standard group.

Another common reason parents give for early introduction of solids is rapid infant weight gain, which they interpret as meaning their fast-growing baby physically "needs" other foods (Savage, Reilly, Edwards, & Durnin, 1998; Wright, Parkinson, & Drewett, 2004). Some baby food manufacturers encourage this belief by advising parents to start solids based on weight rather than age.

In cultures where overweight babies are considered "healthier," introducing solid foods may be considered necessary to insure babies "get enough." If these beliefs cause parents to override their babies' signs of fullness and continue to feed, they may increase the risk of childhood obesity.

• • •

Educational strategies that successfully delay the early introduction of solid foods are most effective when done in a community setting rather than in a health facility.

A 2018 Cochrane Review found that providing education to families about the age at which solid foods are recommended result in up to a 12% improvement in practice (Arikpo et al., 2018). It also concluded that interventions conducted in communities are more effective than those conducted in health facilities.

• • •

To delay solid foods until the recommended age, parents need to know what behaviors are age-appropriate and nonfood strategies for meeting their babies' needs.

Although many parents say that they start solid foods early in response to their babies' "cues" (Crocetti et al., 2004; Wright et al., 2004), in most cases, before a baby is 6 months old, giving solid foods is not the best response. Many parents and family members misinterpret normal infant behaviors or other needs as "hunger for solids."

Suggest parents consider other responses, such as nursing when a baby fusses, holding and playing with their baby, or wearing their baby in a soft baby carrier or sling as they do household chores. Parents need to know that night-waking is common during the first year. For parents struggling with fatigue, discuss strategies for meeting baby's needs at night that maximize their sleep, such as keeping baby near them for night feeds. Sharing experiences with other families, either online or in person, may also be helpful, so they can hear a wide range of strategies that worked for other parents and get a clearer sense of normal baby behavior.

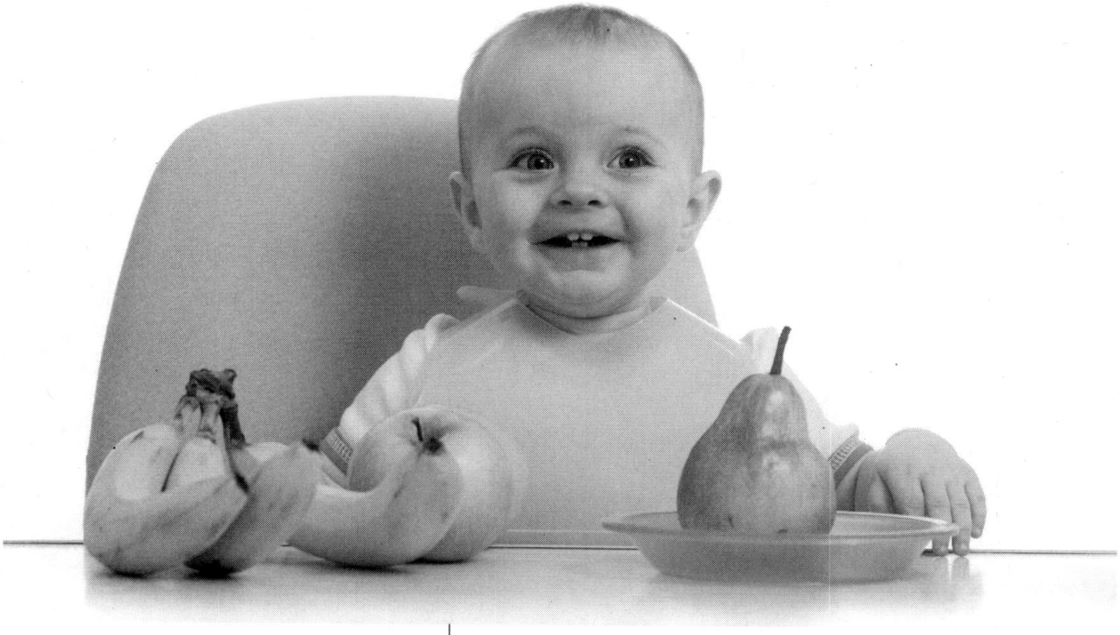

Not Too Late

Some families delay solid foods longer than 6 months in the hopes that this will provide their babies with greater protection from allergy. However, a further delay after 6 months does not appear to offer more protection (Greer et al., 2008). In fact, research findings indicate that even highly allergenic foods should not be delayed longer than 6 months, as was previously recommended (see previous section). See the next section for details about babies' need for iron from solid foods.

Around 6 months of age is a good time to begin offering solid foods, because that's when babies' stores of some minerals start to run low. There's no known advantage to delaying solids longer than 6 months and there may be drawbacks.

Are there drawbacks to delaying solid foods longer than 6 months? A 2018 cross-sectional study of more than 10,000 babies from eight European countries (Papoutsou et al., 2018) found an association between delaying solid foods 7 months or longer and increased risk of later overweight and obesity. This study found the best weight outcomes among children who exclusively nursed for 6 months, started solid foods then, and continued nursing for at least 12 months.

• • •

Of course, not all babies accept solid foods at exactly the same age, and some babies need several exposures to a food before they are willing to swallow it. If a baby rejects attempts to offer solids, see the later section, "Strategies for Giving Solids."

If a 6-month-old baby is not interested in solid foods, suggest the parents try again in a few days.

Iron

Research indicates that the vast majority of babies born full term to well-nourished birthing parents with average or above average birth weights have enough iron stores to last through their first 6 to 9 months of life (Ziegler, Nelson, & Jeter, 2014). The iron in human milk is much better absorbed than iron from other sources, up to 50% absorption from human milk compared with 4% absorption from infant formula (Griffin & Abrams, 2001). This is due at least in part to the vitamin C and lactose in human milk, which enhances iron absorption (Lawrence & Lawrence, 2016, p. 124). But because the amount of iron in human milk is low, nursing babies also need iron from other sources beginning at around 6 to 9 months. For this reason, some suggest introducing foods high in iron, such as meats, beginning at around 6 months (Brown, 2017b; Hong, Chang, Shin, & Oh, 2017).

Most babies begin to need solid foods at around 6 months of age, because that's when their iron stores from birth begin to run low.

One Swedish study (Domellof, Lonnerdal, Abrams, & Hernell, 2002) found that as babies mature, their ability to absorb iron increases. Between 6 and 9 months of age, when babies are on a low-iron diet, developmental changes appear to enhance babies' iron absorption. Breastfed babies who received iron supplements that were added to expressed milk and fed by bottle absorbed a much smaller percentage of the iron than babies who received no iron supplements (17% vs. 37%). These researchers wrote: "…this observation supports the theory that the dietary regulation of iron absorption is immature in the 6-month-old infant and is subject to developmental changes between 8 and 9 months of age….This might prove to be a valuable compensatory mechanism in partially breast-fed infants with low-iron diets and might explain why we found no correlation between complementary food iron intake and iron status in 9-mo-old Swedish infants" (Domellof, Lonnerdal, Abrams, et al., 2002, p. 203).

KEY CONCEPT

Some recommend starting with foods rich in iron.

A 2017 cross-sectional study of babies between 6 and 10 months old conducted in rural Kenya (Uyoga et al., 2017), where iron deficiency and anemia are prevalent, found that babies who were exclusively breastfed for the first 6 months had better iron status and higher hemoglobin levels than babies exclusively breastfed for less than 6 months.

• • •

Healthy iron levels are important, as both too much and too little iron are associated with developmental delays and other negative outcomes.

The effects of too little iron are well known. Too little iron can cause iron deficiency in babies, as well as anemia, which are associated with developmental delays and neurological problems (Lozoff & Georgieff, 2006). If iron levels are too low for too long, it is not always possible to reverse these health issues by giving iron supplements (Lozoff et al., 2006). Some research indicates that boys may be at a greater risk of iron deficiency than girls (Domellof, Lonnerdal, Dewey, et al., 2002).

Too much iron can be problematic, too, as it was linked to slower growth, neurodevelopmental delays, and an increased incidence of some diseases. One study (Dewey et al., 2002) examined growth and health outcomes among 101 Swedish and 131 Honduran babies. It found that when iron-sufficient babies received extra iron, their growth in length and head circumference was significantly less. The researchers concluded that while routine iron supplements provided benefits to babies who were iron deficient, they presented risks for babies who were not. A 2017 systematic review and meta-analysis of the effects of daily iron supplementation of breastfed babies also noted slowed growth during the period of exclusive breastfeeding as a side effect (Cai, Granger, Eck, & Friel, 2017).

Based on the results of just one small study, in 2010, the American Academy of Pediatrics published the recommendation that all breastfeeding babies receive routine iron supplements beginning at 4 months (Baker, Greer, & Committee on Nutrition American Academy of, 2010). However, the AAP Section on Breastfeeding reviewed the literature and concluded (AAP, 2011) that the research that seemed to support the benefits of iron supplementation before 6 months was inadequate both in number and in the clinical importance of the outcome. The Academy of Breastfeeding Medicine wrote in its 2018 protocol on iron, zinc, and vitamin D (S. N. Taylor, 2018, p. 402):

> "There are potential harms of iron supplementation, especially on immune function and in possibly decreasing the bioavailability of iron contained in human milk. In addition, there is potential harm in infant growth and morbidity when iron supplementation is provided to iron-sufficient infants."

A 2012 study (Lozoff, Castillo, Clark, & Smith, 2012) followed 473 healthy, term Chilean babies for 10 years found that feeding babies who are iron-sufficient a high-iron (12 mg/L ferrous sulfate) versus a low-iron infant formula (2.3 mg/L ferrous sulfate) from 6 to 18 months of age resulted in neurodevelopmental delays. At 10 years of age, the children who received as infants the high-iron formula had significantly lower spatial memory, visual-motor integration, arithmetic achievement, visual perception, and motor coordination.

Because iron is a pro-oxidant, supplemental iron is associated with reduced immune function and a reduction in the effects of human milk on pathogens (Campos, Repka, & Falcao, 2013). Too much iron was linked to an increased incidence of malaria (Oppenheimer et al., 1986) and severe sepsis (Barry & Reeve, 1977). When iron is present in the baby's digestive tract—which is not normally the case—it enhances the growth of disease-causing bacteria.

For a review of the literature on the possible drawbacks of iron supplementation in iron-sufficient nursing babies, see the Academy of Breastfeeding Medicine's 2018 Clinical Protocol #29 (S. N. Taylor, 2018), which can be downloaded in multiple languages at: **bfmed.org/protocols**. This protocol's authors wrote: "Iron supplements to the 4-month-old full-term, exclusively breastfed infant is associated with improved hematological indices. However, the long-term benefits of improved hematologic indices at 4-6 months is not known." These authors goes on to say, "If iron supplementation is given before 6 months, it should be given as a 1/mg/kg/day distinct iron supplement" until iron-fortified or iron-rich foods are started.

Rather than recommending iron supplements to all nursing babies, it makes more sense to screen infants and give iron supplements only to those who are iron deficient.

• • •

Other health organizations recommend against routine iron supplements, suggesting instead delayed cord clamping at birth to enhance babies' iron stores.

Supplementing all babies with iron can result in too-high iron levels in some babies, the risks of which are described in the previous point. In its 2017 position paper on complimentary feeding, the European Society for Paediatric Gastroenterology, Hepatology, and Nutrition (ESPHGAN) did not recommend routine iron supplements for breastfeeding babies but suggested enhancing the iron stores of breastfed babies at birth by avoiding early cord clamping (Fewtrell et al., 2017). After the second stage of labor, this involves waiting until the umbilical cord stops pulsing before clamping and cutting it.

In the United States, the estimated percentage of children ages 1 to 5 years with iron deficiency anemia is 1% to 2% (Siu & Force, 2015).

• • •

Low birthweight, preterm babies, and those born to iron-deficient mothers may have low iron stores at birth and need iron supplementation before 6 months.

Babies at risk for low iron stores at birth include babies born preterm or growth-restricted and those born to iron-deficient mothers. For babies needing extra iron for any reason, the American Academy of Pediatrics recommends giving iron supplements while continuing full breastfeeding. As described for full-term babies in the previous point, avoiding early cord clamping after birth is also recommended for preterm babies in order to maximize their iron stores (Katheria, Truong, Cousins, Oshiro, & Finer, 2015).

In areas where pregnant and nursing parents suffer from iron deficiencies, rather than starting solids early, the World Health Organization recommends finding ways to help parents meet their own nutritional needs (WHO, 2001).

• • •

The amount of iron in human milk is not affected by the nursing parent's iron status.

With some nutrients, such as vitamin D, parents can boost the levels in their milk by taking a supplement, but that is not the case with iron (Lawrence & Lawrence, 2016, p. 304). A Turkish study of 168 healthy mothers without anemia who planned to exclusively breastfeed for at least 4 months (Baykan, Yalcin, & Yurdakok, 2006) were randomized to receive 80 mg of daily elemental iron or a placebo. The researchers found no differences in maternal or infant anemia. No differences were found in iron levels in milk or blood.

• • •

If there is concern about a baby's iron levels, the baby's healthcare provider can check them with a simple blood test.

A blood test to check a baby's iron levels can usually be performed in the healthcare provider's office or clinic. Healthy hemoglobin levels in breastfed babies at 4, 6, and 9 months of age are ≥10.5 g/dL at 4 and 6 months and ≥10.0 g/dL at 9 months (Domellof, Dewey, Lonnerdal, Cohen, & Hernell, 2002).

Zinc

Zinc supplements are not beneficial for either the nursing parent or nursing baby.

Zinc deficiency is associated with a variety of health problems, including growth failure, increased susceptibility to infection, and skin inflammation (S. N. Taylor, 2018). However, studies that examined the effects of zinc supplementation on breastfeeding mothers and babies found no benefits. For a review of this literature, see the free, downloadable ABM Clinical Protocol #29 available from the Academy of Breastfeeding Medicine website in multiple languages at: **bfmed.org/protocols**.

STRATEGIES FOR GIVING SOLIDS

How solid foods are introduced is as important as which foods are given.

As with nursing, introducing solid foods tends to go more smoothly if the baby perceives it as a positive experience. When meals are a happy, social time and babies' needs and preferences are respected, they are more likely to accept the foods that are offered (Brown, 2017b; Pelto, Levitt, & Thairu, 2003).

Encourage parents to approach feeding time with patience, encouragement, and eye contact. How much food baby takes is less important. In some cultures, little attention is paid to how much a baby eats unless the baby is sick or refuses to eat (Engle & Zeitlin, 1996).

• • •

Giving baby more control over feeding makes mealtimes more positive and results in more food eaten.

One U.K. study (Farrow & Blissett, 2006) found that when less pressure is used on babies to eat solids, less mealtime negativity is observed at 1 year of age. When mothers used more controlling strategies at mealtimes and were less sensitive to their babies' cues, the babies behaved more negatively at mealtimes at 1 year. Continued nursing was also associated with less controlling behavior at mealtimes, perhaps because nursing itself teaches parents to give their babies more control over their feedings. Longer nursing duration was also associated with less restrictive child-feeding behaviors at 1 year (Taveras et al., 2004).

KEY CONCEPT

Meals should be a happy, social time.

Giving greater control to the child also results in more food eaten. Nursing through the first year was associated with less parental control over feeding, which resulted in more calories from solid foods consumed at 18 months (Fisher, Birch, Smiciklas-Wright, & Picciano, 2000).

• • •

Just as nursing is a part of the relationship between parent and child, so too is their time together at family mealtimes. Responsive feeding of any type involves learning and respecting baby's hunger and satiety cues (Brown & Lee, 2013; Pelto et al., 2003).

Starting solid foods with a "baby-led" approach at about 6 months led to more responsive feeding in the months and years ahead, as well as other positives.

One way to accomplish this is to include babies at family mealtimes and allow babies to take the lead in feeding themselves. Some call this a "baby-led" approach to starting solid foods or ***baby-led weaning*** (Rapley, 2015). This means allowing babies to feed themselves from the start. When using this approach, the adult decides when baby eats and what foods are offered. The baby decides whether to eat and how much food to take. This approach assumes that babies are old enough to sit up by themselves, reach for and grab the food, and bring it to their mouth on their own. In some families, this may mean a spoon is never used to feed baby. In other families, some spoon-feeding may be part of helping baby during this process (D'Auria et al., 2018).

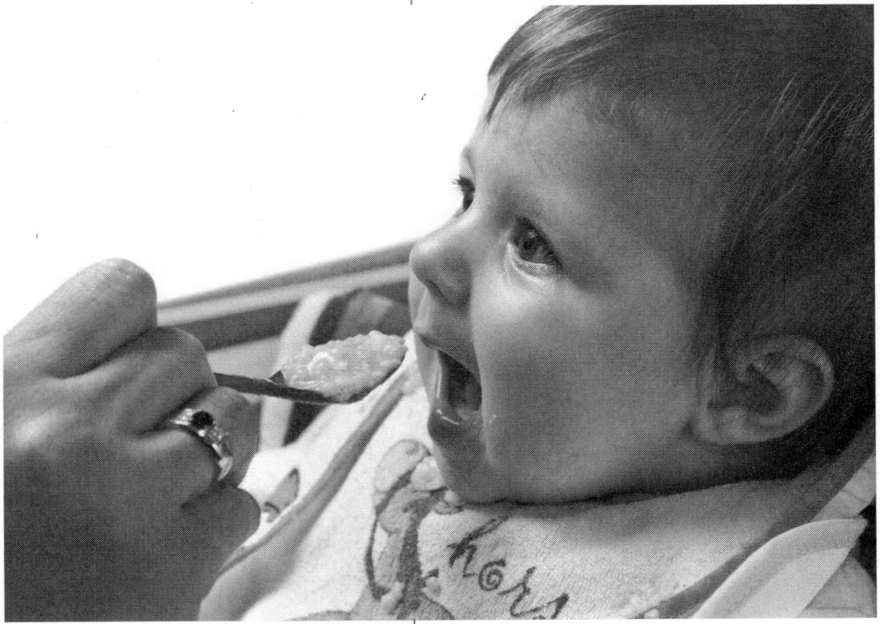

At around 6 months, most babies can handle semi-solid and some finger foods by themselves. There is no need for all of a baby's foods to be pureed or given by spoon. By 8 months, most babies can easily manage many finger foods. Family foods can be used (Dewey & Brown, 2003), as long that they are not too highly seasoned or contain added salt and sugar.

There are advantages to offering firmer rather than pureed foods from the start. Some research indicates that feeding babies only smooth, pureed foods after 10 months increases the risk for feeding difficulties later (Northstone, Emmett, & Nethersole, 2001).

To most easily handle the inevitable mess, many parents undress their babies down to their diapers, use large bibs, and/or use drop cloths or plastic sheets on the floor to catch spills.

• • •

A review of the research on the baby-led approach to solids (Brown, Jones, & Rowan, 2017) noted some distinct differences between the baby-led approach and the more traditional approach in which parents primarily spoon-feed their baby when solids are started.

Families who choose a baby-led approach to starting solids may differ from other families.

- **Timing of introduction to solids.** In one study, around 66% of those using a baby-led approach waited until baby was 6 months old, as compared with only 18% of those who used the traditional spoon-feeding approach (Daniels et al., 2015).
- **Choice of first foods.** Families using a baby-led approach were more likely to start their baby on whole foods from the family diet and they were less likely to choose rice cereal as the first food, compared with

other families. If the first food was pureed, it was more likely to be homemade rather than bought in a jar at a store.

- **Nursing experience.** In families who chose the baby-led approach, the babies were more likely to have nursed, nursed longer, and continued nursing after solids were introduced.
- **Responsiveness to the baby during feeding.** Because the baby-led approach involves baby setting the feeding pace, it's not surprising that families using this approach were found to continue to be more responsive between 18 and 24 months, as well. The families using the baby-led approach were less likely to put pressure on their children to eat, restrict food quantities, monitor food intake, and express concern about their child's weight (Brown & Lee, 2015).

• • •

Many of the concerns and questions from families and professionals about the baby-led approach to starting solids have been examined by research.

A 2018 systematic review of the baby-led weaning research (D'Auria et al., 2018) provided a synopsis of the evidence to date on several common concerns and questions expressed by healthcare providers and parents about a baby-led approach to solid foods.

- **Does a baby-led approach increase risk of choking or gagging?** Some parents and professionals worry that at 6 months a baby may not have enough practice to safely chew and swallow food that is not pureed. Three different studies found no difference between spoon-fed babies and those using the baby-led approach (Brown, 2017a; Cameron, Taylor, & Heath, 2013; Townsend & Pitchford, 2012).
- **Do babies using a baby-led approach eat enough food to grow normally?** None of the children in the baby-led studies showed faltering growth. One study specifically measured growth and found no difference between the two groups (R. W. Taylor et al., 2017). Although some of the studies showed differences in the type of food the babies consumed, this may be due to differences in study design.
- **Does the baby-led approach increase risk for inadequate iron intake?** Fruits and vegetables—both low in iron—are commonly given during baby-led weaning because they are easy for babies to grasp. However, a New Zealand study (Cameron, Taylor, & Heath, 2015), the only one to look at iron intake, specifically, instructed the parents in both groups to provide high-iron foods at every meal, so there was no difference in iron intake between the two groups. The sample size of this study, however, was very small.

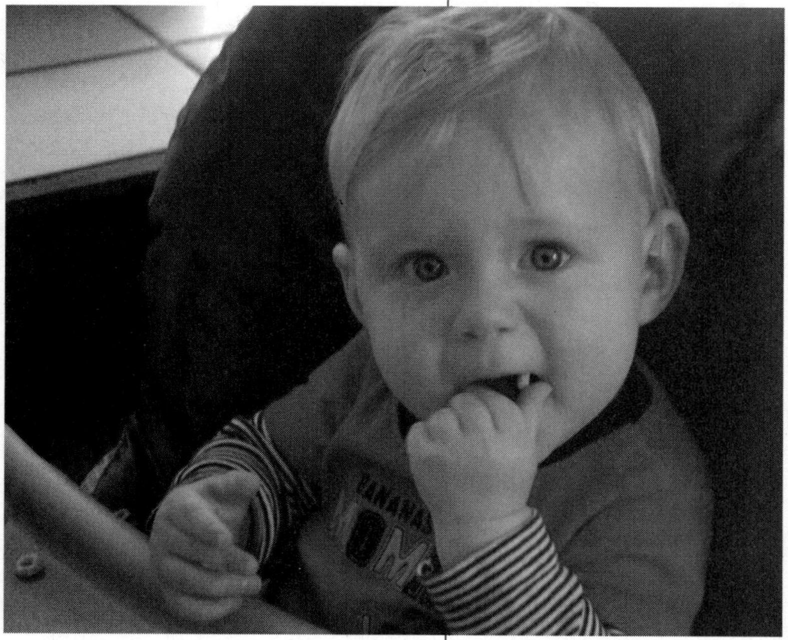

- **How does a baby-led approach affect weight and baby's ability to sense satiety or fullness?** At this writing, research on these issues is mixed, with some research finding the baby-led group less likely to be obese, less motivated by food, and more sensitive to feelings of fullness

(Brown & Lee, 2015) and other research showing the opposite (R. W. Taylor et al., 2017).

- **Does a baby-led approach expose babies to too much salt or sugar too early?** Some studies have found the baby-led groups did consume more salt than those who ate commercially sold baby food (Erickson, 2015). The authors of the systematic review (D'Auria et al., 2018) suggest that parents would benefit from some family nutritional guidance before starting a baby-led approach.
- **Does a baby-led weaning approach have a positive effect on parental anxiety and attitudes about feeding solids?** Mothers using a baby-led approach report lower anxiety levels than mothers who spoon-feed their babies (Brown, 2016). This same study also found the mothers in the baby-led group used fewer restraints during feeding and were also more conscientious. But this may be because more anxious parents are more likely to choose a more conventional approach.

• • •

At about 6 months, suggest continued frequent nursing while offering small meals, increasing the number of daily meals as baby grows. A significant portion of an older baby or toddler's nutrition may come from human milk.

Continued frequent nursing is important, because even babies older than 1 year receive necessary nutrients from human milk. Parents sometimes wonder what portion of an older baby or toddler's diet can be safely assumed to come from their milk. According to researchers, nursing babies 1 to 2 years old getting average amounts of mother's milk receive 35% to 40% of their energy intake from it (Dewey & Brown, 2003). Human milk is an important source of fatty acids and other key nutrients, such as vitamin A, calcium, and riboflavin (PAHO/WHO., 2001).

At 6 months, begin by including baby at family mealtimes 2 or 3 times per day. As baby gets older, suggest parents increase the number of meals and snacks, allowing baby to eat as much as desired at each sitting. Table 4.2 reflects the recommendations of both the U.S. Centers for Disease Control and Prevention (CDC) and the World Health Organization.

TABLE 4.2 Recommended Number of Daily Meals by Age

Baby's Age	Number of Meals/Snacks Per Day
6 to 8 months	2 to 3
9 to 11 months	3 to 4
12 to 24 months	3 to 4 meals, 1 to 2 snacks

Adapted from (CDC, 2018; PAHO/WHO., 2001)

• • •

If a 6-month-old baby rejects solid foods, suggest the parents try again in a few days.

Not all babies are ready to begin solids at exactly the same age, and the family table should never become a battleground. Some children who are prone to food allergies or intolerances may not be interested in solids until they are a little older. An exclusively nursed baby is thriving if iron levels are adequate and weight gain is steady and in the expected range. Even so, encourage parents to continue to offer foods at mealtimes until the baby begins to show an interest in them.

• • •

As babies take more solid foods, they gradually take less mother's milk.

At first, solid foods do not boost a baby's overall food intake. Rather, solids take the place of human milk in a baby's diet (Cohen, Brown, Canahuati, Rivera, & Dewey, 1994). Intake of mother's milk decreases gradually as soon as the first day after babies begin eating solid foods (Islam, Peerson, Ahmed, Dewey, & Brown, 2006). This is a normal stage of nursing, ideally with the baby able to determine the overall amount of food and milk consumed.

SPECIFIC FOODS

Babies grow quickly, so a variety of nutrient-dense foods are recommended.

Specific food choices for babies vary greatly around the world. For this reason, the World Health Organization does not give a list of specific foods but recommends offering babies a variety of nutritious foods to increase the likelihood they will receive the nutrients they need (PAHO/WHO., 2001).

The WHO Multicentre Growth Reference Study (the research used to create the growth standards based on nursing babies) found that the babies at its six international sites (Brazil, Ghana, India, Norway, Oman, and the U.S.) had some aspects of their diets in common. Although the specific foods varied, the diets were nutrient dense, with more than 75% of children receiving milk products and fruits/vegetables and 50% to 95% receiving meat, poultry, or fish ("Complementary feeding in the WHO Multicentre Growth Reference Study," 2006).

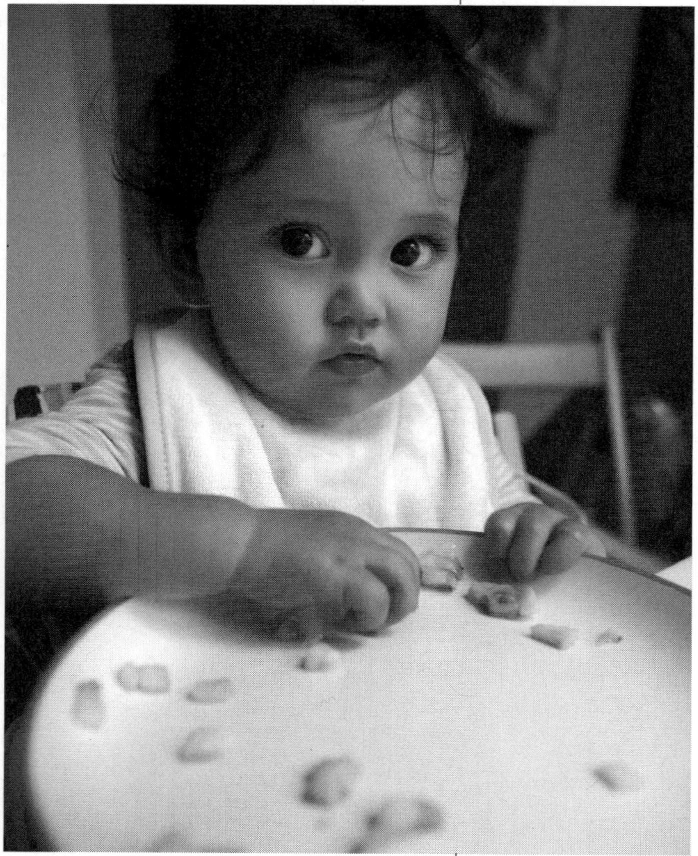

One U.S. study (Krebs et al., 2006) found that meat, which is high in iron, worked well as an early solid food. Examples of nutritious foods by texture that can be given before 12 months include:

Soft and Semi-Soft Foods

- Tender, ground poultry or meat
- Cooked vegetables, such as sweet potatoes, yams, parsnips, carrots, or white potatoes
- Tofu
- Ripe fruit, such as banana, peaches, mangos, avocados
- Cooked cereal, including wheat, rice, oat, and barley
- Cooked eggs
- Grated apples or applesauce

Finger Foods

- Finger-sized slices of toasted or untoasted whole-grain leavened or unleavened breads or crackers
- Tofu cut into slivers
- Fresh or frozen peas

- Soft, ripe, fresh fruit, such as peaches, pears, mangos, etc. cut into slivers
- Tender, cooked, thin slivers of poultry or meat
- Cooked egg yolks cut into slivers or bite-sized pieces

The American Academy of Pediatrics clinical report on preventing iron deficiency (Baker et al., 2010) includes a list of commercially prepared and table foods that are good animal and plant sources of iron. Table foods that are good animal sources of iron include egg yolks, beef and chick liver, canned clams and oysters, shrimp, sardines, turkey, lamb, fish, and chicken. Good plant sources of iron include blackstrap molasses, tofu, wheat germ, soybeans, apricots, lentils, spinach, chickpeas, prunes, lima, navy, and kidney beans.

The U.S. Centers for Disease Control in Prevention launched a website in 2018 (CDC, 2018) that recommends if parents feed their child iron-fortified cereal to offer a variety of grains (oats, barley, multigrain). According to the U.S. Food and Drug Administration, feeding rice cereal exclusively should be avoided, as offering rice alone can expose children to too much arsenic (USFDA, 2017).

• • •

When starting a new food, allow 3 to 5 days before adding another new food.

The U.S. Centers for Disease Control and Prevention (CDC) advises allowing 3 to 5 days between one new food and the next (CDC, 2018). This delay gives parents time to notice if the baby has any allergic reactions to the new food, such as:

- Diarrhea
- Rash
- Vomiting

If the baby has any of these reactions, suggest the parents stop that food for now and give the baby a couple of months to mature before trying that food again.

Once a baby has consumed a food without a reaction for 2 to 3 days, this food can then be served with other foods that have been tried or with a single new food.

• • •

Tell parents to expect changes in baby's stools after solids are started.

Often babies on solids have less frequent stools that smell stronger and are darker in color than they did while the baby was exclusively nursing. Parents may also see bits of undigested food in their baby's stools.

• • •

Babies are more likely to accept foods their nursing parent consumed regularly during pregnancy and nursing.

During pregnancy and nursing, all mammal young are exposed to the flavors of the foods their mothers eat through amniotic fluid (Lipchock, Reed, & Mennella, 2011) and their mother's milk. This helps babies recognize safe foods when they are ready to expand their diet to non-milk foods (Mennella, Reiter, & Daniels, 2016).

Several studies indicate that when parents eat a food regularly during pregnancy and nursing, their babies are more likely to accept its flavor later as a solid food. In one U.S. study (Mennella, Jagnow, & Beauchamp, 2001) mothers drank either carrot juice or water 4 days per week for 3 weeks during pregnancy.

When carrots were introduced as a solid food, the babies' enjoyment of them was rated higher by the mothers who drank the carrot juice than by the mothers who drank the water.

In another U.S. randomized controlled trial (Mennella, Daniels, & Reiter, 2017), lactating mothers began drinking vegetable, beet, celery, and carrot juices for 1 or 3 months, beginning at different time periods after birth. Researchers found that when mothers drank the vegetable juices starting at 2 weeks after birth, this had a much greater effect on their babies' acceptance of carrot-flavored baby cereal at 6 months than if they started drinking the juices at 6 weeks or 10 weeks. One month of juice-drinking after birth had a greater effect on baby's acceptance of that flavor than 3 months of juice drinking, which indicated that the duration of juice-drinking was less important than the timing.

• • •

Suggest that parents avoid adding salt to baby's foods.

This recommendation (Fewtrell et al., 2017) is based on a Dutch study that followed babies for 15 years and found that babies may be more sensitive to salt intake than adults and that salt intake during infancy may lead to high blood pressure later in life (Geleijnse et al., 1997). A later U.S. study of 5- to 10-year-old children found that children have stronger preferences than adults for sweet and salty foods (Mennella, Finkbeiner, Lipchock, Hwang, & Reed, 2014), reinforcing that keeping salt and sugar to a minimum in children's diet is warranted. If parents are giving baby foods from the family table, suggest they add little or no salt or other spices to their food during cooking before they separate the baby's portion (D'Auria et al., 2018).

• • •

Unpasteurized honey is not recommended during a baby's first 12 months.

To help establish healthy eating habits, unsweetened foods are preferred for babies 6 to 12 months old. Because cases of botulism have been reported in babies younger than 1 year who received unpasteurized honey, the American Academy of Pediatrics and other health organizations recommend avoiding unpasteurized honey until a baby is at least 12 months of age (AAP, 2015, pp. 294-295; Fewtrell et al., 2017).

• • •

Foods that could cause choking are not recommended until 3 years of age.

If a food can easily get lodged in a baby's throat and cause choking, it is recommended to wait until the baby is 3 years old before offering it. Examples include:

- Nuts
- Grapes
- Popcorn
- Hot dogs
- Raw carrots

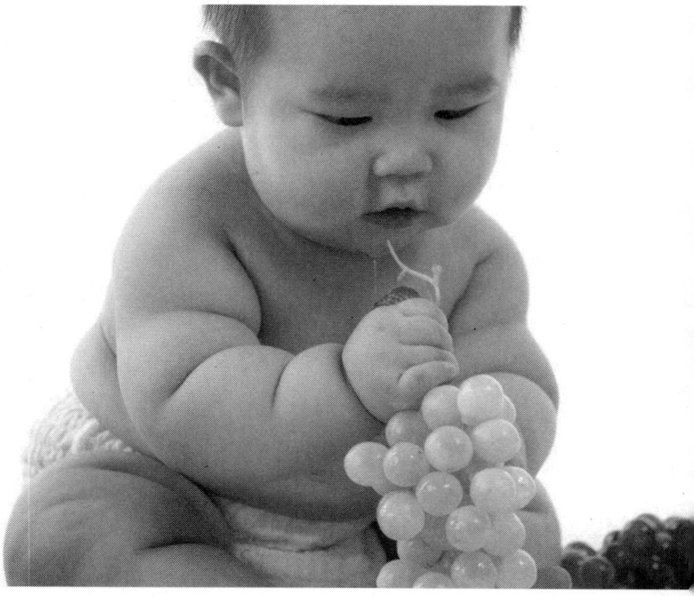

• • •

In the past, the American Academy of Pediatrics suggested that parents wait to introduce highly allergenic foods, such as egg whites, fish, peanuts and other nuts, to babies with a family history of allergy (AAP, 2000). However, in 2008 this recommendation changed based on a review of the literature (Greer et al., 2008) that concluded there is no evidence that delaying highly allergic foods to 1 year has a protective effect against allergies.

It is no longer recommended to delay potentially allergenic foods for the first year of life.

This is consistent with the recommendations of other international health organizations (Fewtrell et al., 2017). For details, see p. 137-138.

• • •

When a baby starts solids, some of the recommended foods include meat, poultry, fish, and eggs (Baker et al., 2010; Dewey & Brown, 2003; Fewtrell et al., 2017; PAHO/WHO., 2001). If a family is vegetarian and chooses not to give their baby these foods, suggest the baby be offered dairy products (Fewtrell et al., 2017).

If babies and young children are fed a vegan diet, nutritional supplements or fortified foods are needed to prevent deficiencies.

If the family diet is vegan, the baby will also need vitamin and mineral supplements or fortified foods containing iron, zinc, and vitamin B_{12}. A vegan diet containing no meat or dairy can lead to nutritional deficiencies in babies (Fewtrell et al., 2017). Dutch babies fed on a vegan diet deficient in protein, vitamin B_{12}, vitamin D, calcium, and riboflavin experienced stunted growth, muscle wasting, and delayed motor development (Dagnelie & van Staveren, 1994). For more details, see p. 568.

BEVERAGES

As babies develop better muscle control, many enjoy drinking from a cup. This could be any time after 6 months or so (Fewtrell et al., 2017). Nutrient-rich drinks that could be offered in a cup include:

Between 6 and 9 months, many babies enjoy drinking from a cup.

- Expressed milk
- Home-cooked broths or thin soups without added salt or spices

Other drinks that could be given in a cup in small amounts include:

- Unsweetened fruit and vegetable juices (see later point on fruit juices)
- Water

The U.S. Centers for Disease Control and Prevention (CDC) recommends children between 6 and 12 months be offered up to 4 to 6 ounces (120 to 180 mL) of water per day (CDC, 2018). Avoid sweetened drinks or any food with added sugar before 24 months.

• • •

Cow's milk is not recommended in significant volumes until after 12 months of age, but other dairy products can be given earlier.

Cow's milk was found to cause intestinal bleeding in babies younger than 9 months old, which can result in lower iron status and vitamin D levels (Maguire et al., 2013). Because cow's milk is also a poor source of iron, giving it as a substitute for mother's milk or infant formula was associated with iron deficiency in babies (Gunnarsson, Thorsdottir, & Palsson, 2004; Thorsdottir, Gunnarsson, Atladottir, Michaelsen, & Palsson, 2003).

For these reasons, most recommend cow's milk not be given to babies younger than 12 months as their main drink (Fewtrell et al., 2017). Some processed dairy products, such as cheese and yogurt are recommended after 6 months.

The U.S. Centers for Disease Control and Prevention (CDC) recommends that children older than 12 months be limited to no more than 24 ounces 720 mL) of fortified, unflavored cow's milk per day (CDC, 2018). Too much milk can make it difficult for a child to get a balanced, diverse diet.

• • •

Fruit juice is best limited to babies older than 1 year, giving no more than 4 oz. (120 ml) per day.

In a U.S. survey of 2,740 children (Grimes, Szymlek-Gay, & Nicklas, 2017), 6% of babies younger than 6 months and 38% of those 6 to 12 months old drank 100% fruit juice daily. In its 2017 policy statement (Heyman, Abrams, 2017), the American Academy of Pediatrics recommended that parents avoid giving any fruit juice before 1 year of age unless medically indicated. After 1 year, if fruit juice is given, they suggest parents:

- Provide children from 1 to 3 years of age no more than 4 ounces (120 mL) of fruit juice per day.
- Limit fruit juice to mealtimes, and give it to children in a cup, not a bottle, as children are at greater risk of dental caries when they carry a bottle of juice around with them or fall asleep with a bottle of juice at night, bathing their teeth in a sugary liquid for long periods.
- Serve whole fruit instead of fruit juice, as it is more nutritious.

Fruit juice fills up a baby or toddler, decreasing interest in nursing and in other foods. Too much juice can also lead to diarrhea in a toddler from carbohydrate overload (Heyman et al., 2017). Although it was once believed that juice could be a risk factor in childhood obesity, a 2017 meta-analysis (Auerbach et al., 2017) found an association between fruit juice consumption and a small weight gain among 1- to 6-year-old children, but this weight gain was not considered clinically significant. There was no association between fruit juice consumption and obesity in children older than 6 years.

• • •

Other drinks, such as tea, coffees, and sodas are not recommended for babies.

In some cultures, teas are commonly given to babies (Wojcicki et al., 2011; Zhang, Fein, & Fein, 2011). Both teas and coffees are not recommended because they interfere with iron absorption (PAHO/WHO., 2001). Teas, coffees, and sodas are best avoided completely, because they have low nutritional value and can decrease a baby's interest in nutritious foods during a time of fast growth.

RESOURCES

bit.ly/BA2-CDCSolids—Webpage for parents on introducing solid foods from the U.S. Centers for Disease Control and Prevention (CDC).

Brown, A. *Why Starting Solids Matters.* London: Pinter & Martin, 2017.

Gonzalez, C. *My Child Won't Eat,* 2nd edition. London: Pinter & Martin, 2012.

Rapley, G & Murkett, T. *Baby-led Weaning: The Essential Guide to Introducing Solid Foods and Helping Your Baby to Grow Up a Happy and Confident Eater.* The Experiment: New York, NY, 2010.

REFERENCES

AAP. (1997). Breastfeeding and the use of human milk. American Academy of Pediatrics. Work Group on Breastfeeding. *Pediatrics, 100*(6), 1035-1039.

AAP. (2000). Hypoallergenic infant formulas. *Pediatrics, 106*(2), 346-349.

AAP. (2011). Concerns with early universal iron supplementation of breastfeeding infants. *Pediatrics, 127,* e1097.

AAP. (2015). *Red Book: 2015 Report of the Committee on Infectious Diseases.* Elk Grove Village, IL: American Academy of Pediatrics.

Alder, E. M., Williams, F. L., Anderson, A. S., et al. (2004). What influences the timing of the introduction of solid food to infants? *British Journal of Nutrition, 92*(3), 527-531.

Anderson, A. S., Guthrie, C. A., Alder, E. M., et al. (2001). Rattling the plate--reasons and rationales for early weaning. *Health Education Research, 16*(4), 471-479.

Arikpo, D., Edet, E. S., Chibuzor, M. T., et al. (2018). Educational interventions for improving primary caregiver complementary feeding practices for children aged 24 months and under. *Cochrane Database of Systematic Reviews, 5,* CD011768.

Armstrong, J., Abraham, E. C., Squair, M., et al. (2014). Exclusive breastfeeding, complementary feeding, and food choices in UK infants. *Journal of Human Lactation, 30*(2), 201-208.

Auerbach, B. J., Wolf, F. M., Hikida, A., et al. (2017). Fruit juice and change in BMI: A meta-analysis. *Pediatrics, 139*(4).

Baker, R. D., Greer, F. R., & Committee on Nutrition American Academy of, P. (2010). Diagnosis and prevention of iron deficiency and iron-deficiency anemia in infants and young children (0-3 years of age). *Pediatrics, 126*(5), 1040-1050.

Barrera, C. M., Hamner, H. C., Perrine, C. G., et al. (2018). Timing of introduction of complementary foods to US infants, National Health and Nutrition Examination Survey 2009-2014. *Journal of the Academy of Nutrition and Dietetics, 118*(3), 464-470.

Barry, D. M., & Reeve, A. W. (1977). Increased incidence of gram-negative neonatal sepsis with intramuscular iron administration. *Pediatrics, 60*(6), 908-912.

Baykan, A., Yalcin, S. S., & Yurdakok, K. (2006). Does maternal iron supplementation during the lactation period affect iron status of exclusively breast-fed infants? *Turkish Journal of Pediatrics, 48(*4), 301-307.

Bentley, A. (2014). *Inventing Baby Food: Taste, Health, and the Industrialization of the American Diet.* Oakland, California: University of California Press.

Black, R. E., & Victora, C. G. (2002). Optimal duration of exclusive breast feeding in low income countries. *British Medical Journal, 325*(7375), 1252-1253.

Brodribb, W., & Miller, Y. (2013). Introducing solids and water to Australian infants. *Journal of Human Lactation, 29*(2), 214-221.

Brown, A. (2016). Differences in eating behaviour, well-being and personality between mothers following baby-led vs. traditional weaning styles. *Maternal and Child Nutrition, 12*(4), 826-837.

Brown, A. (2017a). No difference in self-reported frequency of choking between infants introduced to solid foods using a baby-led weaning or traditional spoon-feeding approach. *Journal of Human Nutrition and Dietetics* (Dec 5).

Brown, A. (2017b). *Why Starting Solids Matters.* London: Pinter & Martin.

Brown, A., Jones, S. W., & Rowan, H. (2017). Baby-led weaning: The evidence to date. *Current Nutrition Reports, 6*(2), 148-156.

Brown, A., & Lee, M. (2013). Breastfeeding is associated with a maternal feeding style low in control from birth. *PLoS One, 8*(1), e54229.

Brown, A., & Lee, M. D. (2015). Early influences on child satiety-responsiveness: the role of weaning style. *Pediatric Obesity, 10*(1), 57-66.

Cai, C., Granger, M., Eck, P., et al. (2017). Effect of daily iron supplementation in healthy exclusively breastfed infants: A systematic review with meta-analysis. *Breastfeeding Medicine, 12*(10), 597-603.

Cameron, S. L., Taylor, R. W., & Heath, A. L. (2013). Parent-led or baby-led? Associations between complementary feeding practices and health-related behaviours in a survey of New Zealand families. *BMJ Open, 3*(12), e003946.

Cameron, S. L., Taylor, R. W., & Heath, A. L. (2015). Development and pilot testing of baby-led introduction to solids--A version of baby-led weaning modified to address concerns about iron deficiency, growth faltering and choking. *BMC Pediatrics, 15,* 99.

Campos, L. F., Repka, J. C., & Falcao, M. C. (2013). Effects of human milk fortifier with iron on the bacteriostatic properties of breast milk. *Jornal de Pediatria (Rio J), 89*(4), 394-399.

CDC. (2018). When, what, and how to introduce solid foods. Retrieved from **cdc.gov/nutrition/infantandtoddlernutrition/foods-and-drinks/when-to-introduce-solid-foods.html**.

Clayton, H. B., Li, R., Perrine, C. G., et al. (2013). Prevalence and reasons for introducing infants early to solid foods: Variations by milk feeding type. *Pediatrics, 131*(4), e1108-1114.

Cohen, R. J., Brown, K. H., Canahuati, J., et al. (1994). Effects of age of introduction of complementary foods on infant breast milk intake, total energy intake, and growth: A randomised intervention study in Honduras. *Lancet, 344*(8918), 288-293.

Complementary feeding in the WHO Multicentre Growth Reference Study. (2006). *Acta Paediatr Suppl, 450,* 27-37.

Crocetti, M., Dudas, R., & Krugman, S. (2004). Parental beliefs and practices regarding early introduction of solid foods to their children. *Clinical Pediatrics (Phila), 43*(6), 541-547.

D'Auria, E., Bergamini, M., Staiano, A., et al. (2018). Baby-led weaning: What a systematic review of the literature adds on. *Italian Journal of Pediatrics, 44*(1), 49.

Dagnelie, P. C., & van Staveren, W. A. (1994). Macrobiotic nutrition and child health: Results of a population-based, mixed-longitudinal cohort study in The Netherlands. *American Journal of Clinical Nutrition, 59*(5 Suppl), 1187S-1196S.

Daniels, L., Heath, A. L., Williams, S. M., et al. (2015). Baby-led introduction to solids (BLISS) study: A randomised controlled trial of a baby-led approach to complementary feeding. *BMC Pediatrics, 15,* 179.

Danowski, L., & Gargiula, L. (2002). Selections from current literature. Attitudes and practices regarding the introduction of solid foods to infants. *Family Practitioner, 19*(6), 698-702.

Dewey, K. G., & Brown, K. H. (2003). Update on technical issues concerning complementary feeding of young children in developing countries and implications for intervention programs. *Food and Nutrition Bulletin, 24*(1), 5-28.

Dewey, K. G., Domellof, M., Cohen, R. J., et al. (2002). Iron supplementation affects growth and morbidity of breast-fed infants: Results of a randomized trial in Sweden and Honduras. *Journal of Nutrition, 132*(11), 3249-3255.

Domellof, M., Dewey, K. G., Lonnerdal, B., et al. (2002). The diagnostic criteria for iron deficiency in infants should be reevaluated. *Journal of Nutrition, 132*(12), 3680-3686.

Domellof, M., Lonnerdal, B., Abrams, S. A., et al. (2002). Iron absorption in breast-fed infants: Effects of age, iron status, iron supplements, and complementary foods. *American Journal of Clinical Nutrition, 76*(1), 198-204.

Domellof, M., Lonnerdal, B., Dewey, K. G., et al. (2002). Sex differences in iron status during infancy. *Pediatrics, 110*(3), 545-552.

Du Toit, G., Roberts, G., Sayre, P. H., et al. (2015). Randomized trial of peanut consumption in infants at risk for peanut allergy. *New England Journal of Medicine, 372*(9), 803-813.

Engle, P. L., & Zeitlin, M. (1996). Active feeding behavior compensates for low interest in food among young Nicaraguan children. *Journal of Nutrition, 126*(7), 1808-1816.

Erickson, L. W. (2015). A baby-led approach to complementary feeding: Adherence and infant food and nutrient intakes at seven months of age. (Masters), University of Otago, Dunedin, New Zealand. Retrieved from **ourarchive.otago.ac.nz/handle/10523/6041**.

Farrow, C., & Blissett, J. (2006). Breast-feeding, maternal feeding practices and mealtime negativity at one year. *Appetite, 46*(1), 49-56.

Fewtrell, M., Bronsky, J., Campoy, C., et al. (2017). Complementary feeding: A position paper by the European Society for Paediatric Gastroenterology, Hepatology, and Nutrition (ESPGHAN) Committee on Nutrition. *Journal of Pediatric Gastroenterology and Nutrition, 64*(1), 119-132.

Fisher, J. O., Birch, L. L., Smiciklas-Wright, H., et al. (2000). Breast-feeding through the first year predicts maternal control in feeding and subsequent toddler energy intakes. *Journal of the American Dietetic Association, 100*(6), 641-646.

Fleischer, D. M., Sicherer, S., Greenhawt, M., et al. (2015). Consensus communication on early peanut introduction and the prevention of peanut allergy in high-risk infants. *Pediatrics.*

Geleijnse, J. M., Hofman, A., Witteman, J. C., et al. (1997). Long-term effects of neonatal sodium restriction on blood pressure. *Hypertension, 29*(4), 913-917.

Gijsbers, B., Mesters, I., Andre Knottnerus, J., et al. (2005). Factors influencing breastfeeding practices and postponement of solid food to prevent allergic disease in high-risk children: Results from an explorative study. *Patient Education and Counseling, 57*(1), 15-21.

Greer, F. R., Sicherer, S. H., & Burks, A. W. (2008). Effects of early nutritional interventions on the development of atopic disease in infants and children: The role of maternal dietary restriction, breastfeeding, timing of introduction of complementary foods, and hydrolyzed formulas. *Pediatrics, 121*(1), 183-191.

Griffin, I. J., & Abrams, S. A. (2001). Iron and breastfeeding. *Pediatric Clinics of North America, 48*(2), 401-413.

Grimes, C. A., Szymlek-Gay, E. A., & Nicklas, T. A. (2017). Beverage consumption among U.S. children aged 0-24 months: National Health and Nutrition Examination Survey (NHANES). *Nutrients, 9*(3).

Gunnarsson, B. S., Thorsdottir, I., & Palsson, G. (2004). Iron status in 2-year-old Icelandic children and associations with dietary intake and growth. *European Journal of Clinical Nutrition, 58*(6), 901-906.

Heyman, M. B., Abrams, S. A., Section On Gastroenterology, H., et al. (2017). Fruit juice in infants, children, and adolescents: Current recommendations. *Pediatrics, 139*(6).

Hoddinott, P., Craig, L. C., Britten, J., et al. (2012). A serial qualitative interview study of infant feeding experiences: Idealism meets realism. *BMJ Open, 2*(2), e000504.

Hollis, J. L., Crozier, S. R., Inskip, H. M., et al. (2016). Age at introduction of solid foods and feeding difficulties in childhood: Findings from the Southampton Women's Survey. *British Journal of Nutrition, 116*(4), 743-750.

Hong, J., Chang, J. Y., Shin, S., et al. (2017). Breastfeeding and red meat intake are associated with iron status in healthy Korean weaning-age infants. *Journal of Korean Medical Science, 32*(6), 974-984.

Illingworth, R. S., & Lister, J. (1964). The critical or sensitive period, with special reference to certain feeding problems in infants and children. *Journal of Pediatrics, 65*, 839-848.

Islam, M. M., Peerson, J. M., Ahmed, T., et al. (2006). Effects of varied energy density of complementary foods on breast-milk intakes and total energy consumption by healthy, breastfed Bangladeshi children. *American Journal of Clinical Nutrition, 83*(4), 851-858. doi:83/4/851 [pii]

Katheria, A. C., Truong, G., Cousins, L., et al. (2015). Umbilical cord milking versus delayed cord clamping in preterm infants. *Pediatrics, 136*(1), 61-69.

Keane, V., et al. (1988). Do solids help baby sleep through the night? *American Journal of Diseases of Childhood, 142*, 404-405.

Kramer, M. S., & Kakuma, R. (2002). Optimal duration of exclusive breastfeeding. *Cochrane Database of Systematic Reviews* (1), CD003517 003510.001002/14651858. CD14003517.

Kramer, M. S., & Kakuma, R. (2012). Optimal duration of exclusive breastfeeding. *Cochrane Database of Systematic Reviews* (8), CD003517.

Krebs, N. F., Westcott, J. E., Butler, N., et al. (2006). Meat as a first complementary food for breastfed infants: Feasibility and impact on zinc intake and status. *Journal of Pediatric Gastroenterology and Nutrition, 42*(2), 207-214.

Lawrence, R. A., & Lawrence, R. M. (2016). *Breastfeeding: A Guide for the Medical Profession (8th ed.)*. Philadelphia, PA: Elsevier.

Lerodiakonou, D., Garcia-Larsen, V., Logan, A., et al. (2016). Timing of allergenic food introduction to the infant diet and risk of allergic or autoimmune disease: A systematic review and meta-analysis. *Journal of the American Medical Association, 316*(11), 1181-1192.

Lipchock, S. V., Reed, D. R., & Mennella, J. A. (2011). The gustatory and olfactory systems during infancy: Implications for development of feeding behaviors in the high-risk neonate. *Clinical Perinatology, 38*(4), 627-641.

Lozoff, B., Beard, J., Connor, J., et al. (2006). Long-lasting neural and behavioral effects of iron deficiency in infancy. *Nutrition Reviews, 64*(5 Pt 2), S34-43; discussion S72-91.

Lozoff, B., Castillo, M., Clark, K. M., et al. (2012). Iron-fortified vs low-iron infant formula: Developmental outcome at 10 years. *Archives of Pediatric & Adolescent Medicine, 166*(3), 208-215.

Lozoff, B., & Georgieff, M. K. (2006). Iron deficiency and brain development. *Seminars in Pediatric Neurology, 13*(3), 158-165.

Macknin, M. L., Medendorp, S. V., & Maier, M. C. (1989). Infant sleep and bedtime cereal. *American Journal of Diseases of Children, 143*(9), 1066-1068.

Maguire, J. L., Lebovic, G., Kandasamy, S., et al. (2013). The relationship between cow's milk and stores of vitamin D and iron in early childhood. *Pediatrics, 131*(1), e144-151.

Manikam, L., Sharmila, A., Dharmaratnam, A., et al. (2018). Systematic review of infant and young child complementary feeding practices in South Asian families: The Pakistan perspective. *Public Health Nutrition, 21*(4), 655-668.

Marriott, B. M., Campbell, L., Hirsch, E., et al. (2007). Preliminary data from demographic and health surveys on infant feeding in 20 developing countries. *Journal of Nutrition, 137*(2), 518S-523S.

Mennella, J. A., Daniels, L. M., & Reiter, A. R. (2017). Learning to like vegetables during breastfeeding: A randomized clinical trial of lactating mothers and infants. *American Journal of Clinical Nutrition, 106*(1), 67-76.

Mennella, J. A., Finkbeiner, S., Lipchock, S. V., et al. (2014). Preferences for salty and sweet tastes are elevated and related to each other during childhood. *PLoS One, 9*(3), e92201.

Mennella, J. A., Jagnow, C. P., & Beauchamp, G. K. (2001). Prenatal and postnatal flavor learning by human infants. *Pediatrics, 107*(6), E88.

Mennella, J. A., Reiter, A. R., & Daniels, L. M. (2016). Vegetable and fruit acceptance during infancy: Impact of ontogeny, genetics, and early experiences. *Advances in Nutritition, 7*(1), 211S-219S.

Munblit, D., Peroni, D. G., Boix-Amoros, A., et al. (2017). Human milk and allergic diseases: An unsolved puzzle. *Nutrients, 9*(8).

Norris, J. M., Barriga, K., Hoffenberg, E. J., et al. (2005). Risk of celiac disease autoimmunity and timing of gluten introduction in the diet of infants at increased risk of disease. *Journal of the American Medical Association, 293*(19), 2343-2351.

Northstone, K., Emmett, P., & Nethersole, F. (2001). The effect of age of introduction to lumpy solids on foods eaten and reported feeding difficulties at 6 and 15 months. *Journal of Human Nutrition and Dietetics, 14*(1), 43-54.

Oppenheimer, S. J., Gibson, F. D., Macfarlane, S. B., et al. (1986). Iron supplementation increases prevalence and effects of malaria: Report on clinical studies in Papua New Guinea. *Transactions of the Royal Society of Tropical Medicine and Hygiene, 80*(4), 603-612.

PAHO/WHO. (2001). *Guiding Principles for Complementary Feeding of the Breastfed Child.* Washington, DC: Pan American Health Organization Retrieved from **iris.paho.org/xmlui/handle/123456789/752**.

Papoutsou, S., Savva, S. C., Hunsberger, M., et al. (2018). Timing of solid food introduction and association with later childhood overweight and obesity: The IDEFICS study. *Maternal and Child Nutrition, 14*(1).

Pelto, G. H., Levitt, E., & Thairu, L. (2003). Improving feeding practices: Current patterns, common constraints, and the design of interventions. *Food and Nutrition Bulletin, 24*(1), 45-82.

Perkin, M. R., Bahnson, H. T., Logan, K., et al. (2018). Association of early introduction of solids with infant sleep: A secondary analysis of a randomized clinical trial. *JAMA Pediatrics,* e180739.

Piescik-Lech, M., Chmielewska, A., Shamir, R., et al. (2017). Systematic review: Early infant feeding and the risk of type 1 diabetes. *Journal of Pediatric Gastroenterology and Nutrition, 64*(3), 454-459.

Rapley, G. (2015). Baby-led weaning: The theory and evidence behind the approach. *Journal of Health Visiting, 3*(3), 144-151.

Rosenbauer, J., Herzig, P., Kaiser, P., et al. (2007). Early nutrition and risk of type 1 diabetes mellitus--A nationwide case-control study in preschool children. *Experimental and Clinical Endocrinology & Diabetes, 115*(8), 502-508.

Sackett, W. (1953). *Bringing Up Babies: A Family Doctor's Practical Approach to Child Care.* New York, NY: Harper & Brothers.

Savage, S. A., Reilly, J. J., Edwards, C. A., et al. (1998). Weaning practice in the Glasgow Longitudinal Infant Growth Study. *Archives of Disease in Childhood, 79*(2), 153-156.

Schiess, S. A., Grote, V., Scaglioni, S., et al. (2010). Intake of energy providing liquids during the first year of life in five European countries. *Clinical Nutrition, 29*(6), 726-732.

Scott, J. A., Dashti, M., Al-Sughayer, M., et al. (2015). Timing and determinants of the introduction of complementary foods in Kuwait: Results of a prospective cohort study. *Journal of Human Lactation, 31*(3), 467-473.

Sicherer, S. H., Munoz-Furlong, A., Godbold, J. H., et al. (2010). US prevalence of self-reported peanut, tree nut, and sesame allergy: 11-year follow-up. *Journal of Allergy and Clinical Immunology, 125*(6), 1322-1326.

Silano, M., Agostoni, C., Sanz, Y., et al. (2016). Infant feeding and risk of developing celiac disease: A systematic review. *BMJ Open, 6*(1), e009163.

Siu, A. L., & Force, U. S. P. S. T. (2015). Screening for iron deficiency anemia in young children: USPSTF recommendation statement. *Pediatrics, 136*(4), 746-752.

Taveras, E. M., Scanlon, K. S., Birch, L., et al. (2004). Association of breastfeeding with maternal control of infant feeding at age 1 year. *Pediatrics, 114*(5), e577-583.

Taylor, R. W., Williams, S. M., Fangupo, L. J., et al. (2017). Effect of a baby-led approach to complementary feeding on infant growth and overweight: A randomized clinical trial. *JAMA Pediatrics, 171*(9), 838-846.

Taylor, S. N. (2018). ABM Clinical Protocol #29: Iron, zinc, and vitamin D supplementation during breastfeeding. *Breastfeeding Medicine, 13*(6), 398-404.

Thorsdottir, I., Gunnarsson, B. S., Atladottir, H., et al. (2003). Iron status at 12 months of age -- Effects of body size, growth and diet in a population with high birth weight. *European Journal of Clinical Nutrition, 57*(4), 505-513.

Togias, A., Cooper, S. F., Acebal, M. L., et al. (2017). Addendum guidelines for the prevention of peanut allergy in the United States: Report of the National Institute of Allergy and Infectious Diseases-sponsored expert panel. *Pediatric Dermatology, 34*(1), e1-e21.

Townsend, E., & Pitchford, N. J. (2012). Baby knows best? The impact of weaning style on food preferences and body mass index in early childhood in a case-controlled sample. *BMJ Open, 2*(1), e000298.

Truby King, M. (1941). *Mothercraft.* Sydney, Australia: Whitecombe & Tombs, Ltd.

USFDA. (2017). For consumers: Seven things pregnant women and parents need to know about arsenic in rice and rice cereal. Retrieved from **fda.gov/consumers/consumer-updates/consumers-seven-things-pregnant-women-and-parents-need-know-about-arsenic-rice-and-rice-cereal**.

Uyoga, M. A., Karanja, S., Paganini, D., et al. (2017). Duration of exclusive breastfeeding is a positive predictor of iron status in 6- to 10-month-old infants in rural Kenya. *Maternal and Child Nutrition, 13*(4).

Wasser, H., Bentley, M., Borja, J., et al. (2011). Infants perceived as "fussy" are more likely to receive complementary foods before 4 months. *Pediatrics, 127*(2), 229-237.

WHO. (2001). *Optimal Duration of Exclusive Breastfeeding: Report of an Expert Consultation.* Geneva, Switzerland: World Health Organization Retrieved from **who.int/nutrition/publications/optimal_duration_of_exc_bfeeding_report_eng.pdf**.

WHO. (2018). Infant and young child feeding. Retrieved from **who.int/mediacentre/factsheets/fs342/en/index.html**.

Wilkinson, P. W., & Davies, D. P. (1978). When and why are babies weaned? *British Medical Journal, 1*(6128), 1682-1693.

Wojcicki, J. M., Holbrook, K., Lustig, R. H., et al. (2011). Infant formula, tea, and water supplementation of Latino infants at 4-6 weeks postpartum. *Journal of Human Lactation, 27*(2), 122-130.

Wright, C. M., Parkinson, K. N., & Drewett, R. F. (2004). Why are babies weaned early? Data from a prospective population based cohort study. *Archives of Disease in Childhood, 89*(9), 813-816.

Zhang, Y., Fein, E. B., & Fein, S. B. (2011). Feeding of dietary botanical supplements and teas to infants in the United States. *Pediatrics, 127*(6), 1060-1066.

Ziegler, E. E., Nelson, S. E., & Jeter, J. M. (2014). Iron stores of breastfed infants during the first year of life. *Nutrients, 6*(5), 2023-2034.

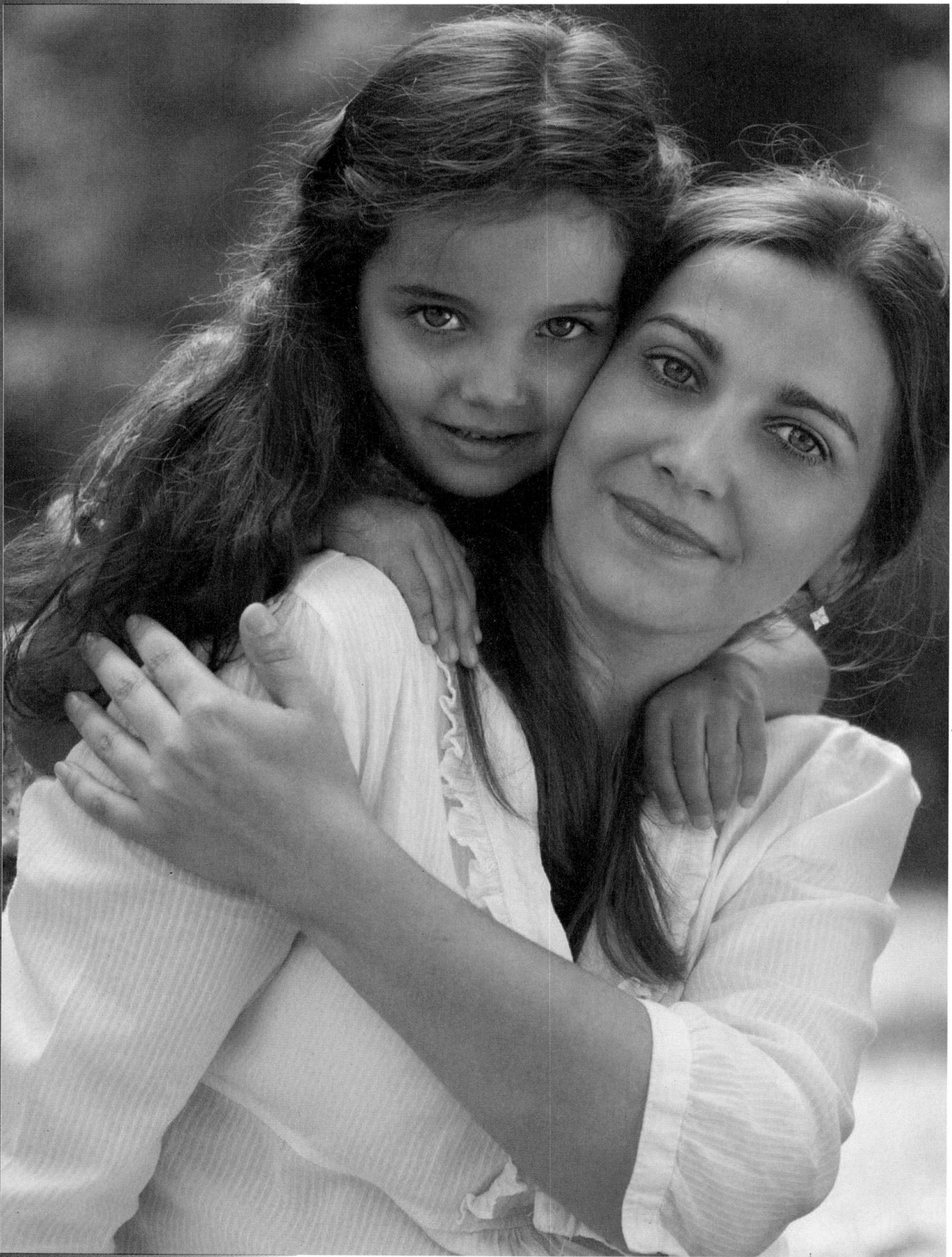

Weaning from Nursing

5

Weaning has different meanings and implications in different cultures.

In some parts of the world, such as the U.K., "weaning" refers to starting solid foods, which are referred to as "weaning foods." In this chapter, weaning is defined as the end of nursing, but it is far more than that. Depending on cultural beliefs, weaning may be considered a time of withdrawal or deprivation or, alternatively, a time of growth and new maturity. But in every culture, weaning is always a time of transition as the child adjusts to new sources of nourishment and comfort and new ways of exploring the world. Weaning is not an act but a process that begins when a baby takes any food other than during nursing and ends with the last nursing session.

RECOMMENDATIONS

Health organizations recommend exclusive breastfeeding for 6 months and continued nursing with other foods until at least 1 to 2 years of age.

In its 2012 policy statement, "Breastfeeding and the Use of Human Milk," the American Academy of Pediatrics (AAP) Committee on Breastfeeding (AAP, 2012, p. e832) wrote:

> "The AAP recommends exclusive breastfeeding for about 6 months, with continuation of breastfeeding for 1 year or longer as mutually desired by mother and infant...."

The World Health Organization recommends continued breastfeeding for 2 years of age or beyond (WHO, 2018). In developing countries, the health risks of early weaning are immense, due to sanitation problems, unreliable food and water supplies, and lack of available health care. However, these recommendations are meant to apply to all babies in all countries.

A 2016 article in *The Lancet* (Victora et al., 2016) estimated that more than 800,000 children worldwide die annually from lack of breastfeeding or early weaning, primarily in the developing world. Earlier research done in developing countries found differences in health outcomes even well after 1 year. For example, weaned children between 16 and 36 months had more types of illness, longer duration of illness, and required more medical care than nursing children the same age (Gulick, 1986). Also, weaned children between 12 and 36 months were 3.5 times more likely to die than those still breastfeeding (Molbak, 1994).

No matter where a child lives, weaning before age two is associated with greater incidence of illness and death. In the U.S., a 2017 analysis of the health effects and healthcare costs of suboptimal breastfeeding (Bartick et al., 2017) found that during the first year of life weaned babies have a higher incidence of:

- Ear infection (otitis media)
- Gastrointestinal infection
- Lower respiratory infection requiring hospitalization
- Sudden Infant Death Syndrome (SIDS)

But the health effects of nursing are not confined to infancy. Later in life, babies who did not nurse or weaned early were more likely to develop severe health problems such as:

- Acute lymphoblastic leukemia
- Crohn's disease and other inflammatory bowel diseases.

In preterm infants, use of formula and early weaning were associated with a greater incidence of necrotizing enterocolitis (NEC), an often-fatal bowel condition that can also lead to lifelong nutrient absorption problems.

This U.S. article (Bartick et al., 2017) defines optimal breastfeeding as at least 90% of families breastfeeding exclusively for the first 6 months and continuing to breastfeed with the addition of solid foods until at least 1 year. Its authors calculated that 721 annual U.S. infant deaths can be attributed to less-than-optimal breastfeeding, with most of these from SIDS (492) and NEC (190).

Annual excess U.S. healthcare costs associated with less-than-optimal breastfeeding are estimated to total $3 billion. But it's not just babies who suffer negative health outcomes from lack of nursing and early weaning. According to this same 2017 U.S. cost analysis, nearly 80% of this $3 billion is from excess maternal healthcare costs plus an estimated $14.2 billion in premature deaths. Women who wean early or don't breastfeed, have a higher incidence of:

- Breast cancer
- Ovarian cancer (premenopausal)
- Type 2 diabetes mellitus
- Hypertension
- Heart attacks (myocardial infarction), the number one killer of women

KEY CONCEPT

Longer and more exclusive nursing is linked to better health outcomes in nursing parents.

The authors concluded that for every 597 women who breastfeed optimally, one infant and one maternal death is prevented.

THE DECISION TO WEAN

When families ask for information on weaning, they may feel vulnerable to criticism. Affirm them and answer any questions.

Many nursing parents consider nursing a central part of their relationship with their child and their expectations of themselves (Hauck & Irurita, 2002). For this reason, when discussing nursing and weaning, the nursing parent may feel vulnerable to criticism and worry about not meeting others' expectations.

When families ask about weaning, first it is important to affirm them and allay their fear of criticism. When parents' concerns about being negatively judged are laid to rest, answer any specific questions to let them know you are willing to help with weaning. Once you provide the requested information about weaning, in the interest of knowing all the options, ask if they are interested in hearing about other alternatives as well.

• • •

Nursing parents often have mixed feelings and unrealistic expectations about weaning. Help them explore their feelings and expectations by asking open-ended questions.

In cultures where early weaning is common, pressure from others may influence a family to consider weaning and raise the expectations for weaning so high that they cannot be met. To get a sense of how parents feel about nursing and their expectations, ask some open-ended questions, such as:

- "How do you think weaning will change your life?"
- "Are there others in your life with strong opinions about nursing?"
- "Describe your relationship with your baby."
- "What are your feelings about weaning?"

• • •

If a family's expectations of weaning are unrealistic, affirm them and then share relevant information.

Some expectations for weaning are unlikely to be met. For example, parents may think weaning will make their baby more independent or decrease his night-waking. If family members' expectations are unrealistic, affirm their underlying need and share the information you have. For example:

- "It's hard to be a good mother or father when you feel exhausted much of the time. But weaning may not help you get more rest. Research found that weaned babies do not sleep longer than babies still nursing (Yilmaz, Gurakan, Cakir, & Tezcan, 2002). Would you like to talk about other ways to get more rest? Are there other reasons you'd like to wean now?"
- "Your mother feels strongly that you should wean because nursing is too stressful for you. She is very lucky you want to be responsive to her feelings. However, there is research your mother might not know about that indicates bottle-feeding is more stressful than nursing (Mezzacappa & Katlin, 2002). Would you like to share this with her?"

Weaning: Culture and History

Depending on cultural norms, weaning may be considered a positive and natural stage of growth or something that is done to a child against his wishes.

Every nursing child eventually weans. However, in different cultures, weaning may be viewed very differently. The word "wean" is derived from a word meaning "satisfaction" or "fulfillment." During most of human history (Tessone, Garcia Guraieb, Goni, & Panarello, 2015) and in many parts of the world, weaning is considered a natural stage of growth, a sign that the child has had his fill and is ready to move into the wider world.

However, in the U.S., the U.K., and some other Western countries, weaning is often not seen as a process to be celebrated or a naturally occurring stage of growth. Weaning is usually considered a time of deprivation and unhappiness, something that is done to a child against his wishes. In cultures where babies tend to wean young, some nursing parents are cautioned to be sure their babies are weaned by a certain age or their babies will nurse "forever." But this does not reflect the broader human experience.

• • •

When viewed cross-culturally, the average age of weaning is between 3 and 4 years.

According to cultural anthropologists, the average age of weaning internationally is between 3 and 4 years of age (Dettwyler, 1995). In 1967, anthropologist Margaret Mead and early breastfeeding researcher Niles Newton published an article describing weaning practices of 64 traditional societies (Mead & Newton, 1967). Among these societies, the average weaning age was 3 years, and only one society weaned their children as early as 6 months.

History tells us that in most times and places it was common practice to nurse for years. The Koran recommends breastfeeding until age two, and the custom of the Egyptian Pharaohs in Moses' time was to nurse for 3 years. Until the 20th century, children in both China and Japan breastfed until age 4 or 5 years. Even in England and the U.S., historical writings tell us that not so long ago 2 to 4 years of breastfeeding was typical. In 1725, authors of child-care texts clearly disapproved of 4-year-olds nursing, which implies there were more than a few of them around. By 1850, nursing for 11 months was recommended and breastfeeding for 2 years was criticized (Bumgarner, 2000).

• • •

To predict the natural age of weaning for humans without the influence of culture, anthropologist Katherine Dettwyler used the same criteria that biologists use to determine the natural age of weaning in other mammals (Dettwyler, 1995). These criteria (followed by the equivalent age for humans) include:

- Age at tripling-quadrupling birth weight (2 to 3 years)
- Age when one third of adult weight is reached (4 to 7 years)
- Age at eruption of permanent teeth (5.5 to 6 years)
- Gestational length (our nearest genetic relative, the chimpanzee, weans at about 6 times its gestational length; which for humans would be 4.5 years)

As a result, Dettwyler concluded that from a biological perspective the natural age of weaning for humans is between 2.5 and 7 years.

Without the influence of culture, the "natural" age of weaning is estimated to be between 2.5 and 7 years.

The Nursing Parent's Perspective

Nursing is a complex social behavior, and feelings about nursing and weaning may vary greatly among families. Feelings about nursing can also vary in the same parent over time. An Australian qualitative study of 25 mothers (Schmied & Barclay, 1999) explored the breastfeeding experience by interviewing these mothers during pregnancy and several times during the first 6 months after birth. In Australia, where more than 90% of families initiate nursing after birth, all of the study mothers considered breastfeeding crucial to their relationship with their baby, and most considered it a part of good mothering. Most were committed to persevering in order "to achieve their identity as a breastfeeding mother."

Feelings about nursing and weaning vary greatly among families.

But not all study mothers felt the same way about nursing. While some enjoyed their breastfeeding baby's dependence on them, others found this difficult and emotionally overwhelming and sought time away from their babies. Although 8 of the 25 mothers (32%) found breastfeeding intimate and pleasurable, 9 (nearly 40%) had mixed feelings and another 8 (32%) experienced "searing pain" during the early weeks and months, and at times considered it "agonizing," "horrendous," and "violent." Rather than feeling in harmony with their babies, as other study mothers did, due to the pain, these mothers at times felt alienated from their babies. Some of these mothers blamed themselves; others blamed their babies. Some also reported feeling restricted from activities they used to enjoy and felt they had to "put their lives on hold."

KEY CONCEPT

Decisions about when to wean may be influenced by nursing problems or deeper issues.

Some of the study mothers weaned early. Others who had early breastfeeding problems continued nursing and eventually enjoyed a connected and intimate breastfeeding relationship with their babies. But all considered breast-feeding central to their experience of motherhood. Of these mothers, 20 of the 25 continued to breastfeed at 3 months and 18 of the 25 were breastfeeding at 6 months.

• • •

The decision to wean may be influenced more by a nursing parent's overall feelings about nursing than by a specific feeding problem.

When researchers ask parents why they chose to wean, many cite specific nursing problems, such as worries about milk production, latching struggles, or nipple pain (Mikami et al., 2018; Newby & Davies, 2016; Odom, Li, Scanlon, Perrine, & Grummer-Strawn, 2013; Perrine, Scanlon, Li, Odom, & Grummer-Strawn, 2012). However, because nursing is a complex social behavior, there are often deeper issues that affect a nursing parent's decisions.

One Canadian study of 80 women who breastfed a baby for 9 months (Rempel, 2004) noted that at every stage of lactation the less control the mothers felt they had over nursing, the weaker their intentions to continue, and the earlier they weaned. This perceived control included three variables: breastfeeding ease, mothers' perception that they could nurse as long as they wanted, and mothers' confidence. At 9 months, the mothers cited biting and maintaining milk production as key issues they faced, and these variables affected whether they weaned their babies then. The mothers also perceived their social support for breastfeeding decreasing the longer they breastfed, which also influenced their weaning decisions. The author suggested that for women to nurse for at least a year, social norms need to change and mothers need to receive support and encouragement for longer nursing. The study author also suggested that understanding how milk production works and the nursing adjustments parents can make as needed may be the key to families' comfort with longer nursing.

In one U.S. study (Isabella & Isabella, 1994), the decision to wean was more strongly associated with a lack of support and difficult adjustment to pregnancy and motherhood than to feeding problems. Another U.S. study that interviewed 52 mothers from the U.S. and Canada (Kelleher, 2006) found that many were surprised by the discomfort they experienced during early nursing, but if they perceived the discomfort as temporary and had support, they were more likely to keep nursing.

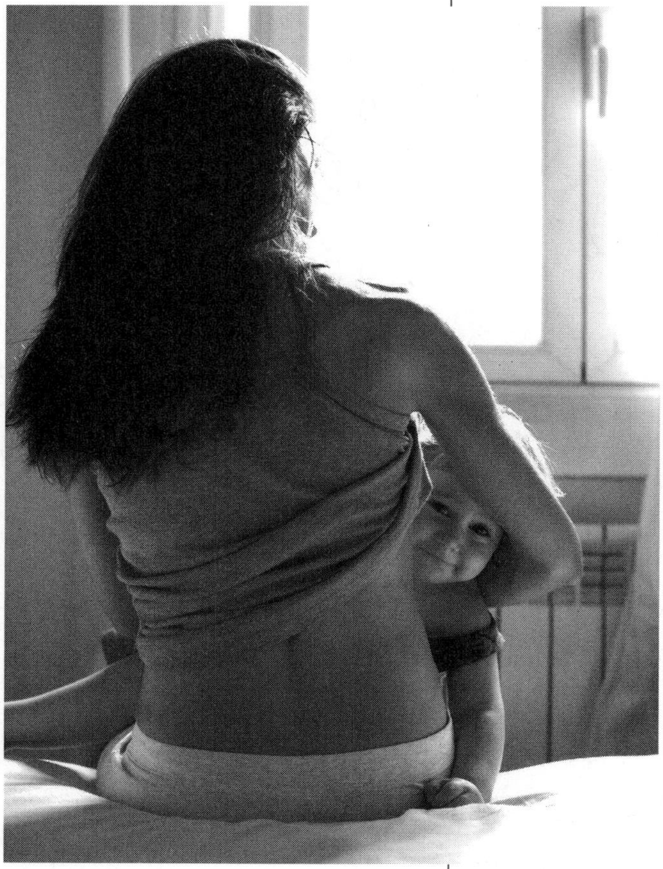

In one Australian study (Cooke, Sheehan, & Schmied, 2003), researchers used the Maternal Breastfeeding Evaluation Scale (Leff, Jefferis, & Gagne, 1994) to rate breastfeeding satisfaction based on answers to a series of questions about adjustment to motherhood, baby's satisfaction, and feelings about lifestyle. The 215 study mothers were surveyed before birth and after birth at 2 weeks, 6 weeks, and 3 months to rate their breastfeeding satisfaction and determine the relationship between their perceived breastfeeding problems and the decision to wean. At 2 and 6 weeks, almost 50% of the mothers reported having breastfeeding problems, such as painful nipples or worries about milk production. By 3 months, the percentage of mothers reporting problems decreased to 28%.

The researchers found the decision to wean was more closely related to the mothers' overall level of breastfeeding satisfaction than to specific problems. For example, more than half of the mothers reported having painful nipples during the first 2 weeks, but less than one third thought it made breastfeeding difficult and at no time did this significantly affect their decision to wean.

TABLE 5.1 Reasons Mothers Gave for Weaning During the First Year

Baby's Age at Weaning (%)	Reasons Mothers Gave for Weaning (%)
<12 weeks (19%)	Not enough milk/My milk alone didn't satisfy baby (91%) Trouble latching (48%) Nipple trauma (30%)
>12 to 26 weeks (10%)	Not enough milk/My milk alone didn't satisfy baby (79%) Trouble latching (14%) Baby lost interest (14%)
>26 to 52 weeks (22%)	Not enough milk/My milk alone didn't satisfy baby (48%) Baby lost interest (29%) Baby biting (16%)

Adapted from (Newby & Davies, 2016)

Mothers who reported engorgement and leaking milk were actually less likely to wean than others. This may be because they perceived engorgement and leaking as indicating abundant milk production, which increased their breastfeeding satisfaction.

• • •

In a 2016 Australian study (Newby & Davies, 2016), researchers categorized the reasons 161 mothers gave for weaning their babies in different time windows during the first year of life (Table 5.1). No matter when they weaned, the most common reason the mothers gave (they were allowed to give more than one reason) related to concerns about their milk production: "not enough milk" and "my milk alone didn't satisfy baby." The researchers also had access to the infants' weight gain data and concluded that most likely most of these women didn't have actual milk production issues, because their babies' weight gains were normal. Only a very small subset of these babies gained weight slowly. It appeared that many of the mothers who believed they didn't have enough milk actually did. The researchers also acknowledged that "not enough milk" is considered a socially acceptable reason for weaning and that some mothers may have given that reason even if it wasn't the primary reason they weaned.

Unrealistic expectations can lead to worries about milk production, which can lead to decreased enjoyment of nursing, which can lead to weaning.

Beginning at around 3 months, another reason given for weaning by the study mothers that became more common was "baby lost interest." This reason is likely also based on faulty assumptions. Nursing babies typically become distractible at 3 months, but they are not physically ready to wean. Parents may mistake this normal baby behavior for weaning readiness. The interventions researchers suggested to prevent unnecessary weaning included developing educational programs to help families learn to recognize normal nursing behaviors at different ages and understand more clearly how milk production works. They also suggested that families need to know that if they use formula, it is still worthwhile to continue nursing, as partial nursing has great value to the nursing parent and child and is a healthier alternative than complete weaning.

Unrealistic expectations of how many minutes nursing babies should stay settled during feeds or how long they should stay satisfied after nursing can affect nursing parents' perception of their ability to nurture their babies, a factor closely linked to their satisfaction with nursing. Although "worries about milk production" is the most common reason women give for weaning and using formula, it is also possible that some study mothers had legitimate milk production issues. But as many qualitative studies found, there is often more going on below the surface. One Canadian researcher (Dennis, 2002, p. 14) wrote:

> "...the most prevalent reason for discontinuing or supplementing breastfeeding has been insufficient milk. Yet it appears unlikely that many women truly experience insufficient milk...Thus, the rationale for discontinuing breastfeeding is a convoluted interplay of factors."

• • •

The decision to wean may occur in several phases.

One Australian qualitative study (Hauck & Irurita, 2002) examined the perspectives of 33 breastfeeding mothers as they made the decision to wean and what came after. The researchers noted the distinct changes in perspective and attitude that occurred as the mothers decided to wean.

- **Shifting focus.** Triggered by the conflicting expectations of others, the mothers described how first their tolerance for this conflict was exceeded, and then how they took charge by deciding what was important to them and making their decision on that basis.
- **Selective focus.** After making their decision, the mothers chose to focus only on those who agreed with their decision and avoided or ignored the rest.
- **Confirming focus.** After weaning, the mothers sought affirmation for their decision by first assessing the impact on their child and then by acknowledging what breastfeeding had meant to them.

A 2018 U.S. qualitative study of 28 women living in Iowa who stopped breastfeeding at least 6 months before the interviews (Schafer, Buch, Campo, & Ashida, 2018) discovered seven common "turning points" in their breastfeeding experiences. Weaning was the final turning point, which involved "letting go" of breastfeeding on an emotional level. Whether the mothers left breastfeeding with a positive feeling of pride and accomplishment or a negative feeling of guilt or regret depended in part on how old their child was at weaning (the older the child, the more likely mothers were to feel positively) and the availability of coping resources, such as people providing emotional support.

The Influence of Others

Timing of weaning is influenced by others and the presence or absence of social support.

Support from others appears to be a crucial ingredient for longer nursing. Conversely, withdrawal of support is associated with the decision to wean (Rempel, 2004).

In one 2013 U.K. study (Dowling & Brown, 2013), researchers combined two qualitative datasets to explore the attitudes and experiences of mothers who breastfed longer than 6 months. In the U.K., at this writing, more than 80% of families nurse after birth, but by 6 months only about one third are still nursing, and by 1 year this has dropped to 1% (McAndrew, 2012). Because it is unusual in the U.K. to see nursing babies older than 6 months, families who want to nurse longer face great social pressure to wean. In this article, the authors categorized the unsupportive comments from

> **KEY CONCEPT**
>
> *Social support is essential for longer nursing duration.*

others that these mothers reported into several main themes:

- Breastfeeding is synonymous with young babies.
- Longer breastfeeding is "pointless."
- Longer-term breastfeeding is bizarre or comical.
- Longer-term breastfeeding is a negative experience for the mother.

The authors concluded that actions are needed in the U.K. to normalize longer nursing, perhaps by providing more education on the positive health effects of longer nursing for parents and children and by featuring images of older babies and toddlers nursing in commonly seen media geared to parents and healthcare providers.

In a 2018 U.K. study (Newman & Williamson, 2018), its authors drew similar conclusions, finding that in the U.K. breastfeeding older babies was routinely stigmatized by sensationalized media accounts and by the overt disapproval expressed by family members and the wider community. This study and a 2017 U.K. article examined the characteristics of families who continue nursing in spite of strong social disapproval (Dowling & Pontin, 2017). They found that most of the mothers were involved in "a range of support networks," which provided the encouragement they needed to keep nursing. These mothers were described as "a group of strong-willed and determined women" with a clear sense of purpose of "doing the right thing" (Dowling & Pontin, 2017, p. 71).

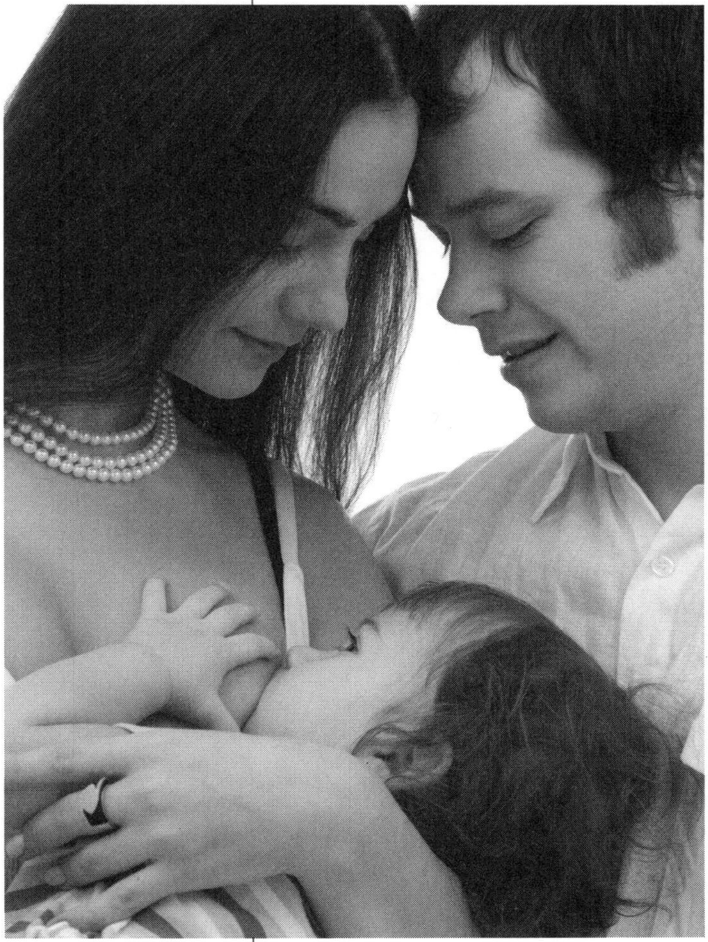

In cultures where early weaning is the norm, the longer babies nurse, in general the less support nursing parents receive, even from healthcare providers. A U.S. study that included surveys from more than 49,000 mothers (Keim, Tchaconas, & Adesman, 2017) found that the 1% of families who used an alternative healthcare provider for their nursing baby, such as a chiropractor or naturopath, rated their healthcare provider more supportive of breastfeeding after 1 year than those families who used a conventional healthcare provider.

The fathers of nursing babies can have a significant effect on breastfeeding duration, either positive or negative. A 2017 U.S. article that examined the findings of two studies (Rempel, Rempel, & Moore, 2017) concluded that the most effective support a father can give to a nursing partner is to use a sensitive, coordinated teamwork approach that is responsive to the partner's needs. Not surprisingly, intimate partner violence was found in another U.S. study (Wallenborn, Cha, & Masho, 2018) to increase the chances of weaning before 8 weeks by 18%.

A 2016 systematic review on the effect of grandmothers on initiation and duration of nursing (Negin, Coffman, Vizintin, & Raynes-Greenow, 2016) found that in many studies a supportive maternal grandmother had a positive effect on nursing.

• • •

Healthcare providers affect families' decisions about nursing. Both a lack of help and encouragement and over-zealousness about nursing are associated with shorter nursing duration.

One U.S. study (Taveras et al., 2003) found that families whose healthcare providers encouraged breastfeeding were about half as likely to wean by 12 weeks compared with those whose healthcare providers did not verbally encourage breastfeeding. Another U.S. study found that mothers were more likely to wean if their healthcare providers recommended formula or didn't think his or her opinion mattered (Taveras et al., 2004). Conversely, a 2016 systematic review of expectant parents (Roll & Cheater, 2016) cautioned that healthcare providers who families perceived as being judgmental or over-zealous about breastfeeding negatively influenced their nursing decisions

WEANING DYNAMICS

The Role of Parent and Child

Even when parents do not actively encourage weaning, children will eventually outgrow nursing on their own.

Babies are born hardwired to breastfeed, but children outgrow nursing as they mature and their need for mother's milk decreases. Just as children get their first tooth, learn to walk, and learn to use the toilet at different ages, children also outgrow nursing at different ages. Factors that may influence the age of weaning include allergies, strength of sucking urge, temperament, and many others.

• • •

Weaning may be driven mostly by the nursing parent, mostly by the child, or it may be a mutual process.

When weaning is perceived by nursing parents as being a mutual process, their emotional adjustment may be easier (Hauck & Irurita, 2002). But weaning is not always mutual. In some cases, the child may decide to wean before the parent feels ready. Then the parent may feel a greater sense of loss. If parents wean before the child is ready, they may worry about the child's emotional and physical adjustment to this transition.

• • •

Where early weaning is common, many families misread normal baby behaviors as signs their babies are ready to wean.

Due to their physiological need for mother's milk, babies younger than 12 months are unlikely to be developmentally ready to wean. However, where early weaning is the cultural norm, many families encourage weaning without realizing it by regularly substituting bottles and pacifiers/dummies for nursing. When the baby shifts his interest from nursing to the nursing substitute, many families think the baby has "weaned himself."

Weaning can also happen inadvertently when parents misinterpret normal infant behavior as signs their baby is ready to wean. One example is the Australian study described in the previous section (Newby & Davies, 2016), in which mothers reported weaning babies as young as 3 to 6 months old because the babies "lost interest." In one Canadian study (Rempel, 2004), 96% of the 80 mothers who weaned their babies between 9 and 12 months said they did so because they were convinced their babies were "ready to wean" by the following behaviors:

- Asking to breastfeed less often
- Shorter breastfeeding sessions
- More distractibility while breastfeeding

All of these behaviors are part of normal growth and development at this age and are not signs of weaning readiness. A baby who "weans himself" before 12 months should be considered on a nursing strike, a solvable feeding problem described on p. 128.

Weaning Basics

Before 1 year, donor milk or infant formula will most likely be recommended as a substitute for nursing, as other milks, such as cow's milk, are not recommended in most parts of the world until after 1 year (Fewtrell et al., 2017).

When weaning before 1 year, consult the baby's healthcare provider about what to substitute for mother's milk.

• • •

In Western cultures, where sanitation is good, if a baby is not nursed, an infant feeding bottle will be most likely used. If the baby is older than 6 to 8 months and is drinking well from a cup, he may be able to forego the bottle and wean directly to a cup. One advantage to this approach is there is no need to wean later from a bottle.

The feeding method chosen will depend on the baby's age and local norms.

In parts of the world where sanitation is poor, infant feeding bottles are not recommended (WHO, 2018). In these areas, safer feeding methods include easy-to-clean containers without crevices, such as small cups with straight sides or spoons. Also, because powdered infant formula is not sterile, it is not the first choice for babies younger than 3 months. ("CDC warns of Cronobacter in powdered milk, infant formula," 2016).

• • •

A sudden weaning is often painful for a nursing parent and difficult for a child. Sometimes a sudden weaning is necessary, such as in case of an emergency medical treatment that is not compatible with nursing. But many families wean abruptly because they aren't aware that there are gentler and more gradual ways to wean. Weaning gradually—with consideration for the feelings and preferences of both parent and child—can make weaning a positive experience, even when a child has not yet outgrown nursing on his own.

The child's age and readiness to wean, as well as the approach used, will affect how easy or difficult weaning is for parent and child.

Approaches to Weaning

Many studies focus on why and when families wean from nursing, but few researchers examine how exactly they do it. In a Canadian study (Williams & Morse, 1989), which is one of the few about the process of weaning, 90 first-time mothers were asked to describe their weaning experiences. Their babies were weaned between 6 weeks and 20 months old, with a median age at weaning of about 9.5 months. As in some other studies (Hauck & Irurita, 2002), this study's authors did not include those who weaned earlier than 6 weeks because full breastfeeding had not yet been established.

Weaning tends to fall into several general categories: gradual, partial, and abrupt.

According to these researchers, the weaning process fell into three categories:

- Gradual weaning (42%), which took 1 to 8 weeks;
- Two-stage weaning (49%), which started over 6 to 8 weeks with a gradual partial weaning until baby was nursing once or twice a day for a while until full weaning occurred;

- Abrupt, sudden, or "cold turkey" weaning (9%), which started and ended within 1 day.

The younger the baby when weaning occurred, the more likely weaning was done abruptly.

The reasons mothers gave for weaning included:

- Return to work (41%)
- It was time (11%)
- Baby lost interest (10%)
- Mother wanted more freedom (9%)
- Pressure from others (9%)
- To have another baby (7%)
- Teeth (5%)
- Illness in mother or baby (4%)
- Mother tired (2%)
- Disliked breastfeeding (2%)

In another U.S. study, all of the 222 mothers weaned before their babies were 5 months old (Neighbors, Gillespie, Schwartz, & Foxman, 2003), and weaning approaches were defined differently. A weaning was considered "gradual" if it took 4 or more days, and "all at once" if the last breastfeeding occurred within 3 days of when weaning began. Using these definitions:

- 67% weaned gradually
- 33% weaned all at once

Half of these mothers weaned within 7 days. The older the baby, the more likely it was to be a gradual approach:

- 0-5 weeks of age—67% weaned ≤3 days
- 21-25 weeks of age—26% weaned ≤3 days

More gradual weaning was associated with returning to work. Women weaning quickly were more likely to be experiencing pain.

Another U.S. study looked at weaning an older child (Sugarman & Kendall-Tackett, 1995). In this study, average age of weaning was 2.5 to 3.0 years of age. The 179 mothers who responded to the survey belonged to La Leche League International and lived in a culture generally unsupportive of breastfeeding after a year.

- More than half (56%) reported that their youngest child weaned gradually, with 53% describing the weaning as "child-led."
- Only about 13% considered the weaning sudden.

Nearly a quarter of these mothers encouraged weaning by talking to their child about it.

Gradual Weaning

A gradual weaning has physical and emotional advantages for nursing parent and child.

A gradual weaning makes it possible for the nursing parent to avoid painful mammary fullness and reduces the risk of mastitis. By reducing nursing gradually and expressing a small amount of milk whenever feelings of fullness occur, the nursing parent can slow milk production comfortably.

A gradual weaning also gives the family some time before the milk is gone to evaluate how well their child tolerates the substitute food. This is more important for a younger baby, who may be more vulnerable to allergies or sensitivities, but it can also be important for some very sensitive older babies and children.

From an emotional standpoint, a gradual weaning allows a child more time to adjust to the loss of the closeness nursing provides.

Gradual Weaning Between Birth and 12 Months

For a gradual weaning of a younger baby, each time a daily nursing session is dropped, before dropping another, suggest allowing at least 3 days for milk production to decrease.

Before a baby is old enough to have strong preferences about his daily routine, weaning usually involves substituting a feeding of infant formula (average volume: 3 to 4 oz. or 89 to 119 mL) for a nursing session. During a gradual weaning, it may take about 2 to 3 weeks for the nursing parent to comfortably go from exclusive nursing to completely weaned. To help accomplish this, suggest the family:

- Note the times each day the baby usually nurses.
- Pick one daily feed (leave the first morning nursing for last, as most nursing parents are fullest then) and instead feed the substitute food by the chosen method.
- Allow at least 3 days before dropping another nursing to give the milk production time to decrease comfortably and gradually.

NOTE: If at any time the nursing parent experiences any uncomfortable feelings of mammary fullness, suggest expressing milk to comfort or allowing the baby to nurse for a short time. Encourage parents to pay attention to their body cues, expressing milk to comfort whenever needed. (For more details, see the last section of this chapter.)

> **KEY CONCEPT**
>
> *Gradual weaning from exclusive nursing takes about 2 to 3 weeks to accomplish.*

• • •

During weaning, suggest the child receive extra focused attention and cuddling.

To help offset the emotional loss of the closeness of nursing, suggest during weaning that the child receive extra focused attention and skin-to-skin contact either from the nursing parent or from someone else. This might include holding, rocking, cuddling, reading stories, or any other activity the child enjoys.

• • •

The weaning child may seek other sucking outlets; suggest the family decide on one that is acceptable to them.

Because children have a strong urge to suck until they outgrow nursing, during or after weaning they may find another outlet, such as thumb-sucking. If the family prefers the child use a bottle or pacifier/dummy, suggest being ready to offer this instead.

Gradual Weaning after 12 Months

For weaning to be a positive experience for the child older than 1 year, suggest respecting his preferences during the process.

At 1 year or older, a child usually has strong preferences about nursing, as he will about all aspects of his daily routine. But even so, weaning can still be a gradual and positive experience. To accomplish this, first allow plenty of time. It may take several weeks to wean, depending on how many times a day he is nursing. It will also be helpful to consider his temperament and opinions, and factor them into the strategies.

• • •

Suggest trying different weaning strategies and use those that work best with the child.

Every child is different and what works for one may not work well for another. Suggest experimenting with the following approaches and see which ones most effectively reduce the child's desire to nurse.

Don't offer, don't refuse. This approach, popularized by La Leche League International, refers to nursing when the child asks but not offering to nurse when he doesn't ask. When used with other strategies, this can speed the process.

Offer regular meals, snacks, and drinks to minimize his hunger and thirst and age-appropriate fun activities to avoid nursing out of boredom.

Change daily routines. Think about the times and places he asks to nurse and how to change their routine, so he will be reminded less often. For example, if he usually asks to nurse when the parent sits in a certain chair, suggest avoiding that chair during weaning.

Get the partner or a support person involved. If the child usually nurses upon waking in the morning, suggest asking the partner or a support person to get him up and make his breakfast. The partner or support person can also help him get back to sleep when he wakes at night and can plan special daytime outings.

Anticipate and offer substitutes and distractions. Be sure to offer substitutes before the child asks to nurse, because once he has asked, he will likely feel rejected and upset if a substitute is offered. As an example, right before a usual nursing time, offer a special snack and drink and then take him to a favorite place, such as a playground as a distraction. Some children nurse more often at home with nothing to do and nurse less often when out and distracted. With this type of child, spend as much of the day as possible out of the house. Some children nurse more often when out of the house and in new surroundings. With this type of child, stay home more and keep distractions to a minimum.

Postpone. This works for a child who nurses at irregular times and places and is old enough to accept waiting. If postponing leaves the child feeling as though the nursing parent is keeping him at arm's length, he may become even more determined to nurse. If so, use other strategies.

Shorten the length of each nursing. This is most effective with children older than 2 years and is a good beginning to the weaning process.

Bargaining can work well with the older child. A child who is close to outgrowing nursing may give up nursing earlier by mutual agreement. But most children younger than 3 years are not mature enough to understand the meaning of a promise.

Adjust the weaning plan as needed based on the child's reactions and preferences. Pick and choose among these strategies based on the child's reactions. One child may be unhappy with postponing but do well with distraction and substitution. Also, certain nursing sessions may be more important to the child than others. If so, suggest continuing those until the end and allow the child to give them up last. If he clings to his bedtime nursing, for example, continue those for a while longer.

Be flexible when unusual situations arise. If the child is ill, allow him to nurse more often for comfort. Return to weaning after he is feeling better.

When to slow down. Even at the same age, some children will be more ready to wean than others. If the child becomes upset and cries or insists upon nursing even when the parent tries to distract or comfort him in other ways, this may mean that weaning is going too fast or that different strategies would be better. Other signs that weaning may be moving too fast are changes or regressions in behavior, such as stuttering, night-waking, an increase in clinginess, a new or increased fear of separation, biting (if he has never bitten before), stomach upsets, and constipation.

• • •

Another way to wean gradually is to simply allow the child to outgrow nursing on his own.

Even in the U.S., where at this writing about 70% of babies are weaned by 1 year, some families allow their children to wean according to their own internal timetable. Some choose it because it feels right to them. Some choose it because it allows their child to grow at his own pace. And some choose it because it is the least work.

Where early weaning is the norm, some assume that nursing past 1 year is an act of martyrdom (Dowling & Brown, 2013; Newman & Williamson, 2018), but in many ways nursing a toddler makes parents' lives easier. The relaxing hormones released during nursing help keep the nursing parent's temper in check, even when under duress, and nursing makes naptimes and bedtimes easy and ends tantrums quickly.

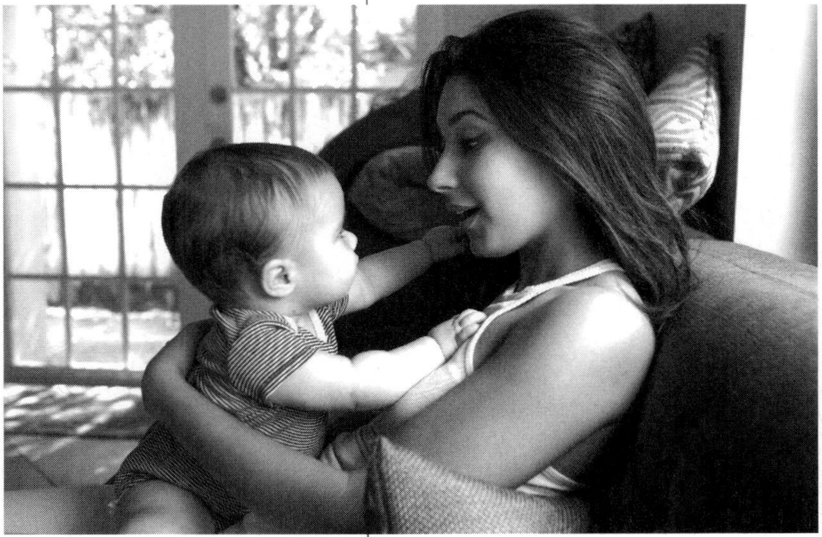

Outgrowing nursing is usually a gradual process, although an occasional child may wean earlier and more abruptly than expected. More commonly, though, milk production reduces slowly and comfortably without any thought or effort as the child's attention becomes more focused on the world around him and less on nursing.

One advantage of going at the child's pace is that families never have to deal with an unhappy child resisting efforts to wean or having to deal later with weaning again from the bottle. As one mother said, "I wouldn't think of limiting or ending the breastfeeding relationship any more than I would think of limiting or ending my love for my children. Gradual weaning allowed us both to grow into other ways of expressing our love" (Kendall-Tackett & Sugarman, 1995, p. 181). Many families who allow their children to outgrow nursing report that the process was so gradual that they are not even sure when their child's last nursing happened.

• • •

The age that children outgrow nursing will vary from child to child.

Children mature at different rates. They learn to walk, talk, and get their first tooth at different ages, and the same is true for weaning. One child may wean at 1 or 2 years old, while another may be avidly nursing at age three. A child with a strong sucking urge, an intense need for closeness, or an unrecognized allergy, sensitivity, or other physical problem may nurse longer than others. As mentioned previously, nursing refusal before 1 year should be considered a nursing strike (p. 128) rather than a sign that the child has outgrown nursing, because at that age the baby still has a physiological need for mother's milk.

• • •

Where early weaning is common, many families find the biggest challenge of allowing their child to outgrow nursing is coping with others' opinions as their children get older.

The older the child, the more challenging dealing with others' opinions can sometimes be (Dowling & Brown, 2013; Dowling & Pontin, 2017; Newman & Williamson, 2018). Yet, in spite of this, some families feel that the positives outweigh the negatives.

One way some families handle the social challenges is to keep nursing private, which is possible because an older child does not usually nurse as often as a young baby. Time-tested strategies for avoiding nursing in less-than-friendly places include:

- Setting limits on where and when the child can nurse.
- Bringing snacks, drinks, toys, and/or books to distract the child when out.
- Choosing a "code word" for nursing that won't be obvious to others.
- Finding private places to nurse away from home, such as clothing fitting rooms or family lounges at shopping malls.
- Carefully choosing clothing. Two-piece outfits allow nursing more easily. So do cover-ups, like ponchos, blankets, or shawls.

Parents who nurse longer than their cultural norm find this easier if they have support. International organizations like La Leche League and national organizations like Breastfeeding USA, the U.K.'s Breastfeeding Network, Ireland's Ciudiú, and the Australian Breastfeeding Association are places families can meet others who value nursing at all ages. The Baby Cafes available in some areas are another place to gather, share stories, and enjoy mutual support.

Partial Weaning

A partial weaning can be an alternative to a complete weaning for some employed nursing parents and those who are feeling overwhelmed.

A nursing parent planning to return to work but not planning to express milk or nurse at work may assume that it's necessary to wean completely. But a partial weaning is another option. A partial weaning may allow nursing to continue at home, while staying comfortable at work.

A partial weaning may also be an alternative to a full weaning for the nursing parent who feels overwhelmed by nursing. For example, some parents with a history of childhood sexual abuse find the intimate contact of nursing difficult (Kendall-Tackett, 2017). More limited nursing may make it possible for someone in this situation to continue. For more details, see p. 840.

After reducing the number of daily feeds, some of the breastfeeding mothers in one Canadian study (Williams & Morse, 1989) decided to breastfeed longer. Discovering they could keep nursing in a more limited way left them feeling better about continuing. This group included employed mothers returning to work, as well as those who wanted to spend more time away from their babies.

• • •

A partial weaning involves eliminating some nursing sessions while continuing others.

A partial weaning usually occurs in several steps. First, decide what the baby will be fed instead of mother's milk.

- If the baby is younger than 1 year, suggest talking to the baby's healthcare provider about what to feed at the missed feeds.
- If the baby is older than 1 year, family foods and other milks or drinks can be substituted for nursing.

To begin a partial weaning, suggest parents take note of their usual nursing times and decide which feeds to drop. If they will be away from the baby for part of the day, suggest starting with a feed during the hours they'll be away (avoid dropping the first morning feed, when parents likely feel full already). After dropping a feed, suggest continuing to give the replacement food at this same feed every day.

Before dropping another feed, suggest allowing at least 3 days for milk production to adjust downward. If at any time uncomfortable feelings of fullness develop, suggest expressing just enough milk to stay comfortable, which will cause milk production to slow gradually while avoiding pain and health risks.

When the desired level of nursing is reached and there is no longer uncomfortable fullness between feeds, the partial weaning is complete. Nursing can continue at this level as long as the parent wishes.

Night Weaning

Night weaning refers to a type of partial weaning in which the number of feeds is reduced so that the child nurses only during the nursing parent's waking hours.

When the nursing parent feels overwhelmed and exhausted from frequent night feeds and the child is old enough to safely sleep for long stretches at night without feeding (after 6 to 9 months or so), some families consider night weaning. This term refers to a partial weaning in which the child nurses only when the nursing parent is awake and doesn't nurse at all while the parent is asleep.

As with any weaning, for the sake of both parent and child, night weaning is best done gradually. Some possible strategies include:

- Encourage the child to cluster feed right before bedtime so he will be less likely to want to nurse from hunger or thirst during the night.
- Have drinks or snacks available if the child awakens.
- Involve the partner or a support person in handling night waking during the weaning process.

• • •

Help keep the family's expectations for night weaning realistic.

Whether the issue is sleep training (p. 82) or night weaning, many families think that once it is done, regular night waking will be a thing of the past. But eliminating nursing at night is not the same as eliminating night wakings. As one U.S. lactation consultant (Shapiro, 2017, p. 18) wrote:

> "...night weaning does not always equal more sleep. Breastfeeding is a highly effective sleep inducer, and removing that tool from the parenting tool box does sometimes mean just as many night wakings, but more time and effort spent getting a child back to sleep."

Many parents are under the impression that the child is only waking at night because he knows the comfort of nursing is available. However, children wake for other reasons, too, and usually only sleep for long stretches at night when they are developmentally mature enough to do so.

If a child is not developmentally ready to sleep longer, night weaning can make nights harder for the whole family. There's also no guarantee that even if the child does start sleeping longer at night after night weaning that this will continue. Teething, developmental changes, family stresses, and other factors may cause night waking to resume later.

Abrupt Weaning

An abrupt weaning is usually most physically and emotionally difficult.

An abrupt weaning is sometimes recommended by healthcare providers who are unaware of other possibilities. A sudden weaning may be necessary in the unusual event that a nursing parent develops a medical condition that requires a treatment that is incompatible with nursing (such as a treatment dose of radioactive iodine). Research (Neighbors et al., 2003) found that when nursing is painful, an abrupt weaning is more likely, perhaps because nursing parents are in a hurry to eliminate the cause of their pain as quickly as possible. Weaning abruptly, though, can add substantially to a parent's discomfort. Weaning too quickly leads to uncomfortable mammary fullness, which can cause intense pain and, as a result, may lead to mastitis. Studies on lactating mice led some researchers (Silanikove, 2014) to suggest that due to the traumatic physical effects of an abrupt weaning on mammary tissue, it may put the nursing parent at greater risk later for breast cancer. A gradual weaning, on the other hand, appears to avoid this possible risk.

Because nursing provides both emotional and physical closeness, an abrupt weaning may be a more difficult emotional adjustment for the child than a gradual weaning.

• • •

During an abrupt weaning, suggest the child receive extra focused attention and touch.

To help offset the emotional loss of the closeness of nursing, as with any type of weaning, suggest during weaning the child receive extra focused attention and skin-to-skin contact. Depending on the child's age, this might involve talking, cuddling, reading stories, rocking, doing art projects together, or any other age-appropriate activities the child enjoys.

• • •

Ask if there is time for a more gradual weaning.

Abrupt weaning is the only approach some families know. It may be a relief to learn that weaning can be done gradually and comfortably. If a sudden weaning can't be avoided, help make it as comfortable as possible by reviewing the comfort measures in the next section.

• • •

A baby younger than 1 year has a physical need for milk. This makes it highly unlikely that a baby this age has outgrown nursing. Most babies who outgrow nursing do so gradually over a period of weeks and months, but some children do wean quickly. If this happens, help the nursing parent use milk expression to reduce milk production comfortably. In a baby older than 12 months, one way to tell whether the child has outgrown nursing or is on a nursing strike is the child's reaction. If the baby seems upset with the change, it is most likely a nursing strike. If the child seems content, he has probably outgrown nursing. In most cases, a nursing strike can be overcome and nursing resumed. For details on overcoming a nursing strike, see p. 128.

If a baby younger than 1 year abruptly stops nursing and seems distressed when it is offered, consider it a possible nursing strike.

Comfort Measures during Weaning

One U.S. study (Neighbors et al., 2003) described the comfort measures used by 222 women who weaned before their babies were 6 months old, including breast-binding, ice packs, milk expression, and over-the-counter pain medications. Women who took 4 days or longer to wean used these comfort measures less often than women who weaned within 3 days.

The more gradual the weaning, the fewer comfort measures are needed.

• • •

Unfortunately, there is little evidence available to help determine the best comfort measures for birthing parents who do not nurse or for parents who wean after establishing nursing (McGee, 1992). A 2012 Cochrane Review on treatments to suppress lactation (Oladapo & Fawole, 2012) found no trials that compared nondrug treatments with no treatments. Those drugs that showed some effectiveness in reducing discomfort in other trials are no longer available (see next point). Practices such as breast-binding, cold compresses, wearing a firm, supportive brassiere, fluid and diet restrictions, and others are commonly recommended, but there is no research to indicate their effectiveness and which are best.

Breast-binding was once recommended during weaning, but this practice—which was never studied—has fallen out of favor.

• • •

In years past, mothers were routinely given bromocriptine (Parlodel), a prolactin suppressor, as "dry-up" medication to suppress milk production either after birth or during weaning. However, serious side effects were reported, including stroke, seizure, even death, and the U.S. Food and Drug Administration withdrew its clearance for this use (FDA, 1994; Hale, 2019, pp. 84-85).

"Dry-up" medication is no longer recommended to suppress milk production.

• • •

Whether weaning is gradual or abrupt, use milk expression to stay comfortable. One milk-expression strategy is called ***pump to comfort***, which means expressing just enough milk to stay comfortable any time uncomfortable mammary fullness develops. When using this strategy, rather than expressing milk long enough to drain the mammary gland well, suggest stopping as soon as the gland feels more comfortable.

Expressing milk while weaning can increase comfort and reduce health risks.

Another milk-expression strategy sometimes recommended during weaning (especially for those with a hardened area in the mammary tissue— plugged, clogged, or a blocked duct—that won't go away) is to remove the milk from both sides as fully as possible then go for longer and longer stretches without nursing or expressing. Encourage nursing parents to use whichever strategies work best for them.

• • •

A variety of other comfort measures are recommended by some authors.

In the book for parents *A Loving Weaning: How to Move Forward Together,* author Winema Wilson Lanoue (Lanoue, 2017, p. 156) suggests:

- Wear a firm bra for support, one size larger than usual if needed.
- Reduce salt intake.
- Massage with warmth to prevent blockage.
- Add foods to the diet that reduce milk production and minimize foods that boost it. According to Lanoue, parsley, mint, and sage can reduce supply, while oats, alfalfa, barley, and sesame seeds can boost it.

Another book for parents, *The Nursing Mother's Guide to Weaning* (Huggins, 2007), offers three other comfort measures intended to relieve the swelling and engorgement that can occur with a quick weaning:

- Wear chilled cabbage leaves inside the bra, replacing them every 4 to 8 hours with fresh chilled leaves.
- For no more than 1 week, every day drink 3 cups (750 mL) of sage tea, made by steeping 1½ teaspoons (6 mL) dry sage leaves in a pint of freshly boiled water for 10 minutes.
- Take two 100 mg vitamin B_6 (pyridoxine) pills 3 times a day for the first day and one tablet daily thereafter; possible side effects include nausea, vomiting, diarrhea, and dark yellow-colored urine.

Physical and Emotional Changes with Weaning

Some nursing parents have no physical or emotional symptoms during weaning, others do.

In one study of 222 U.S. mothers who weaned their babies before 6 months (Neighbors et al., 2003), many physical and emotional changes were reported. This study divided the mothers into two groups, those who weaned their babies within 3 days and those whose weaning took 4 days or longer. Any weaning taking less than a week is more abrupt than gradual, but even so, the incidence of symptoms varied by the time taken to wean (Table 5.2). When parents suffer from depressive symptoms or other mental-health issues, weaning carefully should be an important part of their treatment plan. In some rare cases (Sharma, 2018), weaning may trigger a mental-health crisis.

• • •

If the nursing parent's menstrual cycles have not returned before weaning, expect them to return along with fertility after weaning.

If weaning occurs before the nursing parent's menstrual cycles returned, expect weaning to trigger a return to menstruation and fertility. Menses can be suppressed by the hormones released by frequent nursing (Labbok, 2007). During weaning, as the number of nursing sessions per day decrease and eventually stop, ovulation will occur and menses will resume. For more details, see p. 533-537.

TABLE 5.2 Symptoms Mothers (%) Reported after Weaning

Symptom	Weaned ≤3 days (N=86)	Weaned ≥4 days (N=136)
No symptoms	36	26
Increased energy	15	13
Decreased energy	5	14
Feeling happier overall	23	9
Feeling sadder overall	10	14
Increase in weight	24	28
Decrease in weight	15	15
Change in hair texture or shine	10	24
Increased appetite	4	16
Decreased appetite	13	13
Other	6	9

Adapted from (Neighbors et al., 2003)

• • •

After weaning occurs, many nursing parents experience feelings of loss and sadness.

Even when weaning is a positive experience for parent and child, it is still a kind of "letting go," which can lead to feelings of loss and sadness. Some mothers describe weaning as the loss of a special bond that can "never be recaptured with that child again" (Hauck & Irurita, 2002).

> **KEY CONCEPT**
>
> *Weaning is a time of "letting go," which can trigger feelings of loss and sadness.*

The baby's age at weaning can affect the intensity of a nursing parent's sadness. In one U.S. study (Rogers, Morris, & Taper, 1987), researchers found that 65% of the women who weaned at 3 months or younger wished they had breastfed longer and more than half of the women who weaned at 4 to 6 months were sorry they had weaned their babies so young. One author received correspondence from hundreds of mothers describing their feelings about weaning and noted that those who most consistently described feelings of loss and regret were those who weaned babies younger than 2 years of age (Bumgarner, 2000, p. 288).

> "When nursing continues past 2 or 3, mothers much less frequently describe weaning in the same mixed terms. It seems that a time comes in the growth of the mother-child relationship when it is easier for both to move on and leave baby things behind."

Another U.S. study of mothers who weaned before 6 months (Neighbors et al., 2003) found that even when weaning was done gradually, when it occurred between birth and 5 weeks, it was positively associated with sadness. This study also found that mothers who weaned had less sadness when the baby was 21 to 25 weeks old. One Australian study (Hauck & Irurita, 2002) found that mothers who did not feel ready to wean experienced a longer period of emotional adjustment before they reached acceptance.

RESOURCES

kellymom.com/?s=weaning—The weaning section of the comprehensive website **KellyMom.com**.

Lanoue, W.W. (2017). *A Loving Weaning: How to Move Forward Together.* Amarillo, TX: Praeclarus Press.

Mohrbacher, N. & Kendall-Tackett, K. (2010). *Breastfeeding Made Simple: Seven Natural Laws for Nursing Mothers* 2nd edition. Oakland, CA: New Harbinger Publications.

Robisch, J.E. (2014). *To Three and Beyond: Stories of Breastfed Children and the Mothers Who Love Them.* Amarillo, TX: Praeclarus Press.

REFERENCES

AAP. (2012). Breastfeeding and the use of human milk. *Pediatrics, 129*(3), e827-e841.

Amir, L. H. (1997). Psychological aspects of nipple pain in lactating women. *Breastfeeding Review, 5*(1), 29-32.

Bartick, M. C., Schwarz, E. B., Green, B. D., et al. (2017). Suboptimal breastfeeding in the United States: Maternal and pediatric health outcomes and costs. *Maternal and Child Nutrition, 13*(1).

Bumgarner, N. J. (2000). *Mothering Your Nursing Toddler.* Schaumburg, IL: La Leche League International.

CDC warns of Cronobacter in powdered milk, infant formula. (2016, June 28, 2018). *Food Safety News.* Retrieved from **foodsafetynews.com/2016/04/125714/#.WzWSK7gnaUm**.

Cooke, M., Sheehan, A., & Schmied, V. (2003). A description of the relationship between breastfeeding experiences, breastfeeding satisfaction, and weaning in the first 3 months after birth. *Journal of Human Lactation, 19*(2), 145-156.

Dennis, C. L. (2002). Breastfeeding initiation and duration: A 1990-2000 literature review. *Journal of Obstetric, Gynecologic, & Neonatal Nursing, 31*(1), 12-32.

Dettwyler, K. A. (1995). A time to wean: The hominid bluprint for the natural age of weaning in modern human populations. In P. Stuart-Macadam & K. A. Dettwyler (Eds.), *Breastfeeding: Biocultural Perspectives* (pp. 39-73). New York, NY: Aldine de Gruyter.

Dowling, S., & Brown, A. (2013). An exploration of the experiences of mothers who breastfeed long-term: What are the issues and why does it matter? *Breastfeeding Medicine, 8*(1), 45-52.

Dowling, S., & Pontin, D. (2017). Using liminality to understand mothers' experiences of long-term breastfeeding: 'Betwixt and between', and 'matter out of place'. *Health (London), 21*(1), 57-75.

FDA. (1994). Bromocriptine indication widthrawn. *FDA Med Bulletin, 24*(2), 2.

Fewtrell, M., Bronsky, J., Campoy, C., et al. (2017). Complementary feeding: A position paper by the European Society for Paediatric Gastroenterology, Hepatology, and Nutrition (ESPGHAN) Committee on Nutrition. *Journal of Pediatric Gastroenterology and Nutrition, 64*(1), 119-132.

Gulick, E. (1986). The effects of breastfeeding on toddler health. *Pediatric Nursing, 12*, 51-54.

Hale, T. W. (2019). *Hale's Medications & Mothers' Milk: A Manual of Lactational Pharmacology* (18th ed.). New York, NY: Springer Publishing Company.

Hauck, Y. L., & Irurita, V. F. (2002). Constructing compatibility: managing breast-feeding and weaning from the mother's perspective. *Qualitative Health Research, 12*(7), 897-914.

Huggins, K. a. Z., L. (2007). *The Nursing Mother's Guide to Weaning* (Revised edition ed.). Boston, MA: Harvard Commons Press.

Isabella, P. H., & Isabella, R. A. (1994). Correlates of successful breastfeeding: A study of social and personal factors. *Journal of Human Lactation, 10*(4), 257-264.

Keim, S. A., Tchaconas, A., & Adesman, A. (2017). Comparison of support for breastfeeding beyond 12 months of age from conventional and alternative pediatric primary care providers. *Breastfeeding Medicine, 12*(6), 345-350.

Kelleher, C. M. (2006). The physical challenges of early breastfeeding. *Social Science and Medicine, 63*(10), 2727-2738.

Kendall-Tackett, K. A. (2017). *Depression in New Mothers: Causes, Consequences and Treatment Alternatives.* London and New York: Routledge Taylor& Francis Group.

Kendall-Tackett, K. A., & Sugarman, M. (1995). The social consequences of long-term breastfeeding. *Journal of Human Lactation, 11*(3), 179-183.

Labbok, M. (2007). Breastfeeding, birth spacing, and family planning. In T. W. a. H. Hale, P. (Ed.), *Hale & Hartmann's Textbook of Human Lactation* (pp. 305-318). Amarillo, TX: Hale Publishing.

Lanoue, W. W. (2017). *A Loving Weaning: How to Move Forward Together.* Amarillo, TX: Praeclarus Press.

Leff, E. W., Jefferis, S. C., & Gagne, M. P. (1994). The development of the Maternal Breastfeeding Evaluation Scale. *Journal of Human Lactation, 10*(2), 105-111.

McAndrew, G. (2012). Infant feeding survey: 2010. Retrieved from **data.gov.uk/dataset/infant-feeding-survey-2010**.

McGee, M. L. (1992). Abrupt weaning: Is breast-binding effective? *Journal of Human Lactation, 8*(3), 126.

Mead, M., & Newton, N. (1967). Cultural patterns of perinatal behavior. In S. Richardson & A. Guttmacher (Eds.), *Childbearing: Its Social and Psychological Aspects.* Baltimore, MD: Willliams & Wilkins.

Mezzacappa, E. S., & Katlin, E. S. (2002). Breast-feeding is associated with reduced perceived stress and negative mood in mothers. *Health Psychology, 21*(2), 187-193.

Mikami, F. C. F., Francisco, R. P. V., Rodrigues, A., et al. (2018). Breastfeeding twins: Factors related to weaning. *Journal of Human Lactation, 890334418767382.*

Molbak, K. (1994). Prolonged breastfeeding, diarrhoeal disease, and survival of children. *British Medical Journal, 308,* 1403-1406.

Negin, J., Coffman, J., Vizintin, P., et al. (2016). The influence of grandmothers on breastfeeding rates: A systematic review. *BMC Pregnancy & Childbirth, 16,* 91.

Neighbors, K. A., Gillespie, B., Schwartz, K., et al. (2003). Weaning practices among breastfeeding women who weaned prior to six months postpartum. *Journal of Human Lactation, 19*(4), 374-380; quiz 381-375, 448.

Newby, R. M., & Davies, P. S. (2016). Why do women stop breast-feeding? Results from a contemporary prospective study in a cohort of Australian women. *European Journal of Clinical Nutrition, 70*(12), 1428-1432.

Newman, K. L., & Williamson, I. R. (2018). Why aren't you stopping now?!' Exploring accounts of white women breastfeeding beyond six months in the East of England. *Appetite.* doi:10.1016/j.appet.2018.06.018.

Odom, E. C., Li, R., Scanlon, K. S., et al. (2013). Reasons for earlier than desired cessation of breastfeeding. *Pediatrics, 131*(3), e726-732.

Oladapo, O. T., & Fawole, B. (2012). Treatments for suppression of lactation. *Cochrane Database Syst Rev*(9), CD005937. doi:10.1002/14651858.CD005937.pub3.

Perrine, C. G., Scanlon, K. S., Li, R., et al. (2012). Baby-Friendly hospital practices and meeting exclusive breastfeeding intention. *Pediatrics, 130*(1), 54-60.

Rempel, L. A. (2004). Factors influencing the breastfeeding decisions of long-term breastfeeders. *Journal of Human Lactation, 20*(3), 306-318.

Rempel, L. A., Rempel, J. K., & Moore, K. C. J. (2017). Relationships between types of father breastfeeding support and breastfeeding outcomes. *Maternal and Child Nutrition, 13*(3). doi:10.1111/mcn.12337.

Rogers, C. S., Morris, S., & Taper, L. J. (1987). Weaning from the breast: Influences on maternal decisions. *Pediatric Nursing, 13*(5), 341-345.

Roll, C. L., & Cheater, F. (2016). Expectant parents' views of factors influencing infant feeding decisions in the antenatal period: A systematic review. *International Journal of Nursing Studies, 60,* 145-155.

Schafer, E. J., Buch, E., Campo, S., et al. (2018). From initiation to cessation: Turning points and coping resources in the breastfeeding experience of first-time mothers. *Women and Health.* doi:10.1177/0890334418767382.

Schmied, V., & Barclay, L. (1999). Connection and pleasure, disruption and distress: Women's experience of breastfeeding. *Journal of Human Lactation, 15*(4), 325-334.

Shapiro, S. (2017). *Tandem Nursing: A Pocket Guide.* Chatham, New York: CreateSpace Indepdendent Publishing Platform.

Sharma, V. (2018). Weaning and mixed mania-A case report. *Journal of Human Lactation, 34*(4), 745-748.

Silanikove, N. (2014). Natural and abrupt involution of the mammary gland affects differently the metabolic and health consequences of weaning. *Life Sciences, 102*(1), 10-15.

Sugarman, M., & Kendall-Tackett, K. A. (1995). Weaning ages in a sample of American women who practice extended breastfeeding. *Clinical Pediatrics (Philadelphia), 34*(12), 642-647.

Taveras, E. M., Capra, A. M., Braveman, P. A., et al. (2003). Clinician support and psychosocial risk factors associated with breastfeeding discontinuation. *Pediatrics, 112*(1 Pt 1), 108-115.

Taveras, E. M., Li, R., Grummer-Strawn, L., et al. (2004). Opinions and practices of clinicians associated with continuation of exclusive breastfeeding. *Pediatrics, 113*(4), e283-290.

Tessone, A., Garcia Guraieb, S., Goni, R. A., et al. (2015). Isotopic evidence of weaning in hunter-gatherers from the late holocene in Lake Salitroso, Patagonia, Argentina. *American Journal of Physical Anthropology, 158*(1), 105-115.

Victora, C. G., Bahl, R., Barros, A. J., et al. (2016). Breastfeeding in the 21st century: Epidemiology, mechanisms, and lifelong effect. *Lancet, 387*(10017), 475-490.

Wallenborn, J. T., Cha, S., & Masho, S. W. (2018). Association between intimate partner violence and breastfeeding duration: Results from the 2004-2014 Pregnancy Risk Assessment Monitoring System. *Journal of Human Lactation, 34*(2), 233-241.

WHO. (2018). Infant and young child feeding. Retrieved from **who.int/mediacentre/factsheets/fs342/en/index.html**.

Williams, K. M., & Morse, J. M. (1989). Weaning patterns of first-time mothers. *MCN: American Journal of Maternal and Child Nursing, 14*(3), 188-192.

Yilmaz, G., Gurakan, B., Cakir, B., et al. (2002). Factors influencing sleeping pattern of infants. *Turkish Journal of Pediatrics, 44*(2), 128-133.

PART II

Baby

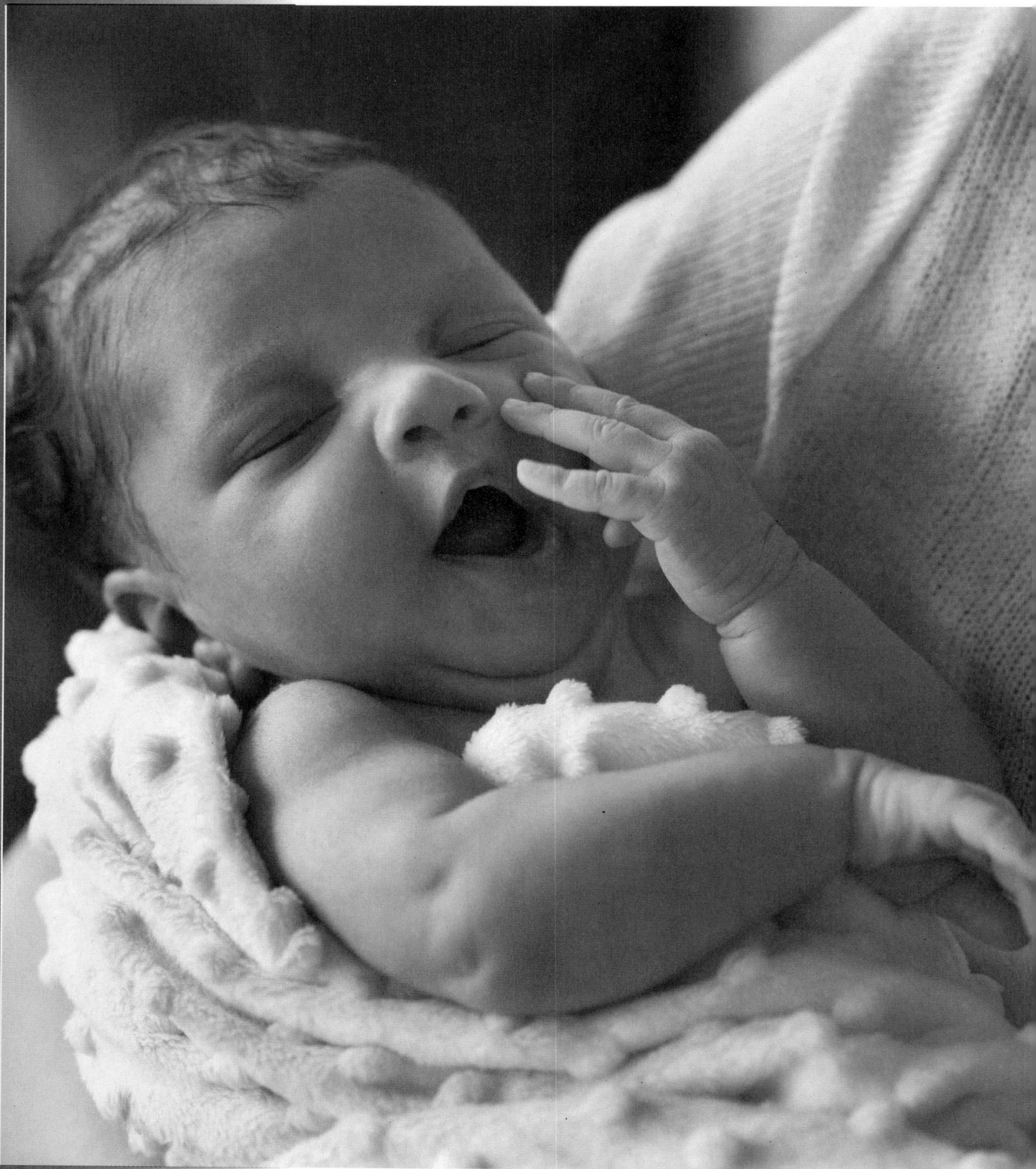

Weight Gain and Growth

6

NORMAL GROWTH

Ages and Stages

Rate of weight gain and growth varies during baby's first year.

It's no secret that babies grow quickly, but it's important when working with families to keep in mind that the rate of weight loss and gain, growth in length, and growth in head circumference changes during the first year. This section describes normal growth during the first 12 months, from the weight loss most babies experience in the first few days after birth, through the very fast growth of the first 3 months, and the slowing of growth that naturally occurs between 3 and 12 months.

Weight Loss after Birth

Most newborns lose weight after birth no matter what and how they are fed, and this weight loss may have beneficial long-term effects.

Weight-loss nomograms. Recent research deepened our understanding of normal weight loss after birth. In 2015, for the first time, U.S. scientists published weight-loss nomograms for both exclusively nursing (Flaherman et al., 2015) and exclusively formula-fed (Miller et al., 2015) newborns, based on weight data collected from many thousands of babies. These nomograms resemble growth charts, with percentiles that allow a newborn's weight to be plotted over the first 3 to 4 days to see how their hourly weight loss compares with other newborns. Comparing a newborn's weight loss to these nomograms can alert healthcare providers when a baby's weight loss warrants concern. From these same weight-loss data, the NEWT app was created to allow clinicians to more easily use this data in busy hospitals (for details, see **newbornweight.com).**

Externally validated (Schaefer et al., 2015), these large studies found that most babies lose weight in the first days after birth, whether they nurse or are formula-fed. When this weight loss is in the normal range (see next point), newborns lose both fat and water, with slightly more fat mass lost than water (Rodriguez et al., 2000; Roggero et al., 2010), so newborns stay well hydrated until milk increase on Day 3 or 4.

Benefits of newborn weight loss. Could this normal newborn weight loss be beneficial? One U.S. longitudinal cohort study followed 653 formula-fed babies for 20 to 30 years (Stettler et al., 2005) and concluded that the first 8 days of life is a critical period during which metabolic programming occurs. They found that greater weight gain during the first 8 days was associated with adult overweight. For every 100 g (3+ ounces) gained during the first week, the risk of adult overweight increased by 28%. Might the fact that nursing newborns lose more weight on average than formula-fed newborns (see next point) during this critical period be one reason many studies found an association between nursing and lower risk of childhood overweight and obesity (Horta, Loret de Mola, & Victora, 2015; Yan, Liu, Zhu, Huang, & Wang, 2014)? For 2 years, a 2018 U.S. study followed 306 mother/baby pairs who used a variety of feeding methods (Feldman-Winter et al., 2018). They found the same association between weight gain during the first week and overweight at 2 years. In this study, babies who gained 100 g (3+ ounces) or more during the first week were 2.3 times more likely to be overweight at 2 years compared with those who gained less. Not surprisingly, the exclusively nursing babies were least likely of all of the groups to gain excess weight during the first week after birth.

• • •

The weight-loss nomograms described in the previous point revealed that the differences in hourly weight-loss patterns after birth varied significantly both by type of birth and by feeding method.

In exclusively nursing babies, the lowest weight is usually on the third or fourth day and average weight loss is 5% to 7% or more, depending on the country and type of birth.

Weight-loss pattern by type of birth. On average, U.S. babies born by cesarean section lost more weight, whether they were nursed or formula-fed. The researchers suggested that the birthing parent's fluid balance (determined in part by IV fluids received during labor, see later point) affected weight loss in formula-fed and nursing babies. Exclusively formula-fed babies born vaginally had a median weight loss of 2.9% compared with 3.7% in formula-fed babies born by cesarean. Exclusively nursed babies born vaginally had a median weight loss of 7.1% compared with 8.6% for those born by cesarean. On average, nursing babies born by cesarean also lost weight for a longer time, as they were still losing weight at 72 hours. Nursing babies born vaginally, on the other hand, on average began gaining weight between 48 and 72 hours.

Weight-loss patterns by feeding method. A 2008 systematic review (Noel-Weiss, Courant, & Woodend, 2008) concluded that when nursing is going well, exclusively nursing babies lose on average between 5% and 7% of birth weight. But that was not true in the U.S. study on which the weight-loss nomograms were based (see above paragraph), nor in other U.S. studies conducted since (DiTomasso & Paiva, 2018).

KEY CONCEPT

On average, exclusively nursing infants lose more weight after birth than those who are formula fed.

Weight loss varies by country of birth. Because birth practices vary, country of birth also affects newborn weight loss. When comparing their own research to two previous studies, U.S. scientists (Dewey, Nommsen-Rivers, Heinig, & Cohen, 2003; Dewey, Nommsen, & Cohen, 2009) noticed that a higher percentage of babies born in the U.S. lost more than 10% of their birth weight compared with babies born elsewhere. Seven to 10% of newborns in both Italy (Manganaro, Mami, Marrone, Marseglia, & Gemelli, 2001) and Peru (Matias, Nommsen-Rivers, Creed-Kanashiro, & Dewey, 2010) lost more than 10% of their birth weight. But in two different U.S. studies, 16% and 18% lost more than 10% of birth weight, and these U.S. statistics were consistent even among different ethnic and socioeconomic groups. The authors suggested that greater weight loss among U.S. babies may be more common in part because (L. A. Nommsen-Rivers & Dewey, 2009, pp. S47-S48):

> "Childbirth is a highly medicalized event in the United States, and this type of birth setting may contribute to additional challenges to successfully establishing lactation."

• • •

When a baby loses more than 7% of birth weight, the first step is not to supplement, even though that's what many birthing facilities do (Thulier, 2017). According to the Academy of Breastfeeding Medicine (Kellams, Harrel, Omage, Gregory, & Rosen-Carole, 2017, p. 190):

If a baby loses more than 7% of her birth weight or continues to lose weight after Day 4, take a closer look at their nursing dynamics to see if there's some way to improve them.

> "...[W]eight loss in the range of 8-10% may be within normal limits if all else is going well and the physical examination is normal, it is an indication for careful assessment and possible breastfeeding assistance."

Making sure that nursing is going as well as possible is always a wise first step. A few adjustments (a deeper latch, more feeds per day) may be enough to improve baby's weight. Also keep in mind (see previous point) that average weight loss is higher than 5% to 7% in some countries, and there are reasons for weight loss unrelated to milk intake (see next point) that need to be considered, too.

• • •

Factors other than milk intake and country of birth affect weight loss after birth.

In addition to birth and post-delivery hospital practices, research found a number of other factors unrelated to milk intake that affect weight loss after birth. One of these factors that commonly influences newborn weight loss is the fluid balance (hydration status) of the birthing parent during labor.

Fluid balance in the hours before delivery. A Canadian observational cohort study of 109 mothers and babies (Noel-Weiss, Woodend, Peterson, Gibb, & Groll, 2011) found that the larger the volume of IV fluids its study mothers received within the final 2 hours before delivery, the greater the effect on their baby's weight loss after birth. IV fluids given during this time window passed through to the fetus, inflating baby's weight and acting as a diuretic after birth that caused more urinations. Babies whose mothers received more IV fluids before birth urinated more during their first 24 hours and as a result lost more weight. Number of wet diapers during the first 24 hours predicted infant weight loss. This was true whether the babies were born vaginally or by c-section. This weight loss is completely unrelated to feeding or milk intake. Another U.S. prospective study of 448 women (Chantry, Nommsen-Rivers, Peerson, Cohen, & Dewey, 2011) had similar findings.

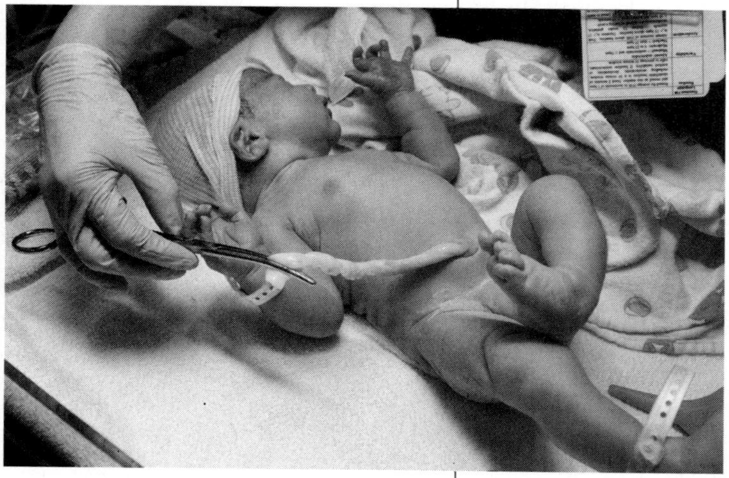

As a result, the Canadian researchers recommended not using baby's birth weight as the reference or baseline. Instead, they suggested that if clinicians want to use weight loss as a gauge of feeding adequacy, they calculate baby's weight loss from their weight at 24 hours. Because the diuretic effect of the IV fluids lasts only 24 hours, using the 24-hour weight as the baseline eliminates the influence of the IV fluids given during labor on baby's weight. An Australian review of the literature on fluid balance and infant weight loss (Tawia & McGuire, 2014) provided an overview of both the research and recommended strategies.

In 2018, a U.S. retrospective chart review of 667 mothers and babies (Deng & McLaren, 2018) examined the impact of using babies' 24-hour weight as the baseline. When they followed these babies through their hospital stay, the researchers found no significant increases in:

- Maximum weight loss
- Length of hospital stay
- Bilirubin levels (a measure of newborn jaundice)
- Percentage of babies who lost ≥10% of birth weight

A positive effect of this change to using the babies' 24-hour weight as the baseline was a significant reduction in the use of formula supplements.

- 44% of the babies received formula before the change
- 27% of the babies received formula after the change

Other factors unrelated to milk intake that affect early weight loss. Canadian researchers conducted a chart review of 812 babies born in six different hospitals in Manitoba (Martens & Romphf, 2007) and found a greater weight loss associated with the use of epidurals for pain relief during labor, most likely due at least in part to extra fluids mother and baby receive. In this same study, other factors associated with percentage of weight loss after birth included:

- **Birth weight**—Heavier babies lost more weight.
- **Cesarean birth**—Babies born surgically lost more weight.
- **Gestational age**—Babies born earlier lost more weight.
- **Gender**—Baby girls lost more weight than baby boys.

• • •

In all cases, a weight loss of more than 10% of birth weight is a red flag to take a close look at nursing. If feeding problems are not overcome quickly or if the baby shows signs of dehydration, supplements may be needed. In an Italian prospective study of 686 full-term babies born over a 6-month period at one hospital (Manganaro et al., 2001), 7.7% (53) of the exclusively breastfed babies lost more than 10% of their birth weight. In 74% of these babies, poor milk transfer was the cause, and after providing lactation help, weight improved. In 26% of these babies, delayed milk production was the cause, which is sometimes a side effect of less-than-optimal nursing (for details, see Chapter 10, "Making Milk"). The researchers recommended all babies be scheduled for a routine weight check at 5 days of age to prevent dehydration.

If a baby loses more than 10% of birth weight, nursing should be evaluated and the baby should be checked for jaundice and dehydration.

KEY CONCEPT

Babies with a weight loss of 8% to 10% are not necessarily at risk.

In some cases, dehydration can lead to hypernatremia, or elevated blood sodium levels, which may require hospitalization to balance the baby's electrolytes in order to prevent seizures and other serious health problems (Lavagno et al., 2016). In addition to excessive weight loss, common symptoms of hypernatremia include fever and dry mouth (Unver Korgali, Cihan, Oguzalp, Sahinbas, & Ekici, 2017). When babies become dehydrated or hypernatremic, families are more likely to give up on breastfeeding (Oddie, Richmond, & Coulthard, 2001).

• • •

One way to prevent weight loss of more than 10% was suggested by U.S. pediatrician Jane Morton (Morton, 2019), who created the website **firstdroplets.com** to encourage families to learn hand expression during the last month of an uncomplicated pregnancy and use it in the early days to feed their newborn extra colostrum by spoon. (See p. 474 for information about the safety of this practice.) U.S. research (Flaherman, et al., 2016) found excess weight loss after birth associated with increased anxiety about milk production and a shorter duration of breastfeeding.

Excess weight loss may be prevented by encouraging families to learn hand expression before birth and using it during the early days to feed extra colostrum by spoon.

• • •

Controversy exists about when exclusively nursing babies should be back to birth weight. In the recent past, the conventional wisdom was that nursing babies should be back to birth weight by 2 weeks (Noel-Weiss et al., 2008). However, the World Health Organization growth standards described in the next section (WHO, 2009) found that when families nurse optimally, most nursing babies are back to birth weight by 5 to 8 days. U.S. scientists reviewed

Most nursing babies begin gaining weight by about Day 4 and regain their birth weight by about Day 10 to 14.

weight-gain data from more than 140,000 newborns and created weight-gain nomograms for the first month (Paul et al., 2016). Nomograms resemble growth charts, with percentiles that allow a newborn's weight to be plotted over the first month to see how their weight compares with other newborns. This very large-scale study found that 50% of newborns were at or above birth weight by 9 days (if born vaginally) and 10 days (if born by cesarean). This, of course, means that 50% of the babies were not at or above birth weight by 9 or 10 days, which indicates a large number had either early or ongoing feeding problems. In this study a significant number of newborns were still not at or above birth weight at 14 days (14%) and 21 days (5%).

Of course, not all newborns nurse optimally. When feeding problems arise, the earlier they are addressed, the faster they are usually resolved. The more weight a baby loses after birth, the longer it takes for her to regain it. Babies who are ill or born preterm (including late preterm babies) may take longer to regain their birth weight than healthy, full-term babies.

If a baby has not regained birth weight by 10 days to 2 weeks, this is another red flag. Take a closer look at how nursing is going and make any needed adjustments. To boost weight gain, a good first step is to help the baby get a deeper latch. Suggest nursing more often or for longer periods and use breast compression (see p. 889) to increase both fat content and milk intake (Bowles, 2011).

Growth from Birth to 12 Months

When a nursing baby starts gaining weight on about Day 3 or 4, an average weight gain is about 8 ounces (245 g) per week.

Weight gain after birth should always be measured from the lowest weight, which is usually on the third or fourth day. But weight checks done around this time can be confusing. For example, if a baby is weighed on Day 2 while she is still losing weight and again on Day 4, her weight may be lower on Day 4 than on Day 2, and it may appear that she is still losing weight. But that may not be the case. She may have reached her lowest weight on Day 3, and then started to gain, but not yet reached her Day 2 level. Another weight check is needed for an accurate gauge of how the baby is doing. If a baby is still losing weight after Day 5, nursing should be closely evaluated.

Average weight gain for the first 2 to 3 months is about 8 ounces (245 g) per week, with boys gaining slightly faster than girls. For the expected weight gains for boys and girls for the entire first year, go to: **who.int/childgrowth/standards/w_velocity/en**.

Look for "1-month increments," click on "percentiles" for boys or girls, then click on the "Simplified field table." (There are 28.35 grams in 1 ounce.) If a baby is gaining weight at well below the 50th percentile, this is a sign nursing needs closer attention. For example, between 1 and 2 months, a weight gain of 4.5 ounces (133 g) per week is below the 5th percentile of expected weight gain for boys and below the 10th percentile for girls. See the later section "Slow Weight Gain" for strategies for increasing weight gain. A weight gain in the higher percentiles is not a problem for an exclusively nursing baby (see the last section, "Rapid Weight Gain").

• • •

Between 3 and 12 months, weight gain gradually slows.

Babies grow rapidly during the first 3 months of life, with growth slowing during months 3 through 12. Slowing growth is normal. If a baby kept growing

TABLE 6.1 Rate of Weight Gain for Exclusively Nursing Babies in the First Year

Age	Weight Gain for Babies in the 25th to 75th Percentiles
Week 1	Loss of up to 7-10% of birth weight (weight at 24 hours may be a more accurate baseline than birth weight)
Week 2	Back to birth weight or now gaining 1 oz (28 g) per DAY
Weeks 3 & 4	Gains 8-9 oz (240-270 g) per WEEK
Month 2	Gains 7-10 oz (210-300 g) per WEEK
Month 3	Gains 5-7 oz (150-210 g) per WEEK
Month 4	Gains 4-6 oz (120-180 g) per WEEK
Month 5	Gains 3-5 oz (90-150 g) per WEEK *or* 12-22 oz (360-660 g) per MONTH
Month 6	Gains 2-4 oz (60-120 g) per WEEK *or* 9-18 oz (270-540 g) per MONTH
Months 7 & 8	Gains 7-16 oz (210-480 g) per MONTH
Months 9-12	Gains 4-13 oz (120-390 g) per MONTH

Adapted from (L. Marasco & West, 2020, p. 28, WHO, 2009)

at her newborn rate, she would be a giant by adulthood. See Table 6.1 for weight gains between the 25th and 75th percentiles by month during the first year (WHO, 2009). The average nursing baby doubles her birth weight by 5 to 6 months of age. When growth charts based on growth data from formula-fed babies are used (see next section), between 3 and 6 months of age, a nursing baby's weight may appear to falter. Growth charts based on normal growth in nursing babies are available from the World Health Organization free and downloadable at: **who.int/childgrowth/standards/en**. For more details, see the next section, "Growth Charts."

During the second 6 months of life, healthy, thriving babies also grow in length and head circumference (see next point). At 12 months, the average nursing baby weighs about 2.5 times her birth weight, has increased in length by 50%, and has increased head circumference by 33%.

• • •

Growing in length and head circumference is an important sign of healthy growth.

Weight gain is not the only important measure of a baby's growth, because weight gain also includes any increase in tissue fluids and fat. During the first 6 months, healthy, thriving babies average a monthly growth in length of about 1 inch (2.5 cm) and head circumference of about 0.5 inch (1.27 cm). No differences in adult height were found between those nursed or formula-fed in infancy (L. Li, Manor, & Power, 2004; Martin, Smith, Mangtani, Frankel, & Gunnell, 2002; Victora, Barros, Lima, Horta, & Wells, 2003).

U.S. research found that babies do not grow consistently in length and head circumference (Lampl, Veldhuis, & Johnson, 1992). Length and head circumference stay static 90% to 95% of the time, with measurable bursts of growth occurring during the remaining 5% to 10%.

Formula-fed babies average a significantly greater weight gain than nursing babies between 3 and 12 months of age, which increases risk of childhood overweight and obesity.

• • •

At all ages, babies fed non-human milks are at greater risk of infection, allergy, and many other illnesses (AAP, 2012). Gaining more weight from 3 to 12 months—which is more likely in formula-fed babies—is also not a good thing, as faster weight gain between 6 and 12 months was associated with an increased risk of childhood obesity (Stocks et al., 2011; Taveras et al., 2011), which has become an epidemic worldwide. According to the World Health Organization, the number of overweight children in lower- and middle-income countries more than doubled between 1990 and 2014 (WHO, 2016). Although many factors influence a child's weight, one of them appears to be infant feeding method.

Meta-analyses and systematic reviews concluded that babies are at higher risk of childhood overweight and obesity when they are formula-fed (Horta et al., 2015; Marseglia et al., 2015; Yan et al., 2014), and risk also increases the more feeds babies receive from a bottle, even bottles containing human milk (Azad et al., 2018; R. Li, Magadia, Fein, & Grummer-Strawn, 2012). What are some of the mechanisms that increase risk of obesity in babies fed formula or human milk by bottle? Here are a few.

- Babies consume more milk per feed and per day from a bottle than while nursing.
- Formula-fed babies consume significantly more protein than nursing babies.
- Formula alters babies' hormonal levels, metabolism, and nutrient use.
- Formula lacks the hormones in human milk that regulate weight and appetite.
- Intestinal bacteria (microbiota) differ in babies fed human milk or formula.

More milk consumed during bottle-feeding. One reason bottle-fed babies average a greater weight gain than nursing babies between 3 and 12 months is that on average they consume much more milk both per feed and per day. One large, prospective randomized controlled trial (17,046 babies in Belarus) compared volume of milk per feed in formula-fed and breastfed babies (Kramer et al., 2004). At each feed, the formula-fed babies averaged 49% more milk at 1 month, 57% more at 3 months, and 71% more at 5 months. Mothers' behaviors also influenced milk intake. Babies whose mothers encouraged them to finish the bottle were heavier than other babies. Using a larger bottle was also associated with greater weight gain in this and other studies (Appleton et al., 2018; Wood et al., 2016). In a U.S. prospective longitudinal study of 119 mothers and their term babies (Heinig, Nommsen, Peerson, Lonnerdal, & Dewey, 1993) researchers compared milk intake in breastfed and formula-fed babies. The researchers found that compared with nursing babies, on average the babies bottle-fed formula consumed per day 15% more milk at 3 months, 23% more at 6 months, 20% more at 9 months, and 18% more at 12 months. But because nursing babies leave milk in the mammary gland after feeds, these U.S. researchers concluded that limited milk availability was not the reason they took less milk (Dewey, Heinig, Nommsen, & Lonnerdal, 1991).

KEY CONCEPT

Formula-fed babies are at greater risk for overweight and obesity for several possible reasons, including feeding dynamics and milk composition.

Another reason bottle-fed babies—even those bottle-fed human milk—consumed more milk and gained more weight may be in part due to differences in milk-flow. During bottle-feeding, milk flows more consistently, unless paced bottle-feeding techniques are used (see p. 902-903). During nursing, however, milk flows faster during milk ejections and slower in between. Experts suggest that adults eat slowly at meals to give their "appetite control mechanism" time to register that they are full before they overeat. The same principle may be true for babies. If so, a fast, consistent milk flow may lead to overfeeding. U.S. researchers analyzed the data from 1,896 babies (R. Li, Fein, & Grummer-Strawn, 2008) and found a link between regular bottle-emptying and faster weight gain. This same data was used to conclude that even babies bottle-fed human milk gain weight faster than those directly nursing (R. Li et al., 2012). A Canadian study of 2,553 concluded (Azad et al., 2018, p. 1):

> "Breastfeeding is inversely associated with weight-gain velocity and BMI. These associations are dose dependent, partially diminished when breast milk is fed from a bottle and substantially weakened by formula supplementation after the neonatal period."

Multiple studies also found that regular overfeeding by bottle contributed to reduced "satiety responsiveness," awareness of feeling full after eating (Azad et al., 2018; Brown & Lee, 2012; Rogers & Blissett, 2017). Formula-feeding on a schedule was also associated with greater weight gain (Mihrshahi, Battistutta, Magarey, & Daniels, 2011).

Formula-fed babies consume significantly more protein. Research found a consistent association between the higher protein levels in many infant formulas and greater weight gain (Escribano et al., 2012; Koletzko et al., 2017). During the first 2 weeks of life, formula-fed babies consume up to 5 times more protein than nursing babies (Hester, Hustead, Mackey, Singhal, & Marriage, 2012). This is due in part to the higher protein content in formula and the greater milk intake described in the previous paragraph. It appears that breaking down the proteins in formula may also affect obesity risk. A 2019 U.S. study used data on 113 diverse formula-fed babies from a double-blind randomized controlled trial (Mennella, Papas, Reiter, Stallings, & Trabulsi, 2019) who were followed for 4.5 months. The babies were randomized into two groups to receive different types of formula: 1) standard cow-milk-based formula (Enfamil), and 2) extensively hydrolyzed formula (Nutramigen), in which the proteins had been partially broken down. The two types of formula had the same number of calories, and the mothers' feeding styles and patterns were the same. But there was a significant difference in the babies' weight gain. Of the babies fed the standard formula, 56% had the kind of rapid early weight gain associated with increased risk of obesity, while only 25% of the babies fed an extensively hydrolyzed formula had this rapid weight gain.

> **KEY CONCEPT**
>
> *Greater intake of both milk and protein contribute to greater weight gain in formula-fed infants.*

Formula alters babies' hormonal levels, metabolism, and nutrient use. In addition to its impact on greater weight gain, the protein in infant formulas is composed of a different combination of amino acids (the building blocks of protein) than the protein in human milk. For example, formula contains higher levels of branched-chain amino acids, which are associated with higher insulin blood levels in babies (Koletzko et al., 2017; Socha et al., 2011). These amino acids stimulate hormonal responses in babies that are linked to low levels of insulin-like growth factor-1 in adulthood, which are associated with increased risk of heart disease, diabetes, and both prostate and breast cancers (Socha et al., 2011). Formula also lacks the components of mother's milk that contribute to better use of food nutrients and healthier metabolic programming (Koletzko et al., 2017). For example, research found that formula-fed babies used more calories during sleep than nursing babies (Butte, Wong, Hopkinson, Heinz, et al., 2000) and formula-fed babies were almost two-fold less efficient in their use of dietary nitrogen (Motil, Sheng, Montandon, & Wong, 1997).

Formula lacks hormones that regulate weight and appetite. Several hormones in human milk—leptin, adiponectin, and ghrelin—are associated with healthy regulation of appetite and metabolism, and they are completely missing from formula. Leptin, for example, sends signals to the brain to control appetite and regulate body weight and energy metabolism (Pico, Jilkova, Kus, Palou, & Kopecky, 2011). Adiponectin appears to affect the metabolism without affecting appetite, and U.S. research found an inverse relationship between adiponectin levels in human milk and the nursing baby's weight-for-height (Newburg, Woo, & Morrow, 2010).

Intestinal bacteria (microbiota) differ in babies fed human milk or formula. Science tells us that the human body contains more bacteria than human cells. The bacteria that live within us interact with our bodies and affect our health, for better or worse. The type of bacteria in a baby's gut is determined in part by whether she is fed human milk or formula (J. H. Savage et al., 2018). Babies who exclusively nurse have more of the "good" *Bifidobacteria*, while partially nursed or formula-fed babies have more *Clostridia* and others, so their gut flora more closely resembles that of an adult (Ho et al., 2018). Although our understanding of the impact of our microbiota on health is still in its infancy, research found links between alterations in gut flora and obesity (Ley, 2010; Paolella & Vajro, 2016).

For a summary of how infant feeding methods affect the risk of obesity in childhood, see the 2018 Appleton systematic review (Appleton et al., 2018). For an overview of other factors that contribute to childhood overweight and obesity, see the next-to-last point in this chapter.

Growth after 12 Months

At 12 months, babies fed non-human milks are typically heavier than nursing babies, but by 24 months there are few differences in growth.

U.S. research on normal growth in healthy babies found that at 12 months nursing babies were on average a little less than 1.5 lbs. (600-650 g) lighter than formula-fed babies (Dewey, Heinig, Nommsen, Peerson, & Lonnerdal, 1992). By 24 months, most differences in weight gain and growth between nursing and formula-fed babies disappeared (Butte, Wong, Hopkinson, Smith, & Ellis, 2000; Dewey et al., 1992). No differences in height have been found in adulthood between those nursed or formula-fed as infants (Dewey, 2009a).

• • •

After 12 months, nursing is still an important source of a baby's nourishment.

Continued, frequent nursing after 12 months provides babies with necessary nutrients. Nursing babies 1 to 2 years old consuming an average volume of mother's milk receive 35% to 40% of their energy intake (Dewey & Brown, 2003), and it provides an important source of fatty acids and other key nutrients, such as vitamin A, calcium, and riboflavin (PAHO/WHO., 2001).

• • •

Research in developing countries (Onyango, Esrey, & Kramer, 1999; Simondon, Simondon, Costes, Delaunay, & Diallo, 2001) found that when babies older than a year continue to nurse and other confounding factors are eliminated, they grow faster in length than their weaned counterparts.

In developing countries, babies who nurse for at least 12 months grow better in length.

Growth Charts

Growth charts can be a useful tool to understand how one baby's growth compares to the growth of other babies the same age, but they can also confuse parents and put the focus in the wrong place.

Growth charts can be helpful, but they can also be confusing. In some cases, their misuse can undermine nursing.

Growth charts plot a baby's growth on a series of percentile lines. An average child will be at the 50th percentile for weight and length. For weight, what this actually means is that out of 100 children, 49 will weigh less and 50 will weigh more. A weight that falls at a higher percentile is not "good," and a weight that falls at a lower percentile is not "bad." By definition, there will be healthy children at every percentile. Some will be chunky and some will be petite, but their percentile does not necessarily reflect their overall health or growth.

The child at the 5th percentile is not necessarily growing poorly, and the child at the 95th percentile is not necessarily growing well. That's because growth can only be evaluated over time, and the evaluation will only be accurate when the chart itself is based on nursing norms (see next point). For example, a preterm baby born very small will likely fall on a low percentile for weight and height at first, even when she is growing and gaining weight well. But her growth should eventually catch up to others born full-term. Also, a large baby's unusually high birth weight may be due more to certain conditions during pregnancy, such as the birthing parent's blood sugar levels, weight gain, and height. According to researcher Lori Nommsen-Rivers (personal communication), after birth, a large baby may "regress to the mean" by falling in percentiles at first as her growth adjusts to her genetic potential.

One point on a baby's growth chart should never be considered in isolation. More important is how this one point compares to the other points on the chart. To accurately evaluate a baby's growth, the answers to the following questions are needed:

- Is the baby gaining weight at a healthy pace?
- Is she growing normally in length and head circumference?

KEY CONCEPT

Nursing provides a significant percentage of the nutrients a baby needs, even after 12 months.

The baby's growth pattern over days, weeks, and months is what provides an accurate picture of how nursing is going. If a baby is growing consistently and well, her actual percentile is irrelevant. However, if over time her percentile drops, this is a red flag to take a closer look (see next section).

One U.K. study examined through multiple interviews at well-baby checkups mothers' and healthcare providers' understanding of growth charts (Sachs, Dykes, & Carter, 2006). The researchers found that many mothers worried about their baby's weight gain between checkups and that both mothers and healthcare providers considered the 50th percentile a goal to be achieved.

When babies fell below the 50th percentile, rather than focusing on optimizing breastfeeding, healthcare providers often recommended the mothers give their babies formula and solid foods to try to boost baby's weight gain to reach this percentile. In their conclusion, the researchers recommended more training for healthcare providers on assessing growth patterns of nursing babies and more training on how to provide families with information that supports rather than undermines nursing.

• • •

Between 3 and 12 months of age, a baby's percentile on the growth chart will vary depending on whether the chart is based on nursing norms.

Some growth charts are based on the growth of mostly formula-fed babies, who have different growth patterns than nursing babies (for details on these differences see the last point in the previous section). For example, the 1977 National Center for Health Statistics (NCHS) growth charts used for many years in the U.S. were based on data from a study conducted in one Ohio town. The data used to create these charts had limitations, including a lack of ethnic diversity, data collection at infrequent, 3-month intervals, sample-size problems, and few nursing babies (Dewey, 2009b).

Unfortunately, the U.S. Centers for Disease Control and Prevention (CDC) charts that replaced them in 2000 also included few nursing babies. The overrepresentation of formula-feeding babies in these studies was a problem, because babies nursed and fed by bottle gain weight differently from 3 to 12 months. When these charts were used, many exclusively nursing babies who were gaining normally were thought to be faltering.

It wasn't until 2006 that the World Health Organization (WHO) released growth charts that accurately reflected the normal growth of the nursing baby. This process began in 1997, when WHO began its ambitious Multicentre Growth Reference Study (WHO, 2006). This study's goal was to define optimal growth in six culturally and ethnically diverse countries (Brazil, Ghana, India, Norway, Oman, and the U.S.) over a 6-year period. About 8,500 children—including about 300 newborns—participated in the study. The mothers of these babies followed healthy practices by breastfeeding exclusively, not smoking, and adding appropriate solid foods to their babies' diet at the recommended age.

Researchers found that no matter where these mothers and children lived, and no matter what their ethnic background, average growth was nearly identical in all six countries. The charts developed from this research for children aged 0-60 months are free and downloadable online at: **who.int/childgrowth/standards/en** and include weight for age, weight for length, body mass index for age, and motor development milestones.

KEY CONCEPT

The WHO growth standards reflect how nursing babies should grow.

These WHO growth standards reflect nursing norms and differ from the previous CDC growth charts in the following ways:

- From birth to 6 months more babies are heavier
- From 6 to 12 months more babies are lighter

Previously used growth charts were a reflection of how mostly formula-fed children grew in a particular time and place. In contrast, the data used to create the WHO growth standards were compiled internationally among families using optimal feeding practices, making them a benchmark of how all children ***should*** grow. They are a standard that can be used to judge childhood growth anywhere in the world.

SLOW WEIGHT GAIN

When a baby is gaining weight slowly, emotions are often intense. Be prepared to listen to and acknowledge these feelings.

When a baby is not gaining well, nursing parents' feelings often run high. They may be frustrated and upset. They may be worried about their ability to care for their baby. They may feel anxious about the baby's health. They may feel guilty, wondering if the baby's slow weight gain is their fault or if they have not provided good care. They may feel like a failure.

Giving the family an outlet to express their worries, fears, and doubts may make it easier for them to discuss and evaluate their situation more objectively. Assure them there is a reason for the slow weight gain and the odds are good that they will be able to overcome this problem.

• • •

The definitions of adequate and slow weight gain have changed since the 2006 release of the WHO growth standards.

For many years, lactation supporters considered weight gain adequate during the first 3 months if a nursing baby gained between a half ounce (14g) and 1 ounce (28 g) per day. After the release of the WHO growth standards in 2006, however, expectations of weight gain in young nursing babies shifted. As described in the last point of the previous section, these WHO growth standards describe how nursing babies ***should*** grow and appear to apply to all ethnicities worldwide. For that reason, most lactation specialists now have higher expectation of weight gain in young babies. Nancy G. Powers wrote in the textbook, *Breastfeeding and Human Lactation* (N.G. Powers, 2016, p. 373):

> "Once over birth weight, the neonate who gains less than 30-40 g per day in the first 2 months of life requires thorough medical and breastfeeding evaluation."

When babies younger than 3 months old gain less than 1 ounce (28 g) per day, it is important to ask relevant questions so that the cause of the slow weight gain can be pinpointed. See the next section for details. See also Table 6.1 for expected weight gain for older babies. Sometimes a weight gain of less than 30 g per day may be an early indicator of a health problem in the baby that needs to be addressed, or perhaps it is a sign that there is room for improvement in how the baby is nursing.

Gathering Basic Information

Before making suggestions, first try to determine the cause(s) of the slow weight gain.

When a baby does not gain well on mother's milk alone, everyone becomes concerned. Something needs to be done, but inappropriate actions can lead to premature weaning. Finding the cause(s) will help determine the best course of action. The cause of slow weight gain usually involves one or more of the following three areas:

- **Nursing dynamics.** Is the baby latched deeply? Is the baby nursing at least eight times each day and nursing until done?
- **Baby's anatomy and health.** Is the baby nursing ineffectively due to anatomical variations or a health problem? Or is a health problem causing slow weight gain despite a healthy milk intake?
- **Nursing parent's milk production.** Is the nursing parent producing enough milk to meet the baby's needs?

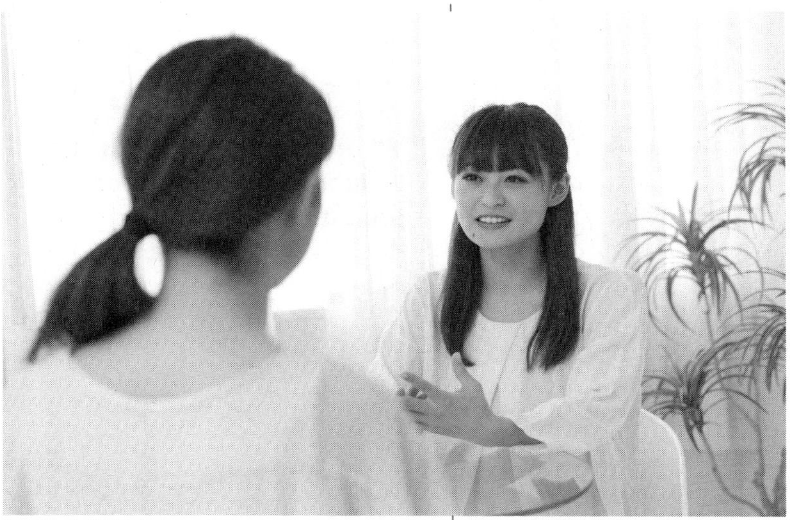

The strategies chosen to improve the baby's weight gain depend on which of these areas are contributing to the problem. Most often, nursing dynamics are the main issue. In this case, an adjustment in feeding pattern or achieving a deeper latch is needed. If the baby has a medical problem, she may need diagnosis and treatment. Variations in oral anatomy, such as tongue-tie, may require assessment and possibly a medical procedure. If the milk production is low, the cause needs to be determined and—if possible—production boosted.

To find the cause(s), some detective work is in order. The answers to the questions in the following sections will provide information that can help get to the root of the problem. Some basic questions should be asked about all slow-gaining babies, but some may not be necessary to explore with all families.

• • •

Ask questions in a calm, relaxed manner and affirm whatever the nursing parent is doing right.

To gather the needed information, listen carefully, take notes, and ask questions calmly to help put the family at ease. Some areas may be sensitive, so try to word questions tactfully. Because nursing parents may worry that the baby's slow weight gain is their fault, emphasize that every nursing couple is different and there are no hard-and-fast rules. Some basic nursing dynamics are good to know (such as drained glands make milk faster and full glands make milk slower), but not all babies respond in the same way. One baby may nurse five times a day and gain weight well (although this is rare), while another may need to nurse every hour or two to gain adequate weight. The nursing parent of a slow-gaining baby may feel vulnerable, and may be criticized for their efforts. Be sure to affirm them for whatever they are doing right and for seeking help.

• • •

Use their answers to guide the conversation.

During the course of the discussion, the answers to certain questions may give clues to the cause of the baby's slow weight gain. When that happens, stop and talk more about this area so parents can expand on their answers and clarify their understanding of nursing and their individual circumstances. If the reasons for the baby's slow weight gain are not obvious after these first three sections, continue to the others. The most common cause of slow weight gain is less-than-optimal nursing dynamics, which includes shallow latch and not nursing often or long enough. Nursing more often may not help if the baby is latched shallowly or nursing ineffectively, for example, so pay careful attention to the answers.

• • •

Be sure the baby is being regularly evaluated by a healthcare provider.

In all cases of slow weight gain, the baby should be seen regularly by her healthcare provider to rule out health problems. Although most cases of slow weight gain are not caused by physical problems, this is a possibility that needs to be considered.

If the baby's healthcare provider recommends supplementing the baby with formula and the nursing parent wants to try other alternatives first, encourage the family to contact him/her to discuss this.

Weight Gain and Loss

How much weight has the baby gained since birth, and how close is her weight gain to the expected range?

Ask for the following information:

- The baby's age
- The baby's current weight
- The baby's birth weight and gestational age at birth (preterm or full-term)
- The baby's lowest weight after birth
- Her age and weights at each of her weight checks

If available, a baby's weight gain should be calculated from its lowest point. For example:

- Birth weight: 7 lbs., 13 ounces (3544 g)
- Lowest weight (age 4 days): 7 lbs., 0 ounces (3175 g)
- Current weight (age 5 weeks): 8 lbs., 13 ounces (3997 g)

Some might mistakenly think this baby girl is gaining slowly because she is only 1 lb. (454 g) over her birth weight at 5 weeks. But when the weight gain is calculated from the lowest point after birth, her weight gain for the last 4 weeks was actually 1 lb., 13 ounces (29 ounces or 823 g). She is not gaining slowly. She is gaining 7.3 ounces (206 g) per week, which is very close to an average weight gain for a girl. The 50th percentile of weight gain from birth to 4 weeks is 879 grams or 220 grams (7.75 ounces) per week.

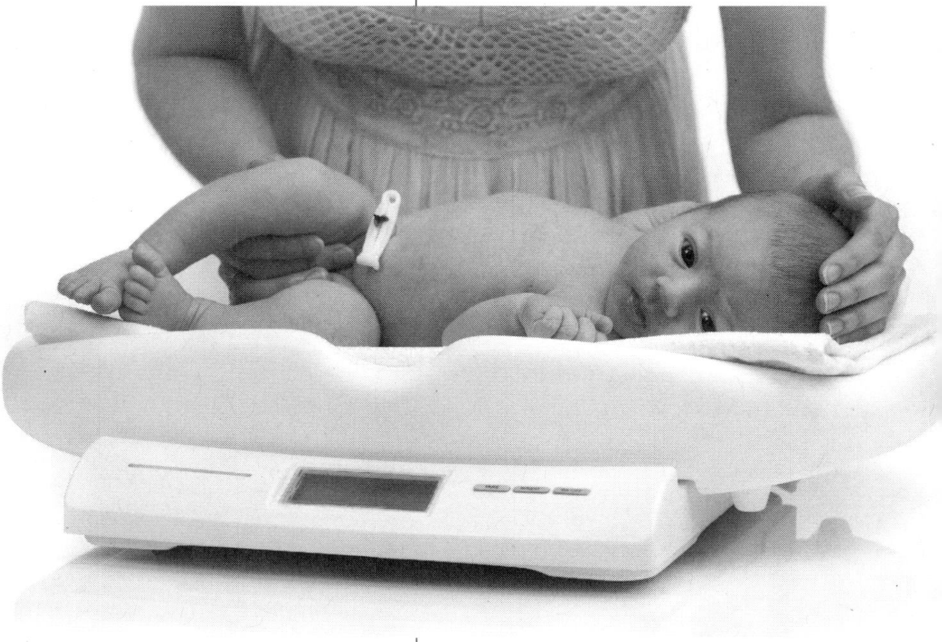

When a baby is born with an elevated birth weight, this can affect perception of weight gain later. For example, IV fluids given during labor can be absorbed by the baby's tissues in utero, boosting her birth weight and causing greater weight loss after birth as these extra fluids are shed (Noel-Weiss et al., 2011; Tawia & McGuire, 2014). Birth weight may also be elevated in babies born to parents with Type 1, Type 2, or gestational diabetes. In these babies, growth after birth is usually slower than average as the baby sheds the excess fluids and fat laid down in utero as a result of their birthing parent's abnormal blood sugar levels.

Growth usually slows with age (see first section), so what is considered slow weight gain will vary by age and stage.

If a baby's weight gain is close to the expected range (in a baby girl younger than 3 months, this is at least about 7 to 8 ounces (198-237 g) per week or about 28 g per day), the baby's healthcare provider will probably be more open to improving nursing dynamics first, rather than insisting the baby be supplemented right away. To have the energy needed to feed effectively, a baby who is continuing to lose weight or is far from a healthy weight gain will need to be supplemented (see later section "When and How to Give Supplements").

• • •

Was the baby's weight an issue from birth, or did the baby gain well at first?

If a baby continues to lose weight after Day 4 or 5 or weight gain is low from the beginning, focus on baby's nursing effectiveness and milk production (see later sections). If the baby's weight loss was in the normal range and baby regained her birth weight by 2 weeks, slow weight gain must have started after that. In this case, focus on nursing dynamics, baby's health, and milk production. A baby's need for milk increases rapidly during the first 5 weeks or so (see the later section "When and How to Supplement"). Therefore, when maximum milk production is limited by breast surgery or underdeveloped mammary tissue, the baby may gain weight well during the first week or two, but weight gain may falter after that.

• • •

Was the same scale used for each of the weight checks? Was the baby's clothing the same when she was last weighed? And when was the scale last calibrated?

Many parents and healthcare providers have assumed at one weight check that a baby was gaining slowly only to discover the problem was actually human error (using the scale incorrectly, misreading the weight, transposing the numbers when writing or typing, plotting the baby's percentile incorrectly, etc.), the scale (low level of accuracy, not properly calibrated), or differences in how the baby was dressed when she was weighed. Before assuming the baby's weight is the problem, suggest the baby be weighed again using the same scale and wearing the same clothing as before. If the baby wears a diaper/nappy during weight checks, the weight difference between one that's dry or full also affects the results. For greater accuracy, some suggest trying to time regular weight checks after baby had a stool and before a feed (L. Marasco & West, 2020, p. 29).

• • •

A healthy weight gain is the most reliable indicator of adequate milk intake, but some babies take adequate milk while nursing, yet still gain slowly.

When an exclusively nursing baby has a healthy weight gain and is growing normally, it is safe to assume she is getting the milk she needs. However, it is possible for a baby to be taking adequate milk during nursing, but still gain weight slowly. That's because there is more to weight gain than milk intake alone.

In addition to consuming enough milk, a baby must also be able to digest the milk, and it must meet her energy needs. Babies with congenital heart disease, for example, usually gain weight slowly no matter how they are fed, because they take more breaths per minute than a healthy baby in order to maintain adequate oxygen levels and circulation (Mangili, Garzoli, & Sadou, 2018). (For more details, see p. 311-313 for the later section, "Slow Weight Gain with Good Milk Intake" and Chapter 8, "Baby's Anatomy and Health Issues"). Other genetic conditions and metabolic, endocrine, and digestive disorders may also require treatment or interventions for normal growth, despite good milk intake.

• • •

How much has the baby grown in length and head circumference?

Growth in length and head circumference is also an important aspect of normal development. During the first 6 months, growth in length averages about 1 inch (2.54 centimeters) per month and head circumference about 0.5 inch (1.27 centimeters) per month. Growth in head circumference indicates brain growth.

• • •

What has the baby's healthcare provider said about the baby's overall health?

The baby's health is an important factor when considering weight gain. If the baby was ill, for example, it is common for weight gain to slow or even stop for a time. Illness can affect a baby's feeding effectiveness and her appetite.

If the baby seems to be otherwise developing well and appears healthy and alert, this means there is probably time to fine-tune nursing to increase baby's weight gain before supplements are needed.

• • •

Is the diagnosis slow weight gain or failure to thrive?

The difference between slow weight gain and failure to thrive is one of degree and definition. The diagnosis of failure to thrive, in addition to indicating the baby is seriously underweight, may also imply abuse or neglect (M. Walker, 2017). A baby identified as failure to thrive is at risk for malnutrition, and immediate intervention is needed. Failure to thrive usually involves feeding problems, continued weight loss after the first week, not reaching birth weight by 3 weeks of age, and depending on birth weight, a weight below the 10th percentile on the growth charts by 1 month of age (Lawrence & Lawrence, 2016). The baby may grow little in length or head circumference, pass concentrated urine and few stools, and have symptoms of malnutrition or dehydration, such as lethargy and a sunken fontanel. A baby older than 1 month with failure to thrive, in addition to most of the previous symptoms, is usually below the 3rd percentile in weight, has fallen at least two standard deviations on the growth chart by 8 weeks, and may be delayed in reaching developmental milestones. In some cases, failure to thrive is due to health problems, such as infection, birth or heart defects, malabsorption, endocrine problems, or other chronic diseases (Homan, 2016). In some cases, the baby may be otherwise healthy and simply have feeding problems (Tolia, 1995). One U.S. report found that underlying illness was the cause in half of babies diagnosed after 1 month (Lukefahr, 1990).

A slow-gaining baby, on the other hand, usually feeds well and often has pale urine and the expected number of stools, appears alert and active, is developing normally, has good skin and muscle tone, and is gaining weight, just gaining slower than average. For this baby, it may be possible to make adjustments to nursing before supplementing.

Other Signs of Milk Intake

How long during feeds can the nursing parent hear the baby swallowing?

How effectively a baby nurses is one important factor in determining milk intake, and swallowing sounds can provide clues to feeding effectiveness. U.S. research (Cote-Arsenault & McCoy, 2012) found that counting baby's swallows during the first few days of life was not a reliable indicator of milk intake, but audible swallowing can be considered a rough indicator of milk intake. When babies swallow, it is usually loud enough to be heard. After milk ejection, most babies swallow after every or every other suck with occasional pauses. As nursing continues, milk flow slows, and as the baby's hunger is satisfied, there is usually more time between swallows and more sucks to swallows. If the baby sucks many times before swallowing right after milk ejection, this is one possible sign of ineffective nursing.

• • •

Are there any other indicators the baby is nursing ineffectively?

Other signs of ineffective nursing include:

- **No swallowing heard at all.** But there are exceptions. Some babies nurse effectively but swallow too quietly to be heard. If so, the baby gains weight well.

- **Baby never seems satisfied.** The family may say the baby nurses "all the time."
- **Shallow latch.** When the baby nurses with the nipple in the front of her mouth (instead of in the "comfort zone" near where her hard and soft palates meet), this can contribute to slower milk flow, less milk intake, and/or difficulty staying latched.
- **Choking during nursing** can occur with very fast milk flow and also with uncoordinated sucking and swallowing or an airway abnormality.
- **Low or high muscle tone.** "Floppy" babies with low tone include those with Down syndrome and other neurological impairments. Babies with high tone may arch away, especially if upright feeding positions are used. For feeding strategies, see p. 327-329 in Chapter 8, "Baby's Anatomy and Health Issues."
- **Cheek dimpling or clicking sounds** during nursing indicate suction is being broken. If baby is gaining weight well, this is not a problem.
- **Nipple pain or trauma** can be due to shallow latch, unusual tongue movements, or anatomical variations, such as tongue-tie.
- **Unrelieved mammary fullness or recurring mastitis** due to ineffective milk removal.

If there is no audible swallowing at all, if it stops early in the feed, or if the baby usually falls asleep quickly, to encourage more active nursing, suggest trying to get a deeper latch and then using breast compression (see p. 889).

• • •

Scales are available in some areas that can measure babies' milk intake during nursing.

Weighing the baby before and after a feed with a very accurate baby scale (to 2 g) can determine a baby's milk intake during nursing at that feed, assuming baby's clothing remains the same at both weights (Rankin et al., 2016). These very accurate scales are available in some hospitals and at many lactation offices or clinics. In some areas, they can be rented for home use at pump rental companies. However, milk intake at one feed does not necessarily reflect a baby's daily milk intake because feeding volumes vary by baby's appetite, how deeply she latches, and other factors. But confirmed good milk intake during one nursing can rule out ineffective nursing at that feed. See the later section, "When and How to Supplement" for average feeding volumes during the first 6 months. After a test-weigh, ask the family if that feed seemed typical.

• • •

Diaper output is not a reliable indicator of milk intake.

During the first day or two of life, daily diaper output is typically one or two wet diapers and stools. After that, some health organizations suggest nursing parents track daily diaper output to determine if baby is getting enough milk. In its 2014 Clinical Protocol #2 (Evans, Marinelli, Taylor, & Academy of Breastfeeding, 2014), the Academy of Breastfeeding Medicine considered one indicator of adequate milk intake 3 to 4 stools per day by the fourth day of life. By Day 5, stools should have turned yellow and baby should have at least 5 to 6 urinations per day.

Three U.S. studies examined whether diaper output accurately reflects adequate milk intake. All three found much room for error. One study of 73 exclusively breastfeeding mother-baby couples (Shrago, Reifsnider, & Insel, 2006) monitored the babies' weight loss and gain, breastfeeding patterns, and diaper output for the first 14 days. The researchers found that more stool output during the first 5 days was associated with positive infant outcomes. The first day of yellow stools was a significant predictor of percentage of weight loss. (The earlier the babies' stools turned yellow, the less weight was lost.) During the first 14 days, the mean number of stools per day was four, but some babies had as many as eight. The average number of daily stools was not an accurate predictor of initial weight loss, but the more stools passed during the entire 14-day study period, the earlier birth weight was regained.

Because some newborns nurse ineffectively, the number of daily feeds was not related to initial weight loss, start of weight gain, regaining of birth weight, or weight at Day 14. (Mean number of daily feeds was 8.5, with a range of 6 to 11.) In fact, the researchers considered unusually frequent feeding with low stool output a red flag to check baby's weight, as the study baby who breastfed the most times per day had the poorest weight outcomes. They found that frequent feeds with good stool output was a sign of effective breastfeeding, but they considered frequent feeds with few stools a possible sign of ineffective feeding.

The second U.S. study followed 242 exclusively breastfeeding mother-baby couples, also for the first 14 days of life (L. A. Nommsen-Rivers, Heinig, Cohen, & Dewey, 2008). These researchers concluded: "diaper output measures, when applied in the home setting, showed too much overlap between infants with adequate versus inadequate breast milk intake to serve as stand-alone indicators of breastfeeding adequacy" (L. A. Nommsen-Rivers et al., 2008, p. 32). The most reliable predictor of poor milk intake was fewer than 4 stools on Day 4, but only when paired with the mothers' perception that their milk had not yet increased. Even when both of these criteria were true, there were many false positives, meaning that many of these babies' weight was in the normal range.

A 2018 prospective observational cohort study of 151 newborns (DiTomasso & Paiva, 2018) divided the babies into two groups: 1) those who lost <7% of birth weight (67 babies) and 2) those who lost ≥7% of birth weight (84 babies). The researchers recorded milk intake, diaper output, and weights in both groups during the first 14 days. The researchers found no significant differences in the number of wet diapers between the two groups. However, the newborns who lost more weight initially averaged slightly fewer stools per day (4.06 versus 4.72) during the first 14 days.

So at best, diaper output can be considered a very rough indicator of milk intake. While it can be helpful when slow weight gain is a concern to track diaper output on a daily basis between regular weight checks, diaper output alone cannot substitute for an accurate weight. Regular weight checks during the first weeks are vital to identifying nursing babies at risk for low milk intake.

KEY CONCEPT

Diaper output is at best a very rough indicator of milk intake.

Also, diaper output patterns change over time. According to one Turkish prospective cohort study of 125 exclusively nursing babies, the average number of stools per day peaked at around 2 weeks at 6 per day and by about 1 month, the average was down to 4 per day. Between 3 and 12 months, 2 per day was average. A French article that described the results of two studies that followed 283 babies total (Camurdan, Beyazova, Ozkan, & Tunc, 2014) found that even during the first month, infrequent stools (fewer than 1 per day) occurred in 37% of the babies in one study. After about 5 weeks or so, some babies stool very infrequently, sometimes less than once per week (Courdent,

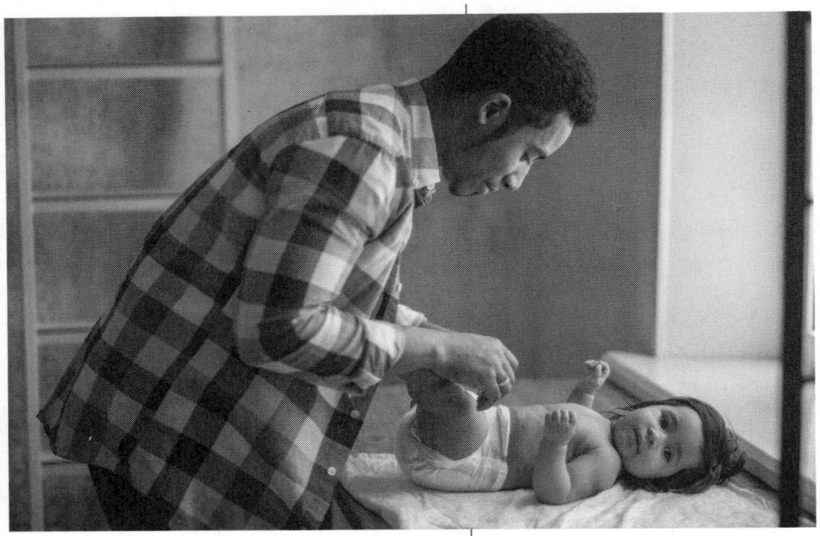

Beghin, Akre, & Turck, 2014; Moretti, Rakza, Mestdagh, Labreuche, & Turck, 2018). As long as the baby's stools are not hard and dry, this is not constipation. And it is not a cause for concern from the perspective of milk intake if the baby is gaining weight well.

Consistently green stools may indicate an overabundant milk production (see p. 457-464) or that the baby is sensitive to a medication taken either by the baby or the nursing parent, or a food in the nursing parent's diet. Mucus or blood in the stool may also be a sign of sensitivity or allergy. For more details, see p. 561-565.

• • •

If the baby's diaper output is low after Day 5 and her stools have not yet turned yellow, is she alert and is her skin resilient?

Normally by Day 5, most nursing babies have at least 5 to 6 wet diapers per day and their stools have changed color from black or greenish to yellow and seedy (Shrago et al., 2006). If not, suggest taking the baby to her healthcare provider to check her weight. As described in the first section, most babies reach their low weight by Day 5 at the latest and then begin gaining weight (Flaherman et al., 2015).

If after Day 3 or 4, the baby still has 2 or fewer wet diapers per day, suggest being alert to the warning signs of dehydration, which indicate the baby needs more fluids immediately:

- The baby acts lethargic and may have a weak cry.
- The baby's skin becomes less resilient (after it's pinched, it stays pinched-looking).
- The baby looks very yellow.
- The baby's eyes and mouth seem dry.
- The baby's fontanel (soft spot) looks sunken.
- The baby has a fever.

If any of these symptoms occur, suggest contacting baby's healthcare provider without delay.

• • •

A baby's temperament and sleep patterns are not reliable indicators of milk intake.

Many parents mistakenly assume that wakefulness, irritability, and fussiness are signs that their baby is not getting enough milk. One of the early studies to describe what is now known as "perceived insufficient milk," was conducted in Sweden (Hillervik-Lindquist, Hofvander, & Sjolin, 1991). It followed 51 breastfeeding mothers and found that many of them went through periods when they were convinced their milk production was low, even though their babies were gaining weight well and their milk intake was comparable to other babies

These kinds of worries about milk production appear to be nearly universal. But as long as an irritable and wakeful baby can nurse effectively (which parents will know for certain from her weight gain), assure the family that this behavior is not a sign of low milk intake. Placid and undemanding babies who do not feed often enough are actually at greater risk of slow weight gain than fussier babies who nurse more often.

Studies from many different countries (Galipeau, Dumas, & Lepage, 2017; Gokceoglu & Kucukoglu, 2017; Otsuka, Dennis, Tatsuoka, & Jimba, 2008) found an association between "perceived insufficient milk" and low breastfeeding self-efficacy (nursing parents' belief in their ability to successfully nurse their baby). A 2017 systematic review found that interventions that raise parents' breastfeeding self-efficacy scores measurably increased nursing exclusivity (Brockway, Benzies, & Hayden, 2017).

• • •

Is the family using a commercial product that claims to measure milk intake during nursing?

In recent years, a variety of products entered the marketplace that claim to provide parents with accurate information about their baby's milk intake during nursing. One includes a device with a small sensor that is placed under baby's tongue during feeds and uses an algorithm to calculate milk intake, which is sent to an app in the parent's smartphone that records the results. Another uses a battery-operated device designed to be used with a scale that hangs from an infant seat to measure changes in the size of the mammary gland and baby's weight during feeds. Anther device uses a nipple shield with sensors attached to measure milk transfer and sends the information to the parent's smartphone where it is recorded. Lactation specialists Lisa Marasco and Diana West wrote in the 2020 2nd edition of their book, *Making More Milk: The Breastfeeding Guide to Increasing Your Milk Production* (L. Marasco & West, 2020, p. 31).

> "Is it worth the money to buy one of these devices? We don't have enough experience to say one way or the other yet, but we're concerned that the technologies may be less accurate in low-supply situations when babies have suck problems, or for mothers with unusually-shaped breasts or nipples."

KEY CONCEPT

Most babies need to nurse at least 8 times per day during the early weeks to gain adequate weight.

Basic Nursing Dynamics

How many times each day does the baby nurse?

To gain weight and thrive, most newborns nurse at least 8 times every 24 hours (Kent et al., 2013). If the slow-gaining baby is nursing fewer than 8 times each day, ask if they are nursing by the clock—feeding at set intervals, limiting number of feeds, or limiting feeding length. If yes, ask why. Some books and parenting programs recommend strict feeding schedules (Ezzo & Bucknam, 2019). If the family believes strongly in scheduled feeds, they may not be open to nursing on cue, because (without evidence) these authors equate frequent feeds with discipline problems later in life. When faced with a slow-gaining baby, however, even some families who believe strongly in feeding schedules may be willing to schedule feeds at shorter intervals and increase the number of feeds per day.

Some families nurse fewer than 8 times per day because the baby is sleepy or doesn't show feeding cues more often. In this case, suggest parents take an active role in initiating nursing, rather than waiting for the baby to indicate a need. For example, if the young baby only shows feeding cues 6 times a day, suggest at least until weight gain is improved, initiating nursing at least 10 or 12 times per day, or 4 to 6 more times than baby shows feeding cues.

• • •

How long does a feed usually take, does the baby take both sides, and who usually ends the feed, parent or baby?

Nursing rhythm varies tremendously from place to place. U.S. researcher Kathleen Kennedy described how a "breastfeeding" means something very different to mothers in different cultures (Kennedy, 2010). A Western mother may consider a "breastfeeding" a lengthy, ritualized activity that may involve changing the baby's diaper, making herself a drink, settling into a certain chair, and then nursing for an extended time. A mother in a developing country, in contrast, may keep her baby on her body, nursing at the slightest cue for just a few minutes 15 to 20 times each day. These two babies may get about the same volume of milk per day, but there are huge cultural differences between their feeding patterns. Consider cultural norms when discussing nursing dynamics.

Finish the first side first. It is helpful to know who decides when the baby is finished on the first side. One recommended strategy is called "finish the first side first," which means the baby determines the length of the feed and feeds on the first side until she comes off on her own, and then the second side is offered. If the baby still wants to nurse after taking the second side, the baby can go back to the first side again.

Some families are erroneously told to limit nursing to a set number of minutes per side to avoid nipple pain or because the baby gets all the milk she needs within a short time. But many years ago U.S. research (de Carvalho, Robertson, & Klaus, 1984) found that limiting nursing time does not prevent nipple pain. (Helping the baby latch deeply is a better strategy.) Ending feeds after a set number of minutes per side is counterproductive for most babies because some are fast feeders and some are slow feeders. For the same reason adults' plates are not removed from the dinner table after a set time, nursing by the clock does not allow for individual differences in feeding pace.

There are also other reasons important to adequate weight gain to let the baby set the feeding pace. One is that the milk's fat content increases during nursing. Limiting length of feeds can decrease the fat and calories the baby receives from the milk, which can slow weight gain. Suggest the family expect most feeds at first to take 10 to 20 minutes per side or longer. If the baby is gaining weight well on shorter feeds, a shorter time is fine. Breast compression may help keep the baby active longer, if needed (see p. 889).

> **KEY CONCEPT**
>
> *It's best not to limit feeds to a set number of minutes.*

One side or more? Australian research on 71 healthy breastfed babies 1 to 6 months old found that at some feeds babies took one side, at some feeds both sides (which the researchers called a "paired breastfeed"), and at some feeds babies took both sides and then fed again from the first side (called a "clustered breastfeed") (Kent et al., 2006). To increase milk intake in a slow-gaining baby, suggest encouraging the baby to take both sides at least once at each feed, and twice if possible, following the baby's lead. Many nursing parents mistakenly think they are "empty" after the baby nurses once on that side. Not likely! On average babies take only about 70% of the available milk before coming off, so there is still milk in both sides if baby takes them again at that feed (Kent, 2007).

• • •

Does the baby latch and quickly fall asleep? Does the nursing parent have nipple pain?

Nipple pain and falling asleep quickly during nursing can both be signs of a shallow latch. See Chapter 1, "Basic Nursing Dynamics," and Appendix A, "Techniques," for strategies for achieving a deeper latch to increase milk intake at feeds. Helping the baby take the nipple deeper in her mouth can help make nursing more effective and more comfortable.

Nipple pain may also be a sign of anatomical variations in the baby or the nursing parent. When a baby is tongue-tied, for example, her restricted tongue movements may cause painful nursing and reduced milk intake (see later sections "Baby's Anatomy and Health" and "Mammary/Nipple Issue").

• • •

What is the baby's sleep/wake pattern, and how long is the baby's longest sleep stretch?

If a baby sleeps so much that she does not wake to nurse at least 8 times per day, the baby may be unusually placid. Or she may be overdressed and overheated, which can make her sleepy. Another possibility is that the family uses soothers that can suppress feeding cues (see the next point). Newborn jaundice can also cause sleepiness during the first few weeks of life. Suggest ruling out physical causes and trying the following strategies:

- **Make sure baby is not too warm.** Unwrap the baby or dress in lighter clothes.
- **Nurse at least once during the night.** If a slow-gaining baby is sleeping longer than about 5 hours at night, suggest rousing her to feed at least once during her longest sleep stretch.
- **Help baby latch during light sleep.** Rather than being fully awakened, many families do "dream feeds" during a baby's light sleep cycle. Signs of light sleep include any movement, such as eyes moving under eyelids.
- **"Cluster" or bunch feeds** during baby's naturally occurring alert periods, rather than waiting for a set interval to nurse again.
- **Spend more time with baby tummy down on the nursing parent's semi-reclined body,** either skin-to-skin or clothed, to trigger baby's inborn feeding behaviors more often.

U.K. research (Colson, 2003) found that newborns—even late preterm babies—can nurse effectively when drowsy and in light sleep. Encourage the nursing parent to take advantage of that to add more daily feeds. Some babies nurse more easily and feed more effectively when drowsy or asleep.

Newborns move in and out of sleep often. A long sleep stretch of up to 4 to 5 hours is not a cause for concern. When discussing their nursing rhythm, make sure the family knows that nursing babies do not usually feed at regular intervals (Benson, 2001). Rather than focusing on maintaining regular feeding intervals, suggest focusing instead on the total number of feeds every 24 hours, which is more important in terms of overall milk intake in an effectively nursing baby. In a slow-gaining baby younger than 6 months, suggest a target goal of at least 10 to 12 feeds per day.

• • •

Is the baby regularly swaddled for long periods or using a soother, such as a pacifier or a baby swing?

For the slow-gaining baby, suggest avoiding products and techniques that mask baby's feeding cues or decrease a baby's interest in feeding.

Routine pacifier/dummy use may decrease the number of feeds per day. Some older observational studies found an association between routine pacifier use and less nursing. One U.S. prospective study (Howard et al., 1999) found that at 2 weeks mothers using pacifiers breastfed on average 8 times per day compared with 9 times per day when the pacifier was not used. An Australian prospective cohort study of 556 mothers and babies (Binns & Scott, 2002) found that mothers using pacifiers breastfed on average 6.9 times per day at 6 weeks compared with 7.4 feeds per day among those not using a pacifier. A Swedish descriptive, longitudinal, prospective study of 506 mothers and babies (Aarts, Hornell, Kylberg, Hofvander, & Gebre-Medhin, 1999) found that at 2, 4, 6, 8, and 10 weeks, babies taking pacifiers breastfed fewer times per day than those who did not. Fewer feeds per day mean less daily milk intake.

Swaddled babies sleep more. U.S. research (Franco et al., 2005) found that swaddled babies aroused less and slept longer. More time asleep can mean less nursing, which can contribute to slow weight gain. A 2017 integrative review of the literature on swaddling (Nelson, 2017) suggested that if newborns are swaddled, they may need to be awakened to nurse often enough.

• • •

Is the nursing baby consuming anything other than mother's milk?

Ask specifically if the baby is receiving water, juice, formula, or solid foods. Also ask if the baby receives expressed milk, and if so, how it is fed. Formula provides calories, but if formula feeds replace nursing, this delays or reduces the time baby spends nursing, which can potentially decrease milk production by decreasing mammary stimulation. A Swedish study (Righard, 1998) found that in some cases, using feeding bottles during the early weeks may interfere with the baby's ability to suck effectively.

KEY CONCEPT

Water or juice supplements can decrease milk production and/or slow weight gain.

If the baby is fed large amounts of low-calorie solid foods when younger than the recommended 6 months, this may potentially reduce the volume of mother's milk baby takes during nursing (Islam, Peerson, Ahmed, Dewey, & Brown, 2006). Low-calorie solids could potentially reduce baby's daily caloric intake and contribute to slow weight gain.

Water and juice are not recommended for nursing babies younger than 6 months (AAP, 2012). They make babies feel full, but do not provide the nutrients needed for healthy weight gain and growth. For the younger baby, suggest gradually replacing other foods or liquids with more frequent nursing. If the baby was not nursing effectively or the supplements are a substantial part of her intake, caution the family to schedule weekly weight checks to monitor the baby's weight gain while the supplements are gradually reduced and baby nurses more.

If the baby is older than 6 months and receiving water or juice, suggest replacing these with expressed milk, if milk production allows, or other, higher-calorie drinks, such as nutritious soups. For the baby older than 12 months, other kinds of milk, such as cow, goat, or nut milks, are an option.

• • •

Are they nursing with a nipple shield?

If they are using a nipple shield, ask why. These thin, silicone nipples have holes in the tip for milk flow during nursing. They are sometimes recommended for babies who nurse ineffectively (Genna, 2017). If this is the reason for the shield's use and the baby is gaining slowly, the shield may not be improving feeding effectiveness enough and the baby may need to be supplemented. If the baby is not getting enough milk through the shield for a healthy weight gain, suggest expressing milk after nursing to boost milk production. Effective nursing with a nipple shield also depends on fit, application, and how deeply the baby latches. For details, see p. 912-917.

BOX 6.1 Factors That May Contribute to Slow Weight Gain in the First 6 Weeks

Nursing Dynamics

- Shallow latch—Can decrease milk transfer and/or cause nipple pain and may be due to positioning issues or poor fit (large nipple, small mouth)
- Too little active nursing time—Scheduled, limited, or infrequent feeds, sleepy baby, overuse of swaddling or soothers (pacifier/dummy, swing), parental depression
- Less-than-optimal early nursing due to birth or hospital practices—Separation, medications, rough suctioning or rough handling during latch
- Feeding low-calorie liquids or solid foods (water, juice, cereal, etc.)—Delays or replaces nursing

Baby Factors

- Temperament—Placid/sleepy baby or fussy and difficult to settle for feeds
- Anatomy or health issues that can cause ineffective nursing—Variations in oral anatomy (tongue-tie, cleft palate, etc.), illness, airway abnormality, neurological impairment (high/low tone)
- Prematurity—Both late preterm and early preterm
- Birth injury—Hematoma, broken bone, torticollis, etc
- Health issues that can cause slow weight gain with healthy milk intake—Illness, cardiac defect, cystic fibrosis (baby tastes salty), metabolic or genetic disorder

Nursing Parent's Anatomy, Health, and Milk Production

- Mammary/nipple issues—Breast or chest surgery or injury (severed milk ducts or nerve damage preventing milk ejection), inadequate glandular tissue (hypoplasia), unusual nipple anatomy or nipple piercing (may decrease or prevent milk transfer)
- Birth-related issues—Delayed nursing, excess blood loss, retained placenta
- Health and medication issues—Serious illness, drugs/herbs that decrease milk production or are incompatible with nursing, obesity, thyroid, pituitary, or hormonal problems, birth injury that makes nursing painful, psychiatric issues, eating disorder, polycystic ovary syndrome (PCOS), gestational ovarian theca lutein cysts

Causes of Slow Weight Gain in the First 6 Weeks

Often there is more than one cause of slow weight gain. See Box 6.1 for a summary of many possible causes of slow weight gain in a baby younger than 6 weeks.

Slow weight gain may be due to a combination of factors.

Other Nursing Dynamics

Excess weight loss and slow weight gain during the first 6 weeks can sometimes begin with birth and early nursing. Questions to ask include:

How did the birth and early nursing go?

- Was the birth difficult? Was it a vaginal or cesarean birth? Was the labor medicated or unmedicated? If medicated, what drugs were used?
- Was there more than usual blood loss? If so, how much?
- Did either the birthing parent or baby suffer any birth-related injuries or receive treatment for any health problems?
- How often did the baby nurse after birth and how much were they separated?
- How did early nursing go?

- Was the baby supplemented in the hospital? If so, what was she fed, how much, and with what feeding method?
- Was the nursing parent engorged or was the baby jaundiced?

When nursing gets off to a slow start due to birth-related difficulties, health problems, hospital practices, or other factors, this can lead to less effective nursing and delayed milk increase, both of which can contribute to greater weight loss and lead to early slow weight gain (Dewey et al., 2003).

A difficult birth or medications during labor and delivery can reduce a baby's nursing effectiveness at first (see p. 40-43). Early separation after birth can also affect weight gain and loss (Bystrova et al., 2007). Supplements can delay or replace nursing, slowing the increase in milk production. If birth-related injuries result in pain during nursing, this can delay or compromise feeds. Babies are sometimes born with broken bones, torticollis (see p. 107), or hematomas (large bruises). Engorgement and exaggerated newborn jaundice can also lead to less effective early nursing. Excess blood loss during delivery can lead to delayed or inhibited milk production (see later section, "The Nursing Parent's Health and Milk Production" and Chapter 10, "Making Milk."). Babies can also develop feeding aversion when handled roughly during latch or when roughly aspirated after birth (Smith, 2017; Svensson, Velandia, Matthiesen, Welles-Nystrom, & Widstrom, 2013).

• • •

When latching, can the baby fit more than just the nipple in her mouth?

"Poor fit" is another aspect of nursing dynamics that can affect early weight gain. This term describes a nursing parent with very large nipples (wide and/or long) and a baby with a very small mouth (most common among small and preterm newborns). No matter how they adjust their positioning and no matter how deeply the baby tries to latch, in some cases, the baby's mouth may only accommodate the nipple, which can lead to nipple pain and/or slow milk flow. For strategies, see p. 103 and 113-114.

Baby's Anatomy and Health

Has the baby been ill? If so, do her symptoms include nasal congestion, vomiting, or diarrhea?

Illness, such as a cold, the flu, or other viruses, may affect a baby's appetite and compromise her weight gain. Because not all sick babies run a fever or have the symptoms common in an older child who is ill, any baby gaining weight slowly should be checked by her healthcare provider for illness. Ear and urinary tract infections can cause slow weight gain, so an ear check and urinalysis should be routine to rule out these easily treated illnesses.

Nasal congestion in the baby can reduce milk intake because when given a choice between breathing and feeding, babies always choose breathing. Struggles with breathing during feeds may be due to a cold, another illness, allergy, inflammation of the mouth or throat from rough suctioning or intubation after birth, spasms, or physical abnormalities of the mouth or throat, such as tracheomalacia and laryngomalacia (softened cartilage that blocks the trachea or larynx) (Genna, 2017). Any baby who consistently struggles with breathing at feeds or who makes high-pitched, squeaky sounds (called "stridor") while nursing, should be checked by her healthcare provider to determine the cause. Between feeds, suggest milk expression to safeguard milk production.

Vomiting and diarrhea can also slow a baby's weight gain because the milk may not stay down long enough to be fully digested and nutrients are not well-absorbed when the milk rushes quickly through the baby's digestive tract during diarrhea. For more details, see p. 300-301.

Ineffective Nursing

A baby who nurses ineffectively may feed "all the time," yet gain weight slowly.

If a baby is nursing long and often, but is still gaining weight slowly or losing weight, this may be a sign of ineffective nursing. The baby may have many wet diapers but few stools because she is getting some of the first rush of milk at milk ejection but is not nursing effectively enough to trigger more milk ejections and reach the fatty hindmilk. Some types of ineffective nursing may cause nipple pain or trauma, while others do not. In the early weeks, regular uncomfortable mammary fullness and recurring mastitis may occur if the baby doesn't drain the mammary glands well. For a more complete list of symptoms, see the point about ineffective nursing in the previous section.

• • •

Has the baby been checked by a lactation specialist or another healthcare provider for variations in lips, palate, tongue, and jaw anatomy?

Effective nursing requires a good anatomical fit between the nursing parent and baby. In some cases, unusual anatomy of the baby's mouth, tongue, lip, or jaw can contribute to ineffective nursing. Examples include cleft lip or palate, tongue-tie, large tongue, high or bubble palate, cleft palate (including submucous clefts), lip-tie, and a small or unusually receded jaw.

If an anatomical variation in the baby is the cause of ineffective nursing, in most cases, this will cause nursing issues right from birth. One U.S. study of 88 tongue-tied babies with nursing problems reported that all the problems were apparent during their hospital stay (Ballard, Auer, & Khoury, 2002). With abundant milk production, though, some babies gain well at first, and it is not until several weeks later that it becomes apparent their nursing effectiveness is low. It's also important to keep in mind that anatomical variations, like tongue-tie, do not always cause ineffective nursing or other feeding problems. A U.K. randomized controlled trial of 201 tongue-tied babies (Hogan, Westcott, & Griffiths, 2005) found that less than half (44%) of its tongue-tied babies had feeding problems. One U.S. study (Messner, Lalakea, Aby, Macmahon, & Bair, 2000) found that only 25% of its tongue-tied babies had difficulty nursing. Another factor that can affect whether the baby with an anatomical variation has trouble nursing is the tautness or looseness of the mammary tissue. For example, a tongue-tied baby might nurse well when her nursing parent's mammary tissue is soft and pliable but struggle when it is firm or taut. For more details, see p. 268.

KEY CONCEPT

Unusual anatomy of the baby's mouth, tongue, or jaws sometimes contributes to ineffective nursing.

• • •

Has the baby been diagnosed with a neurological impairment or other health issue?

Babies with a neurological impairment may have high or low muscle tone, which can also reduce nursing effectiveness and cause inconsistent feeding (some effective, some ineffective). For more details and nursing strategies, see p. 327-329.

• • •

Was the baby born full-term?

Prematurity can affect a baby's nursing effectiveness. Depending on how early the preterm baby was born and her health, she may or may not be ready to nurse exclusively without supplements. For strategies to help the transition to exclusive nursing without compromising a preterm baby's weight gain, see p. 377-382.

Slow Weight Gain with Good Milk Intake

When kissed, does the baby taste salty? Has she been checked for heart, genetic, or metabolic disorders?

By weighing a baby before and after nursing with a very accurate baby scale (to 2 g), a baby's milk intake during nursing can be accurately determined (Rankin et al., 2016). When the scale reveals that a slow-gaining baby is clearly taking enough milk during nursing, keep in mind there is more to weight gain than milk intake alone.

In addition to consuming enough milk, a baby must also be able to digest the milk and it must meet her energy needs. Babies with congenital heart disease, for example, usually gain weight slowly no matter how they are fed because their hearts beat faster and they take more breaths per minute than a healthy baby in order to maintain adequate oxygen levels and circulation (Pados, 2019). Another example is babies with the genetic disease cystic fibrosis, many of whom also gain weight slowly, despite effective nursing and excellent milk intake, because they cannot fully digest the milk (Jadin et al., 2011). For normal weight gain, many of these babies need to receive special enzymes before feeds to aid in digestion. The first sign of this condition is often slow weight gain and salty tasting skin. For more details, see p. 314-315. Other conditions may also require treatment or other interventions for normal growth, despite good milk intake. Examples include congenital hypothyroidism, kidney disease, intestinal malabsorption or obstruction, parasites, neuromuscular disease, and hypoadrenalism. A baby gaining weight slowly despite excellent milk intake should be carefully evaluated by her healthcare provider.

Nursing Parent's Anatomy, Health, and Milk Production

Mammary and Nipple Issues

Does the nursing parent have flat or inverted nipples or unusually large mammary glands?

Because unusual nipple or mammary anatomy may make it more challenging for a newborn to latch deeply, it may also affect milk transfer and weight gain. Flat or inverted nipples were associated with delayed milk increase in one U.S. study (Dewey et al., 2003). An Iranian study of first-time mothers examined the effect of "maternal breast variations" (including flat and inverted nipples and "abnormally large breasts") on weight gain during the first 7 days (Vazirinejad, Darakhshan, Esmaeili, & Hadadian, 2009). At 7 days of life, the mean weight of the babies whose mothers had one or more of these "breast variations" was below birth weight, whereas the mean weight among the babies whose mothers did not have breast variations was above birth weight.

• • •

Is there a history of breast or chest surgery, injury, or nipple piercing?

Some types of surgery or injury, such as breast reduction or trans masculinization chest surgery (MacDonald et al., 2016), put a nursing parent at increased risk of inadequate milk production. A surgical incision near some parts of the areola may damage milk ducts and cause nerve damage, which may inhibit milk ejection and compromise milk transfer. For details, see p. 788-789.

Although there are several case reports of mothers who successfully nursed after nipple piercing (Lee, 1995; Wilson-Clay & Hoover, 2017), there are also mothers whose complications from the piercing caused milk duct obstruction, which resulted in minimal milk transfer during nursing and pumping (Garbin, Deacon, Rowan, Hartmann, & Geddes, 2009). For more details, see p. 742.

KEY CONCEPT

Breast or chest surgery can increase risk of low milk production.

• • •

Are the mammary glands symmetrical in size and shape, and did they grow in size during pregnancy?

In some unusual cases, underdeveloped mammary glands may be incapable of producing enough milk to fully sustain a nursing baby (Arbour & Kessler, 2013). Also known as ***insufficient glandular tissue*** or ***hypoplasia***, according to one estimate, this occurs in about 1 in 1,000 (N. G. Powers, 1999). Some with this condition have bulbous areolae or unusually shaped glands because some normal glandular (milk-making) tissue is missing. One U.S. prospective study of 34 mothers (Huggins, Petok, & Mireles, 2000) found the mothers who were unable to produce enough milk had widely spaced breasts (more than 1.5 inches or about 4 cm apart), had large differences in breast size, or had breasts that were tubular or cone-shaped, rather than rounded. There may be some obvious patches of glandular tissue in a mostly soft breast (Wilson-Clay & Hoover, 2017).

Many of the study mothers with low milk production noticed no breast changes during pregnancy or breast fullness after birth. But it is important never to assume from mammary appearance or lack of changes during pregnancy that low milk production is certain. One Australian study (Cox, Kent, Casey, Owens, & Hartmann, 1999) found that mammary tissue growth continues during nursing throughout the first month post-delivery. However, these physical markers should be considered a red flag to monitor the baby's weight closely after birth. For more details and resources for families, see p. 785-787.

Birth-Related Issues

How much blood loss occurred during delivery?

Severe blood loss (more than 500 cc of blood) after birth increases risk of insufficient milk production (Willis & Livingstone, 1995). In unusually severe cases, extreme blood loss can cause pituitary damage, known as Sheehan syndrome, which can completely inhibit milk production and fertility (Matsuzaki et al., 2017; Schrager & Sabo, 2001). For details, see p. 440.

Never assume, however, that a severe blood loss will definitely reduce milk production. Consider it another red flag to monitor baby's weight closely in the early weeks. With time and sufficient mammary stimulation, many with blood loss during delivery achieve ample milk production.

• • •

Is it possible that some fragments of the placenta were retained after birth?

Was the placenta delivered intact after birth? Did the birth attendant use forceps to remove the placenta? Has post-delivery bleeding continued longer than 6 weeks? The hormonal cascade of events that leads to an increase in milk production after birth begins with the separation of the placenta from the uterus. If placental fragments are retained after birth, this may inhibit milk production as if pregnancy had continued (Anderson, 2001). In this case, removing the fragment will trigger the hormonal changes needed for milk increase.

Nursing Parent's Health and Medications

Has the nursing parent been ill?

Although most illnesses will not affect nursing and milk production, a serious illness may result in separation from the baby and reduce time spent nursing, causing a decrease in milk production. In some extreme cases, severe dehydration or life-threatening illness may cause a decrease in milk production.

• • •

Is the nursing parent using any herbal preparations or prescribed, over-the-counter, or recreational drugs?

Although most medications are compatible with nursing, certain drugs (such as some diuretics and over-the-counter antihistamines and decongestants like pseudoephedrine) were associated with a decrease in milk production (Aljazaf et al., 2003; Hale, 2019). Other drugs may inhibit milk ejection or sedate the baby or make her jittery. If a drug may be affecting any aspect of lactation, ask if the healthcare provider was consulted about taking this drug while nursing. Also ask specifically if hormonal contraception is being used, as some parents receive injectables such as Depo-Provera soon after birth and may not remember that or connect it with nursing. For details, see the next section.

If a drug currently being taken is contraindicated during nursing, unless best practices are used, even a temporary weaning may cause a decrease in milk production. For the latest information on the effects of drugs on milk production, see the LactMed database (available at **bit.ly/BA2-LactMed**) or the current edition of *Hale's Medications and Mothers' Milk* by Thomas Hale (New York: Springer Publishing).

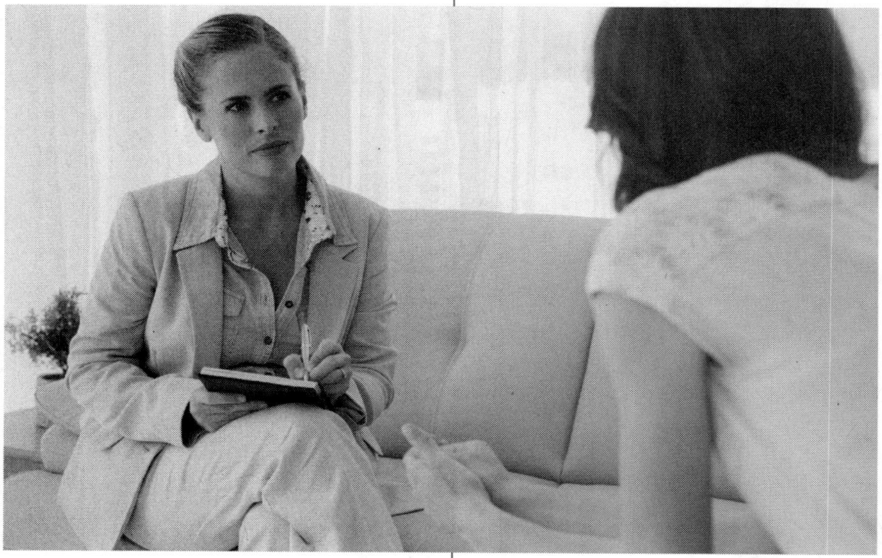

Some herbs, such as sage and peppermint (when consumed in much greater amounts than usual), have been associated with decreased milk production (see p. 464), so ask if the nursing parent is taking any herbal preparations and if so which ones. A reliable resource on the effects of herbals on lactation is the book, *The Nursing Mother's Herbal* by Sheila Humphrey (Humphrey, 2003). Many herbs are also listed in the LactMed database and the book *Making More Milk: The Breastfeeding Guide to Increasing Your Milk Production* (L. Marasco & West, 2020).

• • •

Does the nursing parent have a history of diabetes or pituitary, thyroid, or hormonal problems?

After birth, a history of Type 1 diabetes is associated with a 1-day delay in the increase of milk production. For more details, see p. 844. Research also found an association between suboptimal glucose sensitivity (one of the central issues with diabetes) and milk production problems (Laurie A Nommsen-Rivers, 2016). For more details, see p. 846-847.

Regarding hormonal problems, depending on the hormone involved and whether it is too high or too low, a hormonal imbalance may cause too much milk, too little milk, or inhibit milk ejection. One U.S. article (Hoover, Barbalinardo, & Platia, 2002) described the breastfeeding experiences of two women with gestational ovarian theca lutein cysts who had abnormally high testosterone levels that delayed milk increase after birth. After producing very little milk for 3 weeks with good breast stimulation, their testosterone fell to more normal levels and their milk production finally increased to normal levels.

Polycystic ovary syndrome (PCOS) is another condition that is a risk factor for inadequate milk production. Although some with PCOS produce abundant milk, some do not. One U.S. article (L. Marasco, Marmet, & Shell, 2000) described the breastfeeding experiences of three women with PCOS, all three of whom produced little milk, despite expert help and the use of many strategies to increase milk production. Other hormonal problems, such as low thyroid (hypothyroidism), have also been linked to low milk production or lactation failure. For more details, see p. 856-857.

• • •

Is the nursing parent in the normal weight-for-height range?

Obesity is a risk factor for delay in milk increase after birth (L. A. Nommsen-Rivers, Dolan, & Huang, 2012) and a reduced prolactin response to baby's nursing (Rasmussen & Kjolhede, 2004). Excess body fat contributes to poor metabolic health, which is gauged by extra body fat around the middle, along with high blood sugar, high blood pressure, low HDL, and high cholesterol. Preliminary research (L. Nommsen-Rivers et al., 2017) linked poor metabolic health with increased risk of low milk production. For this and other reasons covered in detail on p. 574-580, a high BMI is another red flag to closely monitor the nursing couple after birth.

• • •

What is the nursing parent's emotional state?

Research found that depressive symptoms can influence interactions between parent and baby, which may also affect how many times each day they nurse and therefore baby's weight gain. For more details, see p. 834-837.

Causes of Slow Weight Gain after 6 Weeks

If a baby gained weight well at first, start by discussing the basics.

If the baby's weight loss during first days after birth was in the normal range and baby regained her birth weight by 2 weeks, the slow weight gain likely started after that. Begin with the "Gathering Basic Information" section to understand the baby's previous weight loss and weight gain patterns, other signs of milk intake, and basic nursing dynamics. In most cases, the cause(s) of the slow weight gain will be found there.

But if not, explore the other possibilities in the previous section, as well as those listed in Box 6.2. Because a baby's milk needs increase rapidly over the first 5 weeks or so (see the later section "When and How to Supplement"), when milk production is limited by breast surgery or underdeveloped milk-making tissue, for example, there may be healthy weight gain during the first few weeks but then weight gain may falter.

Other Nursing Dynamics

Have the baby's feeding or sleeping patterns changed during the last month or so?

Most Western cultures put a high value on babies sleeping for long stretches at night, and many parenting books include strategies to increase babies' nighttime sleep stretch (Ezzo & Bucknam, 2019; Weissbluth, 2015). If a nursing parent has a large storage capacity (see p. 416), long sleep stretches of 7 to 8 hours or more may not compromise the rate of milk production. But with a small or medium storage capacity, these longer night stretches may slow both milk production and the baby's weight gain.

If weight gain slowed within a couple of weeks after the baby began sleeping for longer stretches at night, suggest either waking the baby to nurse at least once during the night or doing a "dream feed," when baby nurses while in a light sleep. (This may be necessary only for those with a medium or small storage capacity.) Another option to try is to nurse more often during the day so that the baby receives more milk during normal waking hours.

• • •

Other than nursing, what foods or drinks does the baby consume?

If low-calorie foods and drinks replace nursing, this can contribute to slow weight gain. See p. 208. Babies who receive only mother's milk well into the second half of their first year may also begin gaining weight slowly. If this is the situation, suggest offering solid foods (see Chapter 4, "Solid Foods").

• • •

Is the nursing parent less available now for nursing or are there any unusual stresses in the household?

Changes that cause significant upheavals in family routines, such as the return to work or school, a household move, marital or relationship problems, major holidays, or even an especially hectic week or two, can decrease nursing frequency and slow milk production.

Stress may slow or inhibit milk ejection, so the baby takes less milk at each nursing. Or with more demands on parents' time and energy, they may nurse less often or for a shorter time. Stress can also affect feelings about nursing and responsiveness to the baby's cues.

If parents are under unusual stress, encourage them to rest when possible and ask for help from their partner, friends, and relatives, or if they aren't available,

BOX 6.2 Factors That May Contribute to Slow Weight Gain After 6 Weeks

Nursing Dynamics

- Too little active nursing time—Scheduled, limited, or infrequent feeds, longer nighttime sleep stretch or sleep training (depending on storage capacity), overuse of swaddling or soothers (pacifier/dummy or swing)
- Feeding baby low-calorie liquids or solid foods (water, juice, cereal, etc.)—Which may delay or replace nursing

Baby Factors

- Issues that can reduce baby's milk intake—Illness, allergy, reflux disease
- Issues that can cause slow weight gain with healthy milk intake—Congenital heart disease, cystic fibrosis (baby tastes salty), other metabolic and genetic disorders

Nursing Parent's Anatomy, Health, and Milk Production

- Health or medications—Serious illness, drugs that decrease milk production or are incompatible with nursing, hormonal, thyroid, or pituitary problems, pregnancy, polycystic ovary syndrome, vitamin B_{12} deficiency from weight-loss surgery or a restricted diet
- Mammary/nipple issues— Nipple piercing, breast or chest surgery, injury, or insufficient glandular tissue (hypoplasia), effect on weight gain may not be obvious until baby needs full milk production to gain weight at about 5 weeks

to consider hiring help. If that's not an option financially, suggest checking into trading time with another family. If the milk ejection seems to be slow, suggest trying semi-reclined starter feeding positions described in Chapter 1 (p. 23-29) to make it easier to relax and rest while nursing.

• • •

Has the baby been more distracted at feeds lately?

A baby's rate of weight gain normally slows after 3 months of age (see Table 6.1 on p. 191), so it is important to gauge an exclusively nursing baby's weight gain on growth charts based on data from nursing babies (see earlier section "Growth Charts."). Normal developmental changes in behavior often affect nursing dynamics, which may affect weight gain. Each stage of development brings new distractions:

2 to 4 months of age. With greater awareness of her surroundings, a baby may pause and come off more often before finishing. Suggest offering to nurse several times before assuming baby is done. If needed, nurse in a quiet or darkened area where there are fewer distractions.

4 to 6 months of age. Teething can cause sore gums, which may lead to fussiness during feeds or chewing on her hands afterwards, which some parents misinterpret as a sign the baby is not getting enough milk. Be sure the family understands that these behaviors indicate teething and suggest offering the baby something cold or hard to chew on to numb her gums before nursing, such as a cold, wet cloth or a refrigerated or frozen teething toy. At this age, for many babies, raised voices lead to interrupted nursing.

6 to 12 months of age. Babies this age are usually easily distracted while nursing. It may help to darken the room and reduce noise. Some 9- to 12-month-olds become so involved in crawling and walking, they forget to nurse. Suggest the family encourage night nursing to help offset missed feeds during the day.

• • •

Is the baby using a pacifier/ dummy or sucking on her fingers or thumb?

Other sucking outlets can reduce time spent nursing and contribute to slow weight gain. Whenever a slow-gaining baby wants to suck on a pacifier, fingers, or thumb, suggest instead offering to nurse. More nursing may be all that's needed to increase baby's weight gain. If an older baby prefers to suck on her thumb or fingers rather than be confined to her parent's lap, suggest putting away the pacifier for now and encourage more night feeds.

Baby's Anatomy and Health

Low Milk Intake

Has the baby been ill?

An illness can slow baby's weight gain by decreasing baby's appetite or the time the milk spends in the baby's gut (i.e., vomiting and diarrhea). For more details, see p. 300-304.

• • •

If the baby is older than 6 months, has a blood test ruled out iron deficiency anemia?

A blood test to measure baby's iron levels is part of many well-baby checkups after 6 months. Iron deficiency anemia is one factor that may contribute to slow weight gain (Dewey et al., 2002).

• • •

Does the baby seem unhappy or in pain during nursing?

Transient pain during nursing may be caused by pain at a recent immunization site when baby is held. But regular pain related to feeding may be caused by the following health problems, both of which can also contribute to slow weight gain, as the baby reduces milk intake to avoid pain.

Allergy, sensitivity, or intolerance. When a nursing baby is allergic or sensitive to either a food her nursing parent eats or something in the environment, symptoms can include gastrointestinal problems, such as vomiting, diarrhea, blood or mucus in stools (ABM, 2011); skin problems, such as eczema, dermatitis, hives, rash, dry skin; respiratory problems, such as congestion, runny nose, wheezing, coughing; crying during or after feeds; and difficulty going to sleep and staying asleep. Pain, vomiting, and diarrhea can lead to slow weight gain. For more details, see p. 300-304.

Reflux disease. Irritability during feeds can be a sign of reflux disease, which is sometimes mistaken for colic. When the washing back of the baby's acidic stomach contents into the esophagus causes damage to its lining, normal gastroesophageal reflux (GER) becomes gastroesophageal reflux disease (GERD). A baby with GERD may have respiratory problems (congestion, coughing, wheezing, bronchitis, pneumonia), inflammation of the esophagus, and pain during feeds (Lightdale, Gremse, Section on Gastroenterology, & Nutrition, 2013). When in pain, baby may limit milk intake, leading to slow weight gain and failure to thrive (McFadden, 2017). Common symptoms include frequent hiccups, sleep problems day and night, back arching and head turning, crying and irritability, and feeding aversion and refusal. For more details, see p. 304-305.

Slow Weight Gain with Good Milk Intake

See the earlier section with the same title on p. 212. Depending on their severity, symptoms of conditions that cause slow weight gain with good milk intake, such as cardiac issues, cystic fibrosis, and other genetic or metabolic disorders may first appear after 6 weeks.

Milk Production

Mammary and Nipple Issues

The effects of surgery and other conditions on milk production may not be obvious until after the first few weeks.

Nursing parents whose mammary and nipple issues cause reduced milk production may produce enough milk for good weight gain during the first few weeks, but as the baby's need for milk exceeds their maximum milk production, weight gain slows. For more details, see Chapter 18, "Breast or Chest Issues."

Nursing Parent's Health and Medications

Does the nursing parent have an acute or chronic illness?

Although most acute illnesses will not affect nursing or milk production, if a parent was seriously ill, that may involve separation from the baby, which can reduce time spent nursing and decrease milk production. In some extreme cases, severe dehydration or life-threatening illness may decrease milk production.

Chronic illnesses, such as diabetes, thyroid problems, congestive heart failure, hormonal imbalances, and anemia, especially if untreated, may affect milk production. With untreated hypothyroidism, treatment may increase milk production significantly. In one U.S. study, anemia was associated with low milk production (Henly et al., 1995). Anemia may also increase feelings of fatigue and susceptibility to infection (Fetherston, 1998). If nursing parents have a history of any of these health problems, suggest seeing their healthcare provider for blood tests to rule out health issues as contributing factors to slow weight gain. For details about specific health problems, see Chapter 19 on p. 806.

• • •

Ask if the parent is taking herbal preparations or any prescribed medications. Ask specifically about hormonal contraceptives.

Illnesses, such as asthma, allergy, depression, hypertension, insomnia, migraine headaches, autoimmune diseases, and heart problems may require the use of medications that may affect milk production (see previous section).

After 6 weeks, one medication that is commonly started is hormonal contraception. Be sure to ask specifically about this and the specific type, as some families may not remember to mention it, especially if they are using a patch, injectables, or hormonal IUDs, which release hormones continuously. The World Health Organization (WHO, 2015) recommended delaying the use of combined oral contraceptives that contain estrogen until the baby is at least 6 months old because earlier versions of these types of birth control were found to decrease milk production significantly (Koetsawang, 1987). Research on progestin-only hormonal contraception, such as the mini-pill, implants, and injectables, have found no significant effect on milk production or infant weight gain when given shortly after birth (Phillips et al., 2016), but anecdotal reports indicate that some women do have a drop in milk production when progestin-only methods are used (Stuebe, Bryant, Lewis, & Muddana, 2016). For more details, see p. 345-347.

• • •

Could the nursing parent be pregnant?

The hormones that maintain a pregnancy also cause milk production to decrease. Between 60% and 65% of pregnant, nursing mothers reported a significant decrease in milk during the fourth or fifth month of pregnancy (Moscone & Moore, 1993; Newton & Theotokatos, 1979). If the baby is younger than 12 months, this naturally occurring decrease in milk production could compromise her nutritional needs. If weight gain slows, supplements may be needed.

• • •

Is the nursing parent on a very restricted diet, or do they have a history of weight-loss surgery?

Vegans, who eat no animal products (meat, fish, cheese, milk, eggs) and those with a history of weight-loss surgery are at greater risk for a vitamin B_{12} deficiency. Because vitamin B_{12} deficiency leads to milk low in vitamin B_{12}, their nursing babies are also at risk of vitamin B_{12} deficiency, which can cause slow weight gain. Symptoms of vitamin B_{12} deficiency in the baby often develop before symptoms in the parent, appearing within the first few months of life or going unrecognized until later. One of the first symptoms is lack of interest in feeding, which can lead to slow weight gain, failure to thrive, and eventually neurological problems (El & Celikkaya, 2019). Although the nursing parent may have no symptoms, blood tests or analysis of milk composition can detect this deficiency.

To avoid vitamin deficiencies after weight-loss surgery and in those on a vegan diet, vitamin B_{12} supplements are recommended (Baroni et al., 2018). Ask nursing parents in either situation if they are taking vitamin B_{12} supplements. An alternative is to eat fortified soy products. For more details, see p. 580-582.

Increasing Weight Gain

The first steps needed to increase baby's weight gain will depend on the baby's condition.

If the baby is so underfed that she cannot nurse effectively, a wise first step is to rule out dehydration. If a baby is dehydrated and at risk of hypernatremia (see the earlier point about this in the "Weight Loss after Birth" section), she needs to be hospitalized and monitored while being safely rehydrated. If dehydration is not a concern, supplements should be started immediately, and she should be encouraged to take as much extra milk as she will accept. Usually within a few days of being well-fed, a baby begins to gain energy and feed more actively. For this situation, see the next section, "When and How to Supplement."

However, if the baby seems alert, and the weight loss or weight gain is not too far from healthy norms, it may make sense to start by improving nursing dynamics. Often, making basic adjustments to feeding technique and patterns can improve weight gain quickly.

• • •

While the nursing parent is taking steps to increase baby's weight gain, suggest keeping a daily record of number of feeds and, if the baby is younger than 4 to 6 weeks, stools.

An "input/output" diary may be helpful in evaluating nursing dynamics, and it doesn't have to be complicated. Over a several-day period, suggest either using an app to record this information or divide a blank piece of paper (a different section or sheet for each day) into two columns:

- Number of feeds
- Number of stools (if the baby is younger than 4 to 6 weeks)

If this is done on paper, mark a line in the appropriate column for every feed at least 5 minutes long and every stool the diameter of a U.S. quarter (2.5 cm) or larger. This will provide a quick, daily count of feeds and stools. Counting wet diapers is unnecessary because research found no association between number of urinations per day and weight gain (DiTomasso & Paiva, 2018; L. A. Nommsen-Rivers et al., 2008). The baby's stools are formed from the fatty hindmilk, which the baby receives after the lower-fat foremilk. During the first 4 to 6 weeks, if baby passes at least 4 stools of this size per day, she has also by default received enough fluids. Although stools are not a reliable stand-alone indicator of milk intake, they can be used as a very rough gauge between weight checks in the baby younger than 4 to 6 weeks.

KEY CONCEPT

Suggest keeping a written or digital record of number of feeds and stools per day.

• • •

Ideally, the strategies chosen to increase weight gain will address the cause(s) of the slow weight gain.

Not all slow weight gain is due to low milk production. Low milk production is sometimes a side effect of infrequent or ineffective nursing.

See Box 6.1 and 6.2 for a summary of the most common cause(s) of slow weight gain before and after 6 weeks, and if possible, tailor the interventions to the cause(s). Although in most cases strategies will include improving nursing dynamics (see next point), there are many unrelated strategies that may be instrumental to addressing underlying causes of a baby's weight gain issues, such as a frenotomy (tongue-tie release) in a tongue-tied baby, vitamin B12 supplementation (for a vitamin B12 deficient baby), replacement thyroid hormones for a nursing parent with hypothyroidism, or medical treatment for a baby with reflux disease, an infection, or other illness. In some cases, such as a very preterm baby or a newborn in pain from a birth injury, patience may also be important.

• • •

Suggest reviewing nursing dynamics to see if improvements can be made and steps implemented to boost milk intake and milk production.

Make sure the baby is latched deeply. A shallow latch can reduce milk transfer and may (but not always) cause nipple pain. Try semi-reclined starter positions, which allow the baby to adjust the latch using her inborn feeding behaviors (see p. 23-29 in Chapter 1). If they prefer an upright feeding position, suggest striving for an asymmetric latch described on p. 878.

Nurse more. If the baby is nursing effectively (audible swallows after every suck or two for at least 5 minutes of active nursing), a good first step is to increase the number of nursing sessions per day, assuming the following are true about the baby:

- She is younger than 6 months old.
- Her healthcare provider considers her at minimal immediate risk.
- She was nursing fewer than 12 times per day.

Under these circumstances, suggest over the next several days increasing the number of feeds to at least 12. (With a baby older than 6 months, doubling number of nursing sessions is a good starting point.) One way to do this is to—as much as possible—keep baby tummy down on the nursing parent's semi-reclined body during normal waking hours to trigger feeding behaviors. Even when in a light sleep, babies can be helped to latch and feed actively. By substantially increasing the number of nursing sessions each day, there is usually a noticeable increase in milk intake and milk production within a week.

Finish the first side first, offer both sides at each feed, and use breast compression as needed to keep baby active. Offer both sides more than once and keep nursing for as long as the baby is willing. Leave the baby on the first side while the baby is nursing actively. Whenever possible, wait until the baby comes off on her own before offering the other side. But if the baby does not suck actively (just lightly mouthing the nipple without swallowing) or falls asleep quickly, use breast compression to keep her active longer and increase the milk's fat content (Bowles, 2011). For a description, see p. 889.

Avoid soothers. As mentioned in the previous section "Basic Nursing Dynamics", pacifiers/dummies may reduce the number of feeds and may contribute to ineffective nursing.

Reduce any formula gradually. Avoid water and juice. If the baby has been fed more than 2 to 3 ounces (59 to 89 mL) of formula per day, it should not be discontinued suddenly. Instead, it should be reduced gradually as milk production increases. Suggest asking the baby's healthcare provider to monitor baby's weight as supplements are being decreased. If the baby is between 6 and 12 months old, suggest offering high-calorie solids after nursing rather than before.

Consider milk expression. Expressing milk after or between feeds can also help increase milk production more quickly, because drained glands make milk faster. As many times per day as practical, use hands-on pumping techniques (see p. 492) to drain each side more fully (Morton et al., 2009). Pumping doesn't have to be at regular intervals around the clock. Unless baby nurses ineffectively, suggest limiting pumping to normal waking hours, with an optional one pump session in the middle of the night.

TABLE 6.2 Create a Plan Based on Baby's Feeding Effectiveness

At Each Feed	Family A with 3-week-old baby nurses effectively (was nursing 6x/day)	Family B with 3-week-old baby nurses ineffectively (was nursing 8x/day)
Nursing	Nurse 12x/day, offer each side at least twice, use compression as needed to keep baby active.	Feed ≥10x/day, nurse 10 min./feed, nurse for comfort between feeds.
Supplement (expressed milk, donor milk, or formula)	Give baby 2-3 days of increased nursing and check weight gain. If no improvement, begin supplements.	After nursing, feed as much supplement as baby will take (≥3 oz, 90 mL)/feed or feed half before and half after nursing.
Milk expression	If desired, add hands-on pumping to speed milk production as often as practical.	Use hands-on pumping technique 8x/24 hr, with one night pump session.

Limit all feeding-related activities to no more than 40 minutes. For a plan to be practical, restrict the total time spent at each feeding session (nursing, milk expression, supplementation) to no more than about 40 minutes. If it takes much longer than that, it becomes difficult to fit in at last 8 feeds per day, which is also critical to improving weight gain. See Table 6.2 for examples of how a plan might vary based on baby's nursing effectiveness.

Discuss galactogogues. See p. 450-455 for a description of galactogogues (milk-boosting foods, herbs, and drugs) that nursing parents can discuss with their healthcare provider in light of their health history.

If a nipple shield is used, be sure baby latches deeply. If the baby is not latching deeply enough, she may be sucking only on the firm tip of the shield rather than its softer brim, which can mean a slower milk flow. For details on application, fit, use and weaning from the shield, see p. 912-917.

Accept all offers of help. Having a slow-gaining baby is stressful. Encourage good self-care to maintain energy and a positive mood. While diet and fluids may not directly affect milk production in most cases, skipping meals and losing sleep can add stress and reduce the ability to cope. Accepting help from others may make this intense time easier.

When and How to Supplement

If the previous section's strategies do not boost the baby's weight gain enough so she is catching up to the weight she should be now, supplements may be needed.

If the baby's healthcare provider does not consider the baby to be at risk, it may be possible to improve nursing dynamics as described in the previous section to achieve a healthy weight gain. But after the family tried these strategies, if the baby's weight gain is not improving or is improving very little, supplements may be needed.

For normal growth and development, it's important for babies who were underfed to have the opportunity to put on the "catch-up weight" needed so that their weight is where it should be at this age. The dynamics of this process are explained in a later point.

• • •

Before starting supplements, be sure the baby's slow weight gain is due to low milk intake.

As mentioned on p. 212, some babies gain slowly despite good milk intake due to health problems, such as a congenital heart disease, a genetic or metabolic disorder, malabsorption, intestinal blockage, parasites, or other conditions that increase their energy needs or prevent them from fully metabolizing the milk. Unless the baby's condition is dire, before starting supplements, be sure these causes are ruled out by the baby's healthcare provider. If one of these conditions is the root cause, supplements will not improve weight gain and will undermine nursing, which may be important to baby's health.

As described in the previous section, a baby's milk intake during nursing can be measured by weighing baby before and after nursing with a very accurate (to 2g) electronic scale, which are available in some hospitals, lactation offices, and for home rental from breast-pump rental companies. For more details, see p. 917-919.

KEY CONCEPT

Suggest baby's provider rule out a health problem as the cause of slow weight gain before starting supplements.

• • •

If supplements are needed and the nursing parent finds this upsetting, talk about these feelings and why the extra calories may help the baby nurse more effectively.

Supplements are sometimes necessary, especially when a baby is underfed. But this can generate strong feelings in some families. The need for supplements can leave a nursing parent feeling inadequate, incompetent, or like a failure. In this case, acknowledge these feelings and explain that supplementation may be important in getting nursing back on track, rather than a sign of failure. When a baby's weight gain is well below borderline, being consistently underfed can cause extreme sleepiness, ineffective or difficult feeds, and even lead to latching struggles. Explain that babies feed better when they are well-nourished. If it is clear the milk production will not increase enough to fully meet the baby's needs, see the points on p. 227 and p. 456-457.

• • •

Discuss the feeding-method options and their advantages and disadvantages.

For the baby older than 6 or 8 months, a cup is the logical first choice for giving extra milk. A baby that age should be able to master the cup (either a straw cup or a sippy cup, whichever the baby takes most easily) and it will not satisfy her need to suck, so it is less likely than a bottle to decrease her desire to nurse.

However, if a younger baby needs to be supplemented, discuss the choices (nursing supplementer, cup, feeding syringe, eyedropper, bottle), describing their advantages and disadvantages. (For details, see p. 896. If the family is open to using it, a nursing supplementer can decrease the time spent feeding (no need to feed again after nursing), and in some cases, it may help improve the baby's effectiveness by giving positive reinforcement during nursing.

• • •

The first choice of a supplement is almost always expressed milk.

If low milk intake has been confirmed, the first priority is to feed the baby. The choice of supplements is the family's to make. From a health perspective, the following options are listed from most to least healthy. Discuss them in light of their practicality for the family and their local availability.

1. Expressed mother's milk
2. Donor human milk
3. Non-human milks, such as infant formula

For the baby older than 6 months, high-calorie solid foods are also an option. Suggest consulting baby's healthcare provider about a choice of supplement.

First choice: expressed milk. If the nursing parent's milk production allows, suggest providing expressed milk as the baby's supplement. If the problem is the baby's nursing effectiveness and there is more than enough expressed milk available, another option is to provide high-fat, high-calorie hindmilk as a supplement. This is done by expressing milk right after the baby nurses. When expressing milk at other times, set aside the milk expressed during the first few minutes (storing it for later use) and using the milk expressed afterward (called "hindmilk feeding") as the supplement. For details on choosing an expression method, see p. 482. If needed, offer to discuss how to fit milk expression into their daily routine.

Second choice: donor milk. In some areas, pasteurized donor human milk from milk banks is available after hospital discharge (Bixby, Baker-Fox, Deming, Dhar, & Steele, 2016). An option becoming more common is donor milk from peer-to-peer milk-sharing networks (O'Sullivan, Geraghty, & Rasmussen, 2018). For details on the four pillars of safe breast milk sharing see the website **EatsonFeets.org** (S. Walker & Armstrong, 2012).

Third choice: formula. If by choice or necessity formula is used as the supplement, encourage following the baby's healthcare provider's preparation recommendations and not to either dilute it or make it too strong, which could be harmful to the baby. If both formula and expressed milk are used, suggest giving them at separate feeds rather than mixing them.

• • •

The volume of extra milk a baby needs per day to gain weight varies by age and by baby.

During the first 5 weeks of life, the volume of milk per day newborns need to grow and thrive increases (Kent, Gardner, & Geddes, 2016). Table 6.3 shows average milk intake per feed and per day for the first 6 months in nursing babies who are gaining weight normally. But not all babies are average, and milk intake needs can vary greatly from one baby to another. An Australian study of 71 healthy, thriving, exclusively breastfed 1- to 6-month-old babies found their daily milk intakes varied by almost threefold, from 15.5 to 43 ounces (440 to 1220 g) per day (Kent et al., 2006).

What this means in practical terms is that the volume of milk needed for a baby to begin gaining weight will vary. However, it is not necessary to know a baby's exact milk-intake needs, because if a baby's weight gain or loss is low

TABLE 6.3 Average Milk Intake by Age for the First 6 Months

Baby's Age	Average Milk Volume Per Feed	Average Milk Intake Per Day
Nursing (after Day 4)	1-2 oz. (30-59 mL)	10-20 oz. (300-600 mL)
Weeks 2 and 3	2-3 oz. (59-89 mL)	15-25 oz. (450-750 mL)
Months 1-6	3-4 oz. (89-118 mL)	25-30 oz. (750-887 mL)

Adapted from (Kent et al., 2016; Kent et al., 2013)

enough to be of concern, she should be given as much extra milk as she will take whenever a supplement is given. With supplementing (as with nursing), it is best to let the baby set the pace. That assumes when a bottle is used for supplementing that paced-feeding techniques (see p. 902-903) are used. As described in a previous section, if bottle-feeds are not slowed down, the consistent flow of the bottle may lead to overfeeding. The goal is to give enough extra milk so baby can catch up, but not so much milk that the number of feeds drops below 8 per day.

Usually, babies who were seriously underfed will start by taking small volumes of supplement. But within a day or two, as their stomachs expand and they gain more energy, they begin taking more and more milk and their weight gain increases markedly until their weight catches up to where it should be. During this catchup phase, babies often take much more milk than typical for their age. When they reach the appropriate weight, their appetite for milk decreases to expected volumes.

If after receiving regular supplements the baby is still not gaining weight, suggest having the baby checked again by her healthcare provider for health problems.

One way to calculate a rough estimate of supplement needed to use as a starting point (see Table 6.4) was suggested by U.S. lactation consultant Catherine Watson Genna (L. Marasco & West, 2020, p. 38) who recommended doubling the baby's weight-gain deficit from the previous week. If the baby should be gaining 7 ounces (210 g) per week but only gained 1 ounce (28 g) the previous week, start with 12 ounces (360 mL) of supplement per day. (The calculation looks like this: 7 ounces target weight minus 1 ounce of actual weight gain equals 6 ounces x 2). Again, see how the baby responds and either increase or decrease the volume of supplement as needed.

• • •

Depending on the baby's weight deficit, the milk production, and the baby's nursing effectiveness, the baby may or may not need a supplement at every feed.

Ideally, the approach to supplementing will be tailored to each situation, but the following general principles may be helpful when formulating a plan.

Supplement only during the nursing parent's waking hours. To make this process more manageable, unless the baby is seriously underfed and at risk, begin by supplementing only during normal waking hours. During sleeping hours, suggest nursing exclusively. If the baby needs a lot of supplement, it may be given while nursing (if a nursing supplementer is used) or after every waking nursing.

Supplement more or less often. If a baby's weight gain is close to borderline, the baby may not need a supplement at every waking nursing session. Every other feed or even less often may be enough. One approach is to offer supplements 2 to 5 times per day, so the baby does not come to expect a supplement after every feed. This might work well if a baby is feeding effectively and the milk production is not too low. The number of times per day the baby needs a supplement depends in part on how much weight she is gaining. If the baby's weight gain is close to borderline, less daily supplement may be needed. If a baby is at risk or weight gain is very low, more supplement may be needed (see Table 6.4 as a starting point). Any plan should be started with the expectation that it may need to be adjusted to better meet the family's needs.

TABLE 6.4 Approximate Supplement Volume Needed Per Day to Increase Weight Gain

Weekly Weight Gain	6 oz. (170 g)	5 oz. (142 g)	4 oz. (113 g)	3 oz. (85 g)	2 oz. (57 g)	1 oz. (28 g)	0 oz. (0 g)
Weekly Weight Deficit	1 oz. (28 g)	2 oz. (57 g)	3 oz. (85 g)	4 oz. (113 g)	5 oz. (142 g)	6 oz. (170 g)	7 oz. (198 g)
Daily Supplement Needed	2 oz. (60 mL)	4 oz. (120 mL)	6 oz. (180 mL)	8 oz. (240 mL)	10 oz. (300 mL)	12 oz. (360 mL)	14 oz. (420 mL)

Adapted from (Genna, 2016)

Smaller rather than larger volumes. In general, it will make the transition to full nursing easier if smaller volumes of the supplement are given more often, rather than a large volume (4 ounces [118 mL] or more) once or twice a day. For this reason, when formula is needed, some clinicians recommend smaller volumes of high-calorie formula as a supplement (Catherine Watson Genna, personal communication). A baby who receives too much supplement at one feed may skip one or more nursing sessions, which can reduce the stimulation needed to boost milk production.

Time of day. The best overall strategy will depend on the circumstances. For example, if the baby feeds effectively and milk production is low, depending on the daily volume of milk produced, the baby may receive a full feed from nursing alone early in the day, with supplements needed only in afternoon and evening, as the volume of milk available at each feed decreases. For most nursing parents, more milk is available in the morning, with diminishing returns as the day goes on.

KEY CONCEPT

Supplementation plans should be tailored to each individual baby.

Effect of feeding method. Whether the supplement is given before, during, or after the nursing will affect the strategy. For example, when a nursing supplementer is used, if the product design allows, the tubing may be clamped shut to prevent milk flow early in the feed while the baby is sucking actively and taking milk well from nursing. As the baby swallows less often or begins to doze, the tubing could then be unclamped to allow the supplement to flow, stimulating longer, more active nursing for more milk production. If the baby is not supplemented during nursing and is sucking effectively, nursing first and giving the supplement afterward is a good strategy for many babies. However, in some cases, a baby may nurse better if she's had some milk first and feels stronger. Encourage the family to experiment to see what works best for them and their baby.

• • •

When it is time to wean from the supplement, suggest doing it gradually as milk production and/or baby's effectiveness improves.

When nursing dynamics are improving—milk production is increasing and baby is feeding effectively—and it is time to begin reducing the volume of supplement, the first step is to make arrangements to carefully monitor the baby's weight during this process. This can be done by either arranging for regular weight checks with the baby's healthcare provider or a lactation specialist or by renting an accurate baby scale (to 5 g) to do daily weight checks at home. Then suggest the following.

- **Decrease the supplement gradually.** Set reasonable goals for decreasing the supplement and increasing nursing. Unless the baby is obviously ready to discontinue the supplement faster, suggest decreasing the supplement by about 2 ounces (59 mL) every other day while increasing time spent nursing.
- **Begin by eliminating supplements at the first morning nursing.** Many babies nurse best at this time, probably due to faster milk flow.
- **Make sure the baby is continuing to gain weight well.** During this process, monitor the baby's weight gain at least once or twice per week using the same scale. Make sure the baby is dressed exactly the same, ideally either naked or wearing a clean, dry diaper. If the baby's weight gain drops to below 5 to 6 ounces (142-177 g) per week, reintroduce the supplement.
- **Expect it to take time before baby is exclusively nursing.** Reassurance and support will make it easier for the family to be patient.

• • •

Some nursing parents do not produce enough milk to exclusively nurse.

Sometimes even extremely dedicated nursing parents are unable to produce enough milk to fully sustain their babies. Chapter 10, "Making Milk" describes physical issues that can compromise milk production, such as breast or chest surgery, post-delivery hemorrhage, hormonal disorders, insufficient glandular tissue, and others. Sometimes the cause is never found.

If it becomes clear that exclusive nursing is not an option for a family, it may help them come to terms with their disappointment if someone helps them understand what happened, sort through their feelings, and acknowledge their disappointment (Williams, 2002).

Feeling like a nursing failure can be a huge blow to a parent's self-esteem, and providing emotional support is vital. Applaud parents' efforts and assure them that even though their baby needs supplements, they are still a nurturing parent. Also ask how their partner (if they have one), their extended family, and others in their social network feel about nursing and supplementation, as their opinions affect parents. Let them know that it is possible to supplement the baby while nursing so that they can continue to share that closeness. If they prefer a bottle, they can continue to comfort the baby by nursing, even if there is little milk. Also, during bottle-feedings, they can still look into their baby's eyes and give skin-to-skin contact so that feedings remain a time of closeness with the baby.

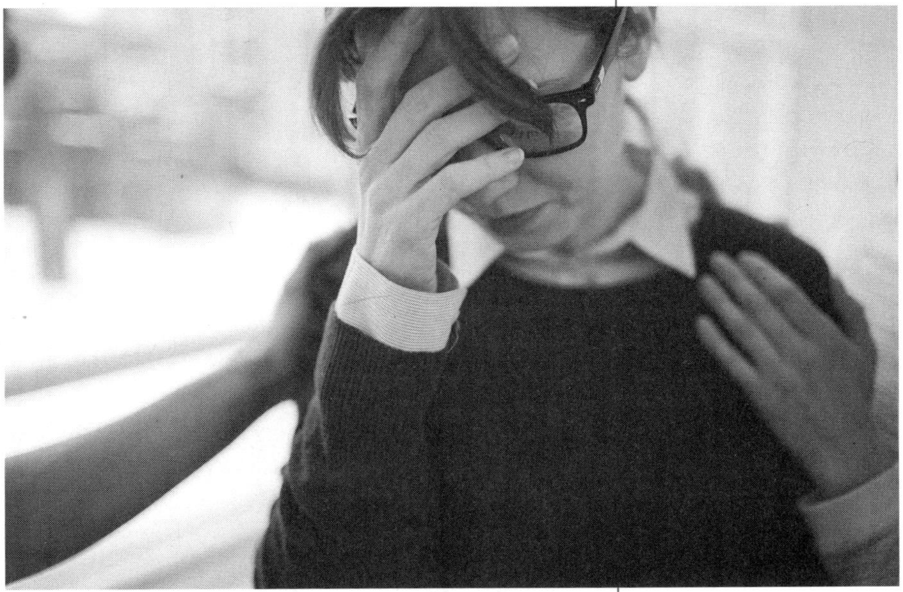

RAPID WEIGHT GAIN

If a family is concerned about overweight in their exclusively nursing baby, ask about baby's weight gain and discuss obesity-prevention strategies.

Weight can be a very emotional subject, especially for parents who are overweight or obese themselves. If a parent expresses concern about future obesity in their nursing baby, begin by asking for some basic information:

- Baby's age
- Exclusively nursing or not, and if not, what other foods their baby is consuming and how much per day
- Current weight, birth weight, and weight at each weight check

The answers should reveal whether the baby's weight gain is within the normal range.

In a nursing baby, rapid weight gain is common during the first few months. However, during months 6 to 12, on average, nursing babies lose more body fat than formula-fed babies, so tell the family to expect their baby will slim down then (WHO, 2009).

Some factors are even stronger predictors of a child's weight than whether she was nursed or formula-fed. The single factor that puts children at greatest risk of overweight and obesity is having overweight or obese parents (Bahreynian et al., 2017). If the parents are overweight or obese, suggest being proactive about helping their child develop healthy eating habits and exercise regularly. If the family expresses concerns about the baby's weight, suggest seeing a dietitian or nutritionist to discuss strategies to minimize the baby's chances of becoming an overweight child or adult.

Attempting to slow a baby's weight gain by limiting nursing time is not an effective strategy. A young child is growing rapidly and needs the nutrients in mother's milk for normal development. Switching to or adding formula, on the other hand, increases risk of overweight and obesity in high-risk families (Carling, Demment, Kjolhede, & Olson, 2015).

• • •

If the baby's weight gain is well above average, assure the family that when a baby is exclusively nursing, this does not necessarily lead to later overweight or obesity.

If the baby is at a high percentile on the growth charts, mention that a baby in the 95th percentile is not necessarily overweight. Most of these babies are also longer than average, and it is the weight-for-length ratio that determines overweight. Weight-for-length growth charts for exclusively nursing babies are available free online from the World Health Organization at: **who.int/childgrowth/standards/en**.

It's also helpful to explain that although some studies found an association between rapid early weight gain and later childhood overweight and obesity (Stocks et al., 2011; Taveras et al., 2011), these studies did not control for feeding method. For many years, clinicians and parents have observed that when fast-gaining, exclusively nursing babies reach the age when they begin rolling over, crawling and eating solid foods, their weight gain slows, and over time they slim down to a normal weight.

Several case reports reflect this same pattern (Grunewald, Hellmuth, Demmelmair, & Koletzko, 2014; Perrella & Geddes, 2016). And research on fast-gaining exclusively nursing babies confirmed these anecdotal accounts and provided more details about the dynamics that contribute to this unusual growth. A 2018 study conducted by researchers from Denmark, the U.K., and Australia (Larsson et al., 2018) followed until 18 months of age a group of 13 exclusively breastfed babies gaining rapidly and compared them with a group of exclusively breastfed babies gaining at the normal rate. They analyzed the milk of the mothers in both groups and measured 24-hour milk intake at different time points. They found that the milk of the fast-gainers was not significantly different from the milk of the other mothers in terms of fat, protein, lactose, or calories. However, at 5 and 9 months of age, the milk consumed by the fast-gainers was significantly lower in the hormone leptin, which regulates appetite. The normal-gainers had about double the blood levels of leptin compared with the fast-gainers. Although fast-gainers gained 60% more weight than the normal-gainers, they consumed an average of only about 15% more milk, an average of 4 ounces (120 mL) per day, and this difference in milk intake was not statistically significant. Their average milk volume per feed and number of feeds per day also did not differ from the normal-gainers. The researchers noted that the rapid weight gain was limited to the babies' first 5 months. After that, the babies went through what the researchers called a "catch-down" phase of weight gain (the opposite of "catch-up" weight in slow-gaining babies).

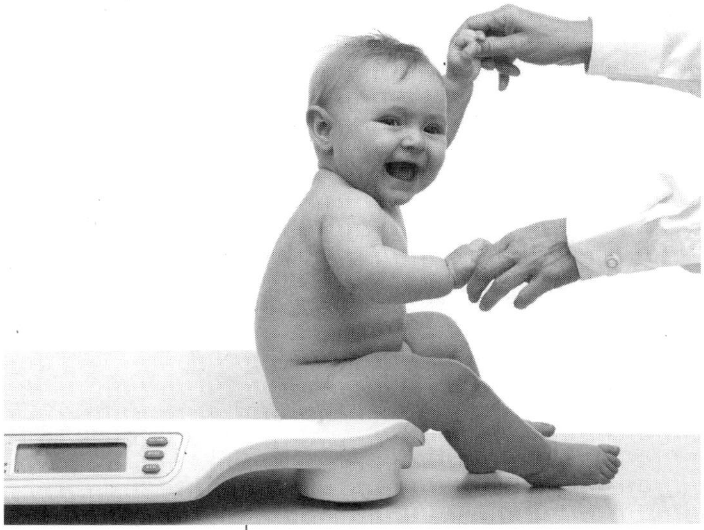

A 2019 article shared case reports of two fast-gaining babies, whom the researchers followed for a much longer time, for 42 months (Larsson, Larnkjaer, Christensen, Molgaard, & Michaelsen, 2019). They noted that at their peak, these two were more than four standard deviations above their peers in terms of weight-for-height. Longer follow-up allowed the authors to record the drops in weight of two standard deviations until the children reached normal weight levels, which is considered to be within two standard deviations of expected weight-for-height.

• • •

The association between nursing and reduced risk of childhood obesity is controversial.

Many observational studies—including meta-analyses and systematic reviews of the literature—found an association between nursing and reduced risk of childhood obesity (Horta et al., 2015; Marseglia et al., 2015; Yan et al., 2014). Lower incidence of obesity in breastfed children was even found in siblings and twins (Metzger & McDade, 2010; Temples et al., 2016). But because it is not ethical to randomize babies to breastfeeding or formula-feeding groups, it's not possible to say for sure that formula-feeding raises risk of obesity and nursing lowers it. The gold standard for determining cause and effect is the randomized controlled trial, and this type of study cannot be done.

Another aspect of this equation that makes it so difficult to solve, is that there are so many confounding factors that affect obesity risk, and these factors interact with one another. Some, such as parental obesity (Bahreynian et al., 2017), have a much greater effect on a child's obesity risk than infant feeding method. For that reason, it's not surprising that one U.S. community-based study that used data from a diverse prospective cohort of 2,172 mothers and babies (Ehrenthal, Wu, & Trabulsi, 2016) found that with the exception of white mothers, in other racial and ethnic groups no difference was found in rates of overweight and obesity in children who were breastfed and formula-fed. While some physical aspects of nursing positively influence a healthy weight (lower protein intake, baby's ability to self-regulate, presence of hormones that regulate appetite, differences in microbiota, etc.), other family or environmental factors—such as parental smoking, poor family diet and exercise, and lower socioeconomic status—may override these positive influences.

When considering the conclusions of a study or a review, it's important to read it critically. One of the primary faults of much of the lactation research published before around 2000 was how breastfeeding was defined. For example, primarily formula-fed babies who nursed once per day were often put into the same study group as babies who nursed exclusively. Along these lines, some of the controversy about the effects of nursing on obesity risk came from the conclusions of a very large prospective study done in Belarus of 17,046 mothers and babies known as the PROBIT study (Kramer et al., 2008). It concluded that breastfeeding had little effect on obesity risk, and this conclusion appeared in commentaries published in two prestigious journals (Casazza et al., 2013; Martin et al., 2013). In a rebuttal, respected Canadian researcher and lactation supporter Patricia Martens explained why these conclusions were suspect (Martens, 2012, p. 340):

> "...[PROBIT] only included women who initiated breastfeeding after giving birth and excluded all non-breastfed infants....[Its results reflect] the effects of slightly longer duration of breastfeeding, as well as much higher exclusive breastfeeding, but [did not compare] any breastfeeding to totally non-breastfed infants."

Although randomized controlled trials cannot be used to determine the impact of nursing on risk of obesity, a number of interesting studies reveal part of the story. One U.S. study examined the effect of nursing on the weight gain of 595 children whose families were at high risk of obesity due to parental obesity, smoking during pregnancy, and low educational levels (Carling et al., 2015). The researchers found that the children who breastfed for less than 2 months were more likely to become obese compared with the children who breastfed for more than 2 months. Another study of 179 sets of Australian twins (31% identical, 69% fraternal) assessed weight gain and feeding history at their 18-month checkup (Temples et al., 2016). The researchers concluded that babies who were supplemented with non-human milks before 4 months of age had higher BMIs at 18 months than those who were exclusively breastfed for the first 4 months. The authors wrote (Temples et al., 2016, p. 481): "The mean BMI decreased from 85% to 65% when infants were breastfeeding for 4 to 6 months compared to breastfeeding for 1 to 3 months." A Swedish prospective longitudinal study that followed its 30,508 babies for 4 years (Wallby, Lagerberg, & Magnusson, 2017), found that at least 4 months of breastfeeding was needed to reduce the risk of childhood obesity.

• • •

If the baby is eating solid foods, discuss feeding strategies and food choices that may affect weight gain.

Early solid foods before 6 months and weight gain. According to the World Health Organization, both babies and nursing parents have better health outcomes when solid foods are delayed until 6 months (see p. 136-139). But rapid weight gain is a common reason for early introduction of solids among U.K. families, who consider this an indication their baby "needs" other foods (S. A. Savage, Reilly, Edwards, & Durnin, 1998; Wright, Parkinson, & Drewett, 2004).

In cultures that believe overweight babies are healthier, parents may consider introducing solid foods early, so their babies "get enough." If this belief causes parents to consistently override their babies' signs of fullness and give more food, this can establish unhealthy feeding habits that increase the risk of childhood obesity later. A 2018 study used the data from a prospective longitudinal cohort study of 346 children living in a socioeconomically disadvantaged region (Mannan, 2018) and found that starting either formula or solid foods before 4 months of age significantly increased the odds of overweight or obesity in these children.

If early solids are being given regularly, ask what solids the baby is fed and how often. Also ask what motivated them to start solids early. Although feeding cereal to babies 3 to 6 months old was associated with lower weights (Kramer et al., 2004), giving large amounts of high-calorie solids may contribute to rapid weight gain. If solids are a substantial part of the baby's diet and the family wants to reduce or eliminate them, encourage them to reduce them gradually and nurse more often to boost milk production and fill the gap.

Solid foods after 6 months and weight gain. Food choices can affect a baby's weight gain. If the baby is gaining weight very rapidly, suggest avoiding "empty calories," such as sweetened foods and drinks, and offer a greater variety of fresh fruits and vegetables. Suggest nursing first, before giving solids. Encourage the family to think of mother's milk as the baby's primary food during the first year and solids as a supplement to nursing. A 2015 U.S. study found that even in families at greater risk for overweight and obesity (Carling et al., 2015), greater intensity and duration of nursing was associated with lower weight gain between 3 and 12 months.

RESOURCES

Cassar-Uhl, D. (2014). *Finding Sufficiency: Breastfeeding with Insufficient Glandular Tissue.* Amarillo, TX: Praeclarus Press.

firstdroplets.com—Videos by Dr. Jane Morton for parents of term and preterm babies show how to prevent excess weight loss after birth by learning hand expression during the last month of pregnancy and using it during the early days.

Marasco, L. & West, D. (2020). *Making More Milk: The Breastfeeding Guide to Increasing Your Milk Production,* 2nd ed. New York: McGraw Hill.

newbornweight.com—Free NEWT app for clinicians incorporates the 2015 newborn weight loss nomograms to make it easy to plot newborn weight loss by percentile, based on the data from more than 108,000 exclusively nursing U.S. babies.

who.int/childgrowth/standards/en/—World Health Organization growth standards based on breastfeeding norms. Free and downloadable charts include length/height for age, weight for age, weight for length/height, BMI for age, head circumference for age, arm circumference for age, subscapular skinfold for age, triceps skinfold for age, motor development milestones, weight velocity, length velocity, and head circumference velocity.

REFERENCES

AAP. (2012). Breastfeeding and the use of human milk. *Pediatrics, 129*(3), e827-e841.

Aarts, C., Hornell, A., Kylberg, E., et al. (1999). Breastfeeding patterns in relation to thumb sucking and pacifier use. *Pediatrics, 104*(4), e50.

ABM. (2011). ABM Clinical Protocol #24: Allergic proctocolitis in the exclusively breastfed infant. *Breastfeeding Medicine, 6*(6), 435-440.

Aljazaf, K., Hale, T. W., Ilett, K. F., et al. (2003). Pseudoephedrine: Effects on milk production in women and estimation of infant exposure via breastmilk. *British Journal of Clinical Pharmacology, 56*(1), 18-24.

Anderson, A. M. (2001). Disruption of lactogenesis by retained placental fragments. *Journal of Human Lactation, 17*(2), 142-144.

Appleton, J., Russell, C. G., Laws, R., et al. (2018). Infant formula feeding practices associated with rapid weight gain: A systematic review. *Maternal and Child Nutrition, 14*(3), e12602.

Arbour, M. W., & Kessler, J. L. (2013). Mammary hypoplasia: Not every breast can produce sufficient milk. *Journal of Midwifery & Women's Health, 58*(4), 457-461.

Azad, M. B., Vehling, L., Chan, D., et al. (2018). Infant feeding and weight gain: Separating breast milk from breastfeeding and formula from food. *Pediatrics, 142*(4).

Bahreynian, M., Qorbani, M., Khaniabadi, B. M., et al. (2017). Association between obesity and parental weight status in children and adolescents. *Journal of Clinical Research in Pediatric Endocrinology, 9*(2), 111-117.

Ballard, J. L., Auer, C. E., & Khoury, J. C. (2002). Ankyloglossia: Assessment, incidence, and effect of frenuloplasty on the breastfeeding dyad. *Pediatrics, 110*(5), e63.

Baroni, L., Goggi, S., Battaglino, R., et al. (2018). Vegan nutrition for mothers and children: Practical tools for healthcare providers. *Nutrients, 11*(1).

Benson, S. (2001). What is normal? A study of normal breastfeeding dyads during the first sixty hours of life. *Breastfeeding Review, 9*(1), 27-32.

Binns, C. W., & Scott, J. A. (2002). Using pacifiers: What are breastfeeding mothers doing? *Breastfeeding Review, 10*(2), 21-25.

Bixby, C., Baker-Fox, C., Deming, C., et al. (2016). A multidisciplinary quality improvement approach increases breastmilk availability at discharge from the neonatal intensive care unit for the very-low-birth-weight infant. *Breastfeeding Medicine, 11*(2), 75-79.

Bowles, B. C. (2011). Breast massage: A "handy" multipurpose tool to promote breastfeeding success. *Clinical Lactation, 2*(4), 21-24.

Brockway, M., Benzies, K., & Hayden, K. A. (2017). Interventions to improve breastfeeding self-efficacy and resultant breastfeeding rates: A systematic review and meta-analysis. *Journal of Human Lactation, 33*(3), 486-499.

Brown, A., & Lee, M. (2012). Breastfeeding during the first year promotes satiety responsiveness in children aged 18-24 months. *Pediatric Obesity, 7*(5), 382-390.

Butte, N. F., Wong, W. W., Hopkinson, J. M., et al. (2000). Energy requirements derived from total energy expenditure and energy deposition during the first 2 y of life. *American Journal of Clinical Nutrition, 72*(6), 1558-1569.

Butte, N. F., Wong, W. W., Hopkinson, J. M., et al. (2000). Infant feeding mode affects early growth and body composition. *Pediatrics, 106*(6), 1355-1366.

Bystrova, K., Widstrom, A. M., Matthiesen, A. S., et al. (2007). Early lactation performance in primiparous and multiparous women in relation to different maternity home practices. A randomised trial in St. Petersburg. *International Breastfeeding Journal, 2,* 9.

Camurdan, A. D., Beyazova, U., Ozkan, S., et al. (2014). Defecation patterns of the infants mainly breastfed from birth till the 12th month: Prospective cohort study. *Turkish Journal of Gastroenterology, 25 Suppl 1,* 1-5.

Çarling, S. J., Demment, M. M., Kjolhede, C. L., et al. (2015). Breastfeeding duration and weight gain trajectory in infancy. *Pediatrics, 135*(1), 111-119.

Casazza, K., Fontaine, K. R., Astrup, A., et al. (2013). Myths, presumptions, and facts about obesity. *New England Journal of Medicine, 368*(5), 446-454.

Chantry, C. J., Nommsen-Rivers, L. A., Peerson, J. M., et al. (2011). Excess weight loss in first-born breastfed newborns relates to maternal intrapartum fluid balance. *Pediatrics, 127*(1), e171-179.

Colson, S., DeRooy, L., Hawdon, J. (2003). Biological Nurturing increases duration of breastfeeding for a vulnerable cohort. *MIDIRS Midwifery Digest, 13*(1), 92-97.

Cote-Arsenault, D., & McCoy, T. P. (2012). Reliability and validity of swallows as a measure of breast milk intake in the first days of life. *Journal of Human Lactation, 28*(4), 483-489.

Courdent, M., Beghin, L., Akre, J., et al. (2014). Infrequent stools in exclusively breastfed infants. *Breastfeeding Medicine, 9*(9), 442-445.

Cox, D. B., Kent, J. C., Casey, T. M., et al. (1999). Breast growth and the urinary excretion of lactose during human pregnancy and early lactation: Endocrine relationships. *Experimental Physiology, 84*(2), 421-434.

de Carvalho, M., Robertson, S., & Klaus, M. H. (1984). Does the duration and frequency of early breastfeeding affect nipple pain? *Birth, 11*(2), 81-84.

Deng, X., & McLaren, M. (2018). Using 24-hour weight as reference for weight loss calculation reduces supplementation and promotes exclusive breastfeeding in infants born by cesarean section. *Breastfeeding Medicine, 13*(2), 128-134.

Dewey, K. G. (2009a). Infant feeding and growth. In G. Goldberg, A. Prentice, P. A., S. Filteau, & K. Simondon (Eds.), *Breast-Feeding: Early Influences on Later Health* (pp. 57-66). New York, NY: Springer.

Dewey, K. G. (2009b). Infant feeding and growth. *Advances in Experimental Medicine and Biology, 639,* 57-66.

Dewey, K. G., & Brown, K. H. (2003). Update on technical issues concerning complementary feeding of young children in developing countries and implications for intervention programs. *Food and Nutrition Bulletin, 24*(1), 5-28.

Dewey, K. G., Domellof, M., Cohen, R. J., et al. (2002). Iron supplementation affects growth and morbidity of breast-fed infants: Results of a randomized trial in Sweden and Honduras. *Journal of Nutrition, 132*(11), 3249-3255.

Dewey, K. G., Heinig, M. J., Nommsen, L. A., et al. (1991). Adequacy of energy intake among breast-fed infants in the DARLING study: Relationships to growth velocity, morbidity, and activity levels. Davis Area Research on Lactation, Infant Nutrition and Growth. *Journal of Pediatrics, 119*(4), 538-547.

Dewey, K. G., Heinig, M. J., Nommsen, L. A., et al. (1992). Growth of breast-fed and formula-fed infants from 0 to 18 months: The DARLING study. *Pediatrics, 89*(6 Pt 1), 1035-1041.

Dewey, K. G., Nommsen-Rivers, L. A., Heinig, M. J., et al. (2003). Risk factors for suboptimal infant breastfeeding behavior, delayed onset of lactation, and excess neonatal weight loss. *Pediatrics, 112*(3 Pt 1), 607-619.

Dewey, K. G., Nommsen, L. A., & Cohen, R. J. (2009). Delayed lactogenesis and excess neonatal weight loss are common across ethnic and socioeconomic categories of primiparous women in northern California. *FASEB Journal, 23,* 344.347 [meeting abstract].

DiTomasso, D., & Paiva, A. L. (2018). Neonatal weight matters: An examination of weight changes in full-term breastfeeding newborns during the first 2 weeks of life. *Journal of Human Lactation, 34*(1), 86-92.

Ehrenthal, D. B., Wu, P., & Trabulsi, J. (2016). Differences in the protective effect of exclusive breastfeeding on child overweight and obesity by mother's race. *Maternal and Child Health Journal, 20*(9), 1971-1979.

El, C., & Celikkaya, M. E. (2019). Infants with vitamin B12 deficiency-related neurological dysfunction and the effect of maternal nutrition. *Annals of Medical Research, 26*(1), 63-67.

Escribano, J., Luque, V., Ferre, N., et al. (2012). Effect of protein intake and weight gain velocity on body fat mass at 6 months of age: The EU Childhood Obesity Programme. *International Journal of Obesity (London), 36*(4), 548-553.

Evans, A., Marinelli, K. A., Taylor, J. S., et al. (2014). ABM Clinical Protocol #2: Guidelines for hospital discharge of the breastfeeding term newborn and mother: "The going home protocol," revised 2014. *Breastfeeding Medicine, 9*(1), 3-8.

Ezzo, G., & Bucknam, R. (2019). *On Becoming Babywise.* Sisters, OR: Hawksflight & Associates.

Feldman-Winter, L., Burnham, L., Grossman, X., et al. (2018). Weight gain in the first week of life predicts overweight at 2 years: A prospective cohort study. *Maternal and Child Nutrition, 14*(1).

Fetherston, C. (1998). Risk factors for lactation mastitis. *Journal of Human Lactation, 14*(2), 101-109.

Flaherman, V. J., Beiler, J. S., Cabana, M. D., et al. (2016). Relationship of newborn weight loss to milk supply concern and anxiety: The impact on breastfeeding duration. *Maternal and Child Nutrition, 12*(3), 463-472.

Flaherman, V. J., Schaefer, E. W., Kuzniewicz, M. W., et al. (2015). Early weight loss nomograms for exclusively breastfed newborns. *Pediatrics, 135*(1), e16-23.

Franco, P., Seret, N., Van Hees, J. N., et al. (2005). Influence of swaddling on sleep and arousal characteristics of healthy infants. *Pediatrics, 115*(5), 1307-1311.

Galipeau, R., Dumas, L., & Lepage, M. (2017). Perception of not having enough milk and actual milk production of first-time breastfeeding mothers: Is there a difference? *Breastfeeding Medicine, 12,* 210-217.

Garbin, C. P., Deacon, J. P., Rowan, M. K., et al. (2009). Association of nipple piercing with abnormal milk production and breastfeeding. *Journal of the American Medical Association, 301*(24), 2550-2551.

Genna, C. W. (2016). *Selecting and Using Breastfeeding Tools: Improving Care and Outcomes.* Amarillo, TX: Praeclarus Press.

Genna, C. W. (2017). The influence of anatomic and structural issues on sucking skills. In C. W. Genna (Ed.), *Supporting Sucking Skills in Breastfeeding Infants* (3rd ed., pp. 209-267). Burlington, MA: Jones & Bartlett Learning.

Gokceoglu, E., & Kucukoglu, S. (2017). The relationship between insufficient milk perception and breastfeeding self-efficacy among Turkish mothers. *Global Health Promotion, 24*(4), 53-61.

Grunewald, M., Hellmuth, C., Demmelmair, H., et al. (2014). Excessive weight gain during full breast-feeding. *Annals of Nutrition and Metabolism, 64*(3-4), 271-275.

Hale, T. W. (2019). *Hale's Medications & Mothers' Milk: A Manual of Lactational Pharmacology* (18th ed.). New York, NY: Springer Publishing Company.

Heinig, M. J., Nommsen, L. A., Peerson, J. M., et al. (1993). Energy and protein intakes of breast-fed and formula-fed infants during the first year of life and their association with growth velocity: The DARLING Study. *American Journal of Clinical Nutrition, 58*(2), 152-161.

Henly, S. J., Anderson, C. M., Avery, M. D., et al. (1995). Anemia and insufficient milk in first-time mothers. *Birth, 22*(2), 86-92.

Hester, S. N., Hustead, D. S., Mackey, A. D., et al. (2012). Is the macronutrient intake of formula-fed infants greater than breast-fed infants in early infancy? *Journal of Nutrition and Metabolism, 2012,* 891201.

Hillervik-Lindquist, C., Hofvander, Y., & Sjolin, S. (1991). Studies on perceived breast milk insufficiency. III. Consequences for breast milk consumption and growth. *Acta Paediatrica Scandinavica, 80*(3), 297-303.

Ho, N. T., Li, F., Lee-Sarwar, K. A., et al. (2018). Meta-analysis of effects of exclusive breastfeeding on infant gut microbiota across populations. *Nature Communications, 9*(1), 4169.

Hogan, M., Westcott, C., & Griffiths, M. (2005). Randomized, controlled trial of division of tongue-tie in infants with feeding problems. *Journal of Paediatrics and Child Health, 41*(5-6), 246-250.

Homan, G. J. (2016). Failure to thrive: A practical guide. *American Family Physician, 94*(4), 295-299.

Hoover, K. L., Barbalinardo, L. H., & Platia, M. P. (2002). Delayed lactogenesis II secondary to gestational ovarian theca lutein cysts in two normal singleton pregnancies. *Journal of Human Lactation, 18*(3), 264-268.

Horta, B. L., Loret de Mola, C., & Victora, C. G. (2015). Long-term consequences of breastfeeding on cholesterol, obesity, systolic blood pressure and type 2 diabetes: A systematic review and meta-analysis. *Acta Paediatrica, 104*(467), 30-37.

Howard, C. R., Howard, F. M., Lanphear, B., et al. (1999). The effects of early pacifier use on breastfeeding duration. *Pediatrics, 103*(3), E33.

Huggins, K. E., Petok, E. S., & Mireles, O. (2000). Markers of lactation insufficiency: A study of 34 mothers. In *Current Issues in Clinical Lactation.* Boston, MA: Jones and Bartlett.

Humphrey, S. (2003). *The Nursing Mother's Herbal.* Minneapolis, MN: Fairview Press.

Islam, M. M., Peerson, J. M., Ahmed, T., et al. (2006). Effects of varied energy density of complementary foods on breast-milk intakes and total energy consumption by healthy, breastfed Bangladeshi children. *American Journal of Clinical Nutrition, 83*(4), 851-858.

Jadin, S. A., Wu, G. S., Zhang, Z., et al. (2011). Growth and pulmonary outcomes during the first 2 y of life of breastfed and formula-fed infants diagnosed with cystic fibrosis through the Wisconsin Routine Newborn Screening Program. *American Journal of Clinical Nutrition, 93*(5), 1038-1047.

Kellams, A., Harrel, C., Omage, S., et al. (2017). ABM Clinical Protocol #3: Supplementary feedings in the healthy term breastfed neonate, revised 2017. *Breastfeeding Medicine, 12*(3), 188-198.

Kennedy, K. I. (2010). Fertility, sexuality, and contraception during lactation. In J. Riordan & K. Wambach (Eds.), *Breastfeeding and Human Lactation* (4th ed., pp. 705-736). Boston, MA: Jones and Bartlett.

Kent, J. C. (2007). How breastfeeding works. *Journal of Midwifery & Women's Health, 52*(6), 564-570.

Kent, J. C., Gardner, H., & Geddes, D. T. (2016). Breastmilk production in the first 4 weeks after birth of term infants. *Nutrients, 8*(12).

Kent, J. C., Hepworth, A. R., Sherriff, J. L., et al. (2013). Longitudinal changes in breastfeeding patterns from 1 to 6 months of lactation. *Breastfeeding Medicine, 8,* 401-407.

Kent, J. C., Mitoulas, L. R., Cregan, M. D., et al. (2006). Volume and frequency of breastfeedings and fat content of breast milk throughout the day. *Pediatrics, 117*(3), e387-395.

Koetsawang, S. (1987). The effects of contraceptive methods on the quality and quantity of breastmilk. *International Journal of Gynaecology and Obstetrics, 25*(suppl), 115-128.

Koletzko, B., Brands, B., Grote, V., et al. (2017). Long-term health impact of early nutrition: The power of programming. *Annals of Nutrition and Metabolism, 70*(3), 161-169.

Kramer, M. S., Fombonne, E., Igumnov, S., et al. (2008). Effects of prolonged and exclusive breastfeeding on child behavior and maternal adjustment: Evidence from a large, randomized trial. *Pediatrics, 121*(3), e435-440.

Kramer, M. S., Guo, T., Platt, R. W., et al. (2004). Feeding effects on growth during infancy. *Journal of Pediatrics, 145*(5), 600-605.

Lampl, M., Veldhuis, J. D., & Johnson, M. L. (1992). Saltation and stasis: A model of human growth. *Science, 258*(5083), 801-803.

Larsson, M. W., Larnkjaer, A., Christensen, S. H., et al. (2019). Very high weight gain during exclusive breastfeeding followed by slowdown during complementary feeding: Two case reports. *Journal of Human Lactation, 35*(1), 44-48.

Larsson, M. W., Lind, M. V., Larnkjaer, A., et al. (2018). Excessive weight gain followed by catch-down in exclusively breastfed infants: An exploratory study. *Nutrients, 10*(9).

Lavagno, C., Camozzi, P., Renzi, S., et al. (2016). Breastfeeding-associated hypernatremia: A systematic review of the literature. *Journal of Human Lactation, 32*(1), 67-74.

Lawrence, R. A., & Lawrence, R. M. (2016). *Breastfeeding: A Guide for the Medical Profession* (8th ed.). Philadelphia, PA: Elsevier.

Lee, N. (1995). More on pierced nipples. *Journal of Human Lactaction, 11*(2), 89.

Ley, R. E. (2010). Obesity and the human microbiome. *Current Opinion in Gastroenterology, 26*(1), 5-11.

Li, L., Manor, O., & Power, C. (2004). Early environment and child-to-adult growth trajectories in the 1958 British birth cohort. *American Journal of Clinical Nutrition, 80*(1), 185-192.

Li, R., Fein, S. B., & Grummer-Strawn, L. M. (2008). Association of breastfeeding intensity and bottle-emptying behaviors at early infancy with infants' risk for excess weight at late infancy. *Pediatrics, 122 Suppl 2,* S77-84.

Li, R., Magadia, J., Fein, S. B., et al. (2012). Risk of bottle-feeding for rapid weight gain during the first year of life. *Archives of Pediatric & Adolescent Medicine, 166*(5), 431-436.

Lightdale, J. R., Gremse, D. A., Section on Gastroenterology, H., et al. (2013). Gastroesophageal reflux: Management guidance for the pediatrician. *Pediatrics, 131*(5), e1684-1695.

Lukefahr, J. L. (1990). Underlying illness associated with failure to thrive in breastfed infants. *Clinical Pediatrics, 29*(8), 468-470.

MacDonald, T., Noel-Weiss, J., West, D., et al. (2016). Transmasculine individuals' experiences with lactation, chestfeeding, and gender identity: A qualitative study. *BMC Pregnancy and Childbirth, 16,* 106.

Manganaro, R., Mami, C., Marrone, T., et al. (2001). Incidence of dehydration and hypernatremia in exclusively breast-fed infants. *Journal of Pediatrics, 139*(5), 673-675.

Mangili, G., Garzoli, E., & Sadou, Y. (2018). Feeding dysfunctions and failure to thrive in neonates with congenital heart diseases. *La Pediatria Medica e Chirurgica, 40*(1).

Mannan, H. (2018). Early infant feeding of formula or solid foods and risk of childhood overweight or obesity in a socioeconomically disadvantaged region of Australia: A longitudinal cohort analysis. *International Journal of Environmental Research and Public Health, 15*(8).

Marasco, L., Marmet, C., & Shell, E. (2000). Polycystic ovary syndrome: A connection to insufficient milk supply? *Journal of Human Lactaction, 16*(2), 143-148.

Marasco, L., & West, D. (2020). *Making More Milk: The Breastfeeding Guide to Increasing Your Milk Production* (2nd ed.). New York, NY: McGraw Hill.

Marseglia, L., Manti, S., D'Angelo, G., et al. (2015). Obesity and breastfeeding: The strength of association. *Women and Birth, 28*(2), 81-86.

Martens, P. J. (2012). What do Kramer's Baby-Friendly Hospital Initiative PROBIT studies tell us? A review of a decade of research. *Journal of Human Lactaction, 28*(3), 335-342.

Martens, P. J., & Romphf, L. (2007). Factors associated with newborn in-hospital weight loss: Comparisons by feeding method, demographics, and birthing procedures. *Journal of Human Lactaction, 23*(3), 233-241, quiz 242-235.

Martin, R. M., Patel, R., Kramer, M. S., et al. (2013). Effects of promoting longer-term and exclusive breastfeeding on adiposity and insulin-like growth factor-I at age 11.5 years: A randomized trial. *Journal of the American Medical Association, 309*(10), 1005-1013.

Martin, R. M., Smith, G. D., Mangtani, P., et al. (2002). Association between breast feeding and growth: The Boyd-Orr cohort study. Archives of Disease in Childhood. *Fetal and Neonatal Edition, 87*(3), F193-201.

Matias, S. L., Nommsen-Rivers, L. A., Creed-Kanashiro, H., et al. (2010). Risk factors for early lactation problems among Peruvian primiparous mothers. *Maternal and Child Nutrition, 6*(2), 120-133.

Matsuzaki, S., Endo, M., Ueda, Y., et al. (2017). A case of acute Sheehan's syndrome and literature review: A rare but life-threatening complication of postpartum hemorrhage. *BMC Pregnancy and Childbirth, 17*(1), 188.

McFadden, H. (2017). Parental concerns on gastroesophageal reflux: When it's more than just a laundry issue--Three case studies. *Clinical Lactation, 8*(4), 169-174.

Mennella, J. A., Papas, M. A., Reiter, A. R., et al. (2019). Early rapid weight gain among formula-fed infants: Impact of formula type and maternal feeding styles. *Pediatric Obesity,* e12503.

Messner, A. H., Lalakea, M. L., Aby, J., et al. (2000). Ankyloglossia: Incidence and associated feeding difficulties. *Archives of Otolaryngology--Head & Neck Surgery, 126*(1), 36-39.

Metzger, M. W., & McDade, T. W. (2010). Breastfeeding as obesity prevention in the United States: A sibling difference model. *American Journal of Human Biology, 22*(3), 291-296.

Mihrshahi, S., Battistutta, D., Magarey, A., et al. (2011). Determinants of rapid weight gain during infancy: Baseline results from the NOURISH randomised controlled trial. *BMC Pediatrics, 11,* 99.

Miller, J. R., Flaherman, V. J., Schaefer, E. W., et al. (2015). Early weight loss nomograms for formula fed newborns. *Hospital Pediatrics, 5*(5), 263-268.

Moretti, E., Rakza, T., Mestdagh, B., et al. (2018). The bowel movement characteristics of exclusively breastfed and exclusively formula fed infants differ during the first three months of life. *Acta Paediatrica.*

Morton, J. (2019). Hands-on or hands-off when first milk matters most? *Breastfeeding Medicine, 14*(5), 295-297.

Morton, J., Hall, J. Y., Wong, R. J., et al. (2009). Combining hand techniques with electric pumping increases milk production in mothers of preterm infants. *Journal of Perinatology, 29*(11), 757-764.

Moscone, S. R., & Moore, M. J. (1993). Breastfeeding during pregnancy. *Journal of Human Lactation, 9*(2), 83-88.

Motil, K. J., Sheng, H. P., Montandon, C. M., et al. (1997). Human milk protein does not limit growth of breast-fed infants. *Journal of Pediatric Gastroenterology and Nutrition, 24*(1), 10-17.

Nelson, A. M. (2017). Risks and benefits of swaddling healthy infants: An integrative review. *MCN American Journal of Maternal and Child Nursing, 42*(4), 216-225.

Newburg, D. S., Woo, J. G., & Morrow, A. L. (2010). Characteristics and potential functions of human milk adiponectin. *Journal of Pediatrics, 156*(2 Suppl), S41-46.

Newton, N., & Theotokatos, M. (1979). Breastfeeding during pregnancy in 503 women: Does a psychobiological weaning mechanism exist in humans? *Emotion & Reproduction, 20B,* 845-849.

Noel-Weiss, J., Courant, G., & Woodend, A. K. (2008). Physiological weight loss in the breastfed neonate: A systematic review. *Open Medicine, 2*(4), e99-e110.

Noel-Weiss, J., Woodend, A. K., Peterson, W. E., et al. (2011). An observational study of associations among maternal fluids during parturition, neonatal output, and breastfed newborn weight loss. *International Breastfeeding Journal, 6,* 9.

Nommsen-Rivers, L., Riddle, S., Thompson, A., et al. (2017). Metabolic syndrome severity score identifies persistently low milk output [abstract]. *Breastfeeding Medicine, 12*(Supplement 1), S22.

Nommsen-Rivers, L. A. (2016). Does insulin explain the relation between maternal obesity and poor lactation outcomes? An overview of the literature. *Advances in Nutrition: An International Review Journal, 7*(2), 407-414.

Nommsen-Rivers, L. A., & Dewey, K. G. (2009). Growth of breastfed infants. *Breastfeeding Medicine, 4 Suppl 1,* S45-49.

Nommsen-Rivers, L. A., Dolan, L. M., & Huang, B. (2012). Timing of stage II lactogenesis is predicted by antenatal metabolic health in a cohort of primiparas. *Breastfeeding Medicine, 7*(1), 43-49.

Nommsen-Rivers, L. A., Heinig, M. J., Cohen, R. J., et al. (2008). Newborn wet and soiled diaper counts and timing of onset of lactation as indicators of breastfeeding inadequacy. *Journal of Human Lactation, 24*(1), 27-33.

O'Sullivan, E. J., Geraghty, S. R., & Rasmussen, K. M. (2018). Awareness and prevalence of human milk sharing and selling in the United States. *Maternal and Child Nutrition, 14 Suppl 6,* e12567.

Oddie, S., Richmond, S., & Coulthard, M. (2001). Hypernatraemic dehydration and breast feeding: A population study. *Archives of Disease in Childhood, 85*(4), 318-320.

Onyango, A. W., Esrey, S. A., & Kramer, M. S. (1999). Continued breastfeeding and child growth in the second year of life: A prospective cohort study in western Kenya. *Lancet, 354*(9195), 2041-2045.

Otsuka, K., Dennis, C. L., Tatsuoka, H., et al. (2008). The relationship between breastfeeding self-efficacy and perceived insufficient milk among Japanese mothers. *Journal of Obstetric, Gynecologic & Neonatal Nursing,* (5), 546-555.

Pados, B. F. (2019). Symptoms of problematic feeding in children with CHD compared to healthy peers. *Cardiology in the Young, 29*(2), 152-161.

PAHO/WHO. (2001). Guiding Principles for Complementary Feeding of the Breastfed Child. Washington, DC: Pan American Health Organization Retrieved from **who.int/nutrition/publications/guiding_principles_compfeeding_breastfed.pdf**.

Paolella, G., & Vajro, P. (2016). Childhood obesity, breastfeeding, intestinal microbiota, and early exposure to antibiotics: What is the link? *JAMA Pediatrics, 170*(8), 735-737.

Paul, I. M., Schaefer, E. W., Miller, J. R., et al. (2016). Weight change nomograms for the first month after birth. *Pediatrics, 138*(6).

Perrella, S. L., & Geddes, D. T. (2016). A case report of a breastfed infant's excessive weight gains over 14 months. *Journal of Human Lactaction, 32*(2), 364-368.

Phillips, S. J., Tepper, N. K., Kapp, N., et al. (2016). Progestogen-only contraceptive use among breastfeeding women: A systematic review. *Contraception, 94*(3), 226-252.

Pico, C., Jilkova, Z. M., Kus, V., et al. (2011). Perinatal programming of body weight control by leptin: Putative roles of AMP kinase and muscle thermogenesis. *American Journal of Clinical Nutrition, 94*(6 Suppl), 1830S-1837S.

Powers, N. G. (1999). Slow weight gain and low milk supply in the breastfeeding dyad. *Clinical Perinatology, 26*(2), 399-430.

Powers, N. G. (2016). Low intake in the breastfed infant: Maternal and infant considerations. In K. Wambach & J. Riordan (Eds.), *Breastfeeding and Human Lactation* (5th ed., pp. 359418). Burlington, MA: Jones & Bartlett Learning.

Rankin, M. W., Jimenez, E. Y., Caraco, M., et al. (2016). Validation of test weighing protocol to estimate enteral feeding volumes in preterm infants. *Journal of Pediatrics, 178,* 108-112.

Rasmussen, K., & Kjolhede, C. (2004). Prepregnant overweight and obesity diminish the prolactin response to suckling. *Pediatrics, 113*(5), 1388.

Righard, L. (1998). Are breastfeeding problems related to incorrect breastfeeding technique and the use of pacifiers and bottles? *Birth, 25*(1), 40-44.

Rodriguez, G., Ventura, P., Samper, M. P., et al. (2000). Changes in body composition during the initial hours of life in breast-fed healthy term newborns. *Biology of the Neonate, 77*(1), 12-16.

Rogers, S. L., & Blissett, J. (2017). Breastfeeding duration and its relation to weight gain, eating behaviours and positive maternal feeding practices in infancy. *Appetite, 108,* 399-406.

Roggero, P., Gianni, M. L., Orsi, A., et al. (2010). Neonatal period: Body composition changes in breast-fed full-term newborns. *Neonatology, 97*(2), 139-143.

Sachs, M., Dykes, F., & Carter, B. (2006). Feeding by numbers: An ethnographic study of how breastfeeding women understand their babies' weight charts. *International Breastfeeding Journal, 1,* 29.

Savage, J. H., Lee-Sarwar, K. A., Sordillo, J. E., et al. (2018). Diet during pregnancy and infancy and the infant intestinal microbiome. *Journal of Pediatrics, 203,* 47-54 e44.

Savage, S. A., Reilly, J. J., Edwards, C. A., et al. (1998). Weaning practice in the Glasgow Longitudinal Infant Growth Study. *Archives of Disease in Childhood, 79*(2), 153-156.

Schaefer, E. W., Flaherman, V. J., Kuzniewicz, M. W., et al. (2015). External validation of early weight loss nomograms for exclusively breastfed newborns. *Breastfeeding Medicine, 10*(10), 458-463.

Schrager, S., & Sabo, L. (2001). Sheehan syndrome: A rare complication of postpartum hemorrhage. *Journal of the American Board of Family Practitioners, 14*(5), 389-391.

Shrago, L. C., Reifsnider, E., & Insel, K. (2006). The Neonatal Bowel Output Study: Indicators of adequate breast milk intake in neonates. *Pediatric Nursing, 32*(3), 195-201.

Simondon, K. B., Simondon, F., Costes, R., et al. (2001). Breast-feeding is associated with improved growth in length, but not weight, in rural Senegalese toddlers. *American Journal of Clinical Nutrition, 73*(5), 959-967.

Smith, L. J. (2017). Impact of birth practices on infant suck. In C. W. Genna (Ed.), *Supporting Sucking Skills in Breastfeeding Infants* (3rd ed., pp. 65-88). Burlington, MA: Jones & Bartlett Learning.

Socha, P., Grote, V., Gruszfeld, D., et al. (2011). Milk protein intake, the metabolic-endocrine response, and growth in infancy: Data from a randomized clinical trial. *American Journal of Clinical Nutrition, 94*(6 Suppl), 1776S-1784S.

Stettler, N., Stallings, V. A., Troxel, A. B., et al. (2005). Weight gain in the first week of life and overweight in adulthood: A cohort study of European American subjects fed infant formula. *Circulation, 111*(15), 1897-1903.

Stocks, T., Renders, C. M., Bulk-Bunschoten, A. M., et al. (2011). Body size and growth in 0- to 4-year-old children and the relation to body size in primary school age. *Obesity Reviews, 12*(8), 637-652.

Stuebe, A. M., Bryant, A. G., Lewis, R., et al. (2016). Association of etonogestrel-releasing contraceptive implant with reduced weight gain in an exclusively breastfed infant: Report and literature review. *Breastfeeding Medicine, 11,* 203-206.

Svensson, K. E., Velandia, M. I., Matthiesen, A. S., et al. (2013). Effects of mother-infant skin-to-skin contact on severe latch-on problems in older infants: A randomized trial. *International Breastfeeding Journal, 8*(1), 1.

Taveras, E. M., Rifas-Shiman, S. L., Sherry, B., et al. (2011). Crossing growth percentiles in infancy and risk of obesity in childhood. *Archives of Pediatrics and Adolescent Medicine, 165*(11), 993-998.

Tawia, S., & McGuire, L. (2014). Early weight loss and weight gain in healthy, full-term, exclusively-breastfed infants. *Breastfeeding Review, 22*(1), 31-42.

Temples, H. S., Willoughby, D., Holaday, B., et al. (2016). Breastfeeding and growth of children in the Peri/postnatal Epigenetic Twins Study (PETS): Theoretical epigenetic mechanisms. *Journal of Human Lactation, 32*(3), 481-488.

Thulier, D. (2017). Challenging expected patterns of weight loss in full-term breastfeeding neonates born by cesarean. *Journal of Obstetric, Gynecologic & Neonatal Nursing, 46*(1), 18-28.

Tolia, V. (1995). Very early onset nonorganic failure to thrive in infants. *Journal of Pediatric Gastroenterology and Nutrition, 20*(1), 73-80.

Unver Korgali, E., Cihan, M. K., Oguzalp, T., et al. (2017). Hypernatremic dehydration in breastfed term infants: Retrospective evaluation of 159 cases. *Breastfeeding Medicine, 12,* 5-11.

Vazirinejad, R., Darakhshan, S., Esmaeili, A., et al. (2009). The effect of maternal breast variations on neonatal weight gain in the first seven days of life. *International Breastfeeding Journal, 4,* 13.

Victora, C. G., Barros, F., Lima, R. C., et al. (2003). Anthropometry and body composition of 18 year old men according to duration of breast feeding: Birth cohort study from Brazil. *British Medical Journal, 327*(7420), 901.

Walker, M. (2017). *Breastfeeding Management for the Clinician: Using the Evidence* (4th ed.). Burlington, MA: Jones & Bartlett Learning.

Walker, S., & Armstrong, M. (2012). The four pillars of safe breast milk sharing. *Midwifery Today International Midwife* (101), 34-37.

Wallby, T., Lagerberg, D., & Magnusson, M. (2017). Relationship between breastfeeding and early childhood obesity: Results of a prospective longitudinal study from birth to 4 years. *Breastfeeding Medicine, 12,* 48-53.

Weissbluth, M. (2015). *Healthy Sleep Habits, Happy Child,* 4th Edition: A Step-by-Step Program for a Good Night's Sleep. New York, NY: Ballantine Books.

WHO. (2006). Breastfeeding in the WHO Multicentre Growth Reference Study. *Acta Paediatrica. Supplement, 450,* 16-26.

WHO. (2009). *WHO Child Growth Standards: Growth Velocity Based on Weight, Length and Head Circumference: Methods and Development.* (2006/07/05 ed. Vol. 450). Geneva, Switzerland: World Health Organization.

WHO. (2015). *Medical Eligibility Criteria for Contraceptive Use.* Geneva, Switzerland: World Health Organization.

WHO. (2016). *Report of the Commission on Ending Childhood Obesity.* Geneva, Switzerland: World Health Organization.

Williams, N. (2002). Supporting the mother coming to terms with persistent insufficient milk supply: The role of the lactation consultant. *Journal of Human Lactation, 18*(3), 262-263.

Willis, C. E., & Livingstone, V. (1995). Infant insufficient milk syndrome associated with maternal postpartum hemorrhage. *Journal of Human Lactation, 11*(2), 123-126.

Wilson-Clay, B., & Hoover, K. (2017). *The Breastfeeding Atlas* (6th ed.). Manchaca, TX: LactNews Press.

Wood, C. T., Skinner, A. C., Yin, H. S., et al. (2016). Bottle size and weight gain in formula-fed infants. *Pediatrics, 138*(1).

Wright, C. M., Parkinson, K. N., & Drewett, R. F. (2004). Why are babies weaned early? Data from a prospective population based cohort study. *Archives of Disease in Childhood, 89*(9), 813-816.

Yan, J., Liu, L., Zhu, Y., et al. (2014). The association between breastfeeding and childhood obesity: A meta-analysis. *BMC Public Health, 14,* 1267.

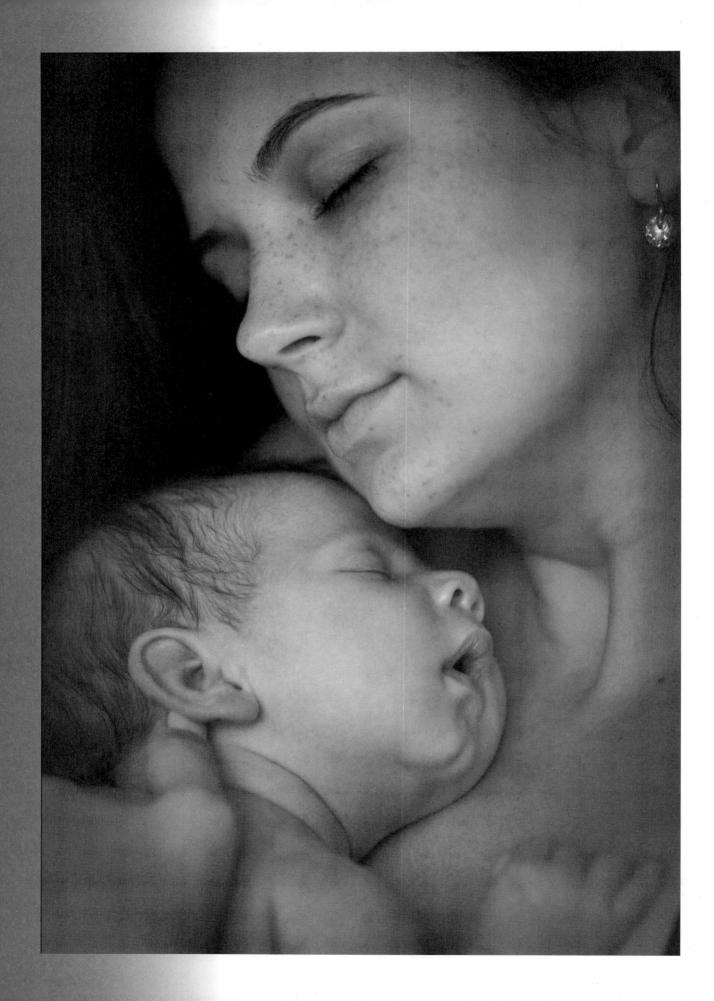

Newborn Hypoglycemia and Jaundice

7

NEWBORN HYPOGLYCEMIA

A newborn's blood sugar levels normally drop after birth and then rise again as he adapts to life outside the womb.

Hypoglycemia is the medical term for low blood glucose levels. Glucose, one type of sugar, is a newborn's primary brain fuel. While in utero, the baby stores glucose in the form of glycogen in his liver and some muscles. After delivery, when the umbilical cord is cut and he no longer receives glucose through the placenta, hormones are released that help him use his glycogen stores for brain fuel while he adapts to life on the outside. About 70% of a baby's brain glucose needs are met this way, with the other 30% coming from alternative fuels (see next point) (Walker, 2017).

In a healthy term newborn, blood sugar levels are usually at their lowest at about 1 to 2 hours after birth. They begin to rise, independent of feeding, within 2 to 4 hours and continue rising until about 96 hours after birth (J. M. Hawdon, Ward Platt, & Aynsley-Green, 1992; WHO, 1997). No short- or long-term benefits have been found to testing and treating newborns for this normal dip in blood-sugar levels they experience during the first hours after birth (N. Wight, Marinelli, & Academy of Breastfeeding, 2014).

KEY CONCEPT

Feeding a nursing newborn formula may compromise his ability to use alternative brain fuels.

By 12 hours after birth, a newborn's glycogen stores are gone, and milk feedings and fat stores provide a baby with the glucose his brain needs (Hagedorn & Gardner, 1999).

• • •

The exclusively nursing baby can access some alternative brain fuels more effectively than a baby fed formula.

For many reasons, nursing within the first 2 hours after birth is important (see p. 45), but this first feed has little effect on baby's blood sugar levels (Sweet, Hadden, & Halliday, 1999; Swenne, Ewald, Gustafsson, Sandberg, & Ostenson, 1994; Zhou, Bai, Bornhorst, Elhassan, & Kaiser, 2017). So from a blood-sugar perspective, if the first nursing is delayed, the baby will not benefit from being fed a supplement. In fact, U.K. research indicates that giving formula may compromise his ability to use alternative brain fuels (de Rooy & Hawdon, 2002; J. Hawdon & Williams, 2000; J. M. Hawdon, Ward Platt, & Aynsley-Green, 1992).

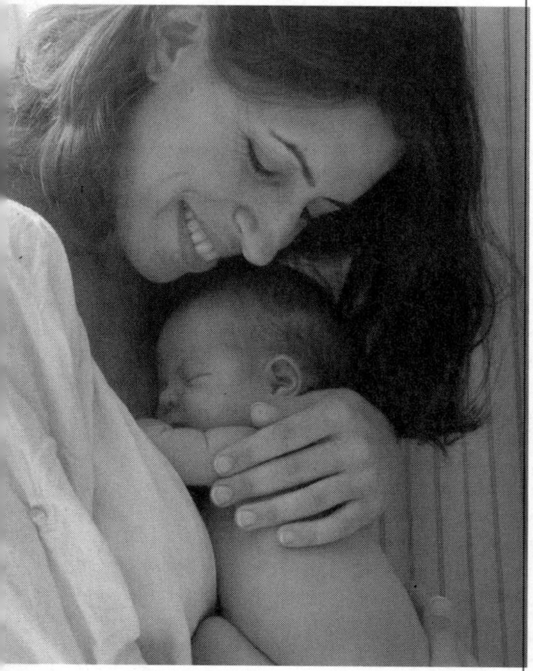

As part of a newborn's natural adaptation from womb to world, in addition to using his glycogen stores for brain fuel, he can access other fuel sources, such as ketone bodies, which are produced by the liver, and lactate. Lactate, also known as lactic acid, is made in muscles and red blood cells when the body breaks down carbohydrates and when oxygen levels are low. (In this context, lactate is unrelated to making milk.) Research found that feeding formula suppressed newborns' ability to use ketone bodies for fuel (Cornblath & Ichord, 2000; de Rooy & Hawdon, 2002; J. M. Hawdon, Ward Platt, & Aynsley-Green, 1992). In an attempt to better understand the role of these alternative brain fuels, a 2015 New Zealand study took blood samples from 35 newborns with hypoglycemia (Harris, Weston, & Harding, 2015) and concluded that in newborns with low blood glucose levels, lactate has a larger role as an alternative brain fuel than ketone bodies.

Full-term, healthy, exclusively nursing babies are not considered at risk for hypoglycemia, in part because they have greater access to these alternative fuels. Routine blood-sugar testing is not recommended, even when a healthy term newborn without symptoms goes 8 hours without nursing (Eidelman, 2001; J. M. Hawdon, Platt, & Aynsley-Green, 1993; WHO, 1997; N. Wight et al., 2014). In fact, researchers recommend against routine blood-sugar testing even for most babies born large-for-gestational-age, as long as they have no symptoms or other risk factors for hypoglycemia (see next point) (Adamkin, Committee on, & Newborn, 2011; N. Wight et al., 2014).

• • •

Hypoglycemia can cause symptoms and serious health problems in at-risk babies.

Symptoms of hypoglycemia include tremors, irritability, jitteriness, a high-pitched cry, irregular breathing, low body temperature, and refusal to feed, as well as low muscle tone, lethargy, and seizures. One of these symptoms, jitteriness, can be difficult to distinguish from normal newborn behavior (N. Wight et al., 2014). One Israeli study of 102 newborns identified as jittery found that 80% stopped acting jittery when they sucked on the clinician's finger (Linder et al., 1989). In its 2019 framework for practice, the British Association of Perinatal Medicine (Levene & Wilkinson, 2019) recommended against checking blood glucose for jitteriness in the absence of other symptoms, because it is common in newborns.

Routine screening of blood sugar—while not recommended for all babies—is recommended for ill and preterm babies and for those born with the risk factors listed in Table 7.1. Routine screening is also recommended for babies born large for gestational age (LGA) in areas where screening for diabetes during pregnancy is not done routinely, because the baby's weight may be a sign of untreated diabetes (N. Wight et al., 2014). Babies also considered at risk are those born small for gestational age (SGA). The definition of SGA, though, varies in different countries. In the U.S., for example, babies are considered SGA if they are born below the 10th percentile for weight, whereas in the U.K., SGA is defined as babies born below the 2nd percentile for weight (N. Wight et al., 2014). Tests exist that can identify which small-for-gestational-age babies are at risk for hypoglycemia (J. M. Hawdon, Ward Platt, McPhail, Cameron, & Walkinshaw, 1992).

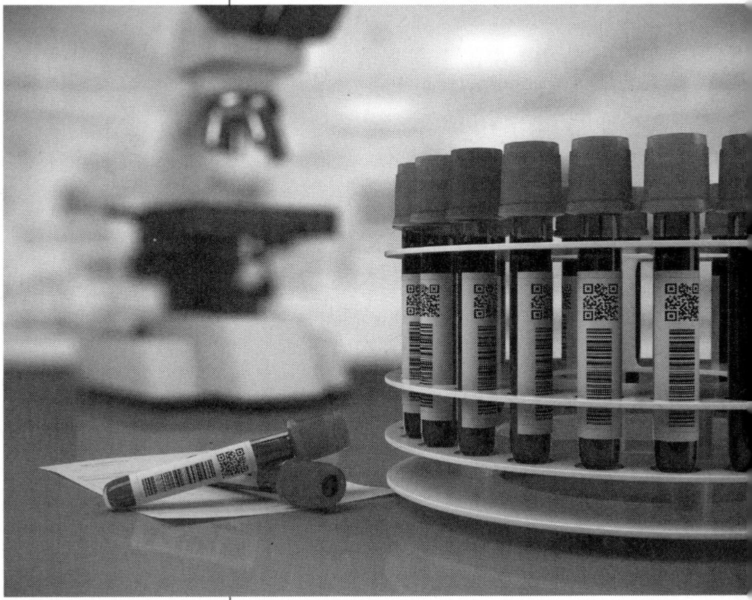

To minimize interference with early nursing, the Academy of Breastfeeding Medicine recommended routine blood-sugar screening for at-risk newborns begin after the first nursing but before the second, no later than 2 hours after birth (N. Wight et al., 2014). Regular monitoring of blood-sugar before feeds is recommended until at least two consecutive measurements are within the healthy range. (The current ABM's Clinical Protocol #1 on hypoglycemia can be downloaded free in multiple language at: **bfmed.org/protocols**.)

The normal and temporary dip in blood sugar after birth that occurs in most mammal species is distinctly different from the more serious type of hypoglycemia that can develop in at-risk newborns. Prolonged and severe if untreated, it can cause brain damage and lead to vision problems, neuromotor retardation, epilepsy, cerebral palsy, and in rare cases, death (J. M. Hawdon, 1999; Inder, 2008).

• • •

Unfortunately, there is no generally agreed-upon definition for hypoglycemia, and many common testing methods are inaccurate.

How is hypoglycemia defined? This varies among healthcare providers and in different parts of the world. One common guideline is less than 40 mg/dL or 2.2 mmol/L (whole blood glucose level lower than 35 mg/dL or 1.9 mmoL). But U.S. research found that when this guideline was used, more than 20% of healthy term newborns with normal blood-sugar levels were misidentified as hypoglycemic (Sexson, 1984). Even so, in many hospitals even higher levels, such as 50 mg/dL (2.8 mmol/L), are now being used.

No matter what specific blood-sugar level is used, there are problems with defining hypoglycemia as one single measurement for all newborns. One blood glucose level does not reflect the many factors that determine the effect of that level on an individual baby, such as his gestational age, his health, his age in hours—which determines where he falls on the normal blood-sugar curve after birth—and his symptoms or lack of symptoms (Thompson-Branch & Havranek, 2017). For this reason, some researchers suggested instead that thresholds be used that take these influencing factors into account (Cornblath et al., 2000; Guemes, Rahman, & Hussain, 2016) (see Table 7.1).

Confusion about the differences among methods of measuring blood sugar also contribute to overtreatment of hypoglycemia. For example, when whole blood is tested, the results are 10% to 18% higher than when plasma is tested (Adamkin et al., 2011). Also, all of the methods of measuring blood sugar levels at the bedside have limited accuracy (Harding, Harris, Hegarty, Alsweiler, & McKinlay, 2017). The American Academy of Pediatrics and World Health Organization recommended against using these as the sole screening method for hypoglycemia (Adamkin et al., 2011; WHO, 1997).

• • •

Post-birth practices, such as skin-to-skin contact and frequent nursing, may reduce a newborn's risk of hypoglycemia.

Post-birth practices can have a profound effect on the incidence of hypoglycemia. One U.S. quality-improvement study examined the impact of improving post-delivery practices on 478 babies born at ≥35 weeks gestation with at least one risk factor for hypoglycemia (LeBlanc et al., 2018). By focusing on ensuring early skin-to-skin contact, early nursing, and doing a blood screen at 90 minutes

TABLE 7.1 When to Treat Hypoglycemia

Baby's Status	Baby's Age in Hours	Glucose Levels Indicating Need for Treatment
No symptoms • Born 35-40 weeks • Healthy	≤24 hours	<30-35 mg/dL (1.7-1.9 mmol/L)
• Taking milk feeds • No risk factors	>24 hours	<40-50 mg/dL (2.2 -2.8 mmol/L)
Symptoms of hypoglycemia	Any age	<45 mg/dL (2.5 mmol/L)
Illness or birth-related issues • Low birth weight • Preterm	≤24 hours	<45-50 mg/dL (2.5-2.8 mmol/L)
• Respiratory distress, failure • Sepsis (blood infection)	>24 hours	<40-50 mg/dL (2.2-2.8 mmol/L)
At risk • Diabetic birthing parent • Low birth weight • Cold stress • Metabolic, endocrine disorder	Any age	<36 mg/dL (2.0 mmol/L)
Low blood glucose levels <20-25 mg/dL	Any age	Start treatment and monitor

Adapted from (Cornblath & Ichord, 2000; Walker, 2017; N. Wight et al., 2014)

for asymptomatic at-risk newborns, the researchers found that admissions to the special-care nursery decreased from 17% to 3%.

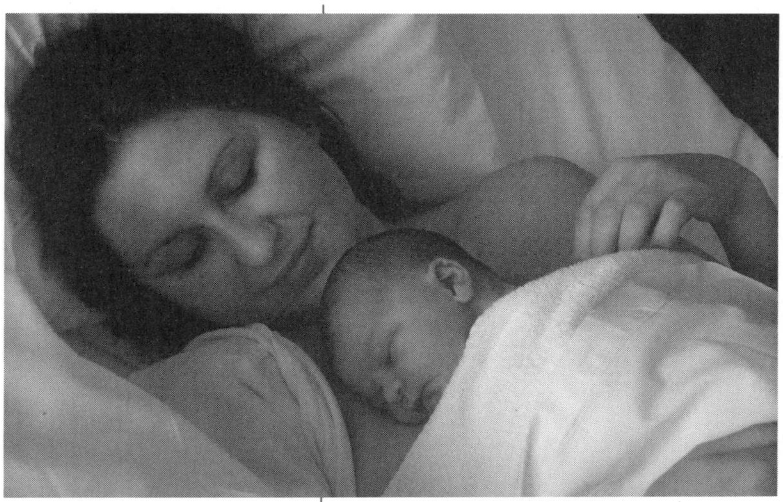

Cold stress is one risk factor for hypoglycemia. Skin-to-skin contact is more effective than mechanical warmers at maintaining newborn body temperature, even among preterm babies (Bergman, Linley, & Fawcus, 2004). A 2016 meta-analysis of at-risk low-birth-weight babies (Boundy et al., 2016) found that early skin-to-skin contact was associated with reduced risk of hypoglycemia. A 2019 quasi-experimental Danish study (Dalsgaard, Rodrigo-Domingo, Kronborg, & Haslund, 2019) found that among babies born to mothers with gestational diabetes, 2 hours of immediate skin-to-skin contact after birth and frequent nursing reduced the incidence of hypoglycemia from 23% to 10%. One Swedish study (Christensson et al., 1992) found that babies separated from their mothers cried 10 times more, had elevated cortisol (a stress hormone), and blood-sugar levels on average 10 mg/dL (55 µmol) lower than babies kept in skin-to-skin contact. Specific practices after delivery that can reduce the risk of hypoglycemia include:

- **Skin-to-skin contact during the first hours** and keep the nursing couple together day and night after that (Dalsgaard et al., 2019).
- **Frequent body contact** to trigger inborn feeding behaviors and early and frequent feeds (Colson, DeRooy, & Hawdon, 2003).
- **Quick response to baby's early signs of hunger** before crying starts. The stress of crying decreases blood-sugar levels (Christensson et al., 1992).

KEY CONCEPT

Immediate and continuous skin-to-skin contact after birth decreases the risk of hypoglycemia.

Another strategy that may reduce the risk of hypoglycemia is to suggest after nursing expressing a little colostrum into a spoon and feeding it to the baby (Morton, 2019; Walker, 2017). Colostrum, either while nursing or expressed and fed, enhances a newborn's ability to use alternative brain fuels and improves gut function, allowing nutrients to be absorbed more quickly. One U.S. prospective pilot study of 84 babies born to mothers with gestational diabetes (Chertok, Raz, Shoham, Haddad, & Wiznitzer, 2009) found that at-risk babies who breastfed in the delivery room were significantly less likely to develop hypoglycemia (10%) than babies whose first breastfeed was later (28%). One U.K. cross-sectional study of 223 full-term, healthy babies with no risk factors (Hoseth, Joergensen, Ebbesen, & Moeller, 2000) found that with frequent nursing even those with very low blood sugar levels at 1 hour developed no symptoms of hypoglycemia.

• • •

Oral dextrose gel with continued nursing is now the recommended first treatment for hypoglycemia.

Dextrose gel. Since the previous edition of this book was published, a new treatment for confirmed hypoglycemia has emerged that is less disruptive of nursing than formula supplements. Now recommended as a first-line treatment (Levene & Wilkinson, 2019), it involves inserting into baby's cheek a 40% dextrose gel, which was found effective in randomized controlled trials worldwide, and a 2016 Cochrane Review (Weston et al., 2016, p. 2) concluded:

"Results suggest that dextrose gel is effective in keeping mothers and infants together and improving the rate of full breast feeding after discharge from hospital. Researchers reported no adverse effects when dextrose gel was given to infants and no effects on development at 2 years of age."

According to research, the use of dextrose gel to treat hypoglycemia reduces hospital treatment costs (Glasgow, 2018) and does not impair later feeds (Weston, Harris, & Harding, 2017). Awareness of this treatment is spreading among clinicians (Alsweiler, Woodall, Crowther, & Harding, 2018). An added benefit of the dextrose-gel treatment is that—unlike formula supplements—its use does not reduce the rate of exclusive nursing during the hospital stay.

IV glucose therapy, an established treatment for hypoglycemia, is recommended in babies who are still hypoglycemic after treatment with dextrose gel or who have very low blood glucose levels. Nursing can continue during IV glucose therapy if baby is willing and able to nurse (N. E. Wight, 2006). Reassure the family that the hypoglycemia is unrelated to the milk and if needed, provide information on how to best keep nursing and milk production going, either through frequent nursing (if the baby is feeding effectively) or frequent milk expression (for details see the section, "Establishing Full Milk Production with Pumping," starting on p. 497).

NEWBORN JAUNDICE

Jaundice Basics

Most newborns become visibly jaundiced during the first week of life.

In utero, babies have extra red blood cells to transport the oxygen they receive through the placenta. After a baby is born and breathing air, however, these extra red blood cells are no longer needed and are broken down and eliminated. Bilirubin, a yellow pigment, is a byproduct of the breakdown of these extra red blood cells. Jaundice occurs as bilirubin accumulates in baby's blood and enters

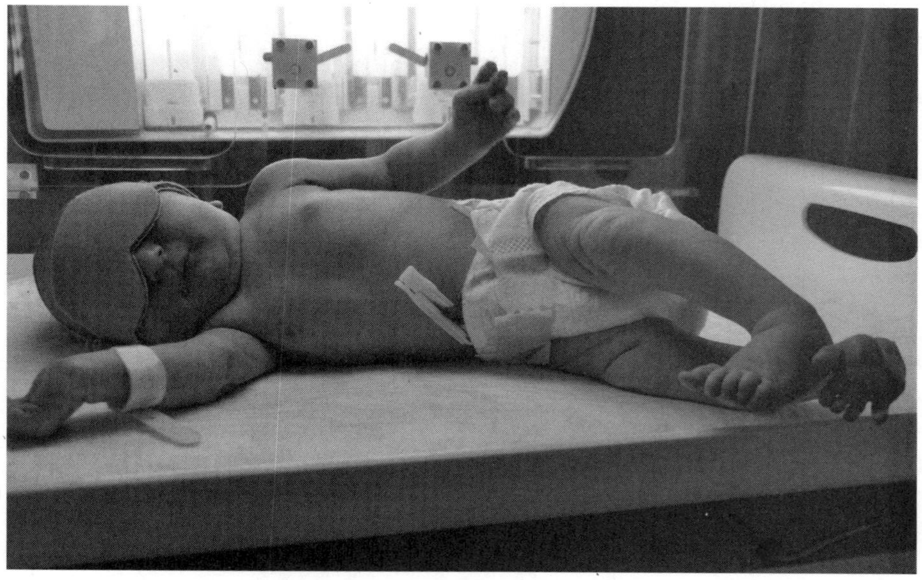

the skin, muscles, and mucous membranes, giving the baby a yellow tinge. Jaundice is more common among newborns than in older children and adults for several reasons:

- Newborns make more bilirubin as extra red blood cells are broken down.
- Newborns process bilirubin more slowly because their liver is immature.
- Newborns absorb bilirubin more easily through their gut.

During the first week of life, more than 80% of newborns become visibly jaundiced, and among nursing babies, bilirubin levels can remain elevated for as long as 12 to 15 weeks (Bhutani et al., 2013; Flaherman, Maisels, & Academy of Breastfeeding Medicine, 2017).

• • •

Bilirubin levels are more likely to become concerning when a nursing baby isn't feeding well.

Before bilirubin can leave the newborn's body, it is first bound to water-soluble proteins in the blood and processed or ***conjugated*** by the baby's liver. From there, his bile carries it to the intestines, and it is excreted from the baby's body in the stool.

It was once thought that because bilirubin leaves a baby's body via the stools, more stooling was vital to lowering high levels of bilirubin. However, the thinking on this has changed. Dutch researchers examined the association between stools and bilirubin levels in healthy term babies during the first 4 days after birth by collecting all the stools from 27 formula-feeding newborns and 33 nursing newborns (Buiter et al., 2008). They discovered that during these first 4 days, formula-fed babies had fewer stools and lower bilirubin levels than the nursing babies. As a result of these findings, experts now believe that to avoid exaggerated newborn jaundice, adequate milk intake is vital. Inadequate feeding, rather than lack of stooling, is a contributing cause of high bilirubin levels. For this reason, in its Clinical Protocol #22 on jaundice (Flaherman et al., 2017), the Academy of Breastfeeding Medicine referred to the most common type of exaggerated newborn jaundice caused by underfeeding as "suboptimal intake jaundice." (This protocol is free and downloadable in multiple languages at: **bfmed.org/protocols**.)

KEY CONCEPT

In healthy term babies, frequent feeds during the first days lead to more milk intake, which keeps bilirubin levels in the safe and moderate range.

Nursing early and often after birth stimulates an earlier increase in milk production, which in healthy term babies keeps bilirubin levels in the safe and moderate range. A 2017 Irani cross-sectional study surveyed the mothers of 634 newborns with elevated bilirubin levels who came to the hospital emergency room or clinic (Boskabadi & Zakerihamidi, 2017). The researchers collected data on the number of nursing sessions per day, and they weighed the babies and measured their bilirubin levels. (Bilirubin is measured in milligrams per deciliter [mg/dL] or in micromoles per liter [µmol/L].) They found an association between the number of nursing sessions per day and the babies' bilirubin levels:

- 11 feeds/day: 1-12 mg/dL (17-205 µmol/L)
- 10 feeds/day: 12-16 mg/dL (205-273 µmol/L)
- 9 feeds/day: 16-20 mg/dL (273-342 µmol/L)
- 7.5 feeds/day: >20 mg/dL (342 µmol/L)

The babies whose bilirubin levels were below 20 mg/dL (342 μmol/L) lost a smaller percentage of their birth weight compared with those with bilirubin levels above 20 mg/dL (342 μmol/L). The researchers concluded that one way to help keep bilirubin levels within the safe range is to encourage frequent nursing, especially during the first days of life.

• • •

Mildly and moderately elevated bilirubin levels may benefit both newborns and adults.

As long as bilirubin levels stay mild to moderate, elevated levels may play an important role in protecting newborn health (McDonagh, 1990; Sedlak & Snyder, 2004). During the early weeks of life, bilirubin acts as an antioxidant while other antioxidants are absent, which can reduce the levels of free radicals that can cause injury to at-risk babies (Baranano, Rao, Ferris, & Snyder, 2002). A 2018 Scottish lab study examined the effects of bilirubin on Group B streptococcus in blood samples of infected babies (Hansen et al., 2018) and concluded that bilirubin also appears to have antibacterial properties. One Dutch study (van Zoeren-Grobben et al., 1994) found that bilirubin reduced free-radical levels in 18 preterm babies, while two U.S. studies found that in preterm babies, higher bilirubin levels (within the safe range) were associated with fewer health problems related to free-radical injury, such as necrotizing enterocolitis and retinopathy of prematurity (Hegyi, Goldie, & Hiatt, 1994; Heyman, Ohlsson, & Girschek, 1989).

Other studies found an association in adults between higher bilirubin levels and lower incidence of coronary heart disease and death from cancer (Djousse et al., 2001; Temme, Zhang, Schouten, & Kesteloot, 2001).

• • •

If a baby becomes visibly jaundiced during the first 24 to 48 hours or if the jaundice quickly becomes severe, this is likely a sign of an underlying health problem.

Although mild to moderate jaundice is common and possibly beneficial in the nursing baby, this normal or ***physiological jaundice*** takes several days to develop and is not usually visible until the second to fifth day of life. When jaundice becomes visible within the first 24 to 48 hours, this is what some call ***pathologic jaundice***, because it is likely due to an underlying physical issue that may require treatment. Another indicator is bilirubin levels rising faster than 5 mg/dL (85 μmol/L) per day and higher than 17 mg/dL (290 μmol/L) in a full-term baby. Possible underlying causes include a variety of diseases or conditions that:

- Cause increased red blood cell breakdown
- Interfere with bilirubin processing in the liver
- Increase reabsorption of bilirubin by the gut

Examples include sepsis (a serious blood infection), blood disease, rubella, Rh or ABO incompatibility, inborn errors of metabolism, congenital thyroid deficiency, serious bruising or cephalohematoma, and intestinal obstruction or defect. One more common condition is the blood disorder G6PD deficiency, which occurs in 11%-13% of those of African descent and is more commonly found among those from Mediterranean countries and southeast Asia (Badejoko et al., 2014; Kaplan, Herschel, Hammerman, Hoyer, & Stevenson, 2004).

KEY CONCEPT

Jaundice appearing in the first 24 to 48 hours may indicate an underlying health problem.

With early and severe jaundice from these causes, with only rare exceptions, nursing can and should continue. Some tests can pinpoint treatable causes, such as identifying blood and Rh type, direct antibody (Coombs) test, complete blood count, and red blood cell smear, as well as both a total bilirubin and a direct-reacting fraction. But underlying causes cannot always be found (there are more than 50 known red blood cell enzyme deficiencies), so some suggest once the usual causes have been ruled out to focus on keeping bilirubin levels within safe levels (Maisels, 2015) (see next section).

• • •

As a baby's bilirubin levels rise, the yellow skin color spreads from the head down.

Jaundice is not usually visible to the eye until bilirubin levels reach at least 4 mg/dL (68 µmol/L). As bilirubin levels rise, the yellow color spreads from the head to the chest (about 10 mg/dL [170 µmol/L]) to the abdomen and finally (usually when levels reach more than 15 mg/dL [255 µmol/L]) to the palms and the soles of the feet (Walker, 2017). Although the color of the baby's body can provide a rough indication of the severity of jaundice, bilirubin levels cannot be reliably gauged visually by checking baby's skin color alone, as room lighting and racial differences affect perception of skin tone (Holland & Blick, 2009).

• • •

Most cases of mild to moderate newborn jaundice do not require treatment.

In most newborns, jaundice is temporary, resolves on its own, and does not require treatment (Adamkin et al., 2011; Flaherman et al., 2017). Bilirubin levels in the full-term, healthy baby usually peak between the third and fifth days of life at less than 12 mg/dl, (204 µmol/L) and rarely go higher than 15 mg/dl (255 µmol/L).

• • •

Even after the first 2 weeks, jaundice is common among nursing babies.

Prolonged jaundice after the first 2 weeks of life was once thought to be a separate and distinct type of jaundice (***late-onset*** or ***breast-milk jaundice***) that affected only a small percentage of nursing babies. However, this is now recognized as an extension of normal newborn jaundice, and bilirubin can remain in the moderate range for many weeks, especially among babies who had higher bilirubin levels earlier.

By 2 to 3 weeks of age, the vast majority of newborns fed non-human milks have adult bilirubin levels of less than 1.3 to 1.5 mg/dL (22 to 26 µmol/L). But at 2 to 3 weeks of age, this is not the case with nursing babies:

- One-third of nursing babies are visibly jaundiced with bilirubin levels above 5 mg/dL (85 µmol/L)
- One-third of nursing babies still have elevated bilirubin levels of between 1.5 and 5 mg/dL (26 to 85 µmol/L), even though their jaundice is not visible

KEY CONCEPT

Bilirubin levels in nursing babies often remain elevated for many weeks.

In healthy term babies, as long as bilirubin levels stay below about 20 mg/dL (342 µmol/L) and are not rising rapidly, this prolonged jaundice will eventually clear without treatment within about 12 to 15 weeks (Flaherman et al., 2017). Sometimes a temporary weaning is recommended in this situation, but as long as bilirubin levels stay moderate, this is neither beneficial nor necessary. If a baby's healthcare provider recommends temporary weaning and the family is unhappy with this, suggest sharing with the healthcare provider the ABM Clinical Protocol #22 on jaundice, which was written for healthcare providers and is available in multiple languages at: **bfmed.org/protocols**.

• • •

With few exceptions, once a baby's bilirubin levels have reached their peak and begun to decline, they are unlikely to rise again.

Whether a baby's bilirubin levels plateau and decline naturally or whether this occurs with treatment (see later section), once the bilirubin levels have peaked and begun to decline, in most cases they are unlikely to increase again. One exception is babies with some inherited hemolytic (blood) disorders, such as G6PD deficiency and spherocytosis. Also, a slight rebound in bilirubin levels is common after phototherapy is stopped or when the baby begins nursing again after a temporary interruption. Any rebound should be slight but should be closely followed.

Monitoring Bilirubin Levels

Monitoring newborn jaundice is vital, because although rare, high bilirubin levels can cause severe health problems.

Although bilirubin may be beneficial if kept at mild to moderate levels, when at the rare times it exceeds 25 mg/dL (425 µmol/L), it may cross the blood-brain barrier, causing a condition known as ***bilirubin encephalopathy***. Its early symptoms include lethargy and feeding refusal and can eventually progress to a high-pitched cry and neurological symptoms, such as seizures, arching back of the head and spine, and even fever. If not treated promptly, the baby may develop ***kernicterus***, a yellow staining of the brain that causes permanent neurological damage and potentially lifelong problems such as cerebral palsy, hearing loss, developmental delays, paralysis, mental retardation, and even death.

Although not all newborns with bilirubin levels higher than 25 mg/dL (425 µmol/L) develop bilirubin encephalopathy, treatment should be started before it becomes a risk. These very high bilirubin levels are rare among full-term, healthy babies in developed countries. A Canadian prospective study of 56,019 mostly Caucasian babies born at least 35 weeks gestation (Jangaard, Fell, Dodds, & Allen, 2008) found that only 0.6% had total serum bilirubin levels of ≥19 mg/dL (325 µmol/L). In this same study, not one of its 56,019 babies developed kernicterus. One expert estimated that in developed countries the incidence of kernicterus is between 1 in 100,000 and 1 in 1,000,000 newborns (Ip et al., 2004).

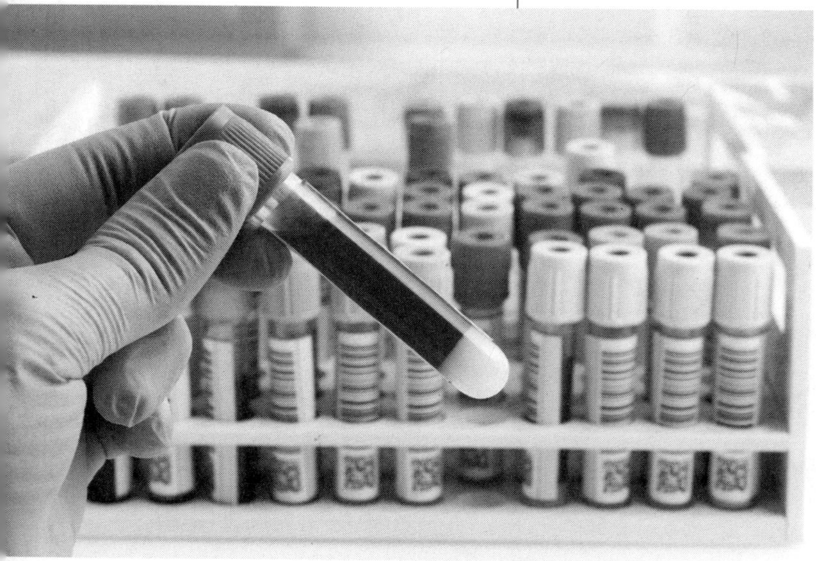

Even in preterm and ill babies, high bilirubin levels are uncommon in developed countries. A 2017 retrospective database analysis examined the medical records of all babies born in England who were admitted to neonatal intensive care units between 2012 and 2015 (Gale et al., 2018). It found that depending on the year, the incidence of kernicterus was very low, between 0.3 to 1.3 per 100,000 births.

However, the outcomes from newborn jaundice are vastly different in the developing world. A 2017 systematic review and meta-analysis (Slusher, Zamora, et al., 2017) concluded that in low- and middle-income countries (where good medical care may be scarce and phototherapy unavailable), bilirubin encephalopathy, exchange transfusions to treat severe jaundice, and death are common and costly.

Several factors, including baby's health and race, affect the course of newborn jaundice. A 2011 study of Egyptian babies admitted to the hospital with severe jaundice (Gamaleldin et al., 2011) found that healthy babies were less likely to develop neurological problems at the same high bilirubin level as at-risk babies with blood disease or ABO incompatibility. Race also plays a role. One study found that Chinese babies were at a 64% higher risk of jaundice compared to non-Chinese babies (Huang, Tai, Wong, Lee, & Yong, 2009). All babies of Asian origin normally have higher bilirubin levels than non-Asian babies.

• • •

Bilirubin levels can be measured with a blood test or by less invasive methods.

As described earlier in this chapter, observing the spread of yellow skin tone from the head down the baby's body gives a rough indication of bilirubin levels, but it is not reliable enough to determine when a baby needs treatment. Not long ago, bilirubin levels could only be confirmed through painful blood tests that often needed to be done repeatedly.

Today, a commonly used initial screening tool for healthy term babies is the less-invasive ***transcutaneous bilirubinometry*** (TcB). This instrument is gently pressed against the baby's skin and reflects light through the skin to the underlying tissues and back into the instrument to calculate the intensity of the skin's yellow color. These instruments are more reliable than the eye alone in gauging the severity of the baby's jaundice, and they are often used first so blood is drawn only from babies in need of medical follow-up. Although not as accurate as blood tests and even less accurate among some races (Kaplan & Bromiker, 2019; Taylor et al., 2015), the use of these devices can help avoid painful blood tests in some babies.

Another initial screening tool is now available, the Bilicam smartphone app, which uses the smartphone's camera. U.S. researchers compared the results of blood tests with the readings from the Bilicam app (Taylor et al., 2017) and found that this handheld technology is reliable enough to use instead of TcB by healthcare providers and parents to assess babies' bilirubin levels in low-risk newborns. At this writing, the Bilicam app is only available on the Android platform.

In 2019, a new tool for measuring bilirubin levels in low-resource areas was validated in the U.S. and Bangladesh (Lee et al., 2019). Its purpose is to prevent delays in identifying babies with high bilirubin levels in parts of the world where many babies die from severe jaundice. The Bili-ruler features six circles of gradually intensifying colors along the ruler with a number above each. The user gently presses the ruler into the bridge of baby's nose to blanch the skin and compares the color of the blanched skin with the six color choices. To see the Bili-ruler and learn about this research, watch the 5-minute video at **bit.ly/BA2-BiliRuler**.

• • •

In many countries, it is recommended that all healthcare institutions routinely screen every newborn for jaundice before hospital discharge.

To prevent dangerously high bilirubin levels, many hospitals are asked to screen all newborns at discharge (Adamkin et al., 2011; Flaherman et al., 2017). This screening often involves a combination of visually checking babies' skin color, determining any risk factors, and/or using one or more of the methods for checking bilirubin levels described in the previous point. Some large hospital systems have successfully implemented screening strategies that have reduced both the number of newborns who developed dangerously high bilirubin levels and the rate of rehospitalizations for jaundice (Darling, Ramsay, Sprague, Walker, & Guttmann, 2014).

• • •

Close follow-up with a healthcare provider after discharge is strongly recommended.

Another way to prevent babies from developing dangerously high bilirubin levels is to arrange for early follow-up after hospital discharge. The American Academy of Pediatrics recommends that all babies be seen by a healthcare provider between 3 and 5 days of age (AAP, 2012). If at this visit the health care provider discovers that a newborn is not nursing well, the family can be referred for skilled lactation help. Babies born at less than 38 weeks gestation are considered at higher risk and require even closer monitoring (Adamkin et al., 2011).

Jaundice Treatments

When newborn jaundice is diagnosed, it can be upsetting, put nursing at risk, and change parents' behaviors and attitudes.

When a baby needs treatment for jaundice, parents may feel worried, anxious, and upset, depending in part on their familiarity with newborn jaundice, how well it is explained, and whether its dangers are overemphasized. If a medical explanation is given while they are upset, they may forget many of the specifics. If so, suggest they contact the baby's healthcare provider to discuss it again when they are feeling calmer. Even something as simple as the healthcare provider encouraging parents to nurse was found to greatly influence their decisions (Willis, Hannon, & Scrimshaw, 2002). Offer moral support with comments like, "You have obviously put a lot of thought into making the best decision for your baby," or, "You are wise to find out more about your options."

If treatment for jaundice involves separation of the nursing couple, feeding formula, or temporary weaning, this can increase anxiety and affect a family's feelings about nursing. If healthcare providers discourage them from spending time with or nursing the baby, they may wonder whether mother's milk might be causing the jaundice or if it has any value to the baby (Hannon, Willis, & Scrimshaw, 2001). If resuming nursing is a challenge, this adds to the stress and worry.

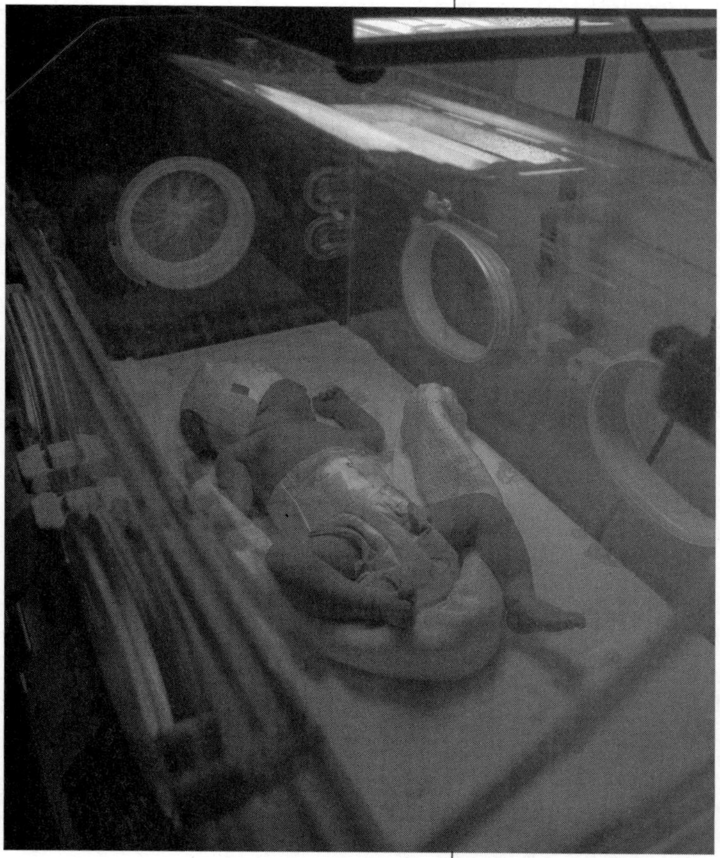

No negative long-term health effects have been associated with mild to moderate newborn jaundice (Draque, Sanudo, de Araujo Peres, & de Almeida, 2011). But even so, treating jaundice can affect a family's behavior and attitudes. U.S. research found that after the jaundice resolved, many of the study mothers considered their baby at risk or "vulnerable." One U.S. study of 209 mothers (K. Kemper, Forsyth, & McCarthy, 1989) found that one month after hospital discharge, mothers whose babies were jaundiced were more likely to have stopped breastfeeding (42% versus 19%), even though more mothers of jaundiced babies started breastfeeding at birth (79% versus 61%). Both the jaundiced and non-jaundiced babies had similar numbers of health problems, but the mothers of the jaundiced babies were more likely to take their baby to well-baby checkups and more than twice as likely to take the baby to his healthcare provider for a sick visit (not counting bilirubin checks) or to the hospital emergency room.

Another U.S. study followed mothers of initially jaundiced and non-jaundiced babies at 6 months (K. J. Kemper, Forsyth, & McCarthy, 1990). The mothers whose babies were jaundiced had more feeding problems, were less likely to be breastfeeding, and were more likely to have tried a special formula. They were also more likely to consider their baby's minor illnesses as serious and to have made at least one trip to the emergency room with their child. The authors concluded that jaundice treatments have adverse effects on breastfeeding and may affect a mother's relationship with her baby.

KEY CONCEPT

Treatments for jaundice and how they are handled can affect a parent's anxiety level and their feelings about nursing.

Optimizing Nursing

While it is true that nursing newborns have naturally higher bilirubin levels than non-nursing babies, as described in an earlier section, this may be a positive rather than a negative. As long as bilirubin stays in the mild to moderate range, it poses no risk to the nursing newborn.

Nursing does not increase a baby's risk for severe jaundice, but inadequate milk intake does.

When best practices are followed after birth (early skin-to-skin contact, nursing within the first hour or two, frequent feeds with a deep latch, 24-hour rooming-in, and no supplements), severe jaundice is much less likely to occur. These strategies are recommended in the Academy of Breastfeeding Medicine's Clinical Protocol #22 on jaundice as a way to prevent or reduce jaundice in the nursing baby (Flaherman et al., 2017).

• • •

Newborn jaundice is one of the most common reasons babies are readmitted to the hospital after discharge (Boubred, Herlenius, Andres, des Robert, & Marchini, 2016), in part because nursing and post-delivery practices are often less-than-optimal, and as a result, many babies do not feed well. As in adults, when babies are deprived of adequate nourishment, bilirubin levels rise. As the Iranian study described in detail in the previous section found (Boskabadi & Zakerihamidi, 2017), more nursing sessions per day during the first 4 days resulted in lower bilirubin levels in the newborns.

Nursing at least 10 to 12 times per day and feeding extra hand-expressed colostrum by spoon can help prevent and resolve jaundice.

Strategies for encouraging early and frequent nursing include:

- Skin-to-skin contact during the first hours after birth
- Keep baby unswaddled and tummy down on the parents' body as much as feels comfortable during the early days to trigger inborn feeding behaviors

KEY CONCEPT

After Day 4, dark meconium stools are a red flag to monitor the nursing couple closely.

See the section "The First Days" in Chapter 2, starting on p. 49, for more details. Optimal nursing helps to prevent high bilirubin levels during the first week of life, which also helps prevent prolonged jaundice at higher levels later (Siu, Chan, & Kwong, 2018). One way to help prevent exaggerated newborn jaundice was recommended by U.S. pediatrician Jane Morton (Morton, 2019). Her website **firstdroplets.com** encourages families to learn hand expression during the last month of an uncomplicated pregnancy and use it after nursing during the early days after birth to feed baby extra expressed colostrum by spoon. This practice may help prevent both severe jaundice and excess weight loss.

• • •

A baby's weight loss after birth and stool color can help gauge early milk intake.

As described on p. 188 in Chapter 6, using baby's 24-hour weight as a baseline (rather than birth weight), the nursing newborn should lose no more than about 10% of this weight before weight gain begins. Weight loss of more than 10% by Day 4 in exclusively nursing newborns or continued weight loss after Day 4 puts a baby at risk for jaundice and indicates the need for skilled lactation help. Dark meconium stools after Day 4 is another red flag to take a closer look at nursing.

• • •

To increase milk intake at feeds, suggest getting a deep latch, nursing more times each day, and using breast compression during feeds to increase milk intake.

The first step in increasing milk intake is to try to get a deep latch. Second is to nurse more times each day during baby's wakeful periods. Between feeds and before latching, make sure baby is in full frontal contact with the nursing parent's body so that his innate feeding behaviors are activated (see Chapter 1). If a baby is swaddled and laid in a separate bed, this can lead to more sleep, suppress feeding behaviors, and decrease overall number of feeds (Nelson, 2017).

If the baby latches but does not nurse actively, suggest trying breast compression, which is described on p. 889. A variation of this is called "alternate breast massage." Both use pressure to stimulate faster milk flow during nursing, keep the baby active and interested for longer periods, and increase the fat content of the milk (Bowles, 2011).

• • •

If high bilirubin levels make the baby lethargic, suggest keeping baby on the nursing parent's body and helping him latch during light sleep.

Some severely jaundiced babies appear sleepy or disinterested in feeding. Does jaundice reduce a newborn's sucking effectiveness? A 2016 Israeli study on infant sucking and jaundice (Bromiker, Medoff-Cooper, Flor-Hirsch, & Kaplan, 2016) used a specially designed infant feeding bottle that measured the babies' ability to transfer milk. These researchers compared the sucking efficiency of two groups of newborns: one group had bilirubin levels of 15 mg/dL (256 μmol/L) or higher and the other group was not jaundiced. The researchers found no significant differences in the newborns' sucking effectiveness.

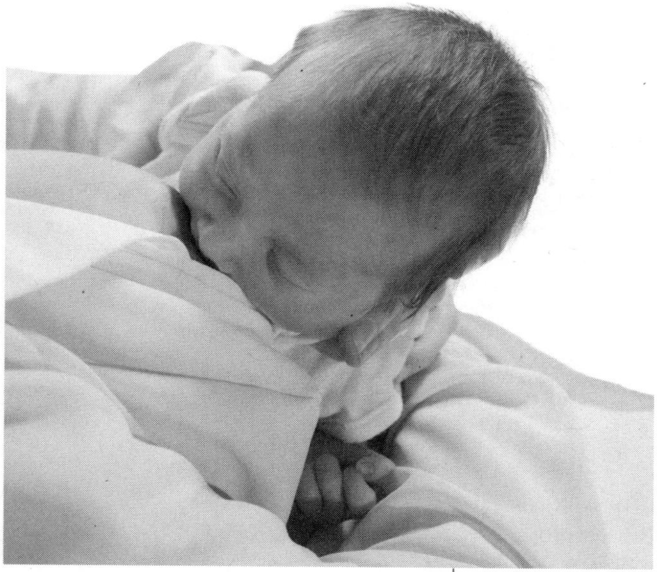

What should parents do if their jaundiced baby is not waking often to nurse? Rather than waiting, encourage them to lean back into a comfortable, well-supported, semi-reclined position and lay baby on top, tummy down (see p. 23-29). When the baby is in a light sleep (any body movement), the feel of the parent's body against his front will trigger inborn feeding behaviors. When baby begins moving and rooting, without changing position, suggest guiding baby to the nipple and helping him latch while asleep, which can stimulate active nursing (Colson et al., 2003).

If despite all efforts the baby is unresponsive and not nursing actively, recommend starting milk expression. The baby's milk intake is important to resolving the jaundice and the stimulation of milk expression is vital for healthy milk production. If the nursing parent needs to initiate milk production primarily with milk expression, for strategies see p. 497 in Chapter 11.

Discuss feeding methods with the family. Expressed milk can be fed using a nursing supplementer, or it can be fed by spoon, cup, eyedropper, feeding syringe, or bottle. For details on the pros and cons of each method, see p. 896.

Feeding Formula

When bilirubin levels rise high enough to be of concern in a healthy term baby, it is usually a result of compromised milk intake, which is likely due to one or more of the following reasons:

Expressed mother's milk and donor milk are the first and second choices if the baby needs more milk than he receives during nursing.

- **Too little time spent nursing effectively,** either too few feeds or too little time actively nursing at each session
- **Nursing ineffectively due to oral variations,** such as tongue-tie, unusual palate, or other infant factors (see the section "Oral Anatomy of the Nursing Baby," starting on p. 262 in Chapter 8.
- **Low milk production,** possibly related to lack of stimulation (above) or other factors (see Box 10.1 on p. 436 in Chapter 10).

Whatever the reason for insufficient milk intake, the baby still needs to be fed. When considering a supplement, the first choice is expressed milk. If the baby is willing to take larger volumes than the nursing parent can express, the second choice, if available, is donor human milk (Flaherman et al., 2017).

• • •

Elemental formula is the third choice for supplementing a jaundiced baby.

When a jaundiced baby needs a supplement and there is not enough expressed milk and donor milk available, elemental (casein–hydrolysate or extensively hydrolyzed) formulas, such as Alimentum and Nutramigen, are recommended over other infant formulas for two reasons:

- They reduce bilirubin levels faster than other formulas, because they contain an ingredient that is more effective at preventing bilirubin in the baby's intestine from being reabsorbed (Gourley, Kreamer, Cohnen, & Kosorok, 1999; He & Pan, 2017).
- They are less likely to sensitize newborns to allergy (Urashima et al., 2019).

If the baby is fed formula, let the family know this is temporary and suggest taking steps to increase milk production by expressing milk and nursing frequently until the baby's needs are met while nursing. Suggest also considering the use of a nursing supplementer (see p. 897) to stimulate milk production while formula is fed.

• • •

Formula may be recommended as a supplement or as a temporary replacement for nursing.

When high bilirubin levels are primarily caused by lack of milk intake, even before the baby's bilirubin reaches the level at which phototherapy is recommended (see next section), some healthcare providers suggest formula supplements or a temporary interruption of nursing, during which baby is fed only formula. Although no short- or long-term ill effects have been associated with phototherapy (Itoh, Okada, Kuboi, & Kusaka, 2017), it can be a costly treatment and lengthen the hospital stay, so some healthcare providers consider this a more cost-effective alternative.

Depending on the baby's bilirubin levels, giving formula supplements while nursing may be recommended as a 12-hour trial or a 24-hour interruption of nursing with or without phototherapy, which may be extended to 48 hours if the baby's bilirubin levels have not decreased significantly.

KEY CONCEPT

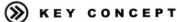

Nursing should continue, if at all possible, during treatment for jaundice.

If the baby's healthcare provider recommends the baby be given formula and the family wants to explore other alternatives, suggest seeking a second opinion.

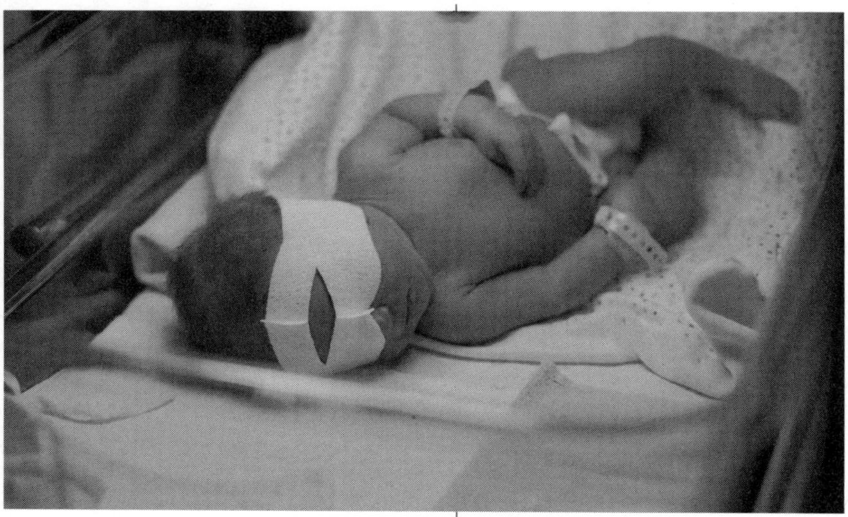

A temporary weaning puts nursing at risk. Whether nursing is interrupted for 12, 24, or 48 hours, suggest expressing milk to stay comfortable and to establish or maintain milk production. For expression strategies to meet the family's goals, see p. 498 in Chapter 11. Also, be sure the family understands the value of mother's milk and the reasons for the interruption. Many families of jaundiced babies assume that formula is recommended because their milk is "bad" for their baby, which can lead to feelings of guilt and undermine continued nursing (Hannon et al., 2001). A 2015 study from China found that providing first-time parents with education about newborn jaundice during pregnancy (Zhang et al., 2015) led to better nursing outcomes when jaundice occurred.

Phototherapy

Phototherapy uses special fluorescent or spotlights to lower bilirubin levels faster.

During phototherapy, typically the baby is laid nearly naked with his eyes covered under a white, blue, or green fluorescent light (called ***bili-lights***). This light is absorbed by the bilirubin under baby's skin, changing it to a water-soluble form that allows the baby to eliminate it without needing to first process it in his liver. Phototherapy can be used for all types of jaundice and is sometimes used along with other treatments. Phototherapy is a relatively safe procedure that has fewer side effects than alternatives like exchange transfusions (Bhutani, Committee on, Newborn, & American Academy of, 2011) (see next section).

• • •

The bilirubin level at which phototherapy should be started depends on the baby's age, his risk factors, and where he lives.

As with hypoglycemia (low blood sugar), one level of bilirubin does not reflect the many factors that determine the effect of that level on an individual baby. With a jaundiced newborn, some of the factors that affect when phototherapy should begin include the baby's gestational age, how soon after birth his jaundice appeared, how fast his bilirubin levels are rising, the compatibility of his blood type with his birthing parent, any bruising, a sibling with a history of jaundice, his race, and the jaundice guidelines in the country where he lives.

The U.K. phototherapy guidelines for jaundiced babies younger than 28 days and born at least 38 weeks (NICE, 2016) are online at: **bit.ly/BA2-UKJaundice**. (The online guidelines are interactive, with the recommended levels for treatment going down when users enter an earlier gestational age.) These guidelines recommend beginning phototherapy at different bilirubin levels, depending on baby's age, and are presented as a line on a graph. The line that indicates at what bilirubin level phototherapy should begin gradually goes up from birth through each 24-hour day during the first 4 days and beyond:

- Birth: 100 μmol/L (5.8 mg/dL)
- 1 day (24 hours): 200 μmol/L (11.7 mg/dL)
- 2 days (48 hours): 250 μmol/L (14.6 mg/dL)
- 3 days (72 hours): 300 μmol/L (17.5 mg/dL)
- 4-28 days: 350 μmol/L (20.5 mg/dL)

The American Academy of Pediatrics' practice guidelines for starting phototherapy on hospitalized newborns born at least 35 weeks gestation first divides newborns by risk into three groups (AAP, 2004):

- Lower risk (≥38 weeks at birth and healthy)
- Medium risk (≥38 weeks at birth with risk factors or 35 to 35 6/7 weeks at birth and healthy)
- Higher risk (35 to 35 6/7 weeks at birth with risk factors)

They define major risk factors as:

- Bilirubin levels in the high-risk zone (if 3 days or older >16 mg/dl)
- Jaundice visible during the first 24 hours
- Blood group incompatibility or other hemolytic (blood) disease
- An older sibling who received phototherapy
- Significant bruising or cephalohematoma
- Exclusive breastfeeding with feeding problems and/or weight loss ≥12%
- East Asian race

Along with the baby's bilirubin level, the rate at which bilirubin is rising is also important. A rise of more than 0.5 mg/dL (8.5 μmol/L) per hour puts the baby at increased risk.

Like the U.S., the Canadian Paediatric Society divided newborns into groups based on risk factors. The Canadian guidelines are available online at: **bit.ly/BA2-CPS.**

• • •

A preterm baby is at greater risk of brain injury at lower bilirubin levels because his immature liver is less effective at processing bilirubin and his blood-brain barrier is less effective at blocking it. Adding illness (such as infection, oxygen deprivation, and blood imbalances) to prematurity increases the risk of injury at lower bilirubin levels. Safe bilirubin levels for the preemie are determined individually based on the baby's gestational age, weight, and health.

Safe bilirubin levels are lower in babies born earlier than 35 weeks.

TABLE 7.2 U.S. Guidelines for Phototherapy in Babies Born ≥35 Weeks Gestation

Baby's Age in Hours	Lower Risk	Intermediate Risk	Higher Risk
24 Hours	12 mg/dL (204 μmol/L)	10 mg/dL (170 μmol/L)	8 mg/dL (136 μmol/L)
48 Hours	15 mg/dL (255 μmol/L)	13 mg/dL (221 μmol/L)	11 mg/dL (187 μmol/L)
72 Hours	17 mg/dL (289 μmol/L)	15 mg/dL (255 μmol/L)	13 mg/dL (221 μmol/L)
96 Hours	20 mg/dL (340 μmol/L)	17 mg/dL (289 μmol/L)	14 mg/dL (238 μmol/L)
5 Days or older	21 mg/dL (357 μmol/L)	18 mg/dL (306 μmol/L)	15 mg/dL (255 μmol/L)

Adapted from (AAP, 2004, p. 304)

• • •

If the nursing couple is separated during phototherapy, discuss alternatives.

If the healthcare providers recommend separation during phototherapy, suggest asking about the following options.

- If phototherapy is given in the hospital nursery, can the nursing parent sit near the baby and nurse when he shows feeding cues?
- Can the bili-lights be set up in the nursing parent's room to make it easier to nurse the baby under the lights or to take the baby out from under the lights to nurse?
- Can a phototherapy unit (a fiberoptic blanket that wraps around the baby) be rented for hospital or home use?

An Indian study of 127 jaundiced newborns (Sachdeva, Murki, Oleti, & Kandraju, 2015) found that in late preterm and term babies who were otherwise healthy, intermittent phototherapy (12 hours on and 12 hours off) was just as effective as continuous phototherapy in reducing bilirubin levels.

> **KEY CONCEPT**
>
> *Phototherapy does not have to be continuous to be effective, so nursing need not be interrupted.*

A 2015 Chinese randomized controlled trial of 56 jaundiced term babies (Lin, Yang, Cheng, & Yen, 2015) found that the babies who were massaged during phototherapy had significantly lower bilirubin levels than the control group.

• • •

Nursing often during phototherapy can help meet the baby's need for extra fluids.

Babies lose more water than usual through their skin and stools during phototherapy. Frequent nursing can help offset this increased water loss. Be sure the family is aware that a baby's stools become looser during phototherapy as the bilirubin in the stools increases.

• • •

In some cases, formula may be recommended as a supplement or a replacement for nursing during phototherapy.

See the previous section "Feeding Formula" for more details. The Academy of Breastfeeding Medicine wrote in its 2017 Clinical Protocol #22 on jaundice (Flaherman et al., 2017, p. 253)

> "Phototherapy can be used while continuing full breastfeeding or it can be combined with supplementation of expressed breast milk or infant formula if maternal supply is insufficient. Only in extenuating circumstances is temporary interruption of breastfeeding with replacement feeding necessary."

Exchange Transfusions

If a baby's bilirubin levels are dangerously high or he has neurological symptoms, an exchange transfusion is recommended.

If a baby is at or near dangerously high bilirubin levels (see Table 7.3 on the next page for U.S. guidelines) or has symptoms of neurological injury, an exchange transfusion is the fastest way to bring down bilirubin levels. During an exchange transfusion, small amounts of the baby's blood are continuously replaced with donor blood. Because safe bilirubin levels are lower in sick or very preterm babies, exchange transfusions may be recommended at lower levels in these at-risk babies.

The U.K. exchange transfusion guidelines for jaundiced babies younger than 28 days born at least 38 weeks (NICE, 2016) are online at: **bit.ly/BA2-UKJaundice**. These guidelines recommend exchange transfusion at different bilirubin levels, depending on baby's age and are presented as a line on a graph. The line for exchange transfusions gradually goes up through the first 42 hours after birth and beyond:

- Birth: 100 μmol/L (5.8 mg/dL)
- 24 hours (1 day): 300 μmol/L (17.5 mg/dL)
- 42 hours-28 days: 450 μmol/L (26.3 mg/dL)

Exchange transfusions are used less often today than in years past due to the use of RhoGAM to prevent severe jaundice from Rh incompatibility. There are more health risks associated with exchange transfusions than phototherapy, so phototherapy is routinely used first to prevent the need for this procedure (AAP, 2004).

• • •

The baby receiving exchange transfusions should continue to nurse because withholding feeds can increase bilirubin levels.

Nursing can continue before and after exchange transfusions.

Other Jaundice Treatments

The drug tin-mesoporphyrin reduces jaundice by preventing hemoglobin from being converted to bilirubin. A 2016 randomized placebo-controlled clinical trial found it to be effective in rapidly reducing bilirubin levels in babies 35 weeks gestation whose TcB screening put them above the 75th percentile in bilirubin levels (Bhutani et al., 2016). At this writing, however, this drug has not yet been approved for use in the U.S. by the Food and Drug Administration (FDA), so is not available for use.

Some medications can bring down bilirubin levels.

Other drugs have been used to treat jaundice. One example is the anti-seizure medication phenobarbital, but it takes about 6 days before it significantly lowers bilirubin levels. Cholestyramine was also used during phototherapy, but it was not found to be very effective.

TABLE 7.3 U.S. Guidelines for Exchange Transfusions in Babies Born ≥35 Weeks Gestation

Baby's Age in Hours	Lower Risk	Intermediate Risk	Higher Risk
24 Hours	19 mg/dL (323 μmol/L)	17 mg/dL (289 μmol/L)	15 mg/dL (255 μmol/L)
48 Hours	22 mg/dL (374 μmol/L)	19 mg/dL (323 μmol/L)	17 mg/dL (289 μmol/L)
72 Hours	24 mg/dL (408 μmol/L)	21 mg/dL (357 μmol/L)	18 mg/dL (306 μmol/L)
96 Hours	25 mg/dL (425 μmol/L)	22 mg/dL (374 μmol/L)	19 mg/dL (323 μmol/L)

Adapted from (AAP, 2004, p. 513)

What to Avoid

Some drugs or other treatments may increase the risk of injury from jaundice when used by the baby or the nursing parent.

Aspirin, other salicylates, ibuprofen, and certain sulfa drugs can increase the risk of injury from jaundice by preventing bilirubin from binding to the protein in the baby's blood (Gartner, 2007; Zecca et al., 2009). Other drugs and treatments that can have this same effect include the antibiotic sulfisoxazole (Gantrisin), benzyl alcohol, and its byproduct, benzoic acid, a preservative in some IV fluids. When a newborn is jaundiced, these treatments in either nursing parent or baby should be avoided and, if needed, a substitute found.

• • •

Glucose or plain water supplements should be avoided, because they do not prevent jaundice and may increase bilirubin levels.

Because only 2% of a baby's bilirubin is excreted in his urine and 98% in his stools, glucose or plain water supplements do not prevent jaundice or bring down a newborn's bilirubin levels. In fact, one classic U.S. study (Nicoll, Ginsburg, & Tripp, 1982) found that water supplements were associated with higher bilirubin levels. This may be because water supplements leave the baby feeling full without providing nourishment. Another U.S. study from the same era (Kuhr & Paneth, 1982) found that babies fed large volumes of glucose water during their first 3 days took less milk per feed by the fourth day and were more likely to be jaundiced than the babies not fed glucose water. U.K. research (de Carvalho, Hall, & Harvey, 1981) found plain water supplements had no effect on bilirubin levels. As a result, health organizations in both the U.S. and Canada recommend against giving plain or glucose water supplements to newborns (AAP, 2004; CPS, 2007).

• • •

Putting the baby in indirect sunlight is not recommended to treat jaundice in developed countries, but filtered sunlight treatments may be an effective strategy in developing nations.

In years past, some families were advised to undress their jaundiced baby to his diaper and lay him near a window, because like phototherapy, indirect sunlight could help bring down bilirubin levels. However, unlike phototherapy, with this home treatment, it is impossible to gauge the amount of light the baby receives and its effect on his bilirubin levels. Another potential downside is that some babies may be put in direct sunlight, which could cause a dangerous increase in body temperature and burn his skin. For these reasons, parents are cautioned against using indirect sunlight as an alternative treatment for jaundice. Some Australian researchers (Harrison, Devine, et al., 2013; Harrison, Nowack, et al., 2013) tested strategies for dissuading families from using indirect sunlight as a substitute for medical treatment. This was also one of the goals of Chinese researchers, who found that providing education to families about newborn jaundice during pregnancy made them more aware of best practices before their baby's birth (Zhang et al., 2015). A jaundiced baby should be promptly seen and evaluated by a healthcare provider.

A different, scientifically validated version of sunlight therapy for jaundice may soon be adopted in some areas where phototherapy (and electricity to power it) are not always available. In these parts of the developing world, many newborns die or suffer permanent neurological damage from severe jaundice (Slusher, Zamora, et al., 2017). An inexpensive, low-tech treatment was developed and researched that uses sunlight passing through a simple canopy—which the baby lies under—to treat jaundice (Slusher et al., 2014). The canopy filters out the harmful UVA and UVB rays from the sun that can cause skin damage but lets through the blue light from sunlight that, like phototherapy, breaks down the bilirubin. A 2015 randomized controlled trial done in Nigeria (Slusher et al.,

2015) randomly assigned its 447 moderately jaundiced babies into two groups: one group received phototherapy and a second group was treated under the filtered sunlight canopies. The study found that these simple canopies provided a safe and effective alternative to phototherapy, and this result was replicated in other studies (Slusher, Day, Ogundele, Woolfield, & Owa, 2017; Slusher et al., 2018). For more details, see the *New England Journal of Medicine* YouTube video about this research at: **bit.ly/BA2-NEJM**.

REFERENCES

AAP. (2004). Management of hyperbilirubinemia in the newborn infant 35 or more weeks of gestation. *Pediatrics, 114*(1), 297-316.

AAP. (2012). Breastfeeding and the use of human milk. *Pediatrics, 129*(3), e827-e841.

Adamkin, D. H., Committee on, F., & Newborn. (2011). Postnatal glucose homeostasis in late-preterm and term infants. *Pediatrics, 127*(3), 575-579.

Alsweiler, J. M., Woodall, S. M., Crowther, C. A., et al. (2018). Oral dextrose gel to treat neonatal hypoglycaemia: Clinician survey. *Journal of Paediatrics and Child Health.* doi:10.1111/jpc.14306

Badejoko, B. O., Owa, J. A., Oseni, S. B., et al. (2014). Early neonatal bilirubin, hematocrit, and glucose-6-phosphate dehydrogenase status. *Pediatrics, 134*(4), e1082-1088.

Baranano, D. E., Rao, M., Ferris, C. D., et al. (2002). Biliverdin reductase: A major physiologic cytoprotectant. *Proceedings of the National Academy of Sciences USA, 99*(25), 16093-16098.

Bergman, N. J., Linley, L. L., & Fawcus, S. R. (2004). Randomized controlled trial of skin-to-skin contact from birth versus conventional incubator for physiological stabilization in 1200- to 2199-gram newborns. *Acta Paediatrica, 93*(6), 779-785.

Bhutani, V. K., Committee on, F., Newborn, et al. (2011). Phototherapy to prevent severe neonatal hyperbilirubinemia in the newborn infant 35 or more weeks of gestation. *Pediatrics, 128*(4), e1046-1052.

Bhutani, V. K., Poland, R., Meloy, L. D., et al. (2016). Clinical trial of tin mesoporphyrin to prevent neonatal hyperbilirubinemia. *Journal of Perinatology, 36*(7), 533-539.

Bhutani, V. K., Stark, A. R., Lazzeroni, L. C., et al. (2013). Predischarge screening for severe neonatal hyperbilirubinemia identifies infants who need phototherapy. *Journal of Pediatrics, 162*(3), 477-482 e471.

Boskabadi, H., & Zakerihamidi, M. (2017). The correlation between frequency and duration of breastfeeding and the severity of neonatal hyperbilirubinemia. *Journal of Maternal-Fetal & Neonatal Medicine, 31*(4), 457-463.

Boubred, F., Herlenius, E., Andres, V., et al. (2016). [Hospital readmission after postpartum discharge of term newborns in two maternity wards in Stockholm and Marseille]. *Archives de Pediatrie, 23*(3), 234-240.

Boundy, E. O., Dastjerdi, R., Spiegelman, D., et al. (2016). Kangaroo Mother Care and neonatal outcomes: A meta-analysis. *Pediatrics, 137*(1).

Bowles, B. C. (2011). Breast massage: A "handy" multipurpose tool to promote breastfeeding success. *Clinical Lactation, 2*(4), 21-24.

Bromiker, R., Medoff-Cooper, B., Flor-Hirsch, H., et al. (2016). Influence of hyperbilirubinemia on neonatal sucking. *Early Human Development, 99,* 53-56.

Buiter, H. D., Dijkstra, S. S., Oude Elferink, R. F., et al. (2008). Neonatal jaundice and stool production in breast- or formula-fed term infants. *European Journal of Pediatrics, 167*(5), 501-507.

Chertok, I. R., Raz, I., Shoham, I., et al. (2009). Effects of early breastfeeding on neonatal glucose levels of term infants born to women with gestational diabetes. *Journal of Human Nutrition and Dietetics, 22*(2), 166-169.

Christensson, K., Siles, C., Moreno, L., et al. (1992). Temperature, metabolic adaptation and crying in healthy full-term newborns cared for skin-to-skin or in a cot. *Acta Paediatrica, 81*(6-7), 488-493.

Colson, S., DeRooy, L., & Hawdon, J. (2003). Biological nurturing increases duration of breastfeeding for a vulnerable cohort. *MIDIRS Midwifery Digest, 13*(1), 92-97.

Cornblath, M., Hawdon, J. M., Williams, A. F., et al. (2000). Controversies regarding definition of neonatal hypoglycemia: Suggested operational thresholds. *Pediatrics, 105*(5), 1141-1145.

Cornblath, M., & Ichord, R. (2000). Hypoglycemia in the neonate. *Seminars in Perinatology, 24*(2), 136-149.

CPS. (2007). Guidelines for detection, management and prevention of hyperbilirubinemia in term and late preterm newborn infants (35 or more weeks' gestation) - Summary. *Paediatrics & Child Health, 12*(5), 401-418.

Dalsgaard, B. T., Rodrigo-Domingo, M., Kronborg, H., et al. (2019). Breastfeeding and skin-to-skin contact as non-pharmacological prevention of neonatal hypoglycemia in infants born to women with gestational diabetes; A Danish quasi-experimental study. *Sexual & Reproductive Healthcare, 19,* 1-8.

Darling, E. K., Ramsay, T., Sprague, A. E., et al. (2014). Universal bilirubin screening and health care utilization. *Pediatrics, 134*(4), e1017-1024.

de Carvalho, M., Hall, M., & Harvey, D. (1981). Effects of water supplementation on physiological jaundice in breast-fed babies. *Archives of Disease in Childhood, 56*(7), 568-569.

de Rooy, L., & Hawdon, J. (2002). Nutritional factors that affect the postnatal metabolic adaptation of full-term small- and large-for-gestational-age infants. *Pediatrics, 109*(3), E42.

Djousse, L., Levy, D., Cupples, L. A., et al. (2001). Total serum bilirubin and risk of cardiovascular disease in the Framingham offspring study. *American Journal of Cardiology, 87*(10), 1196-1200; A1194, 1197.

Draque, C. M., Sanudo, A., de Araujo Peres, C., et al. (2011). Transcutaneous bilirubin in exclusively breastfed healthy term newborns up to 12 days of life. *Pediatrics, 128*(3), e565-571. doi:10.1542/peds.2010-3878

Eidelman, A. I. (2001). Hypoglycemia and the breastfed neonate. *Pediatric Clinics of North America, 48*(2), 377-387.

Flaherman, V. J., Maisels, M. J., & Academy of Breastfeeding, M. (2017). ABM Clinical Protocol #22: Guidelines for management of jaundice in the breastfeeding infant 35 weeks or more of gestation-revised 2017. *Breastfeeding Medicine, 12*(5), 250-257.

Gale, C., Statnikov, Y., Jawad, S., et al. (2018). Neonatal brain injuries in England: Population-based incidence derived from routinely recorded clinical data held in the National Neonatal Research Database. *Archives of Disease in Childhood. Fetal and Neonatal Edition, 103*(4), F301-F306.

Gamaleldin, R., Iskander, I., Seoud, I., et al. (2011). Risk factors for neurotoxicity in newborns with severe neonatal hyperbilirubinemia. *Pediatrics, 128*(4), e925-931.

Gartner, L. M. (2007). Hyperbilirubinemia and breastfeeding. In T. W. Hale & P. E. Hartmann (Eds.), *Hale & Hartmann's Textbook of Human Lactation* (pp. 255-270). Amarillo, TX: Hale Publishing.

Glasgow, M. J., Harding, J. E., Edlin, R., et al. (2018). Cost analysis of treating neonatal hypoglycemia with dextrose gel. *Journal of Pediatrics, 198,* 151-155 e151.

Gourley, G. R., Kreamer, B., Cohnen, M., et al. (1999). Neonatal jaundice and diet. *Archives of Pediatrics and Adolescent Medicine, 153*(2), 184-188.

Guemes, M., Rahman, S. A., & Hussain, K. (2016). What is a normal blood glucose? *Archives of Disease in Childhood, 101*(6), 569-574.

Hagedorn, M. I. E., & Gardner, S. L. (1999). Hypoglycemia in the newborn, part 1: Pathophysiology and nursing management. *Mother Baby J, 4,* 15-21.

Hannon, P. R., Willis, S. K., & Scrimshaw, S. C. (2001). Persistence of maternal concerns surrounding neonatal jaundice: An exploratory study. *Archives of Pediatrics and Adolescent Medicine, 155*(12), 1357-1363.

Hansen, R., Gibson, S., De Paiva Alves, E., et al. (2018). Adaptive response of neonatal sepsis-derived Group B Streptococcus to bilirubin. *Scientific Reports, 8*(1), 6470.

Harding, J. E., Harris, D. L., Hegarty, J. E., et al. (2017). An emerging evidence base for the management of neonatal hypoglycaemia. *Early Human Development,. 104,* 51-56.

Harris, D. L., Weston, P. J., & Harding, J. E. (2015). Lactate, rather than ketones, may provide alternative cerebral fuel in hypoglycaemic newborns. *Archives of Disease in Childhood. Fetal and Neonatal Edition, 100*(2), F161-164.

Harrison, S. L., Devine, S. G., Saunders, V. L., et al. (2013). Changing the risky beliefs of post-partum women about therapeutic sun-exposure. *Women and Birth, 26*(3), 202-206.

Harrison, S. L., Nowack, M., Devine, S. G., et al. (2013). An intervention to discourage Australian mothers from unnecessarily exposing their babies to the sun for therapeutic reasons. *Journal of Tropical Pediatrics, 59*(5), 403-406.

Hawdon, J., & Williams, A. F. (2000). Formula supplements given to healthy breastfed preterm babies inhibit postnatal metabolic adaptation: Results of a randomised controlled trial [Abstract]. *Archives of Disease in Childhood, 82*(Supplement 1).

Hawdon, J. M. (1999). Hypoglycaemia and the neonatal brain. *European Journal of Pediatrics, 158 Suppl 1,* S9-S12.

Hawdon, J. M., Platt, M. P., & Aynsley-Green, A. (1993). Neonatal hypoglycaemia--blood glucose monitoring and baby feeding. *Midwifery, 9*(1), 3-6.

Hawdon, J. M., Ward Platt, M. P., & Aynsley-Green, A. (1992). Patterns of metabolic adaptation for preterm and term infants in the first neonatal week. *Archives of Disease in Childhood, 67*(4 Spec No), 357-365.

Hawdon, J. M., Ward Platt, M. P., McPhail, S., et al. (1992). Prediction of impaired metabolic adaptation by antenatal Doppler studies in small for gestational age fetuses. *Archives of Disease in Childhood, 67*(7 Spec No), 789-792.

He, W., & Pan, J.-H. (2017). Clinical effect of extensively hydrolyzed formula in preterm infants: An analysis of 327 cases. *Chinese Journal of Contemporary Pediatrics, 19*(8), 856-869.

Hegyi, T., Goldie, E., & Hiatt, M. (1994). The protective role of bilirubin in oxygen-radical diseases of the preterm infant. *Journal of Perinatology, 14*(4), 296-300.

Heyman, E., Ohlsson, A., & Girschek, P. (1989). Retinopathy of prematurity and bilirubin. *New England Journal of Medicine, 320*(4), 256.

Holland, L., & Blick, K. (2009). Implementing and validating transcutaneous bilirubinometry for neonates. *American Journal of Clinical Pathology, 132*(4), 555-561.

Hoseth, E., Joergensen, A., Ebbesen, F., et al. (2000). Blood glucose levels in a population of healthy, breast fed, term infants of appropriate size for gestational age. *Archives of Disease in Childhood. Fetal and Neonatal Edition, 83*(2), F117-119.

Huang, A., Tai, B. C., Wong, L. Y., et al. (2009). Differential risk for early breastfeeding jaundice in a multi-ethnic Asian cohort. *Annals of the Academy of Medicine, Singapore, 38*(3), 217-224.

Inder, T. (2008). How low can I go? The impact of hypoglycemia on the immature brain. *Pediatrics, 122*(2), 440-441.

Ip, S., Lau, J., Chung, M., et al. (2004). Hyperbilirubinemia and kernicterus: 50 years later. *Pediatrics, 114*(1), 263-264.

Itoh, S., Okada, H., Kuboi, T., et al. (2017). Phototherapy for neonatal hyperbilirubinemia. *Pediatrics International, 59*(9), 959-966.

Jangaard, K. A., Fell, D. B., Dodds, L., et al. (2008). Outcomes in a population of healthy term and near-term infants with serum bilirubin levels of >or=325 micromol/L (>or=19 mg/dL) who were born in Nova Scotia, Canada, between 1994 and 2000. *Pediatrics, 122*(1), 119-124.

Kaplan, M., & Bromiker, R. (2019). Variation in transcutaneous bilirubin nomograms across population groups. *Journal of Pediatrics.* doi:10.1016/j.jpeds.2019.01.036

Kaplan, M., Herschel, M., Hammerman, C., et al. (2004). Hyperbilirubinemia among African American, glucose-6-phosphate dehydrogenase-deficient neonates. *Pediatrics, 114*(2), e213-219.

Kemper, K., Forsyth, B., & McCarthy, P. (1989). Jaundice, terminating breast-feeding, and the vulnerable child. *Pediatrics, 84*(5), 773-778.

Kemper, K. J., Forsyth, B. W., & McCarthy, P. L. (1990). Persistent perceptions of vulnerability following neonatal jaundice. *American Journal of Diseases of Children, 144*(2), 238-241.

Kuhr, M., & Paneth, N. (1982). Feeding practices and early neonatal jaundice. *Journal of Pediatric Gastroenterology and Nutrition, 1*(4), 485-488.

LeBlanc, S., Haushalter, J., Seashore, C., et al. (2018). A quality-improvement initiative to reduce NICU transfers for neonates at risk for hypoglycemia. *Pediatrics, 141*(3).

Lee, A. C., Folger, L. V., Rahman, M., et al. (2019). A novel icterometer for hyperbilirubinemia screening in low-resource settings. *Pediatrics, 143*(5).

Levene, I., & Wilkinson, D. (2019). Identification and management of neonatal hypoglycaemia in the full-term infant (British Association of Perinatal Medicine-Framework for Practice). *Archives of Disease in Childhood - Education and Practice Edition, 104*(1), 29-32.

Lin, C. H., Yang, H. C., Cheng, C. S., et al. (2015). Effects of infant massage on jaundiced neonates undergoing phototherapy. *Italian Journal of Pediatrics, 41,* 94.

Linder, N., Moser, A. M., Asli, I., et al. (1989). Suckling stimulation test for neonatal tremor. *Archives of Disease in Childhood, 64*(1 Spec No), 44-46.

Maisels, M. J. (2015). Managing the jaundiced newborn: A persistent challenge. *Canadian Medical Association Journal, 187*(5), 335-343.

McDonagh, A. F. (1990). Is bilirubin good for you? *Clinics in Perinatology, 17,* 359-369.

Morton, J. (2019). Hands-on or hands-off when first milk matters most? *Breastfeeding Medicine, 14*(5), 295-297.

Nelson, A. M. (2017). Risks and benefits of swaddling healthy infants: An integrative review. *MCN American Journal of Maternal and Child Nursing, 42*(4), 216-225.

NICE. (2016). Jaundice in the newborn babies under 28 days. *London, UK: National Institute for Health and Care Excellence* (NICE).

Nicoll, A., Ginsburg, R., & Tripp, J. H. (1982). Supplementary feeding and jaundice in newborns. *Acta Paediatrica Scandinavica, 71*(5), 759-761.

Sachdeva, M., Murki, S., Oleti, T. P., et al. (2015). Intermittent versus continuous phototherapy for the treatment of neonatal non-hemolytic moderate hyperbilirubinemia in infants more than 34 weeks of gestational age: A randomized controlled trial. *European Journal of Pediatrics, 174*(2), 177-181.

Sedlak, T. W., & Snyder, S. H. (2004). Bilirubin benefits: Cellular protection by a biliverdin reductase antioxidant cycle. *Pediatrics, 113*(6), 1776-1782.

Sexson, W. R. (1984). Incidence of neonatal hypoglycemia: A matter of definition. *Journal of Pediatrics, 105*(1), 149-150.

Siu, S. L., Chan, L. W., & Kwong, A. N. (2018). Clinical and biochemical characteristics of infants with prolonged neonatal jaundice. *Hong Kong Medical Journal, 24*(3), 270-276.

Slusher, T. M., Day, L. T., Ogundele, T., et al. (2017). Filtered sunlight, solar powered phototherapy and other strategies for managing neonatal jaundice in low-resource settings. *Early Human Development, 114,* 11-15.

Slusher, T. M., Olusanya, B. O., Vreman, H. J., et al. (2015). A randomized trial of phototherapy with filtered sunlight in African neonates. *New England Journal of Medicine, 373*(12), 1115-1124.

Slusher, T. M., Vreman, H. J., Brearley, A. M., et al. (2018). Filtered sunlight versus intensive electric powered phototherapy in moderate-to-severe neonatal hyperbilirubinaemia: A randomised controlled non-inferiority trial. *Lancet Global Health, 6*(10), e1122-e1131.

Slusher, T. M., Vreman, H. J., Olusanya, B. O., et al. (2014). Safety and efficacy of filtered sunlight in treatment of jaundice in African neonates. *Pediatrics, 133*(6), e1568-1574.

Slusher, T. M., Zamora, T. G., Appiah, D., et al. (2017). Burden of severe neonatal jaundice: A systematic review and meta-analysis. *BMJ Paeditrics Open, 1*(1), e000105.

Sweet, D. G., Hadden, D., & Halliday, H. L. (1999). The effect of early feeding on the neonatal blood glucose level at 1-hour of age. *Early Human Development, 55*(1), 63-66.

Swenne, I., Ewald, U., Gustafsson, J., et al. (1994). Inter-relationship between serum concentrations of glucose, glucagon and insulin during the first two days of life in healthy newborns. *Acta Paediatrica, 83*(9), 915-919.

Taylor, J. A., Burgos, A. E., Flaherman, V., et al. (2015). Discrepancies between transcutaneous and serum bilirubin measurements. *Pediatrics, 135*(2), 224-231.

Taylor, J. A., Stout, J. W., de Greef, L., et al. (2017). Use of a smartphone app to assess neonatal jaundice. *Pediatrics, 140*(3).

Temme, E. H., Zhang, J., Schouten, E. G., et al. (2001). Serum bilirubin and 10-year mortality risk in a Belgian population. *Cancer Causes Control, 12*(10), 887-894.

Thompson-Branch, A., & Havranek, T. (2017). Neonatal hypoglycemia. *Pediatrics in Review, 38*(4), 147-157.

Urashima, M., Mezawa, H., Okuyama, M., et al. (2019). Primary prevention of cow's milk sensitization and food allergy by avoiding supplementation with cow's milk formula at birth: A randomized clinical trial. *JAMA Pediatrics.* doi:10.1001/jamapediatrics.2019.3544

van Zoeren-Grobben, D., Lindeman, J. H., Houdkamp, E., et al. (1994). Postnatal changes in plasma chain-breaking antioxidants in healthy preterm infants fed formula and/or human milk. *American Journal of Clinical Nutrition, 60*(6), 900-906.

Walker, M. (2017). *Breastfeeding Management for the Clinician: Using the Evidence* (4th ed.). Burlington, MA: Jones & Bartlett Learning.

Weston, P. J., Harris, D. L., Battin, M., et al. (2016). Oral dextrose gel for the treatment of hypoglycaemia in newborn infants. *Cochrane Database of Systematic Reviews*(5), CD011027. doi:10.1002/14651858.CD011027.pub2

Weston, P. J., Harris, D. L., & Harding, J. E. (2017). Dextrose gel treatment does not impair subsequent feeding. *Archives of Disease in Childhood, Fetal and Neonatal Edition, 102*(6), F539-F541.

WHO. (1997). Hypoglycaemia of the newborn: Review of the literature. Retrieved from **http://whqlibdoc.who.int/hq/1997/WHO_CHD_97.1.pdf**

Wight, N., Marinelli, K. A., & Academy of Breastfeeding, M. (2014). ABM Clinical Protocol #1: Guidelines for blood glucose monitoring and treatment of hypoglycemia in term and late-preterm neonates, revised 2014. *Breastfeeding Medicine, 9*(4), 173-179.

Wight, N. E. (2006). Hypoglycemia in breastfed neonates. *Breastfeeding Medicine, 1*(4), 253-262.

Willis, S. K., Hannon, P. R., & Scrimshaw, S. C. (2002). The impact of the maternal experience with a jaundiced newborn on the breastfeeding relationship. *Journal of Family Practice, 51*(5), 465.

Zecca, E., Romagnoli, C., De Carolis, M. P., et al. (2009). Does Ibuprofen increase neonatal hyperbilirubinemia? *Pediatrics, 124*(2), 480-484.

Zhang, L., Hu, P., Wang, J., et al. (2015). Prenatal training improves new mothers' understanding of jaundice. *Medical Science Monitor, 21,* 1668-1673.

Zhou, Y., Bai, S., Bornhorst, J. A., et al. (2017). The effect of early feeding on initial glucose concentrations in term newborns. *Journal of Pediatrics, 181,* 112-115.

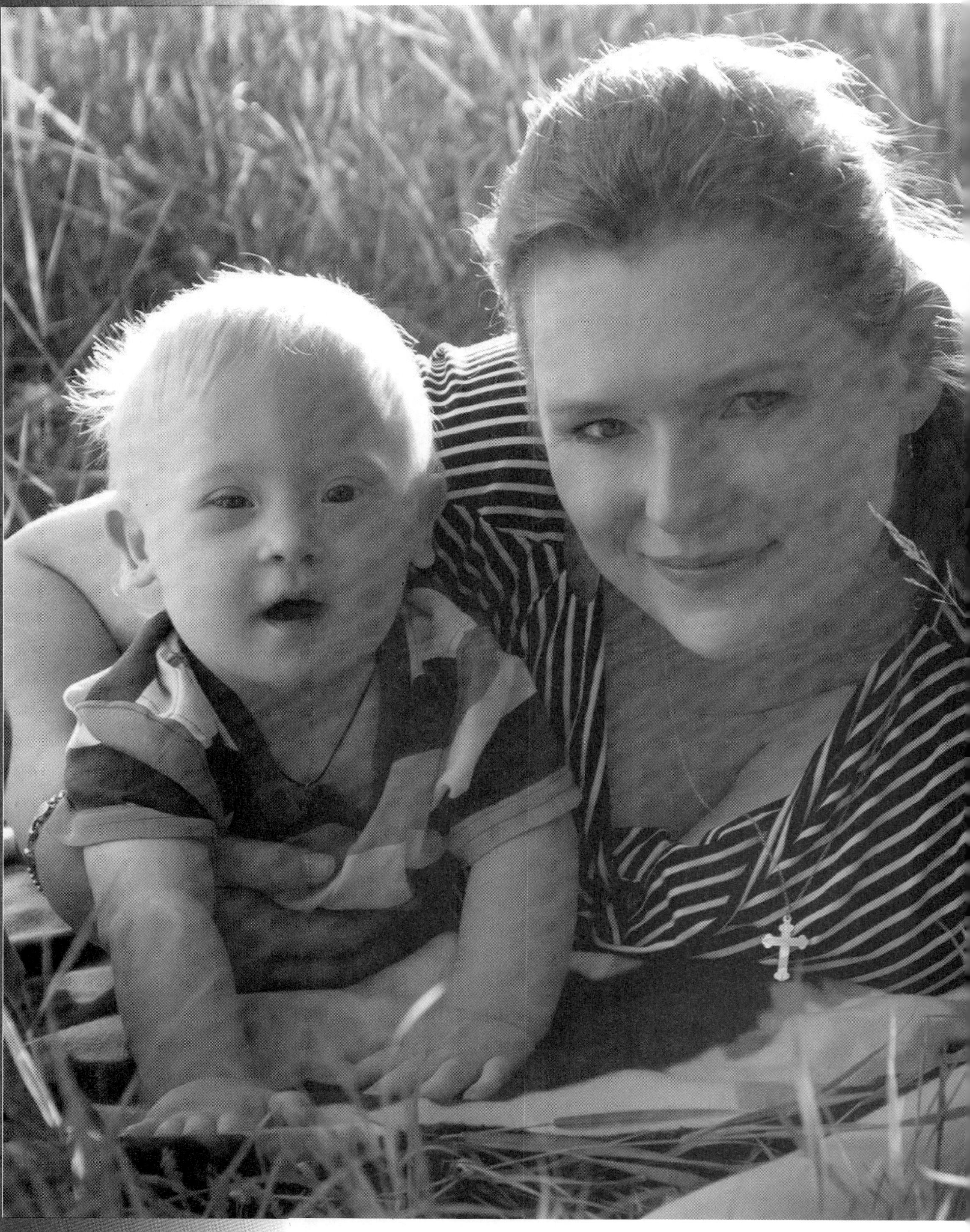

Baby's Anatomy and Health Issues

8

ORAL ANATOMY OF THE NURSING BABY

The baby's tongue, lips, cheeks, palate, and jaws all play vital roles in nursing, and their characteristics are determined by genetics and environment.

Both genetics and environment play a role in some aspects of a baby's oral anatomy. The palate, for example, is molded in utero by the baby's tongue. After birth, babies who are bottle-fed are more likely to have a narrow dental arch than nursing babies (Boronat-Catala, Montiel-Company, Bellot-Arcis, Almerich-Silla, & Catala-Pizarro, 2017). This is due to the regular experience of the firm bottle teat against the baby's palate (Palmer, 1998). Some previously intubated babies develop a groove in their palate as a result (Alves & Luiz, 2012). Some have noted a connection between tongue-tie and an unusually shaped palate (Wilson-Clay & Hoover, 2017). A tongue without a normal range of movement may mold a baby's palate differently.

Baby's Tongue

To nurse effectively, a baby's tongue needs the freedom of movement to extend, lift, lower, and form a groove.

The baby's tongue length, symmetry, and tone may affect feeding, as well as some characteristics of the baby's frenulum, the string-like membrane that attaches the baby's tongue to the floor of her mouth. These include its attachment locations, thickness, consistency and elasticity (see next section).

To suck and swallow effectively, a baby needs the ability to:

- **Extend her tongue past her lower gum** to help cushion the mammary tissue for comfortable nursing
- **Lift the front of her tongue to the roof of her mouth** (Figure 8.1) to keep the nipple in place
- **Lower the back of her tongue** to create the vacuum needed to remove the milk (P. Douglas & Geddes, 2018; Elad et al., 2014)
- **Form a groove with her tongue** to keep the nipple in place and collect the milk for easier swallowing

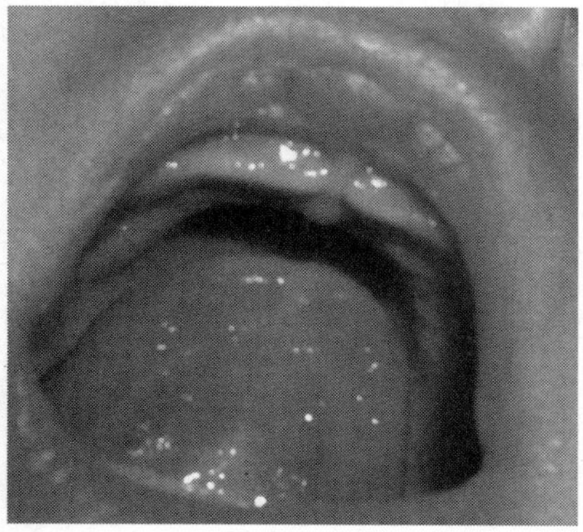

Figure 8.1 Normal tongue elevation. ©2020 Catherine Watson Genna, BS, IBCLC, used with permission.

How much these tongue movements are restricted will determine in part whether or not the baby can nurse effectively. The ability to move the tongue from side to side (called lateralization) does not usually affect nursing (C. W. Genna, 2017b) but it becomes important when a baby eats solid foods (Hiiemae & Palmer, 2003).

In addition to nursing, tongue movements also perform other functions, such as cleaning the teeth, forming speech, bottle feeding, and chewing and moving food.

How the baby moves her tongue can be influenced by her experiences. For example, some babies develop an aversion to anything entering their mouths after being roughly aspirated after birth (L. J. Smith, 2017) or shoved roughly during latch (Svensson, Velandia, Matthiesen, Welles-Nystrom, & Widstrom, 2013). When this happens, babies may use their tongue to block entry to their mouth, contributing to feeding problems.

Tongue-tie (Ankyloglossia)

Tongue-tie or ankyloglossia refers to a lingual frenulum (the membrane under the tongue that attaches it to the floor of the mouth) that is tight, fibrous, or thick enough to restrict normal tongue movement (C. W. Genna, 2017b). Tongue-tie was mentioned by Aristotle as early as 350 B.C. (Patel, Anthonappa, & King, 2018). How do we know if a baby's frenulum is normal in thickness, elasticity, or consistency? Currently, there are no agreed-upon definitions for a normal frenulum. But research is underway. In one U.S. study, scientists took measurements of frenulum attachments in 100 healthy babies (R. D. Walker, Messing, Rosen-Carole, & McKenna Benoit, 2018), while in New Zealand, researchers dissected infant cadavers to better understand the underlying anatomy of the floor of the baby's mouth and how it affects oral function (Mills, Keough, Geddes, Pransky, & Mirjalili, 2019).

Symptomatic tongue-tie restricts tongue movements enough to affect nursing.

KEY CONCEPT

No definition exists of a normal frenulum, so rather than "short," use the term "symptomatic tongue-tie" when feeding problems are not solved with lactation help.

With no definition of a normal lingual frenulum and 99.5% of newborns having one (Haham, Marom, Mangel, Botzer, & Dollberg, 2014), the International Association of Tongue Tie Professionals (IATP, 2019) recommended against using the term "short frenulum" when defining tongue-tie and instead suggested using these terms:

- "Asymptomatic tongue-tie" to describe babies who nurse comfortably and effectively
- "Symptomatic tongue-tie" to describe babies who have nursing problems even after seeing a lactation consultant.

• • •

Symptomatic tongue-tie is more common in males and runs in families. Two U.S. studies found a positive family history of symptomatic tongue-tie in 21% (Ballard, Auer, & Khoury, 2002) and 33% (Pransky, Lago, & Hong, 2015) of the babies identified as tongue-tied. After taking extensive family histories of 149 South Korean patients being surgically treated for tongue-tie, one study (Han, Kim, Choi, Lim, & Han, 2012) found that 39% had a relative with symptomatic tongue-tie. They also found that symptomatic tongue-tie was about twice as common in males as females, the same ratio found in a Canadian population-based study (Joseph et al., 2016) and research from Brazil (Lima et al., 2019). If symptomatic tongue-tie is suspected in a baby, ask if there is a family history.

Incidence of symptomatic tongue-tie is estimated to be between 3% and 13% of all babies

Percentage of babies identified with symptomatic tongue-tie. In the early 2000s, most tongue-tie studies estimated the incidence of tongue-tie as between 3% and 5% (Ballard et al., 2002; Messner, Lalakea, Aby, Macmahon, & Bair, 2000; Ricke, Baker, Madlon-Kay, & DeFor, 2005). However, at that time, only the anterior types of tongue-tie (what some today call "classic tongue-ties" that attach near the baby's tongue tip) were generally recognized. (See later point for a summary of tongue-tie types.) Even in 2005, however, one U.K. randomized, controlled trial that checked all newborn babies for tongue-tie in a region in England over a 5-month period (Hogan, Westcott, & Griffiths, 2005) identified nearly 11% of newborns as tongue-tied. A 2015 Brazilian study of 109 newborns, identified 13% (14) with symptomatic tongue-tie (R. L. Martinelli, Marchesan, Gusmao, Honorio, & Berretin-Felix, 2015).

KEY CONCEPT

Many tongue-tied babies nurse without difficulty.

• • •

Some tongue-tied babies are symptomatic and some are asymptomatic, so when there are nursing problems, it is important to consider other causes, even when tongue-tie is present.

According to research—both old and new—many tongue-tied babies nurse without difficulty.

Percentage of babies with symptomatic tongue-tie. As described in the previous point, during the 2000s many identified only anterior tongue-ties (see later point), which restrict the front of the tongue. So, studies from this period may not reflect all tongue-tied babies. One U.S. prospective controlled study of 50 tongue-tied newborns (Messner et al., 2000) found that only 25% had trouble nursing. In a U.K. randomized, controlled trial of 201 tongue-tied babies (Hogan et al., 2005), researchers reported that about 44% struggled with nursing. A 2015 review of the literature (Power & Murphy, 2015) concluded that about 50% of tongue-tied babies are asymptomatic, or nurse well with no problem. With this in mind, when helping families, it is important to remember:

- When a tongue-tied baby has nursing problems, it is vital to carefully consider other possible causes, because the tongue-tie may not be contributing to the problem.
- Not every tongue-tied baby needs a tongue-tie release (frenotomy, see later point)

To determine which babies may benefit from surgical treatment and which may not, use the tongue-tie assessment tools in a later point.

Nursing problems common among symptomatic tongue-tied babies. One U.K. study of 215 tongue-tied babies who had nursing problems (Griffiths, 2004) found:

- 88% of the babies had difficulty latching
- 77% of the mothers had nipple pain or trauma
- 72% of the babies fed continuously while awake due to inadequate milk intake
- 52% of the nursing couples experienced all three of these symptoms

A clicking sound during nursing, as well as latching struggles and an inability to stay latched are signs a baby is unable to maintain suction during feeds and may not be transferring milk effectively. Any baby who repeatedly breaks the suction during nursing should be checked for tongue-tie. However, if despite the clicking, the baby is gaining weight well, otherwise feeding normally, and nursing is comfortable, this is not necessarily a problem. In one Brazilian prospective longitudinal study of 109 babies, 14 with symptomatic tongue-tie and 95 controls (R. L. Martinelli et al., 2015), the researchers reported that 64% of the symptomatic tongue-tied babies made a clicking sound during nursing as compared with 14% of the control babies.

A 2015 Brazilian prospective longitudinal study that compared 14 babies with symptomatic tongue-tie with 14 asymptomatic controls (R. L. Martinelli et al., 2015) identified other behaviors common among the symptomatic tongue-tied babies but not among the controls:

- No sleep stretches longer than 2 hours
- Alternating between sucking and sleeping during feeds

- Appearing tired after feeds
- Long pauses to rest during feeds
- Slipping off the nipple during feeds
- Frequent coughing during feeds

How does symptomatic tongue-tie contribute to feeding problems? An Australian study of 24 symptomatic tongue-tied babies used ultrasound to examine what occurred inside these babies' mouths during nursing (Geddes, Langton, et al., 2008). They found that the babies fell into two groups. One group had difficulty staying latched and latched shallowly, compressing the end of the nipple. The second group were able to stay latched and latched deeply but compressed the base of the nipple during nursing. The feeding dynamics of both groups caused nipple pain and slowed milk flow.

In babies with symptomatic tongue-tie, nursing problems are often obvious when nursing begins. One U.S. study of 88 symptomatic tongue-tied babies (Ballard et al., 2002) reported that all the problems were apparent during their hospital stay. Another U.S. study (Ricke et al., 2005) found that babies with symptomatic tongue-tie were three times more likely to be exclusively bottle-fed at 1 week compared with a matched control group of asymptomatic babies. But there are exceptions. According to anecdotal reports, some tongue-tied babies seem to nurse fine at first—during the first few weeks when the nursing parent's body is most sensitive to stimulation—but over time, as sucking stays inefficient, weight gain slows.

KEY CONCEPT

In many tongue-tied babies, minor adjustments in technique or positioning will improve the comfort and effectiveness.

Among babies with nursing problems, symptomatic tongue-tie is more common. Lactation specialists who work primarily with families having nursing problems often report that many of these babies have symptomatic tongue-tie. A 2015 U.S. retrospective review study of 290 nursing couples experiencing problems at a breastfeeding clinic (Pransky et al., 2015) found that symptomatic tongue-tie and/or lip-tie were identified in 47%. A 2017 Spanish transversal descriptive study of 302 babies having nursing problems who were seen in a Barcelona hospital (Ferres-Amat et al., 2017) identified nearly 57% as having symptomatic tongue-tie.

• • •

It is unclear whether untreated symptomatic tongue-tie is associated with later issues, such as speech problems.

Some suggest that untreated symptomatic tongue-tie increases the risk of speech problems, difficulty eating solid foods (Hiiemae & Palmer, 2003), dental caries (Koltlow, 2015), the need for orthodontia (Vaz & Bai, 2015), sleep apnea (Huang, Quo, Berkowski, & BGuilleminault, 2015), reflux and colic (Ghaheri, Cole, Fausel, Chuop, & Mace, 2017), and excessive swallowing of air (aerophagia) (L. Kotlow, 2011). One Israeli survey of 183 mothers of children with untreated symptomatic tongue-tie (Riskin et al., 2014) found that by 2 years of age just 12% of these children developed speech problems. A 2013 systematic review (Webb, Hao, & Hong, 2013) found that there was not enough evidence to conclude that untreated tongue-tie contributes to speech problems.

A 2015 systematic review examined the research on tongue-tie and issues other than nursing (Chinnadurai et al., 2015) and concluded there was not enough information to assess the effects of treating symptomatic tongue-tie on non-breastfeeding outcomes.

• • •

Tongue-ties can be classified as one of four or five different types, which are unrelated to whether the tongue-tie is symptomatic or asymptomatic.

Coryllos tongue-tie classification system. Created by the late U.S. pediatric surgeon Elizabeth Coryllos and U.S. lactation consultant Catherine Watson Genna (C. W. Genna, 2017b), this system categorizes tongue-ties into four different types, which are determined by where one end of the frenulum attaches to the baby's tongue and where the other end attaches to the floor of the baby's mouth. Here are the four types with photos of each:

- **Type 1.** Frenulum is attached near the tip of the tongue and on or near the gumline (Figure 8.2).
- **Type 2.** Frenulum is attached 2-4 mm behind tongue tip and just behind the gumline (Figure 8.3).
- **Type 3.** Frenulum is attached to the middle of the tongue and in the middle of the floor of baby's mouth (Figure 8.4).
- **Type 4.** Frenulum is attached behind the mucous membrane of the floor of the mouth, which can make the tongue look short (Figure 8.5).

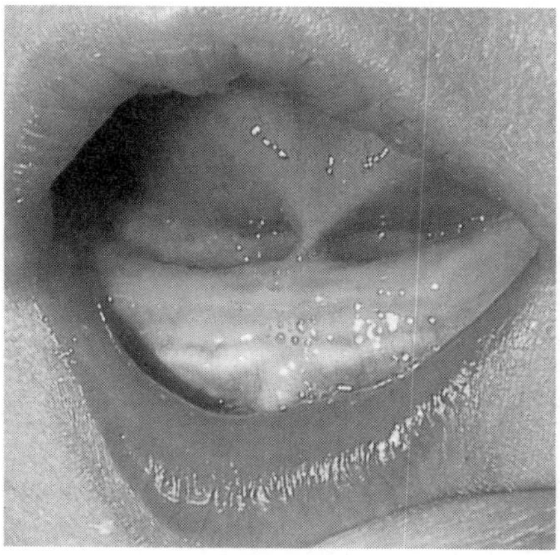

Figure 8.2 Type 1 tongue-tie. ©2020 Catherine Watson Genna, BS, IBCLC, used with permission.

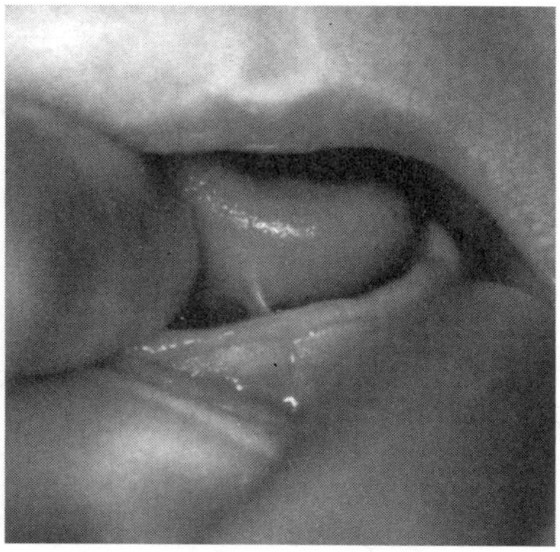

Figure 8.3 Type 2 tongue-tie. ©2020 Catherine Watson Genna, BS, IBCLC, used with permission.

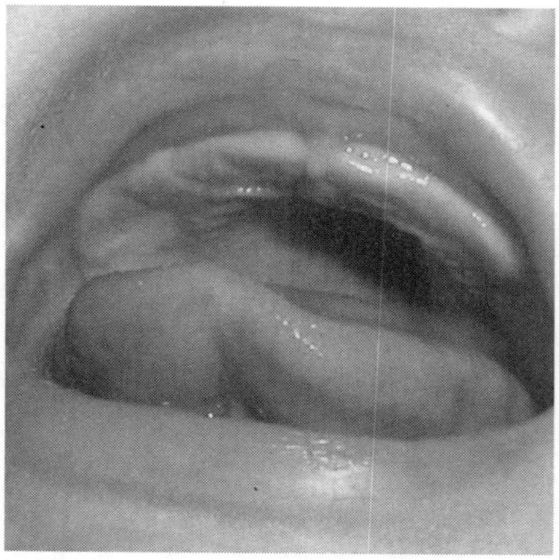

Figure 8.4 Type 3 tongue-tie. ©2020 Catherine Watson Genna, BS, IBCLC, used with permission.

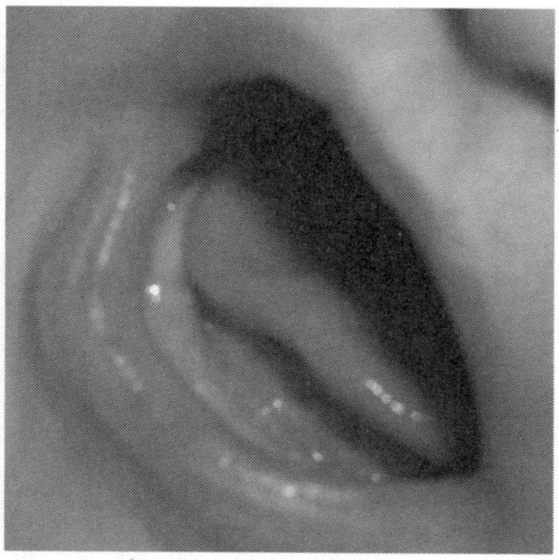

Figure 8.5 Type 4 tongue-tie. ©2020 Catherine Watson Genna, BS, IBCLC, used with permission.

Heart-shaped tongue tip. The most commonly recognized type of tongue-tie (Type 1) pulls on the tongue tip, often making it look notched or heart-shaped rather than rounded. A Type 1 tongue-tie may also prevent the baby from extending her tongue past the lower gumline. The other types of tongue-tie may not cause this heart-shaped appearance.

Anterior and posterior tongue-ties. Although the Coryllos classification system has four types, there are actually two basic types of tongue-tie. Types 1 and 2 are referred to as "anterior" tongue-ties, because the frenulum attaches near the front of the baby's tongue. Types 3 and 4 are referred to as "posterior" tongue-ties, because the frenulum attaches further back on baby's tongue. Signs of posterior tongue-ties include:

- The tongue tip appears to curl down.
- The baby cannot lift the tongue to the roof of the mouth when open wide.
- The tongue looks twisted.
- The tongue tip can elevate while the back of the tongue appears flat.
- The back of the tongue appears pulled down
- Palpable cord under the tongue

Controversy exists about the impact of posterior tongue-tie on nursing. Two U.S. prospective studies that included 237 and 54 babies respectively (Ghaheri et al., 2017; Ghaheri, Cole, & Mace, 2018) found that surgical treatment of posterior tongue-tie resulted in improved nursing outcomes. Some are skeptical about the effects of posterior tongue ties on nursing and suggest that these nursing problems may be due to other factors, such as suboptimal positioning and latch (P. S. Douglas, 2013b).

Submucosal tongue-tie (Type 5?). Some refer to a fifth type of tongue-tie, termed a "submucosal" tongue-tie. According to them, a Type 5 is a posterior tongue-tie in which the frenulum attaches to the floor of the baby's mouth underneath its mucous membrane ("submucosal"). One Australian physician (D. Todd, 2013; D. A. Todd, 2014) wrote that a Type 5 submucosal tongue-tie may involve a portion of the floor of baby's mouth with a broad base above the salivary glands that elevates when the tongue is lifted by a finger. Figure 8.6 shows the percentage of each type of tongue-tie that were released in one Australian hospital in two different years, 2008 and 2011.

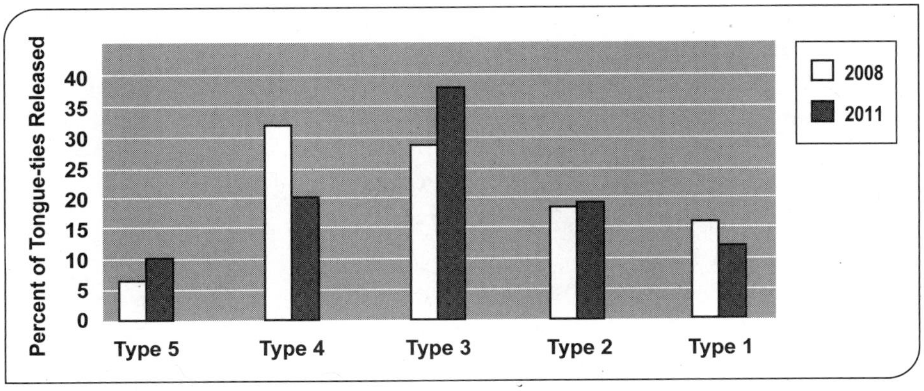

Figure 8.6 Tongue-tie release by type in 2008 and 2011 in one Australian hospital. Adapted from (D. A. Todd & Hogan, 2015).

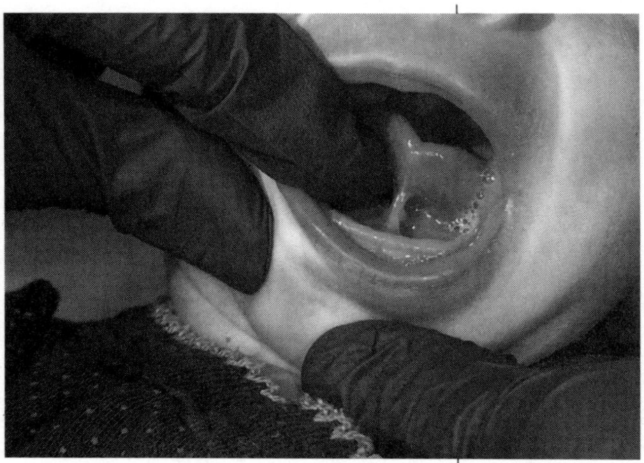

Figure 8.7 Examination of a baby's thick, fibrous frenulum by an Israeli dentist. ©2020 Dr. Gina Weissman, used with permission.

Identifying the type of a tongue-tie is unrelated to whether it is symptomatic or asymptomatic. Tongue appearance and where the frenulum attaches are not the most important factors. A baby may have any of these four or five types of tongue-ties without a feeding problem. Conversely, any of these four or five types of tongue-tie may be symptomatic and contribute to feeding problems. The Coryllos classification system is based only on the appearance of a baby's tongue rather than how much its movements are restricted. And the tongue's function is much more important to nursing than appearance. See the later point for validated tongue-tie assessment tools that assess both appearance and function and can be used to determine if surgically treating the tongue-tie may be beneficial.

• • •

Other factors that may affect nursing in tongue-tied babies include the consistency of the mammary tissue and the floor of baby's mouth, as well as other aspects of the frenulum.

The attachment locations of the frenulum may not affect nursing effectiveness, but the following factors may.

Elasticity and consistency of the baby's frenulum. The thickness and stretchiness of the frenulum matter. The frenulum in Types 1 and 2 tongue-ties are usually thin and elastic, whereas in Types 3 and 4, they are usually thicker and more fibrous (Figure 8.7) (C. W. Genna, 2017b). One U.S. study (Messner et al., 2000) found that of the babies with a very thick, fibrous frenulum, 75% had nursing problems.

The floor of baby's mouth. Another factor vital to nursing effectiveness is the consistency of the floor of the baby's mouth. A loose mouth floor can sometimes help compensate for a tight frenulum by allowing greater tongue movement (C. W. Genna, 2017b).

Consistency of the mammary tissue. The tautness or looseness of the nursing parent's mammary tissue also affects whether a tongue-tie is symptomatic or asymptomatic. One baby might nurse well if the mammary tissue is soft and pliable but struggle if it becomes firm or taut.

• • •

The baby's tongue function is more important to nursing than its appearance, and several validated tongue-tie assessment tools are available that can help gauge tongue function.

In most parts of the world, unless a lactation specialist is also a physician, a midwife, or a nurse-practitioner, diagnosing and treating tongue-tie are outside their scope of practice. However, anyone concerned about whether a baby's tongue-tie is contributing to nursing problems can use one of the following assessment tools that have been validated by research. The diagnosis of tongue-tie, however, needs to come from those with the appropriate credentials.

Assessment Tool for Lingual Frenulum Function (ATLFF). Developed in 1993 by U.S. lactation consultant Alison Hazelbaker (Hazelbaker, 1993), the ATLFF can be used to determine whether a tongue-tie is symptomatic or asymptomatic, in other words, whether or not the baby would benefit from surgical treatment (frenotomy, see later point). This tool (Table 8.1) assigns a score to different aspects of the function and appearance of the baby's tongue, with the function score more heavily weighted than the appearance score. Some researchers found this assessment tool very reliable (Amir, James, & Donath, 2006), while others found that its users did not consistently agree on scoring (Madlon-Kay, Ricke, Baker, & DeFor, 2008). One study found it missed many babies who would benefit from treatment (Ricke et al., 2005).

TABLE 8.1 Hazelbaker Assessment Tool for Lingual Frenulum Function (ATLFF)

FUNCTION ITEMS	***Function Items Score: _______***
Lateralization 2 Complete 1 Body of tongue but not tongue tip 0 None	**Cupping of Tongue** 2 Entire edge, firm cup 1 Side edges only OR moderate cup 0 Poor OR no cup
Lift of Tongue 2 Tip to mid-mouth 1 Only edges to mid-mouth 0 Tip stays at alveolar ridge OR tip rises only to mid-mouth with jaw closure AND/OR mid-tongue dimples	**Peristalsis** 2 Complete anterior to posterior 1 Partial OR originating posterior to tip 0 None OR reverse peristalsis
Extension of Tongue 2 Tip over lower lip 1 Tip over lower gum only 0 Neither of the above OR anterior or mid-tongue humps AND/OR dimples	**Snaps Back** 2 None 1 Periodic 0 Frequent OR with each suck
Spread of Anterior Tongue 2 Complete 1 Body of tongue but not tongue tip 0 None	
APPEARANCE ITEMS	***Appearance Items Score: _______***
Appearance of Tongue when Lifted 2 Round OR square 1 Slight cleft in tip apparent 0 Heart shaped	**Elasticity of Lingual Frenulum** 2 Very elastic (excellent) 1 Moderately elastic 0 Little OR no elasticity
Length of Lingual Frenulum when Tongue Lifted 2 More than 1 cm OR absent frenulum 1 Only 1 cm 0 Less than 1 cm	**Attachment of Lingual Frenulum to Tongue** 2 Occupies less than 50% of the tongue underside in the midline 1 Occupies 50-75% of the tongue underside in the midline 0 Occumpies 75-100% of the tongue underside in the midline
Attachment of Lingual Frenulum to Inferior Alveolar Ridge 2 Attachment to floor of mouth OR well below ridge 1 Attached just below ridge 0 Attached to ridge	
ASSESSMENT	
14 = Perfect Function score regardless of Appearance Items score. Surgical treatment not recommended. **11** = Acceptable Function score only if Appearance Item score is 10. **<11** = Function Score indicates function impaired. Frenotomy should be considered if management fails. Frenotomy necessary if Appearance Item score is <8.	

TABLE 8.2 Bristol Tongue Assessment Tool (BTAT)

	0	1	2	Score
Tongue tip appearance	Heart shaped	Slight cleft/notch	Rounded	
Attachment of frenulum to lower gum ridge	Attached at top of gum ridge	Attached to inner aspect of gum	Attached to floor of mouth	
Lift of tongue with mouth wide (crying)	Minimal tongue lift	Edges only to mid-mouth	Full tongue lift to mid-mouth	
Protrusion of tongue	Tip stays behind gum	Tip over gum	Tip can extend over lower lip	
Total score of 0-3 indicates severe reduction of tongue function				**Total** _______

Adapted from (Ingram et al., 2015)

Bristol Tongue Assessment Tool (BTAT). This streamlined tool (Table 8.2) was developed and validated by U.K. researchers (Ingram et al., 2015) for use in a busy hospital setting. New Zealand researchers (Dixon, Gray, Elliot, Shand, & Lynn, 2018) successfully used the BTAT to provide their multidisciplinary team with consistent criteria for assessing babies with symptomatic tongue-tie for surgical treatment (frenotomy, see later point). These researchers found that when babies with symptomatic tongue-tie had a BTAT score of 4 or less, they benefited from frenotomy. Using the BTAT this way, their New Zealand breastfeeding support program kept rates of exclusive nursing the same while significantly decreasing frenotomy rates from 11% in 2015 to 3.5% in 2017. The BTAT tested as reliable with different users (inter-rater reliability).

Neonatal Tongue Screening Test (NTST). Developed and validated for use in Brazil (R.L. Martinelli et al., 2016), the NTST (Figure 8.8) was mandated by law to be used to assess for symptomatic tongue-tie in all Brazilian newborns. Although an under-powered cohort study challenged this tool's validity (Brandao, de Marsillac, Barja-Fidalgo, & Oliveira, 2018), a 2019 non-probabilistic sample study of 449 nursing couples compared the use of BTAT (see previous paragraph) with its babies and the NTST with the same babies (Lima et al., 2019). It concluded that both of these assessment tools identified the same 14 babies as having symptomatic tongue-tie (3% of the total). All of the identified babies had tongue-tie releases within the first week.

Tongue-tie and Breastfed Baby (TABBY) assessment tool. Developed and evaluated by the same U.K. research team that developed the BTAT (Ingram, Copeland, Johnson, & Emond, 2019), this pictoral assessment tool (Figure 8.9) was created to be more easily translated in non-English-speaking countries. Among the five midwives who who were trained in the use of TABBY, there was nearly 98% agreement in its scoring. It also includes scoring recommendations for frenotomy. The authors recommend a score of 8 means normal tongue function, 6 or 7 borderline and suggest taking a "wait-and see" attitude and giving attention to better positioning and latch, 5 or below indicates impaired tongue function that may or may not affect nursing. If nursing is not affected, no frenotomy is recommended.

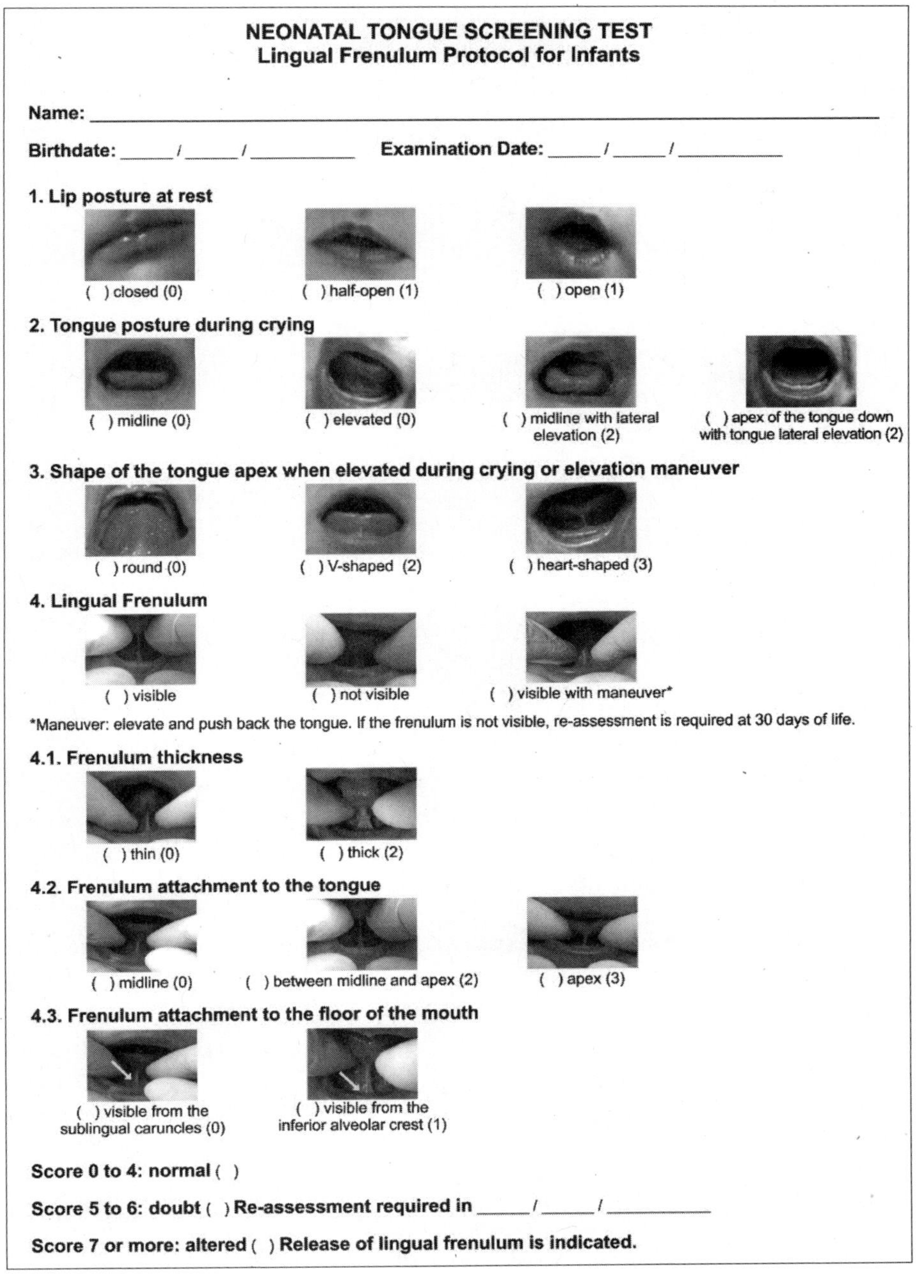

NEONATAL TONGUE SCREENING TEST
Lingual Frenulum Protocol for Infants

Name: ____________________

Birthdate: ____/____/________ **Examination Date:** ____/____/________

1. Lip posture at rest

( ) closed (0) ( ) half-open (1) ( ) open (1)

2. Tongue posture during crying

( ) midline (0) ( ) elevated (0) ( ) midline with lateral elevation (2) ( ) apex of the tongue down with tongue lateral elevation (2)

3. Shape of the tongue apex when elevated during crying or elevation maneuver

( ) round (0) ( ) V-shaped (2) ( ) heart-shaped (3)

4. Lingual Frenulum

( ) visible ( ) not visible ( ) visible with maneuver*

*Maneuver: elevate and push back the tongue. If the frenulum is not visible, re-assessment is required at 30 days of life.

4.1. Frenulum thickness

( ) thin (0) ( ) thick (2)

4.2. Frenulum attachment to the tongue

( ) midline (0) ( ) between midline and apex (2) ( ) apex (3)

4.3. Frenulum attachment to the floor of the mouth

( ) visible from the sublingual caruncles (0) ( ) visible from the inferior alveolar crest (1)

Score 0 to 4: normal ( )

Score 5 to 6: doubt ( ) **Re-assessment required in** ____/____/________

Score 7 or more: altered ( ) **Release of lingual frenulum is indicated.**

Figure 8.8 Neonatal Tongue Screening Test (NTST).

• • •

In many cases, improving nursing technique can help increase comfort and feeding effectiveness. As the authors of a New Zealand study that decreased surgical treatment for tongue-tie while maintaining exclusive nursing rates wrote (Dixon et al., 2018):

> "The clinical challenge with mother and baby dyads experiencing breastfeeding difficulties is to determine how best to support them. The surgical release of a lingual frenulum is only one of many treatments or support options."

Try starter positions and allow baby to self-attach. A logical place to begin is with the starter positions described on p. 23-29. These positions allow the baby to take an active role in latching by first triggering baby's inborn feeding behaviors. As three experienced Australian lactation consultants wrote about tongue-tie (Wattis, Kam, & Douglas, 2017):

If a tongue-tied baby has nursing problems, a good first strategy is to go back to basics and see if working on positioning and latch and other strategies make a difference.

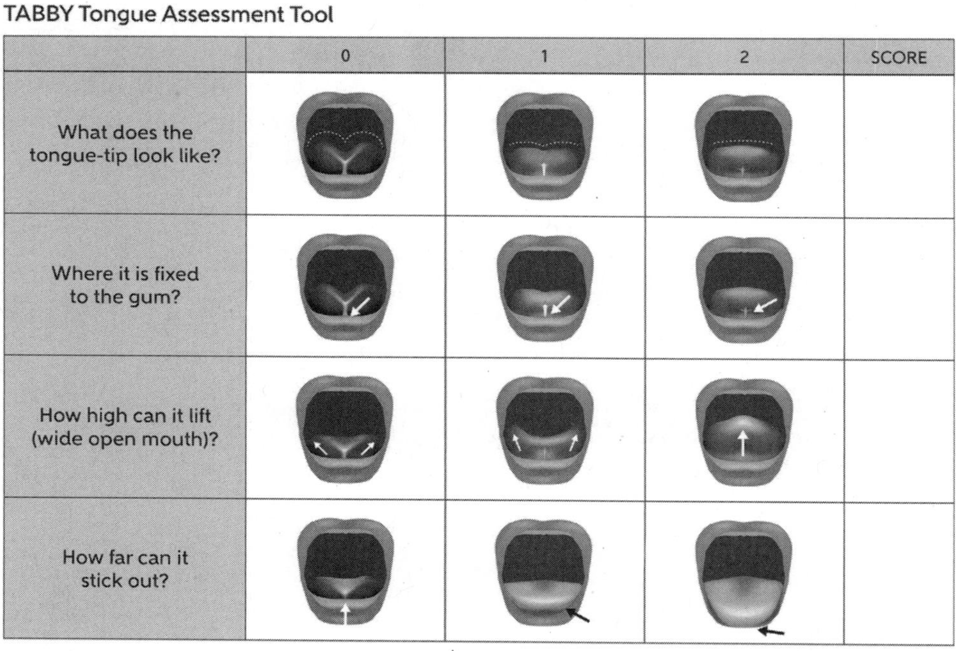

Figure 8.9 TABBY Tongue assessment tool. Reprinted from (Ingram et al., 2019) used with permission.

"The first step should always be to observe a breastfeed and work with the mother to improve her breastfeeding technique....Adjustments of the mother's positioning and attachment technique can enable the baby to respond to his or her instinctive reflexes and achieve a comfortable and effective latch."

Mammary shaping. Shaping the mammary tissue may help the baby latch deeper. For details, see p. 884.

In upright positions, use an asymmetric latch. If using an upright feeding position, encourage the nursing parent to help the baby latch by first aligning the baby nose to nipple, so her lower jaw is as far from the nipple as possible. For details, see p. 878.

Try varying feeding positions. If nursing is very painful, one option is to use a different feeding position at each feed. Depending on the degree of discomfort, some nursing parents find that rotating the area of nipple damage at each feed makes continued nursing without interruption tolerable. See p. 34-35 for ideas.

See if using a nipple shield helps. Using a nipple shield can reduce the sensation enough to make painful nursing bearable. If latching and staying latched is the challenge, a nipple shield may also help a struggling baby. See p. 912-917 for how to choose, fit, and apply a nipple shield. One U.K. study reported that 44% (95) of the mothers of its 215 tongue-tied babies tried a nipple shield with professional guidance, and it helped 41% (39) of these, or 18% of the mothers overall (Griffiths, 2004).

Express milk for some or all feeds. In some cases, nursing parents of symptomatic tongue-tied babies can handle some nursing but may express milk for some feeds. Help create a milk-expression plan to maintain milk production and provide milk for the baby.

Try tongue exercises. Some tongue exercises encourage more normal tongue movements during feeds. Although tongue exercises are not effective for all babies, they may help improve a baby's nursing effectiveness over time. For details, see p. 890.

• • •

If after trying the suggested strategies, feedings are still painful or ineffective or the baby has other concerning symptoms, it's important to rule out other possible causes.

Because about half of tongue-tied babies are asymptomatic and nurse well (Power & Murphy, 2015), it's important to rule out other possible causes of feeding problems.

Normal tongue mobility is not the only important ingredient for effective nursing. Babies also need adequate (not perfect) oral-motor coordination, structural support, nervous system regulation, breathing, and a positive connection with the nursing parent. When ruling out other causes, consider:

- Basic positioning dynamics (see Chapter 1)
- Structural issues, such as asymmetry or torticollis (see p. 107)
- Pain or discomfort from an undiagnosed birth injury or birth trauma, hip dysplasia, a broken bone, a pulled muscle, a hematoma, etc.
- Medical conditions, such as prematurity or neurological, congenital, respiratory, or cardiac abnormalities, nervous system dysregulation
- Digestive issues, such as reflux or food allergy (see p. 304 and 309)
- High palate
- Low muscle tone
- Jaw alignment issues (see later section)
- Aversion from negative experiences, such as deep suctioning, forceful latching attempts, or mental-health issues in the family

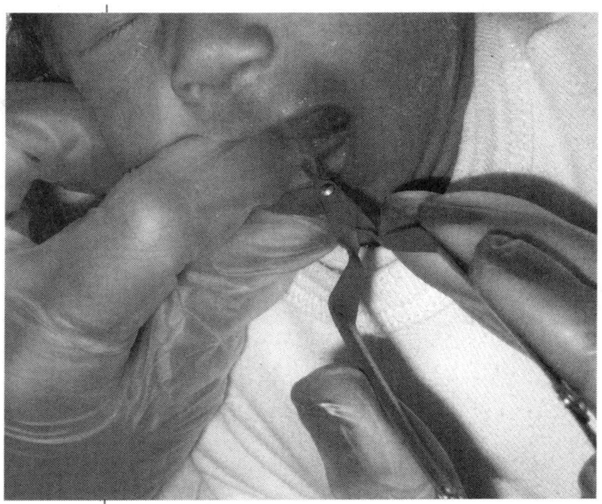

Figure 8.10 An Israeli dentist uses scissors to perform a frenotomy. ©2020 Dr. Gina Weissman, used with permission.

• • •

If nursing effectiveness and comfort do not improve or the baby still has concerning symptoms after trying the previous strategies and ruling out other causes, suggest the family consider seeing an appropriate healthcare provider to evaluate the baby's frenulum for release or division, the procedure known as frenotomy.

After other possible causes of feeding problems are ruled out, discuss the possibility of having the baby evaluated for tongue-tie diagnosis and release (frenotomy).

What is a frenotomy? This procedure (also known as a frenulotomy) is usually uncomplicated and can be done in a provider's office (usually a doctor or dentist). It involves releasing the baby's frenulum, usually with either scissors (Figure 8.10) or a laser, to improve the tongue's range of movement. It involves no stitches. It is usually done without anesthesia. (Sucrose—which is an effective analgesia—is sometimes used.) Because there are few nerves and blood vessels in the frenulum, it involves little discomfort or bleeding.

Who diagnoses a tongue-tie and performs a frenotomy? Not all healthcare providers believe that tongue-tie affects nursing. If the baby's provider discounts this possibility and is unwilling to refer the family to someone who will evaluate and diagnose the baby, it's time to get a second opinion. Lactation supporters should ideally make available a list of skilled local providers. These may include pediatricians, family practice doctors, oral surgeons, dentists, ear-nose-and-throat physicians, and general surgeons. When seeking a provider, suggest the family look for someone who is educated on the possible effects of tongue-tie on nursing and doesn't perform a tongue-tie release on 100% of babies who see them. One U.S. ear-nose-and-throat physician warned against practitioners who charge extra for each type of tie released (tongue, lip, buccal) and don't accept insurance payments so families must pay out of pocket. Suggest the family ask if the provider knows the techniques used to identify and treat Types 3 and 4 tongue-ties, as they differ from those used for Type 1 and 2. With posterior tongue-ties, to provide greater tongue movement, typically a "diamond shape" is seen after frenotomy (Figure 8.11). U.S. physician Elizabeth Coryllos provided a detailed explanation of what healthcare providers need to know to recognize and release posterior or "hidden" tongue-ties in Chapter 9 of the book *Supporting Sucking Skills in Breastfeeding Infants* edited by Catherine Watson Genna (Coryllos, Genna, & LeVan Fram, 2017).

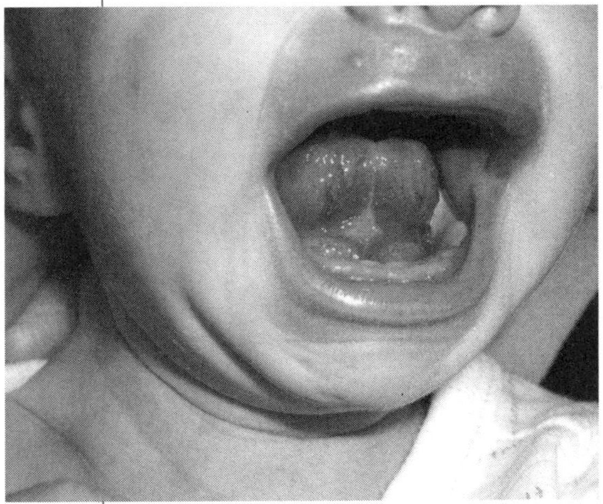

Figure 8.11 The "diamond shape" seen after a frenotomy for a posterior tongue-tie. ©2020 Dr. Gina Weissman, used with permission.

Too many frenotomies? During the last decade, awareness about tongue-tie as a potential cause of nursing problems spread among both parents and professionals. Some questioned whether frenotomies were overdone (Dixon et al., 2018; Kapoor, Douglas, Hill, Walsh, & Tennant, 2018). In many cases, lactation specialists refer babies to providers for tongue-tie evaluation, but often parents read about tongue-tie online and wonder if frenotomy might be the "magic bullet" that will instantly solve their nursing challenges. Some providers report seeing parents who request a frenotomy for their baby without seeing a lactation specialist or considering other possible causes of their nursing problem (Hansen, 2016). Some parents also request a frenotomy, even when nursing is comfortable, their baby has no feeding problems, and is gaining weight normally (Naimer, 2016).

KEY CONCEPT

When improved nursing dynamics do not solve a tongue-tied baby's feeding problems, a frenotomy should be considered.

During the 2000s and 2010s in some parts of the world, the incidence of frenotomy skyrocketed, as well as the number of articles published about tongue-tie (Bin-Nun, Kasirer, & Mimouni, 2017). Population-based studies found huge increases in the number of frenotomies performed:

- **United States.** Between 1997 and 2012, the number of tongue-ties diagnosed increased by 834% and the number of frenotomies performed increased by 866% (Walsh, Links, Boss, & Tunkel, 2017).
- **Australia.** Between 2006 and 2016, the number of frenotomies paid for by healthcare services in children 0 to 4 years rose from 1.22 per 1,000 population to 6.35 in 1,000. (Kapoor et al., 2018).
- **New Zealand.** In one hospital, the percentage of babies undergoing frenotomy increased from a high rate of 7.5% in 2013 to 11.3% in 2015 (Dixon et al., 2018).
- **Canada.** Between 2004 and 2013 in some areas of British Columbia, diagnosis of tongue-tie increased 70% while frenotomy increased 89% (Joseph et al., 2016).

The authors attributed this disconnect between identification and treatment to possible diagnostic bias and questioned whether frenotomies were performed unnecessarily. Another Canadian population-based study examined identification of tongue-tie and rates of frenotomy in all provinces except Quebec between 2002 and 2014 (Lisonek et al., 2017). It found that identification of tongue-tie increased from 6.86 per 1,000 population in 2002 to 22.6 per 1,000 in 2014. Frenotomy rates among babies with tongue-tie increased from nearly 55% in 2002 to 64% in 2014. These rates varied by province. In some provinces the frenotomy rates were three times higher than in others.

Is it possible that tongue-tie was once underdiagnosed and undertreated and is now more likely to be treated appropriately? An Australian study that examined the percentage of babies born in one hospital who underwent frenotomies in 2008 and 2011, (D. Todd, 2013) found that the incidence stayed stable. In both 2008 and 20011, about 5% of the babies born at that hospital had a frenotomy.

Is frenotomy effective in treating tongue-tie? At this writing, the research is mixed. A 2017 Cochrane Review examined five randomized, controlled trials (O'Shea et al., 2017). The total body of evidence was considered of low to moderate quality, and the authors concluded that the research did not find a consistent, long-term positive effect on nursing but that after the frenotomy, breastfeeding mothers experienced less pain in the short term. The U.S. Agency for Healthcare Research and Quality examined the existing research on frenotomy and concluded (AHRQ, 2015, p. 12):

> "A small body of evidence suggests that frenotomy may be associated with improvements in breastfeeding...and potentially in nipple pain, but with small short-term studies, inconsistently conducted, [standard of evidence] is generally low to insufficient."

The Canadian Agency for Drugs and Technologies in Health (CADTH) conducted a systematic review on frenotomy, which concluded (CADTH, 2016, pp. 15-16):

> "The reviewed evidence collectively suggests that tongue-tie division likely has a positive impact on maternally reported or perceived breastfeeding effectiveness in the short-term. Benefit is less clear for long-term outcomes....The evidence underlying these conclusions comes primarily from poor-quality [studies], and does not adequately address the questions of whether frenectomy provides a meaningful incremental benefit over other treatments or procedures to improve breastfeeding, particularly the long-term."

Does the timing of a frenotomy matter? Premature weaning appears to be the greatest risk of delaying frenotomy in a symptomatic tongue-tied baby. A U.K. prospective cohort study of 70 mostly symptomatic tongue-tied babies (Donati-Bourne, Batool, Hendrickse, & Bowley, 2015) found that if the time between assessment and frenotomy was longer than 2 weeks, the likelihood of weaning increased markedly and was significantly higher at 4 weeks. A prospective 2015 Indonesian study of 31 symptomatic tongue-tied babies (Praborini, Purnamasari, Munandar, & Wulandari, 2015) found that babies who had the procedure done before Day 8 had a greater mean weight gain than those whose frenotomy was performed after Day 8. An Australian study compared the rates of frenotomy in one hospital in 2008 and 2011 (D. A. Todd & Hogan, 2015) and found that although the overall percentage of babies receiving frenotomies stayed stable at about 5%, the average age when the frenotomy occurred rose from 2008 to 2011 from 5 to 9 days. In 2011, when more frenotomies were performed later, 17% of the mothers had already switched to exclusive pumping when the frenotomy was done, as compared with only 3.5% in 2008. The author concluded that ideally in babies with symptomatic tongue-tie frenotomies should be performed within the first week of life. But even if a frenotomy is delayed, it may still help. In one case report, after a frenotomy, a 6-month-old exclusively breastfed baby who was diagnosed as failure to thrive began consuming more milk and gaining more weight (Forlenza, Paradise Black, McNamara, & Sullivan, 2010).

Where do we go from here? Another U.S. review article (Walsh & Tunkel, 2017) concluded that what's needed moving forward is consistent terminology, uniform guidelines for assessing tongue-tie, and an emphasis on whether tongue-tie is symptomatic or asymptomatic. In other words, frenotomies should not be performed on babies who are nursing normally and are not showing other signs of problems associated with reduced tongue mobility. A New Zealand article (Dixon et al., 2018) described successful efforts to reduce the rate of frenotomy from 11.3% in 2015 to 3.5% in 2017. Efforts included establishing consistent assessment of tongue-tie across disciplines, clinical education on tongue-tie, and online education for parents and professionals. In addition to reducing the number of frenotomies, these improvements in practice also improved breastfeeding practices. Feeding patterns remained the same in families whose babies received a frenotomy and in those who were declined a frenotomy.

• • •

After a frenotomy, if improvement occurs, it may be immediate or it may take some time.

It is helpful for families to have realistic expectations about what may happen after a frenotomy. Sometimes nursing is immediately more comfortable and effective, but sometimes this takes a while. In cases where tongue-tie was carefully assessed and determined to be contributing to nursing problems (symptomatic), suggest the family expect after a frenotomy at least one better feed each day. It is also helpful to continue working closely with a lactation specialist after the procedure for help and support during the transition.

What does research say about frenotomy and nursing outcomes? In an Israeli study that was one of the rare blinded, randomized controlled trials (Dollberg, Botzer, Grunis, & Mimouni, 2006) 25 tongue-tied babies received either 1) a sham procedure, then breastfed, then had an actual frenotomy, and then breastfed again or 2) had an actual frenotomy, breastfed, and then had a sham procedure and breastfed again. Mothers and healthcare personnel caring for the baby were blinded to what order these procedures occurred. There was a significant difference in pain scores after frenotomy, but not after the sham procedure. In another U.K. randomized controlled trial of 201 symptomatic tongue-tied babies (Hogan et al., 2005), 95% % (54 of 57) of the mothers reported improvement overall, with 79% reporting immediate improvement and 16% within 48 hours.

In the studies listed below, however, there was no control group. What makes these studies weaker is that due to the "placebo effect," simply doing the procedure may influence the parent's perception of nursing comfort and effectiveness. Each study below begins with the percentage of parents who reported improvement after a frenotomy.

- 98% in a U.K. retrospective survey of 63 families (Mettias, O'Brien, Abo Khatwa, Nasrallah, & Doddi, 2013).
- 92% in a Canadian prospective study of 27 symptomatic tongue-tied babies (Srinivasan, Dobrich, Mitnick, & Feldman, 2006)
- 90% in a Canadian study of mothers of 30 babies with posterior tongue-tie (Srinivasan et al., 2018)
- 86% in an Austrian retrospective survey (Ramoser et al., 2019), with 16% unchanged, and 1% with worsened symptoms among 141 tongue-tied babies
- 100% of an Australian study's 24 symptomatic tongue-tied babies, who within 7 days of the procedure latched more easily, took more milk (a mean of 54 g increased to 69 g) and the mothers' mean pain score was reduced from 4.0 to 0.5 (Geddes, Langton, et al., 2008)
- 85% of a New Zealand study's 34 babies with tongue-tie and/or upper lip-tie, with 82% still improved at 2 weeks (Benoiton, Morgan, & Baguley, 2016)
- 79% of a Brazilian study's 14 tongue-tied babies who received frenotomies during the first week of life; at 30 days, 21% did not improve and were losing weight. (Lima et al., 2019)

What care is recommended after a frenotomy? Different practitioners suggest different practices after a frenotomy. At this writing, no research was found on preferred post-frenotomy care practices. But in one 2017 article (Smillie et al., 2017), nine expert clinicians from around the world shared their thoughts and experiences. Some said that nursing alone provided enough "tongue exercise" after a frenotomy to help prevent scarring or reattachment of the frenulum. Others felt that some gentle stretching exercises provided better results. Some expressed concern that any exercise that was painful for the baby could cause nursing aversion.

Tongue Size and Tone

For the baby with a large or low-tone tongue, during latch, suggest triggering the baby's inborn feeding behaviors and allowing time for her to self-attach.

Sometimes, the size or tone of the baby's tongue contributes to nursing struggles. A large tongue or a low-tone tongue (which at rest may stick out of baby's mouth) may present challenges.

If the baby with a large or low-tone tongue also has Down syndrome, for specific strategies, see the later section on p. 327-329. Whatever the cause, using the feeding dynamics described in Chapter 1 makes nursing easier for the baby. If the baby needs encouragement to keep her tongue down while latching, see the tongue exercises described on p. 890-891.

Baby's Lips, Cheeks, and Palate

The baby's upper lip does not need to be flanged out during nursing.

For comfortable and effective feeding, it is not necessary for both the baby's upper and lower lips to be flanged out during nursing. As described in the book *Supporting Sucking Skills in Breastfeeding Infants,* U.S. authors Catherine Watson Genna and Lisa Sandora wrote (C. W. Genna, 2017a, p. 28):

> "The lips are gently applied to the breast with the lower lip flanged completely outward and the upper lip neutral to lightly flanged."

Some nursing parents become over-focused on ensuring both of baby's lips are flanged during feeds and may sometimes even pull out baby's lips after latch. This action may inadvertently turn a deep latch into a shallower latch. What's most important after latch is that the nursing parent is comfortable and the baby is sucking actively. If both of these are present, there is no need to worry about or adjust the position of baby's lips.

Upper Lip-Ties

There is no agreed-upon definition of an upper lip-tie, and little is known about its impact on nursing.

The superior or maxillary labial frenulum (or frenum) is the membrane that connects the upper lip with the upper gumline. As a child grows, a very thick upper lip-tie may create excess space between the two upper front teeth, which in some cases, contributes to gum disease (Delli, Livas, Sculean, Katsaros, & Bornstein, 2013).

When does a normal superior labial frenulum become a "lip-tie?" This is a difficult question to answer because this membrane is not part of the normal newborn exam, so no one knows what characteristics are typical or atypical (Santa Maria et al., 2017). Even its function is unknown. According to one author, a commonly used but vague and subjective definition of lip-tie is: "when it is thought to be contributing to breastfeeding difficulties" (L. S. Merritt, 2019, p. 357). Much like tongue-tie, even without agreed-upon definitions, lip-ties are being identified and surgically released.

What problems are attributed to lip-tie? Anecdotal reports suggested that lip-tie may reduce nursing effectiveness by preventing upper lip flanging, prevent baby from forming a seal on the mammary tissue to complicate latching, and contribute to poor milk transfer, nipple pain, and tooth decay from milk "pooling" around upper front teeth (Koltlow, 2015; L. A. Kotlow, 2013).

What does research say about lip-tie? One of the challenges of determining the effects of lip-tie release on nursing is that it is usually done at the same time as tongue-tie release (frenotomy). This makes it impossible to separate the effects of lip-tie release from tongue-tie release. One U.S. retrospective review of 290 patients with tongue- or lip-ties who were seen at a breastfeeding clinic (Pransky et al., 2015) found that of the 14 babies with upper lip-ties only, the parents reported lip-tie release provided moderate improvement in 50% (7), mild improvement in 29% (4), and no change in 21% (3). A New Zealand prospective study of 34 babies who underwent tongue-tie and/or lip-tie releases included 3 babies with lip-ties only (Benoiton et al., 2016). Two (66%) of the 3 mothers reported improvement after the procedure and improvement continued in these two mothers 2 weeks later. A major problem with all of these studies is that they were done without a control group as a comparison.

Authors of a 2019 systematic review on upper lip-ties (Nakhash et al., 2019) found no randomized controlled trials and concluded that the evidence for routine lip-tie release in babies having nursing problems is poor.

KEY CONCEPT

Two classification systems were developed to identify types of lip-tie, neither of which is reliable.

Kotlow lip-tie classification system. In 2010, U.S. dentist Lawrence Kotlow published a lip-tie classification system (L. A. Kotlow, 2010) with four grades based on the membrane's attachment location. At its debut, this system was not validated, and it was unclear whether there was any association between any of its lip-tie grades and nursing problems.

Stanford lip-tie classification system. In 2017, a team of six researchers from Stanford University took high-resolution, close-up photos of the superior labial frenulum in 100 healthy newborns from the hospital's mother-baby unit. Then they asked each of the six researchers to independently assign each photo a Kotlow grade (Santa Maria et al., 2017). The goal was to test the reliability of the Kotlow system among expert observers. They found this system was not reliable. Only 8 of the 100 photos received the same grade from the six researchers. The Kotlow system was found unreliable both from observer to observer (inter-rater reliability) and within each individual observer's ratings (intra-rater reliability). They noted that 80% of the babies fell into grades 2 and 3, with only 6% in grade 1. Next, they decided to create a new classification system that had only 3 grades (combining Kotlow grades 2 and 3) and after reviewing their responses in light of their new system, they found it was more reliable than the Kotlow system. Even so, the Stanford classification system was still not reliable enough to use in a clinical setting. The reliability among observers rose from 8% to 38% (still not acceptable) and the intra-rater reliability rose from 80% to 90%. In their conclusion, the researchers noted:

- The current debate about lip-ties suffers from a basic lack of knowledge.
- No one knows what is a "normal" upper-lip frenulum, in part because they are examined only when there is a nursing problem.
- We don't know from the available research whether lip-tie release improves nursing.

- Nearly all newborns have this membrane, and research on older children (Bergese, 1966) indicated that this labial frenulum becomes less prominent as children mature, which makes doing a lip-tie release to prevent later problems questionable at best.

In summary, with the dearth of clear evidence on the effects of lip-ties on nursing, it is safe to say that when nursing problems arise, the first priority is to go back to basics. Try other strategies to improve nursing first, before a lip-tie release is considered.

Buccal-ties

Term babies have rounded cheeks because in utero they laid down fat pads in their cheek muscles. Their cheeks support the grooving of baby's tongue during nursing and make it easier to generate the suction needed to nurse effectively (C. W. Genna, 2017a). Depending on gestational age, babies born preterm may lack these fat pads, which can cause their cheeks to collapse during nursing, reducing their ability to generate the needed suction, which may reduce feeding effectiveness.

Babies' cheek muscles and fat pads help stabilize baby's tongue during nursing and play a role in the baby's ability to generate suction.

• • •

Some healthcare providers suggested that in rare cases, abnormal membranes known as "buccal-ties" may extend between the baby's gum and cheeks and cause nursing problems (Chang, 2016; Gatto, 2015; Koltlow, 2015). As with lip-ties (see previous section), data on normal membranes in the cheeks (such as those that create dimples) is scarce. At this writing, little is known about this possibility.

Some say that abnormal membranes in the cheeks ("buccal-ties") may affect nursing.

As with lip-ties, with the dearth of clear evidence on the effects of buccal-ties on nursing, it is safe to say that when nursing problems arise, the first priority is to go back to basics. Try other strategies to improve nursing first, before a buccal-tie release is considered.

Palate Shapes

The palate is the roof of a baby's mouth, and there are different terms for palates of different shapes.

Unusually shaped palates—high, bubble, grooved—sometimes contribute to feeding problems.

Reference palate. An average (or "reference") palate is smooth and sloping. When given a finger pad side up to suck, an average baby will draw it back about 1.5 inches (3.75 cm)—near where her soft and hard palates meet—and the entire length of the finger will stay in contact with the palate.

Grooved palate. With this type of unusual palate, a thin groove runs along its length, which may make it more difficult for a baby to maintain suction during nursing.

High or bubble palate. An average palate slopes upward about 0.25 inches (0.5 cm). A high palate may cause broken suction and a clicking sound during nursing. A high palate's slope is more angled. With a bubble palate, rather than the finger touching the entire palate, a gap (or bubble) can be felt above the finger, which may be shallow or deep, round or oval.

Strong gag reflex. In some cases, a baby with a high or bubble palate may resist drawing in the nipple deeply because she is not used to having the highest part of her palate touched, and this may stimulate the gag reflex. Over several days, gradually help the baby adjust to normal touch on her palate by making it a pleasant game to first touch her lips, wait for an open mouth, and then gently slide a clean finger with a closely trimmed nail back—pad side up— along her hard palate, stopping just before the gag reflex is triggered. By making this a happy time and gradually moving the finger further back, it can help a baby get used to this feel and overcome this sensitivity (C. W. Genna, 2017b, pp. 228-229).

• • •

Suggest any baby with an unusually shaped palate be checked for tongue-tie.

Experienced clinicians noticed an association between unusual palates and tongue-tie. This may be because during the development of the palate, it is "almost as malleable as softened wax" (Palmer, 1998, p. 96) and can be molded by tongue movements, pacifier/dummy, bottle use, and anything else that comes in regular contact with it. For example, babies intubated for long periods may form grooves—or high, narrow arches—in their palates (Wilson-Clay & Hoover, 2017, pp. 136-137; Wolf & Glass, 1992).

Cleft Lip and Palate

A cleft (or opening) of the lip or palate is one of the most common birth defects and is correctable by surgery. Its type, location, and severity will determine its effect on nursing.

Incidence of clefts varies around the world and by race (Saad, Parina, Tokin, Chang, & Gosman, 2014). Clefts may occur alone or as part of a syndrome with other birth defects. Depending on country and race, between about 1 and 3 babies in 1,000 are born with a cleft lip and/or palate, which can occur together or separately and be unilateral (on one side) or bilateral (on both sides). About 20% of cleft-affected babies are born with a cleft lip only, 30% with a cleft palate only, and 50% with both conditions (Boyce, et al., 2019).

With a cleft lip alone, even before surgical repair, some simple feeding strategies (see next section) usually make it possible for babies to nurse directly. With a cleft of the hard palate, however, due to the baby's inability to generate suction inside her mouth, most cannot nurse effectively without significant help in transferring milk. In many cases, milk expression is needed to provide mother's milk for these babies. The more expressed milk these babies receive, the better their development and health outcomes. One Finnish study found that shorter duration of human milk intake (less than 3 months) was associated with poorer school performance among 10-year-old children born with a cleft (Erkkila, Isotalo, Pulkkinen, & Haapanen, 2005).

Time spent sucking is also important to babies with clefts for other reasons. Efforts to nurse promote healthy mouth, tongue, and jaw development. And nursing also enhances the parent-baby relationship (Krol & Grossmann, 2018). In some parts of the world, this relationship may be at risk if an obvious birth defect, such as a cleft lip, causes families to consciously or unconsciously avoid face-to-face contact with their baby. Even if the baby transfers very little milk during nursing, this sensory experience may be important to neurological development (Bergman, 2017) and emotional closeness. Nursing also guarantees time spent cuddling in skin-to-skin contact, which is calming, comforting, and enhances their intimate connection.

• • •

As described in detail on pp. 45-46 in Chapter 2, immediate and uninterrupted skin-to-skin contact for the first 1 to 2 hours after birth is associated with better newborn stability and with an earlier and more successful first nursing (Karimi, Sadeghi, Maleki-Saghooni, & Khadivzadeh, 2019), which is linked to an earlier increase in milk production (Bystrova et al., 2007) and fewer feeding problems (Carberry, Raynes-Greenow, Turner, & Jeffery, 2013). Research also found that allowing baby to do the breast crawl for the first feed (see p. 47) is associated with fewer feeding problems during the hospital stay (Girish et al., 2013). Both early nursing and skin-to-skin contact also nourish the parent-child bond.

Encourage the family of a baby with a cleft to plan for immediate and uninterrupted skin-to-skin contact after birth and early and frequent nursing.

For the baby with a cleft, early frequent nursing also provides the opportunity to learn to latch and nurse when the mammary tissue is still soft and pliable. Early experiences of nursing also make it easier for the baby undergoing early cleft-lip repair to return to nursing afterwards.

Cleft Lip Only

Most babies with only a cleft lip nurse effectively but may need help forming a complete seal around the mammary tissue.

Types of cleft lips. A cleft lip may be either incomplete or complete (all the way up into the baby's nasal cavity), on one side (unilateral), or both (bilateral) and may involve the gum (alveolus) (Figure 8.12). It occurs in utero when parts of the baby's upper lip do not fuse.

Nursing and bottle-feeding. Because mammary tissue is flexible and can be molded to fill gaps more easily than an artificial teat, nursing may be easier than bottle-feeding for a baby with a cleft lip. For nursing families who intend to also use feeding bottles, Alice Farrow, an IBCLC and parent of a cleft-affected child, suggests that for babies with a wide cleft, a wide-base teat may be easier for baby to manage (personal communication, 2018).

Nursing rates in cleft-affected babies. Babies with only a cleft lip have far fewer feeding problems than those with a cleft palate. A Scottish study examined completed questionnaires from 90 families of cleft-affected infants (Britton, McDonald, & Welbury, 2011). In those with a cleft lip only, at 6 months, 67% were nursing compared with 0% of those with a unilateral cleft lip and palate, 9% of those with a bilateral cleft lip and palate, and 7% of those with a cleft palate only. A Brazilian study of 31 babies with cleft lip or palate found that those with a cleft lip only had a rate of exclusive breastfeeding during the first year of life that was higher than those with a cleft palate, and even higher than the babies in the general population without clefts (Garcez & Giugliani, 2005). The researchers concluded that cleft lip is compatible with successful breastfeeding. Another Brazilian study of 881 children with clefts also found higher breastfeeding rates

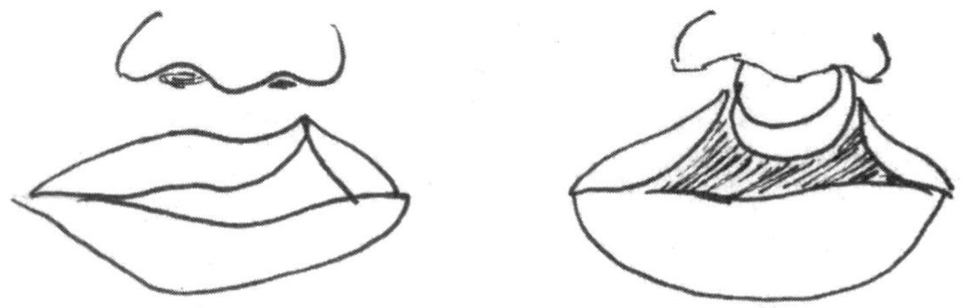

Figure 8.12 Left: unilateral (one-sided) and right: bilateral (two-sided) cleft lip. ©2020 Alice Farrow, used with permission.

among babies with a cleft lip only and found that these babies had better weight gain and growth than the babies with a cleft palate (Montagnoli, Barbieri, Bettiol, Marques, & de Souza, 2005).

Babies with a cleft lip only nurse more effectively than babies with a cleft palate because they can generate suction or negative pressure inside their mouth. In one Australian experimental study of 40 2-week-old bottle-fed babies with cleft lip only (8), cleft palate only (22), and cleft lip and palate (10), the researchers used special equipment to measure suction levels during feeds and confirmed that the babies in the cleft lip only group generated higher suction levels than the other babies (Reid, Reilly, & Kilpatrick, 2007).

Strategies for forming a seal during nursing. During early nursing, suggest experimenting with different feeding positions. Nursing parents may be able to use their thumb or mammary tissue to fill in the lip opening and after latch help the baby form a complete seal, which makes suction possible. This seal is vital because effective nursing requires the baby to generate suction inside her mouth, which is impossible without an air seal (Geddes, Kent, Mitoulas, & Hartmann, 2008; Geddes & Sakalidis, 2016). The location and size of the baby's cleft will affect which feeding position or sealing strategy works best. Some pull up mammary tissue between two fingers and press it into the cleft (Wilson-Clay & Hoover, 2017). With a unilateral cleft lip, some position their nipple to one side of the baby's cleft and use their thumb or a finger to fill the opening.

If after trying these strategies nursing continues to problematic, suggest the baby be checked for a submucous cleft (see later section on p. 290-291), which is much more likely among babies with a cleft lip than other babies (Gosain, Conley, Santoro, & Denny, 1999). Also suggest the baby be checked for tongue-tie (see p. 262 and Chapter 3 to troubleshoot for other problems.

• • •

Surgery to correct a cleft lip may be done as early as the first week or two after birth, or it may be performed months later.

It was once believed that cleft-lip surgery should be delayed until the baby was at least 10 weeks old and weighed at least 10 pounds (4.5 kg), but research found advantages to earlier repair and no differences in outcomes. One Czech retrospective cohort study of 104 cleft-affected babies had cleft-lip repair performed within the first week or two after birth. Its authors (Burianova, Kulihova, Vitkova, & Janota, 2017, p. 504) wrote:

> "Early operation has the following advantages: better wound healing, fewer complications, and a positive psychological effect on the parents (Murray et al., 2016). Early repair has been shown to result in good aesthetic assessments and dental relationships, with adequate growth of the face (Calteux, Schmid, Hellers, Kumpan, & Schmitz, 2013)....Early lip surgery does not result in an increase in mortality during or after surgery or in neonatal morbidity, and results are similar to later surgery (Tse, 2012)....A recent study comparing patients with early repair and patients operated on later in the first 12 months of life showed no anesthetic complications (Petrackova et al., 2015).

This Czech study found the rate of nursing among the babies with cleft lip only who had the early repair surgery (79%) was about the same as the nursing rate of the general population.

After cleft lip repair, nursing may be interrupted for only a few hours (Bessell et al., 2011; Cohen, Marschall, & Schafer, 1992; Boyce, et al., 2019). A 2019 systematic review (Matsunaka, Ueki, & Makimoto, 2019) concluded that there is no increased risk of wound separation if babies nurse or bottle-feed immediately after cleft lip repair. If the surgeon requires a longer interruption, suggest the nursing parent express milk often to stay comfortable and maintain milk production. According to research, after surgery the baby's stitches are not at risk of being disturbed, even if the baby begins nursing again as she leaves the recovery room (Cohen et al., 1992; Weatherley-White, Kuehn, Mirrett, Gilman, & Weatherley-White, 1987). In one Indian study of 40 babies, unrestricted nursing after cleft-lip surgery was also associated with greater weight gain 6 weeks later (Darzi, Chowdri, & Bhat, 1996).

Nursing shortly after surgery needs to be arranged in advance with the baby's surgeon. If the surgeon is uncomfortable with this, suggest sharing the Darzi study citation above. If the surgeon has no personal experience with early nursing after surgery, one option is to arrange for a nurse to stay on hand to observe the baby for signs of damage to the stitches. If the family is not happy with the surgeon's response, encourage them to get a second opinion.

Some babies happily nurse after surgery and some may not. If the baby will not nurse, see p. 129-131 for strategies to help the baby return to nursing.

Cleft Palate With or Without Cleft Lip

A cleft can occur in the hard palate, the soft palate, or both, and its location and size will affect the baby's ability to feed effectively.

A cleft palate occurs when parts of the baby's palate do not fuse in utero, leaving an opening in the roof of her mouth.

Types of cleft palates. The baby may have a cleft of the soft palate, which is comprised of soft muscle covered with mucous membrane and located near the back of the baby's mouth. Or the baby's cleft may include both the soft and hard palates. It is unusual for a cleft to be located only in the hard palate, which is comprised of bone covered with mucous membrane and located near the front of the baby's mouth. As with a cleft lip, a cleft palate can occur in one side (unilateral) or both (bilateral).

Another type is called a "submucous cleft," which refers to an opening of muscle or bone beneath intact skin that may be invisible to the eye or may appear as a depression in the roof of baby's mouth (see later section).

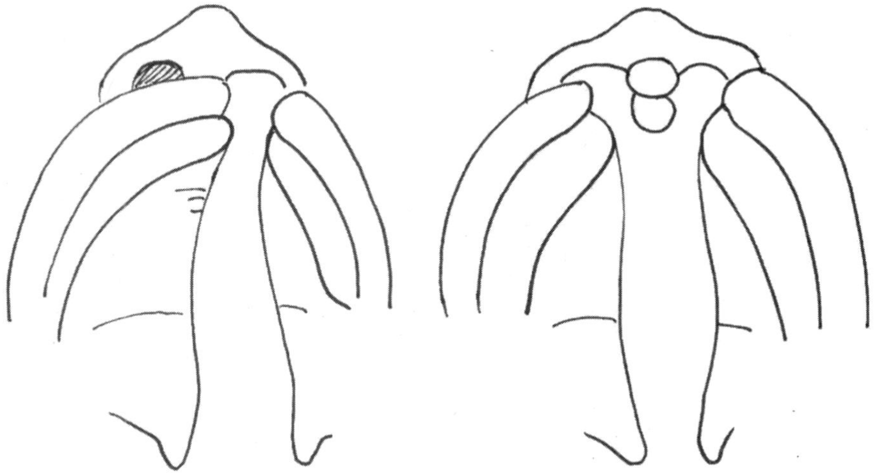

Figure 8.13 Left: unilateral (one-sided) and right: bilateral (two-sided) cleft palate. ©2020 Alice Farrow, used with permission.

Some cleft palates are missed. A U.K. study of 344 individuals with cleft palates (without cleft lip or submucous cleft) found that 28% of these clefts were not detected on the first day of life and five were not detected until after 1 year (Habel, Elhadi, Sommerlad, & Powell, 2006). The researchers suggested that all newborns' mouths be checked for clefts using a light and a tongue depressor.

Part of a syndrome? A cleft palate may be one feature of a genetic syndrome, such as Pierre-Robin sequence (which also includes a small jaw [micrognathia] and a retro-placed tongue). Up to 13% of cleft-affected babies have other birth defects (L. Merritt, 2005). One prospective, longitudinal Australian study of 62 babies with clefts rated their feeding skills at 2 weeks, 3 months, and 14 months (Reid, Kilpatrick, & Reilly, 2006) and found that babies with clefts that were part of a syndrome were 15 times more likely than other babies to have poor feeding skills. A U.K. study of 147 babies with clefts found that 100% of those diagnosed with Pierre-Robin sequence in the study's retrospective arm were failure-to-thrive (Pandya & Boorman, 2001). This led the researchers to institute feeding support for these families in the prospective arm of their study, which reduced the failure-to-thrive rate in babies with Pierre-Robin sequence from 100% to 40%.

Hard and Soft Palate Clefts

To feed effectively, a baby needs a firm surface on which to compress the nipple and the ability to generate suction.

For several reasons, an opening in the roof of a baby's mouth makes feeding challenging.

- It prevents the baby from creating an air seal to keep nipple or bottle teat in place.
- It may make it impossible for the baby to generate suction in her mouth, which is needed to draw milk from the mammary gland or bottle (Geddes & Sakalidis, 2016; Reid et al., 2007).
- It allows milk in the baby's mouth to flow into her nasal cavity, where it can enter the airway.
- Depending on the size and location of the cleft, there may be no firm surface against which the baby can compress a nipple or teat.
- The baby may keep her tongue mostly in the cleft and when she does move it forward, its movements may be uncoordinated rather than smooth.

Due to these physical dynamics, feedings are often very lengthy compared with babies with an intact palate. Families may need to spend most of their baby's waking hours feeding her, especially during her first few weeks. Whether nursed, fed by bottle, or both, a baby with a cleft palate may take up to two or three times longer to feed than other babies. Experimenting with different strategies may help families find ways to make feeds go more smoothly (see the next sections).

• • •

Some babies with a cleft palate may exclusively nurse, either early or later, but may need extra help transferring milk or supplements by another feeding method.

In the 1980s, some parents and providers published reports of babies able to nurse exclusively in spite of their cleft palate. This led to the assumption that with good technique and dedication full nursing was possible for all but a few severe cases (Danner, 1992; Danner & Wilson-Clay, 1986; Grady, 1983). In the 1990s and 2000s, however, this assumption was challenged by parents of cleft-affected babies (J. Miller, 1998) and researchers. One U.K. study (Masarei et al.,

2007), for example, found that only 4% of its 50 cleft-affected babies had normal oral-motor feeding skills during their first month.

In the 2010s, approaches to feeding cleft-affected babies varied in different parts of the world. In one North American Craniofacial Center (Alperovich, Frey, Shetye, Grayson, & Vyas, 2017), after birth, most families established milk production via milk expression and 75% used the specialized feeding bottles such as the Haberman Feeder to feed their babies expressed milk. In this clinic, 67% of 110 families provided some expressed milk and an average of 75% of the feeds were human milk for an average of more than 5 months. The percentage of babies with a cleft palate who consumed human-milk was much lower in many other North American facilities (Gottschlich et al., 2018).

In contrast, in one Thai hospital (Pathumwiwatana, Tongsukho, Naratippakorn, Pradubwong, & Chusilp, 2010), 20 breastfeeding mothers of babies with both cleft lip and cleft palate were taught upright nursing positions and how to express their milk directly into their babies' mouths during nursing, coordinating milk flow with baby's sucking, swallowing, and breathing. Adequate milk intake was gauged by baby's weight, mother's comfort, and baby's diaper output. The researchers reported that 2 of the 20 babies exclusively breastfed for the first 6 months, 16 infants did some breastfeeding for 3 to 4 months, and 2 stopped breastfeeding between 1 and 2 months. According to the researchers, the main reason for weaning in many of these families was unrelated to breastfeeding issues. It was primarily due to the mothers' return to work.

These very different approaches to feeding the baby with a cleft palate illustrate some of the options available to families. Each situation is unique, and a combination of the following physical factors influence cleft-affected babies' ability to nurse effectively:

- Whether or not the mammary tissue is malleable
- Whether milk production is low or abundant
- The location and size of the baby's cleft

Parent-related factors that influence feeding include:

- The adequacy and availability of social and lactation support
- The family's understanding of nursing management and positioning and latch techniques

Nursing usually goes more smoothly if parents know the basics of milk production. It also helps when parents are willing to try the positions, techniques, and devices that allow the baby to keep the nipple far enough back in her mouth to transfer milk with compression and keep the milk flowing down her throat rather than into her nasal cavity. Even if all of these factors are positive and present, some babies may require time (weeks or months) before learning to effectively nurse directly. Some babies may not transition entirely to exclusive direct nursing until after their cleft-palate surgery (McGuire, 2017). Because feeds take so much time, some families who begin by pumping and bottle-feeding stop attempting to latch.

Regarding the location and size of the baby's cleft, if the cleft is small and it's possible to plug it with mammary tissue during nursing, this may allow the baby to seal her mouth and provide the suction needed to keep the nipple in place and the milk flowing in the right direction. One U.K. study compared 50 babies with clefts (some breastfeeding, some bottle-feeding) with 20 babies without clefts (Masarei et al., 2007) and found that the location and size of the cleft made a significant difference in the babies' sucking efficiency. The sucking of all the babies without clefts was rated as normal, but only 2 were rated as normal among the 50 babies with a complete cleft lip and cleft palate or a cleft of the soft palate and at least two-thirds of the hard palate. Of the others in the cleft group who received a rating, all sucked markedly faster (average 109 sucks per minute versus 75 sucks per minute, indicating less milk transfer) and were rated as either disorganized or dysfunctional feeders.

In a U.S. retrospective review study of 143 babies with clefts (Clarren, Anderson, & Wolf, 1987), the researchers found that a baby was more likely to nurse effectively if she could do two things: 1) generate at least some suction and 2) move the tongue appropriately against the nipple. If a baby with a cleft palate could do both of these things, direct nursing was more likely to go well. When one or both were impossible, effective direct nursing was unlikely.

The Academy of Breastfeeding Medicine recommended in its Clinical Protocol #17 on nursing the baby with a cleft lip or palate (Boyce, et al., 2019) that each baby be evaluated for breastfeeding individually. This fully referenced protocol is free and downloadable in multiple languages at: **bfmed.org/protocols**.

• • •

To establish and maintain adequate milk production for the baby with a cleft palate, encourage milk expression from birth.

Learning and practicing hand expression soon after birth will help stimulate milk production and the expressed colostrum can be used to supplement the baby (Morton, 2019). Hand expression and breast compression (p. 889) during direct nursing can also be used to help compensate for a baby's inadequate or incomplete suction. For details on hand expression and the use of a pump to establish and maintain milk production, see p. 498-507 in Chapter 11, "Milk Expression and Storage."

Make sure the family knows that milk expression can provide exclusive mother's milk feeds, even if the baby does not yet nurse effectively. Providing expressed milk will contribute to better health outcomes for both baby and nursing parent. One positive health outcome that is especially significant for cleft-affected babies is reduced incidence of ear infections (otitis media).

Ear infections. With an intact palate, the muscles of the palate open the ear tubes during swallowing to equalize air pressure. A cleft palate interferes with this process, leaving fluid in the middle ear that can become infected. In U.S., Brazilian, and Swedish studies (Aniansson, Svensson, Becker, & Ingvarsson, 2002; Garcez & Giugliani, 2005; Paradise, Elster, & Tan, 1994), babies with cleft palates who were fed only formula developed more ear infections than those receiving some human milk. This greater susceptibility to ear infections continues after cleft-palate surgery (A. T. Wilson, Grabowski, Mackey, & Steinbacher, 2017).

• • •

If exclusive human-milk feeding is important to the family of a baby with a cleft palate, discuss goals and strategies.

When exclusive human-milk-feeding is the goal, discuss possibilities. Some parents prefer to express milk and bottle-feed. Some prefer to express milk into the baby's mouth through compression during direct nursing (p. 889). Both methods are time consuming in different ways. Some parents settle on a combination of methods.

Even without much milk intake, the act of nursing can be soothing to parent and child and promote healthy development of baby's mouth, tongue, and facial muscles. Suggest the family think of nursing as one way to enjoy a closeness and connection with their baby while providing comfort. Nursing may provide more comfort than other sucking outlets because of the skin-to-skin contact and because mammary tissue is more flexible than a silicone nipple and more easily molds to the baby's lips and mouth. Whether the baby finds nursing soothing or difficult depends on the type and location of the baby's cleft.

Every nursing couple is unique, and the way they nurse will be unique, too. With time and practice, some families of babies with a cleft palate eventually exclusively nurse, although—like many other families—most supplement their babies.

Feeding positions. When choosing a nursing position, comfort is important. Suggest first trying the starter positions described on p. 23-29. These positions have some advantages:

- Gravity helps maintain latch in a baby who can't generate suction.
- Baby's tongue is drawn forward and down by gravity, which can be helpful if the baby usually rests her tongue in the cleft.
- Baby's head is positioned higher than the nipple, reducing milk flow into the nose and ear tubes (Boyce, et al., 2019).
- Reduces muscle strain during long feeds, as baby's weight rests on the parent's body.
- It is easier for the baby to use her instinctive feeding behaviors to self-attach (S. D. Colson, Meek, & Hawdon, 2008).

Suggest trying first the slightly more upright version of this position, with the nursing parent's body slope between 55 to 65 degrees. Figure 8.14 illustrates a version of the straddle hold that works well for many babies with cleft palate (C. W. Genna, 2017b).

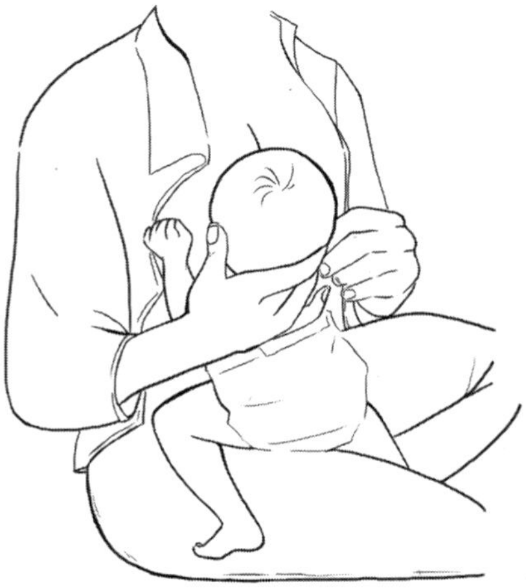

Figure 8.14 Straddle hold. ©2020 Nancy Mohrbacher Solutions, Inc.

In its protocol on breastfeeding cleft-affected babies, the Academy of Breastfeeding Medicine suggested if sitting-up-straight holds are used, to start with a football/rugby hold rather than cross-cradle position (for photos, p. 33 in Chapter 1). The ABM also suggested (Boyce, et al., 2019, p. 4):

> "[I]t may be useful to position the breast toward the 'greater segment' of the palate. That is, the side of the palate that has the most intact bone. This may facilitate better generation of negative pressure and thus milk extraction, while preventing the nipple being pushed into the cleft site."

Mammary support can help keep the nipple in back of the baby's mouth (Boyce, et al., 2019), which is often difficult if the baby cannot generate suction. In the Thai study where 18 of the 20 babies with a cleft lip and palate exclusively nursed for 2 months or longer (Pathumwiwatana et al., 2010), mammary support was one key technique. The authors described how the mothers were taught to hold the baby in a semi-upright position, support their breast during latch, and insert the nipple deeply when the baby opened wide. The mothers then supported their baby's head and neck to keep the nipple deep in baby's mouth. The mothers used part of their breast to seal any gap from the cleft.

Hand express milk while nursing. As described in previous points, in some parts of the world, hand expression is routinely taught to nursing parents of babies with a cleft palate (Pathumwiwatana et al., 2010), which increases their milk intake while nursing. In the Thai study mentioned above, during the hospital stay, when the baby latched, the mothers were taught to wait until the baby began moving her tongue and then compress their mammary tissue firmly with thumb and forefinger. The mothers stopped compressing while the baby swallowed and took a breath. By coordinating hand expressing with the baby's suck-swallow-breathe rhythm, the mothers were able to ensure their babies received the milk they needed while nursing.

Firm/soft mammary tissue. One mother of a baby with a cleft of the soft palate (Grady, 1983) experimented with different positions at different times, keeping careful track of what worked to find an effective approach that worked consistently. She found that her baby breastfed best when her breast was firm and full.

Jaw and chin support. Some babies with a cleft palate need support to hold their jaw and chin steady while nursing (C. W. Genna, 2017b). If the baby's cheeks appear to collapse inward as the baby nurses, try the Dancer Hand position (see p. 890) to provide jaw support. As the baby grows and spends more time nursing, her muscle strength and coordination will improve, and she may need chin support with only an index finger.

Nursing supplementers. A nursing supplementer can provide the cleft-affected baby with an experience similar to that of other babies. At this writing, all commercially manufactured nursing supplementers provide milk flow only when a baby can generate suction, which many of these babies cannot do. However, gravity can be used to speed milk flow for these babies by attaching the supplementer to an object (set the container on a music or hat stand, clip it to a cap brim, etc.) much higher than the baby (Wilson-Clay & Hoover, 2017). Some suggest making a hole near the top of the supplementer container to equalize the internal and external pressure for a faster milk flow (Alice Farrow, personal communication, 2018). Another option is to create a makeshift nursing supplementer that allows the feeder to actively deliver milk to the baby ("suction not required" type, see p. 897), using either a #5 French feeding tube or a butterfly catheter, a port, and a syringe full of milk with the needle removed (C. W. Genna, 2017b). In the book *Selecting and Using Breastfeeding Tools,* U.S. lactation consultant Catherine Watson Genna described easy ways to modify two commercial nursing supplementers made by different manufacturers to give the feeder more control over milk flow and better meet these babies' feeding needs (Genna, 2016). By carefully timing the milk flow with the baby's sucking, swallowing, and breathing, a baby may receive at least a partial feed during nursing.

KEY CONCEPT

Strategies to improve nursing effectiveness need to be tailored to the size and location of the baby's cleft.

Nursing two babies together. Another dynamic that can help ensure adequate milk production is when the cleft-affected baby is a twin. If the other twin has an intact palate and can nurse effectively, by nursing the babies together, the more effective feeder can stimulate milk flow throughout the feed for the cleft-affected baby. This same dynamic may be helpful to the family who is tandem nursing (see Chapter 14).

Patience. Finding ways to make nursing work with cleft-affected babies takes time and patience. Encourage the family to take advantage of all available help.

In some cases, finding good-quality help may not be easy. Research found that many families of cleft-affected babies need to seek information and support outside their birthing facility, especially in rural areas (P. A. Nelson & Kirk, 2013; Snyder & Ruscello, 2018).

• • •

Slow weight gain is a common issue among babies with a cleft palate, but some interventions may enhance weight gain and make feeds easier.

Without help during feeds, the baby with a cleft palate is at risk for inadequate weight gain and growth (Gopinath & Muda, 2005; Montagnoli et al., 2005; Rowicka & Weker, 2014). Some older studies found that babies with a cleft palate gained weight slowly no matter how they were fed (Avedian & Ruberg, 1980), but a later review of the literature found that using a combination of the strategies below improved weight gain and growth (Reid, 2004).

Education and support. Providing parents of cleft-affected babies with education and ongoing counseling is one intervention, when combined with others, that improved weight gain and growth (Reid, 2004). One Danish study of 115 babies with clefts (Smedegaard, Marxen, Moes, Glassou, & Scientsan, 2008) found that when counseling was started at birth by trained health professionals, these babies grew at the same rate as Danish babies without clefts, although they received human milk for a shorter time. A Brazilian study of 26 babies with clefts found that when education was not consistently given to parents, weight gain and growth suffered (Amstalden-Mendes, Magna, & Gil-da-Silva-Lopes, 2007). In many settings, parents of cleft-affected babies want more information and support than they receive (Lindberg & Berglund, 2014; P. A. Nelson & Kirk, 2013; Snyder & Ruscello, 2018).

Feeding bottles and nipples/teats. With today's online marketplace, families have much greater access to a large variety of feeding products, including squeezable bottles and teats. Specialized feeding bottles designed for cleft-affected babies—such as the Haberman and Pigeon Feeders—are not always necessary or helpful. A 2013 Brazilian cross-sectional descriptive study surveyed 211 parents of cleft-affected babies at eight medical centers (Gil-da-Silva-Lopes et al., 2013). When asked which feeding method worked best for their babies with a cleft palate, the largest percentage—36% (cleft palate only) and 32% (cleft lip and palate)—rated ordinary bottle nipples/teats as best. Fewer parents rated the specialized bottles as best. A 2011 Cochrane Review article (Bessell et al., 2011) concluded that squeezable bottles are easier for these babies than rigid bottles but there was no difference in growth. A 2016 systematic review article (Duarte, Ramos, & Cardoso, 2016) also found that squeezable bottles seemed to work better than bottles with rigid sides. These authors noted that the effectiveness of a feeding method will vary depending on the location and size of the baby's cleft.

Palatal obturators. These plastic plates are fitted to the baby's mouth, and some types are used before corrective surgery to keep the cleft in the baby's hard palate from closing improperly. Their use does not enable the baby to generate suction in her mouth, but they do provide a firm surface on which baby can compress mammary tissue or a bottle teat with her tongue during feeds. In some studies, parents felt these devices helped make feeds easier (Goyal, Chopra, Bansal, & Marwaha, 2014; Turner et al., 2001), but a 2011 Cochrane Review (Bessell et al., 2011) concluded that the use of these devices did not affect infant growth. If the nursing baby is fitted with an obturator, suggest the family request one with a smooth surface to reduce friction on the nipple.

Nasogastric (NG) tube. Some studies found that a cleft palate can make feeding so profoundly challenging that the baby needs to be fed for a time by NG tube, a tube that goes through the baby's nose into her stomach. In a Scottish questionnaire study of 90 families (Britton et al., 2011), 29% used the NG tube during or immediately after the hospital stay. In a Brazilian study of 211 families (Gil-da-Silva-Lopes et al., 2013), 20% reported that their baby's first feed was by NG tube.

• • •

Cleft palate repair may be done as early as 3 months and as late as 32 months.

The details of cleft palate repair—such as timing and approach—vary by the surgeon and center. Repair of the cleft palate may be done in stages and is usually scheduled sometime during the baby's first or second year, after the face and mouth have grown more mature, but before the baby has begun to do much talking.

After cleft palate repair, nursing may be uncomfortable for the baby at first. With a newly structured palate, sucking—even if not too painful—will feel different to her, and this new sensation may be unsettling. For some babies, feeling the nipple in their mouth may be comforting. But sometime within a few weeks of the surgery, as nursing becomes easier, she may begin nursing with more enthusiasm than before. In one case report from Australia, a 7-month-old baby who never directly breastfed was able to breastfeed exclusively after the cleft-palate repair (Crossman, 1998). Another Australian case report (McGuire, 2017) followed two mothers of babies with a cleft palate. Both expressed milk until their baby's surgery at 9 and 10 months. One baby successfully transitioned to direct nursing, while the other baby did not. The second mother discovered afterwards that she was pregnant and wondered if that might have been a factor. If the nursing parent expresses milk often enough to maintain milk production, this will increase the chances that the baby will accept nursing after the cleft palate repair surgery.

Submucous Cleft

If milk flows through a baby's nose and feeds are consistently more than 40 minutes long, suggest having the baby checked for a submucous cleft.

A submucous cleft is an opening of muscle or bone beneath the intact skin that is less visible to the eye. It may appear as a depression in the roof of baby's mouth (Figure 8.15). A submucous cleft is much more likely among babies with a cleft lip than in the general population (Gosain et al., 1999).

Depending on which muscles are missing, some babies with a submucous cleft can generate suction inside their mouth, but even so, the cleft alters the muscles of the soft palate, which may affect swallowing. It may also prevent the muscles of the soft palate from closing off the passage to the nose during feeds. As a result, many babies with this condition have feeding problems, such as prolonged nursing (more than 40 minutes), ineffective feeds and regular milk flow through the nose (nasal regurgitation). In one U.K. study (Moss, Jones, & Pigott,

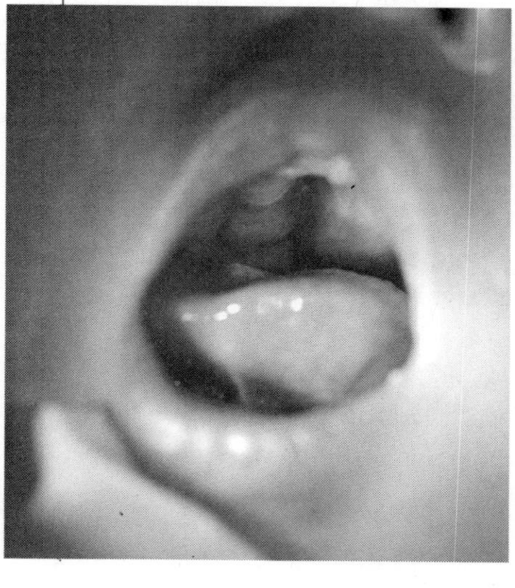

Figure 8.15 A submucous cleft may appear as a depression in the roof of baby's mouth. ©2020 Catherine Watson Genna, BS, IBCLC, used with permission.

1990), 48% of those with confirmed submucous clefts had feeding problem. This condition was also associated with chronic middle ear infections and speech problems later.

• • •

U.S. author and lactation consultant Catherine Watson Genna noted (C. W. Genna, 2017b) that in her lactation practice, babies with submucous clefts seem to feed better while nursing than from the bottle, even specialty bottles. Using the semi-reclined and upright feeding positions described in the previous section can give a baby who finds swallowing difficult more control over milk flow and reduce milk flow through the nose. Some of these babies develop more feeding problems as their head grows, which widens the gap in the muscles of the soft palate and makes feedings more challenging (M. Walker, 2017).

Some semi-reclined and upright feeding positions can give the baby more control over milk flow.

Baby's Lower Jaw and Airway

As described in Chapter 1, a wide-open mouth at latch helps ensure the baby draws in enough mammary tissue for good milk transfer. After latch, the effectively nursing baby has smooth jaw movements with a slight pause as her jaw lowers (C. W. Genna, 2017a). See the next point for how a small or recessed lower jaw can affect tongue placement and feeding effectiveness.

The baby's lower jaw determines in part how far the baby can open her mouth during latch and the placement of the tongue.

Small or Recessed Lower Jaw

All babies are born with receding chins, due in part to their chin-to-chest-position in utero. There is no agreed-upon objective definition for an unusually small lower jaw (mandible), also known as micrognathia (Nemec et al., 2015). But if the baby's lower jaw seems obviously small in relation to the upper jaw (maxilla), the baby may be more likely to have problems nursing.

Babies with an unusually short or recessed lower jaw may have early nursing problems.

A short or recessed jaw (retrognathia) may be problematic due to its effect on tongue placement. A recessed jaw and recessed tongue may restrict baby's tongue movements during nursing. One 2018 Canadian retrospective study (Morice et al., 2018) found no association between severity of jaw and tongue recession in babies with Pierre Robin sequence and feeding or swallowing problems. But according to U.S. lactation consultant Catherine Watson Genna (C. W. Genna, 2017b), a short lower jaw often means the tongue is attached to the jaw closer to the gums, which restricts normal tongue lifting. Micrognathia is also associated with a narrower upper airway. To keep their airway open, these babies may tilt back (extend) their head and position their tongue on the roof of their mouth, which can interfere with nursing.

• • •

Possible strategies for helping babies nurse with a short or recessed jaw include:

Some positioning strategies and tools may help babies with a short or recessed jaw nurse more effectively.

- A very asymmetrical latch (see p. 878) with head tilted back and baby's body pulled in close to the nursing parent's opposite nipple.
- Side-lying positions or semi-reclined starter positions, (see Figure 8.21 and p. 23-29) may help increase the baby's head extension for easier breathing.

If these positioning strategies aren't enough, other options include the use of a nipple shield (see p. 912-917) or finger-feeding (see p. 903-904), as a way to help the baby learn to coordinate sucking, swallowing and breathing and improve her muscle strength.

In babies with multiple challenges, such as Pierre-Robin sequence, a receding chin may be one of several issues that affect nursing (C. W. Genna, 2017b).

Airway Abnormalities

Symptoms of an airway abnormality include fast and noisy breathing, frequent coughing during nursing, and/or a high-pitched squeaky sound.

Consider the possibility of an airway abnormality in a slow-gaining, young baby who struggles to keep up with fast milk flow by coughing or sputtering during nursing (Landry & Thompson, 2012). If a high-pitched squeaky sound known as stridor occurs during nursing or at other times, this may be a sign that the baby has a narrowed airway and is one sign of breathing problems, such as laryngomalacia (narrowing of the upper airway), tracheomalacia (narrowing of the lower airway), vocal cord paralysis, or other respiratory issues. With laryngomalacia, the most common airway abnormality, the airway malformation can cause tissue in the larynx (voice box) to partially block the airway above the vocal cords. With tracheomalacia, which is less common, the cartilage rings in the trachea are misshapen, narrowing the airway.

For effective nursing, a baby needs to coordinate sucking, swallowing, and breathing. A baby with an airway malformation or instability usually breathes faster (more breaths per minute) than other babies to get the oxygen needed. Faster breathing means less time to swallow. When a baby must choose between breathing and eating, breathing always wins.

A baby with laryngomalacia, for example, often nurses in bursts of three to five sucks with longer breathing pauses and may sometimes look bluish during feeds (Nolder & Richter, 2015). Symptoms—which may be mild or severe—may appear at birth or during the first few weeks. Baby's symptoms usually worsen until 6 months and then improve through 18 to 24 months of age.

• • •

Baby's weight gain can help distinguish simple milk-flow issues from breathing issues.

When an airway abnormality compromises a baby's ability to nurse, this can lead to ineffective feeding, coughing and gasping during feeds, and latching struggles. When babies have trouble coping with milk flow, some assume this means overabundant milk production or "hyperlactation" (see p. 457). But babies with airway abnormalities often gain weight slowly, because their faster breathing requires more energy and therefore more calories, while also making milk transfer difficult. Babies struggling with overabundant milk production, on the other hand, usually gain weight faster than average, well above 2 pounds (900 grams) per month.

• • •

Reflux disease is more common among babies with airway abnormalities, and they may benefit from treatment.

The increased airway pressure these babies generate puts them at greater risk for gastroesophageal reflux disease (GERD) (Thottam, Simons, Choi, Maguire, & Mehta, 2016). GERD can cause painful feeds, further complicating nursing. When a baby has a respiratory issue, suggest having the baby evaluated by her healthcare provider for GERD, and if it is diagnosed, consider treatment. For details about GERD, see p. 304.

• • •

Patience and positioning adjustments can make nursing easier for babies with airway abnormalities.

The basic strategies that help nursing babies with respiratory issues include:

- Slow the milk flow (nurse after expressing some milk, paced bottle feeds)
- Help baby relax to slow breathing before feeds (rock, walk, massage, eye contact, babywearing)
- Treat reflux, if present
- Use positioning to keep the airway as open as possible

Although most babies nurse more easily in semi-reclined starter positions (see p. 23-29), these prone positions are particularly helpful for babies with breathing problems because babies have more control when milk flows "uphill." No matter what position is used, another important point for these babies is to allow their head to tilt back (extend) while nursing. Head extension also opens their upper airway and reduces respiratory distress (C. W. Genna, 2017b). Head extension is possible in any feeding position by sliding the baby's body in the direction of her feet. In any position, suggest making sure the baby can release the nipple whenever needed to take a breathing break. (Avoid holding baby's head in place.)

Some babies with an airway abnormality are more comfortable feeding for long periods at a leisurely pace, while others prefer to feed often for a short time.

• • •

If needed, suggest expressing milk as a supplement.

If a baby nurses ineffectively, suggest safeguarding the milk production by expressing milk and supplementing the baby with it. Some babies with airway abnormalities have difficulty bottle-feeding as well. If so, suggest the family consider supplementing with a specialized feeding device, such as a Haberman Feeder set to the slowest flow setting, which may be easier for the baby to manage.

VACCINES AND VITAMIN/MINERAL SUPPLEMENTS

Vaccines

The same immunization schedule is recommended for all babies, nursing or not. Nursing may enhance a baby's immune response to vaccinations.

Not all families choose to have their babies immunized or have that option. However, vaccines are recommended on the same timetable in both nursing and formula-fed babies (AAP, 2015). Nursing does not need to be delayed before, during, or after immunization.

Research in Sweden, Canada, and other countries found that some immunizations produce a more active immune response and, therefore, offer more protection from disease in nursing babies as compared with formula-fed babies (Pabst & Spady, 1990; Pabst et al., 1997; Silfverdal, Ekholm, & Bodin, 2007). One U.S. 12-month randomized, controlled, and blinded multisite feeding trial (Pickering et al., 1998) divided its 311 babies into two groups fed different infant formulas and one group who nursed. The nursing babies had significantly greater antibody response to the polio vaccine than the formula-fed babies.

A 2019 prospective observational study of about 250 Bangladeshi children (Huda et al., 2019) found an association between the abundance of *Bifidobacterium* in babies' gut (this "good bacterium" is at higher levels in exclusively nursing babies) during early infancy and greater T-cell response to vaccines at 2 years of age. These vaccines included tetanus, tuberculosis, polio, and hepatitis B. A 2014 study of Bangladeshi infants by the same research team (Huda et al., 2014) found that the babies who had more of the gut bacteria usually associated with formula feeding (*Enterobacteriales, Pseudmonadales,* and *Clostridiales*) had lower responses to the vaccines.

• • •

Nursing provides effective pain relief during immunizations.

One of the most difficult aspects of immunizations for many families is seeing their baby in pain. Nursing during immunizations is an effective way to soothe babies and reduce pain. As the Academy of Breastfeeding Medicine wrote in its 2016 Clinical Protocol #23 on nonpharmacological pain relief for nursing babies (Reece-Stremtan & Gray, 2016, p. 1): "Breastfeeding should be the first choice to alleviate procedural pain in neonates..." After reviewing 10 studies, a 2016 Cochrane Review (Harrison et al., 2016) concluded that during vaccinations, breastfeeding consistently reduced the time babies spent crying.

Vitamin and Mineral Supplements

Although it may seem counter-intuitive, in some specific cases, nursing babies benefit from vitamin or mineral supplements.

Human milk evolved over many thousands of years to contain just what our babies need. But not all babies are born full term, and changes in both lifestyle and diet mean that some exclusively nursing babies may benefit from a vitamin or mineral supplement.

Vitamin D Supplements

Daily vitamin D supplements are recommended for all exclusively nursing babies and in some parts of the world, for all babies.

Vitamin D is not actually a vitamin; it's a hormone precursor made by the body when the skin is exposed to the ultraviolet rays of the sun. Only about 10% to 20% of our vitamin D intake is meant to come from the food we eat (Papadimitriou, 2017; Wagner, Taylor, & Hollis, 2008). When early humans spent their daylight hours working outdoors with their skin exposed, this guaranteed healthy vitamin D blood levels. With the lifestyle changes that occurred as people moved to northern climates and wore more clothing, by the 17th century, vitamin D deficiency and rickets became a major health problem. In the 1800s, scientists discovered that lack of sunlight exposure was the cause of rickets and began to recommend fish-liver oils to prevent and treat it. In the 1920s, vitamin D was formally identified, and in the 1930s, milk fortified with vitamin D began to be sold. For a time, rickets was virtually eliminated. However, over the past decades as people began spending more time indoors and using sunscreen when outside, the incidence of rickets increased. Also, among some cultures, religious beliefs or climate require women to cover themselves completely when outside the home. In recent years, researchers turned their focus to vitamin D intake recommendations, incidence of vitamin D deficiency, and the effects of vitamin D levels on overall health.

Scientists question current recommended daily allowances of vitamin D. When analyzing current recommendations for vitamin D intake, scientists thought it curious that the same daily allowance (400 IU) was recommended for a tiny preterm baby, an older child, and an adult (Hollis & Wagner, 2004). As they investigated further, they found the less-than-scientific basis for this recommendation. The amount of vitamin D recommended—400 IU—equals the amount in the traditional cod-liver-oil treatment for rickets. Yet U.K. and Turkish research found that 400 IU per day was not enough to increase vitamin D levels in pregnant and breastfeeding mothers (Cockburn et al., 1980; Halicioglu et al., 2012). At 400 IU per day, blood vitamin D levels often decreased, especially during the winter months. Research done internationally found widespread vitamin D deficiency among pregnant women:

> **KEY CONCEPT**
>
> *The current recommendation of 400 IU of vitamin D per day is not sufficient to increase vitamin D levels in pregnant and breastfeeding women.*

- 52% of Black and 23% of white women in the southern U.S. (Burke et al., 2019)
- 63% in Switzerland (Cabaset et al., 2019)
- 84% in northeastern India (Sharma, Nath, & Mohammad, 2019)
- 28% in Australia and New Zealand (R. L. Wilson et al., 2018)
- 60% in Iran (Tabrizi et al., 2018)

When babies are born to vitamin-D deficient parents, they are at increased risk of vitamin D deficiency, which is associated with a greater incidence of cardiovascular problems, Type 1 and 2 diabetes, many types of cancer, and autoimmune diseases, such as lupus and multiple sclerosis (Papadimitriou, 2017; Wagner et al., 2008).

According to one 2016 global consensus (Munns et al., 2016), due to the widespread incidence of vitamin D deficiency during pregnancy, all infants and children should be supplemented with vitamin D. However, the need for extra vitamin D may be even greater among nursing babies. While lactating, the nursing parent's blood vitamin D level determines the level of vitamin D in the milk. In recent decades, the number of reported cases of rickets and vitamin D deficiency among exclusively nursing babies worldwide increased (Beck-Nielsen, Jensen, Gram, Brixen, & Brock-Jacobsen, 2009; Girish & Subramaniam, 2008; Munns et al., 2012). As more birthing parents become vitamin D deficient, so do their nursing babies. A 2016 U.S. cross-sectional study of more than 4,500 healthy children (Darmawikarta et al., 2016) found that when nursing babies were not supplemented with vitamin D, the longer they nursed, the lower their vitamin D blood levels fell.

Risk factors for vitamin D deficiency.. Parents and babies with dark-skin are at greater risk of vitamin D deficiency because darker skin pigmentation acts as a natural filter of ultraviolet light, so they require more sunlight exposure for their body to make vitamin D. Other risk factors for vitamin D deficiency include spending little time outdoors, keeping the skin covered with clothing or sunscreen while outside, and living in areas with heavy air pollution or little sunlight for parts of the year. In temperate climates with cold winters that keep people indoors more, vitamin D levels among people with lighter skin are higher during the summer and lower during the winter (R. L. Wilson et al., 2018). The recommendation to avoid exposure to sunlight to prevent sun damage and skin cancer also contributes to greater risk of vitamin D deficiency (AAP, 1999).

As a result of widespread vitamin D deficiencies and increasing reports of rickets among exclusively nursing babies, in 2008 the American Academy of Pediatrics recommended all exclusively nursing babies be supplemented with 400 IU of vitamin D (one drop) each day, starting within the first 2 months of life and continuing through adolescence (Wagner & Greer, 2008). Some companies make a liquid vitamin supplement with only vitamin D. Because infant formula already contains extra vitamin D, in the U.S., vitamin D supplementation is not recommended for any baby receiving more than 500 mL (17 ounces) of formula per day.

Vitamin D and allergy. One preliminary Swedish study of 206 babies found an association with vitamin D intake during the first year of life and increased incidence of allergy independent of family history (Back, Blomquist, Hernell, & Stenberg, 2009). But due to limited information, a 2018 systematic review (Yepes-Nunez et al., 2018) was unable to confirm this association.

• • •

An alternative to supplementing the nursing baby with vitamin D is to supplement the nursing parent.

Vitamin D blood levels in the nursing parent determine the vitamin D levels in the milk. If the previously recommended 400 IU per day are taken during lactation, research confirmed that this is not enough and puts nursing babies at risk of vitamin D deficiency (Ziegler, Hollis, Nelson, & Jeter, 2006).

One option is to supplement the nursing baby with vitamin D drops. But when only the baby is supplemented, there is still the nursing parent's vitamin D status to consider. Research found that vitamin D deficiency after birth was associated with depression (Abedi, Bovayri, Fakhri, & Jahanfar, 2018; Murphy & Wagner, 2008), as well as the same health problems associated with vitamin D deficiency in the baby mentioned in the previous point.

How much vitamin D do nursing parents need to take to ensure their baby receives healthy levels of vitamin D via their milk? Most prenatal vitamins contain only 400 IU, which results in the parent's vitamin D levels decreasing over time and nursing babies who are vitamin D deficient (Hollis & Wagner, 2004). According to randomized controlled trials conducted in the U.S. and India, the dose that's needed for vitamin D sufficiency in parent and baby depends on how the vitamin D supplement is given.

Oral vitamin D

- 6400 IU per day (Hollis et al., 2015; Wagner, Hulsey, Fanning, Ebeling, & Hollis, 2006)

Injections of vitamin D

- One 60,000 IU injection daily on 10 consecutive days (600,000 IU total) beginning 1 to 2 days after birth (Naik, Faridi, Batra, & Madhu, 2017), which led to vitamin D sufficiency for both through the babies' first 6 months
- A one-time injection of 150,000 IU after birth, which led to vitamin D sufficiency for both through the babies' first 28 days (Oberhelman et al., 2013)

Although concerns about vitamin D toxicity were raised in years past, research into these levels of supplementation laid these concerns to rest (Heaney, Davies, Chen, Holick, & Barger-Lux, 2003; Vieth, 1999; Vieth, Chan, & MacFarlane, 2001).

Vitamin B_{12} Supplements

Vitamin B_{12} supplements are recommended for nursing babies whose nursing parent is vitamin B_{12} deficient.

Nursing parents at risk of a vitamin B_{12} deficiency include those on a diet without animal products (such as a vegan diet) and those with a history of gastric bypass or other bariatric surgery. Others at risk are those with Crohn's disease and other malabsorption disorders. Because nursing parents with a vitamin B_{12} deficiency produce milk low in vitamin B_{12}, their nursing babies are also at risk of vitamin B_{12} deficiency. Symptoms of vitamin B_{12} deficiency in the baby often develop before symptoms in the parent, appearing within the first few months of life or going unrecognized until later. These symptoms include lack of interest in feeding, slow weight gain, failure to thrive, and eventually neurological problems. Although the parent may have no symptoms, a blood test can detect this deficiency. In this case, both parent and baby may need to receive vitamin B_{12} supplements. For more details, see p. 568-569.

Iron Supplements

Healthy iron levels are important for normal development, but routine iron supplements can be detrimental in babies with normal iron levels.

Most babies born full term at average or above average birth weight to well-nourished birthing parents have enough iron stores to last through their first 6 to 9 months of life (Ziegler, Nelson, & Jeter, 2014). The iron in human milk is much better absorbed than iron from other sources, up to 50% absorption from human milk compared with 4% absorption from infant formula (Griffin & Abrams, 2001). But because the amount of iron in human milk is low, nursing babies also need iron from solid foods high in iron beginning at around 6 months (A. Brown, 2017; Hong, Chang, Shin, & Oh, 2017).

Low iron levels are a problem. If they get too low, this puts baby at risk for iron deficiency and anemia, which are associated with developmental delays and neurological problems (Lozoff & Georgieff, 2006). If a baby's blood iron levels stay too low for too long, these neurological problems may become irreversible.

As a precaution, in 2010, the American Academy of Pediatrics began recommending routine iron supplements for all nursing babies starting at 4 months (Baker, Greer, & Committee on Nutrition American Academy of, 2010). However, after reviewing the literature, the AAP Section on Breastfeeding (AAP, 2011) concluded this recommendation was based on inadequate research. Other problems can develop if babies with normal iron levels are routinely supplemented with extra iron. The Academy of Breastfeeding Medicine wrote in its 2018 protocol on iron, zinc, and vitamin D (Taylor, 2018, p. 402):

> "There are potential harms of iron supplementation, especially on immune function and in possibly decreasing the bioavailability of iron contained in human milk. In addition, there is potential harm in infant growth and morbidity when iron supplementation is provided to iron-sufficient infants."

If there is concern about a baby's iron levels, a simple blood test to measure the baby's iron status can usually be done in a healthcare office or clinic. For more details, see p. 143-146.

• • •

Babies born with low iron stores at birth may need extra iron before 6 months.

Babies at risk for low iron stores include some preterm, growth-restricted, and low-birth-weight babies, and babies born to iron-deficient parents. Low iron stores at birth increase the chance that their iron stores may run out before 6 months. In these situations, the American Academy of Pediatrics recommends providing iron supplements while continuing full nursing (AAP, 2012).

Fluoride Supplements

Fluoride supplements are not recommended for the nursing baby younger than 6 months.

Fluoride supplementation in babies younger than 6 months is associated with a permanent discoloration of the teeth called fluorosis. As a result, both the American Academy of Pediatrics and the U.S. Centers for Disease Control and Prevention recommend against fluoride supplements before 6 months (AAP, 2012; CDC, 2001). Fluoride supplements are only recommended in babies older than 6 months when local drinking water contains less than 0.3 ppm of fluoride.

ILLNESS IN THE NURSING BABY

When a child is ill, some parents may be concerned about how the illness will affect nursing.

When talking with families of sick children, ask how they are coping and what the baby's healthcare provider recommended. Continued nursing is almost always the best option, because it comforts a sick baby and helps her recover faster by providing antibodies specific to her illness.

Colds, Flu, Congestion, and Ear Infections

When a nursing baby with nasal congestion struggles to breathe during feeds, provide some basic strategies to make feeding easier.

A congested baby with a cold or the flu usually finds nursing easier than bottle-feeding because—unlike feeds with a fast flowing bottle—during nursing it is easier to coordinate sucking, swallowing, and breathing (Lawrence & Lawrence, 2016). Sometimes, though, when a baby is congested, nursing can become challenging. When a baby's nose is clogged, the following basic strategies may help:

- Before nursing, keep the baby mostly upright (in arms or in a sling or carrier) so that her sinuses can drain.
- If the baby's healthcare provider recommends it, use a soft nasal aspirator to gently clear her nose of mucus.
- Nurse in a position upright enough so that baby's sinuses can drain.
- Nurse more often, as frequent feeds are often easier to manage.
- Nurse where the air is moist; use a cool-mist vaporizer or nurse in the bathroom with the shower running.
- Contact the baby's healthcare provider for other suggestions for easing the baby's symptoms and advice on preventing the spread of illness.

A 2013 U.S. study that included data from 2,833 babies during the first year of life (Soto-Ramirez et al., 2013) concluded that the use of feeding bottles and infant formula were associated with increased risk of coughing and wheezing during the first year of life.

• • •

If during an ear infection or while congested the baby won't nurse, suggest expressing milk and feeding it by spoon or cup.

When babies are so congested they cannot breathe through their nose, it can be difficult to nurse. Nursing can also become painful during an ear infection when sucking creates pressure in the ears. If the baby won't or can't nurse, suggest expressing milk as often as the baby was nursing and offer her the expressed milk in a spoon or cup, offering to nurse every hour or so. This ensures the baby gets the fluids she needs and will help keep the nursing parent comfortable and prevent mastitis. Assure the family that when the baby can breathe through her nose again or the ear infection resolves, she should return to nursing.

• • •

A baby with chronic congestion or trouble breathing during nursing for other reasons should be evaluated by a healthcare provider.

Chronic congestion can be a sign of allergy, gastroesophageal reflux disease, or other physical problems. Breathing always comes before eating, so if breathing is difficult while nursing, a baby will usually pull on and off and may gain weight slowly.

Struggles with breathing during feeds may be due to inflammation in the mouth or throat from rough suctioning or intubation after birth, spasms, or physical abnormalities of the mouth, throat, or airway, such as choanal atresia (a blockage between the nose and pharynx), tracheomalacia, and laryngomalacia (see p. 292-293) (C. W. Genna, 2017b; M. Walker, 2017). Any baby who consistently struggles with breathing at feeds or who makes high-pitched, squeaky sounds (called "stridor") while nursing, should be checked by her healthcare provider to determine and treat the cause.

KEY CONCEPT

A baby with a cold, flu or ear infection usually finds nursing easier but may benefit from some simple strategies.

Gastrointestinal Illness

Nearly all nursing babies with diarrhea and/or vomiting will recover faster if they keep nursing.

If a baby takes anything by mouth, it should be mother's milk, in part because it is absorbed so quickly that some fluids and nutrients will be retained (Heyman, 2006). Permanent weaning is only necessary in the very rare cases where diarrhea and vomiting are symptoms of a metabolic disorder, such as classic galactosemia (see p. 320-322), which usually becomes obvious during the first week of life.

• • •

When a gastrointestinal illness causes diarrhea and/or vomiting, suggest the family be alert to signs of dehydration.

When a nursing baby contracts an illness that causes vomiting and/or diarrhea, it usually passes within a few days. But if prolonged, it can cause more serious problems. Diarrhea occurs when the lining of the intestine becomes inflamed and irritated. Nutrients pass too quickly through the body and fluid is leaked. Either diarrhea alone or diarrhea with vomiting can cause the baby's body to lose water and salt, which may lead to dehydration and eventually to shock.

Whenever a baby shows any of the following signs of dehydration, encourage the family to contact the baby's healthcare provider right away:

- Listlessness, lethargy, and/or sleeping through feeds
- Weak cry
- Baby's skin loses its resiliency (when pinched, it no longer bounces back)
- Dry mouth and eyes
- Fewer tears
- Fewer wet diapers (≤2 in 24 hours)
- Baby's fontanel (soft spot) appears sunken or depressed
- Fever

Dehydration can be prevented by feeding the baby frequently to improve her fluid intake.

Diarrhea

Diarrhea differs from normal nursing stools in frequency, consistency, and/or smell.

Not all frequent and loose stools are diarrhea. A baby's first stool, called meconium, is greenish black and sticky. Usually by about the fourth or fifth day of life, the stools turn yellow, yellow-green, or tan and appear loose and unformed, resembling split pea soup. Occasional green stools are also in the normal range of stool colors. Because of the beneficial bacteria in the exclusively nursing baby's intestine, the odor is usually mild and inoffensive.

On one end of the spectrum, some nursing babies pass frequent stools, sometimes after every feed. Typically, babies younger than 4 to 6 weeks old have at least three to four stools each day (Nommsen-Rivers, Heinig, Cohen, & Dewey, 2008; Shrago, Reifsnider, & Insel, 2006). After 4 to 6 weeks of age, some nursing babies stool less often—as infrequently as once a week—but more profusely. As long as the baby is gaining weight in the expected range (during the first 3 months, an average of 1 ounce or 30 g per day), fewer stools per day are not a cause for concern.

Diarrhea occurs less often among nursing babies (Richard et al., 2018; Santos, Santos, Santos, Leite, & Mello, 2015), but when it occurs, diarrhea may be caused by gastrointestinal illness or as a side effect of a food or medication either consumed directly by the baby or passed to the baby via mother's milk (see later point). The difference between normal nursing stools and diarrhea include:

- More stools, as many as 12 to 16 per day
- Watery stools, often with few "curds"
- A stronger, more offensive smell

• • •

When extended diarrhea occurs after an illness, continued nursing is recommended.

Some healthcare providers recommend weaning babies to formula who are fussy or develop diarrhea because they have "lactose intolerance," but in most cases, weaning is not recommended, and many babies switched to lactose-free formulas do not improve (Heyman, 2006).

Lactose is a sugar abundant in human milk. The enzyme lactase, which is produced in the small intestine, processes lactose by breaking it down into glucose and galactose. Lactose intolerance usually refers to the reactions (bloating, gas, abdominal pain, diarrhea, nausea) that occur when a lack of lactase leaves lactose unprocessed in the gut.

KEY CONCEPT

Most babies with temporary lactose intolerance should continue nursing.

Most cases of lactose intolerance occur only in older children and adults. These are the four main types.

- **Primary lactase deficiency** is the most common. It does not affect young babies but occurs later in life in about 70% of the world's population (with the exception of those of northern European ancestry). Lactase production gradually decreases as early as age three or as late as adulthood. When a nursing parent has this type, the baby will not become lactose intolerant until she is older. This type does not cause diarrhea in babies.
- **Congenital lactase deficiency** (hypolactasia) is a very rare genetic disorder that becomes obvious shortly after birth, causing dehydration, illness, and lack of weight gain (Savilahti, Launiala, & Kuitunen, 1983; Wanes, Husein, & Naim, 2019). Like babies with the metabolic disorder classic galactosemia, the few babies with this condition cannot be safely nursed.
- **Developmental lactase deficiency** describes the temporarily lower level of lactase production common in preterm babies younger than 34 weeks gestation.
- **Secondary lactase deficiency** is the most common type in babies and young children. It is a temporary condition caused by damage to the lining of the small intestine from a medication, infection, celiac disease, or other illness.

To repeat, this last type of lactose intolerance is a temporary condition. Sometimes called "nuisance diarrhea," it usually occurs in a baby or toddler after a gastrointestinal illness, when gut damage temporarily slows or stops the production of lactase. While this damage is healing, diarrhea continues for an average of 2 to 4 weeks and then resolves on its own. When the diarrhea does not immediately resolve, many families are told to switch their nursing babies to formula. However, the American Academy of Pediatrics (AAP) currently recommends continued nursing both during infectious illness with diarrhea and after, as long as the baby has no more than mild dehydration. The AAP wrote (Heyman, 2006, p. 1284): "Breastfed infants should be continued on human milk in all cases". The AAP also concluded that except in severely malnourished formula-fed babies, low-lactose and lactose-free formulas have no clinical advantages.

Other possible causes of "nuisance diarrhea" from intestinal damage include treatment with antibiotics, solid foods that irritate the lining of the child's gut, and excessive fruit juice consumption (Heyman, 2017).

• • •

If the baby seems otherwise healthy, green stools may simply be a normal color variation or may indicate a sensitivity to a food or drug the baby consumed directly or a sensitivity to something the nursing parent ingested that passed into the milk. Two U.S. breastfeeding medicine physicians wrote in their book for

Green watery stools without symptoms of illness may be a sign the baby is sensitive to a food or drug.

medical professionals (Lawrence & Lawrence, 2016, pp. 487-488):

> "Occasionally, an infant will have diarrhea or an intestinal upset because of something in the mother's diet. It is usually self-limited, and the best treatment is to continue to nurse at the breast. If the mother has been taking a laxative that is absorbed or has been eating laxative foods, such as fruits in excess, she should adjust her diet."

Also see "Is Baby Reacting to Something in the Parent's Diet?" on p. 561.

• • •

A foremilk-hindmilk imbalance is unlikely to be the cause of most cases of green, watery stools.

In the 1980s, a theory proposed by two U.K. researchers to explain green, watery stools is referred to as a "foremilk-hindmilk imbalance" (Woolridge & Fisher, 1988). In their 1988 article, these researchers described case reports of irritable, slow-gaining babies with gas and frequent, sometimes explosive green, watery stools, whose symptoms resolved when their mothers changed their breastfeeding pattern by allowing the baby to "finish the first breast first," rather than switching breasts after a set 10-minute period. The researchers suggested that in those with abundant milk production, switching sides before the baby reached the fattier hindmilk might have overloaded the baby's small intestine with more lactose from the low-fat foremilk than it could absorb, causing these symptoms. However, these results have never been replicated. Ideally babies should come off the first side when finished, rather than after a set number of minutes. If a baby has these symptoms and has been fed by the clock, suggest instead allowing the baby to come off the first side on her own before offering the second side. There is no need for most families to be concerned about a foremilk-hindmilk imbalance because according to research (Kent et al., 2006), nursing babies using a wide variety of feeding rhythms easily access the right balance of foremilk and hindmilk.

• • •

A temporary or permanent weaning during a bout of diarrhea is not usually beneficial and may even lead to more problems.

When a baby's illness includes vomiting or diarrhea, the standard advice was once to interrupt nursing and feed instead an oral electrolyte solution, such as Pedialyte, or the more concentrated oral rehydration therapy (ORT). But research found that temporary weaning was associated with more negative health outcomes than continuing to nurse (Ogbo et al., 2019), in part because mother's milk is so easily and rapidly digested. Even in cases of rotavirus, in its Red Book, the American Academy of Pediatrics wrote (AAP, 2015, p. 686): "Breastfeeding is associated with milder disease and should be encouraged". In the developing world, interrupting nursing when an ill baby has diarrhea was found to double the risk of increased severity and death (Clemens et al., 1988; Mahalanabis, Alam, Rahman, & Hasnat, 1991).

KEY CONCEPT

The vast majority of babies with diarrhea should continue nursing.

In developing countries where diarrhea is the number one cause of death in infants and small children, studies found that babies return to health faster when they continue to nurse, with exclusively nursing babies recovering faster than mixed-fed or formula-fed babies (K. H. Brown, 1994; Perin, Carvajal-Velez, Carter, Bryce, & Newby, 2015). To improve health outcomes in babies with diarrhea, in India, Bangladesh, and other developing countries, many non-nursing parents are helped to relactate during their babies' hospital stay (Haider, Kabir, Fuchs, & Habte, 2000).

If the baby's healthcare provider recommends temporary weaning and the family would like to explore other options, suggest telling the baby's healthcare provider they want to continue nursing and ask about reading together some of the references cited in this section. If the healthcare provider is not open to that option, suggest seeking a second opinion.

Vomiting

When a family says that the baby is vomiting, rule out the possibility that the baby is not ill but "spitting up" after feedings.

If a baby is simply bringing up some milk after a feed, otherwise known as "spitting up" or "spilling," she would have no other symptoms of illness. Although most use the term "vomit" to describe a more forceful ejection of milk, some even refer to a dribble of milk in the corner of the baby's mouth that way. In Western cultures where longer nursing intervals are often expected, more than half of babies spit up at least once a day during their first 3 months of life, with spitting up peaking at 4 to 5 months (Hegar et al., 2009; S. P. Nelson, Chen, Syniar, & Christoffel, 1997). Even if a baby appears to be spitting up a lot of milk, what's more important is how she is growing and gaining. It's also important whether she seems generally happy when held or whether she's irritable and fussy most of the time. One possible cause of borderline or slow weight gain and a generally unhappy temperament could be gastroesophageal reflux disease (see next section). If she is a "happy spitter," in other words, gaining weight well and seems content when held, assure the family there is likely no cause for concern.

• • •

If a baby who wasn't spitting up before starts, it may be due to a sensitivity to a food or drug.

If there are no other signs of illness, vomiting that starts after weeks or months of uneventful nursing may be a sign of a sensitivity to a food or drug she receives directly or through her mother's milk. Depending on the type of reaction, spitting up could occur as quickly as right after the exposure or as long as 48 hours later (Heine, 2008). See "Is Baby Reacting to Something in Parent's Diet?" on p. 561.

• • •

If a baby projectile vomits at least once a day, suggest having her checked for pyloric stenosis.

Regular projectile vomiting may be a symptom of pyloric stenosis, an overgrowth of the muscular tube between the stomach and duodenum. In a baby with pyloric stenosis, the milk does not move easily from the baby's stomach into her intestines, which can limit the nutrients the baby absorbs.

One risk factor associated with the development of pyloric stenosis is treatment with certain antibiotics, such as erythromycin, azithromycin, and others known as "macrolides" (Abdellatif et al., 2019; Almaramhy & Al-Zalabani, 2019). Another risk factor is bottle-feeding. One large-population study based on data from the more than 70,000 babies in the Danish National Birth Cohort (Krogh et al., 2012) found that bottle-fed babies were 4.6 times more likely than nursing babies to be diagnosed with pyloric stenosis. But it is possible for nursing babies to develop this condition.

> **KEY CONCEPT**
>
> *Regular projectile vomiting may be a symptom of pyloric stenosis.*

Symptoms of pyloric stenosis usually appear between 2 and 6 weeks of age. The cause of projectile vomiting—often the first symptom—is the contraction of the baby's stomach muscles, which forces the milk up her throat and out of her mouth, sometimes as far as several feet away. At first this may happen only occasionally, but usually it occurs more and more over time until the baby projectile vomits after every feed, which can lead to weight loss and dehydration. Projectile vomiting is not always due to pyloric stenosis, but if it happens at least once a day, suggest having the baby's healthcare provider rule it out.

The treatment for pyloric stenosis is to first evaluate the baby for dehydration and, if needed, restore her electrolyte balance, and then perform a simple surgery called a pyloromyotomy, the most common surgery of the early months (Taghavi, Powell, Patel, & McBride, 2017). During the surgery, suggest expressing milk for comfort and to keep milk production stable. If the surgery is uncomplicated, the baby should be able to nurse after she recovers from the anesthesia. Early feeding post-surgery was associated with decreased hospital stay and reduced stress on the family (Garza, Morash, Dzakovic, Mondschein, & Jaksic, 2002; Puapong, Kahng, Ko, & Applebaum, 2002).

• • •

If an obviously sick baby vomits after every nursing, share strategies that can help keep the baby hydrated and decrease the vomiting.

When a baby has a gastrointestinal illness, the family may worry that because she vomits after every feed that she won't keep enough milk down to prevent dehydration. One way to reduce the vomiting is for the nursing parent to express most of the milk before the baby nurses. This allows the baby to take less milk while sucking for comfort. Offering a little milk more often provides the fluids the baby needs in small doses and keeps vomiting to a minimum until she can handle larger feeds again.

If the baby is 6 months or older, suggest offering ice chips or water from a spoon. Ice goes down slowly and can distract a miserable baby, so the baby's stomach stays emptier longer. Reinforce the value of continued nursing, and share with the family the symptoms of dehydration listed in the previous section so they are aware of the warning signs.

Reflux Disease (GERD)

A baby with gastroesophageal reflux disease (GERD) may or may not spit up, but she may have pain, feeding problems, and other symptoms.

During the first months of life, the sphincter between a baby's esophagus and stomach has low muscle tone and relaxes often. In an average baby, several times each day her stomach contents wash back into her esophagus, also known as gastroesophageal reflux (GER) (Vandenplas et al., 2009). Spitting up (or "spilling") occurs when the stomach contents make it all the way up the esophagus and out the mouth. Spitting up occurs in up to 50% to 70% of babies and peaks around 4 to 5 months of age, occurring less and less often as the digestive system matures (Lightdale, Gremse, Section on Gastroenterology, & Nutrition, 2013). By 12 months, only about 4% to 10% of babies still spit up (Hegar et al., 2009).

When a baby is growing, thriving, and feeding normally, spitting up is a temporary inconvenience. These babies are sometimes referred to as "happy spitters." But when GER causes damage to the lining of the esophagus, normal GER may become gastroesophageal reflux disease (GERD). A baby with GERD may spit up or she may not, because damage to the esophagus can occur even if the stomach contents don't make it all the way to the mouth (called "silent reflux"). GERD can cause health issues, such as respiratory problems (congestion, coughing, wheezing, bronchitis, pneumonia), apnea, esophageal narrowing or stricture, anemia, failure to thrive, and esophagitis, or inflammation of the esophagus, which can cause pain during and after feeds (Semeniuk & Kaczmarski, 2008). GERD can cause behaviors that are upsetting to both babies and parents:

- Crying and irritability
- Poor weight gain
- Sleep problems day and night (Ghaem et al., 1998)
- Back arching and head turning (Frankel, Shalaby, & Orenstein, 2006)
- Feeding aversion, which sometimes leads to feeding refusal (Heine, 2008)

KEY CONCEPT

GERD can cause health problems in babies and be stressful for the whole family.

GERD may be the cause of feeding problems and behaviors sometimes labeled as "colic." In one Belgian study of 60 irritable babies 1 to 6 months old who did not respond to mothers' elimination of cow's milk from their diet, 66% had test results indicating GERD and 43% had esophagitis (Vandenplas, Badriul, Verghote, Hauser, & Kaufman, 2004). One Israeli study confirmed GERD in 16 of 26 babies (62%) thought to have colic; within 2 weeks of treatment with GERD medication, all 16 babies were colic-free (Berkowitz, Naveh, & Berant, 1997). One Belgian study of 700 infants and young children with feeding problems diagnosed 33% with GERD (Rommel, De Meyer, Feenstra, & Veereman-Wauters, 2003). The esophageal damage caused by GERD may lead to other physical problems, such as vocal cord swelling, which can contribute to swallowing and breathing difficulties (Mercado-Deane et al., 2001).

• • •

When a baby is crying and seems to be in pain, it is only natural for parents to want to find the cause and relieve the pain. However, at this writing, most babies treated for GERD by their healthcare providers are diagnosed by symptoms alone, as no diagnostic tests have been found to be completely reliable. In the American Academy of Pediatrics' clinical report on GERD, its authors wrote (Lightdale et al., 2013, p. e1686):

Because some symptoms of reflux disease are common in young babies, GERD may be misdiagnosed and overtreated.

> "For most pediatric patients, a history and physical examination in the absence of warning signs are sufficient to reliably diagnose uncomplicated GER and initiate treatment strategies. Generally speaking, diagnostic testing is not necessary."

According to Australian physician Pamela Douglas (P. S. Douglas, 2013a), many babies younger than 3 to 4 months treated with medications for reflux disease (or treated for "lactose intolerance") were crying and irritable due to undiagnosed feeding problems.

There are many possible causes of spitting up, fussiness, and irritability in young babies, and it is important to rule them out before assuming they are due to reflux disease. For example, allergy to cow's milk protein sometimes mimics symptoms of GERD, as allergy can cause tissue irritation along the gastrointestinal tract (Salvatore & Vandenplas, 2002). This is one reason the basic strategies listed in a later point include exclusively nursing parents eliminating all dairy from their diet for several weeks to rule this out. Also, see the later section on allergy on p. 309. In a 2017 article, an IBCLC described three case reports of infants who were spitting up regularly (McFadden, 2017). The IBCLC determined that one baby was being overfed from a bottle and when the parents began pacing feeds (see p. 902-903), the baby's spitting up subsided. The other two babies needed surgery, one for pyloric stenosis and the other for a bowel obstruction. The IBCLC concluded that it's important not to simply reassure concerned parents about their baby's spitting up without considering all possibilities.

It's not just healthcare providers who sometimes mistake other issues for reflux disease. An Australian mixed-methods study of infants admitted to the hospital during the first 12 months of life examined the medical records of more than 11,500 babies who were hospitalized for reflux and conducted focus groups with providers (Dahlen et al., 2018). The providers reported seeing a huge growth in the number of infants diagnosed and treated for reflux in recent years and admitted to feeling pressured by parents to prescribe reflux medication when babies seemed unsettled. One pediatrician said (Dahlen et al., 2018, p. 7):"You have mums that say they go to the doctor and say, 'I want Losec' (a proton pump inhibitor) and the doctor will write a script." This study found that 38% of the babies admitted to the hospital for reflux disease had "nonspecific symptoms peculiar to infancy" like excessive crying, and irritability. The mothers of the study babies hospitalized for reflux disease were more likely to be first-time mothers, delivered in a private hospital, and have a male baby who was born early and sent to the special-care nursery. They were also 4.6 times more likely to have a psychiatric disorder (anxiety in particular) than mothers of babies who were not hospitalized for reflux disease.

• • •

Weaning to formula can make reflux worse.

When a baby is miserable much of the time and struggles to nurse or has other symptoms of reflux disease, this can demoralize even the most dedicated nursing family. In this situation, parents may wonder if nursing is the problem. They may wonder if the baby is fussy because of inadequate milk intake, something in their diet, or the baby just doesn't like nursing. The baby's healthcare providers may suggest weaning under the mistaken assumption that switching to formula will help. One 2017 U.S. retrospective study based on data from the Infant Feeding Practices Study II found an association between symptoms of reflux at 1 month and weaning the next month (Chen, Soto-Ramirez, Zhang, & Karmaus, 2017).

KEY CONCEPT

Weaning to formula for GERD does not usually bring improvement.

Unfortunately, many families do not discover until their baby is already weaned that giving formula can actually make her discomfort worse. One Australian study that compared 37 breastfed and 37 formula-fed babies with reflux discovered that the episodes of reflux were shorter among the breastfed babies (Heacock, Jeffery, Baker, & Page, 1992). A questionnaire completed by Italian pediatricians from the records of 313 children aged 1 to 12 months who spit up found that nursing babies stopped spitting up earlier than babies fed formula (Campanozzi et al., 2009). A prospective Belgian study of 130 babies followed for 1 year concluded that exclusively nursing babies spit up less than nursing babies who also received formula (Hegar et al., 2009).

• • •

Some basic strategies are effective in minimizing the effects of reflux.

If reflux disease is suspected, in addition to seeing the baby's healthcare provider, a family can try some basic strategies to help keep their baby more comfortable: A study of 6- to 9-month-old babies with reflux disease in Indonesia (Hegar, Satari, Sjarif, & Vandenplas, 2013) found that these strategies improved symptoms by 50%.

Use baby's body position to minimize reflux. Gravity affects the backflow of the baby's stomach contents into the esophagus. To reduce reflux, suggest keeping baby's "head above bottom" when holding, feeding, changing, and sleeping.

- After feeds, keep baby upright for 20 to 30 minutes, either in arms (Figure 8.16) or in an upright baby carrier (Lightdale et al., 2013).
- At diaper changes, avoid lifting baby's legs; instead roll her on her left side to wipe. (see Fig. 8.17).
- Nurse with baby's head higher than bottom at about a 45º angle (Figure 8.18). Nursing parents can lean back with the baby's body tummy down on top (see next point) or hold her with her bottom in their lap or on a pillow (Wolf & Glass, 1992).
- When baby is awake and horizontal, lay her on her left side or on her tummy (prone) (Fig. 8.19). The baby's esophagus connects to the stomach near her back, and lying tummy down triggers less reflux than back-lying (supine) (Ewer, James, & Tobin, 1999).
- Avoid putting baby in a car seat except when riding in the car (Figure 8.20), as this position increases reflux (Carroll, Garrison, & Christakis, 2002).

Eliminate cow's milk and dairy from the nursing parent's diet. An exclusively nursing parent can rule in or out allergy to cow's milk protein, a condition that produces symptoms similar to reflux, by avoiding all forms of cow's milk protein, including milk, yogurt, ice cream, cheese, and butter, and all other sources of casein and whey (Heine, Jordan, Lubitz, Meehan, & Catto-Smith, 2006). It may take up to 4 weeks to notice an improvement in the baby's symptoms (Salvatore & Vandenplas, 2002). During the elimination diet, if formula is given, suggest using a type with the protein at least partially broken down, such as Nutramigen or Alimentum.

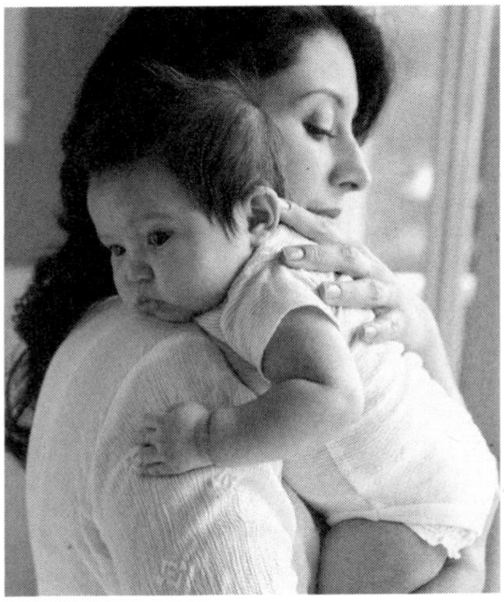

Figure. 8.16 To reduce reflux, keep baby upright after feeds for 20 to 30 minutes.

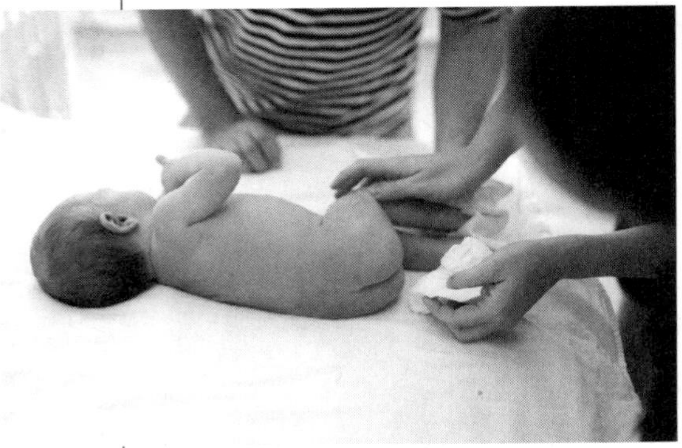

Figure 8.17 To reduce reflux during diaper changes, wipe baby on her left side.

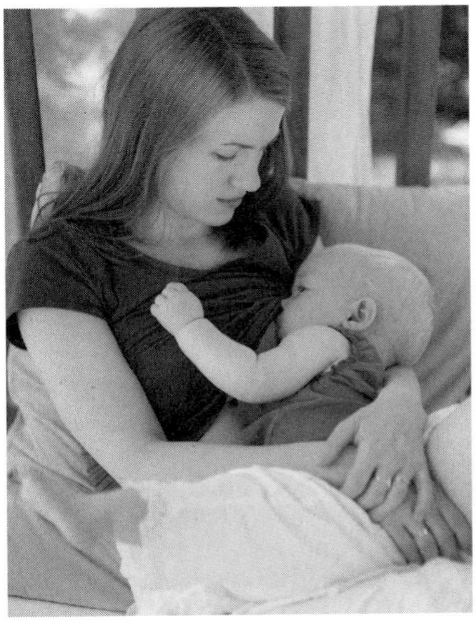

Figure 8.18 To reduce reflux, nurse baby with her "head above bottom".

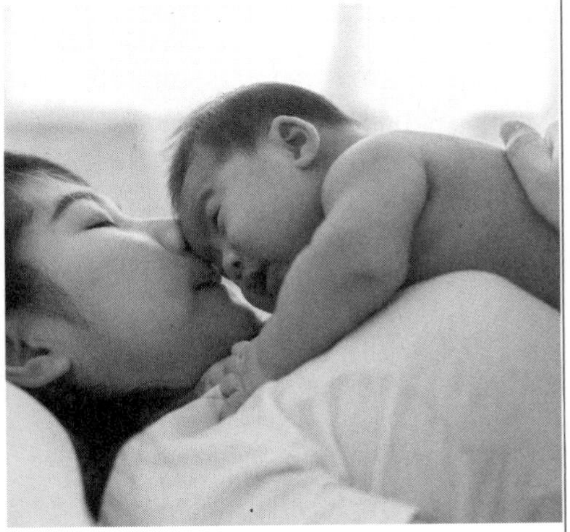

Figure 8.19 To reduce reflux, lay baby on her left side or prone on her tummy.

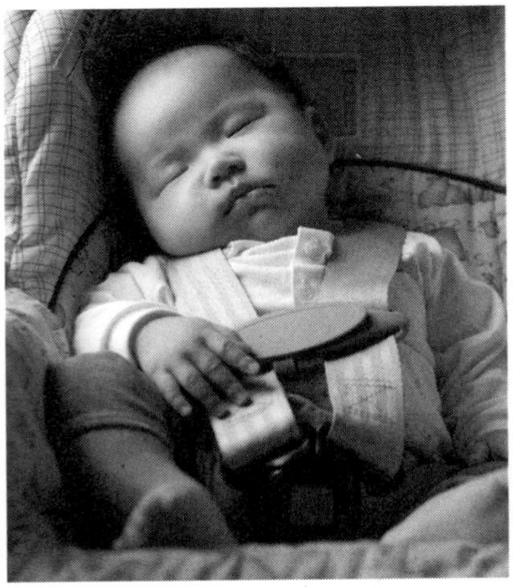

Figure 8.20 To reduce reflux, restrict baby's time in a car seat to car rides.

Feed often. A baby needs a certain volume of milk every 24 hours to grow and thrive (on average 25 oz. [750 mL]). Taking smaller volumes of milk more often means less milk in the stomach to wash back into the esophagus and less time with an empty high-acid-content stomach. One author noted that in the pediatric gastroenterology office where she worked, many mothers of babies with reflux had overabundant milk production (Boekel, 2000). She reported that many of these mothers regularly coaxed their babies to nurse longer because although they seemed finished after 5 to 10 minutes, they worried the baby had not nursed "long enough." As in an adult, an overly full stomach may worsen GERD symptoms.

• • •

Thickening milk is recommended to reduce reflux in formula-fed babies but not in nursing babies.

Formula-fed babies with GERD. Parents of formula-fed babies with GERD may be advised to add cereal or starch to formula to "thicken milk" as a way to reduce the number of reflux episodes (Lightdale et al., 2013). Alternatively, formulas are commercially available that are pre-thickened for this purpose.

Thickening milk is not recommended for nursing babies with GERD. A 2017 Cochrane Review article on the practice of thickening milk for babies with reflux (Kwok, Ojha, & Dorling, 2017) concluded that this practice may be helpful for bottle-feeding babies but found no evidence to support its use in nursing babies. Likewise, the American Academy of Pediatrics' clinical report on reflux (Lightdale et al., 2013) suggested thickeners as an optional strategy for formula-fed babies but not for nursing babies. Direct nursing alone appeared to reduce reflux. Adding solids such as cereal appeared to have no benefit. In 2017, U.S. researchers examined the data from more than 2,800 babies on the effects on reflux of different feeding modes, nursing, formula, combined, and solids (Chen et al., 2017). These authors concluded that feeding solids was not protective of reflux in nursing babies. They also found that the addition of formula and bottle-feeding increased reflux.

The challenges of thickening human milk. Research documented the practical difficulties of trying to thicken expressed human milk. In infants with potential feeding or swallowing disorders, healthcare providers sometimes perform diagnostic tests using barium and thickened liquids to monitor a baby's feeding. When starch-based thickening agents were added to expressed human milk, the results were surprising. The enzymes in human milk (amylase was identified as one) completely digested the thickener (de Almeida, Barker, & Lederer, 2011). In fact, during the 20-minute wait time needed for the thickener to act, the human milk was thinner than before the thickener was added. A 2013 Australian overview article that described the challenges of thickening human milk for feeding and swallowing testing (Cichero, Nicholson, & September, 2013) concluded that starch-based thickeners cannot be used with human milk. Rather, if thickening is necessary for diagnostic tests, gum-based agents made from carob bean gum and guar gum are recommended for use in Australia and New Zealand.

• • •

Most babies outgrow reflux, but in severe cases, they may need treatment to prevent future health problems.

Spitting up is outgrown as the sphincter muscle between stomach and esophagus lengthens with age and increases in muscle tone. But when normal reflux becomes reflux disease, weight gain and growth may slow, pain may lead to feeding struggles, and damage to the esophagus may put babies at risk later in life.

One 2015 U.S. overview article (Baird, Harker, & Karmes, 2015) suggested that the first step in treating suspected reflux disease is to try the basic strategies listed beginning at the bottom of p. 306 for a least 2 to 4 weeks. If there is no improvement, it's time to consider prescription medication. However, studies (Vandenplas et al., 2009) found that proton-pump inhibitors, one of the most commonly prescribed drugs for infant reflux disease, was no more effective than placebos in reducing reflux symptoms. If a baby receives medication and it seems to help, be sure the parents know that the dose of the drug or combination of drugs will probably need to be adjusted as baby grows, because the dose is determined by the baby's weight, which changes quickly. If a drug treatment worked well for a while and the baby's symptoms return, suggest talking to the baby's healthcare provider about possibly adjusting the dose.

CHRONIC CONDITIONS IN THE NURSING BABY

At first, parents of babies with chronic health problems may have conflicting feelings and trouble remembering information.

When a baby is born with special needs, the parents may have mixed emotions, including helplessness, anger, disappointment, and guilt, which may be ongoing. They may need time to grieve the healthy baby they expected before they can accept the baby in their arms. If the baby is diagnosed later, they may worry that something they did caused their baby's health problem. A parent who is wrestling with strong feelings often finds it difficult to remember information. Rather than just providing information verbally, it may be more helpful to give it to the family in writing and go over it with them several different times.

If feeding problems arise, parents may blame themselves and see it as a reflection of their own inadequacy. Or they may interpret normal baby behavior, such as fussiness, as a symptom of the baby's physical problem. When talking to the family:

- Encourage them to talk about their feelings and acknowledge them, which will make it easier for them to think through their situation more clearly.
- Suggest they plan to take life one day at a time, and watch their baby's responses to best determine what will work for them.
- Ask the normal questions all new parents are asked—who the baby looks like and how she responds to those around her.
- Discuss the availability of a support organization, if one exists.

Allergy

When a baby has feeding problems, allergy may be an underlying cause, especially when there is a family history of allergy and the baby has physical symptoms.

Exclusive nursing reduces the odds of babies developing an allergy (Rajani, Seppo, & Jarvinen, 2018), but it is not a guarantee, especially in those with a family history of allergy.

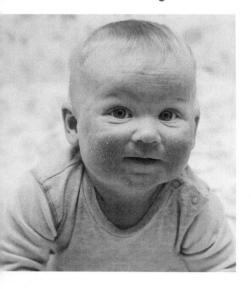

Defining terms. The terms allergy, hypersensitivity, and intolerance are often confused. Most babies who have one of these types of reactions to a food are exposed to it either by consuming it directly, or the nursing parent consumes it and it passes into the milk. Allergy to medications—like penicillin—and environmental triggers—like cat dander and dust mites—are possible, too.

How do allergy and intolerance differ? An ***allergy*** or ***hypersensitivity*** is an immune response, which is often severe, and its symptoms usually affect many organs. Also, these symptoms occur predictably each time the baby is exposed (ABM, 2011). With a food ***intolerance***, on the other hand, there is no immune system reaction. The symptoms are usually not severe and are usually limited to the digestive tract. People with a food intolerance (such as lactose intolerance in older children and adults) are often able to eat small amounts of the food without a problem.

Allergy in children is increasing. The prevalence of allergy varies widely around the world and has increased in recent years in developed countries. Australia, for example, has one of the highest rates of allergy in young children. According to the 2017 population-based HealthNuts cohort study (Peters et al., 2017), at age 1 year, 11% of Australian children were challenge-confirmed positive for food allergy. A 2016 U.S. randomized, cross-sectional survey of a representative sample of more than 40,000 U.S. children (Akinbami, Simon, & Schoendorf, 2016) examined the prevalence of food allergy among U.S. children. It found that 8% of U.S. children between birth and 2 years had at least one confirmed food allergy, and about 30% of these children were allergic to more than one food. It also found that the prevalence of childhood food allergy without asthma increased in the U.S. 1.4% per year between 2001 and 2013. Nearly 39% of the allergic children had severe allergic reactions to a food. The most common U.S. food allergy was to peanut, followed by milk, shellfish, tree nut, egg, fin fish, and strawberry.

Symptoms of allergy. Some parents wonder if their baby's fussiness, wakefulness, or irritability during feeds (which can also be caused by overabundant milk production and reflux disease) are signs of allergy or hypersensitivity. Usually, in addition to these behaviors (especially fussiness during or after feeds), most allergic children also have physical symptoms, such as:

- Skin reactions: eczema, dermatitis, hives, rash, dry skin
- Gastrointestinal issues: vomiting, diarrhea, pain, blood or mucus in stools (ABM, 2011)
- Respiratory problems: congestion, runny nose, wheezing, coughing

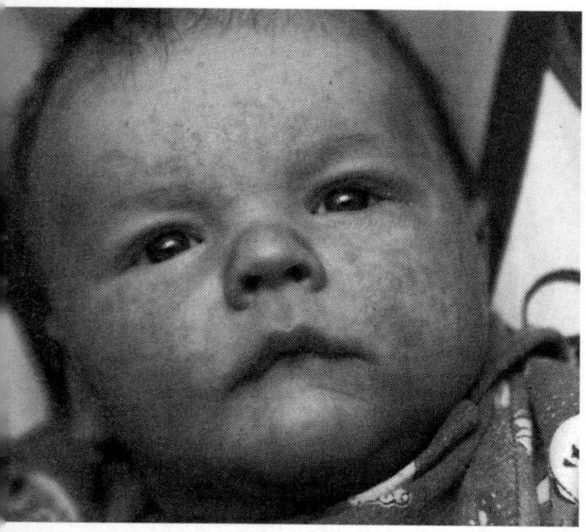

A 2016 Turkish prospective evaluation study that followed during their first year 1,377 children who tested positive for allergy (Dogruel, Bingol, Altintas, Yilmaz, & Guneser Kendirli, 2016) found that skin reactions were the most common physical symptoms of allergy, followed by gastrointestinal reactions, and respiratory problems.

Family history. Allergy occurs more often in children with a family history of allergy. If one parent has an allergy, the baby has a 20% to 40% increased risk of being allergic, and if both parents have an allergy, the baby's risk increases to 50% to 80% (Ferreira & Seidman, 2007).

For strategies to suggest for feeding problems caused by allergy, such as elimination diets, see p. 564.

Cardiac Issues

Heart problems at birth are referred to as congenital heart disease, which includes defects of the heart and major blood vessels. Cardiac issues may occur alone or with Down syndrome, Turner syndrome, or other syndromes (Frommelt, 2004). About 20% of babies with cardiac issues gain weight slowly no matter how they are fed (Costello, Gellatly, Daniel, Justo, & Weir, 2015) because they use more energy than a healthy baby. To maintain adequate oxygen levels and circulation, these babies take more breaths each minute and their hearts beat faster. Adequate weekly weight gain in a healthy newborn is at about 7 oz. (198 g), but because the baby with some cardiac defects has increased energy needs, even with good milk intake, many gain less weight or even lose weight (Daymont, Neal, Prosnitz, & Cohen, 2013; Mangili, Garzoli, & Sadou, 2018).

Some babies with cardiac issues gain weight slowly.

In two U.S. studies (Combs & Marino, 1993; Medoff-Cooper & Irving, 2009), babies with cardiac issues who were fed human milk had better weight-for-age scores compared with the babies fed only formula.

• • •

Some families are discouraged from directly nursing the baby with a cardiac defect due to the misconception that bottle-feeding is "easier" than nursing (Clemente, Barnes, Shinebourne, & Stein, 2001; Lambert & Watters, 1998; Steltzer, Sussman-Karten, Kuzdeba, Mott, & Connor, 2016). Although some babies with cardiac issues have difficulty with both nursing and bottle-feeding (Pados, 2019), direct nursing may actually be easier for them. Just as with preterm babies, oxygen saturation was found to be higher during nursing among both preterm babies and babies with congenital heart issues (Marino, O'Brien, & LoRe, 1995). Research on preterm babies that used the study babies as their own controls (Meier, 1988; Meier & Anderson, 1987) found that coordinating sucking, swallowing, and breathing—a major challenge for babies with cardiac issues—was easier during nursing than during bottle-feeding. The authors of a review article on providing human milk for babies with cardiac disease (Davis & Spatz, 2019, p. 4) wrote:

For the baby with a cardiac issue, direct nursing is easier and results in better health outcomes than bottle-feeding formula.

> "...available research suggests that direct breastfeeding should be viewed as a medical intervention to improve feeding and growth outcomes in this population."

Direct nursing is a better first feed for these babies than bottle-feeding (Steltzer et al., 2016; Torowicz, Seelhorst, Froh, & Spatz, 2015).

As mentioned in the previous point, some babies with cardiac disease struggle with feeding. Direct nursing has several advantages over bottle-feeding. Direct nursing gives families more active participation in their baby's care and enhances their bond. In one U.K. matched case controlled study (Clemente et al., 2001), mothers of babies with cardiac disease who directly breastfed were more likely to describe their baby as "happier" with feeds and having a better appetite than those who were bottle-feeding. Factors important to their nursing success included (Spence, Swinsburg, Griggs, & Johnston, 2011; Steltzer et al., 2016):

- Encouragement and support from healthcare providers
- Consistent and careful lactation management
- Help from lactation specialists
- Maternal motivation

In a U.S. study of 45 babies with congenital heart disease (Combs & Marino, 1993), the severity of the babies' cardiac issue was unrelated to their ability to nurse. Other studies (Lambert & Watters, 1998) also came to this conclusion. This further confirms that all babies with cardiac disease should be given the chance to directly nurse.

One common concern in special-care nurseries is the ability to measure baby's milk intake. Weighing babies before and after nursing with a scale accurate to 2 g allows parents and providers to accurately measure baby's milk intake during nursing, even when baby is wearing leads (Haase, Barreira, Murphy, Mueller, & Rhodes, 2009; Rankin et al., 2016). See p. 917-919 for details.

• • •

Some practical strategies may make nursing easier for the baby with cardiac issues.

Some of the nursing challenges many of these families face include:

- Delayed first feed
- Separation from the baby during the hospital stay
- The need for the baby to fast before some medical procedures
- Inconsistent feeding support from healthcare providers (Barbas & Kelleher, 2004)
- Anxiety about feeding

Families often wonder if their baby is satisfied after coming off the nipple or just worn out (Lobo, 1992) and they have concerns about lack of adequate weight gain, breathlessness, and fatigue during nursing that are unrelated to the severity of their baby's cardiac issue (Clemente et al., 2001).

If a family expresses these concerns, talk about their feelings. Then suggest experimenting with the following strategies (M. Walker, 2017)

- If the baby is facing surgery, suggest spending as much time as possible nursing, which may ease baby's transition back to nursing afterward.
- Try feeding positions, such as the starter positions described on p. 23-29 or side-lying, which allow the baby's head to tilt back slightly (extend) for easier swallowing and breathing.
- If the baby fatigues easily and only nurses well from one side, use breast compression (p. 889), the "milk shake" (see p. 460), or alternate massage to help the baby get fattier milk more quickly (Bowles, 2011).
- Feed often, as a baby with less stamina may do better with smaller, frequent feeds.
- Stop nursing if the baby becomes short of breath, her lips turn blue, or she looks pale or tired.
- If the baby's nursing effectiveness is questionable, express milk after feeds to safeguard milk production.
- If the baby is not feeding well, try the Dancer Hand position (see p. 890) for more support or a nipple shield (see p. 912-917).
- During medical procedures, as needed, request a place to express milk, and arrange for food and drink, a place to rest, and equipment, such as a breast pump, refrigerator, or cleaning supplies.

• • •

Exclusive direct nursing is possible for many babies with cardiac problems, but some need to be supplemented.

Many babies with cardiac defects are able to nurse immediately after birth and exclusively. In some cases, feeding may be delayed after birth or interrupted due to medical procedures. One U.S. study that surveyed the mothers of 68 babies with cardiac disease found that lactation support resulted in improved nursing outcomes among these families (Barbas & Kelleher, 2004).

If the baby gains too little weight while exclusively nursing, some strategies that may help boost weight gain include (M. Walker, 2017):

- Consistently use breast compression (or alternate massage) while nursing to increase the fat content of the milk (see p. 889).
- Add a calorie-rich supplement to expressed milk.
- Nurse during the day and feed baby with a continuous feeding pump at night (Imms, 2001).
- Follow nursing by feeding baby a high-calorie supplement via a nasogastric tube.
- Use a nursing supplementer or other feeding method to feed the baby high-calorie hindmilk as a supplement (see the section starting on p. 894 for details about feeding methods).
- If baby's fluids are restricted, feed only a high-calorie hindmilk (28-30 calories per ounce [30 mL]) or high-calorie preterm formula.

To provide hindmilk (Galloway & Howells, 2015; Ogechi, William, & Fidelia, 2007), suggest the nursing parent express milk after nursing. If exclusively expressing, suggest storing the milk expressed during the first few minutes (or longer to get even higher-calorie milk), and then collect the milk expressed afterward for supplementing. Some hospitals have a device called a creamatocrit that measures the fat content of mother's milk. Expressed milk can also be "fractionated," meaning the fattier milk is separated from the lower-fat-milk in a centrifuge and fed to the baby. Suggest the family ask if the hospital has any of the equipment needed to accomplish this.

Whatever supplement is used, the family and the baby's healthcare provider need to discuss how often and how much supplement should be given. Depending on the baby's weight gain and her feeding effectiveness, the baby may be supplemented after every feed, after every other feed, or less often.

The need for a supplement causes some families to question the value of their milk, their milk production, even their adequacy as parents. Assure them that mother's milk provides the baby with live cells important to her health that are not available elsewhere. Emphasize that cardiac issues mean the baby needs extra nutrients that cannot necessarily be provided simply by increasing her milk intake.

• • •

Time spent nursing, medication, and/or surgery may help the baby with a cardiac issue improve her feeding effectiveness.

A baby's feeding effectiveness may improve with practice, prescribed medication, or if the problem is severe, with surgery (Jadcherla, Vijayapal, & Leuthner, 2009). One case report (Owens, 2002) described a baby born with hypoplastic left heart syndrome who nursed effectively after heart transplant surgery at 30 days of life and continued nursing until he was 13 months old.

Cystic Fibrosis

The first indication a baby has cystic fibrosis may be slow weight gain and a salty taste to her skin.

Cystic fibrosis is a genetic disease that causes the secretion of a thick, gluey mucus that clogs the bronchial tubes, interfering with breathing and blocking the digestive enzymes from leaving the pancreas, which causes incomplete digestion. The sweat glands reabsorb chloride normally, which causes baby's skin to taste salty when kissed.

There are more than 1,000 mutations of the gene responsible for cystic fibrosis, which means the disease may be mild or severe. Cases range from those detectable only by laboratory tests to those that are life-threatening. Depending on the severity, a baby with cystic fibrosis may have breathing problems and regular respiratory infections and may look thin, pale, and undernourished.

The first clue that a baby has cystic fibrosis may be a puzzling slow weight gain in a baby who vigorously nurses and has many wet diapers and stools. In this case, slow weight gain is due to incomplete digestion and is unrelated to the baby's milk intake.

• • •

Babies with cystic fibrosis who do not nurse have poorer health outcomes and earlier onset of symptoms.

Nursing was once promoted in 77% of U.S. cystic fibrosis centers, according to a 2004 survey (Parker, O'Sullivan, Shea, Regan, & Freedman, 2004). This recommendation was due in part to research findings that exclusive formula feeding was associated with an increased incidence of respiratory infections and slow growth (Luder, Kattan, Tanzer-Torres, & Bonforte, 1990). According to studies, there are several downsides to less-than-exclusive nursing in the baby with cystic fibrosis:

- **Slower weight gain and shorter height.** In an Australian study of 65 babies with cystic fibrosis, those who did not exclusively breastfeed gained less weight and were not as tall as those who received only mother's milk (Holliday et al., 1991).
- **More severe disease and earlier onset of symptoms.** A U.S. retrospective survey of 863 people with cystic fibrosis (Parker et al., 2004) found that any formula intake during the first 6 months of life was associated with a more severe form of the disease (based on treatment with IV antibiotics during the previous 2 years) and a trend toward earlier onset of symptoms and poorer lung function.
- **More infections and greater decline in lung function.** A 2015 U.S. prospective study examined the association between gut microbiota and respiratory infections in children with cystic fibrosis (Hoen et al., 2015). It concluded that the "good bacteria" predominant with nursing was associated with better respiratory health over the long term, compared with children fed formula. A Wisconsin prospective study that followed 103 children with cystic fibrosis identified through newborn screening blood tests (Jadin et al., 2011) found that when compared with at least 1 month of exclusive breastfeeding, exclusive formula feeding from birth was associated with more cases during the first 2 years of respiratory infections that are common among those with cystic fibrosis. In an Italian retrospective study of 146 children with cystic fibrosis, weaning before 4 months was associated with more infections during the first 3 years of life and a greater decline in lung function (Colombo et al., 2007).

Since 2004, some fundamental changes occurred that affected rates of nursing in families with cystic fibrosis. According to the U.S. Cystic Fibrosis Foundation, only about 50% of families do any nursing at all (CFF, 2018). One major change is that until the last decade or so, babies were not usually diagnosed with cystic fibrosis until they were at least several months old. Now, newborn blood screening makes it possible to diagnose cystic fibrosis soon after birth (Leung et al., 2017). As a U.K. dietitian wrote (C. Smith, 2019, p. S-18):

> "...breastfeeding rates are low for infants with CF, and most of these infants receive formula as the primary source of nutrition or as a supplement to breastfeeding. Parents may choose not to breastfeed due to the overarching urgency to improve weight and a lack of confidence that breast milk can support good growth. Stress from the diagnosis may also factor into the decision or the success of breastfeeding."

Is there a way to increase nursing rates in babies with cystic fibrosis? A 2019 U.S. study (T. Miller, Antos, Brock, Wade, & Goday, 2019) found that by including an IBCLC at the visit where cystic fibrosis was diagnosed and providing a lactation plan and access to IBCLC support, nursing rates significantly increased. Before the intervention, only 57% of families continued to provide human milk after the first visit, whereas after the intervention, this increased to 94%. The duration of any nursing increased to an average of 7.7 months from 6.4 months.

• • •

In about half of the babies with cystic fibrosis, the flow of digestive enzymes from the pancreas is reduced and replacement enzymes are needed to grow and gain weight appropriately (Koletzko & Reinhardt, 2001). These enzymes can be dissolved in soft foods and given by spoon before nursing. Some of these babies also need extra vitamins, minerals, and salt, especially in hot weather (Gaskin & Waters, 1994; Krebs et al., 2000).

Some nursing babies with cystic fibrosis grow better and stay healthier when they take medications, digestive enzymes, and/or nutritional supplements.

To prevent respiratory infections, the family may be advised to keep the baby upright when possible and to use aerosols, antibiotics, and/or expectorants.

Diabetes

Type 1 diabetes mellitus in small children poses many challenges. But even so, as with nearly all children, nursing is recommended (AAP, 2012). Type 1 diabetes is also known as insulin-dependent diabetes mellitus (or IDDM). Only 5% to 10% of diabetics of all ages have this form of the disease. It occurs when the insulin-producing beta cells in the pancreas are destroyed, leaving the body unable to produce insulin, a hormone needed to convert sugar, starches, and other foods into fuel for the body. Without insulin, blood sugar can rise to dangerous levels and cause health complications and even death.

When babies or toddlers have Type 1 diabetes, encourage families to nurse.

According to the Academy of Breastfeeding Medicine (ABM) Clinical Protocol #27 on breastfeeding the young child with Type 1 diabetes (D. Miller, Mamilly, Fourtner, & Rosen-Carole, 2017), Type 1 diabetes diagnosed in babies younger than 9 months is most likely to be a genetic form of the disease. (ABM Clinical Protocol #27 is available for free download in multiple languages at **bfmed.org/protocols**). Insulin may be used to treat this form of Type 1 diabetes, or after the baby is stabilized, it may be treated with an oral medication, such as sulfonylureas. Babies diagnosed with Type 1 diabetes may also have other neurological issues that sometimes make early nursing more challenging.

In children with Type 1 diabetes, caregivers need to check the child's blood-sugar levels regularly and provide daily medication or insulin replacement therapy via injections or subcutaneous pump, so their blood sugar doesn't become dangerously low or high. The ABM Clinical Protocol #27 suggested whenever possible with young children to use continuous insulin pumps. During infancy and childhood, keeping blood-sugar levels within the normal range is important to healthy brain growth and cognitive development. U.S. research using brain MRIs of 141 children with Type 1 diabetes found an association between blood-sugar variability in young children and variations in brain development (Mazaika et al., 2016).

• • •

Parents of a child with Type 1 diabetes may feel pressure from healthcare providers to wean.

One of the most important tasks parents must do for their child with Type I diabetes is to keep track of their food intake and calculate and provide the needed dose of insulin or other medication to keep the child's blood-sugar levels within the normal range. This is a challenging job, especially when the child is too young to describe symptoms of low blood sugar, which adds to the parents' stress.

When a young child is diagnosed with Type 1 diabetes, some parents report noticing frustration in their healthcare providers because they cannot say exactly how much milk the nursing baby consumes (Hayden-Baldauf, 2016). This can also add to the family's stress and may leave the impression that continuing to nurse is bad for their child's health. There is no evidence to support this point of view. At this writing, there is no research comparing health outcomes in diabetic children who were nursed or formula-fed. But there is evidence that when compared with children who were formula fed, nursing children in general have better brain development (Deoni et al., 2013) and cognitive outcomes independent of the family's means (Horta, Loret de Mola, & Victora, 2015). The infection-fighting aspect of nursing is also very important to a diabetic, who is more prone to infections than those with normal insulin levels.

• • •

Estimating carbohydrate intake in a nursing child is possible.

Parents of diabetic children need to be able to track their child's carbohydrate intake to calculate the dose of insulin needed to keep blood-sugar levels within the normal range.

Carbohydrate content of human milk. Using the recommendations from the U.S. National Guidelines Clearing House, the authors of the ABM protocol (D. Miller et al., 2017) concluded that human milk contains 70 g of carbohydrates per liter (IoM, 2004). This is the same carbohydrate content as infant formula. A difference between human milk and formula is that formula's fat content is about 10 g/L lower than human milk. Because fat modulates glucose absorption into the bloodstream, this difference in fat contact makes it likely that babies fed human milk have less blood-sugar variability than babies fed formula (D. Miller et al., 2017).

Calculating volume of milk consumed during nursing. When nursing directly, the ABM protocol lists different ways to calculate milk intake.

- **Test weights.** In some parts of the world, baby scales accurate to 2 g are available for rent. Using one of these scales to weigh the baby before and after nursing sessions (see p. 917-919) reliably measures milk intake (Rankin et al., 2016). After diagnosis, doing several days of test weights around the clock can provide an accurate idea of baby's intake per feed and per day.

- **Use average milk intake.** Average milk intake per day for nursing babies older than 1 month is about 25 oz. (750 mL) and average milk intake per feed is about 3 to 4 ounces (89 to 118 mL). For an overview of 9 studies of milk intake from different countries, download the latest version of the ABM Clinical Protocol #27 at **bfmed.org/protocols**.

The ABM protocol suggested that for babies who use a "small volume frequent feed" style of nursing to measure baby's blood sugar every 3 hours and give insulin doses as needed to correct high blood sugar.

Another way to check milk intake at a feed over time is to ask to do before- and after-feed weights at regular health checkups.

Down Syndrome

Down syndrome is a genetic birth defect caused by the presence of an extra chromosome that causes developmental delays and other characteristics, such as low muscle tone (hypotonia). With love, care, and support, these babies can lead positive and productive lives.

Some babies with Down syndrome need time and practice to nurse effectively, which promotes better health and development.

Rates of nursing among babies with Down syndrome vary from country to country. In the Netherlands (Hopman et al., 1998), babies born with Down syndrome nursed at the same rate as other babies. Not so in other countries.

- **Croatia.** A 2015 retrospective study examined the medical data from all Croatian births between 2009 and 2012 (Glivetic et al., 2015). It found that of the 120 babies born with Down syndrome, 68% nursed versus 95% of Croatian babies as a whole. The researchers attributed this difference in part to more admissions after birth to special-care, primarily due to heart defects or birth injury.
- **Chile.** In a prevalence study (Genova, Cerda, Correa, Vergara, & Lizama, 2018), 73 mothers completed questionnaires about their baby with Down syndrome. Among this group, 46% exclusively breastfed for 6 months or longer. Child factors, such as hospitalization, were listed as reasons the remaining 64% of the mothers did not breastfeed exclusively for at least 6 months.
- **Italy.** A study compared 560 babies with Down syndrome to a group of control children (Pisacane et al., 2003). Those with Down syndrome were more likely to not breastfeed (57% versus 15% in the general population). Among those whose babies did not go to the special-care nursery at birth, the reasons given for not nursing included depression, perceived insufficient milk, and sucking difficulties.

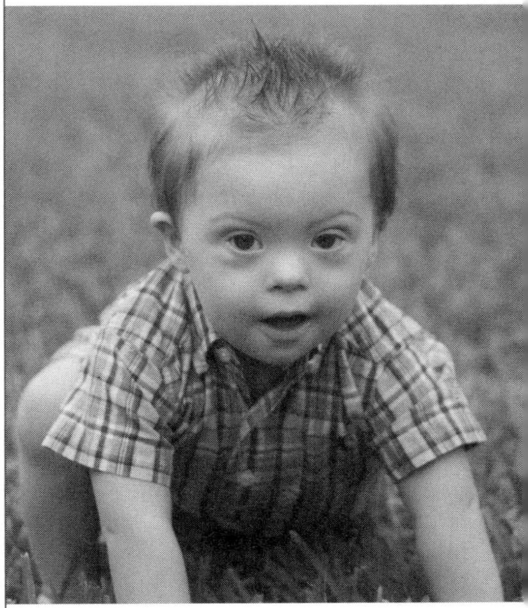

In some babies with Down syndrome, nursing is challenging during the early weeks, but as with any other baby, health outcomes are better with exclusive human-milk feeding. A 2017 Israeli chart review of all 403 babies born with Down syndrome in Jerusalem between 2000 and 2010 (Ergaz-Shaltiel et al., 2017) found that 79% had cardiac anomalies, 32% needed oxygen due to respiratory failure, 23% developed jaundice, 6% had a serious blood infection (sepsis), and

13% had feeding difficulties. Babies with Down syndrome are more prone to respiratory tract infections and heart and bowel problems, and human milk contains components that contribute to immune system development and better bowel health. A Mexican study (Flores-Lujano et al., 2009) found that non-nursing babies with Down syndrome had more infections and rehospitalizations during the first year and a greater incidence of childhood leukemia later. In addition to better health outcomes, nursing strengthens facial muscle tone, promoting mouth and tongue coordination, which is often a challenge for these babies.

KEY CONCEPT

Babies with Down syndrome who breastfeed have better health outcomes than babies who don't.

When a baby is born with Down syndrome, the skin-to-skin contact that occurs during nursing provides physical stimulation that enhances neurodevelopment (Bergman, 2017). The physical contact and hormones released during nursing also promote emotional attachment during the vulnerable time the family is adjusting to the birth of a special-needs baby. As the baby learns to nurse, this process also helps parents become more skilled caregivers. The nursing parent's encouragement and responsiveness to the baby's cues are the same skills families need to help the baby best realize her potential as she grows.

Support is critical to families working to meet their nursing goals. A 2018 Brazilian survey of parents of babies with Down syndrome (Barros da Silva, Barbieri-Figueiredo, & Van Riper, 2018) found that the support of healthcare professionals was vital to nursing success, but that this support was often inconsistent.

• • •

Low muscle tone and time spent in special care contribute to early nursing challenges in some babies with Down syndrome.

Due to low muscle tone, many babies with Down syndrome are "floppy" and may not nurse effectively at first. A low-tone baby may need extra help in finding, latching, and staying attached, especially in upright or side-lying positions. Be sure the family knows the baby's muscle tone and sucking will improve with time and practice.

During the early weeks, suggest allowing extra time for feeds. A baby with low muscle tone may have difficulty cupping her tongue during nursing, and when a baby's tongue stays flat, milk slides to the sides of the mouth rather than being swallowed, requiring extra effort for less milk. A 2019 U.S. retrospective chart review of 174 babies with Down syndrome from birth to 6 months (Stanley et al., 2019) found that 55% had some kind of feeding or swallowing problems. A Japanese study of bottle-feeding babies with Down syndrome (Mizuno & Ueda, 2001) found that ineffective feeding was only partly due to low tone in the mouth, lips, and jaw. Another factor was their uncoordinated tongue movements. Only with time and maturity were they able to master the wave-like coordinated tongue motions needed for effective feeding.

But not all babies with Down syndrome have difficulty nursing. In a U.K. interview study of 59 mothers of breastfed babies with Down syndrome (Aumonier & Cunningham, 1983), these mothers reported that at birth 52% had no trouble breastfeeding effectively. Within the first week, 7% more were sucking well. At 1 week of age, 14% more breastfed effectively. For the remaining 27%, it took longer than 1 week to learn to breastfeed effectively.

Admission to the special-care nursery also affects nursing outcomes in these babies. In the Italian study of 560 babies with Down syndrome (Pisacane et al., 2003), 44% were admitted to the special-care nursery at birth, and of those, only 30% breastfed, with illness given as the main reason for not breastfeeding.

• • •

If the baby is in the special-care nursery or can't yet nurse, offer information on milk expression and strategies for transitioning to nursing.

If due to the respiratory infections and heart and bowel problems common among babies with Down syndrome, the baby is in the special-care nursery, let the family know that by expressing milk, they can provide their milk for their baby. For details, see p. 498-507.

If a baby can feed by mouth, health outcomes are better when she is fed mother's milk. At first, if a baby is tube-fed, she can begin to nurse even before transitioning off the tube (Genna, LeVan Fram, & Sandora, 2017). If extra help is needed in latching, see the later section, "More Strategies for Babies with High/ Low Tone" in "Neurological Impairment."

When the baby begins latching, suggest the family think of early nursing as practice sessions and to focus on enjoying their time together, rather than how much milk the baby takes. Explain that they will have many opportunities to nurse and not to worry if it takes some time for their baby to catch on.

• • •

If the baby seems sleepy most of the time, suggest keeping her on the parent's body as much as possible to trigger feeding behaviors.

Many babies with Down syndrome are sleepy during the first few weeks and can be difficult to rouse for feeding. If so, suggest nursing parents:

- Lean back and lay the baby on their body as much of the day as they're comfortable doing so, which provides the stimulation needed to trigger feeding behaviors, even in light sleep (S. Colson, 2003).
- Help the baby latch whenever she goes from a deep sleep to light sleep. Signs include squirming, eyes moving under eyelids, any body movements.
- Keep the baby skin-to-skin as much as possible, so they will know from the baby's movements and changes in breathing when she may be ready to feed.

• • •

Semi-reclined starter positions give a low-tone baby who coughs during nursing more control over milk flow.

Low muscle tone can leave a baby's airway unprotected during swallowing, which causes the gasping and coughing common among babies with Down syndrome. If this happens, nursing may go more smoothly when the baby feeds in positions with her head higher than the nipple. See Figure 8.21 and pp. 23-29 for illustrations of a variety of starter positions.

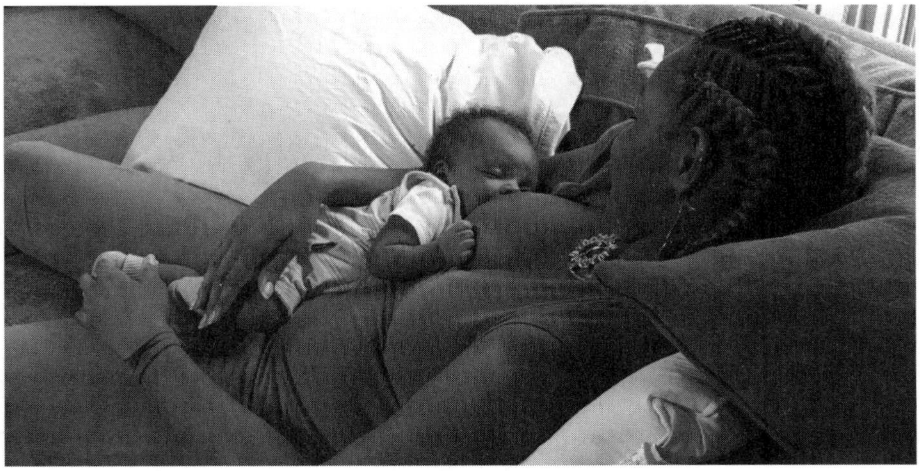

Figure 8.21 A semi-reclined starter position.

• • •

A low-tone, protruding tongue may make latching more challenging.

For suggestions on ways to increase mouth and tongue tone before nursing and techniques and tools that can be used during feeding, see the next section, "Neurological Impairment."

• • •

If the baby gains weight slowly, supplements may be needed.

If despite the nursing parent's efforts, the baby does not nurse effectively or often enough, supplements—ideally expressed milk—may be needed, as gaining weight means gaining strength, too.

Healthy growth in babies with Down syndrome is different from healthy growth in other babies. For this reason, growth charts are available from birth to 18 years specifically for children with Down syndrome based on data in both the U.S. (Zemel et al., 2015) and the U.K. (Styles, Cole, Dennis, & Preece, 2002). The U.S. growth charts are available at: **bit.ly/BA2-USDown** and the U.K. growth charts are available at: **bit.ly/BA2-UKDown**.

A baby who gains weight slowly despite good milk intake needs to be checked for a health problem, such as a heart defect. A baby with a heart defect may use extra energy and calories just to maintain adequate circulation (see the earlier section "Cardiac Issues" on p. 311).

One possible way to boost weight gain is by using high-calorie hindmilk as a supplement. For details, see p. 313 in the earlier section, "Cardiac Issues."

Nursing the baby with Down syndrome is sometimes challenging, but assure the family that with patience and persistence, as the baby grows, gets stronger, and increases in muscle tone, feedings will go more smoothly.

Metabolic Disorders: Galactosemia and PKU

Exclusive nursing is impossible for many babies born with the metabolic disorders galactosemia and phenylketonuria (PKU), but partial nursing is possible for many.

Many babies with the metabolic disorders galactosemia and PKU are unable to break down a component of human milk, either the sugar galactose (in babies with galactosemia) or the amino acid phenylalanine (in babies with PKU). Because these milk components are not metabolized, they accumulate in the baby's body, which can cause serious health problems and eventually become life-threatening. With PKU and some types of galactosemia, it is safe for these babies to do some nursing. (See the later sections on these disorders for details.)

• • •

False positives are common with tests used to screen newborns for PKU and galactosemia, so any baby testing positive should be evaluated and retested before nursing is interrupted.

During the first week of life, newborns in the U.S. and many other countries are routinely screened for both galactosemia and PKU (Kaye et al., 2006; Rubio-Gozalbo et al., 2019). These blood tests are done between 24 and 48 hours of age. For accurate test results for both disorders, the baby must have consumed either galactose or phenylalanine (in other words, be nursing well) and be at least 24 hours old. Babies do not need to be fed formula before these tests.

False positives are common with these tests (Pyhtila, Shaw, Neumann, & Fridovich-Keil, 2015; Welling et al., 2017), although a two-step testing process is used for galactosemia in some countries like Sweden, which reduces false positives (Ohlsson, Guthenberg, & von Dobeln, 2012). For galactosemia, the blood test is designed to detect a liver enzyme that is sensitive to heat. Babies who do not have this disorder sometimes test positive for it, especially during the summer months when blood samples are not always kept cool.

But because exclusive nursing can lead to permanent liver or neurological damage in a baby with galactosemia or PKU, if a baby's test results are positive, encourage the family to first ask the baby's healthcare provider to evaluate the baby for symptoms of the disorder. Then the healthcare provider can advise the family if the baby appears healthy and it seems safe to continue nursing exclusively until they receive the second test results. If the baby has symptoms, they should begin feeding her a lactose-free or phenylalanine-free formula immediately. With galactosemia, symptoms (see the next point) usually begin to appear on about the third day of life.

If nursing is interrupted, suggest expressing milk to stay comfortable and safeguard the milk production until the final results are available.

To speed this testing process, first suggest asking the baby's healthcare provider to do another blood test as soon as possible. Sometimes several retests are needed before these metabolic disorders can be ruled in or out. By being proactive with the healthcare provider and the testing facility, a family may get the second test results faster. For example, the family can ask the baby's healthcare provider to call the testing facility and request special handling of the test. Overnight delivery is an option, or if the family is within driving distance of the testing facility, they may be able to arrange for someone trustworthy to drive the baby's blood sample there. After the sample reaches the testing facility, results should be available within a day or two.

Galactosemia

Nursing is contraindicated when a baby has classic galactosemia, but if the baby has a milder form of galactosemia, full or partial nursing may be possible.

Lactose, or milk sugar, is broken down by a baby's liver enzymes into glucose and galactose, which is then further broken down. Galactosemia is a rare (1 in 47,000), inherited metabolic disorder in which the liver does not produce the enzyme that metabolizes galactose, causing it to accumulate in the baby's system.

Classic galactosemia. Too much galactose usually becomes apparent on about the third day of life as jaundice, enlarged liver, vomiting, and lethargy. If treatment is not begun soon, it can progress to failure-to-thrive, liver and kidney damage, convulsions, and mental retardation. Human milk is high in lactose, so with classic galactosemia, nursing is contraindicated and the baby must be fed a lactose-free formula.

If classic galactosemia is diagnosed, talk to the parents about their feelings and provide strategies for reducing milk production gradually and comfortably. If nursing was important to them, they may need to go through a grieving period. One Dutch questionnaire study of 185 parents of children with galactosemia and PKU (ten Hoedt et al., 2011) found that emotional support was very important to these parents' quality of life.

KEY CONCEPT

Blood tests for galactosemia and PKU sometimes yield false-positive results.

Duarte galactosemia. The term galactosemia covers more than 100 mutations of this disorder. Duarte galactosemia is one type in which the baby may produce varying levels of the liver enzyme needed to break down galactose. Depending on the combination of genes the baby inherited, a carrier of Duarte galactosemia may produce 75% of the enzyme needed to metabolize galactose, while babies who have Duarte galactosemia may produce between 25% and 50%. A blood test can determine the baby's enzyme level. Some of these babies may be able to partially or exclusively nurse. The range of treatment options is broad, from complete removal of human milk from the baby's diet to partial nursing to full nursing (Schmidt, Beebe, & Berg-Drazin, 2013). One 2015 U.S. review article (Pyhtila et al., 2015) found no consensus on diet recommendations for babies with Duarte galactosemia. To keep all options open and to stay comfortable, before a final decision, suggest expressing milk.

PKU (Phenylketonuria)

Partial nursing can continue in the baby with PKU, with the addition of special formula supplements to maintain safe phenylalanine blood levels.

Phenylketonuria (PKU) is a rare metabolic disorder (1 in 14,000) in which the baby lacks the liver enzyme needed to break down the essential amino acid phenylalanine, an ingredient of both human milk and most infant formulas. If untreated, this amino acid accumulates in the blood, causing brain damage. Treatment consists of a lifelong diet of low-phenylalanine foods. However, even when those with PKU maintain their special diet, they may still have cognitive impairments over their lifetime (Manti et al., 2017).

When a baby has PKU, the need for protein must be balanced with the risk of receiving too much phenylalanine. Continued partial nursing works because the baby with PKU needs some phenylalanine for normal growth. So in addition to being fed a special phenylalanine-free formula, the baby also needs protein in her diet.

There are several reasons to consider continuing to nurse the baby with PKU. Because human milk is lower in phenylalanine than regular formula, less of the expensive phenylalanine-free formula is needed, saving the parents significant cost. Mother's milk also provides live cells that protect the baby from illness that are missing in formula. For babies with PKU, the positive effect of human milk on cognitive development is significant (Horta et al., 2015). As one mother of a nursing baby with PKU said in a U.S. interview study (Banta-Wright, Kodadek, Houck, Steiner, & Knafl, 2015, p. 731):

> "I...knew that breastfed babies tended to have higher IQs. I thought that if she is going to be in a position where her IQ would already be lower that it would make more sense for me to do everything that I could to protect her brain. Maybe the breast milk would counter balance it a little bit."

Throughout her life, the baby with PKU must be carefully monitored to avoid unsafe phenylalanine blood levels. After diagnosis, nursing is usually interrupted for a few days to bring the baby's blood levels down to normal. During this time, the nursing parent can express milk to safeguard the milk production. After this, nursing can be combined with special formula in several ways. All of the following strategies have been used successfully:

- Alternate all-nursing with all-formula feeds, allowing baby to take as much of each as desired (van Rijn et al., 2003).

- At each feed, first give the baby a predetermined volume of special formula (65% of the baby's 24-hour milk intake divided by number of feeds) and then nurse unrestrictedly (Motzfeldt, Lilje, & Nylander, 1999).
- At each feed give the baby first a predetermined volume of mother's milk, followed by as much special formula as the baby wants (Ahring et al., 2009).
- Feed the baby a bottle of special formula every 3 hours and nurse as desired during the intervals between (Kanufre et al., 2007).
- Estimate the baby's total daily milk intake by age and calculate the volume of formula needed to maintain safe phenylalanine blood levels. Give the baby this volume of formula every 24 hours (however is most convenient). Schedule biweekly blood tests to monitor baby's blood levels and make adjustments as needed (Greve, Wheeler, Green-Burgeson, & Zorn, 1994).

Some of these feeding routines are simpler than others. The researchers who studied the last routine above concluded that even though more time was needed while establishing nursing to monitor blood levels and assess weight gain, "eventually breastfeeding decreases the need for complicated formula mixtures and can make overall management easier" (Greve et al., 1994, p. 308).

A 2018 review of the early feeding practices after PKU diagnosis in 21 European countries (Pinto et al., 2018) found that nursing rates varied by region. Its authors noted that "the use of breastfeeding in PKU is well established," but there is no consistent approach in the 91 European PKU centers surveyed.

Some studies found that the nursing babies with PKU had better outcomes than those exclusively formula-fed. A 2018 Turkish study that followed 41 babies with PKU (Kose et al., 2018) found that nearly 98% breastfed at birth and 61% continued after diagnosis for a mean duration of more than 7 months. During the babies' first year, the weight gain of the breastfed babies was significantly higher than those not breastfed, and the phenylalanine blood levels were significantly lower in the breastfed group.

Neurological Impairment

A neurological impairment can affect a baby's ability to nurse.

Most babies with a neurological impairment have obvious and serious issues. The baby may have a brain bleed (most common in preterm babies) or have seizures. The baby may have an abnormal brain structure caused by a birth defect, such as macrocephaly (a very large head) or microcephaly (a very small head). Some neurological impairments are caused by substance abuse during pregnancy, such as fetal alcohol spectrum disorders. Other possible causes of neurological impairment are hydrocephaly, autism spectrum disorders, and genetic neurological conditions associated with syndromes such as Down syndrome, Prader-Willi, Williams, Kabuki, Phelan-McDermid, and others. When a baby's brain or nervous system is affected by injury or abnormal development, it may compromise her ability to organize her movements and feed effectively, as well as her ability to learn and stay alert (Genna et al., 2017; Stanley et al., 2019).

But even if nursing does not come easily to the baby, suggest the parents think of nursing as a normal behavior to be encouraged, like walking and talking. Unless the baby has a degenerative neurological disorder, with patience, persistence, and maturity, she will become stronger and more coordinated, which makes nursing easier. Time spent learning to nurse helps improve a baby's neuromuscular coordination. In an experimental study of 23 babies, Finnish researchers found that unlike sucking on a pacifier, the baby's autonomic nervous system responded uniquely to nursing and concluded (Lappi et al., 2007, p. 546): "We consider this response an essential part of the overall psychophysiological maturation of infants." In addition, the baby receives via mother's milk countless components not found in human-milk substitutes that promote the normal development of her immune and digestive systems.

KEY CONCEPT

Even if challenging at first, nursing should be encouraged.

The feelings of closeness associated with nursing also may be important to the family. If the baby is not as responsive to her parents as other babies, this puts their relationship at risk (Clark & Seifer, 1983, 1985). The hormones released by nursing and the regular skin-to-skin contact can help strengthen their attachment and help the parents experience their baby as a person first and a child with a disability second.

If the baby's neurological problem is so severe that it is impossible for her to nurse, emphasize the value of expressed milk and offer to provide details on how to establish full milk production through milk expression (see p. 498-507).

• • •

Encourage the family to seek out healthcare providers supportive of nursing and early intervention programs to prevent or minimize developmental delay.

Feeding problems are sometimes the first sign of a neurological impairment (Mizuno & Ueda, 2005). Some healthcare providers are willing to overlook a nursing problem if a baby can be bottle-fed—even if poorly—rather than seeking the cause. Although some feeding problems are temporary, a neurological impairment may be missed, along with the opportunity for early intervention.

Ideally, when a baby has a feeding problem, the cause will be found, so if it is due to a neurological impairment, the baby can be referred for help. Early intervention programs can be found online with the keywords "early intervention" along with the country or area name. Usually local lactation supporters know individuals, such as lactation-knowledgeable occupational therapists and speech-and-language pathologists, or agencies that provide skilled help. Let the family know that early intervention can help resolve a mild problem quickly and that it does not necessarily mean the baby will need long-term therapy. For a baby with a severe neurodevelopmental impairment, however, early intervention can be vital to the timely development of pre-feeding skills that will allow her to eventually transition to nursing (Morris & Klein, 2001).

Even when a neurological impairment affects a baby's ability to coordinate sucking, swallowing, and breathing, with practice and patience, many of these babies can learn to nurse, and some can learn to feed effectively. The act of bottle-feeding differs fundamentally from nursing, and research found that preterm and term babies with feeding problems experienced higher stress responses and lower oxygen levels when bottle-fed than during nursing (Meier, 1988; Meier & Anderson, 1987; Mizuno & Ueda, 2006). So a baby's ability to bottle-feed should not be used to determine whether the baby can nurse.

If in severe cases the baby needs to be tube-fed, mother's milk should be the first choice. Japanese research (Mizuno & Ueda, 2001) found that even in babies tube-fed for months, feeding competence can improve with maturity and time spent learning to nurse. Nursing can often begin even before tube-feeding ends (Genna et al., 2017).

• • •

Babies with a neurological impairment often have either high or low muscle tone, which can contribute to feeding problems.

Typically, a baby with a neurological impairment has either high or low muscle tone. In some unusual cases, babies may have high muscle tone in their body and low muscle tone in their mouth, and vice versa (Genna et al., 2017). Babies with high tone may arch their bodies, over-respond to stimulation, and bite or clench during nursing. They are often fussy during feeds. Babies with low muscle tone tend to under-respond to feeding triggers. Both high- and low-tone babies may have trouble coordinating sucking, swallowing, and breathing, and they may take very little milk, even after nursing for a long time. The following two sections describe strategies that can help babies achieve a "middle tone" during feeds that enhances both their feeling of well-being and their feeding effectiveness.

High Muscle Tone

A baby with high muscle tone tends to over-respond to sensory stimulation.

During feeds, suggest keeping the environment quiet and dim to avoid overstimulation. Most babies with high muscle tone nurse more effectively if feeds start before they are too hungry. The high-tone baby may have an unusually sensitive mouth, which can cause gagging during feeds. She may arch her body or hyperextend her head. She may clench her jaw muscles or tense her tongue, causing bunching, humping, or retraction.

• • •

Strategies used before and during nursing may help increase milk intake in high-tone babies.

When trying the following strategies with a high-tone baby, suggest using only those that work well and discontinue any that don't or that the baby doesn't like (C.W. Genna, 2017):

- Before feeds, hold baby in the "colic hold" (Figure 8.22) or gently swing from head to foot in a blanket gathered up at the corners (blanket swing) until she relaxes and flexes.
- During feeds, avoid movement, such as rocking or swaying, and try a stable semi-reclined starter position (see p. 23-29), with baby lying tummy down on the parent's body, or try nursing in a snug sling, swaddled, lying on a firm pillow, or side-lying on a firm surface.
- Use deep, firm touch rather than light touch.
- Keep lights and sound low.

If the baby gags easily during nursing, suggest trying a more "baby-driven" approach so baby can take a more active role in latching (pages 23-29).

Skin-to-skin contact helps calm and comfort some high-tone babies. If the baby is so ineffective at feeds that she is not gaining weight adequately, she will need to be supplemented (see later section).

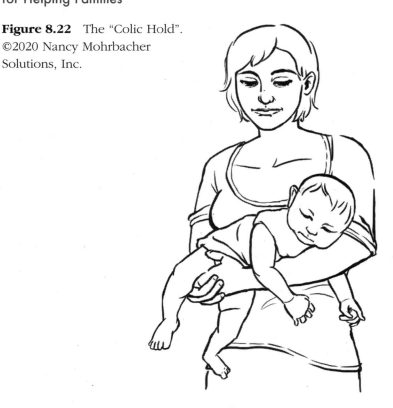

Figure 8.22 The "Colic Hold". ©2020 Nancy Mohrbacher Solutions, Inc.

Low Muscle Tone

A baby with low muscle tone tends to under-respond to sensory stimulation and may nurse ineffectively.

When a neurologically impaired baby with low oral muscle tone nurses, she may suck weakly and dribble milk out of the sides of her mouth. When not nursing, her mouth may stay open and her tongue protrude. Reflux disease is also common among these babies due to the low-tone sphincter muscle that is supposed to keep food down.

• • •

Strategies used before and during nursing may help increase milk intake in low-tone babies.

When trying the following strategies with a low-tone baby, suggest using only those that work well and discontinue any that don't or that the baby doesn't like (C.W. Genna, 2017):

- **Increase muscle tone before feeds** by sitting baby on the nursing parent's knee and bouncing gently or leaning her forward and backward in a non-rhythmic way. If milk was dribbling out of baby's mouth during feeds, try firmly patting her lips before nursing (Wolf & Glass, 1992).
- **Experiment with feeding positions.** Try first the more upright versions of the starter positions (see p. 23-29), which provide the full-body support helpful to low-tone babies. One Japanese study (Mizuno, Inoue, & Takeuchi, 2000) found that compromised babies fed best when positioned tummy down. Or try swaddling the baby with hips and knees flexed, hands positioned near mid-body, and shoulders slightly forward.
- **Use a more "baby-driven" approach to latching,** using the baby's inborn feeding behaviors to trigger a wide-open mouth and gravity to help her latch deeply and maintain a stable position (see p. 23-29).

- **Experiment with the baby's head position.** In neurologically normal babies, nursing with the head slightly tilted back (extended) makes swallowing and breathing easier, but some babies with a neurological impairment or anatomical abnormality find swallowing easier with their chin tucked slightly toward their chest (Genna et al., 2017). Encourage the family to use whichever head position works well for the baby.
- **Try the Dancer Hand position to support the baby's jaw** if an upright or side-lying position is used and the baby has trouble staying latched or if the baby uses unusually wide jaw movements during feeds (see p. 890 for details) (J. Thomas, Marinelli, & Academy of Breastfeeding, 2016).
- **Apply gentle pressure with a fingertip under the baby's chin** if the baby's tongue movements are weak. Do this by gently pressing upward, with a fingertip on the soft tissue behind her baby's jawbone, with a steady, gentle traction toward the mammary gland.

More Nursing Strategies for Babies with High/Low Tone

Even with full milk production, the baby with a neurological impairment may be unable to exclusively nurse.

A baby may feed ineffectively when her neurological impairment causes unusual piston-like tongue movements, wide jaw excursions, low or non-existent vacuum, uncoordinated sucking due to breathing or swallowing problems, and/or other deviations from the norm (Mizuno & Ueda, 2005; Stanley et al., 2019). The nursing parent may express plenty of milk for the baby, but the baby may be unable to transfer enough milk during nursing. Some of these babies take only 10% to 60% of the milk expressed (Genna et al., 2017).

• • •

If the high-tone or low-tone baby cannot yet exclusively nurse, suggest trying a nipple shield.

Until the baby is exclusively nursing, suggest using a silicone nipple shield during feeds to see if that improves the baby's effectiveness. The firmer nipple shield may be able to push past the tensed tongue of the high-tone baby and the protruding tongue of the low-tone baby to provide the right stimulation for more effective sucking. For the low-tone baby, the firmer feel of the shield may trigger a stronger sensory response (J. Thomas et al., 2016).

Because milk flows through the holes in the shield's tip, if the baby's milk intake increases with the use of the shield, the need to supplement may be reduced or eliminated. More milk intake also makes nursing a better experience for the baby. To be effective, the shield must be a good fit for both the baby and the nursing parent. For details on how to choose, fit, apply, use, and wean from a nipple shield, see p. 917.

If the baby is unable to stimulate milk flow through the shield, suggest filling the tip of the shield with expressed milk (either by expressing milk into it or inserting milk with a curved-tip syringe). Getting milk in this way provides the baby with positive reinforcement during the first sucks, which may lead to more interest and effort (Genna et al., 2017).

Until the baby is able to take full feeds while nursing with the shield, to establish or maintain milk production, milk expression is needed. If the shield does not improve the baby's milk intake or help in any other way, suggest discontinuing it.

• • •

If the baby feeds better with a faster milk flow, breast compression or a nursing supplementer may improve feeding effectiveness.

No matter what the baby's neurological issue, she will feed best when the milk flow is fast enough to keep her interested and active, but not so fast that it overwhelms her. The baby's specific issues will determine which milk flow is right for her. For example, a baby with breathing or swallowing problems (dysphagia) may be easily overwhelmed and do best with a very slow milk flow, whereas a baby with low tone who needs more sensory stimulation to stay active during feeds may feed better with a faster flow. Except for the times a baby needs a little squirt of milk to "jumpstart" sucking, ideally the baby should control the milk flow, either through her own efforts or the feeder should coordinate the milk delivered to the baby as she sucks (Genna et al., 2017). Unless a baby's efforts affect the milk flow, a feeding method will not promote more effective nursing.

For a baby who feeds better with a faster milk flow, suggest experimenting with breast compression (see p. 889) while nursing or a nursing supplementer, which uses a thin tube at the nipple to deliver the supplement to the baby during nursing. The baby's natural response to a swallow is to suck. Some babies learn a more effective sucking pattern when the steady milk flow from the tube stimulates more active and consistent sucking and swallowing. When a baby sucks more vigorously, she also takes more milk directly during nursing and stimulates milk production.

Two types of nursing supplementers, "suction required" and "suction not required," can be used. At this writing, all commercial feeding-tube devices (the generic term for nursing supplementers) require suction, which means the baby must actively suck the milk through its thin tubing from the container. Makeshift nursing supplementers that do not require suction can be created using a periodontal syringe or a syringe attached by a port to thin tubing. These "suction not required" devices allow the feeder to push the milk to the baby while she is sucking. Depending on the baby's issue, one or the other may be a more effective tool. For more details, see p. 897.

A nursing supplementer may not improve a baby's nursing effectiveness if the baby learns to take the milk "like a straw" from the supplementer tube without sucking vigorously. In this case, it may help to make the end of the tube flush with the nipple, rather than extending it past the nipple (which is usually recommended). But if this doesn't help, the nursing supplementer may not be a useful tool. In some cases, the baby may do better if the nursing supplementer is used with a nipple shield to provide both a faster milk flow and a firmer feel (J. Thomas et al., 2016). In some cases, a different strategy, such as finger-feeding or oral exercises, may be more effective.

• • •

Mouth and tongue exercises may help, but should be tailored to address the baby's issues.

Some babies become more organized when oral exercises are used, and some become more disorganized. There is a wide range of possible tongue and mouth exercises (such as "Walking Back on the Tongue" described on p. 890-891), but choosing an oral exercise should be done by someone familiar with the underlying cause of the baby's problem and the techniques that best address it (Genna et al., 2017). Unless those providing skilled lactation help are trained in oral-motor evaluation and therapy, they should consider referring the nursing couple to someone with this training, especially if the baby has difficulty nursing and bottle-feeding. These fields include occupational therapy and speech-and-language pathology. The following websites are examples of online resources where local practitioners with this type of training can be found:

- **parentcenterhub.org** Center for Parent Information and Resources
- **asha.org** The American Speech and Hearing Association
- **ndta.org** Neuro-Developmental Treatment Association

Because many in these fields were trained in bottle-feeding norms, suggest the family ask potential providers if they have experience working with nursing babies.

Mouth and tongue exercise should always be enjoyable for everyone. The baby should be actively involved and because her mouth is a private space, the baby should be the one to decide if others can enter it and for how long (Genna et al., 2017). Signs of stress in a baby with a neurological impairment may be subtle, so it is important to model sensitivity to the baby's responses. To avoid overstimulation, in some cases, these exercises may be best timed before the baby shows feeding cues or when switching sides.

• • •

When creating a lactation plan, base the amount of time the baby spends nursing on effectiveness and the baby's interest.

Ideally, when creating a lactation plan, families should plan to spend no more than about 40 minutes on all things feeding-related, which includes nursing, expressing milk, and feeding a supplement. If they spend much more time than that, it becomes impossible to fit in the number of feeds per day baby needs.

If a baby is ineffective during nursing, most parents appreciate some guidance in structuring their day to maximize their milk production, while keeping the rest of their life manageable. How much time a baby spends nursing will depend on how effectively she takes milk. If she consumes little or no milk while nursing, suggest nursing for "practice" whenever the baby seems interested and alert, rather than using a fixed schedule. Then the nursing parent can focus most of the "feeding time" on expressing milk and feeding the baby.

On the other hand, if the baby takes most of her milk while directly nursing, regular nursing time is important. In this case, less time should be spent on milk expression and more time on efforts to maximize the baby's effectiveness during nursing. In these cases, use of a nipple shield and/or a nursing supplementer may increase milk taken during direct nursing, which reduces the need to supplement after feeds.

• • •

As the baby's nursing improves, it's time to gradually reduce supplements.

There are many ways to gradually reduce the volume of supplement the baby receives. If a nursing supplementer is used, the flow can be slowed by lowering the level of the container, the tube can be kinked to stop flow for part of the nursing, or the device can be used at gradually fewer feeds during the day. Usually the first nursing in the morning (or whenever the nursing parent is fullest) is the first feed to stop supplementing.

If other feeding methods are used, less supplement can be given at each feed or supplements can be gradually given fewer and fewer times each day.

HOSPITALIZATION OF THE NURSING BABY

Be prepared to talk about the family's feelings while gathering information.

A baby's hospitalization is stressful for the whole family. Parents may feel vulnerable and badly shaken. They may also be struggling with guilt. Be prepared to offer emotional support during this difficult time.

As the family describes their situation, try to gather the following information:

- The baby's age
- How much she was nursing before the hospitalization (partial/exclusive?)
- The reason the baby was hospitalized
- Estimated length of baby's hospital stay
- How far the nursing parent lives from the hospital and the transportation options
- Any other responsibilities (employment/other children and their ages)

While Baby Is Hospitalized

Ask what the baby's healthcare provider said about nursing and how much time each day the nursing parent can spend with the baby.

Is the baby being fed by mouth? If the baby isn't yet taking oral feeds, make sure the nursing parent has the information needed about milk expression (see next point), in order to safeguard milk production, stay comfortable, and provide the milk baby will need later. If the baby can take anything by mouth, mother's milk is the best first choice. Expressed milk:

- Is most easily digested
- Provides immunities to illness that can help a sick baby get well faster
- Provides protection from other illnesses the baby may be exposed to in the hospital

If the baby's healthcare provider recommends against nursing, encourage the family to discuss their wishes and work with those caring for the baby to find a mutually acceptable solution. A second opinion may be helpful.

How much time each day can the nursing parent spend with the baby? If the hospital is far from home, suggest asking if the baby can be transferred to a closer hospital after her condition is stabilized. Discuss any other responsibilities and help brainstorm ways to spend as much time as possible at the hospital (take sick or vacation time from work, arrange childcare for other children).

Is rooming-in an option? This will depend on the baby's condition, the hospital's policy, and other family responsibilities. Nursing will be easier when the nursing couple is together day and night and can nurse without restrictions, but circumstances (such as other children at home, job responsibilities) may interfere. Some hospitals encourage parents to stay with their children and help care for them, but even if the hospital doesn't usually allow 24-hour rooming-in, they may if the family requests it. If the baby's healthcare provider is supportive, the family can ask for an order for unlimited access. Suggest getting all special orders in writing and have them on hand while at the hospital.

• • •

If the baby is not yet nursing or they cannot be together, ask about the family's feeding goals and help them plan ahead.

When oral feeds begin, is the goal to provide exclusive human milk for the baby, even when they can't be with her? If so, offer to discuss the practical details. For example, talk about a typical day and discuss the times and places milk expression may be possible. For details, see 498-507 in Chapter 11, "Milk Expression and Storage."

If the plan is for baby to be fed formula at missed feeds, be sure the family knows:

1. Depending on the level of milk production, some milk expression may be needed to stay comfortable and prevent mastitis.
2. If the baby was exclusively nursing and the goal is to resume this after the baby is discharged, to maintain milk production, plan to express milk as many times per day as the baby was nursing or if exclusively nursing, at least 6 or 7 times per day.

• • •

A drop in milk production during stressful times is not unusual.

Some families report that during times of unusual stress they have "lost their milk." A temporary drop in milk production or a delay in milk ejection is common (Chatterton et al., 2000). But this does not mean the milk is gone for good. Encourage the use of relaxation techniques and to keep nursing or expressing. With time and regular stimulation, the milk production will return to what it was.

• • •

Offer practical suggestions for making the baby's hospital stay easier.

Attention to details can sometimes make a difficult situation easier to cope with. Here are some examples.

Environment

- If the baby is in a semi-private room, request the bed farthest from the door for more privacy and less traffic.
- Look into the possibility of a private room.

The parent's comfort

- If a large part of each day is spent at the hospital, bring drinks and snacks or ask about receiving hospital meals.
- Bring extra pillows or cushions from home for added comfort.
- Wear comfortable shoes and clothes that make nursing easy.

Medical equipment and procedures

- If the baby is on an IV, ask for longer tubing for more freedom of movement while nursing.
- If the baby needs an oxygen tent, can the parent nurse inside it?

- If painful procedures must be done, ask if the baby can nurse during the procedure (Reece-Stremtan & Gray, 2016). Alternatively, could topical anesthetics be used to numb the site and multiple procedures be done at once, rather than spreading them out over the course of the day (Batton, Barrington, & Wallman, 2006).

• • •

Nursing is a potent pain-reliever, which can help speed baby's recovery.

Helping to reduce a baby's pain is always a kindness, but pain-relief can also be an important aspect of a faster recovery. In their joint policy statement on pain management in newborns, the American Academy of Pediatrics and the Canadian Paediatric Society explained that better pain management improves health outcomes after surgery by "minimizing the endocrine and metabolic responses" to pain (Batton et al., 2006). It was once thought that newborns did not feel pain and that their pain didn't matter because they wouldn't remember it later. But research has clearly demonstrated that pain is felt by preterm and term newborns and has profound negative physical effects (Bartocci, Bergqvist, Lagercrantz, & Anand, 2006; Bembich et al., 2015).

When a baby undergoes a painful medical procedure, nursing is the most effective non-drug pain reducer (Carbajal, Veerapen, Couderc, Jugie, & Ville, 2003; Codipietro, Ceccarelli, & Ponzone, 2008; Gray, Miller, Philipp, & Blass, 2002). This may be due to body responses unique to nursing. Finnish research found that unlike sucking on a pacifier, breastfeeding produces measurable changes in a baby's autonomic nervous system, which were reflected as changes in heart rate variability (Lappi et al., 2007).

In its 2016 protocol on non-drug pain management in nursing babies, the Academy of Breastfeeding Medicine wrote (Reece-Stremtan & Gray, 2016, p. 1):

> "Breastfeeding should be the first choice to alleviate procedural pain in neonates undergoing a single painful procedure..."

Other effective non-drug pain relievers listed in the ABM protocol are skin-to-skin contact, warmth, the scent of human milk, and sucrose (with or without a pacifier). For a complete overview of options in preterm and term newborns and older babies, download ABM Protocol #23 at: **bfmed.org/protocols**.

• • •

A baby's usual nursing rhythms may change during illness or injury.

Some babies want to nurse more often—sometimes almost constantly—when very sick or injured. Other babies, such as those whose illness makes them lethargic, may be less interested. If a baby loses interest in nursing, suggest expressing milk to stay comfortable and to maintain milk production for later, when the baby is feeling better. A lethargic baby can be fed mother's milk by tube (gavage feeding) if necessary.

Coping with Surgery

Suggest asking how close to surgery the child can nurse and how soon after surgery nursing can resume.

One of the most stressful aspects of surgery on a nursing child is the period before the surgery when all food and drink stops, so that her stomach will be empty during the procedure. Described as "preoperative fasting" or being

"NPO," this practice is meant to decrease the risk of the child's stomach contents entering her lungs (aspiration) during and after surgery.

Over the years, the length of time recommended for preoperative fasting decreased, from "no food or drink after midnight" to much shorter periods, which vary by food, depending on how quickly that food leaves the stomach. While this timing was being debated, one aspect that sometimes led to inconsistencies was disagreement about which food category human milk fell into, which affected fasting time. In 1999 44 U.S. hospitals were surveyed (Ferrari, Rooney, & Rockoff, 1999), and there was little agreement. Some considered human milk a clear liquid (23%), some concluded it was somewhere between a clear liquid and formula (36%), some thought it was a solid (34%), and some decided it was the same as formula (7%).

In 2012, the Academy of Breastfeeding Medicine published its Clinical Protocol #25 (ABM, 2012), which listed preoperative fasting times for different foods:

- Light meal: 6 hours
- Non-human milks: 6 hours
- Infant formula: 6 hours
- Human milk: 4 hours,
- Clear liquids: 2 hours

Some European authors questioned this 2-hour guideline for clear liquids and recommended for elective pediatric surgery 1 hour be the fasting time for clear liquids (M. Thomas, Morrison, Newton, & Schindler, 2018). However, the American Society of Anesthesiologists' Task Force on Preoperative Fasting recommended a 2-hour fasting time for clear liquids in its 2017 practice guidelines (ASA, 2017)

Encourage the family to talk to the baby's surgeon and anesthesiologist before the day of the surgery to reach an agreement on the fasting time. During those difficult hours before surgery, one possible option suggested by a respected U.S. physician (Lawrence & Lawrence, 2016, p. 517) is to ask about pumping first and then nursing the baby for comfort up to 2 hours before the surgery. Help the family plan strategies for comforting and distracting the baby while nursing is restricted.

In the case of emergency surgery, Canadian research (Bhatt et al., 2018) found there was no benefit to delaying surgery to meet the fasting guidelines

After surgery, it may be possible to nurse in the recovery room. Suggest talking to the baby's healthcare provider about this option. Whenever the baby is ready to be fed by mouth, nursing should resume.

• • •

Discuss possible milk-expression strategies based on the baby's need for milk and how long nursing will be restricted.

Sometimes stress temporarily decreases milk production or delays milk ejection, so depending on the child's age and need for milk, suggest the possibility of expressing some extra milk to tide them over. If there is advance notice of at least several days before the baby's surgery, suggest the possibility of expressing and storing extra milk in case stress reduces the milk expressed before and after the surgery.

RESOURCES

bfmed.org/protocols—To download the current versions of the Academy of Breastfeeding Medicine Clinical Protocols, most available in multiple languages:

- #11 Neonatal ankyloglossia
- #16 Breastfeeding the hypotonic infant
- #17 Guidelines for breastfeeding infants with cleft lip or palate
- #23 Non-pharmacologic management of procedure-related pain in the breastfeeding infant
- #24 Allergic proctocolitis in the exclusively breastfed infant
- #25 Preprocedural fasting for the breastfeeding infant
- #27 Breastfeeding an infant or young child with insulin-dependent diabetes
- #29 Iron, zinc, and vitamin D supplementation during breastfeeding

Cullen, E. , Ed. (2019). *Breastfeeding and Down Syndrome: A Comprehensive Guide for Mothers and Medical Professionals.* Hanover, MA: Julia's Way. Free download for noncommercial use at: **juliasway.org**

Genna, C.W., ed. (2017). *Supporting Sucking Skills in Breastfeeding Infants*, 3rd. ed. Burlington, MA: Jones & Bartlett Learning.

REFERENCES

AAP. (1999). Ultraviolet light: A hazard to children. American Academy of Pediatrics. Committee on Environmental Health. *Pediatrics, 104*(2 Pt 1), 328-333.

AAP. (2011). Concerns with early universal iron supplementation of breastfeeding infants. *Pediatrics, 127,* e1097.

AAP. (2012). Breastfeeding and the use of human milk. *Pediatrics, 129*(3), e827-e841.

AAP. (2015). *Red Book: 2015 Report of the Committee on Infectious Diseases.* Elk Grove Village, IL: American Acadmy of Pediatrics.

Abdellatif, M., Ghozy, S., Kamel, M. G., et al. (2019). Association between exposure to macrolides and the development of infantile hypertrophic pyloric stenosis: A systematic review and meta-analysis. *European Journal of Pediatrics, 178*(3), 301-314.

Abedi, P., Bovayri, M., Fakhri, A., et al. (2018). The relationship between vitamin D and postpartum depression in reproductive-aged Iranian women. *Journal of Medicine and Life, 11*(4), 286-292.

ABM. (2011). ABM Clinical Protocol #24: Allergic proctocolitis in the exclusively breastfed infant. *Breastfeeding Medicine, 6*(6), 435-440.

ABM. (2012). ABM Clinical Protocol #25: Recommendations for preprocedural fasting for the breastfed infant: "NPO" Guidelines. *Breastfeeding Medicine, 7*(3), 197-202.

Ahring, K., Belanger-Quintana, A., Dokoupil, K., et al. (2009). Dietary management practices in phenylketonuria across European centres. *Clinical Nutrition, 28*(3), 231-236.

AHRQ. (2015). *Treatments for Ankyloglossia and Ankyloglossia with Concomitant Lip-Tie.* Rockville, MD: Agency for Healthcare Research and Quality.

Akinbami, L. J., Simon, A. E., & Schoendorf, K. C. (2016). Trends in allergy prevalence among children aged 0-17 years by asthma status, United States, 2001-2013. *Journal of Asthma, 53*(4), 356-362.

Almaramhy, H. H., & Al-Zalabani, A. H. (2019). The association of prenatal and postnatal macrolide exposure with subsequent development of infantile hypertrophic pyloric stenosis: A systematic review and meta-analysis. *Italian Journal of Pediatrics, 45*(1), 20.

Alperovich, M., Frey, J. D., Shetye, P. R., et al. (2017). Breast milk feeding rates in patients with cleft lip and palate at a North American craniofacial center. *Cleft Palate-Craniofacial Journal, 54*(3), 334-337.

Alves, P. V., & Luiz, R. R. (2012). The influence of orotracheal intubation on the oral tissue development in preterm infants. *Oral Health and Preventive Dentistry, 10*(2), 141-147.

Amir, L. H., James, J. P., & Donath, S. M. (2006). Reliability of the Hazelbaker Assessment Tool for Lingual Frenulum Function. *International Breastfeeding Journal, 1*(1), 3.

Amstalden-Mendes, L. G., Magna, L. A., & Gil-da-Silva-Lopes, V. L. (2007). Neonatal care of infants with cleft lip and/or palate: Feeding orientation and evolution of weight gain in a nonspecialized Brazilian hospital. *Cleft Palate-Craniofacial Journal, 44*(3), 329-334.

Aniansson, G., Svensson, H., Becker, M., et al. (2002). Otitis media and feeding with breast milk of children with cleft palate. *Scandanavian Journal of Plastic and Reconstructive Surgery and Hand Surgery, 36*(1), 9-15.

ASA. (2017). Practice guidelines for preoperative fasting and the use of pharmacologic agents to reduce the risk of pulmonary aspiration: Application to healthy patients undergoing elective procedures: An updated report by the American Society of Anesthesiologists Task Force on Preoperative Fasting and the Use of Pharmacologic Agents to Reduce the Risk of Pulmonary Aspiration. *Anesthesiology, 126*(3), 376-393.

Aumonier, M. E., & Cunningham, C. C. (1983). Breast feeding in infants with Down's syndrome. *Child: Care, Health and Development, 9*(5), 247-255.

Avedian, L. V., & Ruberg, R. L. (1980). Impaired weight gain in cleft palate infants. *Cleft Palate Journal, 17*(1), 24-26.

Back, O., Blomquist, H. K., Hernell, O., et al. (2009). Does vitamin D intake during infancy promote the development of atopic allergy? *Acta Dermato-Venereologica, 89*(1), 28-32.

Baird, D. C., Harker, D. J., & Karmes, A. S. (2015). Diagnosis and treatment of gastroesophageal reflux in infants and children. *American Family Physician, 92*(8), 705-714.

Baker, R. D., Greer, F. R., & Committee on Nutrition American Academy of, P. (2010). Diagnosis and prevention of iron deficiency and iron-deficiency anemia in infants and young children (0-3 years of age). *Pediatrics, 126*(5), 1040-1050.

Ballard, J. L., Auer, C. E., & Khoury, J. C. (2002). Ankyloglossia: Assessment, incidence, and effect of frenuloplasty on the breastfeeding dyad. *Pediatrics, 110*(5), e63.

Banta-Wright, S. A., Kodadek, S. M., Houck, G. M., et al. (2015). Commitment to breastfeeding in the context of phenylketonuria. *Journal of Obstetric, Gynecologic & Neonatal Nursing, 44*(6), 726-736.

Barbas, K. H., & Kelleher, D. K. (2004). Breastfeeding success among infants with congenital heart disease. *Pediatric Nursing, 30*(4), 285-289.

Barros da Silva, R., Barbieri-Figueiredo, M. D. C., & Van Riper, M. (2018). Breastfeeding experiences of mothers of children with Down syndrome. *Comprehensive Child and Adolescent Nursing,* 1-15.

Bartocci, M., Bergqvist, L. L., Lagercrantz, H., et al. (2006). Pain activates cortical areas in the preterm newborn brain. *Pain, 122*(1-2), 109-117.

Batton, D. G., Barrington, K. J., & Wallman, C. (2006). Prevention and management of pain in the neonate: An update. *Pediatrics, 118*(5), 2231-2241.

Beck-Nielsen, S. S., Jensen, T. K., Gram, J., et al. (2009). Nutritional rickets in Denmark: a retrospective review of children's medical records from 1985 to 2005. *European Journal of Pediatrics, 168*(8), 941-949.

Bembich, S., Brovedani, P., Cont, G., et al. (2015). Pain activates a defined area of the somatosensory and motor cortex in newborn infants. *Acta Paediatrica, 104*(11), e530-533. doi:10.1111/apa.13122.

Benoiton, L., Morgan, M., & Baguley, K. (2016). Management of posterior ankyloglossia and upper lip ties in a tertiary otolaryngology outpatient clinic. *International Journal of Pediatric Otorhinolaryngology, 88,* 13-16.

Bergese, F. (1966). [Research on the development of the labial frenum in children of age 9-12]. *Minerva Stomatologica, 15*(10), 672-676.

Bergman, N. (2017). Breastfeeding and perinatal neuroscience. In C. W. Genna (Ed.), *Supporting Sucking Skills in Breastfeeding Infants* (3rd ed., pp. 49-63). Burlington, MA: Jones & Bartlett Learning.

Berkowitz, D., Naveh, Y., & Berant, M. (1997). "Infantile colic" as the sole manifestation of gastroesophageal reflux. *Journal of Pediatric Gastroenterology and Nutrition, 24*(2), 231-233.

Bessell, A., Hooper, L., Shaw, W. C., et al. (2011). Feeding interventions for growth and development in infants with cleft lip, cleft palate or cleft lip and palate. *Cochrane Database of Systematic Reviews*(2), CD003315. doi:10.1002/14651858.CD003315.pub3.

Bhatt, M., Johnson, D. W., Taljaard, M., et al. (2018). Association of preprocedural fasting with outcomes of emergency department sedation in children. *JAMA Pediatrics, 172*(7), 678-685.

Bin-Nun, A., Kasirer, Y. M., & Mimouni, F. B. (2017). A dramatic increase in tongue tie-related articles: A 67 years systematic review. *Breastfeeding Medicine, 12*(7), 410-414.

Boekel, S. (2000). *Gastro-esophageal Reflux Disease (GERD) and the Breastfeeding Baby.* Raleigh, NC: International Lactation Consultant Association.

Boronat-Catala, M., Montiel-Company, J. M., Bellot-Arcis, C., et al. (2017). Association between duration of breastfeeding and malocclusions in primary and mixed dentition: A systematic review and meta-analysis. *Scientific Reports, 7*(1), 5048.

Bowles, B. C. (2011). Breast massage: A "handy" multipurpose tool to promote breastfeeding success. *Clinical Lactation, 2*(4), 21-24.

Boyce, J.O., Reilly, S., Skeat, J., et al. (2019). ABM Clinical Protocol #17: Guidelines for breastfeeding infants with cleft lip, cleft palate, or cleft lip and palate--revised 2019. *Breastfeeding Medicine, 14*(7), 1-8.

Brandao, C. A., de Marsillac, M. W. S., Barja-Fidalgo, F., et al. (2018). Is the Neonatal Tongue Screening Test a valid and reliable tool for detecting ankyloglossia in newborns? *International Journal of Paediatric Dentistry, 28*(4), 380-389.

Britton, K. F., McDonald, S. H., & Welbury, R. R. (2011). An investigation into infant feeding in children born with a cleft lip and/or palate in the West of Scotland. *European Archives of Paediatric Dentistry, 12*(5), 250-255.

Brown, A. (2017). *Why Starting Solids Matters.* London: Pinter & Martin.

Brown, K. H. (1994). Dietary management of acute diarrheal disease: Contemporary scientific issues. *Journal of Nutrition, 124*(8 Suppl), 1455S-1460S.

Burianova, I., Kulihova, K., Vitkova, V., et al. (2017). Breastfeeding after early repair of cleft lip in newborns with cleft lip or cleft lip and palate in a baby-friendly designated hospital. *Journal of Human Lactation, 33*(3), 504-508.

Burke, N. L., Harville, E. W., Wickliffe, J. K., et al. (2019). Determinants of vitamin D status among Black and White low-income pregnant and non-pregnant reproductive-aged women from Southeast Louisiana. *BMC Pregnancy and Childbirth, 19*(1), 111.

Bystrova, K., Widstrom, A. M., Matthiesen, A. S., et al. (2007). Early lactation performance in primiparous and multiparous women in relation to different maternity home practices. A randomised trial in St. Petersburg. *International Breastfeeding Journal, 2,* 9.

Cabaset, S., Krieger, J. P., Richard, A., et al. (2019). Vitamin D status and its determinants in healthy pregnant women living in Switzerland in the first trimester of pregnancy. *BMC Pregnancy and Childbirth, 19*(1), 10.

CADTH. (2016). Frenectomy for the correction of ankyloglossia: A review of clinical effectiveness and guidelines. Retrieved from Ottawa, ON Canada: **cadth.ca/frenectomy-correction-ankyloglossia-review-clinical-effectiveness-and-guidelines**.

Calteux, N., Schmid, N., Hellers, J., et al. (2013). [Neonatal cleft lip repair: Perioperative safety and surgical outcomes]. *Annales de Chirurgie Plastique Esthetetique, 58*(6), 638-643.

Campanozzi, A., Boccia, G., Pensabene, L., et al. (2009). Prevalence and natural history of gastroesophageal reflux: Pediatric prospective survey. *Pediatrics, 123*(3), 779-783.

Carbajal, R., Veerapen, S., Couderc, S., et al. (2003). Analgesic effect of breast feeding in term neonates: Randomised controlled trial. *British Medical Journal, 326*(7379), 13.

Carberry, A. E., Raynes-Greenow, C. H., Turner, R. M., et al. (2013). Breastfeeding within the first hour compared to more than one hour reduces risk of early-onset feeding problems in term neonates: A cross-sectional study. *Breastfeeding Medicine, 8*(6), 513-514.

Carroll, A. E., Garrison, M. M., & Christakis, D. A. (2002). A systematic review of nonpharmacological and nonsurgical therapies for gastroesophageal reflux in infants. *Archives of Pediatrics and Adolescent Medicine, 156*(2), 109-113.

CDC. (2001). Recommendations for using fluoride to prevent and control dental caries in the United States. Centers for Disease Control and Prevention. *MMWR Recommendations and Reports, 50*(RR-14), 1-42.

CFF. (2018). Cystic Fibrosis Foundation Patient Registry: 2017 Annual Data Report. Retrieved from **cff.org/Research/Researcher-Resources/Patient-Registry/2017-Patient- Registry-Annual-Data-Report.pdf**.

Chang, C. Y. (2016). Buccal ties and breastfeeding. Retrieved from **blog.fauquierent.net/2016/04/buccal-ties-and-breastfeeding.html**.

Chatterton, R. T., Jr., Hill, P. D., Aldag, J. C., et al. (2000). Relation of plasma oxytocin and prolactin concentrations to milk production in mothers of preterm infants: Influence of stress. *Journal of Clinical Endocrinology and Metabolism, 85*(10), 3661-3668.

Chen, P. L., Soto-Ramirez, N., Zhang, H., et al. (2017). Association between infant feeding modes and gastroesophageal reflux: A repeated measurement analysis of the Infant Feeding Practices Study II. *Journal of Human Lactation, 33*(2), 267-277.

Chinnadurai, S., Francis, D. O., Epstein, R. A., et al. (2015). Treatment of ankyloglossia for reasons other than breastfeeding: A systematic review. *Pediatrics, 135*(6), e1467-1474.

Cichero, J. A., Nicholson, T. M., & September, C. (2013). Thickened milk for the management of feeding and swallowing issues in infants: A call for interdisciplinary professional guidelines. *Journal of Human Lactation, 29*(2), 132-135.

Clark, G., & Seifer, R. (1983). Facilitating mother-infant communication: A treatment model for high-risk and developmentally-delayed infants. *Infant Mental Health Journal, 4*(2), 67-81.

Clark, G., & Seifer, R. (1985). Assessment of parents' interactions with their developmentally delayed infants. *Infant Mental Health Journal, 6*(4), 214-225.

Clarren, S. K., Anderson, B., & Wolf, L. S. (1987). Feeding infants with cleft lip, cleft palate, or cleft lip and palate. *Cleft Palate Journal, 24*(3), 244-249.

Clemens, J. D., Harris, J. R., Sack, D. A., et al. (1988). Discontinuation of breast-feeding during episodes of diarrhoea in rural Bangladeshi children. *Transactions of the Royal Society of Tropical Medicine and Hygiene, 82*(5), 779-783.

Clemente, C., Barnes, J., Shinebourne, E., et al. (2001). Are infant behavioural feeding difficulties associated with congenital heart disease? *Child: Care, Health, and Development, 27*(1), 47-59.

Cockburn, F., Belton, N. R., Purvis, R. J., et al. (1980). Maternal vitamin D intake and mineral metabolism in mothers and their newborn infants. *British Medical Journal, 281*(6232), 11-14.

Codipietro, L., Ceccarelli, M., & Ponzone, A. (2008). Breastfeeding or oral sucrose solution in term neonates receiving heel lance: A randomized, controlled trial. *Pediatrics, 122*(3), e716-721.

Cohen, M., Marschall, M. A., & Schafer, M. E. (1992). Immediate unrestricted feeding of infants following cleft lip and palate repair. *Journal of Craniofacial Surgery, 3*(1), 30-32.

Colombo, C., Costantini, D., Zazzeron, L., et al. (2007). Benefits of breastfeeding in cystic fibrosis: A single-centre follow-up survey. *Acta Paediatrica, 96*(8), 1228-1232.

Colson, S. (2003). Biological nurturing increases duration of breastfeeding for a vulnerable cohort. *MIDRIS Midwifery Digest, 13*(1), 92-97.

Colson, S. D., Meek, J. H., & Hawdon, J. M. (2008). Optimal positions for the release of primitive neonatal reflexes stimulating breastfeeding. *Early Human Development, 84*(7), 441-449.

Combs, V. L., & Marino, B. L. (1993). A comparison of growth patterns in breast and bottle-fed infants with congenital heart disease. *Pediatric Nursing, 19*(2), 175-179.

Coryllos, E., Genna, C. W., & LeVan Fram, J. (2017). Minimally invasive treatment for posterior tonuge-tie (the hidden tongue-tie). In C. W. Genna (Ed.), *Supporting Sucking Skills in Breastfeeding Infants* (3rd ed., pp. 269-278). Burlington, MA: Jones & Bartlett Learning.

Costello, C. L., Gellatly, M., Daniel, J., et al. (2015). Growth restriction in infants and young children with congenital heart disease. *Congenital Heart Disease, 10*(5), 447-456.

Crossman, K. (1998). Breastfeeding a baby with a cleft palate: A case report. *Journal of Human Lactation, 14*(1), 47-50.

Cullen, E.G. (2019). *Breastfeeding & Down Syndrome: A Comprehensive Guide for Mothers and Medical Professionals.* Julia's Way: Hanover, MA.

Dahlen, H. G., Foster, J. P., Psaila, K., et al. (2018). Gastro-oesophageal reflux: A mixed methods study of infants admitted to hospital in the first 12 months following birth in NSW (2000-2011). *BMC Pediatrics, 18*(1), 30.

Danner, S. C. (1992). Breastfeeding the infant with a cleft defect. *NAACOGS Clinical Issues in Perinatal and Womens Health Nursing, 3*(4), 634-639.

Danner, S. C., & Wilson-Clay, B. (1986). *Breastfeeding the Infant with a Cleft Lip/Palate.* In Lactation Conultant Series Unit 10. Franklin Park, IL: La Leche League International.

Darmawikarta, D., Chen, Y., Lebovic, G., et al. (2016). Total duration of breastfeeding, Vitamin D supplementation, and serum levels of 25-hydroxyvitamin D. *American Journal of Public Health, 106*(4), 714-719.

Darzi, M. A., Chowdri, N. A., & Bhat, A. N. (1996). Breast feeding or spoon feeding after cleft lip repair: A prospective, randomised study. *British Journal of Plastic Surgery, 49*(1), 24-26.

Davis, J. A., & Spatz, D. L. (2019). Human milk and infants with congenital heart disease: A summary of current literature supporting the provision of human milk and breastfeeding. *Advances in Neonatal Care, 19*(3), 212-218.

Daymont, C., Neal, A., Prosnitz, A., et al. (2013). Growth in children with congenital heart disease. *Pediatrics, 131*(1), e236-242.

de Almeida, M. B., Barker, E., & Lederer, C. L. (2011). Adequacy of human milk viscosity to respond to infants with dysphagia: Experimental study. *Journal of Applied Oral Science, 19*(6), 554-559.

Delli, K., Livas, C., Sculean, A., et al. (2013). Facts and myths regarding the maxillary midline frenum and its treatment: A systematic review of the literature. *Quintessence International, 44*(2), 177-187.

Deoni, S. C., Dean, D. C., 3rd, Piryatinsky, I., et al. (2013). Breastfeeding and early white matter development: A cross-sectional study. *Neuroimage, 82,* 77-86.

Dixon, B., Gray, J., Elliot, N., et al. (2018). A multifaceted programme to reduce the rate of tongue-tie release surgery in newborn infants: Observational study. *International Journal of Pediatric Otorhinolaryngology, 113,* 156-163.

Dogruel, D., Bingol, G., Altintas, D. U., et al. (2016). Clinical features of food allergy during the 1st year of life: The ADAPAR Birth Cohort Study. *International Archives of Allergy and Immunology, 169*(3), 171-180.

Dollberg, S., Botzer, E., Grunis, E., et al. (2006). Immediate nipple pain relief after frenotomy in breast-fed infants with ankyloglossia: A randomized, prospective study. *Journal of Pediatric Surgery, 41*(9), 1598-1600.

Donati-Bourne, J., Batool, Z., Hendrickse, C., et al. (2015). Tongue-tie assessment and division: A time-critical intervention to optimise breastfeeding. *Journal of Neonatal Surgery, 4*(1), 3.

Douglas, P., & Geddes, D. (2018). Practice-based interpretation of ultrasound studies leads the way to more effective clinical support and less pharmaceutical and surgical intervention for breastfeeding infants. *Midwifery, 58,* 145-155.

Douglas, P. S. (2013a). Diagnosing gastro-oesophageal reflux disease or lactose intolerance in babies who cry a lot in the first few months overlooks feeding problems. *Journal of Paediatrics and Child Health, 49*(4), E252-256.

Douglas, P. S. (2013b). Rethinking "posterior" tongue-tie. *Breastfeeding Medicine, 8*(6), 503-506.

Duarte, G. A., Ramos, R. B., & Cardoso, M. C. (2016). Feeding methods for children with cleft lip and/or palate: A systematic review. *Brazilian Journal of Otorhinolaryngology, 82*(5), 602-609.

Elad, D., Kozlovsky, P., Blum, O., et al. (2014). Biomechanics of milk extraction during breast-feeding. *Proceedings of the National Academy of Sciences U.S.A., 111*(14), 5230-5235.

Ergaz-Shaltiel, Z., Engel, O., Erlichman, I., et al. (2017). Neonatal characteristics and perinatal complications in neonates with Down syndrome. *American Journal of Medical Genetics Part A, 173*(5), 1279-1286.

Erkkila, A. T., Isotalo, E., Pulkkinen, J., et al. (2005). Association between school performance, breast milk intake and fatty acid profile of serum lipids in ten-year-old cleft children. *Journal of Craniofacial Surgery, 16*(5), 764-769.

Ewer, A. K., James, M. E., & Tobin, J. M. (1999). Prone and left lateral positioning reduce gastro-oesophageal reflux in preterm infants. *Archives of Disease in Childhood. Fetal and Neonatal Edition, 81*(3), F201-205.

Ferrari, L. R., Rooney, F. M., & Rockoff, M. A. (1999). Preoperative fasting practices in pediatrics. *Anesthesiology, 90*(4), 978-980.

Ferreira, C. T., & Seidman, E. (2007). Food allergy: A practical update from the gastroenterological viewpoint. *Jornal de Pediatria (Rio J), 83*(1), 7-20.

Ferres-Amat, E., Pastor-Vera, T., Rodriguez-Alessi, P., et al. (2017). The prevalence of ankyloglossia in 302 newborns with breastfeeding problems and sucking difficulties in Barcelona: A descriptive study. *European Journal of Paediatric Dentistry, 18*(4), 319-325.

Flores-Lujano, J., Perez-Saldivar, M. L., Fuentes-Panana, E. M., et al. (2009). Breastfeeding and early infection in the aetiology of childhood leukaemia in Down syndrome. *British Journal of Cancer, 101*(5), 860-864.

Forlenza, G. P., Paradise Black, N. M., McNamara, E. G., et al. (2010). Ankyloglossia, exclusive breastfeeding, and failure to thrive. *Pediatrics, 125*(6), e1500-1504.

Frankel, E. A., Shalaby, T. M., & Orenstein, S. R. (2006). Sandifer syndrome posturing: Relation to abdominal wall contractions, gastroesophageal reflux, and fundoplication. *Digestive Diseases and Sciences, 51*(4), 635-640.

Frommelt, M. A. (2004). Differential diagnosis and approach to a heart murmur in term infants. *Pediatric Clinics of North America, 51*(4), 1023-1032, x.

Galloway, C., & Howells, J. (2015). Harnessing breastmilk composition to improve a preterm infant's growth rate--A case study. *Breastfeeding Review, 23*(1), 17-21.

Garcez, L. W., & Giugliani, E. R. (2005). Population-based study on the practice of breastfeeding in children born with cleft lip and palate. *Cleft Palate-Craniofacial Journal, 42*(6), 687-693.

Garza, J. J., Morash, D., Dzakovic, A., et al. (2002). Ad libitum feeding decreases hospital stay for neonates after pyloromyotomy. *Journal of Pediatric Surgery, 37*(3), 493-495.

Gaskin, K. J., & Waters, D. L. (1994). Nutritional management of infants with cystic fibrosis. *Journal of Paediatrics and Child Health, 30*(1), 1-2.

Gatto, K. (2015). Tethered oral tissue: What is that? Retrieved from **http://www.agesandstages.net/blog.php?**

Geddes, D. T., & Sakalidis, V. S. (2016). Ultrasound imaging of breastfeeding--A window to the inside: Methodology, normal appearances, and application. *Journal of Human Lactation, 32*(2), 340-349.

Genna, C. W. (2016). *Selecting and Using Breastfeeding Tools: Improving Care and Outcomes.* Amarillo, TX: Praeclarus Press.

Genna, C. W. (2017a). Breastfeeding: Normal sucking and swallowing. In C. W. Genna (Ed.), *Supporting Sucking Skills in Breastfeeding Infants* (3rd ed., pp. 1-48). Burlington, MA: Jones & Bartlett Learning.

Genna, C. W. (2017b). The influence of anatomic and structural issues on sucking skills. In C. W. Genna (Ed.), *Supporting Sucking Skills in Breastfeeding Infants* (3rd ed., pp. 209-267). Burlington, MA: Jones & Bartlett Learning.

Genna, C. W. (2017). Sensory integration and breastfeeding. In C. W. Genna (Ed.), *Supporting Sucking Skills in Breastfeeding Infants* (3rd ed., pp. 309-333). Burlington, MA: Jones & Bartlett Learning.

Genna, C. W., LeVan Fram, J., & Sandora, L. (2017). Neurological issues and breastfeeding. In C. W. Genna (Ed.), *Supporting Sucking Skills in Breastfeeding Infants* (3rd ed., pp. 335-397). Burlington, MA: Jones & Bartlett Learning.

Genova, L., Cerda, J., Correa, C., et al. (2018). Good health indicators in children with Down syndrome: High frequency of exclusive breastfeeding at 6 months. *Revista Chilena de Pediatria, 89*(1), 32-41.

Ghaem, M., Armstrong, K. L., Trocki, O., et al. (1998). The sleep patterns of infants and young children with gastro-oesophageal reflux. *Journal of Paediatrics and Child Health, 34*(2), 160-163.

Ghaheri, B. A., Cole, M., Fausel, S. C., et al. (2017). Breastfeeding improvement following tongue-tie and lip-tie release: A prospective cohort study. *Laryngoscope, 127*(5), 1217-1223.

Ghaheri, B. A., Cole, M., & Mace, J. C. (2018). Revision lingual frenotomy improves patient-reported breastfeeding outcomes: A prospective cohort study. *Journal of Human Lactation, 34*(3), 566-574.

Gil-da-Silva-Lopes, V. L., Xavier, A. C., Klein-Antunes, D., et al. (2013). Feeding infants with cleft lip and/or palate in Brazil: Suggestions to improve health policy and research. *Cleft Palate-Craniofacial Journal, 50*(5), 577-590.

Girish, M., Mujawar, N., Gotmare, P., et al. (2013). Impact and feasibility of breast crawl in a tertiary care hospital. *Journal of Perinatology, 33*(4), 288-291.

Girish, M., & Subramaniam, G. (2008). Rickets in exclusively breast fed babies. *Indian Journal of Pediatrics, 75*(6), 641-643.

Glivetic, T., Rodin, U., Milosevic, M., et al. (2015). Prevalence, prenatal screening and neonatal features in children with Down syndrome: A registry-based national study. *Italian Journal of Pediatrics, 41,* 81.

Gopinath, V. K., & Muda, W. A. (2005). Assessment of growth and feeding practices in children with cleft lip and palate. *Southeast Asian Journal of Tropical Medicine and Public Health, 36*(1), 254-258.

Gosain, A. K., Conley, S. F., Santoro, T. D., et al. (1999). A prospective evaluation of the prevalence of submucous cleft palate in patients with isolated cleft lip versus controls. *Plastic and Reconstructive Surgery, 103*(7), 1857-1863.

Gottschlich, M. M., Mayes, T., Allgeier, C., et al. (2018). A retrospective study identifying breast milk feeding disparities in infants with cleft palate. *Journal of the Academy of Nutrition and Dietetics, 118*(11), 2154-2161.

Goyal, M., Chopra, R., Bansal, K., et al. (2014). Role of obturators and other feeding interventions in patients with cleft lip and palate: A review. *European Archives of Paediatric Dentistry, 15*(1), 1-9.

Grady, E. (1983). *Nursing my baby with a cleft of the soft palate.* Franklin Park, IL: La Leche League International.

Gray, L., Miller, L. W., Philipp, B. L., et al. (2002). Breastfeeding is analgesic in healthy newborns. *Pediatrics, 109*(4), 590-593.

Greve, L. C., Wheeler, M. D., Green-Burgeson, D. K., et al. (1994). Breast-feeding in the management of the newborn with phenylketonuria: A practical approach to dietary therapy. *Journal of the American Dietetic Association, 94*(3), 305-309.

Griffin, I. J., & Abrams, S. A. (2001). Iron and breastfeeding. *Pediatric Clinics of North America, 48*(2), 401-413.

Griffiths, D. M. (2004). Do tongue-ties affect breastfeeding? *Journal of Human Lactation, 20*(4), 409-414.

Haase, B., Barreira, J., Murphy, P. K., et al. (2009). The development of an accurate test weighing technique for preterm and high-risk hospitalized infants. *Breastfeeding Medicine, 4*(3), 151-156.

Habel, A., Elhadi, N., Sommerlad, B., et al. (2006). Delayed detection of cleft palate: An audit of newborn examination. *Archives of Disease in Childhood, 91*(3), 238-240.

Haham, A., Marom, R., Mangel, L., et al. (2014). Prevalence of breastfeeding difficulties in newborns with a lingual frenulum: A prospective cohort series. *Breastfeeding Medicine, 9*(9), 438-441.

Haider, R., Kabir, I., Fuchs, G. J., et al. (2000). Neonatal diarrhea in a diarrhea treatment center in Bangladesh: Clinical presentation, breastfeeding management and outcome. *Indian Pediatrics, 37*(1), 37-43.

Halicioglu, O., Sutcuoglu, S., Koc, F., et al. (2012). Vitamin D status of exclusively breastfed 4-month-old infants supplemented during different seasons. *Pediatrics, 130*(4), e921-927.

Han, S. H., Kim, M. C., Choi, Y. S., et al. (2012). A study on the genetic inheritance of ankyloglossia based on pedigree analysis. *Archives of Plastic Surgery, 39*(4), 329-332.

Hansen, J. (2016, March 26, 2016). Doctors warning parents to stop new fad of operating on their baby's tongues. Daily Telegraph. Retrieved from **dailytelegraph.com.au/news/doctors-warning-parents-to-stop-new-fad-of-operating-on-their-babys-tongues/news-story/bdc5a7fe78e74da01b3290d85ab14655**

Harrison, D., Reszel, J., Bueno, M., et al. (2016). Breastfeeding for procedural pain in infants beyond the neonatal period. *Cochrane Database of Systematic Reviews,* 10, CD011248. doi:10.1002/14651858.CD011248.pub2

Hayden-Baldauf, E. (2016). Breastfeeding the Type-1 diabetic child. Retrieved from **kellymom.com/health/baby-health/breastfeeding-type-1-diabetes-child**.

Hazelbaker, A. (1993). *The assessment tool for lingual frenulum function: Use in a lactation consultant private practice (Master's thesis).* Pacific Oaks College, Pasadena, CA.

Heacock, H. J., Jeffery, H. E., Baker, J. L., et al. (1992). Influence of breast versus formula milk on physiological gastroesophageal reflux in healthy, newborn infants. *Journal of Pediatric Gastroenterology and Nutrition, 14*(1), 41-46.

Heaney, R. P., Davies, K. M., Chen, T. C., et al. (2003). Human serum 25-hydroxycholecalciferol response to extended oral dosing with cholecalciferol. *American Journal of Clinical Nutrition, 77*(1), 204-210.

Hegar, B., Dewanti, N. R., Kadim, M., et al. (2009). Natural evolution of regurgitation in healthy infants. *Acta Paediatrica, 98*(7), 1189-1193.

Hegar, B., Satari, D. H., Sjarif, D. R., et al. (2013). Regurgitation and gastroesophageal reflux disease in six to nine months old indonesian infants. *Pediatric Gastroenterology, Hepatology & Nutrition, 16*(4), 240-247.

Heine, R. G. (2008). Allergic gastrointestinal motility disorders in infancy and early childhood. *Pediatric Allergy and Immunology, 19*(5), 383-391.

Heine, R. G., Jordan, B., Lubitz, L., et al. (2006). Clinical predictors of pathological gastro-oesophageal reflux in infants with persistent distress. *Journal of Paediatrics and Child Health, 42*(3), 134-139.

Heyman, M. B. (2006). Lactose intolerance in infants, children, and adolescents. *Pediatrics, 118*(3), 1279-1286.

Heyman, M. B., Abrams, S. A., Section On Gastroenterology, H., et al. (2017). Fruit juice in infants, children, and adolescents: Current recommendations. *Pediatrics, 139*(6).

Hiiemae, K. M., & Palmer, J. B. (2003). Tongue movements in feeding and speech. *Critical Reviews in Oral Biology and Medicine, 14*(6), 413-429.

Hoen, A. G., Li, J., Moulton, L. A., et al. (2015). Associations between gut microbial colonization in early life and respiratory outcomes in cystic fibrosis. *Journal of Pediatrics, 167*(1), 138-147 e131-133.

Hogan, M., Westcott, C., & Griffiths, M. (2005). Randomized, controlled trial of division of tongue-tie in infants with feeding problems. *Journal of Paediatrics and Child Health, 41*(5-6), 246-250.

Holliday, K. E., Allen, J. R., Waters, D. L., et al. (1991). Growth of human milk-fed and formula-fed infants with cystic fibrosis. *Journal of Pediatrics, 118*(1), 77-79.

Hollis, B. W., & Wagner, C. L. (2004). Assessment of dietary vitamin D requirements during pregnancy and lactation. *American Journal of Clinical Nutrition, 79*(5), 717-726.

Hollis, B. W., Wagner, C. L., Howard, C. R., et al. (2015). Maternal versus infant vitamin D supplementation during lactation: A randomized controlled trial. *Pediatrics, 136*(4), 625-634.

Hong, J., Chang, J. Y., Shin, S., et al. (2017). Breastfeeding and red meat intake are associated with iron status in healthy Korean weaning-age infants. *Journal of Korean Medical Science, 32*(6), 974-984.

Hopman, E., Csizmadia, C. G., Bastiani, W. F., et al. (1998). Eating habits of young children with Down syndrome in The Netherlands: Adequate nutrient intakes but delayed introduction of solid food. *Journal of the American Dietetic Association, 98*(7), 790-794.

Horta, B. L., Loret de Mola, C., & Victora, C. G. (2015). Breastfeeding and intelligence: A systematic review and meta-analysis. *Acta Paediatrica, 104*(467), 14-19.

Huang, Y.-S., Quo, S., Berkowski, J. A., et al. (2015). Short lingual frenulum and obstructive sleep apnea in children. *International Journal of Pediatric Research, 1,* 003.

Huda, M. N., Ahmad, S. M., Alam, M. J., et al. (2019). Bifidobacterium abundance in early infancy and vaccine response at 2 years of age. *Pediatrics, 143*(2).

Huda, M. N., Lewis, Z., Kalanetra, K. M., et al. (2014). Stool microbiota and vaccine responses of infants. *Pediatrics, 134*(2), e362-372.

IATP. (2019). About tongue-tie. Retrieved from **tonguetieprofessionals.org/about-tongue-tie**. Accessed June 27, 2019.

Imms, C. (2001). Feeding the infant with congenital heart disease: An occupational performance challenge. *American Journal of Occupational Therapy, 55*(3), 277-284.

Ingram, J., Copeland, M., Johnson, D., et al. (2019). The development and evaluation of a picture tongue assessment tool for tongue-tie in breastfed babies (TABBY). *International Breastfeeding Journal, 14,* 31.

Ingram, J., Johnson, D., Copeland, M., et al. (2015). The development of a tongue assessment tool to assist with tongue-tie identification. *Archives of Disease in Childhood. Fetal and Neonatal Edition, 100*(4), F344-348.

IoM. (2004). Composition of infant formulas and human milk for feeding term infants in the United States. *In Infant Formula: Evaluating the Safety of New Ingredients.* Washington, DC: National Academies Press.

Jadcherla, S. R., Vijayapal, A. S., & Leuthner, S. (2009). Feeding abilities in neonates with congenital heart disease: A retrospective study. *Journal of Perinatology, 29*(2), 112-118.

Jadin, S. A., Wu, G. S., Zhang, Z., et al. (2011). Growth and pulmonary outcomes during the first 2 y of life of breastfed and formula-fed infants diagnosed with cystic fibrosis through the Wisconsin Routine Newborn Screening Program. *American Journal of Clinical Nutrition, 93*(5), 1038-1047.

Joseph, K. S., Kinniburgh, B., Metcalfe, A., et al. (2016). Temporal trends in ankyloglossia and frenotomy in British Columbia, Canada, 2004-2013: A population-based study. *Canadian Medical Association Journal Open, 4*(1), E33-40.

Kanufre, V. C., Starling, A. L., Leao, E., et al. (2007). Breastfeeding in the treatment of children with phenylketonuria. *Jornal de Pediatria (Rio J), 83*(5), 447-452.

Kapoor, V., Douglas, P. S., Hill, P. S., et al. (2018). Frenotomy for tongue-tie in Australian children, 2006-2016: An increasing problem. *Medical Journal of Australia, 208*(2), 88-89.

Karimi, F. Z., Sadeghi, R., Maleki-Saghooni, N., et al. (2019). The effect of mother-infant skin to skin contact on success and duration of first breastfeeding: A systematic review and meta-analysis. *Taiwanese Journal of Obstetrics & Gynecology, 58*(1), 1-9.

Kaye, C. I., Accurso, F., La Franchi, S., et al. (2006). Introduction to the newborn screening fact sheets. *Pediatrics, 118*(3), 1304-1312.

Kent, J. C., Mitoulas, L. R., Cregan, M. D., et al. (2006). Volume and frequency of breastfeedings and fat content of breast milk throughout the day. *Pediatrics, 117*(3), e387-395.

Koletzko, S., & Reinhardt, D. (2001). Nutritional challenges of infants with cystic fibrosis. *Early Human Development, 65 Suppl,* S53-61.

Koltlow, L. (2015). TOTS--Tethered oral tissues: The assessment and diagnosis of the tongue and upper lip ties in breastfeeding. *Oral Health and Preventive Dentistry(March),* 64-70.

Kose, E., Aksoy, B., Kuyum, P., et al. (2018). The effects of breastfeeding in infants with phenylketonuria. *Journal of Pediatric Nursing, 38,* 27-32.

Kotlow, L. (2011). Infant reflux and aerophagia associated with the maxillary lip-tie and ankyloglossia (tongue-tie). *Clinical Lactation, 2*(4), 25-29.

Kotlow, L. A. (2010). The influence of the maxillary frenum on the development and pattern of dental caries on anterior teeth in breastfeeding infants: Prevention, diagnosis, and treatment. *Journal of Human Lactation, 26*(3), 304-308.

Kotlow, L. A. (2013). Diagnosing and understanding the maxillary lip-tie (superior labial, the maxillary labial frenum) as it relates to breastfeeding. *Journal of Human Lactation, 29*(4), 458-464.

Krebs, N. F., Westcott, J. E., Arnold, T. D., et al. (2000). Abnormalities in zinc homeostasis in young infants with cystic fibrosis. *Pediatric Research, 48*(2), 256-261.

Krogh, C., Biggar, R. J., Fischer, T. K., et al. (2012). Bottle-feeding and the risk of pyloric stenosis. *Pediatrics, 130*(4), e943-949.

Krol, K. M., & Grossmann, T. (2018). Psychological effects of breastfeeding on children and mothers. *Bundesgesundheitsblatt Gesundheitsforschung Gesundheitsschutz, 61*(8), 977-985.

Kwok, T. C., Ojha, S., & Dorling, J. (2017). Feed thickener for infants up to six months of age with gastro-oesophageal reflux. *Cochrane Database of Systematic Reviews,* 12, CD003211. doi:10.1002/14651858.CD003211.pub2.

Lambert, J. M., & Watters, N. E. (1998). Breastfeeding the infant/child with a cardiac defect: An informal survey. *Journal of Human Lactation, 14*(2), 151-155.

Landry, A. M., & Thompson, D. M. (2012). Laryngomalacia: Disease presentation, spectrum, and management. *International Journal of Pediatrics, 2012,* 753526. doi:10.1155/2012/753526.

Lappi, H., Valkonen-Korhonen, M., Georgiadis, S., et al. (2007). Effects of nutritive and non-nutritive sucking on infant heart rate variability during the first 6 months of life. *Infant Behavior and Development, 30*(4), 546-556.

Lawrence, R. A., & Lawrence, R. M. (2016). *Breastfeeding: A Guide for the Medical Profession* (8th ed.). Philadelphia, PA: Elsevier.

Leung, D. H., Heltshe, S. L., Borowitz, D., et al. (2017). Effects of diagnosis by newborn screening for cystic fibrosis on weight and length in the first year of life. *JAMA Pediatrics, 171*(6), 546-554.

Lightdale, J. R., Gremse, D. A., Section on Gastroenterology, H., et al. (2013). Gastroesophageal reflux: Management guidance for the pediatrician. *Pediatrics, 131*(5), e1684-1695.

Lima, M. G. S., Araujo, M., Freitas, R. L., et al. (2019). Evaluation of the lingual frenulum in newborns using two protocols and its association with breastfeeding. *Jornal de Pediatria (Rio J).* doi:10.1016/j.jped.2018.12.013.

Lindberg, N., & Berglund, A. L. (2014). Mothers' experiences of feeding babies born with cleft lip and palate. *Scandinavian Journal of Caring Sciences, 28*(1), 66-73.

Lisonek, M., Liu, S., Dzakpasu, S., et al. (2017). Changes in the incidence and surgical treatment of ankyloglossia in Canada. *Paediatrics & Child Health, 22*(7), 382-386.

Lobo, M. L. (1992). Parent-infant interaction during feeding when the infant has congenital heart disease. *Journal of Pediatric Nursing, 7*(2), 97-105.

Lozoff, B., & Georgieff, M. K. (2006). Iron deficiency and brain development. *Seminars in Pediatric Neurology, 13*(3), 158-165.

Luder, E., Kattan, M., Tanzer-Torres, G., et al. (1990). Current recommendations for breast-feeding in cystic fibrosis centers. *American Journal of Diseases of Children, 144*(10), 1153-1156.

Madlon-Kay, D. J., Ricke, L. A., Baker, N. J., et al. (2008). Case series of 148 tongue-tied newborn babies evaluated with the assessment tool for lingual frenulum function. *Midwifery, 24*(3), 353-357.

Mahalanabis, D., Alam, A. N., Rahman, N., et al. (1991). Prognostic indicators and risk factors for increased duration of acute diarrhoea and for persistent diarrhoea in children. *International Journal of Epidemiology, 20*(4), 1064-1072.

Mangili, G., Garzoli, E., & Sadou, Y. (2018). Feeding dysfunctions and failure to thrive in neonates with congenital heart diseases. *La Pediatria Medica e Chirugica, 40*(1).

Manti, F., Nardecchia, F., Paci, S., et al. (2017). Predictability and inconsistencies in the cognitive outcome of early treated PKU patients. *Journal of Inherited Metabolic Disease, 40*(6), 793-799.

Marino, B. L., O'Brien, P., & LoRe, H. (1995). Oxygen saturations during breast and bottle feedings in infants with congenital heart disease. *Journal of Pediatric Nursing, 10*(6), 360-364.

Martinelli, R. L., Marchesan, I. Q., Gusmao, R. J., et al. (2015). The effects of frenotomy on breastfeeding. *Journal of Applied Oral Science, 23*(2), 153-157.

Martinelli, R. L., Marchesan, I. Q., Lauris, J. R., et al. (2016). Validity and reliability of the neonatal tongue screening test. *Revista Cefac, 18*(6), 1323-1331.

Masarei, A. G., Sell, D., Habel, A., et al. (2007). The nature of feeding in infants with unrepaired cleft lip and/or palate compared with healthy noncleft infants. *Cleft Palate-Craniofacial Journal, 44*(3), 321-328.

Matsunaka, E., Ueki, S., & Makimoto, K. (2019). Impact of breastfeeding and/or bottle-feeding on surgical wound dehiscence after cleft lip repair in infants: A systematic review. *Journal of Cranio-Maxillofacial Surgery, 47*(4), 570-577.

Mazaika, P. K., Weinzimer, S. A., Mauras, N., et al. (2016). Variations in brain volume and growth in young children with Type 1 diabetes. *Diabetes, 65*(2), 476-485.

McFadden, H. (2017). Parental concerns on gastroesophageal reflux: When it's more than just a laundry issue--Three case studies. *Clinical Lactation, 8*(4), 169-174.

McGuire, E. (2017). Cleft lip and palates and breastfeeding. *Breastfeeding Review, 25*(1), 17-23.

Medoff-Cooper, B., & Irving, S. Y. (2009). Innovative strategies for feeding and nutrition in infants with congenitally malformed hearts. *Cardiology in the Young, 19 Suppl 2,* 90-95.

Meier, P. (1988). Bottle- and breast-feeding: Effects on transcutaneous oxygen pressure and temperature in preterm infants. *Nursing Research, 37*(1), 36-41.

Meier, P., & Anderson, G. C. (1987). Responses of small preterm infants to bottle- and breast-feeding. *MCN American Journal of Maternal and Child Nursing, 12*(2), 97-105.

Mercado-Deane, M. G., Burton, E. M., Harlow, S. A., et al. (2001). Swallowing dysfunction in infants less than 1 year of age. *Pediatric Radiology, 31*(6), 423-428.

Merritt, L. (2005). Part 1. Understanding the embryology and genetics of cleft lip and palate. *Advances in Neonatal Care, 5*(2), 64-71.

Merritt, L. S. (2019). The effect of tongue-tie and lip-tie on breastfeeding. *Journal for Nurse Practitioners, 15,* 356-360.

Messner, A. H., Lalakea, M. L., Aby, J., et al. (2000). Ankyloglossia: Incidence and associated feeding difficulties. *Archives of Otolaryngology--Head & Neck Surgery, 126*(1), 36-39.

Mettias, B., O'Brien, R., Abo Khatwa, M. M., et al. (2013). Division of tongue tie as an outpatient procedure. Technique, efficacy and safety. *International Journal of Pediatric Otorhinolaryngology, 77*(4), 550-552.

Miller, D., Mamilly, L., Fourtner, S., et al. (2017). ABM Clinical Protocol #27: Breastfeeding an infant or young child with insulin-dependent diabetes. *Breastfeeding Medicine, 12,* 72-76.

Miller, J. (1998). *The Controversial Issue of Breastfeeding Cleft-Affected Infants.* Innisfall: Alberta: InfoMed Publications.

Miller, T., Antos, N. J., Brock, L. A., et al. (2019). Lactation consultation sustains breast milk intake in infants with cystic fibrosis. *Journal of Pediatric Gastroenterology and Nutrition.* doi:10.1097/MPG.0000000000002415.

Mills, N., Keough, N., Geddes, D. T., et al. (2019). Defining the anatomy of the neonatal lingual frenulum. *Clinical Anatomy.* doi:10.1002/ca.23410.

Mizuno, K., Inoue, M., & Takeuchi, T. (2000). The effects of body positioning on sucking behaviour in sick neonates. *European Journal of Pediatrics, 159*(11), 827-831.

Mizuno, K., & Ueda, A. (2001). Development of sucking behavior in infants with Down's syndrome. *Acta Paediatrica, 90*(12), 1384-1388.

Mizuno, K., & Ueda, A. (2005). Neonatal feeding performance as a predictor of neurodevelopmental outcome at 18 months. *Developmental Medicine and Child Neurology, 47*(5), 299-304.

Mizuno, K., & Ueda, A. (2006). Changes in sucking performance from nonnutritive sucking to nutritive sucking during breast- and bottle-feeding. *Pediatric Research, 59*(5), 728-731.

Montagnoli, L. C., Barbieri, M. A., Bettiol, H., et al. (2005). Growth impairment of children with different types of lip and palate clefts in the first 2 years of life: A cross-sectional study. *Jornal de Pediatria (Rio J), 81*(6), 461-465.

Morice, A., Soupre, V., Mitanchez, D., et al. (2018). Severity of retrognathia and glossoptosis does not predict respiratory and feeding disorders in Pierre Robin Sequence. *Frontiers in Pediatrics, 6,* 351.

Morris, S., & Klein, M. (2001). *Pre-feeding Skills.* Tucson, AZ: Therapy Skill Builders.

Morton, J. (2019). Hands-on or hands-off when first milk matters most? *Breastfeeding Medicine, 14*(5), 295-297.

Moss, A. L., Jones, K., & Pigott, R. W. (1990). Submucous cleft palate in the differential diagnosis of feeding difficulties. *Archives of Disease in Childhood, 65*(2), 182-184.

Motzfeldt, K., Lilje, R., & Nylander, G. (1999). Breastfeeding in phenylketonuria. *Acta Paediatrica. Supplement, 88*(432), 25-27.

Munns, C. F., Shaw, N., Kiely, M., et al. (2016). Global consensus recommendations on prevention and management of nutritional rickets. *Journal of Clinical Endocrinology and Metabolism, 101(*2), 394-415.

Munns, C. F., Simm, P. J., Rodda, C. P., et al. (2012). Incidence of vitamin D deficiency rickets among Australian children: An Australian Paediatric Surveillance Unit study. *Medical Journal of Australia, 196*(7), 466-468.

Murphy, P. K., & Wagner, C. L. (2008). Vitamin D and mood disorders among women: An integrative review. *Journal of Midwifery & Women's Health, 53*(5), 440-446.

Murray, L., De Pascalis, L., Bozicevic, L., et al. (2016). The functional architecture of mother-infant communication, and the development of infant social expressiveness in the first two months. *Scientific Reports, 6,* 39019.

Naik, P., Faridi, M. M. A., Batra, P., et al. (2017). Oral supplementation of parturient mothers with vitamin D and its effect on 25OHD status of exclusively breastfed infants at 6 months of age: A double-blind randomized placebo controlled trial. *Breastfeeding Medicine, 12*(10), 621-628.

Naimer, S. A. (2016). To cut or not to cut? Approach to ankyloglossia. *Canadian Family Physician, 62*(3), 231-232.

Nakhash, R., Wasserteil, N., Mimouni, F. B., et al. (2019). Upper lip tie and breastfeeding: A systematic review. *Breastfeeding Medicine, 14*(2), 83-87.

Nelson, P. A., & Kirk, S. A. (2013). Parents' perspectives of cleft lip and/or palate services: A qualitative interview. *Cleft Palate-Craniofacial Journal, 50*(3), 275-285.

Nelson, S. P., Chen, E. H., Syniar, G. M., et al. (1997). Prevalence of symptoms of gastroesophageal reflux during infancy. A pediatric practice-based survey. Pediatric Practice Research Group. *Archives of Pediatrics and Adolescent Medicine, 151*(6), 569-572.

Nemec, U., Nemec, S. F., Brugger, P. C., et al. (2015). Normal mandibular growth and diagnosis of micrognathia at prenatal MRI. *Prenatal Diagnosis, 35*(2), 108-116.

Nolder, A. R., & Richter, G. T. (2015). The infant with noisy breathing. *Current Treatment Options in Pediatrics, 1*(3), 224-233.

Nommsen-Rivers, L. A., Heinig, M. J., Cohen, R. J., et al. (2008). Newborn wet and soiled diaper counts and timing of onset of lactation as indicators of breastfeeding inadequacy. *Journal of Human Lactation, 24*(1), 27-33.

O'Shea, J. E., Foster, J. P., O'Donnell, C. P., et al. (2017). Frenotomy for tongue-tie in newborn infants. *Cochrane Database of Systematic Reviews, 3,* CD011065. doi:10.1002/14651858.CD011065.pub2.

Oberhelman, S. S., Meekins, M. E., Fischer, P. R., et al. (2013). Maternal vitamin D supplementation to improve the vitamin D status of breast-fed infants: A randomized controlled trial. *Mayo Clinic Proceedings, 88*(12), 1378-1387.

Ogbo, F. A., Okoro, A., Olusanya, B. O., et al. (2019). Diarrhoea deaths and disability-adjusted life years attributable to suboptimal breastfeeding practices in Nigeria: Findings from the global burden of disease study 2016. *International Breastfeeding Journal, 14,* 4.

Ogechi, A. A., William, O., & Fidelia, B. T. (2007). Hindmilk and weight gain in preterm very low-birthweight infants. *Pediatrics International, 49*(2), 156-160.

Ohlsson, A., Guthenberg, C., & von Dobeln, U. (2012). Galactosemia screening with low false-positive recall rate: The Swedish experience. *JIMD Reports, 2,* 113-117.

Owens, B. (2002). Breastfeeding an infant after heart transplant surgery. *Journal of Human Lactation, 18*(1), 53-55.

Pabst, H. F., & Spady, D. W. (1990). Effect of breast-feeding on antibody response to conjugate vaccine. *Lancet, 336*(8710), 269-270.

Pabst, H. F., Spady, D. W., Pilarski, L. M., et al. (1997). Differential modulation of the immune response by breast- or formula-feeding of infants. *Acta Paediatrica, 86*(12), 1291-1297.

Pados, B. F. (2019). Symptoms of problematic feeding in children with CHD compared to healthy peers. *Cardiology in the Young, 29*(2), 152-161.

Palmer, B. (1998). The influence of breastfeeding on the development of the oral cavity: A commentary. *Journal of Human Lactation, 14*(2), 93-98.

Pandya, A. N., & Boorman, J. G. (2001). Failure to thrive in babies with cleft lip and palate. *British Journal of Plastic Surgery, 54*(6), 471-475.

Papadimitriou, D. T. (2017). The big vitamin D mistake. *Journal of Preventive Medicine & Public Health, 50*(4), 278-281.

Paradise, J. L., Elster, B. A., & Tan, L. (1994). Evidence in infants with cleft palate that breast milk protects against otitis media. *Pediatrics, 94*(6 Pt 1), 853-860.

Parker, E. M., O'Sullivan, B. P., Shea, J. C., et al. (2004). Survey of breast-feeding practices and outcomes in the cystic fibrosis population. *Pediatric Pulmonology, 37*(4), 362-367.

Patel, J., Anthonappa, R. P., & King, N. M. (2018). All tied up! Influences of oral frenulae on breastfeeding and their recommended management strategies. *Journal of Clinical Pediatric Dentistry, 42*(6), 407-413.

Pathumwiwatana, P., Tongsukho, S., Naratippakorn, T., et al. (2010). The promotion of exclusive breastfeeding in infants with complete cleft lip and palate during the first 6 months after childbirth at Srinagarind Hospital, Khon Kaen Province, Thailand. *Journal of the Medical Association of Thailand, 93 Supplement 4,* S71-77.

Perin, J., Carvajal-Velez, L., Carter, E., et al. (2015). Fluid curtailment during childhood diarrhea: A countdown analysis. *BMC Public Health, 15,* 588.

Peters, R. L., Koplin, J. J., Gurrin, L. C., et al. (2017). The prevalence of food allergy and other allergic diseases in early childhood in a population-based study: HealthNuts age 4-year follow-up. *Journal of Allergy and Clinical Immunology, 140*(1), 145-153 e148.

Petrackova, I., Zach, J., Borsky, J., et al. (2015). Early and late operation of cleft lip and intelligence quotient and psychosocial development in 3-7 years. *Early Human Development, 91*(2), 149-152.

Pickering, L. K., Granoff, D. M., Erickson, J. R., et al. (1998). Modulation of the immune system by human milk and infant formula containing nucleotides. *Pediatrics, 101*(2), 242-249.

Pinto, A., Adams, S., Ahring, K., et al. (2018). Early feeding practices in infants with phenylketonuria across Europe. *Molecular Genetics and Metabolism Reports, 16,* 82-89.

Pisacane, A., Toscano, E., Pirri, I., et al. (2003). Down syndrome and breastfeeding. *Acta Paediatrica, 92*(12), 1479-1481.

Power, R. F., & Murphy, J. F. (2015). Tongue-tie and frenotomy in infants with breastfeeding difficulties: Achieving a balance. *Archives of Disease in Childhood, 100*(5), 489-494.

Praborini, A., Purnamasari, H., Munandar, A., et al. (2015). Early frenotomy improves breastfeeding outcomes for tongue-tied infants. *Clinical Lactation, 6*(1), 9-15.

Pransky, S. M., Lago, D., & Hong, P. (2015). Breastfeeding difficulties and oral cavity anomalies: The influence of posterior ankyloglossia and upper-lip ties. *International Journal of Pediatric Otorhinolaryngology, 79*(10), 1714-1717.

Puapong, D., Kahng, D., Ko, A., et al. (2002). Ad libitum feeding: Safely improving the cost-effectiveness of pyloromyotomy. *Journal of Pediatric Surgery, 37*(12), 1667-1668.

Pyhtila, B. M., Shaw, K. A., Neumann, S. E., et al. (2015). Newborn screening for galactosemia in the United States: Looking back, looking around, and looking ahead. *JIMD Reports, 15,* 79-93.

Rajani, P. S., Seppo, A. E., & Jarvinen, K. M. (2018). Immunologically active components in human milk and development of atopic disease, with emphasis on food allergy, in the pediatric population. *Frontiers in Pediatrics, 6,* 218.

Ramoser, G., Guoth-Gumberger, M., Baumgartner-Sigl, S., et al. (2019). Frenotomy for tongue-tie (frenulum linguae breve) showed improved symptoms in the short- and long-term follow-up. *Acta Paediatrica.* doi:10.1016/j.jped.2018.12.013

Rankin, M. W., Jimenez, E. Y., Caraco, M., et al. (2016). Validation of test weighing protocol to estimate enteral feeding volumes in preterm infants. *Journal of Pediatrics, 178,* 108-112.

Reece-Stremtan, S., & Gray, L. (2016). ABM Clinical Protocol #23: Nonpharmacological management of procedure-related pain in the breastfeeding infant, Revised 2016. *Breastfeeding Medicine, 11,* 425-429.

Reid, J. (2004). A review of feeding interventions for infants with cleft palate. *Cleft Palate-Craniofacial Journal, 41*(3), 268-278.

Reid, J., Kilpatrick, N., & Reilly, S. (2006). A prospective, longitudinal study of feeding skills in a cohort of babies with cleft conditions. *Cleft Palate-Craniofacial Journal, 43*(6), 702-709.

Reid, J., Reilly, S., & Kilpatrick, N. (2007). Sucking performance of babies with cleft conditions. *Cleft Palate-Craniofacial Journal, 44*(3), 312-320.

Richard, S. A., McCormick, B. J. J., Seidman, J. C., et al. (2018). Relationships among common illness symptoms and the protective effect of breastfeeding in early childhood in MAL-ED: An eight-country cohort study. *American Journal of Tropical Medicine and Hygiene, 98*(3), 904-912.

Ricke, L. A., Baker, N. J., Madlon-Kay, D. J., et al. (2005). Newborn tongue-tie: Prevalence and effect on breast-feeding. *Journal of the American Board of Family Practice, 18*(1), 1-7.

Riskin, A., Mansovsky, M., Coler-Botzer, T., et al. (2014). Tongue-tie and breastfeeding in newborns-Mothers' perspective. *Breastfeeding Medicine, 9*(9), 430-437.

Rommel, N., De Meyer, A. M., Feenstra, L., et al. (2003). The complexity of feeding problems in 700 infants and young children presenting to a tertiary care institution. *Journal of Pediatric Gastroenterology and Nutrition, 37*(1), 75-84.

Rowicka, G., & Weker, H. (2014). Nutritional standard for children with orofacial clefts. *Developmental Period Medicine, 18*(1), 102-109.

Rubio-Gozalbo, M. E., Haskovic, M., Bosch, A. M., et al. (2019). The natural history of classic galactosemia: Lessons from the GalNet registry. *Orphanet Journal of Rare Diseases, 14*(1), 86.

Saad, A. N., Parina, R. P., Tokin, C., et al. (2014). Incidence of oral clefts among different ethnicities in the state of California. *Annals of Plastic Surgery, 72 Suppl 1,* S81-83.

Salvatore, S., & Vandenplas, Y. (2002). Gastroesophageal reflux and cow milk allergy: Is there a link? *Pediatrics, 110*(5), 972-984.

Santa Maria, C., Aby, J., Truong, M. T., et al. (2017). The superior labial frenulum in newborns: What is normal? *Global Pediatric Health, 4,* 2333794X17718896.

Santos, F. S., Santos, F. C., Santos, L. H., et al. (2015). Breastfeeding and protection against diarrhea: An integrative review of literature. *Einstein (Sao Paulo), 13*(3), 435-440.

Savilahti, E., Launiala, K., & Kuitunen, P. (1983). Congenital lactase deficiency. A clinical study on 16 patients. *Archives of Disease in Childhood, 58*(4), 246-252.

Schmidt, D., Beebe, R., & Berg-Drazin, P. (2013). Galactosemia and the continuation of breastfeeding with variant form. *Clinical Lactation, 4*(4), 148-154.

Semeniuk, J., & Kaczmarski, M. (2008). Acid gastroesophageal reflux and intensity of symptoms in children with gastroesophageal reflux disease. Comparison of primary gastroesophageal reflux and gastroesophageal reflux secondary to food allergy. *Advances in Medical Sciences, 53*(2), 293-299.

Sharma, N., Nath, C., & Mohammad, J. (2019). Vitamin D status in pregnant women visiting a tertiary care center of North Eastern India. *Journal of Family Medicine and Primary Care, 8*(2), 356-360.

Shrago, L. C., Reifsnider, E., & Insel, K. (2006). The Neonatal Bowel Output Study: Indicators of adequate breast milk intake in neonates. *Pediatric Nursing, 32*(3), 195-201.

Silfverdal, S. A., Ekholm, L., & Bodin, L. (2007). Breastfeeding enhances the antibody response to Hib and Pneumococcal serotype 6B and 14 after vaccination with conjugate vaccines. *Vaccine, 25*(8), 1497-1502.

Smedegaard, L., Marxen, D., Moes, J., et al. (2008). Hospitalization, breast-milk feeding, and growth in infants with cleft palate and cleft lip and palate born in Denmark. *Cleft Palate-Craniofacial Journal, 45*(6), 628-632.

Smillie, C., Genna, C. W., Murphy, J., et al. (2017). Post-revision instruction and pain relief. *Clinical Lactation, 8*(3), 107-109.

Smith, C. (2019). Supporting optimal growth in infants with chronic conditions: How are we doing and what can we do? *Breastfeeding Medicine, 14*(S1), S18-S19.

Smith, L. J. (2017). Impact of birth practices on infant suck. In C. W. Genna (Ed.), *Supporting Sucking Skills in Breastfeeding Infants* (3rd ed., pp. 65-88). Burlington, MA: Jones & Bartlett Learning.

Snyder, M., & Ruscello, D. M. (2018). Parent perceptions of initial feeding experiences of children born with cleft palate in a rural locale. *Cleft Palate-Craniofacial Journal, 1055665618820754.*

Soto-Ramirez, N., Karmaus, W., Zhang, H., et al. (2013). Modes of infant feeding and the occurrence of coughing/wheezing in the first year of life. *Journal of Human Lactation, 29*(1), 71-80.

Spence, K., Swinsburg, D., Griggs, J. A., et al. (2011). Infant well-being following neonatal cardiac surgery. *Journal of Clinical Nursing, 20*(17-18), 2623-2632.

Srinivasan, A., Al Khoury, A., Puzhko, S., et al. (2018). Frenotomy in infants with tongue-tie and breastfeeding problems. *Journal of Human Lactation, 890334418816973.*

Srinivasan, A., Dobrich, C., Mitnick, H., et al. (2006). Ankyloglossia in breastfeeding infants: The effect of frenotomy on maternal nipple pain and latch. *Breastfeeding Medicine, 1*(4), 216-224.

Stanley, M. A., Shepherd, N., Duvall, N., et al. (2019). Clinical identification of feeding and swallowing disorders in 0-6 month old infants with Down syndrome. *American Journal of Medical Genetics Part A, 179*(2), 177-182.

Steltzer, M. M., Sussman-Karten, K., Kuzdeba, H. B., et al. (2016). Creating opportunities for optimal nutritional experiences for infants with complex congenital heart disease. *Journal of Pediatric Health Care, 30*(6), 599-605.

Styles, M. E., Cole, T. J., Dennis, J., et al. (2002). New cross sectional stature, weight, and head circumference references for Down's syndrome in the UK and Republic of Ireland. *Archives of Disease in Childhood, 87*(2), 104-108.

Svensson, K. E., Velandia, M. I., Matthiesen, A. S., et al. (2013). Effects of mother-infant skin-to-skin contact on severe latch-on problems in older infants: A randomized trial. *International Breastfeeding Journal, 8*(1), 1.

Tabrizi, R., Moosazadeh, M., Akbari, M., et al. (2018). High prevalence of vitamin D deficiency among Iranian population: A systematic review and meta-analysis. *Iranian Journal of Medical Sciences, 43*(2), 125-139.

Taghavi, K., Powell, E., Patel, B., et al. (2017). The treatment of pyloric stenosis: Evolution in practice. *Journal of Paediatrics and Child Health, 53*(11), 1105-1110.

Taylor, S. N. (2018). ABM Clinical Protocol #29: Iron, zinc, and vitamin D supplementation during breastfeeding. *Breastfeeding Medicine, 13*(6), 398-404.

ten Hoedt, A. E., Maurice-Stam, H., Boelen, C. C., et al. (2011). Parenting a child with phenylketonuria or galactosemia: Implications for health-related quality of life. *Journal of Inherited Metabolic Disease, 34*(2), 391-398.

Thomas, J., Marinelli, K. A., & Academy of Breastfeeding, M. (2016). ABM Clinical Protocol #16: Breastfeeding the hypotonic infant, revision 2016. *Breastfeeding Medicine, 11*(6), 271-276.

Thomas, M., Morrison, C., Newton, R., et al. (2018). Consensus statement on clear fluids fasting for elective pediatric general anesthesia. *Paediatric Anaesthesiology, 28*(5), 411-414.

Thottam, P. J., Simons, J. P., Choi, S., et al. (2016). Clinical relevance of quality of life in laryngomalacia. *Laryngoscope, 126*(5), 1232-1235.

Todd, D. (2013). Tongue ties in newborns at the Centenary Hospital in 2008 and 2011 [abstract]. *Journal of Paediatrics and Child Health, 49*(52), 74.

Todd, D. A. (2014). Tongue-tie in the newborn: What, when, who and how? Exploring tongue-tie division. *Breastfeeding Review, 22*(2), 7-10.

Todd, D. A., & Hogan, M. J. (2015). Tongue-tie in the newborn: Early diagnosis and division prevents poor breastfeeding outcomes. *Breastfeeding Review, 23*(1), 11-16.

Torowicz, D. L., Seelhorst, A., Froh, E. B., et al. (2015). Human milk and breastfeeding outcomes in infants with congenital heart disease. *Breastfeeding Medicine, 10*(1), 31-37.

Tse, R. (2012). Unilateral cleft lip: Principles and practice of surgical management. *Seminars in Plastic Surgery, 26*(4), 145-155.

Turner, L., Jacobsen, C., Humenczuk, M., et al. (2001). The effects of lactation education and a prosthetic obturator appliance on feeding efficiency in infants with cleft lip and palate. *Cleft Palate-Craniofacial Journal, 38*(5), 519-524.

van Rijn, M., Bekhof, J., Dijkstra, T., et al. (2003). A different approach to breast-feeding of the infant with phenylketonuria. *European Journal of Pediatrics, 162*(5), 323-326.

Vandenplas, Y., Badriul, H., Verghote, M., et al. (2004). Oesophageal pH monitoring and reflux oesophagitis in irritable infants. *European Journal of Pediatrics, 163*(6), 300-304.

Vandenplas, Y., Rudolph, C. D., Di Lorenzo, C., et al. (2009). Pediatric gastroesophageal reflux clinical practice guidelines: Joint recommendations of the North American Society for Pediatric Gastroenterology, Hepatology, and Nutrition (NASPGHAN) and the European Society for Pediatric Gastroenterology, Hepatology, and Nutrition (ESPGHAN). *Journal of Pediatric Gastroenterology and Nutrition, 49*(4), 498-547.

Vaz, A. C., & Bai, P. M. (2015). Lingual frenulum and malocclusion: An overlooked tissue or a minor issue. *Indian Journal of Dental Research, 26*(5), 488-492.

Vieth, R. (1999). Vitamin D supplementation, 25-hydroxyvitamin D concentrations, and safety. *American Journal of Clinical Nutrition, 69*(5), 842-856.

Vieth, R., Chan, P. C., & MacFarlane, G. D. (2001). Efficacy and safety of vitamin D3 intake exceeding the lowest observed adverse effect level. *American Journal of Clinical Nutrition, 73*(2), 288-294.

Wagner, C. L., & Greer, F. R. (2008). Prevention of rickets and vitamin D deficiency in infants, children, and adolescents. *Pediatrics, 122*(5), 1142-1152.

Wagner, C. L., Hulsey, T. C., Fanning, D., et al. (2006). High-dose vitamin D3 supplementation in a cohort of breastfeeding mothers and their infants: A 6-month follow-up pilot study. *Breastfeeding Medicine, 1*(2), 59-70.

Wagner, C. L., Taylor, S. N., & Hollis, B. W. (2008). Does vitamin D make the world go 'round'? *Breastfeeding Medicine, 3*(4), 239-250.

Walker, M. (2017). *Breastfeeding Management for the Clinician: Using the Evidence* (4th ed.). Burlington, MA: Jones & Bartlett Learning.

Walker, R. D., Messing, S., Rosen-Carole, C., et al. (2018). Defining tip-frenulum length for ankyloglossia and its impact on breastfeeding: A prospective cohort study. *Breastfeeding Medicine, 13*(3), 204-210.

Walsh, J., Links, A., Boss, E., et al. (2017). Ankyloglossia and lingual frenotomy: National trends in inpatient diagnosis and management in the United States, 1997-2012. *Otolaryngology—Head and Neck Surgery, 156*(4), 735-740.

Walsh, J., & Tunkel, D. (2017). Diagnosis and treatment of ankyloglossia in newborns and infants: A review. *JAMA Otolaryngology—Head & Neck Surgery, 143*(10), 1032-1039.

Wanes, D., Husein, D. M., & Naim, H. Y. (2019). Congenital lactase deficiency: Mutations, functional and biochemical implications, and future perspectives. *Nutrients, 11*(2).

Wattis, L., Kam, R., & Douglas, P. (2017). Three experienced lactation consultants reflect upon the oral tie phenomenon. *Breastfeeding Review, 25*(1), 9-15.

Weatherley-White, R. C., Kuehn, D. P., Mirrett, P., et al. (1987). Early repair and breast-feeding for infants with cleft lip. *Plastic and Reconstructive Surgery, 79*(6), 879-887.

Webb, A. N., Hao, W., & Hong, P. (2013). The effect of tongue-tie division on breastfeeding and speech articulation: A systematic review. *International Journal of Pediatric Otorhinolaryngology, 77*(5), 635-646.

Welling, L., Boelen, A., Derks, T. G., et al. (2017). Nine years of newborn screening for classical galactosemia in the Netherlands: Effectiveness of screening methods, and identification of patients with previously unreported phenotypes. *Molecular Genetics and Metabolism, 120*(3), 223-228.

Wilson-Clay, B., & Hoover, K. (2017). *The Breastfeeding Atlas* (6th ed.). Manchaca, TX: LactNews Press.

Wilson, A. T., Grabowski, G. M., Mackey, W. S., et al. (2017). Does type of cleft palate repair influence postoperative eustachian tube dysfunction? *Journal of Craniofacial Surgery, 28*(1), 241-244.

Wilson, R. L., Leviton, A. J., Leemaqz, S. Y., et al. (2018). Vitamin D levels in an Australian and New Zealand cohort and the association with pregnancy outcome. *BMC Pregnancy Childbirth, 18*(1), 251.

Wolf, L., & Glass, R. (1992). *Feeding and Swallowing Disorders in Infancy.* Tucson, AZ: Therapy Skill Builders.

Woolridge, M. W., & Fisher, C. (1988). Colic, "overfeeding", and symptoms of lactose malabsorption in the breast-fed baby: A possible artifact of feed management? *Lancet, 2*(8607), 382-384.

Yepes-Nunez, J. J., Brozek, J. L., Fiocchi, A., et al. (2018). Vitamin D supplementation in primary allergy prevention: Systematic review of randomized and non-randomized studies. *Allergy, 73*(1), 37-49.

Zemel, B. S., Pipan, M., Stallings, V. A., et al. (2015). Growth charts for children with Down syndrome in the United States. *Pediatrics, 136*(5), e1204-1211.

Ziegler, E. E., Hollis, B. W., Nelson, S. E., et al. (2006). Vitamin D deficiency in breastfed infants in Iowa. *Pediatrics, 118*(2), 603-610.

Ziegler, E. E., Nelson, S. E., & Jeter, J. M. (2014). Iron stores of breastfed infants during the first year of life. *Nutrients, 6*(5), 2023-2034.

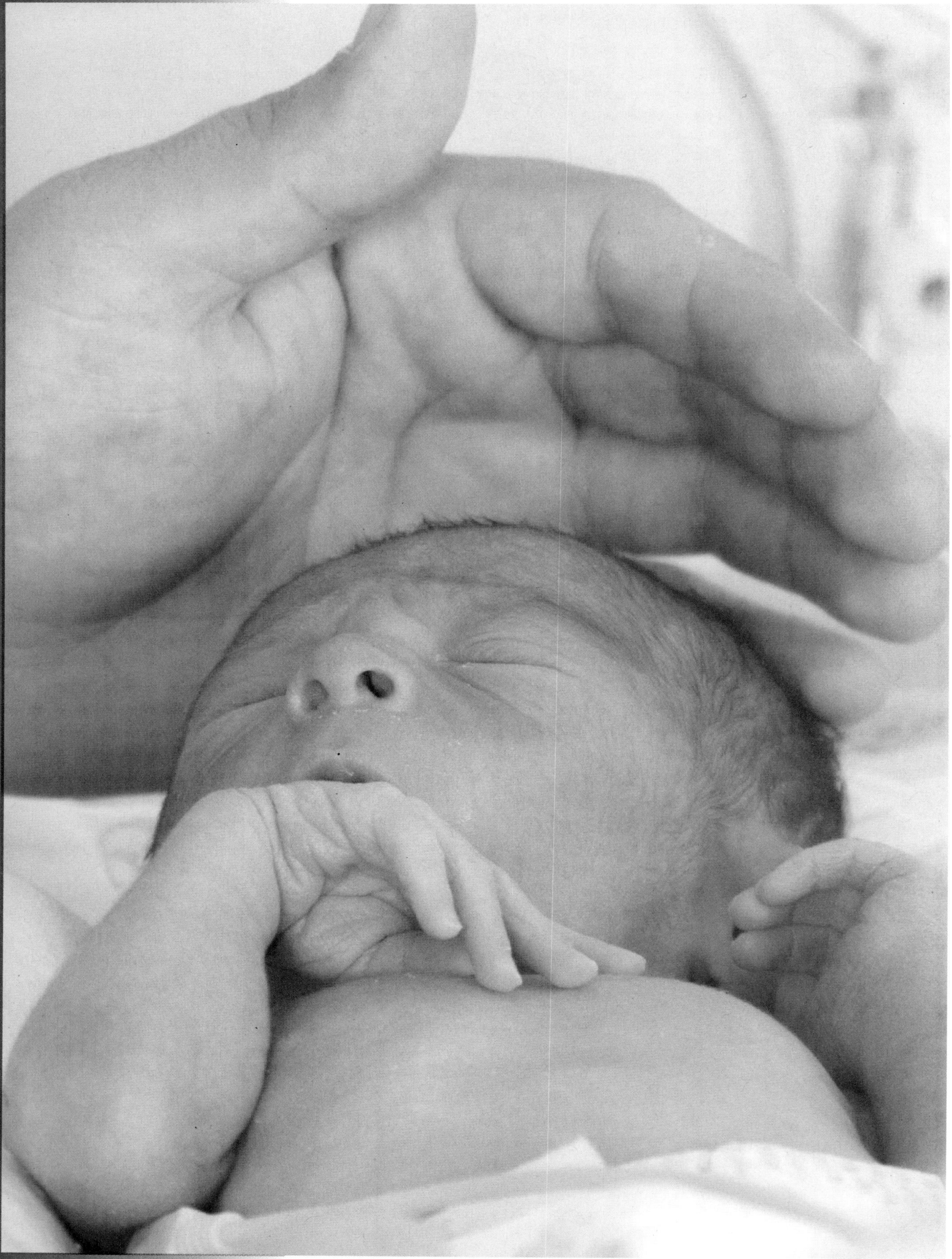

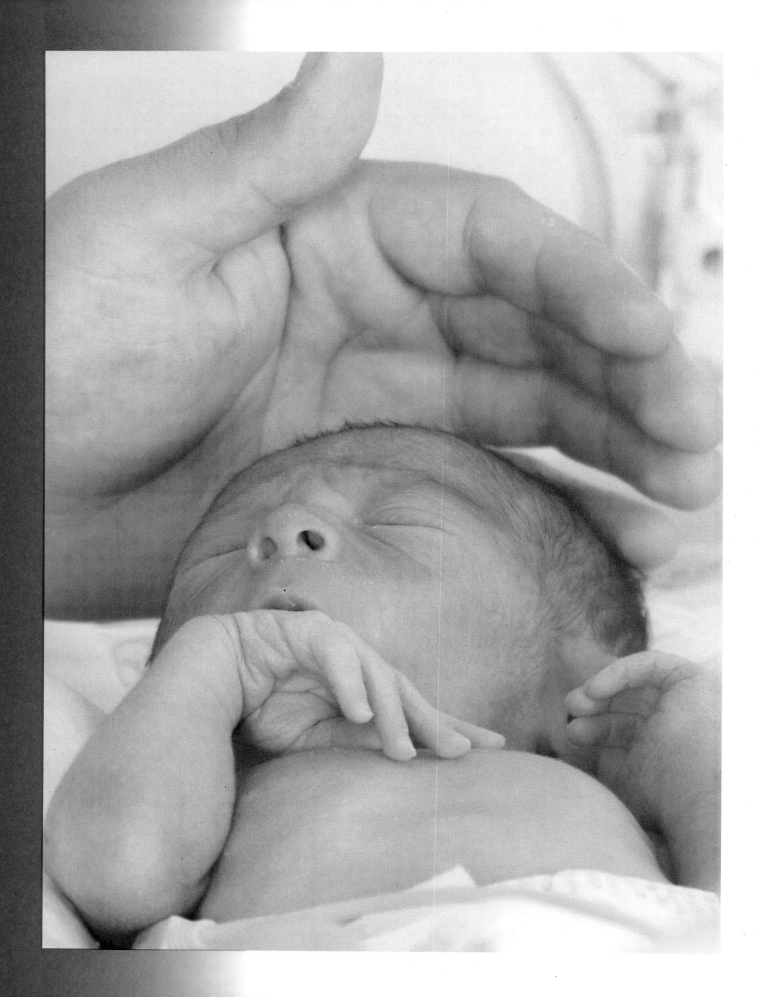

The Preterm Baby

9

Prematurity covers a wide range of gestational ages, feeding abilities, and health issues.

A baby is considered preterm when he is born more than 2 weeks before his due date. This covers a broad spectrum of gestational ages, feeding abilities, and health issues, from tiny, fragile infants born months early to healthy, robust late preterm babies.

FEELINGS ABOUT NURSING

Grieving the Expected Birth

After a preterm birth, grief may affect parents' ability to process and remember information.

Before parents can come to terms with a very premature birth, they may first need to mourn the loss of the expected healthy term baby and normal pregnancy. This is especially true if the baby was born very early or has health problems. Parents' first reactions may include shock and denial or worry and anxiety. A lack of parental feelings is also common (Lucas, Paquette, Briere, & McGrath, 2014). During this emotional adjustment, it may be impossible to accept and understand information unless it is repeated several times and given in written form.

Once the initial shock passes and the reality of the baby's condition sinks in, other intense feelings may surface. The family may refuse to believe the baby's medical caregivers and search for a specialist who will solve the baby's problems. They may be overly optimistic or overly pessimistic. If the baby has serious health problems, they may feel anger, guilt, or depression. Anger may be directed at the hospital staff or the baby's healthcare provider. The parents may feel helpless and isolated. They may have crying bouts and develop physical symptoms, such as insomnia, eating problems, or fatigue.

Encourage them to express their feelings and let them know that these feelings are normal. The parents may experience different stages of grief, impairing their ability to communicate with and comfort each other. Acknowledge that if their baby is in special care, bonding with their baby is being interrupted, which may feel unnatural (N. Hurst, Engebretson, & Mahoney, 2013). Congratulate them for what they are doing for their baby, such as providing milk and any contact with the baby. Touch is comforting to both parents and baby and can help reduce anxiety. Encourage skin-to-skin contact as soon as it's possible.

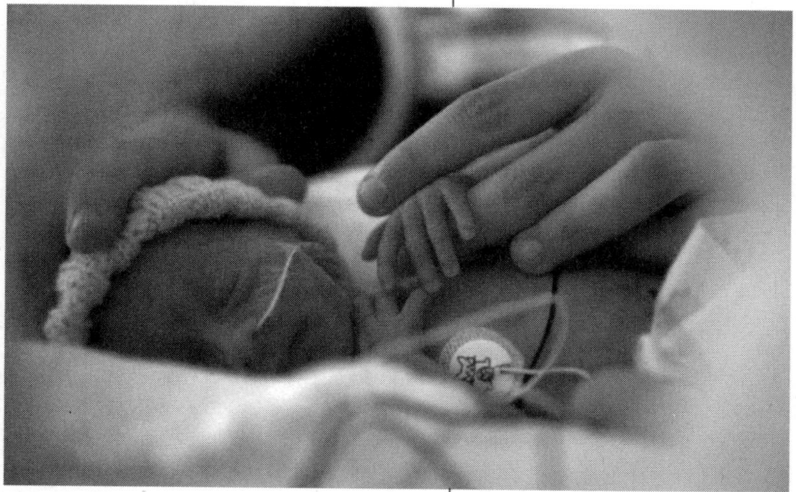

Suggest they ask if there is a lactation specialist available to them and if the healthcare facility has a support group for parents with babies in the special-care nursery. Contact with others with similar experiences can be comforting and provide realistic expectations and practical information (P. P. Meier, Engstrom, Mingolelli, Miracle, & Kiesling, 2004; P. P. Meier, Engstrom, & Rossman, 2013). U.S. research found that ongoing peer support significantly increased nursing duration among low-income mothers of preterm babies (Gharib, Fletcher, Tucker, Vohr, & Lechner, 2018; Merewood et al.,

2006). If the facility has both dedicated lactation help and peer support available, this leads to better lactation outcomes (Oza-Frank, Bhatia, & Smith, 2014).

• • •

A preterm birth may be traumatic, and as described on p. 40, a traumatic birth can affect the intention to nurse. What happens after birth affects nursing, too. A 2016 U.S. study of 172 women with high-risk pregnancies (Cordero, Oza-Frank, Moore-Clingenpeel, Landon, & Nankervis, 2016) found that even those planning to nurse were 2.3 times more likely to not initiate nursing after delivery, especially if they did not have contact with their baby during the first hour and there was limited lactation help.

Giving birth prematurely may affect a family's feelings about nursing.

Previous Feeding Goals

Even if nursing was not part of the original plan, the family needs to know the importance of expressed milk to the preterm baby's health.

Ask the family about their feeding goals. Even if they did not plan to exclusively nurse their preterm baby after discharge, all families should be encouraged to provide the milk their preterm baby needs during the hospital stay.

If a parent has mixed or negative feelings about nursing, emphasize that the first few weeks are the most critical for a baby's health and to approach nursing or milk expression as a temporary commitment. One 2019 U.S. review (Johnson et al., 2019) concluded that every 10 mL (0.3 ounce) of human milk a baby in the NICU receives during his first 14 days of life was associated with fewer rehospitalizations and specialized therapies needed during the first year of life. Assure parents that even if they decide to wean after a week or two, the baby will receive protection from infection. Explain that it is much easier to stop nursing or expressing milk than it is to start later. If a family's goal is to express milk short-term, encourage the nursing parent to do so at whatever level of milk expression will meet the baby's short-term needs and that the parent finds acceptable. Let the family know that with gradual weaning they can discontinue expressing whenever desired without experiencing pain. To help them formulate a plan, see p. 498-507 in Chapter 11.

KEY CONCEPT

Telling parents about the importance of their milk to the preterm baby's health does not cause guilt or increase anxiety.

Because preterm babies have significantly better health outcomes when they receive mother's own milk (see later section "Health Risks of Non-Human Milks"), parents need to know the importance of their milk to their baby. One U.S. study of 880 preterm babies (Romaine et al., 2018) found that racial and economic disparities affected if and for how long human milk was provided, so it is vital that all medical centers make human milk for preterm babies a priority.

In some birthing facilities, healthcare providers hesitate to ask families to provide expressed milk for fear of putting pressure on them during a crisis or making them feel "guilty." One U.S. study examined this dynamic among 21 women, 76% of whom were African American or Latina and 62% were low-income (Miracle, Meier, & Bennett, 2004). All had decided during pregnancy not to breastfeed, but when they delivered a preterm baby, hospital staff asked them to provide their milk and explained why it was important to their baby from a medical standpoint. When asked if they felt pressured or coerced, the mothers all said no. Two of these mothers were transferred from another hospital, which

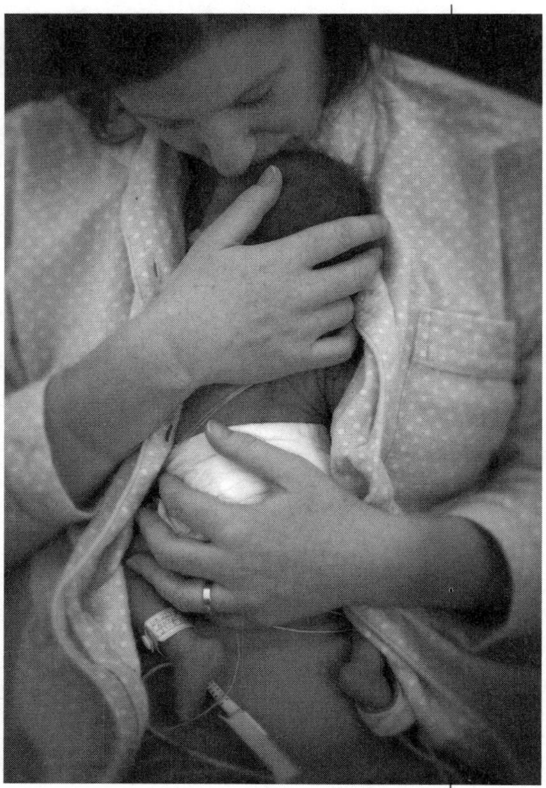

had given them no encouragement to breastfeed or express milk. Rather than feeling pressured, both mothers were unhappy that the staff at the first hospital hadn't told them the importance of their milk to their babies. A 2015 Australian prospective cohort study (Sharp, Campbell, Chiffings, Simmer, & French, 2015) reported that nursing initiation rates rose from 66% to 97% among families of preterm babies born before 32 weeks when parents consistently received information about how important their milk was to their preemie.

Another larger U.S. study (Sisk, Lovelady, Dillard, & Gruber, 2006) examined the effects of providing lactation counseling to mothers of very-low-birth-weight preterm babies. Among its 196 mothers, 115 had intended to breastfeed and 81 had not. After being told the importance of their milk to their babies, 100% of the mothers intending to breastfeed began expressing their milk, as did 85% of those who had not. Those with a prior intention to breastfeed provided more milk for a longer time, but all of the mothers surveyed reported they were glad they did, and study questionnaires found no increase of stress or anxiety among either group. For suggestions on how to present this information to parents, see these cited articles: (P. P. Meier, Patel, Bigger, Rossman, & Engstrom, 2013; Rodriguez, Miracle, & Meier, 2005).

PARENTS' ROLE IN BABY'S CARE

Taking an active role in the baby's care can decrease parents' anxiety and feelings of helplessness and over time build a closer bond with their baby.

Building a Relationship

While the baby is in the NICU, the parents may need to work at building their relationship with their baby.

Love between a parent and a baby does not always happen automatically, especially when they are separated after birth. Feelings develop and are reinforced through touch, behaviors, and cues, and it may take extra time and effort to create a relationship with a preterm baby and for the parents to feel like parents.

Other aspects of giving birth to a preterm baby can also make forming a close relationship more difficult. For example, if the baby's life is at risk, parents may be afraid to feel close to the baby for fear of making themselves vulnerable to a greater trauma if the baby dies. Once they feel sure the baby will live, it may be easier to let their feelings for him grow. Also, depending on how early the baby was born, parents may find the baby's appearance upsetting. A very preterm baby is thin, with little fat under translucent skin, and has a protruding abdomen and low muscle tone. Seeing the baby surrounded by medical paraphernalia, with tubes and wires coming from his body, can also be upsetting.

Cultivating a relationship involves two people who are open and responsive to one another, but depending on his condition and his environment, a preemie may be unresponsive. In a bright, noisy, and busy NICU, many preemies spend much of their time sleeping to protect themselves from overstimulation. Many hospitals changed their intensive-care nurseries to reduce the stimulation preterm babies receive by combining medical procedures to minimize disruptions, draping blankets over incubators to reduce glare, providing tactile boundaries for the babies, and holding and positioning them in special ways. If the baby seems "shut down" much of the time, suggest requesting these approaches be tried. Even for very preterm babies, encourage skin-to-skin contact as soon and for as long a time as possible, as it enhances parents' interactions with their baby, provides better health outcomes (Box 9.1), and helps establish nursing (see next section).

• • •

Encourage the parents to spend as much time as possible with their baby and try other ways to feel closer to him.

In addition to touching and holding the baby as much as possible (see next section), other strategies for feeling closer include:

- Use the baby's name when talking about him and to him.
- Take an active role in the baby's care (see next point).
- Share the family's goals, feelings, observations, and suggestions with the NICU staff.
- If they are apart, leave a recording of their voice and a family photo for the baby.
- Take photos of the baby and keep a journal or album to record his progress.

• • •

In some hospitals, parents are encouraged to take an active role in their preterm baby's care.

In Sweden, where 98% of babies nurse at birth, many NICUs consider parents their preterm baby's primary caregivers and encourage them to be active in all aspects of their baby's care. As part of family-centered maternity care, the healthcare providers teach parents to do routine medical procedures and support them as they learn (Nyqvist & Engvall, 2009). One aspect of the national culture that makes this possible is that Swedish parents receive government-paid parental leave from their jobs after birth. Space is set aside for parents to move into the hospital to more easily be with their babies and care for them around the clock. They also promote early nursing as a developmental skill to be facilitated. As a result, many preterm babies are exclusively nursing at much earlier gestational ages than they are in the U.S. (Nyqvist, 2008; Nyqvist, Sjoden, & Ewald, 1999). The adoption of family-centered maternity care is spreading. Research was done in Canada (Brockway, Benzies, & Hayden, 2017), where it improved nursing rates among moderately preterm and late-preterm babies, and the U.K. (Lv et al., 2019), where a quasi-experimental study found an association between its use and improved health outcomes in very-low-birth-weight babies.

At this writing, in most U.S. NICUs, parents' primary role is as providers of milk because direct nursing is not as high a priority as in other parts of the world. The most common U.S. goal is for the preemies to gain enough weight to be discharged as soon as possible. To accomplish this, bottle-feeding is often suggested, even though there is no evidence this will lead to earlier discharge (Briere, 2015). In some U.S. NICUs, expressed milk is valued as a "medicine" for the baby and mothers' efforts to express milk are a priority (P. P. Meier, Johnson, Patel, & Rossman, 2017). At this writing, it is unusual in the U.S. for a baby born very preterm to directly nurse exclusively before hospital discharge.

Milk Expression

For many preterm babies, expressed milk is life-saving, so parents need to know about best practices, although following them can feel overwhelming at times.

Ongoing support and information on best practices are critical to parents expressing milk for their preemie. For better milk volumes long term, parents exclusively pumping need to start expressing milk as soon as possible after delivery (ideally within the first hour), express at least 8 times every 24 hours during the first 2 weeks, and incorporate hands-on pumping techniques. For details, see p. 492.

Following best milk-expression practices to establish significant milk production can feel like an overwhelming task (Bujold, Feeley, Axelin, & Cinquino, 2018). But this can be more difficult for some families than for others. According to U.S. research, a family's income level, education, and neighborhood demographics affect whether they provide milk for their preemie through the first 30 days (Romaine et al., 2018).

U.S. and Finnish reviews on milk expression in mothers of preterm babies (Ikonen, Paavilainen, & Kaunonen, 2015; Lucas et al., 2014) noted common challenges and feelings. Many parents described frequent pumping as:

- Difficult and exhausting
- Degrading, with some "feeling like a cow"
- A paradox, both a link to their baby and a wedge between them

In one U.S. qualitative study, mothers described pumping for their baby in the NICU as being like a "full-time job" (Bower, Burnette, Lewis, Wright, & Kavanagh, 2017). In another U.S. qualitative study (Rossman, Kratovil, Greene, Engstrom, & Meier, 2013), some mothers were able to focus on the deeper meaning of their milk, describing it as having healing properties for their baby, which gave them faith in the value of the milk. Expressing milk is a learned skill, and milk yields are influenced by emotions as well as frequency and technique.

• • •

When pumping exclusively for a preterm baby, parents appreciate knowing what to expect and how to handle possible problems.

With frequent pumping, problems commonly arise. A U.S. review article (Dowling, Blatz, & Graham, 2012) reported that during the course of pumping for babies in special care, about half of parents experienced difficulties, such as nipple pain, pumping pain, and engorgement, along with struggles with milk ejection and milk production. One U.S. review article described the importance of sharing with pumping parents what's normal and possible problems (Lucas et al., 2014). When parents learned in advance about these problems and how to resolve them, they were more likely to keep pumping. If they were unaware of these problems before they developed, they were more likely to quit.

• • •

Even if donor milk is available, parents need to know that infant health outcomes are better when mother's own expressed milk is provided.

In most countries, donor milk consists of pooled mature milk mostly from mothers of term babies. While this is a better choice for preterm babies than formula (see later section, "Health Risks of Non-Human Milks"), mother's own expressed milk is better suited to these babies' needs. Preterm colostrum is higher than donor milk in components that protect the baby from infection, such as anti-infectives, anti-inflammatories, growth factors, and others (Paduraru et al., 2018; Xavier et al., 2018). This is why—even before tiny preemies are ready to be fed by mouth—many special-care nurseries apply small volumes of expressed colostrum to the inside surfaces of baby's mouth to help prevent illness and prepare his digestive tract for oral feeds (Garofalo & Caplan, 2019). Preterm milk is higher in protein, sodium, chloride, iron, and fatty acids than term milk (Boyce et al., 2016). The preterm baby needs more of these nutrients than the term baby, as well as the live cells , which are killed when donor milk is pasteurized. For more details, see the later section, "The Use of Donor Milk."

Skin-to-Skin Contact

Keeping preemies in skin-to-skin contact after birth saves many lives around the world.

Skin-to-skin contact, originally called "kangaroo care," was introduced as a post-delivery alternative to incubators in 1978 by Dr. Edgar Rey Sanabria in a hospital in Bogota, Colombia (Charpak et al., 2005). Death from infection was common—babies born at less than 1350 grams (3 lbs.) usually died—and abandonment of preterm babies by their families was a serious problem. In the years since, kangaroo care (which when practiced 8 to 24 hours per day is referred to as "kangaroo mother care") has been studied internationally and used widely (Cattaneo et al., 2018). The World Health Organization estimated that the universal practice of kangaroo mother care worldwide could save the lives of more than 450,000 babies each year (WHO, 2013).

KEY CONCEPT

Skin-to-skin contact after birth could save the lives of more than 450,000 premature babies.

"Kangaroo mother care" originated in the early 1990s in rural Zimbabwe, when Nils Bergman, a South African public-health physician and researcher, joined the staff of a missionary hospital. When Bergman arrived, there was no high-tech care available for preterm babies, and as a result, there was a high death rate. After charting survival rates using the previous practice of separating mothers and preterm babies at birth, Bergman and Swedish nurse midwife Agneta Jurisoo began using a new approach inspired by the work in Colombia. Early kangaroo mother care involved keeping mothers and their preemies in skin-to-skin contact from birth for 23 hours per day by wrapping babies against their mothers' body. Mothers could move around by day and sleep by night at a 30-degree angle with their babies on their bodies. With this intervention, survival rates improved from 70% to 90% among babies born between 1500 g and 2000 g, and from 10% to 50% among babies born between 1000 g and 1500 g—an increase in survival of 400% among the smallest preemies (N. J. Bergman & Jurisoo, 1994).

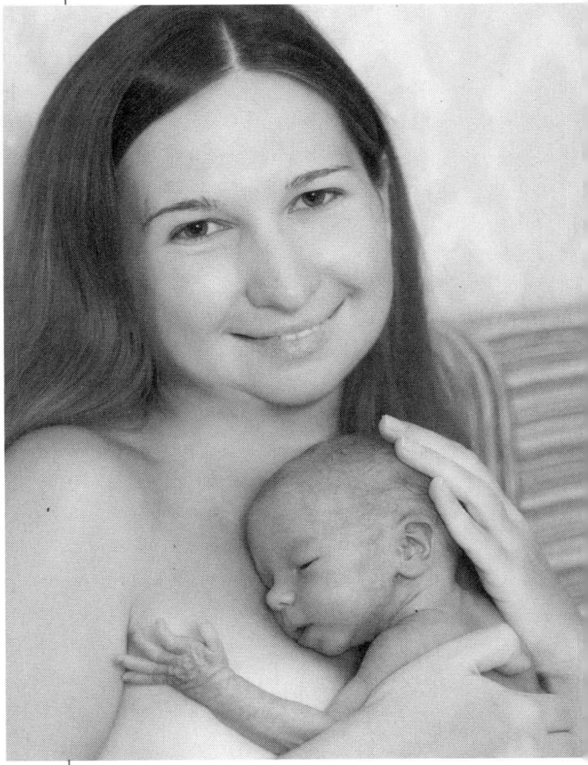

From birth, these kangaroo-mother-care babies were given small feeds of mother's milk by nasogastric tube at 2-hour intervals. By Day 7 to 10, as they learned to nurse, they received full feeds of mother's milk by dropper or cup. Among this population, babies born at less than 31 weeks gestation did not usually survive, but those who did typically regained birth weight by 1 week, gaining on average 30 g (1 oz) per day. Of those who stabilized during the first day, 98% survived.

A 2016 Cochrane Review examined 21 quality studies (some randomized controlled trials) that included 3,042 low-birth-weight infants (Conde-Agudelo & Diaz-Rossello, 2016). Some of these babies experienced kangaroo mother care before and some after they stabilized. Its authors concluded that the evidence supported the use of kangaroo mother care in low-birth-weight babies—especially in limited-resource areas—where it reduces incidence of illness and death. When kangaroo mother care was started within a baby's first 24 hours, it was associated with a shorter hospital stay.

• • •

Skin-to-skin contact improves preemies' stability, reduces their stress, and promotes health and growth.

After the dramatic results of Bergman's Zimbabwe study (see previous point), he began to investigate the mechanisms responsible for the dramatic increase in preemie survival rates. After reviewing the scientific literature, Bergman discovered that human newborns—like other mammals—have inborn physiological programming vital to survival and growth (N. Bergman, 2017). Separation of parent and baby triggers physiological changes that stress preemies, making them more vulnerable to illness and death. In contrast, extended skin-to-skin contact decreases physiological stress, normalizes heart rate and breathing, triggers behaviors that lead to nursing, and elicits the nurturing behaviors in parents that enhance their bond. For details, see p. 45-46 in Chapter 2.

Kangaroo mother care is more effective than an incubator. After decades of research and experience, kangaroo mother care—extended skin-to-skin contact after birth—is practiced in many countries, with many lessons learned (Cattaneo et al., 2018). In high-income areas, where high-tech equipment is available, skin-to-skin contact is often encouraged on a more limited basis (intermittent periods of a few hours or less each day) after the preterm baby's temperature, breathing, and heart rate have stabilized in an incubator (Davanzo et al., 2013). But randomized controlled trials indicated that in many cases, preterm babies stabilize more quickly when in skin-to-skin contact than in an incubator. In one Swedish prospective, unblinded, randomized clinical trial of 34 preemies (born between 1200 g and 2199 g) (N. J. Bergman, Linley, & Fawcus, 2004), 12 of the 13 babies cared for in incubators exceeded the stability parameters, while only 3 of 18 babies kept in skin-to-skin contact did. Eight of the 13 incubator babies experienced hypothermia (low body temperature); none of the 20 babies in skin-to-skin care did. The babies in the incubators had more temperature fluctuations and cardio-respiratory instability. A 2016 randomized controlled trial conducted in Vietnam (Chi Luong, Long Nguyen, Huynh Thi, Carrara, & Bergman, 2016) reached similar conclusions. Its authors found that when the babies were in extended skin-to-skin contact, they had significantly less need for respiratory support, IV fluids, and antibiotics for the rest of their hospital stay.

Benefits of kangaroo mother care. KMC is life-saving in developing countries, but it is also important in the developed world. Box 9.1 lists the advantages of extensive skin-to-skin contact for babies born in high-tech settings.

A 2016 systematic review and meta-analysis of kangaroo mother care and health outcomes among low-birth-weight preterm babies (Boundy et al., 2016) concluded after reviewing 124 high-quality studies that compared to conventional care after birth, kangaroo mother care was associated with a 36% lower risk of infant mortality and a decreased risk of

- Serious blood infections (sepsis)
- Low blood sugar (hypoglycemia)
- Hospital readmission

The positive outcomes associated with kangaroo mother care included:

- Lower respiratory rates
- Higher levels of oxygen in the blood (higher oxygen saturation)
- Greater growth in head circumference
- More exclusive breastfeeding

BOX 9.1 Benefits of Extended Skin-to-Skin Contact in High-Tech Settings

Better for the Preemie
• Prevents hypothermia, is more effective than artificial warmers at keeping baby warm • More stable heart rate and breathing, even in very preterm babies • Lower levels of cortisol, a stress hormone • Healthier sleep patterns, which improves brain development • Better neurobehavioral and psychomotor development • Decreased pain response during painful procedures
Better for the Preemie's Parents
• Better interactions between parents and preemie • Easier adjustment to parenthood after preterm birth • Faster recovery from depression, better mood • Better sleep quality • Lower levels of cortisol, a stress hormone • Preemie discharged sooner from the hospital
Better for Nursing
• Increases milk production • Makes responsive nursing easier, as the parent can feel the preemie's movements • More likely to meet family nursing goals

Adapted from (Angelhoff et al., 2018; Davanzo et al., 2013)

Kangaroo mother care may affect children for decades. A 2017 article charted the outcomes of those who participated 20 years earlier in a randomized controlled trial of babies born at 1800 g or less (Charpak et al., 2017). One of the two groups received kangaroo mother care (KMC) after delivery and the other group received conventional care. The researchers found that the neurological advantages associated with kangaroo mother care at 1 year were still measurable 20 years later. Those in the KMC group had fewer school absences, less hyperactivity, less aggression, and less deviant conduct as young adults. Neuroimaging found that parts of the brain were larger in the KMC group. The researchers concluded that KMC has positive long-term social and behavioral effects.

• • •

Any parent can provide their preemie with skin-to-skin-contact. A 2016 integrative review of the research on fathers and skin-to-skin contact (Shorey, He, & Morelius, 2016) found that—as with mothers—both babies and fathers benefited. In father and child, skin-to-skin contact reduced stress and anxiety and improved the quality of their interactions.

Any parent can provide a preemie with skin-to-skin contact using simple strategies.

How to practice skin-to-skin contact. Wearing only a diaper and often a hat, the preemie is held chest-to-chest against his parent's bare skin and is covered by a shirt, a blanket, or a binder that is tight enough to support the baby in the kangaroo position (Kledzik, 2005). The baby is supported with his head turned to one side, his chin slightly raised, and arms and legs flexed.

• • •

Skin-to-skin contact promotes both feeding competence and milk production.

When held in skin-to-skin contact, the baby can look at his parent, respond to their voice, nurse at will (if nursing has begun), or relax and sleep peacefully. As he rests against the parent's body, the parent learns the baby's feel, sounds, and responses. This close body contact triggers a baby's inborn feeding behaviors (see Chapter 1). In one Swedish NICU, frequent and extended skin-to-skin contact was associated with earlier exclusive breastfeeding (Nyqvist, 2004). See also the later section, "Transitioning to Full Nursing."

The baby's touch also affects the parent hormonally. Even an hour per day of skin-to-skin contact was found to increase expressed milk volumes (N. M. Hurst, Valentine, Renfro, Burns, & Ferlic, 1997).

• • •

Early and extensive skin-to-skin contact was associated with greater milk production and better nursing outcomes.

Early preterm birth is associated with a shorter duration of nursing, even in countries such as Sweden, where nursing is near universal (Akerstrom, Asplund, & Norman, 2007; Flacking, Nyqvist, Ewald, & Wallin, 2003). But skin-to-skin contact can help to partly offset this dynamic. Many studies from around the world have found an association between skin-to-skin contact and increased incidence and duration of nursing (Bonnet et al., 2018; Jayaraman, Mukhopadhyay, Bhalla, & Dhaliwal, 2017; Oras et al., 2016). In a randomized, controlled trial that followed 66 preterm babies from birth through 18 months (Hake-Brooks & Anderson, 2008), one U.S. NICU found that early and unlimited skin-to-skin contact was associated with significantly greater nursing exclusivity between birth and 6 months and duration through 18 months.

• • •

In some situations, skin-to-skin contact is not possible.

The vast majority of preterm babies will benefit from skin-to-skin contact. But in some specific situations, skin-to-skin contact may need to be delayed. This can happen when the preemie (Davanzo et al., 2013):

- Is less than 28 weeks gestation or born at less than 750 g
- Is unstable or very sick
- Is on mechanical ventilation for a serious illness
- Is being treated with vasopressor drugs
- Has a catheter in the umbilical artery, jugular or femoral vein, or his chest or abdomen is being drained
- Had surgery within the past week
- Underwent a major procedure within the previous 6 to 12 hours.

• • •

If parents are unable to spend time with their preemie in skin-to-skin contact, encourage them to find other ways to touch their baby, such as infant massage.

Although skin-to-skin contact is the first choice, if it is not possible, encourage the parents to sit beside the baby's incubator, look into his eyes, and stroke him. Knowing that someone loves him is important to his progress. One U.S. study found that mothers' depression and anxiety scores were lower after they gave their preemies massage therapy in the NICU (Feijo et al., 2006). Other U.S. studies found that with infant massage, babies had increased temperature, better digestion, fewer stress behaviors, and better weight gain and growth (Ang et al., 2012; Diego, Field, & Hernandez-Reif, 2008; Diego et al., 2007).

NURSING THE PRETERM BABY

Human milk can be lifesaving for preemies, but direct nursing is important for other reasons, too.

When a preemie is born very early, it makes sense for parents to make milk expression a major priority. Providing the very tiny preemie with an exclusive human-milk diet can make the difference between life and death (see the later section, "Health Risks of Non-Human Milks").

Making the transition to direct nursing is important, too, but it may feel daunting. As families become accustomed to precisely measured feeds and strict feeding schedules, some question whether the act of direct nursing matters to their baby and even wonder if direct nursing might be risky. Why does it matter? Direct nursing in the NICU is associated with a greater likelihood of:

- Human-milk feeding at discharge (Casavant, McGrath, 2015)
- Human-milk feeding after discharge (Briere, McGrath, Cong, Brownell, & Cusson, 2016)
- Direct nursing at discharge (Casey, Fucile, & Dow, 2018)

But there are other reasons it's important for direct nursing to begin in the hospital. For one, families can receive guidance and support during this process. It also sends the message from the healthcare team that direct nursing is important to the preemie, that nursing is about more than just the milk (R. Pineda, 2011).

Enhanced neurological development and bonding. During direct nursing, hormones such as oxytocin are released that enhance the bond between parent and child, and all of a preemie's senses are stimulated in a comforting way. As one researcher described it (R. G. Pineda, 2016), nursing is a complex skill that contributes to a baby's social, motor, sensory and neurological development. As another researcher emphasized (N. Bergman, 2017), nursing provides positive sensory input that wires the newborn brain in a healthy, calming way. Baby's vision is stimulated as he looks into his parent's eyes. His skin is warmed by skin-to-skin contact. As the baby's body and hands are pulled in close to his parent's body and he feels his parent's hands and arms around him, his body moves with his parent's movements. This positive, loving touch offsets the negative touch of medical procedures. His senses of taste and smell are stimulated by the milk, and his hearing is stimulated by his parent's voice. Whether or not the baby consumes measurable volumes of milk during early nursing sessions, this sensory stimulation enhances his neurological development and his relationship with the nursing parent.

> **KEY CONCEPT**
>
> *Even with no milk intake, direct nursing positively stimulates all of baby's senses, enhancing both his neurological development and his bond with his nursing parent.*

Exclusive pumping is more difficult to maintain long term. Even when the milk is the uppermost concern, families who exclusively express are much more likely to stop earlier than families who make the transition to direct nursing. One U.S. retrospective chart review of 34 mothers and babies who were born at less than 1500 g (Smith, Durkin, Hinton, Bellinger, & Kuhn, 2003) found that 4 months after the preterm birth, 72% of those who made the transition to direct nursing were still nursing, whereas among those who continued to exclusively express, only 10% were still expressing. A 2017 multi-ethnic cohort Singapore study of 500 Asian mothers (Pang et al., 2017) found that those who exclusively expressed were 2.4 times more likely to wean before 3 months compared with those who directly nursed or mixed fed.

What to Expect

Preterm babies go through predictable stages as they mature and their nursing effectiveness improves.

Premature birth covers a wide range of gestational ages, from the tiniest preemies born at 22 or 23 weeks through larger late preterm babies born just before 37 weeks. The weeks between a very early preterm and a late preterm baby make a huge difference in terms of brain development (Figure 9.1), which profoundly affects their ability to feed (Kelly et al., 2016; Walsh, Doyle, Anderson, Lee, & Cheong, 2014).

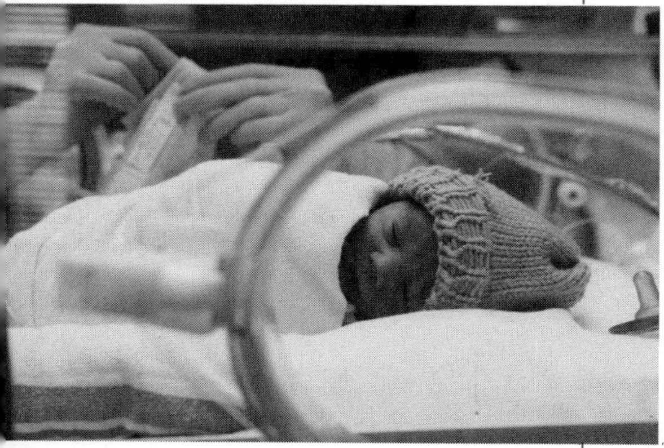

Preterm babies are different. In terms of feeding, preemies differ from full-term babies in several key ways. Preemies have a small mouth without fat pads in their cheeks, which may decrease feeding effectiveness (see p. 279). Less body fat makes staying warm more challenging and increases risk for low blood sugar (hypoglycemia). Their heart rate and breathing may be unstable. Many have low muscle tone (hypotonia). Because their brains are smaller and less developed (Figure 9.1), it is more difficult for them to control their head and limbs, and as compared with term babies, they spend much more time asleep or drowsy.

Predictable stages of preterm nursing. With practice and growing maturity, preemies' feeding effectiveness improves. Creating a supportive environment for feeding (see later section) also makes a difference in how effectively they nurse. Swedish researcher Kerstin Hedberg Nyqvist, who extensively studied preterm nursing, developed a "road map" of the predictable stages preemies experience as they move to effective direct nursing (Box 9.2).

When a preemie doesn't yet feed effectively enough to get all the milk he needs via direct nursing, this overview provides parents with realistic expectations and a positive perspective. So rather than thinking direct nursing is a hopeless cause, parents and professionals can chart the preemie's progress through these stages with confidence that effective, direct nursing is in their future.

Not all preterm babies start at the first stage. Those who are born healthier and closer to term may start at a later stage. But no matter where on the road map a

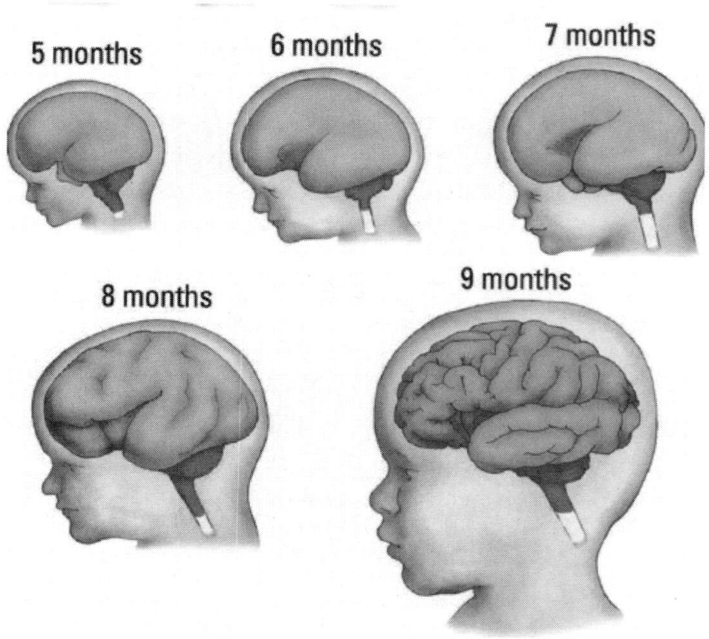

Figure 9.1 Fetal brain development by month. ©2020 Bryan Kolb, used with permission.

BOX 9.2 The "Road Map"

7 Stages of Preterm Nursing
Babies born closer to term or healthier may start at a later stage

Stage 1	Frequent milk expression, baby is tube-fed, lots of skin-to-skin contact
Stage 2	Nursing begins: rooting, licking, or mouthing the nipple with no milk intake yet
Stage 3	Single sucks, short bursts, long pauses, baby stays latched for a short time, some milk intake
Stage 4	Longer sucking bursts, baby stays latched longer, milk intake variable but baby takes more milk more often, need to plan supplementation strategy
Stage 5	Milk intake increases with occasional larger volumes
Stage 6	More milk intake with immature sucking pattern, short bursts, long pauses, full nursing possible with semi-demand feeding
Stage 7	Effective, mature sucking pattern of a term baby, can now nurse on cue

Adapted from (Nyqvist, 2017, p. 201)

preemie starts, with regular opportunities to latch and suck, his ability to nurse will improve until he reaches the last stage, where he can feed as effectively as a full-term newborn.

When a preemie starts nursing before stage 6 or 7, even if he consumes some milk, in addition to nursing, he will likely need to be supplemented at many feeds. Assure the family that is normal until the baby is feeding more effectively. If the goal is to exclusively nurse, continued milk expression is needed until the baby can take all the milk he needs via direct nursing. (See later section, "Supplementing Nursing."

• • •

A preterm baby's progress through the nursing stages may be slower if he was born earlier than 28 weeks and/or has health problems.

For healthy preemies born at 28 weeks or later, gestational age is not always related to feeding effectiveness. Some very early preemies nurse surprisingly well. Swedish researcher Kerstin Hedberg-Nyqvist wrote about the babies in a study she conducted on 71 healthy preemies (Nyqvist, 2017, p. 190):

> "The first breastfeed occurred at 27 weeks [post-menstrual age]...all infants rooted (the majority showed obvious rooting) and latching on, half of them efficiently. Most infants stayed fixed for short periods, 5 minutes or less. Nearly all infants engaged in single sucks or short sucking bursts. Obvious rooting, efficient areolar grasp and staying fixed at the breast for long periods were observed as early as 28 weeks. Some infants sucked in long sucking bursts, even bursts of 30 or more sucks, at 32 weeks. The larger sucking bursts data showed large variation. Mothers perceived repeated audible swallowing at 31 weeks at the earliest."

When to Start Nursing

Rather than thinking in terms of "readiness," in some countries, nursing is considered a normal behavior to be facilitated as early as possible.

In some neonatal intensive care nurseries, arbitrary criteria, such as gestational age or weight (see next point) are used to decide when it is safe for a preemie to begin nursing. However, in Sweden, where 98% of families nurse, it is considered a normal activity to be facilitated. As Swedish researcher Kerstin Hedberg Nyqvist wrote (Nyqvist, 2017, p. 181): "In settings where breastfeeding is considered the norm for infant and young child feeding, mothers and personnel in neonatal

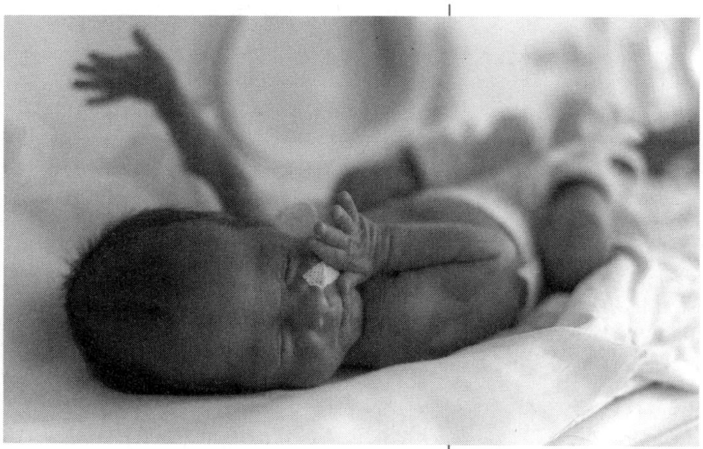

units strive for 'normalcy'." In the innovative Swedish NICU where she worked and did her research, gestational age and weight were not considered. Nursing began as soon as the baby was weaned off the ventilator and continuous positive airway (CPAP) and had no severe instability. Rather than trying to gauge a baby's "readiness," their philosophy was instead to modify the environment and observe each baby to facilitate their ability to nurse. That's why—as described in the previous point—some babies latched on and nursed as early as 28 weeks gestation. According to a 2018 European population-based cohort study (Bonnet et al., 2018), about half of babies born very preterm in Sweden were still nursing at 6 months. In the U.S., on the other hand, direct nursing is often unnecessarily delayed and nursing rates among preterm babies are much lower. One 2018 article that used data from two large national studies (Campbell & Miranda, 2018) concluded that only about 26% of very preterm American babies were nursing at 6 months.

• • •

Direct nursing is less stressful for preterm babies than bottle-feeding, so direct nursing should ideally be baby's first oral feed.

A 2015 U.S. retrospective review of 88 babies born at less than 34 weeks gestational age (Briere, McGrath, Cong, Brownell, & Cusson, 2015) found that 59% nursed for their first oral feed. They concluded that in the NICU parents should be supported to nurse before using bottles. In some areas, however, parents of preemies are told to delay nursing until the baby reaches a certain weight or gestation age or until bottle-feeding is going well. These recommendations were based on the following commonly held but incorrect assumptions:

- Nursing is too physically stressful for babies who weigh less than 1500 g (3.3 pounds).
- The ability to coordinate sucking, swallowing, and breathing does not occur until 34 to 35 weeks gestation.
- Babies should be bottle-fed before nursing, because nursing is more difficult.

Research proved these assumptions wrong. Two of the earliest studies to compare nursing to bottle-feeding in preemies used five preterm babies serving as their own controls (P. Meier, 1988; P. Meier & Anderson, 1987). The babies were about 32 weeks gestation, weighed on average 1300 g (about 2.9 pounds), and were 20 to 50 days old before they began nursing. Body temperature, breathing, heart rate, and transcutaneous oxygen pressure were used to measure stress. The researchers found that nursing was less physically stressful than bottle-feeding, and the smaller the babies, the greater the difference. These early studies found that preterm babies could organize sucking, swallowing, and breathing more easily during nursing than bottle-feeding and that the ability to nurse develops well before the ability to bottle-feed. These babies were able to suck and swallow regularly and predictably while nursing, but when given a bottle—presumably due to the faster, more consistent flow—their sucking and swallowing patterns became disorganized.

Other studies also found that oxygen desaturation (low blood oxygen levels) was more common during bottle-feeding and that a preterm baby's oxygen saturation levels remain higher during nursing (Blaymore Bier et al., 1997; Chen, Wang, Chang, & Chi, 2000; Dowling, 1999).

• • •

If the family thinks the NICU practices are not evidence-based and supportive of their nursing goals, encourage the parents to:

If the preemie's healthcare providers do not follow best practices, suggest the family make their wishes known.

- Be tactful and respectful and expect this in return.
- Acknowledge everyone's good intentions.
- Be honest with all healthcare providers.
- Be clear about their goals, the reasons for them, and be ready to repeat them if needed.
- Seek out the most supportive healthcare providers for moral support and help.
- Ask for more information if they are uncomfortable with suggested treatments or strategies.
- Offer research citations when suggesting alternatives.
- Practice what they want to say before talking to the healthcare team.
- Be friendly and project confidence.
- Be aware that the parents have the ultimate responsibility for the baby's health.
- If the parents are not satisfied, seek a second opinion.

In 2013, experts compiled the Ten Steps designed to expand the Baby Friendly Hospital Initiative to include NICUs (Nyqvist et al., 2013). If needed, suggest parents share this citation with their healthcare providers.

How to Start Nursing

Although some recommend starting nursing by offering very small preemies an "emptied" breast, this strategy is based on bottle-feeding studies.

Some recommend starting preemies with "an emptied breast" (Spatz, 2021). This recommendation is based on research done with bottle-feeding preemies that found restricting milk flow made bottle-feeding more manageable (Lau, Sheena, Shulman, & Schanler, 1997). However, during nursing, preterm babies have more control over milk flow (Nyqvist, 2017). Other research cited to support this strategy suggested that nursing with low milk flow could provide "non-nutritive sucking" as a substitute for a pacifier during tube-feeding (Narayanan, 1990). Pacifer use during tube feeds was found to improve weight gain in preemies (Measel & Anderson, 1979). Swedish research (Nyqvist, 2008; Nyqvist et al., 1999), however, found that even very tiny preemies could nurse well from a full mammary gland without the need for this intermediate step.

• • •

Expect early nursing to be a learning process.

Learning to nurse usually requires time and patience. The nursing parent may feel awkward and frustrated at times. To help create realistic expectations, mention that it will probably take some time and practice before the baby begins to take milk, but with patience, he will learn. The baby may begin by simply licking or mouthing the nipple. Many preemies suck in short bursts and fall asleep quickly (see Box 9.2). Make sure the family knows that it is okay if the baby does not take milk during these early nursing sessions because, if needed, he will be supplemented with milk afterwards.

• • •

Emotional support is vital when a preemie begins direct nursing, as families often experience distress, which can negatively affect nursing outcomes.

A 2016 U.S. exploratory and descriptive study of 34 mothers with hospitalized preterm babies (Park et al., 2016) found the highest levels of emotional distress occurred shortly before their baby began oral feeds. Understandably, worry about their baby's health was high at that time, as well as depression. Mothers also experienced stress over their caregiving role. When others act as baby's primary caregivers, it takes time for parents to build a relationship with their baby. Younger mothers experienced more intense depression, and those who had other children worried most about their relationship with their baby. If a family expresses these feelings, assure them they are not alone. Let them know, too, that as parents master feeding, these negative feelings decrease. With time, their bond will grow and they will grow in confidence.

Emotional distress made it more difficult for the study mothers to respond appropriately to their preemie's special needs during feeds (see next point). Preemies feed best when stimulation is kept low and touch steady. The study mothers who were depressed stroked their babies more during feeds and used light rather than steady touch, which made feeds challenging. The researchers suggested that providing emotional support to reduce parents' distress may help ease the transition to oral feeds.

Creating a Supportive Environment

A supportive environment makes early nursing easier.

When creating a supportive nursing environment for a preemie, keep these factors in mind.

Privacy is ideal, preferably a separate room with a door. If the baby is very preterm, he may be on a monitor, oxygen, and an IV. If so, it may not be possible to go to a private room. But a private area can be created, even in a busy NICU, by using a curtain, partition wall, or screen. If that is not possible, position the parent's chair with its back to the room.

Comfort. A comfortable chair with good back and arm support that can recline is ideal. Extra pillows may be helpful. Suggest the nursing parent choose clothing that allows the baby easy access to the nipple. Make sure the baby is not too warm or overheated, which can make him drowsy. Close contact with the parent's body will provide warmth, and a hat and a blanket over him may be all that's needed to maintain his body temperature.

Sound and light. A calm, quiet environment helps keep stimulation manageable for baby, so encourage others to talk quietly. Try to position the nursing couple away from flashing lights and, if possible, dim the room lights and protect the baby's eyes from direct light.

Relaxed time together. Suggest the family ask not to be rushed or interrupted. In a relaxed environment, body contact is soothing and can reduce stress.

• • •

At first, arrange for skilled lactation help and support.

Encourage the family to ask for skilled lactation help during the first few nursing sessions to help boost their confidence while they learn baby's cues. During the first sessions, offer practical suggestions on how to help the baby latch deeply and positions they may find comfortable. In a Swedish study (Weimers,

Svensson, Dumas, Naver, & Wahlberg, 2006) demonstrating these strategies with a doll was better accepted than hands-on help.

In Swedish NICUs, if the baby has a history of breathing or heartbeat irregularities (apnea, bradycardia, oxygen desaturation), a healthcare provider monitors the baby during early feeds. If the baby remains stable during the first few feeds, then the nursing parent is taught to observe the baby's breathing and skin color and can contact a healthcare provider if needed (Nyqvist, 2017). It may help the family to know that as part of an immature sucking pattern, when a very preterm baby begins to latch, he may hold his breath while sucking, which can cause a temporary drop in his oxygen levels. This is not a cause for concern and the oxygen levels return to normal quickly (K. H. Nyqvist, 2017).

• • •

Avoid stressful events or procedures right before nursing.

Because preterm babies are so sensitive to stimulation, even washing, bathing, and a diaper change may be stressful (Morelius, Hellstrom-Westas, Carlen, Norman, & Nelson, 2006). Suggest if possible, these and any medical procedures be done after nursing.

Helping Baby Latch and Feed

To encourage nursing, start with unrestricted skin-to-skin contact.

When baby spends time in skin-to-skin contact under the nursing parent's clothing, it is easy to tell from the baby's movements when he is arousing and ready to feed. Other cues include changes in his breathing, sounds, eyes opening, and sucking movements.

• • •

Encourage the family to use whatever feeding positions work best for them.

To latch deeply and feed well, good body and head support are vital for the preterm baby. This can happen in a number of ways. For example, the starter positions described on pp. 23-29 were used in one U.K. study of 11 late preterm babies (35 to 37 weeks gestation) and one small-for-gestational-age baby born at 38 weeks (Colson, DeRooy, & Hawdon, 2003). Similar to positions used during skin-to-skin contact, when using these semi-reclined positions, baby lies tummy down on the parent's body. The baby's head is supported by the parent's arm, and after latching, gravity helps keep the nipple deeply in baby's mouth.

One Japanese study examined the effect of the body position during feeds on 14 babies (some term, some preterm) who were having trouble maintaining oxygen levels during bottle-feeds (Mizuno, Inoue, & Takeuchi, 2000). The researchers found that the babies had better oxygenation, exerted more sucking pressure, and took more milk when they fed prone (tummy down).

If upright feeding positions are used, the nursing parent needs to provide the baby with body and head support.

- Make sure the parent has good back, neck, and arm support.
- Hold the baby with the entire front of his body facing and touching the parent's body.
- Help guide the baby to the nipple with the parent's palm on his back, thumb and index finger supporting the base of his head (see Figure 9.2).

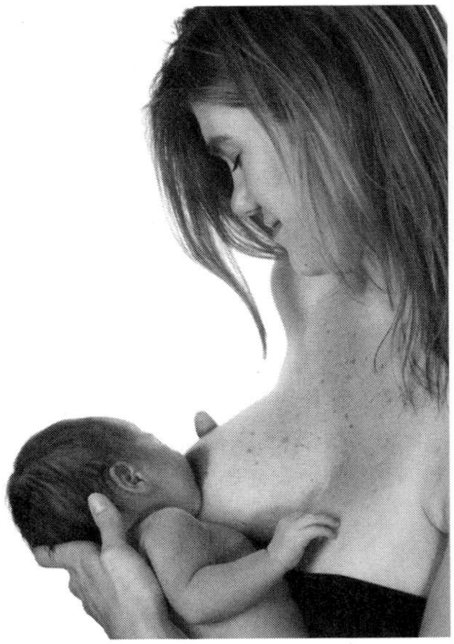

Figure 9.2 One possible upright feeding position with a preterm baby.

- Align the baby nose to nipple, so that he can approach the mammary gland chin first, with a wide-open mouth and head slightly tilted back to make swallowing easier.
- Apply gentle pressure on the baby's shoulders as he latches to ensure he takes a big mouthful and throughout the feed, so he stays deeply latched.
- Consider putting a pillow or cushion under baby to support him at nipple height.

• • •

In upright feeding positions, it may help to support the mammary tissue.

Tiny babies sometimes have trouble staying attached. If this happens in an upright position, suggest supporting the weight of the mammary gland, so it doesn't rest on the baby's chin. Depending on its size, it may help to support it throughout the feed. If the baby needs more help, suggest trying the Dancer Hand position described on p. 890 and see the later point on p. 363 on using a nipple shield.

• • •

After choosing a comfortable position, suggest avoiding too much movement or extra touching.

Preterm babies are so sensitive to stimulation that the natural movements a parent makes during nursing, like patting and rocking, may overstimulate him. Until nursing is established, suggest nursing with "still hands" (Nyqvist, 2017).

• • •

It is not unusual at first for milk ejection to take longer.

The first time a nursing parent uses a breast pump, it often takes a couple of minutes for the milk ejection to occur and the milk to flow, because the feel of a pump is very different from the feel of a baby nursing. The same can be true in reverse when the milk was flowing well with the feel of the pump, but the nursing parent's body is not yet conditioned to the feel of the nursing baby.

When nursing begins after a time of exclusive pumping, it often takes a little longer for the milk ejection to occur. The baby may suck for several minutes and fall asleep before the milk starts to flow. Although this can be frustrating, assure the family that soon the parent's body will become conditioned to the feel of the baby nursing and the milk will flow more quickly. In the meantime, the best way to speed up the process is to spend some time in skin-to-skin contact before nursing. If this doesn't help, before baby latches, suggest stimulating milk ejection with the breast pump or hand expression. Another alternative is to use the pump (or ask a helper to hold the pump) on the opposite side after latch, so the pump can trigger the milk ejection sooner.

• • •

Suggest the family learn to recognize the signs it is safe for the baby to continue nursing and the signs that he needs to stop.

Because of preemies' sensitivity to stimulation, suggest watching for baby's cues to determine which sounds and touches work best, so he does not get more stimulation than he can handle. Swedish researcher Kerstin Hedberg Nyqvist described "Cues of Approach" and "Cues of Avoidance" that can help interpret preterm babies' needs during nursing (Nyqvist, 2017). "Cues of Approach" are signs the baby wants to continue nursing and "Cues of Avoidance" indicate the baby wants to stop. These cues come from the work of Als and colleagues as part of the Newborn Individual Developmental Care and Assessment Program (NICAP), which was created to encourage care for preterm babies in harmony with their health and development (Als et al., 1994; Ross & Browne, 2002). These cues include physiological changes, movements, state changes, and ways of interacting, some of which are listed in Table 9.1.

TABLE 9.1 Preterm Babies' Cues During Nursing

CUES OF APPROACH	CUES OF AVOIDANCE
Changes in Physiology	
Regular heartbeat and breathing	Fast, slow or irregular heartbeat or breathing
Skin color unchanged	Skin color changes (pale, mottled, flushed)
Digestion stable	Spits up, gags, grunts while passing stool
Occasional startles or twitches	Hiccups, startles, tremors
Movements	
Stable muscle tone	Low tone in hands, arms, legs, trunk, face
Shows signs of wanting more:	Flexes arms, legs, trunk and maintains this
• Tucks himself closer	Shows tongue
• Brings hands to face or mouth	Extends arms/legs
• Smiles	Arches head and/or trunk away or turns
• Mouths, licks, laps milk	Spreads out fingers
State	
Stable sleep or alertness	Light sleep
Deep sleep	Drowsy, movements with closed eyes
States easy to distinguish	Little alertness, fast shifting between states
Oriented to parent with focused look	Looks glassy-eyed, tense, surprised, scared
Calm state changes	Difficult to calm, irritable, overactive
Blocks stimuli easily	Limited ability to shut out stimuli
Interactions	
Orients toward parent's face, voice	Looks away, stares in another direction
Frowns	Eyes "float" from side to side or roll
Forms "oh" with lips	Fusses, cries, becomes drowsy, closes eyes
Mimics facial expressions, coos	Yawns, sneezes

Adapted from (Nyqvist, 2017)

Gauging Nursing Effectiveness

Although not completely reliable, some signs of milk intake during nursing include audible swallowing, milk around the baby's mouth, and fresh milk when the feeding tube is aspirated. In some NICUs, the appearance of these signs mean it is time to begin regular test weighing (see next point).

Some simple signs are rough indicators a baby may be transferring milk during nursing.

• • •

Knowing how much milk a baby consumes during nursing can be important for several reasons. It can prevent over-supplementation, which can delay the transition to full nursing (N. M. Hurst, Meier, Engstrom, & Myatt, 2004). It can also prevent delays in initiating direct nursing, as some healthcare providers are reluctant to allow early nursing if they think they cannot accurately chart baby's milk intake. Knowing how effectively a baby is nursing can also affect discharge plans, as in some places, feeding competence is one of the determining criteria (McCain, Gartside, Greenberg, & Lott, 2001; Nye, 2008).

A reliable way to measure milk intake during nursing is weighing baby before and after feeds with a baby scale accurate to 2 g.

Unreliable indicators. One classic U.S. study (P. P. Meier, Engstrom, Fleming, Streeter, & Lawrence, 1996) found that neither mothers nor experienced lactation consultants could accurately estimate preterm babies' milk intake during nursing sessions using the same behaviors sometimes used to gauge milk intake in full-term babies, such as audible swallowing and wide jaw movements.

Pre- and post-feed weights. According to several U.S. studies (Juliano, Puchalski, & Walsh, 2019; P. P. Meier & Engstrom, 2007; P. P. Meier et al., 1994; Rankin et al., 2016), a reliable way to gauge milk intake during nursing is by using a very accurate (to 2 g) baby scale for pre- and post-feed weights. Even when babies wear leads that connect them to medical equipment, test-weighing was found to be reliable (Haase, Barreira, Murphy, Mueller, & Rhodes, 2009). Very accurate scales are available in many hospitals and lactation clinics, and in some areas, they can be rented for home use. (For details on how to do test-weights, see p. 919.) However, if the family finds test-weighing stressful or low milk intake leaves them feeling discouraged, an alternative is to reduce the baby's supplement gradually, while carefully monitoring his growth (Flacking et al., 2003).

Early Nursing Rhythms

Once a preterm baby starts nursing, ideally, he should be encouraged to nurse often and without time restrictions.

Sometimes families are told to restrict nursing to a specific number of feeds per day or a specific number of minutes.

Energy expenditure during nursing. At this writing, there is no evidence to support the practice of limiting number of nursing sessions or cutting sessions short. A 2009 Israeli study compared resting energy expenditure (REE) in 19 preemies at 32 weeks gestation who served as their own controls (Berger, Weintraub, Dollberg, Kopolovitz, & Mandel, 2009). Although these babies spent more minutes nursing than bottle-feeding (an average of 20 minutes versus 8 minutes), there were no differences in the REE measured after nursing or bottle-feeding. Suggest the family ask that the baby nurse as long as he is handling it well and to expect that feeding time will vary a lot at first. A preterm baby usually has periods of rest and activity during nursing, and restricting the time may substantially cut down on the volume of milk he consumes.

If baby falls asleep early in the feed, suggest holding him while he sleeps, keeping him close to the nipple and offering it to him while he is in a light sleep (eyes moving under eyelids, any body movement). If needed, tube-feeding can ideally be done while baby is nursing to provide him with positive reinforcement for his efforts.

• • •

There is no need to offer both sides at feeds unless the baby wants both.

At first, very tiny preemies may do better staying on one side per feed. Movement, repositioning, and latching to the other side may be too much stimulation. Just like a full-term baby, a preemie may get all the milk he needs from one side, and it is better to feed well from one side than to nurse less effectively on both. Encourage the family to watch the baby's cues to avoid overtiring or stressing him.

If the baby is still awake and alert after the first side and is interested, it is fine to offer the other side.

• • •

At first, suggest watching for feeding cues, and if possible, nurse at least every 2 hours or even more often during the day.

Although in many countries, preterm babies are fed much less often than every 2 hours, small babies can better handle smaller, more frequent feeds. Frequent feeds are closer to a typical newborn nursing rhythm, and are part of ensuring adequate milk intake in preemies who have reached the sixth stage (see Box 9.2) of nursing effectiveness (Nyqvist, 2017). (See also the later point on "semi-demand feeding.") After hospital discharge, one Swedish study asked 24 exclusively breastfeeding mothers to keep a 24-hour feeding diary (Oras et al., 2015) and found that these preemies nursed between 8 and 26 times per day, with a median of 14 breastfeeds per day (see Table 9.3). Their nursing frequency decreased over time.

In most cases, before a preterm baby is ready for exclusive nursing, he will need to be supplemented (see next section). The volume given and the feeding pattern should be based on each baby's individual needs, so that he gets enough milk each day to gain weight well (see next section) as he learns to nurse.

Once the baby is taking significant milk volumes during nursing, if the family is not rooming in at the hospital, encourage them to work out a schedule with the hospital staff, so they can nurse freely during the time they are with their baby. When they are not available, the hospital staff will use other feeding methods (see next section).

• • •

If the baby has trouble staying latched or is not taking much milk, try using a nipple shield to see if it helps.

The research on the use of nipple shields with preterm babies is mixed, but in some specific cases, a nipple shield may be a useful tool.

More milk intake with nipple shields in preemies with latching problems. In one U.S. study of 34 preemies who were having trouble latching, were slipping off the nipple during pauses, or were falling asleep quickly during nursing (P. P. Meier et al., 2000), these babies were able to take significantly more milk when the shield was used than when it wasn't. Milk transfer per feed was greater for all 34 babies, with a mean increase of 14.4 ml or about half an ounce. With the shield, the babies had longer sucking bursts and stayed awake longer during nursing. These preemies used the shield for a mean of 32.5 days (with a range of 2 to 171 days) out of a mean nursing duration of 169 days (with a range of 14 to 365 days), so overall, the mothers used the shield for about 24% of the time they nursed. The researchers noted that the babies who were unable to transfer milk without the shield used the shield longer than the babies who transfered milk when nursing without the shield. There was no association between the length of time the shield was used and duration of nursing. The researchers suggested that the shields helped because they increased suction during nursing. However, a 2017 ultrasound prospective cross-sectional observational study of 38 preterm babies (Geddes et al., 2017) found that when using a nipple shield, their suction was weaker and that the increased milk intake was unrelated to suction strength.

KEY CONCEPT

Nipple shields are not helpful for all preemies, but they may improve milk intake in some specific situations.

If using a nipple shield increases milk intake, eliminates the need to supplement, or shortens the time to exclusive nursing, encourage the family to use it as long as needed. The U.S. study described above found that preemies nursed better with the shield on average until they reached term corrected age of about 40 weeks.

Nipple shield use associated with failure to exclusively nurse. In a Danish prospective cohort survey of more than 1,200 mothers of preemies born between 24 and 36 weeks gestation (Maastrup et al., 2014), 68% were exclusively breastfeeding and 17% partially breastfeeding at hospital discharge. This survey found an association between the use of nipple shields and a failure to exclusively nurse.

Nipple shield use associated with earlier use of formula. A 2017 Danish study based on data from 4,815 Danish mothers (Kronborg, Foverskov, Nilsson, & Maastrup, 2017) found that nipple shield use was associated with lower infant gestational age and birth weight and a threefold increase in earlier cessation of exclusive nursing.

For details on fitting, applying, and weaning from the shield, see p. 912-917.

• • •

Until the baby is exclusively nursing, encourage continued milk expression.

If the baby is not yet nursing effectively enough to get all his milk at nursing sessions, to maintain milk production, continued milk expression is needed. Abundant milk production improves milk flow, making nursing easier for the baby.

Weight Gain and Supplementation

In most cases, after nursing begins, the preterm baby will both nurse and receive supplements. Being well fed is vital to healthy growth and feeding effectiveness.

How Should Preterm Babies Grow?

Experts are uncertain about optimal weight gain for very preterm babies.

In the U.S. and Europe, medical organizations recommend that preterm babies gain and grow at about the same rate expected in utero (AAP, 2014; Agostoni et al., 2010). The focus on maintaining intrauterine growth rates began more than 40 years ago and originated from charts based on the growth patterns of the larger preterm babies of that time. Preemies today, however, are being saved earlier and earlier, and these tiny preemies have different nutritional needs. Preemies who also suffer from health problems grow more slowly, so this goal may be difficult for many tiny babies to achieve. In addition, disagreement exists on which growth curves to use for very-low-birth-weight babies (Fenton et al., 2017). The quality improvement toolkit developed by the California Perinatal Quality Care Collaborative (downloadable at: **bit.ly/BA2-VLBW** provides several different growth charts that may be used with very-low-birth-weight preemies.

For very tiny preemies, one reason meeting intrauterine weight-gain goals is challenging is because their immature digestive system is less able to absorb and digest food, as compared with a full-term baby. Also, any extra nutrients must be given in a digestible and absorbable form in just the right amounts, so the baby's kidneys and other organs are not stressed.

Developing universal nutritional guidelines for very preterm babies is difficult because these babies vary so much in birth weight, gestational age, nutritional status, and health. Many tiny preemies fed exclusively mother's milk do not grow at intrauterine rates. In this case, some recommend fortifying mother's milk or using higher-calorie hindmilk to increase weight gains (see later section). The most important focus for any preterm baby is a healthy weight gain and positive long-term health outcomes. The Academy of Breastfeeding Medicine (L. M. Noble, Okogbule-Wonodi, & Young, 2018) recommends a daily weight gain of 15 g to 30 g (0.5 to 1 ounce). Gaining too much weight and not enough weight both have the potential to result in poorer long-term outcomes.

• • •

Adequate nourishment is vital for healthy neurological development and to prevent newborn hypoglycemia and jaundice.

Due to preterm babies' physical immaturity at birth, they are at greater risk for hypoglycemia and jaundice, and also due to their immaturity, a more moderate drop in blood-sugar levels and lower levels of bilirubin are more risky for them. Adequate nourishment helps prevent health complications from these conditions. This is true, too, with late preterm babies, who may look mature but not feed vigorously at birth (see later section).

Adequate nutrition, especially during the first 2 weeks after birth, is also important to very preterm babies' neurological development. Malnutrition was linked to slower growth in head circumference (Regev et al., 2016) and the growth of white matter in the brain (Schneider et al., 2018) and other indicators of neurodevelopment (Belfort et al., 2011).

• • •

If the baby is gaining slowly on expressed milk alone and weight gain is a concern, discuss possible adjustments that might boost weight gain.

If a preemie's healthcare providers are concerned about the baby's weight gain, ask the family about their baby's target weight gain. Sometimes the target is not a daily weight gain but rather a body mass index (BMI) or a weight-for-height z-score. Acceptable weight gain may be 15 to 30 g or 0.5 to 1 ounce per day, but if the baby fell behind in expected weight gain, healthcare providers may want to try to boost it faster to catch up to where the baby should be.

If the preterm baby's weight gain is slow enough to be of concern and the baby is receiving mostly expressed mother's milk, some adjustments in how the milk is expressed, handled, or fed may help. Suggest asking first if the baby might be ready to handle more milk per feed or if the same volume could be given more times per day. With rapid growth, sometimes feeding volumes are not increased quickly enough. An Australian randomized clinical trial (Kuschel et al., 2000) found that giving more milk to preemies born at less than 30 weeks gestation resulted in faster weight gain by 35 weeks, but there were no differences in overall growth or health outcomes at 1 year. See also the later section "Fortification and Hindmilk Feeding" on increasing the fat content of mother's milk and its fortification with protein and other nutrients.

In a 2017 overview article (P. P. Meier et al., 2017), U.S. NICU expert Paula Meier described some milk-expression, storage, and handling factors that can unintentionally slow a preemie's weight gain:

- During milk expression, not draining the mammary gland as thoroughly as possible. To remedy this, suggest the hands-on pumping techniques described on p. 492.
- Changing containers during a pump session and providing the first, low-fat milk. To remedy this, ask for larger containers.
- Not realizing that the layer of fat at the top of the expressed milk is normal and discarding it. Parents need to know its impact on weight gain.

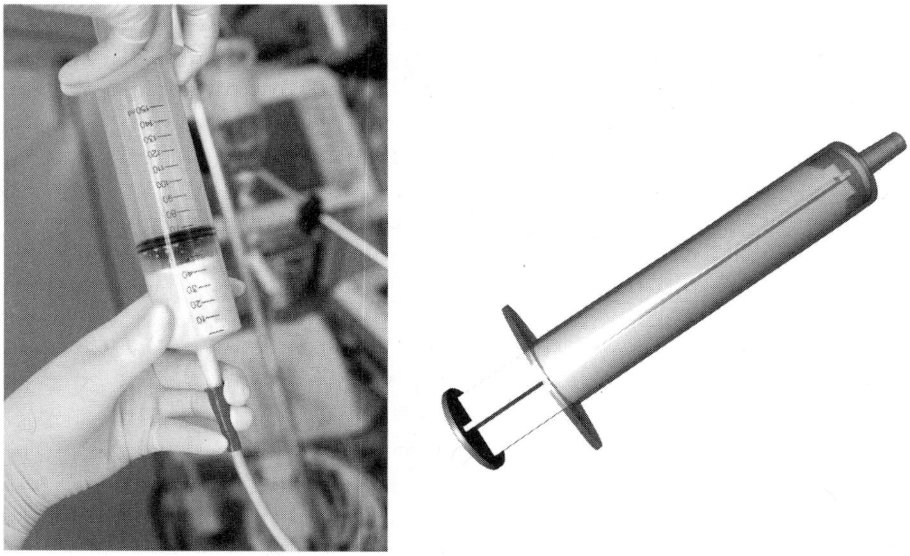

Figure 9.3 If a preemie is tube-fed using an infusion syringe, instead of positioning it vertically (left), inverting it (right) causes milk fat to rise to the top, preventing fat loss.

- Transferring the milk into another container and leaving milk fat behind in the original container's crevices. Review mixing and transferring instructions.
- Baby is fed with a slow, continuous gavage tube system that traps the milk fat in the tubing. Suggest switching to intermittent feeds.
- Infusion syringes used to tube-feed the baby are positioned so that the fat rises away from the tubing. Suggest changing the syringe position so that the milk fat rises to the tubing (Figure 9.3).

If the baby is exclusively nursing and gaining weight slowly despite taking significant milk volumes, Meier suggests avoiding switching sides often and supplement baby with milk expressed after nursing.

Supplementing Nursing

Until they reach stage 6 or 7 of the stages of preterm nursing (Box 9.2 on p. 355), most preterm babies will need to be supplemented.

Milk Issues

It may be upsetting if expressed milk volumes fall short or if the baby's provider says that expressed milk needs to be fortified.

Too little expressed milk or the need for its fortification may leave a family feeling discouraged, demoralized, and upset. Some consider giving up, even when exclusive nursing was their original goal. A family in this situation needs to talk about their feelings and to receive reassurance and support. See the later section "Risks of Non-Human Milks" for some of the many reasons any volume of mother's own milk is important to a preemie's health. Be sure the family knows that some expressed milk is always better than none and that any fortification will be temporary.

Milk Production Challenges

Parents' age and other factors affect their risk of low milk production and weaning.

In some countries, family demographics influence the odds of both giving birth to a preterm baby and of meeting—or not meeting—milk-production goals (Romaine et al., 2018). Parents more likely to meet milk-production goals are older, white, live in safer neighborhoods, and have more income, education, and support for nursing. These families are also more likely to produce higher milk volumes, to nurse their preemie after NICU discharge, and to nurse for a longer time. Conversely, parents at greater risk for inadequate milk production for their preemie and giving up during the NICU stay are younger, non-white (in the U.S., especially African-American), live in unsafe neighborhoods, and have less income, education, and family support for nursing (M. G. Parker et al., 2019). Some researchers concluded that families at-risk due to racial, ethnic, and economic disparities need more targeted interventions (such as staff and patient education, free home breast-pump use, and easy access to lactation consultants and peer counselors) than other families (Dereddy, Talati, Smith, Kudumula, & Dhanireddy, 2015).

• • •

Families cope more easily with milk expression when they know what to expect at each stage and how their actions affect their ability to meet their long-term goals.

The experience of exclusive milk expression varies at different stages of lactation. For example, during the first few days after birth, it is common to express only drops or even no milk at all. But there is no milk volume too small to save for the baby, and the time spent expressing during those early days quickly leads to much more milk. See p. 500-503 for a description of what to expect at each stage.

Early and frequent milk expression is vital to adequate milk production later (Morton et al., 2009; L. A. Parker, Sullivan, Krueger, Kelechi, & Mueller, 2012). Nearly half of those expressing for babies in the NICU experience common problems, such as nipple pain, low milk production, and engorgement (Dowling et al., 2012). Families are more likely to give up if they are unaware of these common problems and how to solve them (Lucas et al., 2014). In other words, talking to families about possible problems and their solutions can help them continue to provide expressed milk for their at-risk baby.

If a family finds it difficult to express milk often enough or if there are other challenges, offer to brainstorm. If fitting in enough milk expressions is the problem, talk to them about their daily routine, emphasizing that the daily expression total is the top priority and the intervals between milk expressions are not as important. For example, some find it easier to meet their daily milk-expression totals if they express every hour for the part of the day they are more available or have help.

• • •

The factors that affect milk volumes most during the first 2 weeks are the number of milk expressions per day and how effectively the milk is removed.

How early baby was born does not appear—in some studies—to have a major effect on overall milk production. For example, one Canadian secondary analysis of data from 90 mothers (Asztalos et al., 2019) found that when these mothers followed best milk-expression practices, the milk volumes produced by mothers who gave birth before 30 weeks was comparable to those who delivered their preemies later. Another small Canadian study of 24 mothers (Bishara, Dunn, Merko, & Darling, 2009), however, found that those who delivered before 26 weeks produced milk with a different proportion of foremilk and hindmilk than mothers who delivered later. Two small studies conducted in the U.S. and China (Hoban, Patel, et al., 2018; Yu, Li, Lin, & Luan, 2019) found that giving birth very preterm can delay milk increase during the first week.

The first 2 weeks is a critical period for milk production. As Chapter 10 describes, during the first 14 days, mammary stimulation triggers higher levels of blood prolactin (a hormone linked to milk production) than the levels triggered by stimulation after the first 2 weeks. During this early time window, the birthing parent's body is most responsive to stimulation, producing the most milk with the least effort. (See also p. 425 on the "lactation curve.") Milk production of ≥500 mL (17 oz.) per day at 2 weeks is one predictor that a preemie will still be receiving mother's-own-milk feeds at NICU discharge (Hoban, Bigger, et al., 2018).

Hands-on pumping yields on average 50% more milk. A U.S. prospective study compared milk volumes of 67 mothers of babies born at less than 31 weeks gestation who were taught hands-on pumping techniques (Morton et al., 2009). These study mothers did not rely on the pump alone to remove milk. They also used manual techniques of breast massage, compression during pumping, and hand expression after pumping (see p. 492). This study concluded:

- To establish abundant milk production, pumping 7 or more times each day during the first 2 weeks after birth is necessary.
- Those using hands-on techniques averaged nearly 50% higher milk volumes than comparable mothers using the pump alone.
- Milk-fat content was nearly double that of those who used the pump alone (Morton et al., 2012).
- After the first 2 weeks, removing the milk more fully each time with the hands-on techniques was more important to maintaining and even increasing milk production than the number of pump sessions per day.

Some of the study mothers saw an increase in their milk volumes after 2 weeks, even though they dropped to an average of 6 pump sessions per day.

• • •

It is common for milk volumes to fluctuate with the baby's condition.

When the family is very worried about the baby's health or survival, milk ejection may be delayed or inhibited (see p. 480-481), decreasing the volume of milk expressed (Chatterton et al., 2000). Times of crisis may cause a temporary decrease in milk expressed, which can also affect production. During this time, unsupportive comments from others may convince the family to give up entirely unless they have a source of support. Assure them that this decrease is only temporary and milk production will rebound as the baby's condition improves. It may also be comforting to talk to another family who has had a similar experience.

• • •

A healthy milk production is one factor associated with nursing at and after NICU discharge.

Several studies found—not surprisingly—that producing inadequate volumes of milk was associated with shorter duration of human-milk feeding and lower likelihood of direct nursing after discharge (Casey et al., 2018; Fleurant et al., 2017; Gianni et al., 2018).

Health Risks of Non-Human Milks

Preterm babies fed formula are at greater risk for many complications of prematurity, some life-threatening.

All babies, preterm included, benefit from the bioactive components of mother's milk, such as anti-oxidants, cytokines, growth factors, and others that contribute to healthy growth and development (Gila-Diaz et al., 2019). But non-human milks, including infant formula, are problematic for very-low-birth-weight preterm babies in ways that differ from other babies. Formula is not risky for tiny preemies just because these bioactive components are missing. Formula contains inflammatory factors that may damage their fragile organs (Ginovart, Gich, & Verd, 2016). In fact, in some cases, mother's milk can make the difference between life and death. That's why some researchers (P. P. Meier, 2019) strongly recommend making "high-dose long exposure to mother's own milk" a high priority in NICUs and why many NICUs make donor human milk available when mother's own milk is in short supply. Here are some of the ways non-human milks like formula increase health risks in tiny preemies.

Digestive tract. One of the most dangerous complications of prematurity is necrotizing enterocolitis, or NEC for short. When a baby contracts NEC, part of his bowel becomes inflamed and dies. The earlier a baby is born, the more vulnerable he is to NEC. Of the tiniest babies born between 500 and 750 g, 12% developed NEC in the hospital and 42% of those died from it (Knell, Han, Jaksic, & Modi, 2019). One of the most effective ways to prevent NEC is to completely avoid formula, which causes gut inflammation, at least until a baby is 33 or 34 weeks gestation (Patel & Kim, 2018). One U.S. study found that digested formula but not digested fresh human milk caused the death of intestinal cells (Penn et al., 2012), which could be a precursor to NEC.

Brain. A U.S. experimental study of preemies born at 28 to 32 weeks gestation (Amin, Merle, Orlando, Dalzell, & Guillet, 2000) found the use of formula was associated with slower maturation of the babies' brainstem. A 2016 Australian longitudinal cohort study (Belfort et al., 2016) found that at 7 years of age, 180 children born at less 30 weeks gestation for whom human milk comprised less than half of their total intake had measurably less nuclear gray brain matter, lower IQ scores, and poorer motor function than those whose milk intake was more than half human-milk.

Eyes. Formula may also contribute to a vision problem in preemies known as retinopathy of prematurity, or ROP. A 2015 meta-analysis examined 5 studies of 2,208 preemies (Zhou, Shukla, John, & Chen, 2015) and concluded that in very preterm newborns, formula-fed babies were more likely to develop ROP and human-milk feeding plays a protective role in preventing it.

Lungs. Breathing problems, such as bronchopulmonary dysplasia, are another complication of prematurity. A U.S. 5-year prospective cohort study of 254 very-low-birth-weight preemies (Patel et al., 2017) concluded that mother's-own-milk feeds from birth to 36 weeks were associated with a reduction in the odds of developing this condition.

Infections. Immune factors in both colostrum and mature milk (macrophages, leukocytes, secretory IgA, and more) bind microbes and prevent them from entering the baby's delicate tissues. They kill microorganisms, block inflammation, and promote normal growth of the baby's thymus, an organ devoted solely to developing normal immune function. At age 4 months, the thymus of formula-fed babies is half the size of nursing babies (Hasselbalch, Jeppesen, Engelmann, Michaelsen, & Nielsen, 1996). As a result, the more human milk a preemie consumes, the lower the risk of serious infection, such as late-onset sepsis (a life-threatening blood infection). A 2019 Dutch multicenter case-control study of 755 preterm infants, 194 with late-onset sepsis (El Manouni El Hassani et al., 2019), concluded that formula-feeding was an independent risk factor and human milk was protective of late-onset sepsis. A 2013 U.S. prospective cohort study of 175 very-low-birth-weight preemies found a dose-response relationship between human milk and decreased risk of sepsis (Patel et al., 2013) and concluded that for every extra 10 mL (0.3 ounce)

KEY CONCEPT

Human milk prevents many complications of prematurity.

per day of human milk, a very-low-birth-weight preemie received, his risk of sepsis decreased by 19%.

The Use of Donor Milk

Donor human milk from milk banks is more available now than in the past in NICUs internationally.

During the last decade, donor human milk from nonprofit and for-profit milk banks became more readily available in NICUs around the world (Kantorowska et al., 2016; Perrine & Scanlon, 2013). The donor milk provided by most milk banks consists of term mother's milk that is pooled from many carefully screened donors. In Muslim countries, however, milk banks limit the number of donors whose milk is pooled, because Muslim children who share milk from the same nursing parent are not allowed to marry (Ghaly, 2018). For this reason, recipients of donor milk from these milk banks are provided with the names of the milk donors. Guidelines in Europe, North America, and Brazil (which has more than 200 milk banks) require pasteurization of donor milk before distribution (HMBANA, 2018; Langland, 2019; Weaver et al., 2019). Pasteurizing reduces some of the protective components of human milk, but also kills any viruses and bacteria (Silvestre, Ruiz, Martinez-Costa, Plaza, & Lopez, 2008).

• • •

Feeding preemies with mother's own milk leads to better health outcomes, but donor human milk is a good second choice.

Several aspects of banked donor milk make it less desirable than mother's own milk:

- Most donor milk consists of term milk, so it is lower than preterm milk in many of the extra nutrients small preemies need
- When donor milk is substituted for mother's own colostrum and transitional milk, the preemies do not receive the unique components that prepare their digestive and immune systems.
- Pasteurization decreases the milk's bioactivity, so although it prevents NEC (see previous point), it is not as effective in preventing infection or promoting healthy growth as mother's own milk (Hard et al., 2019; Kantorowska et al., 2016).

Even so, for preemies, donor milk offers health advantages over formula. A 2019 Cochrane Review (Quigley, Embleton, & McGuire, 2019) concluded that preterm babies fed donor milk rather than formula (which increases inflammation in the gut) had significantly lower rates of necrotizing enterocolitis, or NEC, which can be lifesaving. On the negative side, weight gain and growth were slower with donor milk as compared with formula. At this writing, some milk banks, such as the Mothers' Milk Bank in Austin, Texas, provide donor milk higher in calories and can provide donor milk fortified with specific nutrients for preemies with special needs. When a preemie is gaining weight slowly with donor milk, it is also vital to make sure milk fat is not being lost when donor milk is fed to the baby (see previous point) or to consider the use of fortification of donor milk (see next section).

A U.K. systematic review of the use of donor milk in NICUs and its effect on nursing and the use of mother's own milk (Williams, Nair, Simpson, & Embleton, 2016) found that introducing donor milk into NICUs increased any nursing at discharge but had no effect on exclusive nursing. It noted that in one single-center study, there was a significant decrease in mother's-own-milk feeds over time, so it's important to emphasize to families that even when donor milk is available, their expressed milk is still vital to their baby's health (P. Meier, Patel, & Esquerra-Zwiers, 2017).

Fortification and Hindmilk Feeding

Parents who give birth prematurely produce milk higher in several key nutrients (Boyce et al., 2016). But within a month after delivery, their preterm milk gradually changes to term milk, even though their babies' need for extra nutrients remains high. Some preterm babies grow and develop well when fed exclusively human milk (Jarvenpaa, Raiha, Rassin, & Gaull, 1983; Ramasethu, Jeyaseelan, & Kirubakaran, 1993). But despite the low quality of evidence available, it has become standard practice in many parts of the world to add extra protein, calcium, phosphorus, and sometimes other nutrients to mother's milk for extremely early and small preemies (Arslanoglu et al., 2019). A 2016 Cochrane Review on fortification of mother's milk for tiny preemies (Brown, Embleton, Harding, & McGuire, 2016) concluded that adding these extra nutrients increased only short-term weight gain, length and head growth during the NICU stay, but had no long-term benefits. NICU lactation expert Diane Spatz wrote (Spatz, 2017, p. 117):

Very early and small preemies may grow faster in the short term—but not necessarily in the long term—when extra protein and other nutrients are added to mother's milk.

KEY CONCEPT

Fortification of expressed milk for very early preemies appears to improve weight gain in the short term but may not have long-term benefits.

> "This routine fortification of human milk can lead mothers to question why their milk is 'not good enough for their infant'....In many NICUs, the expectation is that infants gain 15 to 30 g/day. It is evident from the meta-analysis that adding fortifiers to milk is not solving the concern of weight gain. One must question if the small gains in head circumference and length are clinically significant."

A Swedish study found that although the babies who received fortifiers grew faster, there was also more illness in the fortified group and that exclusive breastfeeding led to later improvement in growth (Funkquist, Tuvemo, Jonsson, Serenius, & Hedberg-Nyqvist, 2006). A 2019 review that compared the results of studies on early versus delayed fortification (Alyahya, Simpson, Garcia, Mactier, & Edwards, 2019) found there were no consistent definitions of these terms and no significant impact on growth of early versus delayed fortification.

The term "lacto-engineering" refers to adding extra human-milk protein or fat to mother's milk. Over the last decade, commercial companies have developed and released human-milk-based fortifiers for use in NICUs (Czank, Simmer, & Hartmann, 2010; Hair et al., 2016; Oliveira et al., 2019). One drawback of the cow-milk-based fortifiers many NICUs currently use is that exposure to cow-milk protein was found to cause gut inflammation in very-low-birth-weight babies (Panczuk et al., 2016), which has the potential to increase the risk of NEC.

• • •

Rather than giving every preterm baby of the same gestational age and weight the same amount of standard fortifier, fortification can be tailored to the individual needs of each preemie. Two ways of individualizing milk fortification are

According to research, there are benefits to tailoring any fortification to preemies' individual needs.

- Adjustable fortification, which is based on blood tests
- Targeted fortification, which is based on an analysis of the milk (either mother's milk or donor milk)

Some randomized controlled trials indicated that targeted fortification may be more effective than standard or adjustable fortification at improving preemies' short-term weight gain (Bulut, Coban, Uzunhan, & Ince, 2019; Kadioglu Simsek et al., 2019; Rochow, Landau-Crangle, & Fusch, 2015).

• • •

Some slow-gaining preterm babies may benefit from receiving more hindmilk.

Another form of lacto-engineering known as "hindmilk feeding" helps some preemies gain weight faster. This may involve adding extra high-fat hindmilk to expressed milk or storing the first milk expressed for future use, keeping the fattier milk at the end of the expression to feed the baby now, as hindmilk averages double or triple the fat content of foremilk and can boost the calories consumed. Of course, this strategy is practical only for parents expressing more milk than their baby is consuming. In one Canadian experimental study (Bishara et al., 2009), 82% of its 39 mothers who delivered at less than 28 weeks gestation expressed enough milk to provide hindmilk feeds for their preterm babies. In some NICUs, the milk's fat content is measured with a device called a creamatocrit. The results are used to make adjustments to parents' expression routine, and the higher-fat, higher-calorie milk is fed to the baby (P. P. Meier et al., 2017).

Hindmilk feeding was used successfully to increase preterm weight gain in both developed and developing countries (Galloway & Howells, 2015; Ogechi, William, & Fidelia, 2007; Valentine, Hurst, & Schanler, 1994). Foremilk and hindmilk contain about the same amount of protein, so if extra protein is recommended, hindmilk alone will not provide it (Valentine et al., 1994). In some cases, fortifiers may be used in combination with hindmilk feeding. One Canadian experimental study found that because vitamins A and E are concentrated in fat, preterm babies receiving both hindmilk feeding and fortifiers may receive more than the recommended amounts (Bishara, Dunn, Merko, & Darling, 2008).

Milk Handling and Safety

Colostrum and mature milk should ideally be fed fresh in the order they were expressed.

Many hospitals make it a priority to use freshly expressed mother's own milk, because it contains more of the components (immunomodulatory proteins) that protect babies from infection than frozen or pasteurized milk (Akinbi et al., 2010). If the baby is not yet ready to directly nurse, first treating the baby's mouth with fresh colostrum or tube-feeding the colostrum to him helps promote healthy gut flora and prepare his digestive system for oral feeds (Garofalo & Caplan, 2019). In some NICUs, mother's milk containers are given color-coded labels to distinguish colostrum from transitional and mature milk, so colostrum can be given first (P. P. Meier et al., 2017). After the baby receives all of the expressed colostrum, suggest that for the first month, the fresh or frozen mature milk be given in the order in which it was expressed.

• • •

If formula is given, suggest giving it separately, rather than mixing it with mother's milk, especially previously frozen expressed milk.

In some cases, mother's milk and donor milk are in short supply, so formula may be needed. Although there is limited information about mixing human milk and formula, there may be some advantages to feeding them separately, especially when previously frozen milk is used (Jones, 2019, p. 110). One U.S. study (Quan et al., 1994) found that when cow-milk-based formula was mixed with previously frozen expressed milk before feeds, this reduced lysozyme activity in the expressed milk by 41% to 74%. Lysozyme in human milk fights infection by destroying the cell walls of bacteria. Other studies found an association between the decrease in anti-infective activity in human milk and an increase in the harmful bacteria *E. coli* (Narayanan, Prakash, Murthy, & Gujral, 1984; Quan et al., 1992). One U.S. study (Schanler & Abrams, 1995) recommended alternating feeds of human milk with feeds of formula, because mineral absorption was greater.

Does mixing the formula available today with fresh milk have these same effects? At this writing, we don't know.

• • •

Guidelines for milk collection and storage for hospitalized babies may be different from those used by parents of healthy term babies at home.

In years past, parents expressing milk for preemies often received a long list of procedures thought to reduce contamination of the milk. Later, though, these procedures were found to be unnecessary. They included breast/nipple cleansing before pumping, nipple lubrication during pumping, sterilizing pump parts after each use, discarding the first milk expressed, routine bacterial screening of the expressed milk, and pasteurizing mother's own milk. Pasteurization of mother's own milk, while unnecessary for parents expressing milk for their own baby, may be important for donor milk (for details, see the next section).

Research-based guidelines used by many North American hospitals to set their protocols are available in the book *Best Practice for Expressing, Storing and Handling Human Milk in Hospitals, Home and Child Care Settings* (Jones, 2019), published by the Human Milk Banking Association of North America (HMBANA). It recommended the following hygiene practices for all pumping parents of preemies.

- Wash hands well before touching pump parts and containers.
- After each use, wash the pump parts and containers as instructed.
- Keep fingers away from the inside of milk-storage containers.

Because preemies are more vulnerable than babies born at term, some hospitals create their own independent expression and storage guidelines for parents expressing milk for babies in the NICU. Suggest the family talk to their hospital staff for instructions. Guidelines for healthy term babies at home are on p. 514.

• • •

If fortifier is added to expressed milk, it should be used within 24 hours.

A U.S. experimental study (Santiago, Codipilly, Potak, & Schanler, 2005) found that adding cow-milk-based fortifiers to mother's milk did not affect bacteria counts, and even with the fortifier added, expressed milk continued to reduce bacterial levels for the first 72 hours. Another U.S. experimental study (Jocson, Mason, & Schanler, 1997) found that neither bacteria counts nor IgA levels in the milk were affected by adding cow-milk-based fortifier, but the milk's osmolality (number of dissolved particles in a fluid) increased with storage over time. For that reason, a maximum storage time of 24 hours is recommended by the Human Milk Banking Association of North America (Jones, 2019) for human milk with fortifier added.

• • •

Mother's milk is not sterile and no standards have yet been set for acceptable bacterial levels, so routine screening of expressed milk is not helpful.

Some hospitals culture expressed milk due to the mistaken assumption that milk bacterial levels indicate how hygienically families express and collect milk. But a 2013 Malaysian study found no link between hygiene during milk expression and bacterial counts (Dahaban, Romli, Roslan, Kong, & Cheah, 2013). Also, expressed milk is not sterile, so some bacteria in the milk is normal. Milk is usually judged acceptable if it does not contain certain disease-causing organisms and contains low levels of other types of bacteria, such as skin flora. But currently, there are no accepted, research-based standards for "safe" milk, so the results of this testing are often inconclusive. The Human Milk Banking Association of North America recommended against routine bacterial screening of expressed mother's own milk, except in the rare event a high-risk infant receiving expressed milk develops signs of infection (Jones, 2019, p. 19). In this situation, a milk culture may indicate whether the expressed milk contributed to the infection.

Cytomegalovirus (CMV) and Other Maternal Illnesses

In some situations, the CMV virus in mother's milk may put tiny preterm babies at risk of serious illness.

Cytomegalovirus (CMV) is the most widespread of the herpes viruses that infect humans. By 40 years of age, more than half of U.S. adults are infected with CMV for life (CDC, 2019). When infected, few experience symptoms of CMV, which include fatigue, fever, and swollen lymph glands.

If the birthing parent is CMV-positive during pregnancy, the baby is exposed to both the virus and its antibodies in utero. The CMV virus and its antibodies are also shed into the milk of CMV-positive parents (Schleiss, 2006). In full-term healthy babies, mother's milk acts like a vaccine, with more than two-thirds of the full-term babies of CMV-positive parents born positive for CMV but without symptoms.

For preterm babies, the risk of developing severe illness from CMV in expressed milk is low. In one 2014 U.S. prospective cohort study of 539 preemies born at ≤1500 g (Josephson et al., 2014), blood tests found that 7% acquired CMV from expressed milk but only 17% of those babies (1% of the total) developed symptoms of CMV. Unlike babies born at term, babies are born very preterm with an immature immune system, making them more vulnerable to infections of all kinds (Bryant, Morley, Garland, & Curtis, 2002).

• • •

When there is a possibility of CMV transmission via expressed milk, processing the expressed milk may reduce or eliminate any risk.

When tiny preterm babies are born CMV-negative and their birthing parents are CMV-positive or the parents' CMV status is unknown, there is no international consensus on the best course of action (Eidelman, 2016).

The American Academy of Pediatrics wrote (AAP, 2012, p. e833):

> "The value of routinely feeding human milk from [CMV] seropositive mothers to preterm infants outweighs the risk of clinical disease…fresh mother's own milk is preferable."

In other parts of the world, though, recommendations vary. One article (Eidelman, 2016) summarized:

- France: Raw expressed milk is fed only to preemies older than 32 weeks gestation.
- Sweden: In CMV-positive mothers, previously frozen milk is fed to babies born <32 weeks.
- Australia: In CMV-positive mothers, Holder pasteurized milk is fed until 35 weeks.
- Germany: In CMV-positive mothers of babies born at <1,000 g or <30 weeks, many neonatologists recommend feeding only heat-treated expressed milk.

Processing mother's expressed milk can kill CMV or reduce the virus levels before feeding the milk to tiny preemies. Using Holder pasteurization to treat mother's milk (heating it to 62.5°C [145°F] for 30 minutes) kills the virus and eliminates the risk of infection, but it also destroys or reduces some of the milk's protective components. A 2019 review article described the published research on many milk-processing options (Wesolowska et al., 2019). For example, heating mother's milk briefly at a high temperature (short-term pasteurization of 72°C [162°F] for 10 to 15 seconds) kills the CMV virus and also preserves more of the milk's protective components. Freezing mother's milk reduces virus levels, but does not completely eliminate it (Ben-Shoshan, Mandel, Lubetzky, Dollberg, & Mimouni, 2016; Buxmann et al., 2009). Even microwaving the milk—long cautioned against—was studied and found effective at killing 100% of the CMV in the milk (Mikawa et al., 2019). But more research is needed. After reviewing these and other milk-processing options, the authors of the 2019 overview article wrote (Wesolowska et al., 2019, p. 12):

> "Data evaluating the effectiveness of interventions with thermal pasteurized donor milk are not clear, and there are no clinical trials concerning new techniques. Therefore, studies with human participants are needed to be carried out with the most promising new techniques of human milk processing in comparison to Holder pasteurization."

In each situation, the family and baby's healthcare providers need to weigh the risk of active CMV disease with the risks associated with processing mother's own milk.

• • •

Few maternal illnesses contraindicate feeding mother's milk to a preterm baby.

The very few illnesses in the nursing parent that would contraindicate providing expressed milk to the preterm baby include HIV (only in developed countries), HTLV-1 and 2, and active tuberculosis before treatment. For details, see p. 824-827 in Chapter 19.

There are also few illnesses the nursing parent of a preemie could have that require temporarily expressing and discarding milk. These include varicella-zoster (chickenpox), measles, and herpes sores on or near the nipple. If a herpes sore comes in contact with the nursing parent's hands or pump parts, the milk needs to be discarded until the herpes sore heals.

Nursing Parent's Diet and Medications

In most cases, dietary restrictions are unnecessary.

Diet does not usually have a major effect on the quality or quantity of mother's milk, unless the nursing parent's diet is very restricted, which may contribute to vitamin deficiencies (for details see p. 555-556). It's not necessary to eat a perfect diet to produce good quality milk. Milk production aside, however, a poor diet, may negatively affect other aspects of a nursing parent's life, such as mood, energy levels, and resistance to illness.

• • •

Before taking any prescribed or over-the-counter medications, suggest discussing it with the baby's healthcare provider.

A preterm baby is more vulnerable than a term baby to drugs taken by the nursing parent that pass into the milk. The preemie is more vulnerable due to his small size and immature ability to process and excrete them. For this reason, the baby's healthcare provider should evaluate any drug's compatibility in light of the baby's size and condition before the nursing parent begins taking it.

However, even when a specific drug is problematic, a substitute compatible with continued nursing and/or expressed milk feedings is likely available.

• • •

Suggest talking to the baby's healthcare provider before smoking cigarettes, drinking alcohol, and/or using other legal or illegal substances.

Alcohol, nicotine, cannabis, and other substances all pass into mother's milk to some extent. Because a preterm baby is less able to process these substances than a healthy, term baby, it is vital to discuss this with the baby's healthcare provider, even if it involves an occasional cigarette or alcoholic drink. Legal and illegal substances may pose significant risk to a very preterm baby.

Feeding Methods

Depending on a preterm baby's gestational age and condition, at first, he may be fed intravenously or by tube.

If the baby is very small or ill, he may first be fed a nutrient-rich solution via IV (called "parenteral nutrition"). When milk feeds by mouth begin, in some parts of the world, they may be given continuously by tube. In other parts of the world, continuous feeds are not used and milk feeds are begun with small or larger volumes (called a "bolus") fed every couple of hours, often through a nasogastric (or NG) tube, also called "gavage feeding." Whenever possible, encourage the family to put the baby in skin-to-skin contact during these feeds to help him better digest the milk. Skin-to-skin contact during feeds also increases expressed milk volumes and may lead to earlier nursing (N. M. Hurst et al., 1997).

• • •

When the baby begins taking oral feeds, suggest starting with nursing, but if supplements are needed or the parent will not be present for all feeds, discuss the other feeding methods.

The previous section "When to Start Nursing" described why nursing is a preemie's best first oral feed. However, as preterm babies transition from gavage (tube) feeding to oral feeds, most require extra milk after direct nursing. In some NICUs, tube-feeding provides needed supplements (see next point). When supplements are needed along with nursing, see the section "Alternative Feeding Methods," starting on p. 894 for the pros and cons of each. Some parents have strong preferences about feeding methods, which should be honored and supported, but all parents deserve to receive the information needed to make an informed choice.

Bottle-feeding. Although the use of feeding bottles is common in many developed countries, research (Blaymore Bier et al., 1997; Chen et al., 2000; P. Meier & Anderson, 1987; Poets, Langner, & Bohnhorst, 1997) found that due to the fast, consistent flow, bottle-feeding preemies can cause breathing and heart-rate irregularities, as well as oxygen desaturation. A 2016 Cochrane Review (Collins, Gillis, McPhee, Suganuma, & Makrides, 2016) concluded that with preterm babies, avoiding bottles and using cups instead increased the extent and duration of nursing.

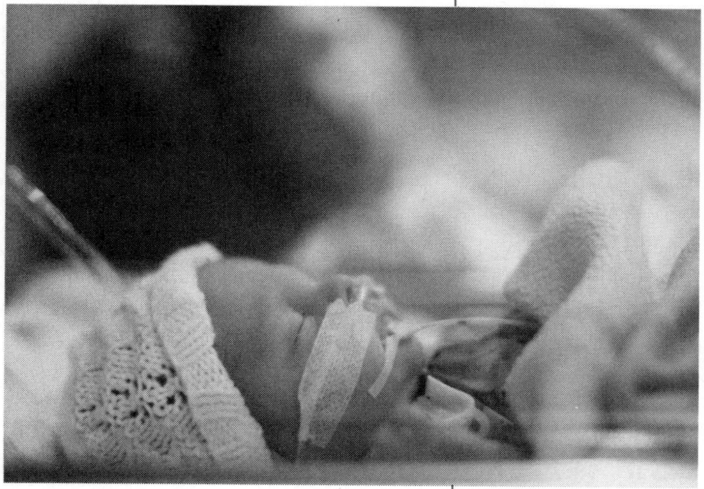

NG tube (gavage feeding). One U.S. randomized controlled trial (Kliethermes, Cross, Lanese, Johnson, & Simon, 1999) found that babies who were supplemented only by nasogastric (NG) tube were 4.5 times more likely to be nursing at hospital discharge and more than 9.0 times more likely to be exclusively nursed than the babies who were supplemented by bottle. At 3 months, the babies supplemented by NG tube were 3.0 times more likely to be nursing and 3.0 times more likely to be fully breastfeeding than the preemies who were supplemented by bottle.

Cup-feeding is used routinely in some developed countries (Nyqvist, 2017). Brazilian research found the muscles used and feeding behaviors in babies while cup-feeding were closer to nursing than other feeding methods (Franca, Sousa, Aragao, & Costa, 2014; Gomes, Trezza, Murade, & Padovani, 2006). In parts of the developing world, cup-feeding is used where an unsafe water supply makes bottle-feeding dangerous (N. J. Bergman & Jurisoo, 1994). A cup-like device called a paladai is used traditionally in India to supplement preterm babies (Aloysius & Hickson, 2007; Malhotra, Vishwambaran, Sundaram, & Narayanan, 1999). One early U.K. study on cup-feeding compared 85 preterm babies and found that babies could successfully feed by cup as young as 30 weeks gestation, earlier than they could bottle-feed (Lang, Lawrence, & Orme, 1994). More of the babies fed by cup were fully nursing at hospital discharge than those fed by bottle (81% vs. 63%). A 2018 integrative review of the literature on cup-feeding preterm babies (Penny, Judge, Brownell, & McGrath, 2018) concluded that when fed by cup, preterm babies had more stable heart rates and oxygen saturation than when fed by bottle. A 2016 Cochrane Review on cup feeding (Flint, New, & Davies, 2016) compared babies fed by cup and bottle and concluded there was no difference in weight gain or gestational age at discharge, but those fed by cup were more likely to be exclusively nursing at discharge and were more likely to be directly nursing at some feeds at 3 and 6 months, compared to the preemies fed by bottle. For more details on cup-feeding, see p. 894-896.

Transitioning to Full Nursing

How long the process to full nursing takes depends on many factors: how early the baby was born, the baby's health, the level of milk production, how much time the baby spends nursing, and the cultural norms. This transition may happen in the NICU or at home.

• • •

When a preterm baby sometimes takes large volumes of milk while nursing, it may be time to begin the transition to full nursing.

The seven stages of preterm nursing developed by Swedish researcher Kerstin Hedberg-Nyqvist (Box 9.2 on p. 355) comprise the "road map" parents can use to chart their preemie's nursing progress. In Sweden, preemies are not discharged from the NICUs until they are fully nursing, which usually happens during the sixth stage. During that stage, preemies still have an "immature sucking pattern," which Nyqvist describes as short sucking bursts with the baby holding his breath and breathing during pauses (Nyqvist, 2013). These preemies are not yet ready to nurse on cue. But with help from the nursing parent, preemies in this sixth stage can nurse fully using a strategy called "semi-demand feeding" (see next point).

• • •

Good health and experience with nursing improves feeding effectiveness, so if it is possible, encourage frequent direct nursing.

Some researchers suggested that most preterm babies cannot feed effectively until they reach term age of 40 weeks gestation (P. P. Meier et al., 2017), but the Swedish experience indicates otherwise.

Experience matters. In studies conducted in Sweden, nursing experience has a greater impact on nursing effectiveness than gestational age alone. Swedish researcher Kerstin Hedberg-Nyqvist described one of her many studies, in which

94% of the preemies were breastfeeding at hospital discharge, 80% exclusively and 14% partially (Nyqvist, 2017, p. 190):

> "Infants with…a longer period of separation from their mothers (number of days when the mother was not living in a parent room in the unit) established breastfeeding at a higher [postmenstrual age] and postnatal age. Low [gestational age] at birth was associated with early efficient breastfeeding behavior and a high incidence of full breastfeeding. This supports the theory that infant motor development occurs with experience. Oral motor competence is triggered when the nipple touches the infant's lips, the nipple touches the hard palate, and milk flows into the infant's mouth."

Preemies' sucking patterns are different from those of full-term babies, but this does not necessarily make them less effective. Nyqvist noted that preterm babies' nursing effectiveness should not be gauged by how closely their sucking pattern resembles that of a full-term baby. Rather (Nyqvist, 2013, p. 298), "Breastfeeding success in preterm infants should be defined only as the ability to take a sufficient daily milk volume for having a sustained growth." Where preterm babies were given lots of nursing time, two Swedish studies found that 85% of the babies were exclusively breastfeeding at 36 weeks gestation, with some fully breastfeeding as young as 32 weeks gestation (Nyqvist, 2008; Nyqvist et al., 1999). In one of these studies, the median age of exclusive breastfeeding was 35 weeks (Nyqvist, 2008). Many started nursing at 27 or 28 weeks, and at an average of 30.6 weeks, these preemies began to take milk while breastfeeding. With regular nursing, by 36 weeks, 57 of the 67 babies were exclusively breastfeeding (Nyqvist et al., 1999).

Health problems decrease preemies' nursing effectiveness. Health problems were associated with less effective nursing, and these babies took longer to nurse exclusively than healthy preemies. Neurological issues, among others, can delay effective nursing, which requires an intact and well-functioning central nervous system (Radzyminski, 2005). One Japanese study found that very-low-birthweight preterm babies with the respiratory problem bronchopulmonary dysplasia had more feeding problems than those without it (Mizuno et al., 2007). The more severe the breathing problem, the less sucking pressure the babies could generate, the fewer the babies' sucking bursts and swallows, and the lower their oxygen levels during feeds.

• • •

Suggest the parent plan to be available to nurse at as many feeds as possible.

Giving preterm babies ample nursing experience can be easy or difficult, depending on the cultural climate. In Sweden where nursing is the norm, parents are encouraged to stay at the hospital to feed and care for their preterm babies. With 1-year paid maternity leave, there is no financial pressure to return to work, even when a baby is hospitalized for months. In this breastfeeding-friendly environment, most parents are encouraged to nurse often with support from their healthcare providers and their families. Learning their babies' feeding and sleeping rhythms before discharge makes this transition easier.

However, in countries like the U.S., where financial pressures force many parents to return to work before their baby's hospital discharge, availability for feeds may be more limited. In situations like this, nursing may be delayed, and at first the parent may nurse only once or twice a day, with other feeds given by tube, cup, or bottle. In this case, encourage the family to do the best they can,

TABLE 9.2 Preterm Infant Breastfeeding Behavior Scale (PIBBS)

Breastfeeding Behavior Observed					Points Awarded
Rooting	1. No rooting	2. Some rooting	3. Obvious rooting		
Amount of nipple/areola in baby's mouth	1. Mouth just touched nipple	2. Part of the nipple in baby's mouth	3. Whole nipple in baby's mouth	4. Nipple and part of areola in baby's mouth	
Latched and stayed on	1. Did not stay on	2. Stayed on for <1 minute	3. Number of minutes baby stayed on		
Number of consecutive sucks	1. No activity while latched	2. No sucking, only licked/tasted milk	3. Single sucks, occasional short bursts	4. 2 or more short sucking bursts >10 sucks	
Longest sucking burst	Maximum number of consecutive sucks before a pause				
Swallowing	1. Noticed no swallowing	2. Occasional swallowing	3. Repeated swallowing		
				Total Points	________

Adapted from (Nyqvist, 2017)

perhaps devoting some days off to staying at the hospital and keeping the baby in skin-to-skin contact and frequent feeds.

Encourage the family to make sure the hospital staff knows when they will be at the hospital and post a sign on the baby's bed as a reminder, so they won't arrive to find the baby was just fed. One Swedish study found that feeding the baby just before the mother's arrival felt "devastating" to some mothers and caused them to doubt their importance to their baby's care (Nyqvist, Sjoden, & Ewald, 1994).

• • •

A Swedish researcher developed and tested the Preterm Infant Breastfeeding Behavior Scale (PIBBS), (Table 9.2), which can be used by both parents and professionals (Nyqvist, Rubertsson, Ewald, & Sjoden, 1996; Nyqvist et al., 1999). When using the PIBBS, parents rate six aspects of each nursing session. A higher score indicates greater nursing competence, which raises families' awareness of their preemie's progress.

Tools can help raise the parent's awareness of the baby's nursing behaviors and provide strategies for improving nursing effectiveness.

Based on the answers, suggestions to improve feeding effectiveness were provided (Nyqvist, 2017):

Rooting. If no rooting, trigger it by touching baby's lips with the nipple or a finger. Crying is a late hunger cue and touching the baby's cheek causes term babies to root but may cause only restless movements in a preterm baby.

Amount of the nipple/areola in the baby's mouth. If baby does not latch, takes part of the nipple, or the nipple without any areola, follow the suggestions in the previous section "Helping Baby Latch and Feed" on p. 359 to help baby take in more mammary tissue.

Staying latched. If the baby does not stay on or only stays on for a short time, if using an upright position, pull in the baby's body closer.

Sucking. If the baby does not start sucking or takes very long pauses while awake and breathing calmly, talk to the baby or touch his feet or palm.

Swallowing. If no swallowing sounds are heard, the baby may be a quiet swallower.

• • •

As the baby becomes more adept at nursing, some strategies may ease the transition to full nursing.

From scheduled to semi-demand feedings. In innovative Swedish NICUs, as soon as test-weighing indicates that babies are taking about half the milk needed at a feed, the 1- to 2-hour feeding schedule used at first is replaced with a "semi-demand" feeding plan (Davanzo, Strajn, Kennedy, Crocetta, & De Cunto, 2014; Nyqvist, 2017). This involves offering to nurse whenever the baby shows subtle feeding cues, which are also the signs baby is in a light sleep (any body movement, including eyes moving under eyelids) and whenever it has been at least 3 hours since the baby last fed. If the baby is asleep, his mouth is touched to the nipple. Test-weighing is done at each feed and milk volumes totaled. If the family finds test-weighing stressful, the daily milk volumes given as a supplement are gradually reduced over time, with the baby's weight gain carefully monitored. The healthcare provider determines how much daily milk volume the baby needs by weight, and the parents and healthcare provider decide how any needed supplement is given and how often.

Once exclusive nursing is achieved, many families continue this semi-demand routine until the baby is at around term corrected age. Many Swedish babies go home at this semi-demand stage and make the transition to cue-based feedings there. Until the baby can self-regulate his feeds, parents must remain vigilant about avoiding long intervals between feeds day and night and keeping track of number of daily feeds to ensure adequate milk intake.

From semi-demand to feeding on cue. When the baby's sucking pattern becomes more mature—long, rhythmic sucking bursts interspersed with breathing—he has matured enough to regulate his own feeds and move to cue-based feeding, where baby determines when to feed and for how long Test-weighing is stopped, and for a time the baby is weighed every 1 to 3 days to make sure he gains weight well.

In some parts of the U.S., this transition happens differently. As the baby becomes more adept at nursing, the parent will begin to nurse more times per day. Once all baby's feeds are by mouth, an individual plan can be created with help from baby's healthcare provider, including how much supplement to give and when, based on baby's weight and feeding skill. In one U.S. hospital, for example, if a 1700 g baby needs 300 mL of milk in 24 hours, the baby's intake is monitored by test weighing to be sure the baby gets at least 100 mL (3.3 oz) every 8 hours from all sources. By doing test-weights, the family can see how much the baby takes while nursing and feed him on cue. At the end of each 8-hour period, if he did not yet take 100 mL, he can be supplemented (Spatz, 2021). Thus, baby begins to set the pace and gains experience nursing even before he is exclusively nursing, while the parents begin to learn their baby's cues.

• • •

An important aspect of transitioning to full nursing is monitoring the baby's milk intake and weight gain.

A baby making this transition is at risk of inadequate milk intake, so parents need to be sure the baby is getting enough milk. If while in the hospital the parents have access to an accurate electronic scale (to 2 g) for test weights, suggest using it to monitor how much milk the baby takes during nursing. They can use this information to gauge how much supplement is needed.

In a U.S. study in which babies were transitioned from NG tube feeds to direct nursing (Kliethermes et al., 1999), a scale was not used. The volume and frequency of supplementation after nursing was determined by how long the babies nursed actively and if swallows were heard. If these signs were seen, no supplement was given. If a baby's nursing was considered only fair—he latched but didn't suck actively for very long and few swallows were heard—baby received half of a usual feed via NG tube. If the baby rooted or licked the nipple but did not latch or suck, he received a full feed via NG tube. The babies made the transition to full nursing gradually without using any other feeding method. However, research found that gauging milk intake by observation alone is unreliable (P. P. Meier et al., 1996). Baby's milk intake may be overestimated or underestimated. But what's ultimately most important is making sure baby is well fed while helping the family meet its feeding goal, rather than the time it takes to get there.

One U.S. study examined mothers' reactions to either using or not using a scale as they transitioned their preterm babies to nursing (N. M. Hurst et al., 2004). All the mothers who used the scale found it either very or extremely helpful, and 75% of those who didn't use the scale reported that it would have been somewhat to extremely helpful to them to know exactly how much milk their baby was taking during nursing. Another U.S. study (Hall, Shearer, Mogan, & Berkowitz, 2002) found that there was no significant difference in confidence among mothers who transitioned to direct nursing using a scale for test-weighs and those who didn't.

Whether or not the family uses a scale for test-weighing, frequent weight checks are important to be sure the baby is gaining daily at least 0.5 to 1 ounce (15 g to 30 g).

• • •

Until the baby is able to exclusively nurse on cue, suggest the family continue milk expression.

Until the exclusively nursing preemie can self-regulate his milk intake without needing to be awakened or stimulated to feed often enough, suggest the nursing parent continue expressing to keep up milk production. Healthy milk production is an important aspect of effective nursing, as faster flow keeps a baby interested and actively nursing. If the milk production slows and baby gets little milk during nursing, suggest taking steps to increase it. For details see p. 442. If milk production is low and the baby seems to lose interest easily, suggest trying a nursing supplementer to increase milk flow at feeds (see next point).

• • •

If the baby was supplemented by bottle and is not nursing well, for an easier transition, suggest strategies to make the bottle more like nursing.

To make the transition easier from bottle-feeding to direct nursing, try these strategies for making bottle-feeding more like nursing.

Bait and switch involves starting bottle-feeding in a nursing position, with the baby's cheek touching the exposed mammary gland. As the baby gets into a sucking-and-swallowing pattern, quickly remove the bottle teat and insert the nipple (Wilson-Clay & Hoover, 2017).

Latch to the bottle teat like nursing. One U.S. lactation consultant (Kassing, 2002) suggested that parents hold the baby in a semi-upright position, touch his lips with the bottle nipple/teat, and wait until he opens wide. Then allow him to draw the bottle teat well back into his mouth, rather than pushing it in. Hold the bottle horizontally rather than vertically, so the flow is not as fast, and keep the baby in a semi-upright upright position, rather than on his back. Suggest the feeder avoid letting the baby take just the tip of the teat with a tightly closed mouth. (For more details on paced bottle-feeding, see p. 902-903.)

Firmer feel and/or faster flow. When a baby seems to prefer the bottle, assume there is something he is looking for during nursing that is he is not finding—most likely the firm feel of the teat or the consistent, immediate flow of the bottle. If it's possible to provide one or both of these during nursing, it may help. For example, a nipple shield will provide the baby with a firmer feel and a helper dripping milk or a nursing supplementer can provide instant flow. (For details on using these tools, see p. 912-917 and 897-900.) These tools can be used either individually or together to help the baby find what he is looking for and begin to form positive associations with nursing. If they are used together, this may be difficult for parents to manage by themselves. If so, encourage them to get help, as an extra pair of hands can make it easier. As baby learns, the family can wean him from these transitional aids.

Keep nursing attempts positive. Most important is not to allow nursing to become a negative experience. If a baby is fussing or crying during attempts, suggest stopping and comforting him, so that the baby does not associate nursing with frustration and unhappiness. Relaxed skin-to-skin time near the nipple will help the baby develop positive associations and make him more open to nursing.

Going Home

Preparing for Discharge

Before hospital discharge, encourage the parents to get actively involved in their baby's care and check on any available post-discharge services.

The more time the parents spend with their baby before discharge, the easier the transition to home will be. In some hospitals, parents are encouraged to room-in with their preemie and take over all his care before they go home. If that is an option, suggest they take advantage of it (L. M. Noble et al., 2018). Also, if the parents have not yet been spending lots of time in skin-to-skin contact with their baby, suggest they start now to help bring them closer, reduce stress, increase their confidence in their relationship, and to become familiar with their baby's sleep-wake rhythms.

Some hospitals provide parents with follow-up care when discharged; others do not. Encourage the parents to find out what services the hospital offers before discharge, so they will know what to expect and can make arrangements. One New Zealand study found that when good follow-up support was provided to families whose preterm babies were discharged fully nursing, nursing rates did not suffer, even when they were discharged earlier than routine (Gunn et al., 2000).

• • •

Parents who had little time to care for their baby may have mixed emotions about discharge.

If a baby is not nursing well and the parents have not cared for their baby during most of his hospitalization, they may experience a second crisis at hospital discharge that brings similar feelings as the birth. Even after the healthcare providers pronounce a baby healthy and growing well, earlier fears and

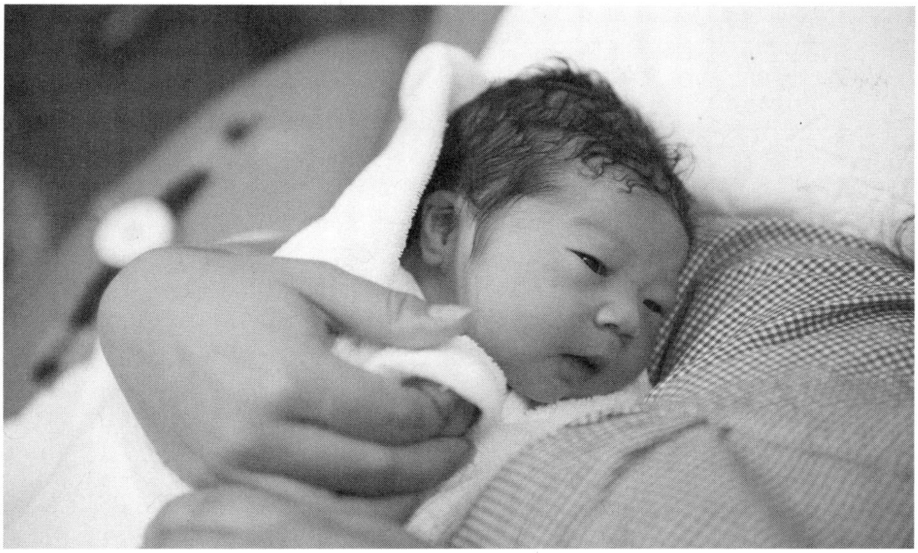

difficulties may linger. It is common to feel helpless and apprehensive mixed with joy and happiness. The parents may feel overwhelmed that they will have to care for their special-needs baby at home, while at the same time feel eager to be like a "normal" family and start enjoying their baby.

• • •

Suggest the family arrange for household help.

If baby comes home before full nursing is well established, parents may have a lot to juggle at home. Some families bring their baby home doing what some refer to as "triple feeding"—nursing, supplementing, and then expressing. Many find this intense routine unsustainable over time (Boies & Vaucher, 2016).

Although the birthing parent may have at least partly recovered physically from childbirth before the baby comes home, no matter how well the baby is nursing, the constant, 24-hour demands of caring for a small baby can be exhausting. Encourage the family—if possible—to spend their first week at home with their baby doing nothing but nursing and caring for him. Many parents who were separated from their baby crave time alone with him. Also suggest considering getting household help from family or friends, or if not available, hire help to do laundry, clean, and cook for at least the first week. If the nursing parent's partner was thinking of working during this time, suggest their homecoming would be easier if they are both home for that first week. Suggest limiting visitors who are not there to help and ask those who do come not to stay long.

If there are older children, suggest the family consider making arrangements with relatives or friends to entertain them on some days during the first week. One Swedish study (Flacking et al., 2003) found that for mothers of preterm babies, having older children was one risk factor for shorter nursing duration.

Feeding Considerations

After discharge, parents need to know how to gauge whether their preemie is getting enough milk.

One U.S. descriptive study of 27 mothers of preterm babies (Reyna, Pickler, & Thompson, 2006) reported that during the first few weeks at home, most of the study mothers found feeding a struggle and then gradually began to feel comfortable with their new routine. These mothers said it would have been helpful to be told how their baby's feeding would progress over time. Even those whose

TABLE 9.3 Median Nursing Sessions/Night Feeds after Discharge in Preemies Born 28 to 33 Weeks

CA = Corrected Age	1st Week after NICU Discharge	2 Months CA	6 Months CA	12 Months CA
Exclusive Nursing				
Median # Nursing/24 hr. (Range)	14 (8-26)	10 (6-25)	11.5 (9-14)	N/A
Median # Night Feeds (Range)	4 (1-9)	2 (0-5)	2 or 3	
Nursing & Human Milk Supplements				
Median # Nursing/24 hr. (Range)	12.5 (6-28)	9 (7-14)	N/A	N/A
Median # Night Feeds (Range)	2 (2-10)	2 (2-5)		
Partial Nursing				
Median # Nursing/24 hr. (Range)	8.5 (1-15)	6 (1-12)	5 (1-14)	5.5 (1-12)
Median # Night Feeds (Range)	2.5 (1-15)	1 (0-3)	2 (0-4)	2 (0-3)

Adapted from (Oras et al., 2015)

preemies nursed well in the hospital reported being worried about their baby's milk intake at home (Kavanaugh, Mead, Meier, & Mangurten, 1995). In a 2015 Swedish prospective questionnaire study of families whose preemies were born between 28 and 33 weeks gestation (Oras, 2015), at NICU discharge, researchers sent home with mothers a feeding diary to record their babies' nursing patterns at home. The researchers were struck by the greater frequency of nursing sessions than is typically described, especially at first (Table 9.3). They noted that some of the mothers nursed at regular intervals while others nursed irregularly.

Regular weight checks. The most reliable sign of good milk intake is a daily weight gain of at least 0.5 to 1 ounce (15 g to 30 g) (Boies & Vaucher, 2016). One way to monitor the baby after discharge is to schedule frequent weight checks, so the parents know for sure how their baby is doing with their new routine. The American Academy of Pediatrics recommends pediatricians schedule a visit with high-risk babies within 72 hours of hospital discharge (AAP, 2008). If the baby's weight gain is within the expected range, this will ease any worries and if not, parents will know they need to adjust their routine.

Test weights. Another way to monitor milk intake after discharge is for the family to rent an accurate (to 2 g) electronic scale for short-term home use. This could be used either to monitor the baby's weight gain from day to day, or if the parents are concerned about milk intake at nursing sessions, they can use it to do pre- and post-feed test weights. This will give them an accurate measure of whether or not supplements are needed and if so, how much (Rankin et al., 2016). If parents feel anxious about the baby's milk intake during nursing and have no way to measure it, the natural tendency is to over-supplement rather than taking a chance that the baby is not getting enough milk (N. M. Hurst et al., 2004). For some families, having an accurate gauge of baby's milk intake during nursing can make the transition to full nursing faster and less anxiety-producing. Other families do fine without it (Hall et al., 2002).

• • •

Encourage the parents to keep their baby on their bodies as much as possible, take the lead by offering to nurse often, and seek out support.

Once the baby is home, parents will need a feeding strategy that works well for everyone. Depending on the baby's gestational age, he may not yet be ready to feed on cue (see previous section). At first, it is wise for parents to make sure nursing happens more often than the baby shows feeding cues. If the baby is sleepy, the parents can keep him on their body and offer to nurse frequently, as preterm babies can nurse even when in a light sleep (Colson et al., 2003). Waking baby often to feed may also help.

• • •

Suggest creating a comfortable nursing area at home.

Especially at first, it may be helpful for the nursing parent to find a comfortable place to nurse, away from activity and possible overstimulation, with plenty of pillows to support parent and baby. Suggestions from the previous section, "Helping Baby Latch and Feed," may help in finding a comfortable and effective position and helping baby latch. Also see Chapter 1.

• • •

Suggest keeping baby nearby for night feeds.

Most health organizations recommend parents keep their baby in their room at night for at least the baby's first 6 months, because it is protective for Sudden Infant Death Syndrome (AAP, 2016). Many parents find nursing easier at night when the baby is in their room, that their sleep is less disrupted, and they more easily rest during feeds. The baby might sleep in a crib, a bassinette, in a co-sleeper attached to their bed, or on the floor on a mattress or pallet. If the parent has not yet mastered nursing lying down, suggest leaning back in bed to nurse, with extra pillows for back and elbow support, with baby lying tummy down on their body.

When a night feed is over, parents can either return the baby to his own bed or keep him next to them, so they won't have to get out of bed for the next feed. If the parents decide to keep the baby in bed with them, see safe sleep recommendations on p. 84-87.

• • •

In some cases, continued fortification of mother's milk is recommended after discharge.

For tiny preemies born at less than 1500 g (3.3 lbs.), after discharge, the baby's healthcare provider may recommend fortifying mother's milk at some feeds (Boies & Vaucher, 2016). Before making this recommendation, ideally a detailed nutritional assessment would be done. For an overview of the current thinking on fortification of mother's milk after discharge, download the current version of the Academy of Breastfeeding Medicine's Clinical Protocol #12, "Transitioning the Preterm Baby from the NICU to Home" at **bfmed.org/protocols.** Also, because preemies are born without the iron stores full-term babies have, iron supplements are often recommended.

Practical details for managing milk fortification at home. Usually fortification is recommended at only some feeds. This can be done by providing the fortified milk with a nursing supplementer during nursing sessions or via other feeding methods. One Canadian study (O'Connor et al., 2008) found that when mothers were provided with extensive breastfeeding support from a lactation consultant, this daily fortification did not shorten nursing duration, despite the extra time and effort involved. Overall, the babies who did not receive the fortifier and self-regulated their milk intake during direct nursing took more milk daily overall. At 12 weeks, the babies who received fortified milk at half their daily feeds grew longer and those smallest at birth (≤1250 g) had larger head circumferences than those not receiving fortified milk. The researchers wrote: "The estimated energy intakes of infants in our study did not differ between feeding groups, suggesting that human milk-fed [low birth weight] infants are able to compensate to some degree for the energy and/or nutrient density of their feeding" (O'Connor et al., 2008, p. 773).

THE LATE PRETERM AND EARLY TERM BABY

Early term and late preterm births are a significant proportion of the babies born worldwide.

Many newborns are considered early term—born between 37 and 38 completed weeks gestation. Early-term babies comprised one third of all births in one Hong Kong prospective cohort study of 2,704 families (Fan, Wong, Fong, Lok, & Tarrant, 2019). Late preterm babies—those born between 34 and 36 completed weeks gestation—on the other hand, are a smaller proportion of births, but the largest group of preterm babies (Lapillonne et al., 2019). In a study that included one third of all babies born in Portugal (Barros, Clode, & Graca, 2016), slightly more than 5% were born late preterm. Once referred to as "near-term," the label "late preterm" was adopted to more accurately reflect a vulnerability that is not always obvious (Raju, 2017).

The Late Preterm Baby

A late preterm baby may look healthy but needs careful monitoring during the hospital stay and may not yet be ready to nurse on cue.

Although most babies born between 34 and 36 completed weeks are mature enough at birth to breathe on their own, the late preterm baby should not be treated like a full-term healthy baby. Due to his immaturity, he is at greater risk of low body temperature, jaundice, hypoglycemia, apnea, and many other health problems (Adamkin & AAP, 2011; Boies & Vaucher, 2016).

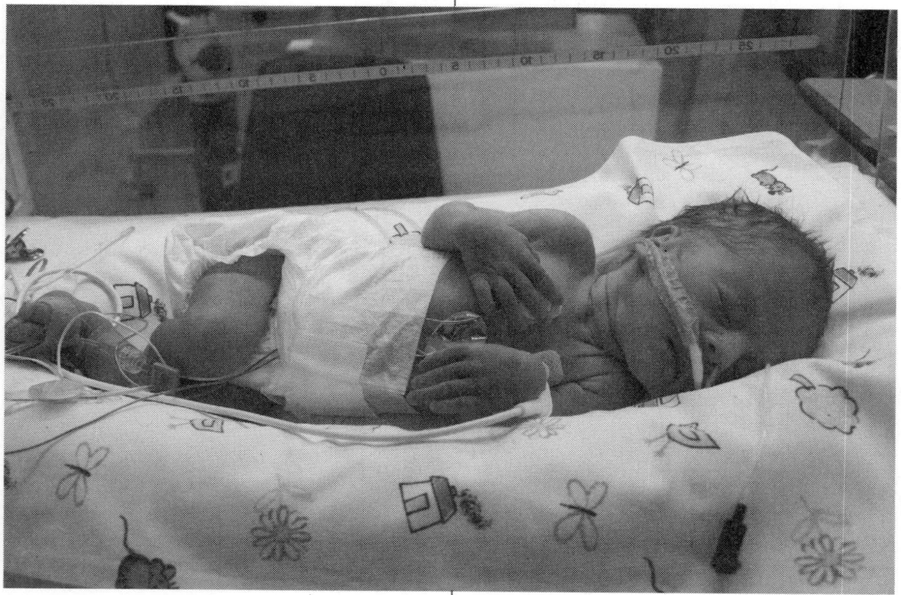

Vulnerable and immature. Depending on the late preterm baby's gestational age at birth, his brain may be only 60% to 80% the size and maturity of the brain of a full-term baby (Kinney, 2006). This brain immaturity (see Figure 9.1) affects his arousal, sleep-wake cycles, breathing, and his ability to self-regulate feeding. U.S. research (Dewey, Nommsen-Rivers, Heinig, & Cohen, 2003) found prematurity to be significantly associated with suboptimal early nursing. Late preterm babies are also four times more likely than term babies to have other medical problems (Wang, Dorer, Fleming, & Catlin, 2004), which also affect nursing.

At risk for delayed first nursing and less exclusive nursing. One U.S. study that included more than 68,000 late preterm babies (Demirci, Sereika, & Bogen, 2013) found that when compared with term newborns, late preterm babies were less likely to nurse within the first hour of life. An Australian retrospective populations-based study (Ayton, Hansen, Quinn, & Nelson, 2012) found the same, as well as a lower likelihood (compared with babies born at 37 weeks) of exclusive nursing at hospital discharge. After discharge, these babies were more likely to be readmitted to the hospital (Escobar, Clark, & Greene, 2006; Tomashek et al., 2006).

Early challenges parents reported. During the hospital stay, some of the challenges parents of late preterm babies reported in one U.K. interview study of 14 mothers of late preterm babies (Cescutti-Butler, Hemingway, & Hewitt-Taylor, 2019) included:

- Separation from the baby
- Over-supplementing, which left baby too full to nurse
- Inconsistent lactation support
- Confusing feeding regimens

Swedish researcher Kerstin Hedberg Nyqvist described seven breastfeeding stages (Box 9.1) through which preterm babies may pass (Nyqvist, 2017). A late preterm baby will likely begin further along this continuum than a preemie born earlier, but at birth he may not yet be ready to set his own feeding rhythm. At birth, many late-preterm babies have an immature sucking pattern and feed well at some feeds but not at others. Nursing parents also report latching challenges due to their baby's small mouth (Dosani et al., 2016). Full nursing may be possible for many with the "semi-demand feeding" pattern described on p.380, in which the nursing parent takes charge of ensuring the baby has the required number of feeds each day.

• • •

Some strategies help late preterm babies master nursing during the hospital stay.

In addition to the semi-demand feeding strategy described in the previous point, a 2017 integrative review of hospital strategies to promote nursing in late preterm babies (Cartwright, Atz, Newman, Mueller, & Demirci, 2017) described those that had a positive impact on nursing exclusivity and duration.

Skin-to-skin contact. According to this literature review, more time spent in skin-to-skin contact per day was associated with nursing significantly longer and more time spent directly nursing. According to a 2019 review of the literature (Evans, Hilditch, & Keir, 2019), immediate skin-to-skin contact after birth is effective at improving nursing outcomes.

Avoid separation. The Clinical. Protocol #10 of the Academy of Breastfeeding Medicine (ABM) (Boies & Vaucher, 2016) on nursing the late preterm baby (downloadable at **bfmed.org/protocols**) recommended 24-hour rooming-in during the hospital stay. Late preterm babies are at greater risk of jaundice, so to keep families together, instead of providing phototherapy in the NICU, the authors of the ABM protocol suggested making it available in the baby's room, so nursing can continue without restrictions.

Close monitoring, education, and support. As described previously, late preterm babies are vulnerable and physically immature, so it's vital to keep a close eye on their blood-sugar and bilirubin levels, body temperature, and weight loss. If greater milk intake during nursing is needed, the authors of the ABM protocol (Boies & Vaucher, 2016) suggested using breast compression (see p. 889) for faster milk flow, which may help keep the baby actively nursing longer. A 2018 Spanish quasi-experimental study of 373 late preterm babies (Estalella, et al., 2018) found that staff education had a major impact on both breastfeeding support during the hospital stay and rates of breastfeeding at hospital discharge. The parents in the control group received a one-page printed instruction sheet at hospital admission and were asked once a day during their stay if they had any breastfeeding questions. The intervention group received this same instruction sheet and were asked to complete a feeding diary every day about nursing, pumping, supplements, diaper output, and baby behaviors. The baby's healthcare provider and charge nurse also completed a feeding evaluation separately. If the baby needed phototherapy for jaundice, this was done in the baby's room. At hospital discharge, 51% of the control group was exclusively nursing compared with 68% of the intervention group.

Spending time tummy down on the parents' body. This practice, whether done in skin-to-skin contact or lightly dressed, stimulates the baby's inborn feeding reflexes for more frequent feeding cues and helps parents get to know their newborn more quickly. When late preterm newborns are swaddled and laid in a separate bed, they are more likely to sleep longer and show fewer feeding cues (Nelson, 2017), which can lead to underfeeding. One small U.K. study of 12 babies (11 late-preterm and one small for gestational age) examined the effects of keeping babies tummy down on their mothers' semi-reclined bodies for extended periods during the first 3 days after birth (Colson et al., 2003). During the first 24 hours, the babies had a mean of 12 of these periods, which resulted in from 4 to 16 hours of close body contact and a mean total of 2 hours and 35 minutes of active breastfeeding. In some cases, the mothers moved the babies to their nipple while the babies were in a light sleep, and they fed well. At hospital discharge, all babies were exclusively breastfeeding, with 58% (7) exclusively breastfed from birth. Five received supplements of mother's milk and formula, two for borderline blood sugar levels during the first 2 days and three for jaundice on the third or fourth day.

The long-term nursing outcomes for these mothers and babies were much better than the U.K. norm at that time, with 11 of the 12 mothers still breastfeeding at 4 months and more than half at 6 months, three of them exclusively. The researchers suggested that extensive early body contact may be a factor.

Nipple shields. If the baby's weight loss confirms that he is feeding ineffectively, the ABM protocol suggests trying a nipple shield. However one integrative review (Cartwright et al., 2017) concluded that interventions like syringe feeding, nursing supplementers, and nipple shields may lead to shorter nursing duration.

If supplements are needed, the authors of the ABM protocol recommended avoiding overfeeding by providing late preterm babies only 5 to 10 mL of supplement on the first day and 10 to 30 mL during the following few days. When choosing a supplement, it recommended expressed milk as the first choice, donor milk as the second choice, and formula as the third choice. As described on p. 895, cup feeding as opposed to bottle-feeding was associated with greater likelihood of full nursing. For a list of pros and cons of each alternative feeding method, see p. 896. A 2017 U.S. prospective interview study of 54 mothers of late preterm babies and 51 controls (Tully, Holditch-Davis, Silva, & Brandon, 2017) found that the nursing mothers whose babies were supplemented with formula in the hospital suffered from more severe anxiety at 1 month compared with other mothers. The authors recommended that families receive more information on possible problems and their solutions.

• • •

Just a few weeks of maturity and growth can turn an ineffective late preterm baby into an effective nurser. One U.S. prospective interview study of 2,772 mothers (Hackman, Alligood-Percoco, Martin, Zhu, & Kjerulff, 2016) found that gestational age was significantly associated with nursing at 1 month after birth. At 1 month, 76% of term babies, 73% of early term babies, and 57% of late preterm babies were nursing. A U.K. secondary analysis of the 2010 Infant Feeding Survey, which included more than 15,000 families (Rayfield, Oakley, & Quigley, 2015), found that providing families with a phone number for breastfeeding support after hospital discharge was associated with more nursing at 1 month in term babies and more nursing at 10 days in late preterm babies.

With the late preterm baby, careful monitoring and ongoing lactation help and support after hospital discharge are vital to meeting feeding goals.

What do nursing parents of late preterm babies need? Those interviewed in several studies (Cescutti-Butler et al., 2019; Dosani et al., 2016) described lactation support in the hospital as inconsistent. In one U.S. study (Kair, Flaherman, Newby, & Colaizy, 2015), parents said they could have used more help with latching, access to donor milk, and providers who were better educated about nursing.

The Early Term Baby

As described in the previous point, a U.S. prospective interview study of 2,772 mothers (Hackman et al., 2016) found a difference in nursing rates among early term babies who were born just 2 to 3 weeks early. At 1 month after birth, 76% of term babies and 73% of early term babies were nursing. Compared with late preterm babies, the early term babies were much closer to the term babies in nursing outcomes, but they still lagged by a little.

Being born just 2 or 3 weeks early affects nursing outcomes in early term babies.

Lower rates of exclusive nursing by gestational age. A 2019 U.S. secondary analysis of 743 geographically and ethnically diverse women (Keenan-Devlin et al., 2019) found that while women who gave birth to early term babies began nursing at the same rate as those who gave birth to full-term babies (85.8% versus 85.5%), fewer early term babies nursed exclusively. The percentage of babies who exclusively nursed varied by gestational age at birth:

- 35% born at 37 weeks
- 36% born at 38 weeks
- 42% born at 39 weeks
- 55% born at 40 weeks
- 57% born at 41+ weeks

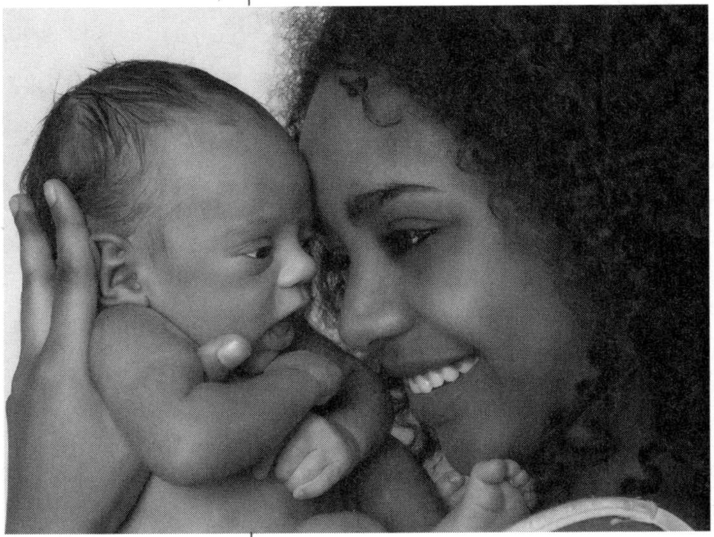

Fewer nursed during the first hour. A 2019 U.S. prospective cohort study of 358 mothers of early term babies (A. Noble et al., 2019) found that compared with babies born at full term, significantly fewer early term babies nursed during the first hour.

Lower rates of exclusive and high-intensity nursing. This same U.S. study (A. Noble et al., 2019) found that the early term babies had lower rates of exclusive nursing in the hospital at 1 month of age, and lower rates of higher nursing intensity. The early term babies also had more visits to the emergency room during the first month, and all of the babies who went to the emergency room were exclusively nursing.

PRETERM TWINS, TRIPLETS, AND MORE

The milk made by nursing parents of preterm multiples differs in composition from the milk made by parents of preterm singletons.

A 2019 Italian study analyzed expressed milk from 19 mothers of twins and 5 mothers of triplets who were born before 28 weeks at less than 1500 g and compared it with the milk expressed by 28 mothers of preterm singleton babies (Congiu et al., 2019). The researchers found that the milk made by mothers of preterm multiples was higher in protein (1.53 g versus 1.29 g per 100 mL) and lower in lactose (6.34 g versus 6.72 g per 100 mL) compared with the milk expressed by the mothers of preterm singleton babies.

• • •

Multiples—twins, triplets, and more—are often born preterm, so during pregnancy suggest the family prepare for this possibility.

There are several ways a family can prepare for the preterm birth of multiple babies:

Take an early lactation class, spend time with nursing families, and meet the hospital lactation staff. Suggest meeting both the lactation consultants on the maternity unit and those in the special care nursery. Discuss services (hours and days of availability) and options that promote nursing. Learning how milk production works is also vital for families of multiples. Both a 2018 Brazilian secondary data analysis of 28 women who gave birth to twins (Mikami et al., 2018) and a 2016 prospective survey of 30 twin mothers in Iran (Cinar, Kose, Alvur, & Dogu, 2016) found that, like other families, the most common reason cited for weaning among families of multiples was insufficient milk. Encourage the family to check their local area to see if meetups with other nursing families are available or whether they can find online groups for parents of multiples.

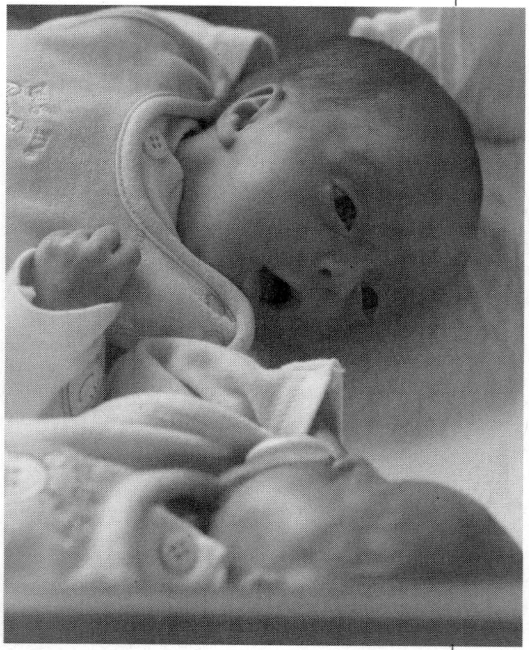

Learn about milk expression. There's a good chance the family will need to express milk during the early weeks, and it is much easier to absorb new information before the babies are born than after. Recommend families view the videos on Dr. Jane Morton's website, **firstdroplets.com**, which teach hand expression during pregnancy. If all of the babies are not yet ready to nurse at birth, discuss why starting early and expressing often is important to milk production. Describe hands-on pumping technique (p. 492) and the research (Morton et al., 2009) that found using this technique stimulates on average 50% greater milk yields than using the pump alone.

Discuss skin-to-skin contact. As described in Box 9.1 on p. 351, immediate skin-to-skin contact after birth improves health and lactation outcomes in low-birth-weight babies.

Plan to begin nursing as soon as possible after delivery. If the babies are healthy at birth, they can nurse right away. A 2016 South Korean retrospective survey (Kim, 2016) found that early nursing of twins was associated with greater likelihood of nursing throughout the hospital stay. If the babies nurse effectively, most nursing parents of multiples can produce enough milk for all the babies from the beginning. Many families have fully nursed twins, triplets, and even quadruplets (Berlin, 2007; Gromada, 2007)

Arrange for help at home, for at least the first month, but ideally for the first 3 months. If hiring help is not an option, suggest enlisting family and friends.

• • •

If milk expression is needed to bring in full milk production, suggest a goal of 750 mL (25 oz.) per baby per day, ideally within the first few weeks.

For the most effective research-based milk-expression strategies, see the section "Establishing Full Milk Production with Pumping" starting on p. 497. For a parent exclusively expressing for multiples, suggest staying in Stage 2 (described on p. 501) until reaching about 750 mL (25 ounces) per day per baby. As described in that section, during the first 2 weeks after birth, mammary stimulation has the most profound effect on milk production, so the sooner milk production is increased to that level, the less work is required.

• • •

It is not unusual for one baby to nurse more effectively than another or for babies to go home at different times.

If the nursing parent notices that one baby is more effective at feeds, assure the family this is common (Nyqvist, 2002). It may help to nurse two babies together (see p. 35 for positioning ideas), so the more effective baby can trigger milk ejection for the less effective baby.

Some families of multiples bring one baby home before the others are ready for discharge. This may mean nursing at home and continuing to express milk for one or more babies in the hospital. Extra help at home can be invaluable during this hectic time. Once all of the babies are home, one Swedish study found that after sharing a womb, sharing a sleep surface can help them keep their sleep cycles coordinated, so that both are awake and asleep at the same time (Nyqvist & Lutes, 1998).

RESOURCES

bfmed.org/protocols—To download the current versions of the Academy of Breastfeeding Medicine Clinical Protocols, most available in multiple languages:

- #10 Breastfeeding the late preterm baby
- #12 NICU graduate going home

bit.ly/BA2-VLBW—Wight, N., Kim, J., Rhine, W. Mayer, O., Morris, M., Sey, R., Nisher,C. (2018). *Nutritional Support of the Very Low Birth Weight Infant (VLBW): A Quality Improvement Toolkit.* Stanford, CA: California Perinatal Quality Carae Collaborative.

Nyqvist, K. H. (2017). Breastfeeding preterm infants. In C. W. Genna (Ed.), *Supporting Sucking Skills in Breastfeeding Infants* (3rd ed., pp. 181-208). Burlington, MA: Jones & Bartlett Learning.

REFERENCES

AAP. (2008). Hospital discharge of the high-risk neonate. *Pediatrics, 122*(5), 1119-1126.

AAP. (2012). Breastfeeding and the use of human milk. *Pediatrics, 129*(3), e827-e841.

AAP. (2014). Nutritional needs of preterm infants. *Pediatric Nutrition Handbook* (7th ed.). Elk Grove Village, IL: American Academy of Pediatrics.

AAP. (2016). SIDS and other sleep-related infant deaths: Updated 2016 recommendations for a safe infant sleeping environment. *Pediatrics, 138*(5).

Adamkin, D. H., & AAP. (2011). Postnatal glucose homeostasis in late-preterm and term infants. *Pediatrics, 127*(3), 575-579.

Agostoni, C., Buonocore, G., Carnielli, V. P., et al. (2010). Enteral nutrient supply for preterm infants: Commentary from the European Society of Paediatric Gastroenterology, Hepatology and Nutrition Committee on Nutrition. *Journal of Pediatric Gastroenterology and Nutrition, 50*(1), 85-91.

Akerstrom, S., Asplund, I., & Norman, M. (2007). Successful breastfeeding after discharge of preterm and sick newborn infants. *Acta Paediatrica, 96*(10), 1450-1454.

Akinbi, H., Meinzen-Derr, J., Auer, C., et al. (2010). Alterations in the host defense properties of human milk following prolonged storage or pasteurization. *Journal of Pediatric Gastroenterology and Nutrition, 51*(3), 347-352.

Aloysius, A., & Hickson, M. (2007). Evaluation of paladai cup feeding in breast-fed preterm infants compared with bottle feeding. *Early Human Development, 83*(9), 619-621.

Als, H., Lawhon, G., Duffy, F. H., et al. (1994). Individualized developmental care for the very low-birth-weight preterm infant. Medical and neurofunctional effects. *Journal of the American Medical Association, 272*(11), 853-858.

Alyahya, W., Simpson, J., Garcia, A. L., et al. (2019). Early versus delayed fortification of human milk in preterm infants: A systematic review. *Neonatology,* 1-9.

Amin, S. B., Merle, K. S., Orlando, M. S., et al. (2000). Brainstem maturation in premature infants as a function of enteral feeding type. *Pediatrics, 106*(2 Pt 1), 318-322.

Ang, J. Y., Lua, J. L., Mathur, A., et al. (2012). A randomized placebo-controlled trial of massage therapy on the immune system of preterm infants. *Pediatrics, 130*(6), e1549-1558.

Angelhoff, C., Blomqvist, Y. T., Sahlen Helmer, C., et al. (2018). Effect of skin-to-skin contact on parents' sleep quality, mood, parent-infant interaction and cortisol concentrations in neonatal care units: Study protocol of a randomised controlled trial. *BMJ Open, 8*(7), e021606.

'Arslanoglu, S., Boquien, C. Y., King, C., et al. (2019). Fortification of human milk for preterm infants: Update and recommendations of the European Milk Bank Association (EMBA) Working Group on Human Milk Fortification. *Frontiers in Pediatrics, 7,* 76.

Asztalos, E. V., Kiss, A., daSilva, O. P., et al. (2019). Role of days postdelivery on breast milk production: A secondary analysis from the EMPOWER trial. *International Breastfeeding Journal, 14,* 21.

Ayton, J., Hansen, E., Quinn, S., et al. (2012). Factors associated with initiation and exclusive breastfeeding at hospital discharge: Late preterm compared to 37 week gestation mother and infant cohort. *International Breastfeeding Journal, 7*(1), 16.

Barros, J. G., Clode, N., & Graca, L. M. (2016). Prevalence of late preterm and early term birth in Portugal. *Acta Medica Portuguese, 29*(4), 249-253.

Belfort, M. B., Anderson, P. J., Nowak, V. A., et al. (2016). Breast milk feeding, brain development, and neurocognitive outcomes: A 7-year longitudinal study in infants born at less than 30 weeks' gestation. *Journal of Pediatrics, 177,* 133-139 e131.

Belfort, M. B., Rifas-Shiman, S. L., Sullivan, T., et al. (2011). Infant growth before and after term: Effects on neurodevelopment in preterm infants. *Pediatrics, 128*(4), e899-906.

Ben-Shoshan, M., Mandel, D., Lubetzky, R., et al. (2016). Eradication of cytomegalovirus from human milk by microwave irradiation: A pilot study. *Breastfeeding Medicine, 11,* 186-187.

Berger, I., Weintraub, V., Dollberg, S., et al. (2009). Energy expenditure for breastfeeding and bottle-feeding preterm infants. *Pediatrics, 124*(6), e1149-1152.

Bergman, N. (2017). Breastfeeding and perinatal neuroscience. In C. W. Genna (Ed.), *Supporting Sucking Skills in Breastfeeding Infants* (3rd ed., pp. 49-63). Burlington, MA: Jones & Bartlett Learning.

Bergman, N. J., & Jurisoo, L. A. (1994). The 'kangaroo-method' for treating low birth weight babies in a developing country. *Tropical Doctor, 24*(2), 57-60.

Bergman, N. J., Linley, L. L., & Fawcus, S. R. (2004). Randomized controlled trial of skin-to-skin contact from birth versus conventional incubator for physiological stabilization in 1200- to 2199-gram newborns. *Acta Paediatrica, 93*(6), 779-785.

Berlin, C. M. (2007). "Exclusive" breastfeeding of quadruplets. *Breastfeeding Medicine, 2*(2), 125-126.

Bishara, R., Dunn, M. S., Merko, S. E., et al. (2008). Nutrient composition of hindmilk produced by mothers of very low birth weight infants born at less than 28 weeks' gestation. *Journal of Human Lactation, 24*(2), 159-167.

Bishara, R., Dunn, M. S., Merko, S. E., et al. (2009). Volume of foremilk, hindmilk, and total milk produced by mothers of very preterm infants born at less than 28 weeks of gestation. *Journal of Human Lactation, 25*(3), 272-279.

Blaymore Bier, J. A., Ferguson, A. E., Morales, Y., et al. (1997). Breastfeeding infants who were extremely low birth weight. *Pediatrics, 100*(6), E3.

Boies, E. G., & Vaucher, Y. E. (2016). ABM Clinical Protocol #10: Breastfeeding the late preterm (34-36 6/7 weeks of gestation) and early term infants (37-38 6/7 weeks of gestation), second revision 2016. *Breastfeeding Medicine, 11,* 494-500.

Bonnet, C., Blondel, B., Piedvache, A., et al. (2018). Low breastfeeding continuation to 6 months for very preterm infants: A European multiregional cohort study. *Maternal and Child Nutrition,* e12657.

Boundy, E. O., Dastjerdi, R., Spiegelman, D., et al. (2016). Kangaroo Mother Care and neonatal outcomes: A meta-analysis. *Pediatrics, 137*(1).

Bower, K., Burnette, T., Lewis, D., et al. (2017). "I had one job and that was to make milk". *Journal of Human Lactation, 33*(1), 188-194.

Boyce, C., Watson, M., Lazidis, G., et al. (2016). Preterm human milk composition: A systematic literature review. *British Journal of Nutrition, 116*(6), 1033-1045.

Briere, C. E. (2015). Breastfed or bottle-fed: Who goes home sooner? *Advances in Neonatal Care, 15*(1), 65-69.

Briere, C. E., McGrath, J. M., Cong, X., et al. (2015). Direct-breastfeeding premature infants in the neonatal intensive care unit. *Journal of Human Lactation, 31*(3), 386-392.

Briere, C. E., McGrath, J. M., Cong, X., et al. (2016). Direct-breastfeeding in the neonatal intensive care unit and breastfeeding duration for premature infants. *Applied Nursing Research, 32,* 47-51.

Brockway, M., Benzies, K., & Hayden, K. A. (2017). Interventions to improve breastfeeding self-efficacy and resultant breastfeeding rates: A systematic review and meta-analysis. *Journal of Human Lactation, 33*(3), 486-499.

Brown, J. V., Embleton, N. D., Harding, J. E., et al. (2016). Multi-nutrient fortification of human milk for preterm infants. *Cochrane Database of Systematic Reviews*(5), CD000343. doi:10.1002/14651858.CD000343.pub3.

Bryant, P., Morley, C., Garland, S., et al. (2002). Cytomegalovirus transmission from breast milk in premature babies: Does it matter? *Archives of Disease in Childhood. Fetal and Neonatal Edition, 87*(2), F75-77.

Bujold, M., Feeley, N., Axelin, A., et al. (2018). Expressing human milk in the NICU: Coping mechanisms and challenges shape the complex experience of closeness and separation. *Advances in Neonatal Care, 18*(1), 38-48.

Bulut, O., Coban, A., Uzunhan, O., et al. (2019). Effects of targeted versus adjustable protein fortification of breast milk on early growth in very low-birth-weight preterm infants: A randomized clinical trial. *Nutrition in Clinical Practice.*

Buxmann, H., Miljak, A., Fischer, D., et al. (2009). Incidence and clinical outcome of cytomegalovirus transmission via breast milk in preterm infants </=31 weeks. *Acta Paediatrica, 98*(2), 270-276.

Campbell, A. G., & Miranda, P. Y. (2018). Breastfeeding trends among very low birth weight, low birth weight, and normal birth weight infants. *Journal of Pediatrics, 200,* 71-78.

Cartwright, J., Atz, T., Newman, S., et al. (2017). Integrative review of interventions to promote breastfeeding in the late preterm Infant. *Journal of Obstetric, Gynecologic & Neonatal Nursing, 46*(3), 347-356.

Casavant, S. G., McGrath, J. M., Burke, G., et al. (2015). Caregiving factors affecting breastfeeding duration within a neonatal intensive care unit. *Advances in Neonatal Care, 15*(6), 421-428.

Casey, L., Fucile, S., & Dow, K. E. (2018). Determinants of successful direct breastfeeding at hospital discharge in high-risk premature infants. *Breastfeeding Medicine, 13*(5), 346-351.

Cattaneo, A., Amani, A., Charpak, N., et al. (2018). Report on an international workshop on kangaroo mother care: Lessons learned and a vision for the future. *BMC Pregnancy & Childbirth, 18*(1), 170.

CDC. (2019). Cytomegalovirus (CMV) and congenital CMV infection. Retrieved from **cdc.gov/cmv/index.html**.

Cescutti-Butler, L., Hemingway, A., & Hewitt-Taylor, J. (2019). "His tummy's only tiny" - Scientific feeding advice versus women's knowledge. Women's experiences of feeding their late preterm babies. *Midwifery, 69,* 102-109.

Charpak, N., Ruiz, J. G., Zupan, J., et al. (2005). Kangaroo mother care: 25 years after. *Acta Paediatrica, 94*(5), 514-522.

Charpak, N., Tessier, R., Ruiz, J. G., et al. (2017). Twenty-year follow-up of kangaroo mother care versus traditional care. *Pediatrics, 139*(1).

Chatterton, R. T., Jr., Hill, P. D., Aldag, J. C., et al. (2000). Relation of plasma oxytocin and prolactin concentrations to milk production in mothers of preterm infants: influence of stress. *Journal of Clinical Endocrinology and Metabolism, 85*(10), 3661-3668.

Chen, C. H., Wang, T. M., Chang, H. M., et al. (2000). The effect of breast- and bottle-feeding on oxygen saturation and body temperature in preterm infants. *Journal of Human Lactation, 16*(1), 21-27.

Chi Luong, K., Long Nguyen, T., Huynh Thi, D. H., et al. (2016). Newly born low birthweight infants stabilise better in skin-to-skin contact than when separated from their mothers: A randomised controlled trial. *Acta Paediatrica, 105*(4), 381-390.

Cinar, N., Kose, D., Alvur, M., et al. (2016). Mothers' attitudes toward feeding twin babies in the first six months of life: A sample from Sakarya, Turkey. *Iranian Journal of Pediatrics, 26*(5), e5413.

Collins, C. T., Gillis, J., McPhee, A. J., et al. (2016). Avoidance of bottles during the establishment of breast feeds in preterm infants. *Cochrane Database of Systematic Reviews, 10,* CD005252. doi:10.1002/14651858.CD005252.pub4.

Colson, S., DeRooy, L., & Hawdon, J. (2003). Biological nurturing increases duration of breastfeeding for a vulnerable cohort. *MIDIRS Midwifery Digest, 13*(1), 92-97.

Conde-Agudelo, A., & Diaz-Rossello, J. L. (2016). Kangaroo mother care to reduce morbidity and mortality in low birthweight infants. *Cochrane Database of Systematic Reviews*(8), CD002771. doi:10.1002/14651858.CD002771.pub4.

Congiu, M., Reali, A., Deidda, F., et al. (2019). Breast milk for preterm multiples: More protein, less lactose. *Twin Research and Human Genetics, 1-7.*

Cordero, L., Oza-Frank, R., Moore-Clingenpeel, M., et al. (2016). Failure to initiate breastfeeding among high risk obstetrical patients who intended to breastfeed. *Journal of Neonatal-Perinatal Medicine, 9*(4), 401-409.

Czank, C., Simmer, K., & Hartmann, P. E. (2010). Design and characterization of a human milk product for the preterm infant. *Breastfeeding Medicine, 5*(2), 59-66.

Dahaban, N. M., Romli, M. F., Roslan, N. R., et al. (2013). Bacteria in expressed breastmilk from mothers of premature infants and maternal hygienic status. *Breastfeeding Medicine, 8*(4), 422-423.

Davanzo, R., Brovedani, P., Travan, L., et al. (2013). Intermittent kangaroo mother care: A NICU protocol. *Journal of Human Lactation, 29*(3), 332-338.

Davanzo, R., Strajn, T., Kennedy, J., et al. (2014). From tube to breast: The bridging role of semi-demand breastfeeding. *Journal of Human Lactation, 30*(4), 405-409.

Demirci, J. R., Sereika, S. M., & Bogen, D. (2013). Prevalence and predictors of early breastfeeding among late preterm mother-infant dyads. *Breastfeeding Medicine, 8*(3), 277-285.

Dereddy, N. R., Talati, A. J., Smith, A., et al. (2015). A multipronged approach is associated with improved breast milk feeding rates in very low birth weight infants of an inner-city hospital. *Journal of Human Lactation, 31*(1), 43-46.

Dewey, K. G., Nommsen-Rivers, L. A., Heinig, M. J., et al. (2003). Risk factors for suboptimal infant breastfeeding behavior, delayed onset of lactation, and excess neonatal weight loss. *Pediatrics, 112*(3 Pt 1), 607-619.

Diego, M. A., Field, T., & Hernandez-Reif, M. (2008). Temperature increases in preterm infants during massage therapy. *Infant Behavior and Development, 31*(1), 149-152.

Diego, M. A., Field, T., Hernandez-Reif, M., et al. (2007). Preterm infant massage elicits consistent increases in vagal activity and gastric motility that are associated with greater weight gain. *Acta Paediatrica, 96*(11), 1588-1591.

Dosani, A., Hemraj, J., Premji, S. S., et al. (2016). Breastfeeding the late preterm infant: Experiences of mothers and perceptions of public health nurses. *International Breastfeeding Journal, 12,* 23.

Dowling, D. A. (1999). Physiological responses of preterm infants to breast-feeding and bottle-feeding with the orthodontic nipple. *Nursing Research, 48*(2), 78-85.

Dowling, D. A., Blatz, M. A., & Graham, G. (2012). Mothers' experiences expressing breast milk for their preterm infants: Does NICU design make a difference? *Advances in Neonatal Care, 12*(6), 377-384.

Eidelman, A. I. (2016). Postnatal acquired cytomegalovirus infection from feeding raw breastmilk to the preterm infant. *Breastfeeding Medicine, 11,* 157-158.

El Manouni El Hassani, S., Berkhout, D. J. C., Niemarkt, H. J., et al. (2019). Risk factors for late-onset sepsis in preterm infants: A multicenter case-control study. *Neonatology, 116*(1), 42-51.

Escobar, G. J., Clark, R. H., & Greene, J. D. (2006). Short-term outcomes of infants born at 35 and 36 weeks gestation: We need to ask more questions. *Seminars in Perinatology, 30*(1), 28-33.

Estalella, I., San Milan, J., Trincado, M.J., et al. (2018). Evaluation of an intervention supporting breastfeeding among late preterm infants during in-hospital stay. *Women and Birth.* doi: 10.1016/j.wombi.2018.11.003.

Evans, L., Hilditch, C., & Keir, A. (2019). Are there interventions that improve breastfeeding and the use of breast milk in late preterm infants? *Journal of Paediatrics and Child Health, 55*(4), 477-480.

Fan, H. S. L., Wong, J. Y. H., Fong, D. Y. T., et al. (2019). Breastfeeding outcomes among early-term and full-term infants. *Midwifery, 71,* 71-76.

Feijo, L., Hernandez-Reif, M., Field, T., et al. (2006). Mothers' depressed mood and anxiety levels are reduced after massaging their preterm infants. *Infant Behavior and Development, 29*(3), 476-480.

Fenton, T. R., Chan, H. T., Madhu, A., et al. (2017). Preterm infant growth velocity calculations: A systematic review. *Pediatrics, 139*(3).

Flacking, R., Nyqvist, K. H., Ewald, U., et al. (2003). Long-term duration of breastfeeding in Swedish low birth weight infants. *Journal of Human Lactation, 19*(2), 157-165.

Fleurant, E., Schoeny, M., Hoban, R., et al. (2017). Barriers to human milk feeding at discharge of very-low-birth-weight Infants: Maternal goal setting as a key social factor. *Breastfeeding Medicine, 12,* 20-27.

Flint, A., New, K., & Davies, M. W. (2016). Cup feeding versus other forms of supplemental enteral feeding for newborn infants unable to fully breastfeed. *Cochrane Database of Sysematict Reviews*(8), CD005092. doi:10.1002/14651858.CD005092.pub3.

Franca, E. C., Sousa, C. B., Aragao, L. C., et al. (2014). Electromyographic analysis of masseter muscle in newborns during suction in breast, bottle or cup feeding. *BMC Pregnancy & Childbirth, 14,* 154.

Funkquist, E. L., Tuvemo, T., Jonsson, B., et al. (2006). Growth and breastfeeding among low birth weight infants fed with or without protein enrichment of human milk. *Upsala Journal of Medical Sciences, 111*(1), 97-108.

Galloway, C., & Howells, J. (2015). Harnessing breastmilk composition to improve a preterm infant's growth rate--A case study. *Breastfeeding Review, 23*(1), 17-21.

Garofalo, N. A., & Caplan, M. S. (2019). Oropharyngeal mother's milk: State of the science and influence on necrotizing enterocolitis. *Clinical Perinatology, 46*(1), 77-88.

Geddes, D. T., Chooi, K., Nancarrow, K., et al. (2017). Characterisation of sucking dynamics of breastfeeding preterm infants: A cross sectional study. *BMC Pregnancy & Childbirth, 17*(1), 386.

Ghaly, M. (2018). Human milk-based industry in the Muslim world: Religioethical challenges. *Breastfeeding Medicine, 13*(S1), S28-S29.

Gharib, S., Fletcher, M., Tucker, R., et al. (2018). Effect of dedicated lactation support services on breastfeeding outcomes in extremely-low-birth-weight neonates. *Journal of Human Lactation, 34*(4), 728-736.

Gianni, M. L., Bezze, E. N., Sannino, P., et al. (2018). Maternal views on facilitators of and barriers to breastfeeding preterm infants. *BMC Pediatrics, 18*(1), 283.

Gila-Diaz, A., Arribas, S. M., Algara, A., et al. (2019). A review of bioactive factors in human breastmilk: A focus on prematurity. *Nutrients, 11*(6).

Ginovart, G., Gich, I., & Verd, S. (2016). Formula feeding is independently associated with acute kidney injury in very low birth weight infants. *Journal of Human Lactation, 32*(4), NP111-NP115.

Gomes, C. F., Trezza, E. M., Murade, E. C., et al. (2006). Surface electromyography of facial muscles during natural and artificial feeding of infants. *Jornal de Pediatria (Rio de Janeiro), 82*(2), 103-109.

Gromada, K. K. (2007). *Mothering Multiples: Breastfeeding & Caring for Twins or More!* (3rd ed.). Schaumburg, IL: La Leche League International.

Gunn, T. R., Thompson, J. M., Jackson, H., et al. (2000). Does early hospital discharge with home support of families with preterm infants affect breastfeeding success? A randomized trial. *Acta Paediatrica, 89*(11), 1358-1363.

Haase, B., Barreira, J., Murphy, P. K., et al. (2009). The development of an accurate test weighing technique for preterm and high-risk hospitalized infants. *Breastfeeding Medicine, 4*(3), 151-156.

Hackman, N. M., Alligood-Percoco, N., Martin, A., et al. (2016). Reduced breastfeeding rates in firstborn late preterm and early term infants. *Breastfeeding Medicine, 11,* 119-125.

Hair, A. B., Bergner, E. M., Lee, M. L., et al. (2016). Premature infants 750-1,250 g birth weight supplemented with a novel human milk-derived cream are discharged sooner. *Breastfeeding Medicine, 11,* 133-137.

Hake-Brooks, S. J., & Anderson, G. C. (2008). Kangaroo care and breastfeeding of mother-preterm infant dyads 0-18 months: A randomized, controlled trial. *Neonatal Network, 27*(3), 151-159.

Hall, W. A., Shearer, K., Mogan, J., et al. (2002). Weighing preterm infants before & after breastfeeding: Does it increase maternal confidence and competence? *MCN American Journal of Maternal and Child Nursing, 27*(6), 318-326; quiz 327.

Hard, A. L., Nilsson, A. K., Lund, A. M., et al. (2019). Review shows that donor milk does not promote the growth and development of preterm infants as well as maternal milk. *Acta Paediatrica, 108*(6), 998-1007.

Hasselbalch, H., Jeppesen, D. L., Engelmann, M. D., et al. (1996). Decreased thymus size in formula-fed infants compared with breastfed infants. *Acta Paediatrica, 85*(9), 1029-1032.

HMBANA. (2018). *Guidelines for the Establishment and Operation of a Donor Human Milk Bank* (10th ed.). Fort Worth, TX: Human Milk Banking Association of North America.

Hoban, R., Bigger, H., Schoeny, M., et al. (2018). Milk volume at 2 weeks predicts mother's own milk feeding at neonatal intensive care unit discharge for very low birthweight infants. *Breastfeeding Medicine, 13*(2), 135-141.

Hoban, R., Patel, A. L., Medina Poeliniz, C., et al. (2018). Human milk biomarkers of secretory activation in breast pump-dependent mothers of premature infants. *Breastfeeding Medicine, 13*(5), 352-360.

Hurst, N., Engebretson, J., & Mahoney, J. S. (2013). Providing mother's own milk in the context of the NICU: A paradoxical experience. *Journal of Human Lactation, 29*(3), 366-373.

Hurst, N. M., Meier, P. P., Engstrom, J. L., et al. (2004). Mothers performing in-home measurement of milk intake during breastfeeding of their preterm infants: Maternal reactions and feeding outcomes. *Journal of Human Lactation, 20*(2), 178-187.

Hurst, N. M., Valentine, C. J., Renfro, L., et al. (1997). Skin-to-skin holding in the neonatal intensive care unit influences maternal milk volume. *Journal of Perinatology, 17*(3), 213-217.

Ikonen, R., Paavilainen, E., & Kaunonen, M. (2015). Preterm infants' mothers' experiences with milk expression and breastfeeding: An integrative review. *Advances in Neonatal Care, 15*(6), 394-406.

Jarvenpaa, A. L., Raiha, N. C., Rassin, D. K., et al. (1983). Preterm infants fed human milk attain intrauterine weight gain. *Acta Paediatrica Scandinavica, 72*(2), 239-243.

Jayaraman, D., Mukhopadhyay, K., Bhalla, A. K., et al. (2017). Randomized controlled trial on effect of intermittent early versus late kangaroo mother care on human milk feeding in low-birth-weight neonates. *Journal of Human Lactation, 33*(3), 533-539.

Jocson, M. A., Mason, E. O., & Schanler, R. J. (1997). The effects of nutrient fortification and varying storage conditions on host defense properties of human milk. *Pediatrics, 100*(2 Pt 1), 240-243.

Johnson, T. J., Patra, K., Greene, M. M., et al. (2019). NICU human milk dose and health care use after NICU discharge in very low birth weight infants. *Journal of Perinatology, 39*(1), 120-128.

Jones, F. (2019). *Best Practice for Expressing, Storing, and Handling Human Milk in Hospitals, Homes, and Child Care Settings* (4th ed.). Fort Worth, TX: Human Milk Banking Association of North America.

Josephson, C. D., Caliendo, A. M., Easley, K. A., et al. (2014). Blood transfusion and breast milk transmission of cytomegalovirus in very low-birth-weight infants: A prospective cohort study. *JAMA Pediatrics, 168*(11), 1054-1062.

Juliano, G. M., Puchalski, M. L., & Walsh, S. M. (2019). Inplementation of pre-/post-weight to enhance direct breastfeeding in the NICU. *Clinical Lactation, 10*(1), 29-39.

Kadioglu Simsek, G., Alyamac Dizdar, E., Arayici, S., et al. (2019). Comparison of the effect of three different fortification methods on growth of very low birth weight infants. *Breastfeeding Medicine, 14*(1), 63-68. doi:3.

Kair, L. R., Flaherman, V. J., Newby, K. A., et al. (2015). The experience of breastfeeding the late preterm infant: A qualitative study. *Breastfeeding Medicine, 10*(2), 102-106.

Kantorowska, A., Wei, J. C., Cohen, R. S., et al. (2016). Impact of donor milk availability on breast milk use and necrotizing enterocolitis rates. *Pediatrics, 137*(3), e20153123.

Kassing, D. (2002). Bottle-feeding as a tool to reinforce breastfeeding. *Journal of Human Lactation, 18*(1), 56-60.

Kavanaugh, K., Mead, L., Meier, P., et al. (1995). Getting enough: Mothers' concerns about breastfeeding a preterm infant after discharge. *Journal of Obstetric, Gynecologic & Neonatal Nursing, 24*(1), 23-32.

Keenan-Devlin, L. S., Awosemusi, Y. F., Grobman, W., et al. (2019). Early term delivery and breastfeeding outcomes. *Maternal and Child Health Journal.* doi: 10.1007/s10995-019-02787-4.

Kelly, C. E., Cheong, J. L., Gabra Fam, L., et al. (2016). Moderate and late preterm infants exhibit widespread brain white matter microstructure alterations at term-equivalent age relative to term-born controls. *Brain Imaging and Behavior, 10*(1), 41-49.

Kim, B. Y. (2016). Factors that influence early breastfeeding of singletons and twins in Korea: A retrospective study. *International Breastfeeding Journal, 12,* 4.

Kinney, H. C. (2006). The near-term (late preterm) human brain and risk for periventricular leukomalacia: A review. *Seminars in Perinatology, 30*(2), 81-88.

Kledzik, T. (2005). Holding the very low birth weight infant: Skin-to-skin techniques. *Neonatal Network, 24*(1), 7-14.

Kliethermes, P. A., Cross, M. L., Lanese, M. G., et al. (1999). Transitioning preterm infants with nasogastric tube supplementation: Increased likelihood of breastfeeding. *Journal of Obstetric, Gynecologic & Neonatal Nursing, 28*(3), 264-273.

Knell, J., Han, S. M., Jaksic, T., et al. (2019). Current status of necrotizing enterocolitis. *Current Problems in Surgery, 56*(1), 11-38.

Kronborg, H., Foverskov, E., Nilsson, I., et al. (2017). Why do mothers use nipple shields and how does this influence duration of exclusive breastfeeding? *Maternal and Child Nutrition, 13*(1). doi:10.1111/mcn.12251.

Kuschel, C. A., Evans, N., Askie, L., et al. (2000). A randomized trial of enteral feeding volumes in infants born before 30 weeks' gestation. *Journal of Paediatrics and Child Health, 36*(6), 581-586.

Lang, S., Lawrence, C. J., & Orme, R. L. (1994). Cup feeding: an alternative method of infant feeding. *Archives of Disease in Childhood, 71*(4), 365-369.

Langland, V. (2019). Expressing motherhood: Wet nursing and human milk banking in Brazil. *Journal of Human Lactation, 35*(2), 354-361.

Lapillonne, A., Bronsky, J., Campoy, C., et al. (2019). Feeding the late and moderately preterm infant: A position paper of the European Society for Paediatric Gastroenterology, Hepatology and Nutrition Committee on Nutrition. *Journal of Pediatric Gastroenterology and Nutrition.* doi:10.1097/MPG.0000000000002397.

Lau, C., Sheena, H. R., Shulman, R. J., et al. (1997). Oral feeding in low birth weight infants. *Journal of Pediatrics, 130*(4), 561-569.

Lucas, R., Paquette, R., Briere, C. E., et al. (2014). Furthering our understanding of the needs of mothers who are pumping breast milk for infants in the NICU: An integrative review. *Advances in Neonatal Care, 14*(4), 241-252.

Lv, B., Gao, X. R., Sun, J., et al. (2019). Family-centered care improves clinical outcomes of very-low-birth-weight infants: A quasi-experimental study. *Frontiers in Pediatrics, 7,* 138.

Maastrup, R., Hansen, B. M., Kronborg, H., et al. (2014). Factors associated with exclusive breastfeeding of preterm infants. Results from a prospective national cohort study. *PLoS One, 9*(2), e89077.

Malhotra, N., Vishwambaran, L., Sundaram, K. R., et al. (1999). A controlled trial of alternative methods of oral feeding in neonates. *Early Human Development, 54*(1), 29-38.

McCain, G. C., Gartside, P. S., Greenberg, J. M., et al. (2001). A feeding protocol for healthy preterm infants that shortens time to oral feeding. *Journal of Pediatrics, 139*(3), 374-379.

Measel, C. P., & Anderson, G. C. (1979). Nonnutritive sucking during tube feedings: Effect on clinical course in premature infants. *Journal of Obstetric, Gynecologic & Neonatal Nursing, 8*(5), 265-272.

Meier, P. (1988). Bottle- and breast-feeding: effects on transcutaneous oxygen pressure and temperature in preterm infants. *Nursing Research, 37*(1), 36-41.

Meier, P., & Anderson, G. C. (1987). Responses of small preterm infants to bottle- and breast-feeding. *MCN; American Journal of Maternal Child Nursing, 12*(2), 97-105.

Meier, P., Patel, A., & Esquerra-Zwiers, A. (2017). Donor human milk update: Evidence, mechanisms, and priorities for research and practice. *Journal of Pediatrics, 180,* 15-21.

Meier, P. P. (2019). Prioritizing high-dose long exposure to mothers' own milk during the neonatal intensive care unit hospitalization. *Breastfeeding Medicine, 14*(S1), S20-S21.

Meier, P. P., Brown, L. P., Hurst, N. M., et al. (2000). Nipple shields for preterm infants: Effect on milk transfer and duration of breastfeeding. *Journal of Human Lactation, 16*(2), 106-114; quiz 129-131.

Meier, P. P., & Engstrom, J. L. (2007). Test weighing for term and premature infants is an accurate procedure. *Archives of Disease in Childhood. Fetal and Neonatal Edition, 92*(2), F155-156.

Meier, P. P., Engstrom, J. L., Crichton, C. L., et al. (1994). A new scale for in-home test-weighing for mothers of preterm and high risk infants. *Journal of Human Lactation, 10*(3), 163-168.

Meier, P. P., Engstrom, J. L., Fleming, B. A., et al. (1996). Estimating milk intake of hospitalized preterm infants who breastfeed. *Journal of Human Lactation, 12*(1), 21-26.

Meier, P. P., Engstrom, J. L., Mingolelli, S. S., et al. (2004). The Rush Mothers' Milk Club: Breastfeeding interventions for mothers with very-low-birth-weight infants. *Journal of Obstetric, Gynecologic & Neonatal Nursing, 33*(2), 164-174.

Meier, P. P., Engstrom, J. L., & Rossman, B. (2013). Breastfeeding peer counselors as direct lactation care providers in the neonatal intensive care unit. *Journal of Human Lactation, 29*(3), 313-322.

Meier, P. P., Johnson, T. J., Patel, A. L., et al. (2017). Evidence-based methods that promote human milk feeding of preterm infants: An expert review. *Clinical Perinatology, 44*(1), 1-22.

Meier, P. P., Patel, A. L., Bigger, H. R., et al. (2013). Supporting breastfeeding in the neonatal intensive care unit: Rush Mother's Milk Club as a case study of evidence-based care. *Pediatric Clinics of North America, 60*(1), 209-226.

Merewood, A., Chamberlain, L. B., Cook, J. T., et al. (2006). The effect of peer counselors on breastfeeding rates in the neonatal intensive care unit: Results of a randomized controlled trial. *Archives of Pediatrics and Adolescent Medicine, 160*(7), 681-685.

Mikami, F. C. F., Francisco, R. P. V., Rodrigues, A., et al. (2018). Breastfeeding twins: Factors related to weaning. *Journal of Human Lactation*, 890334418767382.

Mikawa, T., Mizuno, K., Tanaka, K., et al. (2019). Microwave treatment of breast milk for prevention of cytomegalovirus infection. *Pediatrics International.*

Miracle, D. J., Meier, P. P., & Bennett, P. A. (2004). Mothers' decisions to change from formula to mothers' milk for very-low-birth-weight infants. *Journal of Obstetric, Gynecologic & Neonatal Nursing, 33*(6), 692-703.

Mizuno, K., Inoue, M., & Takeuchi, T. (2000). The effects of body positioning on sucking behaviour in sick neonates. *European Journal of Pediatrics, 159*(11), 827-831.

Mizuno, K., Nishida, Y., Taki, M., et al. (2007). Infants with bronchopulmonary dysplasia suckle with weak pressures to maintain breathing during feeding. *Pediatrics, 120*(4), e1035-1042.

Morelius, E., Hellstrom-Westas, L., Carlen, C., et al. (2006). Is a nappy change stressful to neonates? *Early Human Development, 82*(10), 669-676.

Morton, J., Hall, J. Y., Wong, R. J., et al. (2009). Combining hand techniques with electric pumping increases milk production in mothers of preterm infants. *Journal of Perinatology, 29*(11), 757-764.

Morton, J., Wong, R. J., Hall, J. Y., et al. (2012). Combining hand techniques with electric pumping increases the caloric content of milk in mothers of preterm infants. *Journal of Perinatology, 32*(10), 791-796.

Narayanan, I. (1990). Sucking on the "emptied" breast--A better method of non-nutritive sucking than the use of a pacifier. *Indian Pediatrics, 27*(10), 1122-1124.

Narayanan, I., Prakash, K., Murthy, N. S., et al. (1984). Randomised controlled trial of effect of raw and holder pasteurised human milk and of formula supplements on incidence of neonatal infection. *Lancet, 2*(8412), 1111-1113.

Nelson, A. M. (2017). Risks and benefits of swaddling healthy infants: An integrative review. *MCN American Journal of Maternal and Child Nursing, 42*(4), 216-225.

Noble, A., Eventov-Friedman, S., Hand, I., et al. (2019). Breastfeeding intensity and exclusivity of early term infants at birth and 1 month. *Breastfeeding Medicine.* doi:10.1089/bfm.2018.0260.

Noble, L. M., Okogbule-Wonodi, A. C., & Young, M. A. (2018). ABM Clinical Protocol #12: Transitioning the breastfeeding preterm infant from the neonatal intensive care unit to home, revised 2018. *Breastfeeding Medicine, 13*(4), 230-236.

Nye, C. (2008). Transitioning premature infants from gavage to breast. *Neonatal Network, 27*(1), 7-13.

Nyqvist, K. H. (2002). Breast-feeding in preterm twins: Development of feeding behavior and milk intake during hospital stay and related caregiving practices. *Journal of Pediatric Nursing, 17*(4), 246-256.

Nyqvist, K. H. (2004). How can kangaroo mother care and high technology care be compatible? *Journal of Human Lactation, 20*(1), 72-74.

Nyqvist, K. H. (2008). Early attainment of breastfeeding competence in very preterm infants. *Acta Paediatrica, 97*(6), 776-781.

Nyqvist, K. H. (2013). Lack of knowledge persists about early breastfeeding competence in preterm infants. *Journal of Human Lactation, 29*(3), 296-299.

Nyqvist, K. H. (2017). Breastfeeding preterm infants. In C. W. Genna (Ed.), *Supporting Sucking Skills in Breastfeeding Infants* (3rd ed., pp. 181-208). Burlington, MA: Jones & Bartlett Learning.

Nyqvist, K. H., & Engvall, G. (2009). Parents as their infant's primary caregivers in a neonatal intensive care unit. *Journal of Pediatric Nursing, 24*(2), 153-163.

Nyqvist, K. H., Haggkvist, A. P., Hansen, M. N., et al. (2013). Expansion of the baby-friendly hospital initiative ten steps to successful breastfeeding into neonatal intensive care: Expert group recommendations. *Journal of Human Lactation, 29*(3), 300-309.

Nyqvist, K. H., & Lutes, L. M. (1998). Co-bedding twins: A developmentally supportive care strategy. *Journal of Obstetric, Gynecologic & Neonatal Nursing, 27*(4), 450-456.

Nyqvist, K. H., Rubertsson, C., Ewald, U., et al. (1996). Development of the Preterm Infant Breastfeeding Behavior Scale (PIBBS): A study of nurse-mother agreement. *Journal of Human Lactation, 12*(3), 207-219.

Nyqvist, K. H., Sjoden, P. O., & Ewald, U. (1994). Mothers' advice about facilitating breastfeeding in a neonatal intensive care unit. *Journal of Human Lactation, 10*(4), 237-243.

Nyqvist, K. H., Sjoden, P. O., & Ewald, U. (1999). The development of preterm infants' breastfeeding behavior. *Early Human Development, 55*(3), 247-264.

O'Connor, D. L., Khan, S., Weishuhn, K., et al. (2008). Growth and nutrient intakes of human milk-fed preterm infants provided with extra energy and nutrients after hospital discharge. *Pediatrics, 121*(4), 766-776.

Ogechi, A. A., William, O., & Fidelia, B. T. (2007). Hindmilk and weight gain in preterm very low-birthweight infants. *Pediatrics International, 49*(2), 156-160.

Oliveira, M. M., Aragon, D. C., Bomfim, V. S., et al. (2019). Development of a human milk concentrate with human milk lyophilizate for feeding very low birth weight preterm infants: A preclinical experimental study. *PLoS One, 14*(2), e0210999.

Oras, P., Blomqvist, Y. T., Nyqvist, K. H., et al. (2015). Breastfeeding patterns in preterm infants born at 28-33 gestational weeks. *Journal of Human Lactation, 31*(3), 377-385.

Oras, P., Thernstrom Blomqvist, Y., Hedberg Nyqvist, K., et al. (2016). Skin-to-skin contact is associated with earlier breastfeeding attainment in preterm infants. *Acta Paediatrica, 105*(7), 783-789.

Oza-Frank, R., Bhatia, A., & Smith, C. (2014). Impact of peer counselors on breastfeeding outcomes in a nondelivery NICU setting. *Advances in Neonatal Care, 14*(4), E1-8.

Paduraru, L., Dimitriu, D. C., Avasiloaiei, A. L., et al. (2018). Total antioxidant status in fresh and stored human milk from mothers of term and preterm neonates. *Pediatrics and Neonatology, 59*(6), 600-605.

Panczuk, J. K., Unger, S., Francis, J., et al. (2016). Introduction of bovine-based nutrient fortifier and gastrointestinal inflammation in very low birth weight infants as measured by fecal calprotectin. *Breastfeeding Medicine, 11*(1), 2-5.

Pang, W. W., Bernard, J. Y., Thavamani, G., et al. (2017). Direct vs. expressed breast milk feeding: Relation to duration of breastfeeding. *Nutrients, 9*(6).

Park, J., Thoyre, S., Estrem, H., et al. (2016). Mothers' psychological distress and feeding of their preterm infants. *MCN American Journal of Maternal and Child Nursing, 41*(4), 221-229.

Parker, L. A., Sullivan, S., Krueger, C., et al. (2012). Effect of early breast milk expression on milk volume and timing of lactogenesis stage II among mothers of very low birth weight infants: A pilot study. *Journal of Perinatology, 32*(3), 205-209.

Parker, M. G., Burnham, L. A., Melvin, P., et al. (2019). Addressing disparities in mother's milk for VLBW infants through statewide quality improvement. *Pediatrics.*

Patel, A. L., Johnson, T. J., Engstrom, J. L., et al. (2013). Impact of early human milk on sepsis and health-care costs in very low birth weight infants. *Journal of Perinatology, 33*(7), 514-519.

Patel, A. L., Johnson, T. J., Robin, B., et al. (2017). Influence of own mother's milk on bronchopulmonary dysplasia and costs. *Archives of Disease in Childhood. Fetal and Neonatal Edition, 102*(3), F256-F261.

Patel, A. L., & Kim, J. H. (2018). Human milk and necrotizing enterocolitis. *Seminars in Pediatric Surgery, 27*(1), 34-38.

Penn, A. H., Altshuler, A. E., Small, J. W., et al. (2012). Digested formula but not digested fresh human milk causes death of intestinal cells in vitro: Implications for necrotizing enterocolitis. *Pediatric Research, 72*(6), 560-567.

Penny, F., Judge, M., Brownell, E., et al. (2018). Cup feeding as a supplemental, alternative feeding method for preterm breastfed infants: An integrative review. *Maternal and Child Health Journal, 22*(11), 1568-1579.

Perrine, C. G., & Scanlon, K. S. (2013). Prevalence of use of human milk in US advanced care neonatal units. *Pediatrics, 131*(6), 1066-1071.

Pineda, R. (2011). Direct breast-feeding in the neonatal intensive care unit: Is it important? *Journal of Perinatology, 31*(8), 540-545.

Pineda, R. G. (2016). Feeding: An important, complex skill that impacts nutritional, social, motor and sensory experiences. *Acta Paediatrica, 105*(10), e458.

Poets, C. F., Langner, M. U., & Bohnhorst, B. (1997). Effects of bottle feeding and two different methods of gavage feeding on oxygenation and breathing patterns in preterm infants. *Acta Paediatrica, 86*(4), 419-423.

Quan, R., Yang, C., Rubinstein, S., et al. (1994). The effect of nutritional additives on anti-infective factors in human milk. *Clinical Pediatrics (Philadelphia), 33*(6), 325-328.

Quan, R., Yang, C., Rubinstein, S., et al. (1992). Effects of microwave radiation on anti-infective factors in human milk. *Pediatrics, 89*(4 Pt 1), 667-669.

Quigley, M., Embleton, N. D., & McGuire, W. (2019). Formula versus donor breast milk for feeding preterm or low birth weight infants. *Cochrane Database of Systematic Reviews, 7,* CD002971. doi:10.1002/14651858.CD002971.pub5.

Radzyminski, S. (2005). Neurobehavioral functioning and breastfeeding behavior in the newborn. *Journal of Obstetric, Gynecologic & Neonatal Nursing, 34*(3), 335-341.

Raju, T. (2017). The "late preterm" birth-Ten years later. *Pediatrics, 139*(3).

Ramasethu, J., Jeyaseelan, L., & Kirubakaran, C. P. (1993). Weight gain in exclusively breastfed preterm infants. *Journal of Tropical Pediatrics, 39*(3), 152-159.

Rankin, M. W., Jimenez, E. Y., Caraco, M., et al. (2016). Validation of test weighing protocol to estimate enteral feeding volumes in preterm infants. *Journal of Pediatrics, 178,* 108-112.

Rayfield, S., Oakley, L., & Quigley, M. A. (2015). Association between breastfeeding support and breastfeeding rates in the UK: A comparison of late preterm and term infants. *BMJ Open, 5*(11), e009144.

Regev, R. H., Arnon, S., Litmanovitz, I., et al. (2016). Association between neonatal morbidities and head growth from birth until discharge in very-low-birthweight infants born preterm: A population-based study. *Developmental Medicine & Child Neurology, 58*(11), 1159-1166.

Reyna, B. A., Pickler, R. H., & Thompson, A. (2006). A descriptive study of mothers' experiences feeding their preterm infants after discharge. *Advances in Neonatal Care, 6*(6), 333-340.

Rochow, N., Landau-Crangle, E., & Fusch, C. (2015). Challenges in breast milk fortification for preterm infants. *Current Opinion in Clinical Nutrition and Metabolic Care, 18*(3), 276-284.

Rodriguez, N. A., Miracle, D. J., & Meier, P. P. (2005). Sharing the science on human milk feedings with mothers of very-low-birth-weight infants. *Journal of Obstetric, Gynecologic & Neonatal Nursing, 34*(1), 109-119.

Romaine, A., Clark, R. H., Davis, B. R., et al. (2018). Predictors of prolonged breast milk provision to very low birth weight infants. *Journal of Pediatrics, 202,* 23-30 e21.

Ross, E. S., & Browne, J. V. (2002). Developmental progression of feeding skills: An approach to supporting feeding in preterm infants. *Seminars in Neonatology, 7*(6), 469-475.

Rossman, B., Kratovil, A. L., Greene, M. M., et al. (2013). "I have faith in my milk": The meaning of milk for mothers of very low birth weight infants hospitalized in the neonatal intensive care unit. *Journal of Human Lactation, 29*(3), 359-365.

Santiago, M. S., Codipilly, C. N., Potak, D. C., et al. (2005). Effect of human milk fortifiers on bacterial growth in human milk. *Journal of Perinatology, 25*(10), 647-649.

Schanler, R. J., & Abrams, S. A. (1995). Postnatal attainment of intrauterine macromineral accretion rates in low birth weight infants fed fortified human milk. *Journal of Pediatrics, 126*(3), 441-447.

Schleiss, M. R. (2006). Acquisition of human cytomegalovirus infection in infants via breast milk: Natural immunization or cause for concern? *Reviews in Medical Virology, 16*(2), 73-82.

Schneider, J., Fischer Fumeaux, C. J., Duerden, E. G., et al. (2018). Nutrient intake in the first two weeks of life and brain growth in preterm neonates. *Pediatrics, 141*(3).

Sharp, M., Campbell, C., Chiffings, D., et al. (2015). Improvement in long-term breastfeeding for very preterm infants. *Breastfeeding Medicine, 10*(3), 145-149.

Shorey, S., He, H. G., & Morelius, E. (2016). Skin-to-skin contact by fathers and the impact on infant and paternal outcomes: An integrative review. *Midwifery, 40,* 207-217.

Silvestre, D., Ruiz, P., Martinez-Costa, C., et al. (2008). Effect of pasteurization on the bactericidal capacity of human milk. *Journal of Human Lactation, 24*(4), 371-376.

Sisk, P. M., Lovelady, C. A., Dillard, R. G., et al. (2006). Lactation counseling for mothers of very low birth weight infants: Effect on maternal anxiety and infant intake of human milk. *Pediatrics, 117*(1), e67-75.

Smith, M. M., Durkin, M., Hinton, V. J., et al. (2003). Initiation of breastfeeding among mothers of very low birth weight infants. *Pediatrics, 111*(6 Pt 1), 1337-1342.

Spatz, D. L. (2021). The use of human milk and breastfeeding in the neonatal intensive care unit. In K. Wambach & B. Spencer (Eds.), *Breastfeeding and Human Lactation* (6th ed., pp. 397-441). Burlington, MA: Jones & Bartlett Learning.

Spatz, D. L. (2017). Is routine fortification of human milk for babies in the neonatal intensive care unit indicated? *MCN American Journal of Maternal and Child Nursing, 42*(2), 117.

Tomashek, K. M., Shapiro-Mendoza, C. K., Weiss, J., et al. (2006). Early discharge among late preterm and term newborns and risk of neonatal morbidity. *Seminars in Perinatology, 30*(2), 61-68.

Tully, K. P., Holditch-Davis, D., Silva, S., et al. (2017). The relationship between infant feeding outcomes and maternal emotional well-being among mothers ofl late preterm and term infants: A secondary, exploratory analysis. *Advances in Neonatal Care, 17*(1), 65-75.

Valentine, C. J., Hurst, N. M., & Schanler, R. J. (1994). Hindmilk improves weight gain in low-birth-weight infants fed human milk. *Journal of Pediatric Gastroenterology and Nutrition, 18*(4), 474-477.

Walsh, J. M., Doyle, L. W., Anderson, P. J., et al. (2014). Moderate and late preterm birth: Effect on brain size and maturation at term-equivalent age. *Radiology, 273*(1), 232-240.

Wang, M. L., Dorer, D. J., Fleming, M. P., et al. (2004). Clinical outcomes of near-term infants. *Pediatrics, 114*(2), 372-376.

Weaver, G., Bertino, E., Gebauer, C., et al. (2019). Recommendations for the establishment and operation of human milk banks in Europe: A consensus statement from the European Milk Bank Association (EMBA). *Frontiers in Pediatrics, 7,* 53.

Weimers, L., Svensson, K., Dumas, L., et al. (2006). Hands-on approach during breastfeeding support in a neonatal intensive care unit: A qualitative study of Swedish mothers' experiences. *International Breastfeeding Journal, 1,* 20.

Wesolowska, A., Sinkiewicz-Darol, E., Barbarska, O., et al. (2019). Innovative techniques of processing human milk to preserve key components. *Nutrients, 11*(5).

WHO. (2013). What kind of care do preterm babies need? Retrieved from **who.int/features/qa/preterm_baby_care/en/**.

Williams, T., Nair, H., Simpson, J., et al. (2016). Use of donor human milk and maternal breastfeeding rates: A systematic review. *Journal of Human Lactation, 32*(2), 212-220.

Wilson-Clay, B., & Hoover, K. (2017). *The Breastfeeding Atlas* (6th ed.). Manchaca, TX: LactNews Press.

Xavier, A. A. O., Diaz-Salido, E., Arenilla-Velez, I., et al. (2018). Carotenoid content in human colostrum is associated to preterm/full-term birth condition. *Nutrients, 10*(11).

Yu, X., Li, J., Lin, X., et al. (2019). Association between delayed lactogenesis and early milk volume among mothers of preterm infants. *Asian Nursing Research (Korean Society of Nursing Science), 13*(2), 93-98.

Zhou, J., Shukla, V. V., John, D., et al. (2015). Human milk feeding as a protective factor for retinopathy of prematurity: A meta-analysis. *Pediatrics, 136*(6), e1576-1586.

PART III

The Nursing Parent

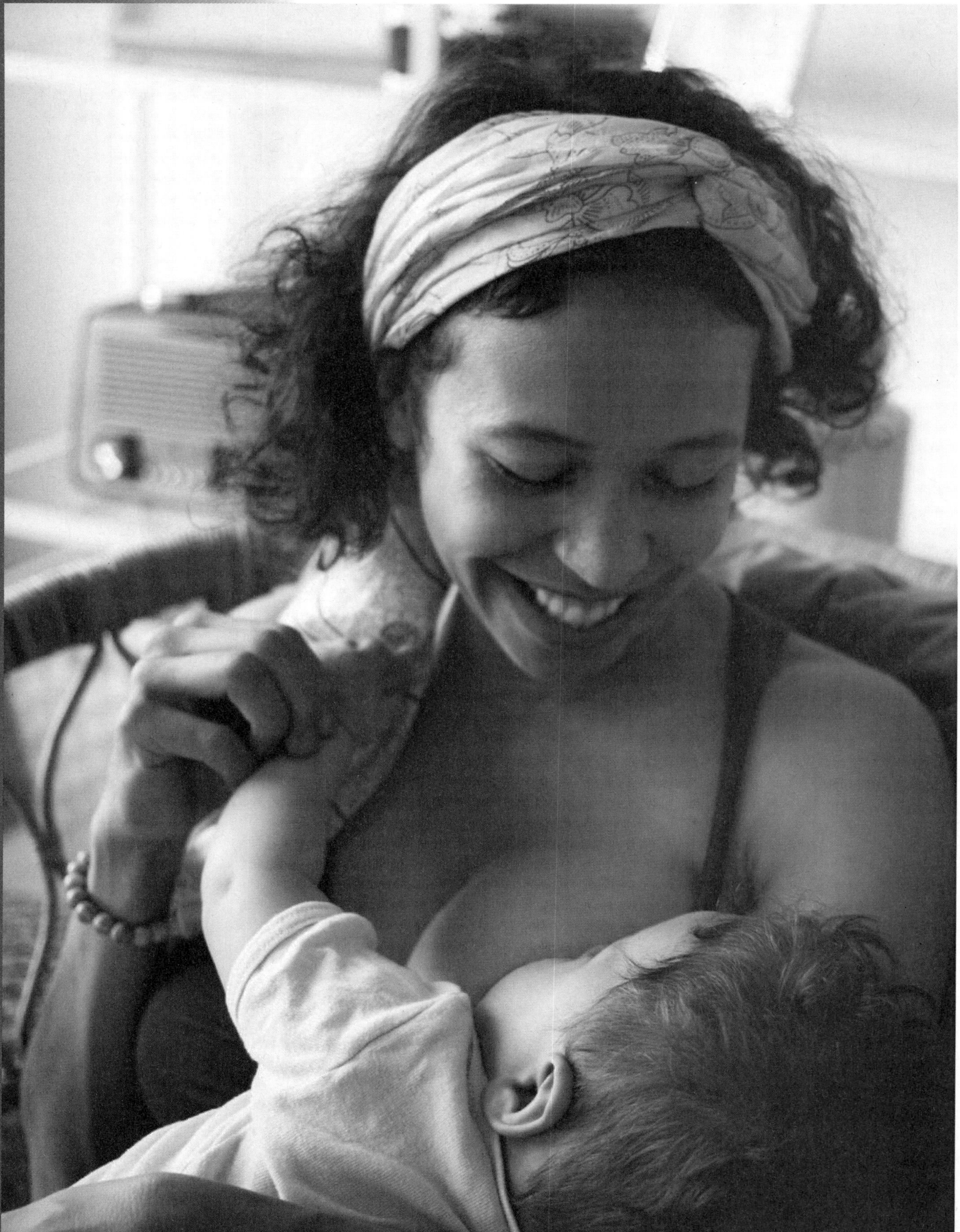

Making Milk

10

ANATOMY OF THE MAMMARY GLAND

Basic familiarity with the anatomy of the mammary gland offers insights into some of the physical dynamics that affect milk production.

Development of the mammary gland begins while a baby is still in the womb, but this gland doesn't become fully functional until lactation begins. The mammary gland changes throughout the lifespan: during menstrual cycles, pregnancies, births, nursing, weaning, aging, and menopause, when the gland begins to atrophy, one aspect of a process called involution. The mammary growth during pregnancy and during the first month of nursing is one indicator of functional tissue (Cox, Kent, Casey, Owens, & Hartmann, 1999; Thanaboonyawat, Chanprapaph, Lattalapkul, & Rongluen, 2013). A deeper understanding of the dynamics affecting nursing starts with an awareness of this gland's anatomy.

• • •

The mammary gland consists of several basic types of tissues and fluids.

Each part of the mammary gland (Figure 10.1) falls into one of several basic categories:

- Glandular tissue, which makes milk and transports it to the nipple
- Connective (muscle) tissue, including Cooper's ligaments, which provides mechanical support to the gland
- Adipose (fatty) tissue, which supports the growth of milk ducts during puberty and provides protection from outside injury (Geddes, 2007a)
- Nerves, which provide the sensitivity to touch and temperature important for milk ejection
- Blood, which provides nourishment and the ingredients needed to make milk
- Lymph, which transports waste products away from the gland

The size of the mammary gland is determined mainly by the amount of fatty tissue present, which is unrelated to milk production. The proportion of glandular tissue to fatty tissue during lactation varies greatly among nursing parents, but on average, there is about twice as much glandular tissue as fatty tissue (63% vs. 37%), and they tend to be intermixed, rather than separated within the gland (Ramsay, Kent, Hartmann, & Hartmann, 2005). On average, about 70% of the glandular tissue is located within a 30 mm radius (a little more than an inch) of the nipple. No relationship was found between proportion of glandular to fatty tissue and storage capacity (see later section) or volume of milk produced (Geddes, 2007b)

• • •

Each aspect of the glandular tissue has a specific function.

The glandular or milk-making tissue is composed of the following components (Figure 10.1):

Alveoli are milk-making factories where cells called lactocytes, also known as mammary epithelial cells, draw the needed nutrients from the bloodstream. Resembling clusters of grapes, they are surrounded by a network of muscular myoepithelial cells that squeeze the alveoli during milk ejection, pushing the milk into the ductules and on into the ducts (Berry, Thomas, Piper, & Cregan, 2007).

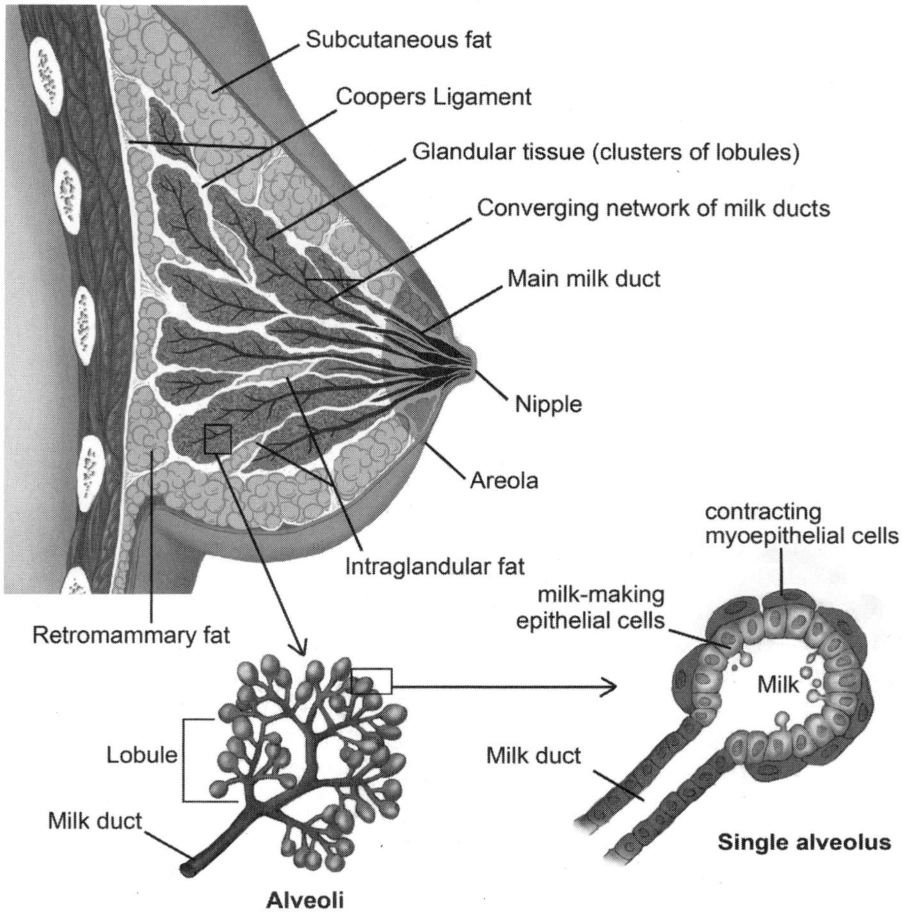

Figure 10.1 Anatomy of the lactating mammary gland. ©2019 Taina Litwin, used with permission.

Ducts and ductules are the small tubes that carry the milk from the alveoli to the nipple. The smaller ductules lead from the clusters of alveoli to the larger ducts, which join with other ducts before reaching the nipple. Ultrasound research revealed that the branching of the major ducts is close the nipple (Ramsay, Kent, et al., 2005).

It was once thought that wider ducts known as "milk sinuses" or "lactiferous sinuses" were located under the areola and that these reservoirs of milk needed to be compressed during nursing and milk expression for best milk flow. However, ultrasound research found the ducts in this area are no larger than the ducts elsewhere in the mammary gland, challenging the existence of these milk reservoirs (Ramsay, Kent, et al., 2005).

> **KEY CONCEPT**
>
> *On average, about 70% of the glandular tissue is located within a 30 mm radius of the nipple.*

At rest, milk ducts average 2 mm in diameter and increase in diameter during milk ejection by about 58% (Ramsay, Kent, Owens, & Hartmann, 2004). Some milk ducts are so close to the surface that expanded ducts can be seen on the surface of the unused side when milk ejection occurs. Being easily compressible and close to the surface explains why consistent pressure on the gland may cause plugged or blocked ducts. Rather than radiating symmetrically from the nipple, as illustrated in many older diagrams, milk ducts appear more like tangled tree roots intermixed with the fatty tissue, which makes them difficult to avoid during mammary surgery.

Lobes and lobules are segments of the mammary gland. A lobule consists of a single branch of alveoli and milk ducts that deliver milk to a lobe, which leads to a single nipple pore. Until the 2000s, it was thought there were 15 to 20 lobes in a mammary gland, but ultrasound research discovered that most have between 4 and 17 lobes per side, with an average of 9 (Going & Moffat, 2004; Love & Barsky, 2004; Ramsay, Kent, et al., 2005). Japanese research (Mizuno et al., 2008) found that how deeply the baby latches affects how evenly the mammary gland is drained, with a deep latch draining the lobes more evenly and shallow latch leaving some lobes well-drained and others full.

The nipple includes on its outer surface between 4 and 18 nipple openings (or pores) that measure on average 0.4 to 0.7 mm in diameter and are connected to the lobes (Jutte, Hohoff, Sauerland, Wiechmann, & Stamm, 2014; Ramsay, Kent, et al., 2005). There may be many more nipple pores that are not connected to functional ducts (Geddes, 2007a; Going & Moffat, 2004; Love & Barsky, 2004). Very little fat is located under the skin near the nipple. The nipple and areola contain smooth muscle erectile tissue that contracts with stimulation, such as touch or cold, causing the nipple to become firm and protrude. The nipple's flexibility allows it to stretch and conform to the inside of the baby's mouth during nursing.

The areola, which can be pronounced "a RE ola" or "air e O la" (both are correct), is the darker pigmented area from which the nipple protrudes and where the Montgomery glands are located. Some suggested that this darkened area may act as a "target" to help the baby find the nipple. The plural of areola is areolae.

Montgomery glands are a combination of sebaceous and mammary glands located on the areola that enlarge and become more prominent during pregnancy. Their number varies from 1 to 15 (Geddes, 2007b). The fluid they secrete may serve several purposes:

- Protect the skin from sucking friction
- Reduce bacterial counts by altering the pH of the skin
- Help the baby find the nipple after birth via their fluid's odor (Doucet, Soussignan, Sagot, & Schaal, 2009)

Research of 64 French mothers found that having more Montgomery glands was associated with greater infant weight gain between birth and Day 3 (Schaal, Doucet, Sagot, Hertling, & Soussignan, 2006). Washing the nipples with soap or disinfecting fluids, including alcohol, can remove the fluids secreted by the Montgomery glands. Unless the mother has nipple trauma (see p. 722), the usual bathing routine is all that's needed to keep the nipples clean and maintain this fluid's lubricating and anti-bacterial effects.

• • •

Research indicates that nursing does *not* cause the mammary glands to sag.

In one U.S. survey (Rinker, Veneracion, & Walsh, 2008), many women considering cosmetic breast surgery attributed their loss of breast shape to nursing. Surveys done worldwide (Hull, Thapa, & Pratomo, 1990; McLennan, 2001; Pisacane & Continisio, 2004) found that people of all ages believed that nursing causes sagging breasts.

Three U.S. plastic surgeons examined whether nursing is a risk factor for loss of breast shape ("breast ptosis") by doing a chart review and phone interviews with all 132 women seeking cosmetic breast surgery (breast implants or breast lifts) at one clinic between 1998 and 2006 (Rinker et al., 2008). Of the 91 women who had at least one term pregnancy, 58% had a history of nursing. They found that a history of nursing, number of children nursed, how long each child nursed, and how much weight was gained during pregnancy were not associated with loss of breast shape. Significant predictors for loss of breast shape included number of pregnancies, age, a history of smoking, larger prepregnancy bra cup size, and higher body mass index (BMI). Neither "any breastfeeding" nor duration of breastfeeding was an independent risk factor for loss of breast shape.

Italian researchers also concluded that nursing did not alter breast shape after surveying 500 first-time mothers at three health centers in Italy (Pisacane & Continisio, 2004). Similar percentages of women who never breastfed reported breast changes as women who breastfed. The researchers concluded that changes in breast appearance occur as a result of pregnancy, not nursing, and occur whether or not the mother breastfed.

A South Korean study measured breast volumes in 250 premenopausal women between age 20 and 50 (S. J. Kim, Kim, & Kim, 2014) and concluded that breast size increased with age, but this size increase was due to increasing body weight with aging, not type of birth or nursing.

MILK EJECTION

Milk ejection is triggered by the release of the hormone oxytocin and is responsible for most of the milk removal during nursing and milk expression.

During nursing and milk expression, significant milk removal occurs only after milk ejection, sometimes referred to as "let-down." Without it, only the small volume of milk (0.1 to 10 mL) located in the ducts near the nipple can be accessed, with most milk remaining in the mammary gland (Ramsay et al., 2004; Ramsay, Mitoulas, Kent, Larsson, & Hartmann, 2005). Milk ejection occurs when the hormone oxytocin is released by the posterior pituitary gland into the bloodstream, travels to the mammary gland and binds to oxytocin receptors, which causes the band-like muscles around the milk-producing alveoli (Figure 10.1) to squeeze and the milk ducts to shorten and dilate, pushing the milk out of the nipple pores. Because its trigger is hormonal, milk ejection occurs in both glands within about 10 seconds of each other (Gardner, Kent, Hartmann, & Geddes, 2015) and lasts for an average of 2 minutes (D.K. Prime, Geddes, & Hartmann, 2007).

When a baby nurses, her sucking sends nerve impulses to the parent's brain, where the hypothalamus signals the posterior pituitary to release oxytocin in bursts into the bloodstream (Rossoni et al., 2008). In addition to the physical sensations of the baby's sucking, her softness and warmth may also promote milk ejection. The nursing parent's emotional state (relaxed or tense) can also affect milk ejection. During early nursing sessions, it may take a few minutes for milk ejection to occur until the parent's body becomes conditioned to this response. But with time and conditioning, milk ejection becomes faster and more automatic, sometimes occurring even without a baby nursing (see later point).

• • •

Most nursing parents have several milk ejections per feed, but most feel only one and some feel none.

Number of milk ejections per nursing. According to Australian research (Cobo, 1993; Kent et al., 2008; Ramsay, Mitoulas, et al., 2005), the average number of milk ejections at each nursing session is 3 to 4, with a range of 1 to 17.

Perceptions of milk ejection. Australian researchers used ultrasound to observe milk ejection with 45 mothers during 166 breastfeeding sessions (Ramsay et al., 2004) and found that 88% of the study mothers felt their first milk ejection, but none felt subsequent milk ejections. In another Australian study of 11 breastfeeding mothers (Ramsay, Mitoulas, et al., 2005), four reported feeling more than one milk ejection. Pumping produced the same number of milk ejections as nursing. In one Australian study (Ramsay, Mitoulas, et al., 2005), mothers had multiple milk ejections during 95% of their pumping sessions.

Some nursing parents feel milk ejection as a tingling, pressure, a pins-and-needles sensation, a feeling of "drawing" or "rushing down," increased thirst, milk leakage from the other side, even pain, while others feel nothing (Ramsay et al., 2004; Ramsay, Mitoulas, et al., 2005). During the first week or two after birth, milk ejection may also be felt as uterine cramping or as tension across the shoulder blades. Parents feel milk ejection at varying levels of intensity. Some consider the feelings mild and others very intense. Feelings of nausea, intestinal pain, and vaginal bleeding were associated with milk ejection in some (D.K. Prime et al., 2007).

When milk ejection occurs. On average, during a nursing session, it takes about a minute or so of baby's sucking for a milk ejection to occur (Gardner, Kent, Lai, et al., 2015; Ramsay et al., 2004). The most reliable indicators of milk ejection during nursing are longer, slower jaw movements or audible swallowing by the baby. During milk expression, visibly faster milk flow is a reliable sign milk ejection occurred. As nursing becomes more routine, milk ejection may occur sooner. U.K. researchers (McNeilly, Robinson, Houston, & Howie, 1983) found that oxytocin was released when the baby began to fuss and as the nursing couple got ready to nurse. Japanese research (Kimura & Matsuoka, 2007) found that mammary skin temperature began to rise even before nursing began.

KEY CONCEPT

On average, milk ejection occurs after about a minute of active nursing.

• • •

Some sensations and emotions can trigger or inhibit milk ejection.

Milk ejection outside of nursing sessions. It is not unusual for milk ejections to occur in lactating parents in response to sensory stimuli other than nursing, such as hearing another baby cry or having loving thoughts about the baby. This is because milk ejection is in part a conditioned response, so other familiar sights, smells, sounds, touch, and thoughts can sometimes trigger it. One Australian lactation researcher told the story of one of his exclusively-pumping study mothers who covered her pump with a towel because otherwise whenever she saw it, this triggered a milk ejection. Researchers from Colombia and the U.K. (Cobo, 1993; McNeilly & McNeilly, 1978) reported cases of "spontaneous milk ejection," which were likely due to triggers other than nursing. A Canadian article described the experiences of three women with cervical spinal-cord injuries and damaged nerve pathways between breast and brain (Cowley, 2005, 2014). Because they were unable to feel the sensations of nursing, they learned to trigger milk ejections with mental imagery while their babies nursed.

Emotions that trigger or inhibit milk ejection. The parent's emotions can also trigger or inhibit milk ejection. For example, feeling upset, frustrated, stressed, or angry releases the stress hormone epinephrine (adrenaline), which may delay milk ejection (D.K. Prime et al., 2007). It is not unusual for parents

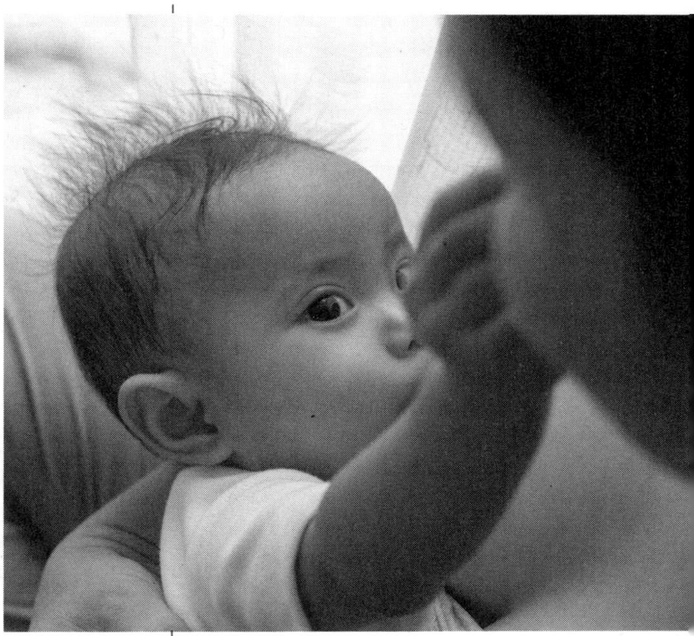

of preterm babies to express less milk after receiving bad news about their baby's condition (Chatterton et al., 2000). Anticipating pain can also delay milk ejection, which can happen in those experiencing nipple or mammary pain.

Sensations and substances that inhibit milk ejection. The feeling of ice against skin (Newton & Newton, 1948), excessive alcohol intake, and some medications (Lawrence & Lawrence, 2016) were found to block milk ejection.

Strategies to speed a delayed milk ejection. A U.S. study of 95 women exclusively pumping for preterm babies and 98 mothers nursing term babies (Hill, Aldag, Chatterton, & Zinaman, 2005) found that the normal stresses of parenthood, fatigue, and lack of sleep did not affect milk ejection or milk volumes. But if milk ejection is inhibited for any reason, suggest trying relaxation techniques (such as childbirth breathing), warm compresses, or mammary massage. If strong negative emotions may be a factor, try waiting a little while, until the parent feels calmer. In a crisis, if the milk ejection is consistently delayed, this may temporarily slow milk production. If so, encourage continued nursing and/or milk expression. Assure the family that with time and stimulation, milk ejection and production will quickly return to normal.

• • •

Just before milk ejection, a small percentage of nursing parents report feeling strong negative emotions, known as D-MER.

Dysphoric milk ejection reflex, or D-MER, is described as an abrupt emotional drop just before milk ejection that continues for no more than a few minutes (Heise & Wiessinger, 2011). The 9% of nursing parents who reported D-MER in a retrospective chart review of 115 mothers (Ureno, Berry-Caban, Adams, Buchheit, & Hopkinson, 2019) describe these feelings—including wistfulness, hopelessness, dread, anxiety, anger—as ranging from mild to severe (Ureno, Buchheit, Hopkinson, & Berry-Caban, 2018). In some, the intensity of these feelings increased as more milk accumulated in the mammary glands.

At this writing, although there seems to be general agreement that D-MER is a physical response rather than a symptom of psychological issues, the source of this physical response is unknown. Some suggested it may be related to a drop in dopamine (Heise & Wiechmann, 2018; Heise & Wiessinger, 2011), while others suggested it may relate to the oxytocin spike that occurs during milk ejection (Uvnas-Moberg & Kendall-Tackett, 2018).

Strategies for parents experiencing D-MER. When parents find these negative feelings upsetting, U.S. IBCLC, Alia Heise—who experienced D-MER and created the website **d-mer.org**—suggested lactation supporters convey these points to families (Heise & Wiechmann, 2018):

- Visit the D-MER website and read the personal stories. Just knowing that this condition has a name and that others have experienced it is helpful.
- Try the approaches these other families reported worked for them.
- Know that D-MER seems to be physical rather than psychological.
- Post experiences on the website to increase the general knowledge about this condition.

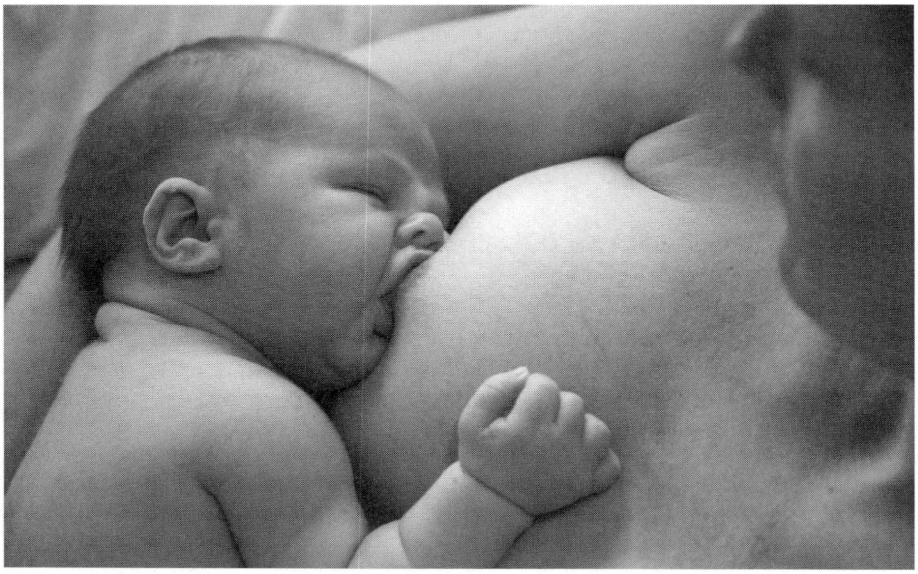

MILK PRODUCTION

Basic Dynamics of Milk Production

Each mammary gland produces milk independently from the other, and milk volume can vary greatly between left and right sides.

After birth, milk production in each side is regulated independently based on milk removal. It's possible to establish or maintain milk production in just one side, even after milk production in the unused side ceases. (This is one alternative to complete weaning when there is recurring mastitis or abscess in one mammary gland.) U.S. and Australian studies (Engstrom, Meier, Jegier, Motykowski, & Zuleger, 2007; Ramsay, Mitoulas, et al., 2005) measured milk production by side and found that the left and right sides rarely produce the same volume of milk, and these differences are often significant. Only about 1 in 4 lactating parents produce about the same volume of milk from both sides.

If the exclusively nursing baby is gaining weight normally but the parent is concerned because one side produces much more milk, explain that what matters to the baby is getting enough milk overall, not whether milk production in each side is the same. In some cases, differences in production may be due to usage, especially if a parent or baby often favors one side over the other. In most cases, though, differences in output are more likely because one mammary gland is just a naturally larger milk producer. One U.S. study of 95 exclusively expressing mothers (Hill, Aldag, Zinaman, & Chatterton, 2007) found that 70% produced more milk from their right side and that milk output by side was not associated with the mother's dominant hand, number of children, or previous nursing experience. If there are concerns about obvious differences in size due to uneven but full milk production, reassure the family that both sides usually return to prepregnancy size after nursing ends or even sooner (Kent, Mitoulas, Cox, Owens, & Hartmann, 1999).

• • •

Several basic dynamics affect milk production.

In the book, ***Making More Milk*** (L. Marasco & West, 2020), U.S. lactation consultants Lisa Marasco and Diana West described what they call the "Milk Supply Equation" (paraphrased below), which listed the basic forces affecting milk production. If any of the following are missing, milk production may be compromised:

Sufficient glandular tissue

+ Enough intact nerve pathways and milk ducts

+ Adequate normal hormones and receptors

+ Adequate lactation-critical nutrients

+ Frequent and effective milk removal/transfer and mammary stimulation

+ No lactation inhibitors

= Ample milk production

The following sections examine each of these dynamics in detail.

Amount of Glandular Tissue

Some parents lack the milk-producing glands needed to achieve full milk production.

Some parents have a condition called mammary hypoplasia or insufficient glandular tissue, in which much of their glandular tissue is missing (Diana Cassar-Uhl, 2014; Wilson-Clay & Hoover, 2017). Physical characteristics of this condition may include widely spaced mammary glands (more than 1.5 inches or about 4 cm apart); large differences in size (asymmetry); tubular, irregular, or cone-shaped glands rather than rounded, especially in the lower quadrants; and bulbous-looking areolae (K Huggins, Petok, & Mireles, 2000). Many of these parents report no tissue changes or mammary growth during pregnancy. For more details, see p. 785.

There is great variability among nursing parents in mammary size and shape, as well as how much of it is glandular tissue (Geddes, 2007b), and it is important never to assume from mammary shape or lack of tissue changes during pregnancy that a parent will not produce enough milk for the baby. A 2018 Polish study that measured mammary growth during pregnancy in 93 women and analyzed their milk after delivery (Zelazniewicz & Pawlowski, 2019) found no correlation between tissue growth and successful lactation and no differences in milk composition after birth. However, it is wise to consider this a risk factor for insufficient milk production, and whenever possible, babies whose parents have these physical characteristics should be monitored closely during their first month without planting seeds of doubt. One way to explain it is that "not all parents with mammary glands of this shape have challenges with milk production, but some do, so let's plan to keep a careful eye on your baby's weight gain during the first few weeks."

> **KEY CONCEPT**
>
> *If a parent has physical signs of insufficient glandular tissue, monitor closely the baby's weight gain during the first month without planting seeds of doubt.*

• • •

Some parents have too much glandular tissue.

In addition to the lack of glandular tissue described in the previous point, some parents have the opposite issue: called "hyperplastic" or "hypertrophic" mammary glands, meaning overdevelopment of glandular tissue. This may occur in one side or both (Lawrence & Lawrence, 2016). Not all types of hyperplasia cause problems, but for details on one that does (called "gestational gigantomastia"), see p. 787.

Condition of Nerves and Milk Ducts

Breast or chest surgery or injury can damage nerves and may affect milk production.

If the nursing parent has a history of surgery or injury (including nipple or areola scarring) to the breast or chest, this could potentially affect milk ejection by damaging nerve pathways between brain and mammary gland. Intact nerve pathways allow nerve impulses to trigger the release of the hormone oxytocin, which is needed for milk ejection (see previous section). Those with a history of surgery or injury will know they have nerve damage because some or all sensation in the nipple and areola is lost. If the nursing parent can feel both touch and temperature on the nipple and areola, problems with milk ejection during nursing are unlikely (West & Hirsch, 2008). For more details on the impact of surgery or injury on nursing, see p. 788-799.

When nerve pathways are damaged, until they grow back, or ***reinnervate***, milk ejection may only be possible with the help of techniques like mental imagery (Cowley, 2005, 2014), touch on other areas of the mammary glands and body, acupressure (see p. 789 and 865-866), the use of a synthetic oxytocin nasal spray, or by applying pressure to the gland during nursing or pumping via compression or other manual techniques.

• • •

Severe engorgement, surgery, and/or injury could damage or sever milk ducts, which may affect milk production.

In rare cases, prolonged, severe engorgement can cause enough damage to a mammary gland to affect long-term milk production. If there is a history of surgery or injury to the breast or chest, the following factors may affect the impact on milk production.

Location of any incision or injury. Surgical incisions or injuries on the lower outer area of the areola are more likely to cause nerve damage and severed milk ducts than incisions on other areas of the areola, in the fold under the mammary gland, in the armpit, or in the navel. For more details, see p. 794-795.

Anatomical differences. The previous section "Anatomy of the Mammary Gland" described research on 21 fully lactating women (Ramsay, Kent, et al., 2005) that found between 4 and 17 lobes in the gland. With breast or chest surgery or injury, the number of working ducts and lobes may partly determine whether it has a major or minor effect on milk production. For example, if two milk ducts are cut during surgery in a parent with four working milk ducts, this could significantly affect milk production, but cutting two milk ducts in a parent with 15 working ducts may have little noticeable effect (Geddes, 2007b). Milk ducts can eventually grow back or ***recannalize***, but this takes time. Parents and healthcare providers will not know how many working lobes and ducts the parent has, but this might be one reason milk production is affected after surgery when the parent was told it should not affect lactation.

Hormonal Levels and Receptor Function

For adequate milk production, the necessary hormones should be in balance and these hormones and their receptors should interact well.

After birth, hormones become a more minor player in milk production (see next section). But if a parent's hormonal levels are far enough out of the normal range, this can lead to too much or too little milk (Edge & Segatore, 1993; L.. Marasco, 2006). But there is more to know about hormonal dynamics. A body's response to any hormone will be partly determined by how many receptors exist for that hormone and how many of these receptors are ***upregulated***, or activated and responsive. As described in more detail later, during the first few weeks after birth, milk removal is responsible for upregulating prolactin receptors, and the more receptors upregulated, scientists theorize, the greater the milk-making potential for that lactation (De Carvalho, 1983).

Another aspect of the hormonal influence on lactation is whether each hormone and its receptor work together normally. In their book ***Making More Milk,*** U.S. lactation consultants Lisa Marasco and Diana West (L. Marasco & West, 2020) liken the relationship between the hormone and its receptor to that of a lock and key, with both being necessary. Even if hormonal levels are in the normal range, if there are too many locks and not enough keys or vice versa, the hormone will not have the expected effect. And if the hormone and its receptor do not work well together (i.e., the lock is rusty and the key can't open it), this can blunt the effect of that hormone. For example, the ***insulin resistance*** that occurs with Type 2 diabetes refers to the "resistance" of the insulin receptors to binding with the insulin produced by the body. In this case, the body makes enough insulin; it just can't be used appropriately.

• • •

The hormones affecting lactation play different roles during pregnancy, birth, and nursing.

Although we still don't completely understand all the hormonal intricacies affecting mammary development and milk production, we know that the hormones described below play a role.

Before birth. During pregnancy, high blood levels of estrogen, placental lactogen, prolactin, and progesterone stimulate the growth and development of the milk-making parts of the mammary glands, preparing the body to produce milk. The production of colostrum, the first milk, begins mid-pregnancy. Another role progesterone plays is to inhibit significant milk production until after birth (Czank, Henderson, Kent, Tat Lai, & Hartmann, 2007). This growth of glandular tissue and the beginning of milk production is called ***secretory differentiation*** or ***lactogenesis I***. Hormones that regulate the parent's metabolism, such as growth hormone, glucocorticoids, thyroid hormone, and insulin also prepare the mammary glands during pregnancy (Neville, McFadden, & Forsyth, 2002).

After birth. The delivery of the placenta triggers the hormonal chain of events that causes milk production to rapidly increase, called ***secretory activation***, ***"lactogenesis II***, or the milk "coming in" or "coming to volume." Secretion of placental lactogen ends with the delivery of the placenta that produced it. Estrogen and progesterone blood levels also fall quickly and stay low for the first months of nursing, while prolactin (the "milk-producing hormone") levels start high and then decrease over the weeks but remain higher overall (Pang & Hartmann, 2007; Stuebe, Meltzer-Brody, Pearson, Pedersen, & Grewen, 2015). Other hormones crucial to regulating the parent's metabolic changes, such as cortisol, thyroid-stimulating hormone, and insulin, are also important to milk production (Czank, Henderson, et al., 2007; Laurie A Nommsen-Rivers, 2016; Thayer, Agustin Bechayda, & Kuzawa, 2018).

A parent's blood prolactin levels rise and fall with each nursing and milk expression (see next point). According to research, sleep can increase prolactin levels (Freeman, Kanyicska, Lerant, & Nagy, 2000). The release of prolactin and oxytocin together may contribute to the intense feeling of oneness with the baby that many nursing parents experience (Uvnas-Moberg, 2014).

KEY CONCEPT

Prolactin, cortisol, thyroid-stimulating hormone and insulin are all important in milk production.

Oxytocin is released during labor, causing the muscles of the uterus to contract, leading to the delivery of the baby. After birth, oxytocin release triggers delivery of the placenta. During nursing, oxytocin release triggers milk ejection by causing contractions of the band-like cells surrounding the alveoli (see previous section). Oxytocin release after birth also causes the uterus to contract, returning it more quickly to its prepregnancy size, which is why uterine cramps may occur during milk ejection in the first week after birth.

After the hormonal chain of events that occurs during the first days after birth, hormones play a more minor role in establishing and maintaining milk production (Cox, Owens, & Hartmann, 1996; De Coopman, 1993). The hormonal influence on milk production is sometimes referred to as ***endocrine control***. After birth, the most important aspect of establishing ample milk production is removing milk early, often, and well, which is sometimes referred to as ***autocrine*** or local control of milk production.

• • •

The first 2 weeks after birth may be a critical period for activating enough prolactin receptors in the mammary gland for adequate long-term milk production.

Each time the baby nurses or milk is expressed, the nursing parent's blood prolactin levels rise. During the early months, blood prolactin levels peak about 10 to 15 minutes after the end of a nursing or pumping session and return to baseline levels within 3 hours or so.

During the first 10 days after birth, the parent's prolactin response to mammary stimulation is at its peak (Cox et al., 1996). Within 45 minutes of the start of a nursing session, blood prolactin levels may be double or triple baseline levels, sometimes rising as much as 20 to 30 times higher (Noel, Suh, & Frantz, 1974). As the weeks and months pass, even with ample milk production, baseline prolactin blood levels and prolactin surges after nursing gradually decrease (Stuebe et al., 2015). Months after birth, the prolactin levels of nursing parents are still higher than those of non-nursing parents, but the difference is not nearly as great (Table 10.1).

TABLE 10.1 Prolactin Levels Expected During Full or Nearly Full Lactation

Stage	Baseline (ng/mL)	After Nursing (ng/mL)
During childbearing years (not lactating or pregnant)	2-20	N/A
Third trimester of pregnancy	150-250	N/A
Pregnant at term	200-500	N/A
First 10 days after birth	200	400
1 month	100-140	260-310
2 months	100-140	195-240
4 months	60-80	120-155
6 months	50-65	80-100
7-12 months	30-40	45-80

From Marasco & West, 2020; collated from (Cox et al., 1996; Lawrence & Lawrence, 2016; Lopez, Rodriguez, & Garcia, 2020)

According to the ***prolactin receptor theory***, the higher and more often a parent's blood prolactin levels rise during this critical first 2 weeks after birth, the more prolactin receptors are upregulated, increasing cellular activity and milk production potential for that baby (De Carvalho, 1983). This upregulation of prolactin receptors starts anew with each birth. If for whatever reason a parent does not remove milk often and well during these first 2 weeks, fewer prolactin receptors may be upregulated and the milk production potential may be more limited. After the first 2 weeks, when the parent's hormonal levels naturally decline, most parents find it requires much more time and work to boost milk production. In rare cases, it may even be impossible. During these first 2 weeks, encourage the family to use this hormonal advantage to set milk production potential at "abundant." Prolactin also works to keep the milk-making alveoli open and prevent involution, or reverting back to their prepregnancy state.

• • •

Some aspects of nursing parents' metabolic function and health can affect their hormonal levels or responses, which may affect milk production.

We are still learning about how hormonal interactions influence each other and milk production. Conditions like obesity, diabetes, insulin resistance, thyroid dysfunction, polycystic ovary syndrome (PCOS), gestational ovarian theca lutein cysts, excessive blood loss during delivery, and anemia may affect milk production. (See Table 10. 3 on p. 435 for a more complete list.)

Nurse early, often, and effectively. Some parents with these conditions make ample milk, but when one or more of these conditions are present, consider this a red flag for possible problems with milk production and encourage the family to use best practices, such as nursing early, often, and effectively (see Figure 10.3 on p. 425) and chapters 1 and 2).

Learn hand expression during pregnancy and use it after birth. Another strategy to optimize milk production is to follow the suggestions on **firstdroplets.com** and learn hand expression during the last month of pregnancy. During the first few days after birth, follow nursing with hand expression. Express colostrum into a spoon and feed baby this "dessert." These practices both stimulate healthy milk production and help prevent excess weight loss in baby (Bertini, Breschi, & Dani, 2015). Encourage close monitoring of the baby's weight gain after birth without planting the seeds of doubt.

• • •

Hormonal disruption during puberty may affect mammary development and milk production later.

If normal hormonal levels are disrupted during puberty, this may lead to abnormal development of the mammary glands, which may lead to low milk production after birth. When taking a history, be sure to ask about whether the nursing parent experienced any of the health or metabolic issues listed in the previous point during puberty.

• • •

The nursing parent's emotions and the baby's touch have a hormonal effect on milk production.

Mammary stimulation and milk removal are important to milk production (see next section), but so too are the "softer" aspects of nursing: the parent's emotions and the baby's touch. The earlier section on milk ejection described the impact of emotions on milk ejection, which can affect milk removal and therefore production.

Research also found that the hormonal response to milk-making is affected by the presence or absence of the baby's touch. Skin-to-skin contact after birth, for example, was associated with increased oxytocin blood levels, which is important to milk production and was associated with long-term effects on nursing duration and the parent-baby relationship (Matthiesen, Ransjo-Arvidson, Nissen, & Uvnas-Moberg, 2001; Uvnas-Moberg, 2014). One Swedish study measured the hormonal levels of 63 mothers during the first 2 days after delivery (Handlin et al., 2009) and found that the more minutes these mothers and babies spent in skin-to-skin contact before nursing, the lower the mothers' blood levels of the stress hormone cortisol, which is associated with greater relaxation. Chapter 2 described on p. 45-46 the effects on nursing dynamics of an intimate, private environment after birth, where the family can relax together and get in sync (Hauck, Summers, White, & Jones, 2008). This intimate connection enhances the family's hormonal response to nursing and milk production. A U.S. study (Hurst, Valentine, Renfro, Burns, & Ferlic, 1997) found that even 1 hour of skin-to-skin contact per day with preterm babies and their exclusively expressing mothers increased milk output during pumping.

Lactation-Critical Nutrients

Consuming adequate calories matters to milk production.

A perfect diet is not necessary for making lots of good quality milk (see p. 555), but the process of lactation requires some calories, and making milk means giving some calories to the baby. Over the years, studies (Butte, Garza, Stuff, Smith, & Nichols, 1984; Strode, Dewey, & Lonnerdal, 1986) found that a minimum of 1,500 to 1,800 calories per day are important for lactating parents. Anecdotally, some parents report increased milk production when they consume more calories (L. Marasco & West, 2020). When considering factors that may affect milk production, include diet.

• • •

For adequate milk production, some nursing parents may benefit from reviewing their diet and considering making changes.

When low milk production is an issue and the usual strategies don't seem to help, take a closer look at diet. U.S. lactation consultants Lisa Marasco and Diana West (L. Marasco & West, 2020) suggest focusing on the following lactation-critical nutrients, which research on both animals and humans (S. Lee & Kelleher, 2016) found may affect lactation.

Protein. Even in developed countries, it's possible for nursing parents to rely on high-carbohydrate snack foods rather than eating the 65 g to 100 g per day of protein recommended during lactation. One Norwegian cross-sectional study of 98 women (Torris et al., 2013) found an association between lower-protein intake and shorter duration of nursing. A Thai randomized controlled trial of 120 poorly nourished mothers of term newborns (Achalapong, 2016) found that during the first days after birth, those supplemented with the high-protein foods eggs, milk, or both produced more milk at 48 and 72 hours compared with those fed the regular diet.

Vitamin B_{12} deficiency should be considered with vegan families, some vegetarians, those with a history of weight-loss surgery, and anyone with a digestion/absorption problem like Crohn's disease. Also, some medications when taken long term deplete vitamin B_{12} stores. In animal studies (Dangat, Kale, & Joshi, 2011), a link was found between vitamin B_{12} deficiency and low milk production. A Russian study on human mothers gave one group of mothers vitamin B_{12} shots during the first 2 weeks after birth (Chubukov, Belentseva, & Makarov, 1973) and found these mothers had higher milk volumes at this time than those who didn't receive the shots. Vitamin B_{12} is better absorbed when taken with omega-3 fatty acids.

Calcium assists with many body processes, including prolactin release (Lamberts & Macleod, 1990). Recommended daily intake of calcium is 1,000 mg (Kolasa, Firnhaber, & Haven, 2015). If calcium stores are low during lactation, some (VanHouten et al., 2004) believe that the body limits milk production to protect the bones from losing too much calcium. Animal studies (Weisstaub, Zeni, de Portela, & Ronayne de Ferrer, 2006) found a link between low calcium intake and reduced milk production.

Iron. As mentioned earlier, anemia (usually caused by low iron levels) is considered a risk factor for low milk production (Mathur, Chitranshi, Mathur, Singh, & Bhalla, 1992; Rioux, Savoie, & Allard, 2006) and delayed milk increase after birth (Salahudeen, Koshy, & Sen, 2013). In one study (Toppare et al., 1994), hemoglobin levels below 9.5 g/dL were associated with a shorter nursing duration. Blood loss during birth can cause or worsen anemia (Henly et al., 1995).

Zinc is involved in many aspects of lactation: the development of glandular tissue during pregnancy, milk increase after birth, keeping the milk-making cells working, and assisting in involution after weaning (S. Lee & Kelleher, 2016). A Russian study analyzed blood samples from 514 mothers (Scheplyagina, 2005) and more than three-quarters of them were zinc deficient. They found that these zinc-deficient mothers were more likely to have low milk production than those who were zinc-sufficient.

Iodine is essential to the normal function of the thyroid gland, which is critical to making abundant milk (Leung, Pearce, & Braverman, 2011). With pregnancy and lactation, the iodine requirements of the parent nearly double, from 150 µg/L to 250 to 290 µg/L, and many fall short (Fisher, Wang, George, Gearhart, & McLanahan, 2016), which increases the risk of thyroid problems and low milk production. It's important, though, not to overdo iodine, as too much can also reduce thyroid function and the release of prolactin (Miyai, Tokushige, & Kondo, 2008; Serrano-Nascimento et al., 2017).

Omega-3 fatty acids and healthy fats in the nursing parent's diet increases their content in the milk but can also increase the total fat content in lean women (N. K. Anderson et al., 2005). Higher fat milk can make the difference between a baby who is gaining weight well and one who isn't.

Fiber. The same Norwegian study that found an association between low protein and shorter duration of nursing (Torris et al., 2013) found the same association among mothers who ate a low-fiber diet. Adding more fiber to the diet may not increase milk production in every family, but it may be worth a try.

• • •

Dietary restrictions or medical conditions that compromise nutrient intake or absorption may affect milk production.

The following situations can compromise the intake or absorption of some of the lactation-critical nutrients described in the previous point.

- Vegan and some vegetarian diets may lead to a vitamin B_{12} deficiency unless supplements are taken. For details, see p. 568.
- Eating disorder, past or present, may cause vitamin or nutrient deficiencies. For details, see p. 571.
- Weight-loss surgery can reduce nutrient absorption. For research on its effect on lactation, see p. 580.
- Nutrient malabsorption due to Crohn's disease or other health issues.

How Well and Often Milk Is Removed

After birth, milk removal is the primary driver of milk production.

The physical characteristics described in the previous sections—how much glandular tissue the nursing parent has, the condition of the nerves and milk ducts, and hormonal levels and receptors—may significantly inhibit milk production when there are major deviations from the norm. But under some circumstances, milk removal can provide the stimulation needed to overcome these and other issues. Hormones, for example, prepare the mammary glands for milk production during pregnancy and cause the cascade of events that lead to milk increase, or "coming to volume," after birth (the endocrine control of milk production mentioned earlier). But with mammary stimulation and milk removal, even parents who have never been pregnant can make milk, or induce lactation (see p. 666).

• • •

Focusing on "rate of milk production" rather than "milk supply" may make it easier to understand how to use milk production's underlying dynamics.

Some people refer to "milk supply," a concept that implies a set volume of milk that is either there or it isn't. But milk production is not static. It can vary from day to day and even over the course of a day. A more useful concept for understanding milk-making is "rate of milk production," which puts the focus on how fast or slow a parent makes milk.

• • •

Patterns of milk removal can vary greatly by culture, which influences milk production.

Cultural differences in feeding patterns. Nursing rhythm—the heart of local control of milk production—varies tremendously from place to place. As U.S. researcher Kathleen Kennedy once noted, a "nursing" means something very different to parents in different cultures (Kennedy, 2010). A Western parent, for example, may consider a "nursing" a lengthy, ritualized activity that involves changing the baby's diaper, making a drink, turning off their phone, settling into a certain chair, and then nursing baby for an extended time. In contrast, a parent in a developing country may keep the baby on their body, nursing her at the slightest cue for just a few minutes 15 to 20 times each day. These two babies may have about the same daily milk intake, but the immense cultural differences in their feeding rhythms may affect the rate of milk production.

Nursing norms differ from bottle-feeding norms. Many Western attitudes about feeding are based on bottle-feeding norms, such as the belief that babies should feed at set intervals, every few hours. Another is the belief that as babies get older, they should take fewer and larger feeds. However, there are basic differences between nursing and bottle-feeding and between human milk and infant formulas, so the same expectations cannot be applied to both. For example, U.S. research (Heinig, Nommsen, Peerson, Lonnerdal, & Dewey, 1993) found significant differences in the volume of milk taken by nursing and formula-fed babies. On average, babies fed formula consume 15% more milk at 3 months, 23% more at 6 months, 20% more at 9 months, and 18% more at 12 months. And Australian research (Kent et al., 2013; Kent et al., 2006) found that among exclusively nursing babies the number of feeds per day did not change significantly between 1 and 6 months of age. If a Western parent disregards their nursing baby's feeding cues and manipulates her feeding pattern based on formula-feeding norms, this can sometimes lead to milk production issues.

KEY CONCEPT

Milk removal is the primary driver of milk production.

Milk production is best regulated without "rules" by encouraging the family to be responsive to their baby's feeding cues. If the baby drives the process, they are more likely to avoid both milk-production extremes:

low milk production and overabundant milk production. Efforts to manipulate the process are more likely to create these challenges (Smillie, Campbell, & Iwinski, 2005).

Degree of Mammary Fullness

Our knowledge about milk production increased dramatically during the 1990s and 2000s, thanks in large part to the work of a Western Australian research team led by Peter Hartmann. With the help of local nursing parents who volunteered to be part of their studies, this team used a high-tech approach to learn more about how the mammary gland makes milk. In some studies, they used techniques from the field of topography, which measures mountain terrains, to chart physical changes in the mammary glands and determined how much milk they hold (Cregan & Hartmann, 1999). They used sensitive scales (to 2 g) to weigh babies before and after feeds to determine exactly how much milk a baby takes at each side, at each feed, and during a 24-hour period (Daly, Owens, & Hartmann, 1993). And they used ultrasound to learn more about milk ejection during feeds (Ramsay et al., 2004). According to their findings, one of the primary factors that affects how quickly or slowly milk is made is how full or well drained the glands are, otherwise known as ***degree of mammary fullness***.

One of the main dynamics affecting rate of milk production is how full the mammary glands become or how well drained they are.

• • •

Full glands make milk slower. As the mammary gland becomes full of milk, two potential dynamics cause its rate of milk production to slow.

Drained glands make milk faster and full glands make milk slower.

1. *FIL.* As the volume of milk in the gland increases—according to some—so, too, does the amount of the substance known as "feedback inhibitor of lactation" (FIL for short), which slows milk production (Knight, Peaker, & Wilde, 1998; A. Prentice, 1989; Wilde, Addey, Boddy, & Peaker, 1995).
2. *Internal pressure from the milk* can slow milk production by reducing blood flow to the gland and compressing the milk-making cells, which can cause them to temporarily shut down production.

As the glands fill with more and more milk, it is the combination of increasing FIL and increasing internal pressure that causes milk production to become slower and slower. At this writing, research (Hernandez et al., 2008; Pai, Hernandez, Stull, & Horseman, 2015; Stull et al., 2007) indicated that FIL may be serotonin, which is produced in the milk-making lactocytes and whose presence is linked to a decrease in milk synthesis.

Drained glands make milk faster. The opposite is also true. Milk production speeds when the mammary glands are drained more fully. This is how a baby adjusts her parent's milk production as needed. If she wants more milk, she nurses more often and drains the mammary glands more fully, taking a larger percentage of the available milk, which causes the milk to be produced faster and faster.

Although many assume that babies take all of the available milk when they nurse, Australian research (Kent, 2007) found that, on average, babies take 67% (or two thirds) of the milk in the glands. This means that after an average feed, 33% (or a third of the milk) is left in the gland. One way to increase the rate of milk production is to drain the glands more fully, perhaps 90% to 95% instead of 67%. This can be done by nursing the baby more than once from each side, by expressing milk after nursing, or by doing both. The more fully drained the glands are at the end of a feed and the more times a day they are more fully drained, the faster the rate of milk production. If a parent has overabundant milk production, they can also use this dynamic for the opposite effect. As described in the last section of this chapter, feeding less often on one side and allowing that side to stay fuller for longer periods can slow the rate of milk production and resolve overabundant milk production.

Within one day and even from feed to feed, rate of milk production can change dramatically. For example, in one Australian study (Daly, Kent, Owens, & Hartmann, 1996), after one study mother's breasts became full after 6 hours without milk removal, her rate of milk production per breast was measured at 22 mL (about 2/3 oz.) per hour. By nursing from that breast every 90 minutes and draining her breasts more completely, her rate of production per breast increased quickly to 56 mL (nearly 2 oz.) per hour—more than double the previous rate. As researchers wrote in a review article (Daly & Hartmann, 1995, p. 30):

> "...[T]he breast can rapidly change its rate of milk synthesis from one interfeed interval to the next. This is a newly discovered property of the human mammary gland. In the past, it has been assumed that the rate of milk synthesis of a breast could change significantly only over a period of days."

This review article also noted that the average rate of milk production over 24 hours in these mothers was only 64% of the fastest milk production measured, which meant that these parents had a much greater milk-making potential.

• • •

With frequent milk removal, three different physical processes act to speed milk production.

The short-term increase in milk-production described in the previous point is only part of the picture. Scientists described several processes stimulated by frequent milk removal that work together over time to speed milk production even more (Czank, Henderson, et al., 2007):

1. **Short-term:** Frequent milk removal minimizes FIL and pressure in the gland, leading to faster milk production.

2. **Medium-term:** Faster milk production speeds the metabolic activity of key enzymes used in milk-making, speeding milk production more.

3. **Long-term:** Over time frequent milk removal stimulates the growth and development of more glandular, milk-making tissue (why induced lactation works), also increasing the speed of milk production.

Storage Capacity

Storage capacity is the maximum volume of milk available to the baby when the mammary gland is at its fullest and is unrelated to mammary size.

In addition to "degree of mammary fullness" described in the previous section, a parent's mammary storage capacity also influences the rate of milk production. Storage capacity is defined as the maximum volume of milk available to the baby when the mammary gland is at its fullest time of the day, and it can vary greatly from person to person and from baby to baby in the same nursing parent. This individual difference helps explain why feeding rhythms can vary so greatly from one nursing couple to another. An Australian study of 71 breastfeeding mothers and babies (Kent et al., 2006) found a storage capacity range among its mothers of 74 to 382 g (2.6 to 12.9 oz.) per breast. Another Australian study (Daly et al., 1993) found an even broader range among its mothers, from 81 to 606 mL (2.7 to 20.5 oz.). The mother in this second study with the largest storage capacity accumulated up to 90% of her baby's daily milk intake in both breasts, while the one with the smallest storage capacity accumulated at most up to 20% of her baby's daily milk intake in both breasts.

KEY CONCEPT

Milk storage capacity is unrelated to mammary size.

Storage capacity is not related to the size of the mammary gland, so those with small mammary glands may have a large capacity and those with large mammary glands may have a small capacity.

• • •

Parents with both large and small storage capacities can make ample milk for their babies, but their feeding rhythms will likely vary.

Depending on cultural practices, after about the first month post-delivery, parents with a large storage capacity often have far different feeding rhythms than those with a small storage capacity. Because by definition the mammary glands of a parent with a large storage capacity can hold more milk, the baby may be satisfied with one side at most feeds, may feed fewer times per day overall, and may sleep longer at night. The mammary glands of a parent with a small storage capacity hold less milk, so to achieve the same daily milk intake, the baby may take both sides at each feed, nurse more times per day, and feed more often at night. For more details on how storage capacity affects feeding rhythm, see p. 71.

Although storage capacity affects feeding rhythm, it does not affect parents' ability to produce ample milk for their baby. In the study of 71 babies mentioned in the previous point (Kent et al., 2006), Australian researchers found that all of the study babies whose mothers had a small storage capacity had healthy weight gains. There were no issues with low milk supply or slow weight gain. These babies just fed more times each day than the babies whose mothers had a large capacity.

• • •

Mammary storage capacity determines how long it takes for mammary glands to become full enough for the rate of milk production to slow.

While "full glands make milk slower," the time it takes to become full varies by both rate of milk production and storage capacity. A parent with a small storage capacity may feel full with 3 ounces (89 mL) of milk in each side, and this fullness could cause the rate of milk production to slow. Whereas a parent with a larger storage capacity would not yet feel full with this same 3 ounces (89 mL) in the glands, allowing this parent to go longer between feeds without the rate of milk production slowing.

The term "intercept time" was used by researchers (Daly et al., 1996) to describe the point at which mammary fullness causes milk production to slow to a below-average rate. In this Australian study, rate of milk production was measured in four breastfeeding women with full milk production, and their "intercept time" ranged from 6 to 12 hours.

• • •

Some clues may make it possible to estimate a parent's storage capacity.

Australian researchers use sophisticated technology to determine mammary storage capacity (Cregan & Hartmann, 1999; Kent et al., 1999). But simple observations can provide clues. For example, in parents who exclusively express their milk and do not get up at night to express, in general, those with larger storage capacities can express 300 mL (10 oz.) or more at their first morning expression. The parent with a small storage capacity, on the other hand, may awaken before morning with mammary discomfort, yet be unable to express more than 89 to 150 mL (3 to 5 oz.) or so (Mohrbacher, 1996). When test-weighing is used before and after nursing, a baby's maximum intake at one nursing will also provide clues.

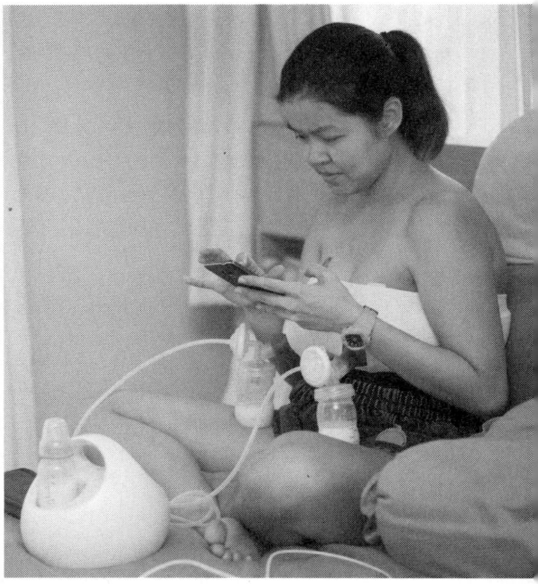

Nursing patterns also provide clues to storage capacity. For example, if an exclusively nursing baby is gaining weight at average or above-average rates (during the first 3 months this would be at least 1 ounce or 30 g per day) with fewer than 7 to 8 feeds per day, this may be a sign of a large storage capacity. Another sign of a large capacity is the baby who sleeps for many hours at night without nursing with excellent weight gain

• • •

A parent's capacity can vary from baby to baby and change as the rate of milk production increases or decreases.

Australian research (Kent et al., 1999) found that there was a relationship between the peak volume of milk that could be stored in a mammary gland and overall milk production. This means, for example, that while nursing twins, a parent's storage capacity would probably be greater than when nursing a single baby.

Lactation Inhibitors

Even with all other milk-making dynamics working well, exposure to a lactation suppressant can undermine milk production.

Taking a medication used to suppress lactation will likely cause milk-production issues. Two dopamine agonist medications given after birth to "dry up" milk production in families who are not nursing are bromocriptine (Parlodel) and cabergoline (Dostinex). Bromocriptine is no longer recommended in the U.S. to suppress lactation due to severe side effects, including stroke, heart attack, and death (FDA, 1994; Hale, 2019). Although cabergoline is considered safer because it has fewer side effects (Aydin, Atis, Kaleli, Uludag, & Goker, 2010), its lactation-inhibiting effects last longer than bromocriptine. However, according to ***Hale's Medications & Mothers' Milk*** (Hale, 2019, p. 98), some mothers treated with cabergoline in the early post-delivery period successfully recovered their milk production through "heavy pumping."

• • •

Some medications, vitamins, and herbs may slow milk production in some users but not others.

Individual biochemistry varies. This means that some parents may experience slowed milk production from exposure to the substances listed in Table 10.2 while others may not. Although many substances used to boost milk production (galactogogues, see later section) raise parents' blood prolactin levels, doctor of pharmacology Phillip O. Anderson noted in his 2017 article (P. O. Anderson,

TABLE 10.2 Lactation Suppressants and Potential Lactation Inhibitors

Dopamine-agonist lactation suppressants	Bromocriptine (Parlodel) Cabergoline (Dostinex)
Hormones that slow milk production in some users	Estrogen Progesterone Testosterone
Drugs that slow milk production in some users	Buproprion (Wellbutrin, Zyban) Aripiprazole (Abilify) Promethazine Pseudoephedrine (Sudafed, not Sudafed PE) Ergot alkaloids, e.g., methylergonovine maleate (Methergine) Injections of high-dose corticosteroids (triamcinolone, depo methylprednisolone)
Vitamins (in large doses) that slow milk production in some users	B_6 (pyridoxine)
Herbs or foods (in large doses) that slow milk production in some users (anecdotal)	Sage leaves Parsley Peppermint Jasmine Chasteberry
Other substances that slow milk production in some users	Alcohol (may delay milk ejection) Tobacco (shorter duration of nursing) Cannabis (shorter duration of nursing)

Adapted from (P. O. Anderson, 2017b, 2017c; Eglash, 2014; L. Marasco & West, 2020)

2017c) that no direct link has yet been found between blood prolactin levels and milk production. This may only be partly true, however. As U.S. associate professor of pharmacology, Thomas Hale explained (personal communication, 2017), this lack of association between prolactin levels and milk production is only true in lactating parents whose prolactin levels are 75 ng/mL or higher. When prolactin levels fall below 75 ng/mL, there may be an association with low milk production.

In some lactating parents taking drugs known to lower prolactin levels had no obvious effect on milk production. In other words, it is important not to assume that the substances listed in the last five categories of Table 10.2 will definitely slow milk production in every family. But in cases when low milk production is an issue and no other contributing factors can be identified, it may be worth asking about their use.

• • •

The use of alcohol, tobacco, and cannabis by the nursing parent may negatively affect milk production.

Substances socially acceptable in many cultures, such as alcohol, tobacco, and cannabis, are not directly linked to milk production, but they affect the hormones of lactation. A literature review (Haastrup, Pottegard, & Damkier, 2014) noted an association between alcohol use and reduced milk intake at feeds and delayed milk ejection. Nicotine reduced levels of prolactin and oxytocin (Napierala et al., 2017). Associations were also found between the use of tobacco and cannabis and shorter duration of nursing (Crume et al., 2018; Napierala, Mazela, Merritt, & Florek, 2016). For more details, see p. 585 on alcohol, 589 on tobacco, and 594 on cannabis.

Misconceptions about Milk Production

Contrary to popular belief, drinking more fluids is not associated with greater milk production.

When a family expresses concern about milk production, often the first advice they receive is to drink more fluids. Although severe dehydration could potentially reduce milk production, mild dehydration does not. A classic 1940 study examined the effect on milk production of reducing nursing mothers' daily fluid intake by 1 liter (Olsen, 1940), with no change found in their milk production. One U.S. study (Dusdieker, Booth, Stumbo, & Eichenberger, 1985) found that when mothers drank 25% more fluids than when they "drank to thirst," there was no statistically significant difference in milk production. In fact, during the "more fluids" period, the mothers produced slightly less milk.

• • •

Worries about low milk production often arise from misinterpreting baby's behavior and other "false alarms," which is known as "perceived insufficient milk."

The most common reason for premature weaning is "not enough milk" (Kair & Colaizy, 2016). As research worldwide indicates, this concern seems to be universal (Galipeau, Dumas, & Lepage, 2017; Gokceoglu & Kucukoglu, 2017; Lou et al., 2014; Otsuka, Dennis, Tatsuoka, & Jimba, 2008; Reza, Rahmani, Mohsen, & Saeedeh, 2013).

Some of the first studies on "perceived insufficient milk" from the U.S. and Sweden (Hill & Humenick, 1989; Hillervik-Lindquist, 1991) found that these crises of confidence over milk production were not due to actual low milk production. The concerned parents produced just as much milk as those who were not concerned. What were the root causes of these worries? U.S. focus groups and surveys (Bartick & Reyes, 2012; DaMota, Banuelos, Goldbronn, Vera-Beccera, & Heinig, 2012) found that among many low-income and Latina mothers, lack of knowledge about nursing and newborn norms were the underlying cause. Many were unaware that giving formula supplements affected milk production, and they assumed that any time their baby woke up or cried this was due to hunger. Of course, most newborns have some fussy periods when they are irritable, wakeful at night, and want to nurse often or even constantly for part of the day. These behaviors are not reliable signs of low milk production. Especially during the first month, when milk production is increasing to meet a baby's growing needs, these baby behaviors are normal aspects of infancy. As long as a baby is gaining weight normally, milk production is adequate.

Other research done in different parts of the world (Galipeau et al., 2017; Mannion & Mansell, 2012; Otsuka et al., 2008) found a strong link between "perceived insufficient milk" and low breastfeeding self-efficacy (BSE), or parents' lack of confidence in their ability to fully nurse their baby (Dennis, 2003). Nearly every study on the variables that affect exclusivity and duration of nursing finds an association with BSE, with more confident parents nursing longer and more exclusively than less confident parents. One 2017 systematic review and meta-analysis (Brockway, Benzies, & Hayden, 2017) concluded that interventions that improve BSE had the greatest impact on nursing rates.

False alarms that sometimes lead to concerns about milk production are:

- **An inability to express as much milk as expected (Yamada, Rasmussen, & Felice, 2019):** milk expression is a learned skill that improves with practice
- **Mammary tissue feels softer and less full:** this usually occurs after the first few weeks when the hormones of childbirth settle down

- **No milk leakage:** not all nursing parents leak
- **Not feeling milk ejections:** many parents do not
- **Expressed milk looks thin:** this is how human milk is supposed to look after the change from transitional to mature milk after the first 2 weeks or so
- **Baby will take a bottle after nursing:** this can happen even if baby received enough milk during nursing

It's important to always take a family's concerns about milk production seriously. A U.S. study that analyzed milk composition for physical indicators of milk increase after birth (Murase, Wagner, C, Dewey, & Nommsen-Rivers, 2017) found that among parents with concerns about milk production on Day 7, 41% produced milk whose composition reflected a delay in milk increase, compared with only 21% of those without milk-production concerns. Another U.S. study of 1,107 mothers (Flaherman, Beiler, Cabana, & Paul, 2016) noted an association between more anxiety about milk production in those whose newborns lost excess weight (≥10% of birthweight) after delivery compared to those whose newborns lost <10% of birth weight (42% versus 20%). Mothers with more anxiety about milk production at 2 weeks were much less likely to be nursing at 6 months. The researchers concluded that efforts to reduce infant weight loss after birth (such as early milk expression and supplementing expressed colostrum by spoon) may be effective at preventing anxiety about milk production in many families and increase duration of nursing.

KEY CONCEPT

Newborn weight loss of more than 10% is associated with greater anxiety about milk production and shorter duration of nursing.

Milk Production Norms

Making Milk During the First Year and Beyond

Knowing average milk production can be useful in some situations, but the best gauge of adequate production is the baby's weight gain and growth.

This section includes the milk production averages and ranges during the first 6 months for parents exclusively nursing. The range of milk production norms is large, but keep in mind it's not the number of ounces or milliliters a baby consumes per day that determines whether milk production is too low, too high, or just right. The best gauge of milk adequacy is the baby's weight gain and growth. In one Australian study of 71 healthy, thriving nursing babies from 1 to 6 months of age (Kent et al., 2006), the difference in daily milk intake was nearly threefold (between 15.5 and 43 oz. [440 to 1220 g]). For details on healthy growth in exclusively nursing babies, see Figure 6.1 on p. 191.

• • •

Around mid-pregnancy, production of colostrum begins.

Production of colostrum begins about mid-pregnancy, but the high blood levels of progesterone during pregnancy inhibit significant milk production until after birth. During pregnancy, colostrum may leak. It may also be possible to express small volumes. As yet, no one has examined the relationship between the volume of colostrum leaked or expressed during pregnancy and milk production after birth. After 16 weeks, if pregnancy ends, milk increase will occur (Geddes, 2007a).

• • •

During their first day of life, nursing newborns consume on average, 37 to 56 mL (1.2-1.9 oz.) of colostrum, with milk intake doubling on the second day.

The volume of colostrum consumed on the first day of life varies greatly from one nursing couple to another. A newborn may receive a larger volume of colostrum if her first nursing is within 1 hour after birth as compared with later. Research found that mothers exclusively expressing milk for very preterm babies express significantly more milk if their first expression is within the first hour after delivery (Parker, Sullivan, Krueger, Kelechi, & Mueller, 2012). An Australian study of 9 babies (Saint, Smith, & Hartmann, 1984) found that 24-hour milk intake on the first day of nursing ranged from 7 to 123 mL (0.25 to 4.2 oz.), with an average daily intake of 37 mL (1.2 oz.) and average intake per feed of 7 mL (0.25 oz.). A U.S. study of 13 mothers (Neville et al., 1988) found 24-hour milk production on the first day of life averaged 56 mL (1.9 oz.) and on the second day increased to 185 mL (6.2 oz.), with a range of 12 to 379 mL (0.4-12.8 oz.). By the second day, a Dutch study of 18 mothers and babies (Houston, Howie, & McNeilly, 1983) estimated the average milk intake per feed was 14 mL (0.5 oz.), with a range of daily intake from 44 to 335 mL (1.5 to 11.3 oz.). When nursing is going well, the baby's milk intake increases as milk production increases and starting after the first 24 hours, the baby's stomach expands in size (Zangen et al., 2001).

• • •

Within 30 to 40 hours after birth, milk production begins to increase dramatically.

The delivery of the placenta triggers the hormonal chain of events that causes milk production to rapidly increase, referred to as secretory activation, lactogenesis II, or the milk "coming in" or "coming to volume" (Pang & Hartmann, 2007). With the placenta delivered, levels of placental lactogen, progesterone, and estrogen fall quickly, while prolactin levels remain high, causing a dramatic upswing in milk production (Pang & Hartmann, 2007). Although this process begins about 30 to 40 hours after birth, nursing parents don't usually perceive their milk as "coming to volume" until a little later—50 to 60 hours after birth (Smith, 2021).

One classic U.S. study (Neville et al., 1988) documented the milk output of 13 mothers and included in its daily totals the milk the baby took during nursing (measured by test-weighing) plus milk spilled, spit up, or leaked. The following mean daily milk outputs illustrated the amazing increase in milk production during the first 4 days after birth:

- Day 1: 56 mL
- Day 2: 185 mL
- Day 3: 393 mL
- Day 4: 580 mL

According to a U.S. study (L. A. Nommsen-Rivers, Heinig, Cohen, & Dewey, 2008), the nursing parent's perception of milk increase after birth (feelings of fullness and heaviness) is a reliable indicator that milk increase occurred.

First time nursing? The rapid milk increase after birth happens faster if the nursing parent lactated for a previous baby (Dewey, Nommsen-Rivers, Heinig, & Cohen, 2003). One U.K. study (J. C. Ingram, Woolridge, Greenwood, & McGrath, 1999) estimated that those who nursed a previous baby were about 1 day ahead of first-time nursing parents, who produced about 3 to 4 ounces (89-142 mL) less milk on Day 3 than the experienced nursing parents. See the later section, "Inhibited Milk Increase After Birth" for other conditions that can inhibit or delay in this process.

Milk removal drives early milk production. Beginning at birth, the primary driver of milk production is how early, often, and effectively baby nurses or milk is expressed (Neville et al., 2002). Each of these dynamics is critical.

- ***Early.*** More frequent early milk removal (nursing or milk expression) is associated with greater milk production during the first week and beyond. One U.S. study of mothers exclusively expressing milk for their very preterm babies (Parker et al., 2012) found that those who began expressing milk within 1 hour of delivery produced significantly more milk at the first expression and at every other evaluation point. At 6 weeks, when the study ended, those who began expressing within the first hour expressed an average of 132% more milk than those who began expressing between 2 and 6 hours after birth.
- ***Often.*** The more often the baby nurses effectively or milk is effectively expressed during the first 10 days to 2 weeks, the greater the impact on later milk production. A 2017 Iranian study (Boskabadi & Zakerihamidi, 2017) found an association between more nursing sessions per day and lower bilirubin levels in the study newborns, which the researchers ascribed to greater milk intake. A U.S. study of women exclusively expressing for very preterm babies (Morton et al., 2009) found that during the first 2 weeks, a minimum of 7 to 8 expressions per day were necessary to reach full milk volume.
- ***Effective.*** If a baby is not latched deeply or nurses ineffectively, she may nurse often but fail to stimulate adequate milk production. A study of U.S. women exclusively expressing milk for very preterm babies (Morton et al., 2009) found that those who used their hands in addition to the pump to extract more milk at each session expressed on average nearly 50% more milk by 8 weeks compared with those who used the pump alone. The more effectively and fully milk is removed, the more milk production is stimulated. That is the idea behind U.S. pediatrician Jane Morton's initiative to encourage parents to learn hand expression during the last month of pregnancy and to hand express after each early nursing, feeding that expressed milk "dessert" to the baby by spoon (**firstdroplets.com**). According to research, parents who learn hand expression during pregnancy are less likely to supplement with formula in the hospital (Casey, Banks, Braniff, Buettner, & Heal, 2019), and even first-time parents gain confidence in their ability to fully nurse their baby (J. R. Demirci, Glasser, Fichner, Caplan, & Himes, 2019). Also, early hand expression and supplementation by spoon can prevent excess weight loss and low milk production (Bertini et al., 2015).

• • •

When nursing is going well, by the end of the first week, milk production increases from an average of 37 to 56 mL (1.2-1.9 oz.) on the first day to a mean of 610 mL (20.6 oz.) per day by Day 7 (Kent, Gardner, & Geddes, 2016; Neville et al., 1988).

By the end of the first week, average milk production increases more than tenfold over the first day.

• • •

Although many consider colostrum, transitional milk, and mature milk three separate and distinct types of milk, they actually reflect a continuum of changes that occur after birth when hormones shift and the mammary gland begins making more milk.

During the first 2 to 3 weeks, the milk changes gradually from colostrum to transitional milk to mature milk.

Even before a nursing parent notices an increase in milk production, the milk has already started to change. A steep drop in blood progesterone levels with stable blood prolactin levels causes the spaces between the milk-making cells (lactocytes) to close, so the milk and its components can no longer leak out of the alveoli (Figure 10.2). With these "tight junctions" in place, as milk production ramps up, the milk stays in the alveoli and its composition begins to change. As more of some components (fat, lactose, citrate, and potassium) remain in the alveoli rather than leaking out, their concentrations increase, causing other components (immunoprotective proteins, sodium, and chloride) to decrease in concentration. Increase in milk volume also changes the concentrations of some milk components. Scientists can gauge when milk increase occurs by measuring the concentrations of specific milk components, such as the ratio of sodium to potassium (Galipeau, Goulet, & Chagnon, 2012; Murase et al., 2017).

KEY CONCEPT

After birth, the number of milk removals per day is associated with milk volume at 6 weeks.

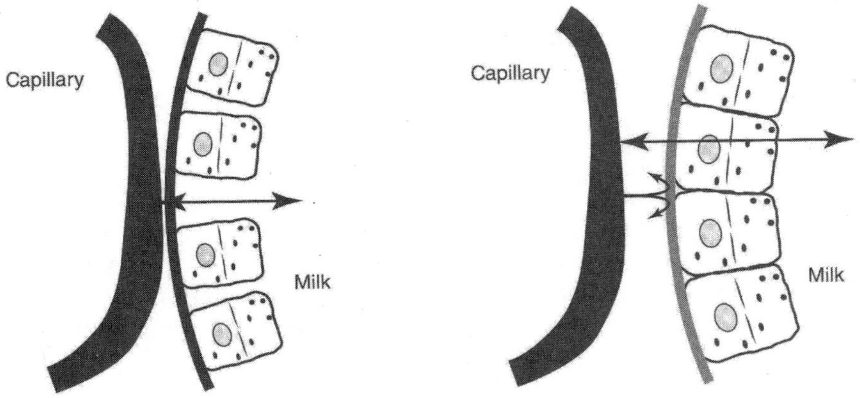

Figure 10.2 As the junctions between the milk-making cells close in the days after birth, milk composition changes. ©2020 Thomas W. Hal, PhD, Infant Risk Center, Texas Tech University, used with permission.

Over the first 2 to 3 weeks, as the milk undergoes these changes, the nursing parent may notice the milk becoming whiter and thinner-looking. There is a wide range of colors and consistencies considered normal for colostrum, transitional milk, and mature milk. Colostrum, for example, may be clear, golden, white, and other colors. As many as 24% of nursing parents have blood in their colostrum (known as "rusty-pipe syndrome," see p. 782). It may appear very thick or it may be thinner. Colostrum is a concentrated form of immunities and nourishment that provides the baby with protection from illness and infection and prepares her digestive system for the greater volumes of milk to come. For the normal range of colors for mature milk, see p. 517-518 in the next chapter.

• • •

In most parents, milk production continues to increase from weeks 1 through 5.

With frequent and effective feeds or milk expression, milk production continues to increase. Babies 2 to 3 weeks old usually take about 2 to 3 ounces (59 to 89 mL) during nursing sessions, taking daily about 20 to 25 ounces (591 to 750 mL) of milk (Kent et al., 2016). To increase milk production to meet their growing needs, babies often have periods of longer, more frequent feeds, which are sometimes termed "growth spurts" or "frequency days."

During weeks 4 and 5, many babies continue to take more milk per feed as their stomachs grow in size. An average nursing is about 3 to 4 ounces (89 to 118 mL), with daily milk intake increasing to an average of about 25 to 30 ounces (750 to 887 mL) per day (Kent et al., 2013; Kent et al., 2006). In one U.S. study, 98 mothers of term breastfeeding babies did test-weights to measure milk intake at every feed around the clock for the first 6 weeks of life (Hill et al., 2005), and researchers found that babies' milk intake increased rapidly during the first 3 weeks of life, increasing slightly during Weeks 4 and 5, and staying relatively stable from Weeks 5 to 6.

When working with individual families, however, keep in mind that not every nursing couple is average. One Australian study of 71 exclusively breastfed babies between 1 and 6 months (Kent et al., 2006) found a large range of daily milk intake among healthy, thriving babies, from 15.5 to 43 ounces or 440 to 1,220 g.

• • •

As mentioned earlier, according to the prolactin receptor theory, the higher and more often a parent's blood prolactin levels rise (surge) during the critical first 2 weeks after birth, the more prolactin receptors are upregulated, increasing milk production potential for that lactation (De Carvalho, 1983). This process starts anew with each birth. If for whatever reason a parent does not remove milk early, often, and well during these first 2 weeks, fewer prolactin receptors may be upregulated, and the milk production potential may be more limited. After the first 2 weeks, when the parent's response to prolactin naturally decreases, it is still possible to boost milk production, but it usually requires much more time and work. In rare cases, it may even be impossible.

Early, frequent, and effective milk removal during the first 2 weeks after birth is key to long-term milk production.

During these first 2 weeks, encourage families to remove milk early, often, and effectively to set milk production potential at "abundant." U.S. lactation consultants Lisa Marasco and Diana West compared the rise in milk production during the early weeks to a rocket launch (Figure 10.3) and described how the trajectory of milk production (called the lactation curve in dairy science) varies depending on early milk removal patterns. In this analogy, the rocket fuel is hormones (which start the countdown and lift-off process) and mammary stimulation (L. Marasco & West, 2020, p. 58), which:

> "...work together to blast the rocket off the launch pad and into outer space. The rocket has a limited amount of fuel and it needs to get up high enough into the atmosphere where gravity is lower and less power is needed to keep it going in order to the complete its mission....When the prolactin levels start their natural decline, having lots of receptors in place ensures that milk production can be maintained to meet baby's needs. Launching is the most critical stage of a successful mission. If things go wrong at the start, the potential for a compromised mission is high."

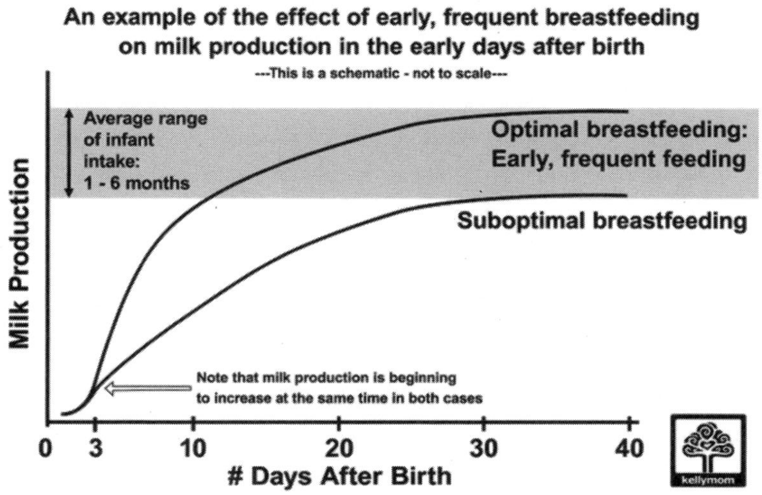

Figure 10.3 How early, often, and effective milk removal affects long-term production. ©2020 KellyMom.com, used with permission.

• • •

After milk production reaches its peak at about 5 weeks, it stays relatively stable until it begins to decline when the baby starts other foods at around 6 months.

On average, at about 5 weeks after birth, most nursing parents produce nearly as much milk per day as their nursing baby will ever need (Allen, Keller, Archer, & Neville, 1991). After 5 weeks of age, a baby's daily milk intake reaches a plateau (Kent et al., 2013). At about 6 months, when the baby starts solid foods, milk production starts to decline because solid foods take the place of mother's milk in baby's diet (Islam, Peerson, Ahmed, Dewey, & Brown, 2006). The reason nursing babies don't need increasing volumes of milk between 1 and 6 months is because their rate of growth (along with their metabolism) slows during this period (Butte, 2005). So even though babies grow bigger and heavier at this time, their slowing growth rate offsets the need for more milk. For more details, see p. 498.

• • •

Milk composition varies among nursing parents and may vary by baby's sex.

Milk composition varies in different ways among nursing parents.

Milk fat and caloric content. Milk fat content can vary as much as tenfold among nursing parents (Agostoni et al., 2001). A 2017 U.S. study that analyzed five milk samples from 24 mothers (Sauer, Boutin, & Kim, 2017) found a wide range of caloric content, with an average of just under 18 kcal/oz. This challenged the rule of thumb that human milk is 20 kcal/oz. In this study, only 34% of the milk samples were within 10% of the expected caloric density. However, an Australian study (S. Khan et al., 2013) noted that the fat content (and therefore its calories) varies greatly over the course of a day and that only averaging the fat content of 24-hour milk samples along with the milk volume would provide an accurate gauge of the milk's adequacy. A 2016 Dutch study that analyzed hindmilk samples from 614 mothers (P. Prentice et al., 2016) found that the more exclusively the mothers nursed, the higher their milk's caloric content.

The type of fat in mother's milk may also vary, depending on diet. A 2016 systematic review (Bravi et al., 2016) noted that in some studies, nursing parents who ate fish regularly had higher levels of the omega-3 fatty acid DHA in their milk than those who didn't eat fish.

Milk metabolites and the milk microbiome. A 2018 international study examined milk samples at 1 month from 109 mothers who lived in five different countries (Australia, Japan, the U.S., Norway, and South Africa) and analyzed these samples using nuclear magnetic resonance (Gay et al., 2018). The researchers found subtle differences in the milk's metabolites, the components that interact with the bacteria in the human body to promote growth and development. These metabolites varied by ethnicity and country, and by whether or not the country was industrialized. The authors noted that some components of human milk are produced by the bacteria present in the milk's microbiome, and the type of bacteria in the milk microbiome varied among countries.

Different milk for boys and girls? A 2018 review of animal and human studies (Galante et al., 2018) noted that male and female infants in all mammal species grow and develop differently. (The World Health Organization provides different growth charts for boys and girls.) The authors noted that to maximize growth and development, non-human mammal mothers produce milk of different composition for male and female newborns. Some evidence exists that there may be sex differences in the milk humans produce, too. At this writing, more research is needed to confirm the specifics of these differences and their importance to health outcomes.

• • •

Over the course of lactation, as baby grows, milk composition changes in several ways.

Milk composition changes over time.

Whey-casein ratios. One aspect of milk that changes over time is its ratio of whey proteins to casein proteins (Gridneva et al., 2018). Unlike most mammal milks, at birth, human milk is higher in whey proteins than casein. Whey proteins (which include lysozyme, lactoferrin, and secretory IgA) are easily and quickly digested by human babies and are responsible for the soft curds in babies' stools (Czank, Mitoulas, & Hartmann, 2007). Cow's milk (and most infant formulas) was once about 80% casein proteins, which is good for calves' multi-stomach digestive system but difficult for human babies to digest. In recent years, some infant formulas have adjusted their products for a greater whey-to-casein ratio, however these ratios do not change over time like human milk. During the first month or so, when the baby's digestive system is most immature, the ratio of whey proteins to casein proteins in human milk is about 90:10 (Kunz & Lonnerdal, 1992). Over time, as the baby's digestive system matures, this ratio changes. By about 6 weeks, the ratio is 80:20. By about 6 months, this ratio is 60:40. In later lactation, it is 50:50.

Day and night variations in milk melatonin levels. In an overview article about changes in milk composition by day, week, and month (Hahn-Holbrook, Saxbe, Bixby, Steele, & Glynn, 2019), its U.S. authors described human milk as ***chrononutrition***, meaning that when a baby nurses directly (rather than receiving previously expressed milk) the needed variations are delivered at the right time. For example, a 2016 study analyzed milk samples expressed at different times of day and night by 14 mothers of preterm babies and 7 mothers of term babies (Katzer et al., 2016). It found that milk concentrations of melatonin (a hormone associated with better sleep) were higher at night.

Changes in milk composition during the second year and beyond. Many families are told by the uninformed that after the first year, human milk has "no nutritional value." Not so, according to several studies. Average percentage of fat in mother's milk changes over time, with milk received by older nursing babies significantly higher in fat than the milk received by younger nursing babies. One U.S. study (Mandel, Lubetzky, Dollberg, Barak, & Mimouni, 2005) compared the milk fat content of 34 mothers with nursing babies older than a year (12 to 39 months) and 27 mothers with nursing babies 2 to 4 months old. The researchers found that the milk the older babies received was about 50% higher in fat than the milk received by the younger babies, the same result as other studies (Dewey, Finley, & Lonnerdal, 1984).

Another U.S. study analyzed monthly milk samples from 19 lactating women between 11 and 17 months after birth and compared them with pooled milk samples from donors to a local milk bank whose babies were younger than 1 year (Perrin, Fogleman, Newburg, & Allen, 2017). Between 11 and 17 months, the concentrations of some components increased, including total protein, lactoferrin, lysozyme, IgA, sodium, and oligosaccharides (a milk sugar that feeds the "good bacteria" in a baby's digestive system). However, from 11 to 17 months some components decreased, including zinc and calcium. The researchers concluded (Perrin et al., 2017, p. 2):

> "Human milk between 11 and 17 months postpartum provides equal or greater concentrations of macronutrients and key bioactive proteins compared with mature milk bank samples donated in the first year postpartum..."

To better understand the changes in milk composition during longer lactation, a 2018 Polish study examined milk samples from 137 mothers from the 1st to the 48th months of lactation (Czosnykowska-Lukacka, Krolak-Olejnik, & Orczyk-Pawilowicz, 2018). In those who nursed longer than 18 months, milk fat and protein content increased and carbohydrate content decreased. They attributed these changes to the changing needs at each stage in the rapidly growing child. Between the 24th and the 48th months of nursing, the level of fat, protein, and carbohydrates remained stable. The researchers suggested that the calories in the milk consumed by the older children primarily came from fat, while carbohydrates played a larger role in nutrition during early infancy.

• • •

After 1 year, milk production varies, depending on how often the baby nurses, while the mammary tissue decreases.

In Australia, by the time the nursing baby is 15 months old and is eating many other foods, daily milk production was measured at between 95 and 315 mL (about 3 to 10 ounces) per day (Kent et al., 1999; Neville et al., 1991). But milk production at this stage is determined by how many times per day baby nurses. Research done in Zaire (where nursing older babies is the norm) found mothers' producing, on average, 300 mL (10 oz.) per day at 30 months (Hennart, Delogne-Desnoeck, Vis, & Robyn, 1981).

Mammary tissue is at its peak when baby's milk intake is at its peak, between 1 and 6 months after birth. As the baby starts eating other foods, mammary tissue usually decreases significantly between 6 and 9 months (Kent, 2007). By 15 months, in most cases, the mammary glands return to their prepregnancy size, even when they are producing significant volumes of milk (Kent et al., 1999).

• • •

With weaning, the glandular tissue involutes and milk production stops.

As a baby weans, the glandular tissue involutes, when the mammary glands stop producing milk, and the tissue reverts to its prepregnancy state. First the milk-making cells (lactocytes) die, and then the fat cells in the glands differentiate to fill the spaces they occupied (Bosschaart et al., 2019). Blood vessels recede, changing the internal landscape of the mammary gland (Watson, 2006). As milk production slows and stops, the milk increases in sodium, chloride, fat, and protein and decreases in lactose and potassium (Hartmann & Kulski, 1978).

After involution is complete, it is usually possible to express drops of milk for at least 6 weeks (Kent, 2007). Anecdotally, parents reported being able to express a little milk even years after their baby stopped nursing.

Making Milk for Twins, Triplets, and More

Most nursing parents can produce enough milk for twins, triplets, and even quadruplets.

The same milk-production dynamics described earlier apply equally to parents of multiples. The only real difference is the volume of milk needed. To exclusively nurse, the parents of twins, triplets, and quadruplets will need double, triple, or quadruple the milk needed by the parent of one baby.

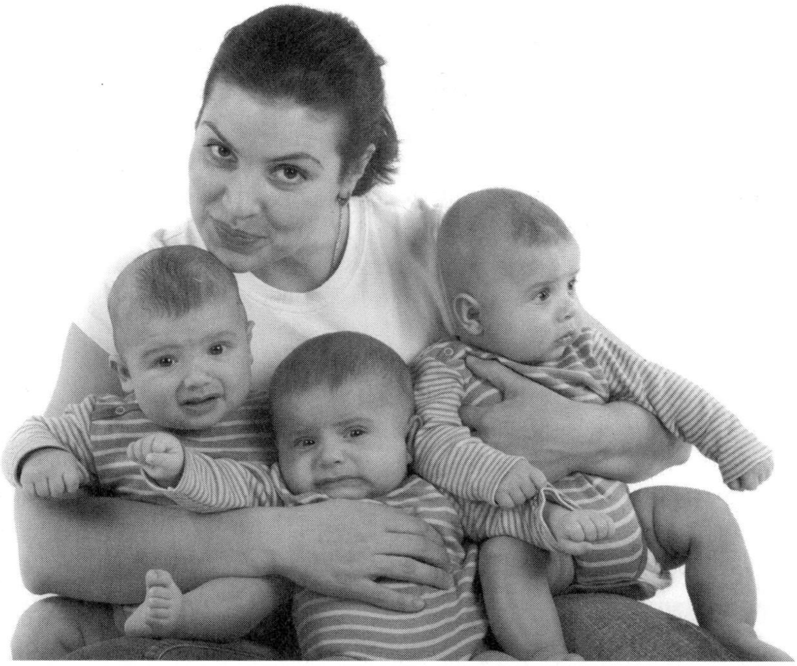

If babies from a multiple pregnancy are born healthy and nursing effectively, the most important thing the average parent needs to know is that by nursing on cue, it is most likely possible to produce enough milk for all of the babies. In general, parents who give birth to multiple babies have the advantage of more placenta, which means the release of more mammary-stimulating hormones and the growth and development of more glandular tissue during pregnancy. One Australian study of eight mothers of twins and one mother of triplets (Saint, Maggiore, & Hartmann, 1986) found that all of the twin mothers except one produced double the milk of mothers of one baby. The mother of triplets in this study produced 3.08 kg (109 oz.) of milk per day, or more than enough milk for all three babies. In one amazing U.S. case report, a mother of quadruplets "exclusively" nursed her four babies for 6 months, starting solids at the appropriate age and continuing to breastfeed in addition to other foods for 12 months (Berlin, 2007). The word "exclusively" is in quotation marks because one of the quadruplets had the metabolic disorder PKU, and as a result, needed a small amount of phenylalanine-free formula each day. (For details on nursing the baby with PKU, see p. 322.

One U.S. mother of quadruplets born at 34 weeks by cesarean section reported that within the first month she produced so much milk that when her babies slept for 2-hour stretches, she could express enough milk for their supplemental feeds, which were primarily mother's milk (Mead, Chuffo, Lawlor-Klean, & Meier, 1992). These babies breastfed until they were 12, 15, 15, and 18 months old.

A 2013 case report described the experience of a U.S. mother of twins who had previously had a mastectomy to treat breast cancer and by nursing from the one remaining breast achieved exclusive breastfeeding of her twins at 3 months (Michaels & Wanner, 2013). She delivered her two boys at 37.5 weeks and received ongoing help and support from an IBCLC, who recommended immediate skin-to-skin contact after delivery, frequent nursing and pumping after nursing. It took a period of formula supplementation and the use of domperidone to boost her milk production to finally meet her goal at 3 months of exclusive nursing. She nursed her twins for 2 years 10 months and served as a support person for other parents nursing after mastectomy.

• • •

Families nursing multiples benefit from getting off to a good start, receiving extra help and support, and having realistic expectations.

Even when milk production is no problem, finding the time to nurse and manage the rest of life's demands can be daunting. Suggest the family expect each baby will need to nurse at least 8 times every 24 hours during the early weeks. See the next point for strategies. Getting off to a good start—nursing early, often, and effectively—is also critical. A 2016 South Korean prospective survey (B. Y. Kim, 2016) found that twins were more likely to nurse throughout the hospital stay when their first feed was nursing and they started nursing early.

Having support and help is also vital. A 2018 Brazilian secondary analysis (Mikami et al., 2018) found that lack of support and low birth weight were two factors associated with premature weaning among 128 mothers of twins. A Japanese study of 1,529 mothers of twins, 234 mothers of triplets, 20 mothers of quadruplets, and 4 mothers of quintuplets (Yokoyama & Ooki, 2004) found that mothers of multiples had a significantly shorter duration of nursing than parents of single babies and that they were 1.83 times more likely to decide not to nurse when their husband did not help with child-rearing.

A 2019 Indonesian questionnaire study of 184 mothers of twins (Anjarwati, Waluyanti, & Rachmawati, 2019) found that the single most significant factor associated with exclusive nursing of twins was the mothers' level of breastfeeding self-efficacy (BSE)—her confidence in her ability to fully nurse her babies—which the researchers found could be boosted by counseling from healthcare providers.

• • •

There is no one right way to nurse multiples; encourage each family to work out their own system.

Deciding which babies nurse when. Some parents of multiples prefer as a time-saver to always nurse two babies at once (see an illustration of possible positions on p. 35). Most, however, prefer to nurse their babies separately at some feeds to enjoy some one-on-one time with each baby or because one baby needs extra help. Babies' feeding patterns may vary, with one baby nursing more often than the other. If one baby does not nurse as effectively as her sibling(s), suggest nursing both babies together. The more effective baby may better stimulate milk ejection, and the faster flow of milk may help the less effective baby get more milk more quickly. If that doesn't help, try to determine the cause of the baby's ineffective feeding. (Is she preterm? Does she have a tongue-tie? Is she ill? Does she have a neurological impairment?) After finding the cause, provide suggestions addressing that issue.

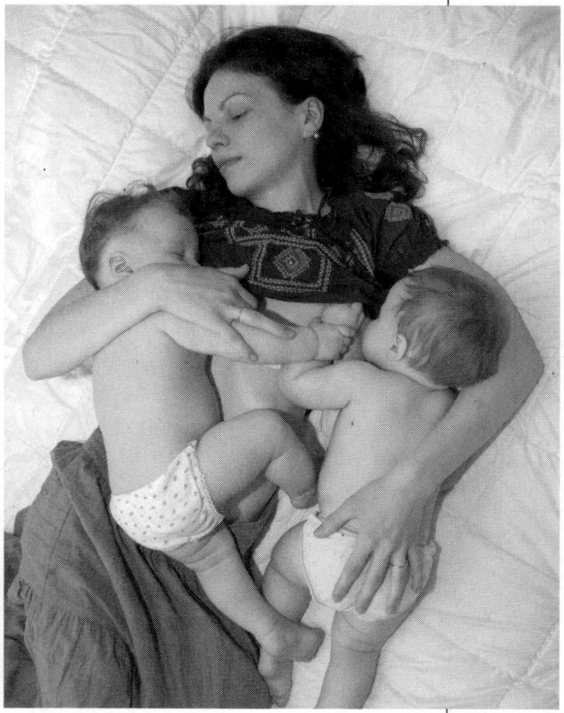

Which baby gets which side when. There are different ways to decide which baby gets which side. Some parents nurse with no particular plan, offering whichever side feels fuller to whichever baby seems hungriest at the moment. Other parents keep each baby on the same side for an entire day, alternating sides every day. Some parents of twins assign each baby a particular side that she receives at every feed and never varies. If one baby nurses less effectively, alternating sides ensures both sides are well stimulated to maintain milk production.

Keeping track of nursing. Some parents of multiples keep a daily written or digital log of which baby nursed when and on which side along with diaper output. Other parents don't keep track of either feeds or diapers. If both babies gain weight well, no record-keeping is needed. If a baby is not gaining weight well, suggest recording frequency and length of feeds and diaper output for a few days. Life with multiples can be unbelievably hectic, and if a baby is placid or sleepy, she may not be nursing often or long enough to meet her needs.

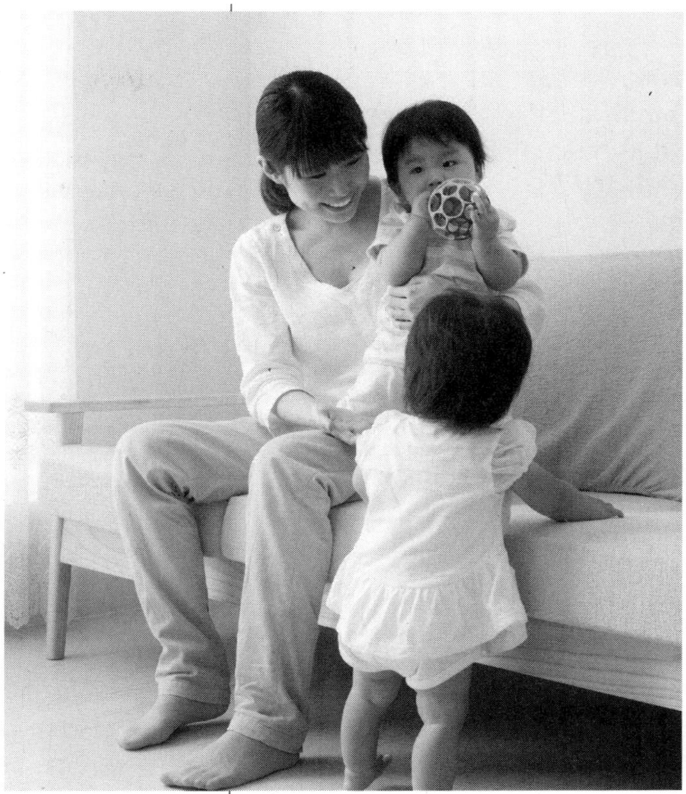

Night nursing. Encourage the parent to find well-supported feeding positions that allow resting during nursing. For positioning ideas, see Chapter 1. Many multiples sleep in one crib or bed because they sleep better when they are touching. If a crib is used, it may make night feeds easier if it is in the parent's room. One option is to fasten the crib to the side of the parent's bed, adjust the mattress levels to the same height, and remove the side rail closest to the adult bed for easy access to the babies at night. The parent can then pull into the adult bed whichever baby wants to nurse, feed her, and return her to the crib after she's finished, or—if the parent falls asleep—when another baby awakens to feed.

Another alternative, which is common in Japan, is for the parent to sleep on a mattress or futon on the floor. The sleeping surface could be in the babies' room or the parent's room so that the parent can lie down with the babies and sleep during feeds. If the parent wants to bring the babies into the adult bed, discuss safe sleeping options (see p. 84-87).

• • •

If due to health issues one or more babies aren't nursing or aren't nursing effectively, discuss milk expression.

When one or more babies are not yet nursing, the nursing parent can provide milk for her/them by expressing milk. For details, see p. 498-507.

• • •

Nursing multiples does not have to be all or nothing; partial nursing is almost always a better option than no nursing.

Either by choice or by circumstance, some families partially nurse twins, triplets, and higher order multiples. One case report (Auer & Gromada, 1998) described a mother who partially breastfed all four of her quadruplets until one baby weaned abruptly at 12 months. The other three continued breastfeeding a couple times each day until 30 months of age.

If a nursing parent is feeling overwhelmed or believes sharing feeds with others would make life easier, discuss the option of partial nursing. In one U.S. study of 123 mothers of twins (Damato, Dowling, Madigan, & Thanattherakul, 2005), after birth 110 (89%) initiated either breastfeeding or milk expression, and the mothers who persisted continued to provide a high percentage of mother's milk feeds through 28 weeks. Another article based on this study data reported that of those mothers who weaned by 9 weeks, the most common reason given (by 40%) was their perceptions of inadequate milk production (Damato, Dowling, Standing, & Schuster, 2005). Of the mothers who weaned between 9 and 28 weeks, the most common reason given (by 32%) was the extra time and/or burden involved in breastfeeding and/or milk expression. However, illness in the mother and/or babies was mentioned as one reason for weaning by 33% at 9 weeks and 8% at 28 weeks.

LGBTQ Nursing

When gender-diverse families ask for information on nursing, tailor strategies to their situation.

Since the first edition of this book, many Western societies increasingly acknowledge gender diversity and families that do not conform to cisgender expectations. Although at this writing, the science on LGBTQ nursing is scarce, the same basic principles apply to these families. To read more about nursing in transgender and non-binary families, see La Leche League International's webpage: **bit.ly/BA2-LLLITransgender**.

• • •

In families with same-sex female partners, breastfeeding can happen in different ways, including co-nursing, which requires thought and planning about milk production.

Breastfeeding can occur in several ways in families with same-sex female partners who were both assigned as female at birth and both identify as female (cisgender). If the pregnant partner plans to do all the breastfeeding, there are no special considerations. However, in some families the non-gestational parent may plan to do all of the breastfeeding and either relactate or induce lactation to bring in her milk (see Chapter 16 for details). However, if both partners decide to co-nurse the baby, this can also happen in different ways.

- Both women go through pregnancy and give birth within a short time of each other and breastfeed both babies.
- One partner gives birth and the other relactates or induces lactation (Koning, 2011).
- Neither woman gives birth, and the couple adopts a baby or the baby is born via surrogacy, with both women inducing lactation.

In one case report (Wilson, Perrin, Fogleman, & Chetwynd, 2015), a lesbian couple adopted a baby and both induced lactation. During the early weeks, this couple co-nursed the baby along with the baby's birth mother.

One aspect of co-nursing that the family needs to sort out is how to balance milk production between the co-nursing partners. For more on the benefits of co-nursing and specific suggestions and approaches, see the section "Co-Nursing with Partners" on p. 688.

• • •

Transgender female parents can produce milk, with one reported case of exclusive nursing for the first 6 weeks.

Transgender women were assigned as male at birth but identify as female and transitioned to female. Their transition may involve undergoing hormone therapy to suppress male traits and enhance female traits. They may or may not have "bottom surgery" to further physically transform themselves. For those planning to breastfeed, induced lactation is an option. A 2018 case report (Reisman & Goldstein, 2018) described the experience of a transgender woman who received female hormone therapy (spironolactone, estradiol, and progesterone) for 6 years and developed breast tissue before her partner (who did not want to breastfeed) became pregnant. During the pregnancy, the estradiol and progesterone were increased and her healthcare provider added domperidone to mimic the hormones of pregnancy. She pumped a few times each day. After 1 month, she began to express drops of milk and the medications were increased again along with more intensive pumping. At 3 months, she produced 8 oz (240 mL) per day. About 2 weeks before the baby was born, the estradiol and progesterone were reduced. After the baby was born, she breastfed exclusively, producing enough milk to fully sustain the baby for the first 6 weeks. According to research (Sonnenblick, Shah, Goldstein, & Reisman, 2018), estrogen therapy grows mammary tissue. In another case report, a transgender woman induced lactation and shared breastfeeding with her female partner, who was also the baby's birth mother (Sperling & Robinson, 2018). Here is a link to this case report: **bit.ly/BA2-BFTransWoman**.

A transgender woman who decides to breastfeed may produce more milk if she has undergone female hormone therapy. Another option is following the induced lactation protocols described on p. 679. If she is interested in using herbal galactogogues, U.S. lactation consultants Lisa Marasco and Diana West (L. Marasco & West, 2020) suggest using those herbs thought to stimulate the growth of mammary tissue, such as goat's rue, or anti-androgen herbs, such as saw palmetto and fennel. If milk production is not the top priority, she may want to consider ***dry nursing***, which is described on p. 689 as an option for parents who produce no milk, such as fathers, wanting to experience nursing.

• • •

Nursing is an option for transgender male parents, who—depending on previous surgeries and hormone treatments—may produce milk.

Transgender men were assigned as female at birth but identify as male and transitioned to male. As with transgender women, the transition from female to male may involve hormone treatments and surgery. "Top surgery" has similarities to breast reduction surgery, as it involves the removal of mammary tissue. But not all transgender men have this surgery. Some instead bind their mammary tissue to appear more masculine, which needs to be done carefully to avoid plugged ducts and mastitis.

In some families, transgender men get pregnant, give birth, and nurse their babies, which some refer to as ***chestfeeding*** (MacDonald et al., 2016). Going through the biologically female experiences of pregnancy, mammary growth, birth, and nursing, however, can be stressful, leading to a type of distress or anxiety known as ***gender dysphoria***. Because each transgender man falls on a different point of the gender spectrum, how pregnancy and nursing fit into his gender identity will vary from person to person. (For more details, see p. 797.) The use of male hormones, such as testosterone, which enhances male traits such as facial hair, may also suppress mammary growth during lactation and milk production. In some cases, transgender men prefer to nurse in private and if milk production is less than full, use a feeding-tube device or supplement in other ways. To read about the experiences of 22 transgender men who became pregnant and gave birth, go to: **bit.ly/BA2-Transmasculine**.

Low Milk Production

Slow weight gain is not always due to low milk production.

Low milk production is not always the cause of excess weight loss after birth or slow weight gain later. Some health problems cause babies to gain weight slowly even with ample milk intake. (For details, see p. 212.) In other cases, the mammary glands produce abundant milk but the baby doesn't nurse effectively due to anatomical variations, airway abnormalities, neurological impairment, prematurity, or other issues. Before assuming low milk production is the cause of slow weight gain, be sure to rule out other factors. (See Chapter 6, "Weight Gain and Growth.") Before suggesting strategies, it is best to first determine the cause, making sure in the meantime the baby gets the milk she needs and that steps are taken to safeguard milk production.

Determining Milk Production

When there is concern about a baby's weight after Day 3 or 4, test-weighing and milk expression can help gauge milk production.

If a baby's weight loss after birth is in the normal range and after that she gains weight and grows well, it is safe to assume that milk production is ample. If baby's weight loss within the first few days is more than 10%, the first step is to help the baby latch deeper, use massage and compression, and make sure baby nurses at least 10 to 12 times per day. If the baby's weight doesn't improve, supplements may be needed (see the section starting on p. 222).

Watching for signs of milk intake as a baby nurses is not a reliable gauge of milk production. One U.S. study found that neither mothers nor experienced lactation consultants could accurately estimate preterm babies' milk intake during nursing by listening for swallowing and watching for wide jaw movements (P. P. Meier, Engstrom, Fleming, Streeter, & Lawrence, 1996). However, the following two strategies may be useful to determine milk production after milk increase on Day 3 or 4. They are not usually helpful before then because milk production and intake are relatively small.

KEY CONCEPT

Milk expression can rule out low milk production, but it cannot necessarily confirm it.

Test-weighing. One reliable gauge of milk intake during nursing is by using a very accurate (to 2 g) electronic baby scale for pre- and post-feed weights (P. P. Meier & Engstrom, 2007; Rankin et al., 2016). These scales are available in many hospitals and lactation clinics and in some areas can be rented for home use from breast pump rental businesses. For average milk intake per nursing session by age, see Table 6.3 on p. 224, keeping in mind that feeding volumes vary at different times of day. One test-weight does not provide enough information to gauge a baby's daily milk intake. So although it can rule out ineffective nursing at that feed and low milk production, it does not reveal whether a baby is consistently effective during nursing. Doing 24-hour test-weights provides much more information. For more details on accurate test-weighing, see p. 919.

Milk expression. Expressing milk can rule out low milk production as a cause of slow weight gain if the nursing parent can express ample milk at several sessions. (The first session should not be used as a final gauge because milk may have accumulated in the mammary gland.) However, milk expression is a less reliable way to confirm low milk production because not all parents can express milk effectively, especially at first. For example, one Australian study of 28 breastfeeding mothers with established and ample milk production (Kent, Ramsay, Doherty, Larsson, & Hartmann, 2003) found 11% were unable to express much milk using any of the seven pump cycling patterns tested. For many parents, milk expression is a learned skill that takes time and practice to master. Even when the most effective type of pump (usually a multi-user rental-grade pump) is used, factors unrelated to milk production—such as fit and responsiveness—can affect milk yield. For details, see p. 907-908.

In a research setting, where the parents' responsiveness to the pump was verified first, one technique found accurate in measuring 24-hour milk production (Kent et al., 2018) was draining the mammary glands as fully as possible once per hour for 4 consecutive hours with a multi-user rental-grade pump then multiplying this combined volume from the last pump session by 24. For example, if after combining the milk from both sides at the fourth session, the parent pumped a total of 1 oz. (29 mL), multiplying this volume by 24 estimates the 24-hour milk production to be 24 oz. (696 mL).

Commercial devices that claim to measure milk intake. In recent years, a variety of products entered the marketplace that claim to accurately measure baby's milk intake at a nursing session. One includes a device with a small sensor that is placed under baby's tongue during feeds and uses an algorithm to calculate milk intake, which is sent to an app in the parent's smartphone that records the results. Another uses a battery-operated device designed to be used with a scale that hangs from an infant seat to measure changes in the size of the mammary gland and baby's weight during feeds. Another device uses a nipple shield with sensors attached to measure milk transfer and sends the information to the parent's smartphone where it is recorded. Lactation specialists Lisa Marasco and Diana West wrote in their book, ***Making More Milk*** (L. Marasco & West, 2020, p. 31):

> "Is it worth the money to buy one of these devices? We don't have enough experience to say one way or the other yet, but we're concerned that the technologies may be less accurate in low-supply situations when babies have suck problems, or for mothers with unusually-shaped breasts or nipples."

Inhibited Milk Increase after Birth

Milk production is considered delayed when the nursing parent notices no mammary changes or fullness by about 72 hours after delivery.

When milk production does not increase within the first 3 days after birth, U.S. researchers (Neville & Morton, 2001) suggest three categories of possible causes:

1. **Hormonal issues** preventing the mammary gland from responding normally, such as retained placenta, ovarian tumor, or subnormal pituitary function
2. **Mammary issues** that could limit milk production, such as a history of breast or chest surgery or underdeveloped mammary tissue
3. **Ineffective or infrequent milk removal.**

See Box 10.1 for a more detailed list of possible causes.

Delays in milk increase are common in cultures where childbirth is managed using a medical model and early feeding practices are suboptimal. See Table 10.3 for differences in practices and outcomes found in two 2015 studies done in Italy and the U.S.

TABLE 10.3 Delays in Milk Increase with Vaginal Births in Italy and the U.S.

Italy	U.S.
1,760 "natural births," all nursed ≤1st hour	83,433 vaginal births, "routine care"
Low threshold for spoon-feeding newborns with hand-expressed colostrum	Rarely spoon-fed newborns with hand-expressed colostrum
Average weight loss 5.95%	Average weight loss 7.1%
Lowest weight at 44 hr.	Lowest weight at 48-72 hr.
No babies with weight loss of ≥10%	10% of babies with weight loss of ≥10%

Adapted from (Bertini et al., 2015; Flaherman et al., 2015)

BOX 10.1 Factors that May Inhibit Milk Increase after Birth

Parent Factors

- First time nursing
- Overweight, obese, or excessive weight gain during pregnancy
- Mammary/nipple issues, such as underdeveloped glandular tissue, a history of surgery or injury, or unusual mammary or nipple anatomy
- Health conditions that may affect hormonal levels or the body's response to hormones, such as diabetes, polycystic ovary syndrome (PCOS), thyroid or pituitary issues, pregnancy hypertension, prolactin resistance, gestational ovarian theca lutein cysts
- Medications that suppress or inhibit lactation

Baby Factors

- Any condition that reduces baby's nursing effectiveness (variations in oral anatomy, birth injury, airway abnormalities, health or neurological issues, etc.)

Birth-Related Factors

- Long labor or traumatic or unusually stressful birth, which increases cortisol levels
- Preterm birth
- Retained placenta or other placental issues, which may affect hormonal levels or mammary tissue development
- Blood loss of more than 1,000 mL (more than 2 pints), affecting hormonal levels and possibly pituitary function

Post-delivery Factors

- A late start or little or no nursing or milk expression
- Separation, little or no skin-to-skin or body contact

• • •

Hormonal and health issues may affect the timing of milk increase and long-term milk production.

The following conditions, which may affect the nursing parent's hormonal levels and therefore milk production, should be considered red flags, and arrangement should be made to closely monitor these nursing couples after birth.

First time nursing. As described in an earlier point, milk increase after birth in parents who nursed a previous child averages about 1 day earlier than those nursing for the first time (J. C. Ingram et al., 1999).

Overweight and obesity. Excess fatty tissue in the body produces hormones, which can interact with other hormones and affect milk production. Several studies found obesity, overweight, and excessive weight gain during pregnancy were associated with inhibited milk increase after birth (Hilson, Rasmussen, & Kjolhede, 2004; Preusting, Brumley, Odibo, Spatz, & Louis, 2017; K. Rasmussen, 2007). However, a U.S. secondary analysis (Haile, Chavan, Teweldeberhan, & Chertok, 2017) found the association between weight gain during pregnancy and a delay in milk increase was only statistically significant among white women, not among women of other ethnicities. Obesity was also associated with a decreased prolactin response to baby's sucking (K. M. Rasmussen & Kjolhede, 2004). Obesity should be considered a red flag to closely monitor the nursing couple after birth. For more details, see the section starting on p. 574.

Diabetes and insulin resistance. As mentioned previously, insulin is one of the hormones involved in milk production. Like first time nursing, Type

1 diabetes was associated with a delay of milk increase after birth of about 1 day. If the nursing parent has a family history of diabetes, tested as borderline diabetic, or had gestational diabetes, it may helpful for the family to request the following tests to see if they might benefit from treatment: hemoglobin A1C and a 2-hour glucose tolerance test (see also Table 10.4 on p. 443).

Thyroid dysfunction, either too high or too low, increases risk for low milk production. Pregnancy and birth disrupt thyroid function in some parents (see p. 855). If there is a family or personal history of thyroid problems, extreme fatigue, unexplained weight gain or weight loss with jitteriness, suggest requesting their healthcare provider test TSH, T3, T4, and TPO antibodies. See Table 10.4 and p. 856-857 for more details.

Polycystic ovary syndrome (PCOS) is not consistently associated with low milk production. Some with this condition have overabundant milk production, some have average milk production, and some have low milk production. When PCOS occurs with insulin resistance and/or high levels of male hormones, such as testosterone, this may increase risk of low milk production. If the nursing parent has excess facial or body hair or reports thinning of head hair, this may indicate excess male hormones. In this case, suggest seeing their healthcare provider about a possible test for bioavailable testosterone. For more details, see Table 10.4 and p. 852.

Pregnancy-induced hypertension was found in several studies (J. Demirci, Schmella, Glasser, Bodnar, & Himes, 2018; Leeners, Rath, Kuse, & Neumaier-Wagner, 2005; Salahudeen et al., 2013) to be linked to a delay in milk increase after birth.

Gestational ovarian theca lutein cysts, which can cause a jump in testosterone levels during pregnancy, inhibiting milk production after birth until levels fall, which usually takes weeks (Betzold, Hoover, & Snyder, 2004; Hoover, Barbalinardo, & Platia, 2002).

Risk factors for low prolactin levels. Some of the following aspects of a parent's health history are worth noting, as they may affect prolactin levels, which may influence the course of lactation.

- Cranial radiotherapy (CRT), a treatment for childhood cancer associated with low prolactin production (Follin et al., 2013; Johnston, Vowels, Carroll, Neville, & Cohn, 2008)
- A family history of alcoholism, which was found to reduce responsiveness to prolactin (Mennella & Pepino, 2010)

Infertility may occur in part due to hormonal issues, which may also affect lactation. Research has noted an association between the use of assisted reproductive technology and a shorter duration of nursing (Cromi et al., 2015; Wiffen & Fetherston, 2016).

Medications that suppress or inhibit lactation. See Table 10.2 on p. 419 for drugs that suppress lactation and other drugs that may inhibit lactation in some users, including hormonal birth control containing estrogen and progesterone (see p. 547).

• • •

Mammary and nipple issues may be a factor in delayed milk increase.

In some cases, physical aspects of the nipple or the mammary gland may affect milk production.

Underdeveloped mammary glands. In some unusual cases, the mammary glands did not develop fully. Also known as ***insufficient glandular tissue***, or ***mammary hypoplasia***, some with this condition have bulbous areolae or widely spaced mammary glands (more than 1.5 inches or about 4 cm apart), large differences in gland size, or tubular or cone-shaped glands rather than rounded (Diana Cassar-Uhl, 2014; K Huggins et al., 2000). When the glands are examined, there may be some obvious patches of glandular tissue in a mostly soft gland (Wilson-Clay & Hoover, 2017, p. 69). Parents with this condition often notice no mammary changes during pregnancy or feelings of fullness after birth. Although the change to mature milk happens on schedule, the volumes are too low to be felt as fullness. Consider these physical signs a red flag to monitor the nursing couple closely after birth. Depending on how much functional milk-making tissue a parent has and the nursing dynamics, it may be possible to increase milk production over time (nursing stimulates the growth of glandular tissue) and eventually exclusively nurse later babies (K Huggins et al., 2000; Wilson-Clay & Hoover, 2017). For more details, see p. 785.

A history of breast or chest surgery or injury. Any surgery performed on the chest before puberty or one that removed mammary tissue (reduction mammaplasty or the top surgery performed on some transgender men) increases risk of inadequate milk production. This is not a delayed milk increase, but overall low milk production. For details, see p. 788.

Unusual nipple anatomy. Because variations in nipple anatomy may make latching more challenging, it may affect milk transfer. Flat or inverted nipples were associated with delayed milk increase in one U.S. study (Dewey et al., 2003) and an Iranian study of first-time mothers (Vazirinejad, Darakhshan, Esmaeili, & Hadadian, 2009). Also, those missing nipple pores (sometimes called "blind nipples") may have obstructed milk flow.

Nipple piercing can also affect milk transfer. Although there are several case reports of successful nursing after a nipple piercing (N. Lee, 1995; Wilson-Clay & Hoover, 2017), there are also case reports of complications from the piercing that caused milk duct obstruction and reduced milk transfer during nursing and milk expression (Garbin, Deacon, Rowan, Hartmann, & Geddes, 2009). For more details, see p. 742.

• • •

Some aspects of the pregnancy, labor, and birth may delay milk increase after birth.

Medications used during pregnancy and childbirth. Some studies found an association between the use of drugs used during pregnancy and childbirth that either delayed milk increase or contributed to low milk production:

- ***Anti-contraction drugs*** known as tocolytics were associated with shorter duration of nursing and low milk production in one study (Bjelakovic et al., 2016).
- ***Betamethasone,*** for hastening lung maturity before preterm birth, was associated with delayed milk increase only when given between 3 and 9 days before delivery (P. O. Anderson, 2017b) but not at other times.
- ***SSRI anti-depressants*** were associated with a delay in milk increase after birth in one small U.S. study (Marshall et al., 2010) that included 8 women taking SSRIs during pregnancy but not in an Australian study that included 86 women exposed to SSRIs during pregnancy (Grzeskowiak, Leggett, Costi, Roberts, & Amir, 2018).

- ***Insulin*** to treat either Type 2 or gestational diabetes was associated with a delay in milk production (P. O. Anderson, 2017b).
- ***Pyridoxin*** (vitamin B_6) is sometimes used to treat pregnancy-related vomiting. When taken in large doses (150-600 mg) long term during lactation, it was associated with lactation suppression in some studies (Everett, 1982) but not others (Oladapo & Fawole, 2012).
- ***Labor pain medications*** (Lind, Perrine, & Li, 2014) and epidurals (French, Cong, & Chung, 2016) were associated with a delayed milk increase in some studies.
- Synthetic oxytocin (Pitocin) during and after delivery was associated with shorter duration of nursing and may negatively affect oxytocin receptors (Erickson & Emeis, 2017).

Long labor or traumatic birth. Stress increases the level of cortisol in the bloodstream, affecting the hormonal balance. One Guatemalan study found high levels of cortisol in mothers after a difficult birth (Grajeda & Perez-Escamilla, 2002). U.S., Greek and New Zealand research found an association between an exhausting labor or physically or psychologically traumatic birth and a delayed milk increase (Beck & Watson, 2008; Dewey, 2001; Dimitraki et al., 2016).

Cesarean birth. A large (>108,000 newborns) U.S. study (Flaherman et al., 2015) found a significant association between cesarean birth and delayed increase in milk production. Why? Clues can be found in two studies. A 2019 Chinese study of more than 600 newborns compared those born vaginally with those born by cesarean and found differences in their early feeding patterns. A 2003 Australian study (Evans, Evans, Royal, Esterman, & James, 2003) compared 88 mothers who delivered vaginally with 97 who delivered by cesarean. Although the babies born vaginally and by cesarean had the same number of nursing sessions per day, there were other significant differences in feeding patterns.

- Delayed first feed (41 min. vaginal, 75 min. cesarean)
- Shorter first feed (18 min. vaginal, 15 min. cesarean)
- Even with the same number of feeds per day, babies born by cesarean fed for a consistently shorter time per feed
- Birth weight regained by Day 6 (40% vaginal, 20% cesarean)

According to the results of one small Turkish study (Sozmen, 1992), it may not be the surgery itself that delays milk increase but rather the timing of the first nursing session and the frequency of feeds. These researchers compared among its 20 women who gave birth by caesarean the timing of the first feed and nursing frequency. Not surprisingly, they found that those whose first feed was earlier and nursed more often had an earlier increase in milk production than those whose first feed was later.

Preterm birth. Older studies (Hill et al., 2005) found low milk production to be a consistent issue among exclusively expressing parents who gave birth to a very preterm baby. We know now that the timing of the first milk expression is vital to both early and later milk production. One U.S. study of mothers exclusively expressing milk for their very preterm babies (Parker et al., 2012) found that those who began expressing milk within the first hour after delivery produced significantly more milk at the first expression and at every evaluation point until the study ended at 6 weeks. At the 6-week point, those who began expressing within the first hour produced an average of 132% more milk than those who began expressing between 2 and 6 hours after birth. Expressing milk early, often, and effectively is key for parents of preemies. For many families, the pump alone is not enough to effectively remove the milk. Hands-on pumping techniques (p. 492) can boost milk yields nearly 50% (Morton et al., 2009).

Retained placenta or other placental issues. Two U.S. authors wrote "Anything that compromises placental function can also affect breast development during pregnancy" (L. Marasco & West, 2020, p. 103). This is because some of the hormones needed for mammary development are released by the placenta. In some cases, a baby born small for gestational age (SGA) or a diagnosis of intrauterine growth restriction (IUGR) may be a sign of placental issues. If placental fragments stay attached after birth, they can continue to release progesterone, preventing the hormonal chain of events needed for milk increase (A. M. Anderson, 2001; Neifert, McDonough, & Neville, 1981; Pieh-Holder, Scardo, & Costello, 2012). This is more likely if the placenta was slow to deliver or the birth attendant used tension to speed its delivery. Ask if the placenta was delivered intact or if the birth attendant manually removed it, as manual removal increases the risk of retained fragments. One way to rule out retained placenta is for the healthcare provider to do a blood test for beta human chorionic gonadotropin (β-hCG).

Excessive blood loss. Losing no more than 1,000 mL (2 pints) of blood (500 mL after a vaginal birth) is considered within normal limits. Research (Thompson, Heal, Roberts, & Ellwood, 2010; Willis & Livingstone, 1995) found a blood loss of more than 1,500 mL (3 pints) during the 24 hours after birth or a drop in hemoglobin of 4 g/dL or a hemoglobin level of less than 7 g/dL was associated with low milk production.

Extreme blood loss during delivery—or at other times—can cause a serious condition known as Sheehan's syndrome. This condition is caused by a lack of blood flow to the pituitary, rendering it nonfunctional and making both lactation and future pregnancy impossible (Du et al., 2015). Sheehan's syndrome is rare in developed countries and some pituitary function may remain in some cases. There are now multiple reports of women diagnosed with Sheehan's syndrome who later conceived and delivered another baby (Jain, 2013). In one case (Laway, Mir, & Zargar, 2013), a woman was able to lactate after giving birth to her second baby post-diagnosis.

An Indian review article reported some reduction of pituitary function in nearly one third of parents who experienced severe hemorrhage during childbirth (Shivaprasad, 2011). Most, though, who experience excess post-birth bleeding get off to a slow start with lactation, but with careful attention to good nursing dynamics and milk removal, they eventually produce ample milk.

• • •

Post-delivery practices and early nursing dynamics play a significant role in how quickly milk increases.

How soon after birth and how often a baby nurses on the first day of life affects how quickly milk production increases. That's why to safeguard milk production and prevent excess newborn weight loss, U.S. pediatrician Jane Morton recommends in the free videos on her website **firstdroplets.com** that parents learn to hand express during the last month of pregnancy and beginning at birth hand express after nursing during the early days, spoon-feeding this expressed colostrum to the baby (Morton, 2019). A Russian study (Bystrova et al., 2007) found a positive association between the timing of the first feed and milk intake on Day 4. Newborns who nursed for the first time within 2 hours of birth took, on average, 55% more milk on Day 4 (284 mL or 9.6 oz.) as compared with the babies whose first feed occurred more than 2 hours after birth (184 mL or 6.2 oz.). A U.S. study randomized mothers who gave birth to very preterm babies into two groups: 1) those who began expressing milk within the first hour after birth and 2) those who began expressing milk 1 to 6 hours after giving birth (Parker et al., 2012). At every time point of this 6-week study, those who began expressing within 1 hour of birth pumped significantly more milk than those who began expressing later. A Japanese study of 140 mothers and babies (Yamauchi & Yamanouchi, 1990) found that the babies who nursed 7 to 11 times on their first day consumed 86% more milk on Day 3 than the babies who nursed less than 7 times. The difference in milk intake between these two groups continued to be significant through the fifth day of life. See Figure 10.3 on p. 425 for an illustration of impact of feeding early and often on long-term milk production.

Low Milk Production after 1 Week

Many factors can contribute to low milk production after 1 week.

For some of the many factors that can contribute to low milk production after 1 week, see Box 10.2 (below) and the section "Slow Weight Gain" in Chapter 6, "Weight Gain and Growth." Keep in mind that before attempting to boost milk production, it is important to rule out causes of slow weight gain that are unrelated to milk production.

BOX 10.2 Factors That May Contribute to Low Milk Production after 1 Week

Less-Than Optimal Feeding Dynamics

- A late start to nursing or milk expression
- Shallow latch—Can decrease milk transfer; may be due to positioning issues or poor fit (large nipple, small mouth)
- Too little active nursing time—Scheduled, limited, or infrequent feeds, sleepy baby (overdressed?), overuse of swaddling or soothers (pacifier/dummy, swing), parental mental health issues
- Delay in early milk production due to less-than-optimal milk-removals
- Supplementing baby with other liquids or solid foods (formula, water, juice, cereal, etc.)—Which delay or replace direct nursing

Baby Factors

- Temperament—Placid, sleepy, or difficult to settle for feeds
- Anatomy or health issues contributing to ineffective sucking—Variations in oral anatomy (tongue-tie, unusually shaped or cleft palate, etc.), illness, preterm birth, birth injury (hematoma, broken bone, torticollis), airway abnormalities, neurological impairment (high/low tone)
- Health issues contributing to slow weight gain with healthy milk intake—Cardiac defect, cystic fibrosis (baby tastes salty), metabolic, respiratory, other disorders

Parent Factors

- Mammary/nipple issues—History of breast or chest surgery or injury (severed milk ducts or nerve damage), insufficient glandular tissue, unusual nipple anatomy or nipple piercing
- Health or medication issues—Serious illness, drugs/herbs that suppress or inhibit milk production or are incompatible with nursing, any conditions that may affect a parent's hormonal levels (obesity, thyroid, pituitary, infertility, ovarian cyst), hormonal contraceptives

Strategies for Making More Milk

Before parents can absorb information about boosting milk production, first discuss their feelings.

A parent struggling with milk-production issues needs an empathetic ear. As U.S. lactation consultant Lisa Marasco (L. Marasco, 2005, p. 28) wrote:

> "Some mothers may initially be in denial that their breasts may not be doing their expected job and may need gentle help in facing the reality of their situation. For others, there may be feelings of guilt and self-condemnation, especially if the problem first becomes evident by the baby's inadequate growth. Tears of grief are common, and there is sometimes anger at the healthcare providers and educators who taught her how important breastfeeding was but did not warn her about such potential problems.
>
> "So often the resources brought to the situation concentrate largely on the physical aspects of breastfeeding to the neglect of the emotions of the mother. Women experiencing any degree of lactation failure are facing a loss that is not generally appreciated in our culture, and we are in a key position as breastfeeding supporters to extend empathy and help assuage some of the grief. Sometimes, affected women need to hear that they are not at fault for what has happened and that they have indeed done their very best, whatever the outcome."

Listening and acknowledging the parents' feelings can help them feel ready to take the next step: sorting through their choices and deciding how they want to proceed.

• • •

With low milk production, the first priority is to feed the baby and the second is to safeguard the milk production.

No matter what the cause of low milk production, the first priority is to make sure the baby is adequately fed. How this is done will depend on the situation. For example, some expressed milk in a cup and solid foods may be all an older baby on a nursing strike needs while her parent is working to get her back to nursing. For the more vulnerable newborn, however, if nursing is not meeting all of her needs for milk, the next best option is to feed her expressed milk. If there is not enough to meet her needs, donor human milk is the next best choice. According to a cross-sectional study from an internet survey of 475 women producing insufficient milk (D. Cassar-Uhl & Liberatos, 2018), nearly one third (29%) fed their babies expressed milk provided by another mother. Of those who used shared milk, nearly 60% continued to provide human milk to their babies at 6 months compared with 40% of those who did not use shared milk. If there is not enough human milk of any kind available for the baby younger than 6 months, feeding infant formula is the third option.

Supplementing with extra milk can be critical to supporting nursing. When a baby is underfed, she can become weak and feed ineffectively. The strategy of withholding milk until the baby "gets hungry enough" can put a small baby at risk for dehydration and electrolyte imbalance (hypernatremia), which may require hospitalization to balance electrolytes before supplements are given.

When a baby nurses ineffectively, milk expression may be necessary to safeguard milk production. The number of expressions per day will depend on the baby's age, the volume of milk needed, and how far the parent is from full milk production (see next section). In general, any parent needing to express milk to boost production should choose the most effective method available, which in developed countries is a multi-user rental-grade pump. For details on expression methods, see p. 487.

• • •

Finding the cause(s) of low milk production will help determine the most effective strategies for making more milk.

The most common cause of low milk production is too little time spent actively nursing, but when low production has another cause, increasing the time spent nursing will not necessarily be an effective solution. In nursing parents with hormonal issues, such as thyroid imbalance, polycystic ovary syndrome, retained placenta, and other physical conditions, medical treatment may be the best milk-enhancing strategy. (See Table 10.4 for medical tests to determine possible hormonal causes.) But it's not necessary to test for all possible hormonal causes. As U.S. lactation consultants Lisa Marasco and Diana West (L. Marasco & West, 2020, p. 168) wrote:

> "Breastfeeding medicine physicians approach the question by taking an in-depth health and lactation history and then ordering any lab tests based on suspicions that need to be validated or ruled out....If you've identified possible problems, share this information and ask for testing to rule them out. That's a fair and defensible request and more likely to happen than if you drag in a long list of hormones to check."

TABLE 10.4 Tests for Hormonal Causes of Low Milk Production

	Reasons to Test	Tests to Consider	Levels
Prolactin	• Insufficient milk with normal mammary tissue, no other risk factors • History of excess blood loss, pituitary tumor, head injury	Test levels before and 10-15 min. after nursing to check for prolactin surge	See Table 10.1
Testosterone	• Excess hair on face or body, thinning head hair, and acne are signs of excess male hormoness that tests may not find	Bioavailable testosterone	If elevated, an ultrasound can confirm presence of gestational ovarian theca lutein cysts
Thyroid	• Personal or family history of thyroid issues • Extreme fatigue (hypothyroidism) • Weight gain (hypothyroidism) • Weight loss and jittery (hyperthyroidism)	TSH T4 T3 levels may reveal a T4 to T3 conversion issue: TPO antibody test may reveal a problem before it becomes obvious	Ideal: 0.5-2.5 Okay: 0.3-3.5
Retained Placenta	• No milk increase in 1st week • Vaginal birth in which tension was applied to umbilical cord during delivery of placenta	β-hCG (beta human chorionic gonadotropin)	High levels may indicate retained placenta
Insulin Resistance	• Family history of diabetes • Borderline glucose tolerance test or gestational diabetes • High birth weight baby	Hemoglobin A1C 2-hr glucose tolerance test	

Adapted from (L. Marasco & West, 2020, p. 167)

If milk production is compromised by surgery or underdeveloped mammary tissue, using the basic strategies described in the next section may not be enough to stimulate full milk production, but they may help provide a greater percentage of daily milk intake.

If the baby's feeding effectiveness is compromised by tongue-tie, other variations in oral anatomy, airway abnormalities, neurological impairment, prematurity, or other health conditions, treating or addressing the baby's health issue directly while using milk expression to boost production may be the best option.

• • •

Encourage the family working to boost milk production to accept all offers of help and practice good self-care.

For most nursing parents, getting more rest, eating a more nutritious diet, and drinking more fluids will not be the most effective strategies for boosting milk production. But these can be important to a nursing parent's morale and coping skills. Encourage the parents to accept all offers of assistance and offer to help them formulate a daily plan that will maximize the time spent boosting milk production while giving them time needed to nurture their relationship with their baby, care for other children, and handle any other responsibilities.

Using Basic Dynamics to Boost Milk Production

When milk production is low or faltering, first review the basics.

When considering strategies to boost milk production, start with these questions:

- **How many times per day does the baby nurse and is milk expressed?** Rather than discussing how many hours apart baby's feeds are (e.g., every 3 hours), ask the parent to describe about what time nursing or milk expression happens during a typical day and add them together for the daily total.
- **About how long does baby nurse or is milk expressed on each side at each session?** Is the baby nursing effectively? Has this changed recently? If using a pump, is the parent single or double pumping?
- **What is the longest stretch between milk removals?** For most parents, depending on storage capacity, stretches longer than about 8 hours (sometimes less) cause production to slow over time (Mohrbacher, 2011).
- **If expressing milk, what method or pump is being used?** If using a pump, ask the brand and model to decide whether it is well suited for the situation. Also ask about the pump fit. Even with a good fit at first, fit can change with time and pumping (E. Jones & Hilton, 2009; P. Meier, 2004; Wilson-Clay & Hoover, 2017). For details about checking pump fit, see p. 907-908.
- **How much time each day does the baby spend in skin-to-skin contact?** Time spent touching can enhance milk-making (Acuna-Muga et al., 2014; Hurst et al., 1997).
- **Discuss other factors that might affect milk production** (see Box 10.2 on p. 441).

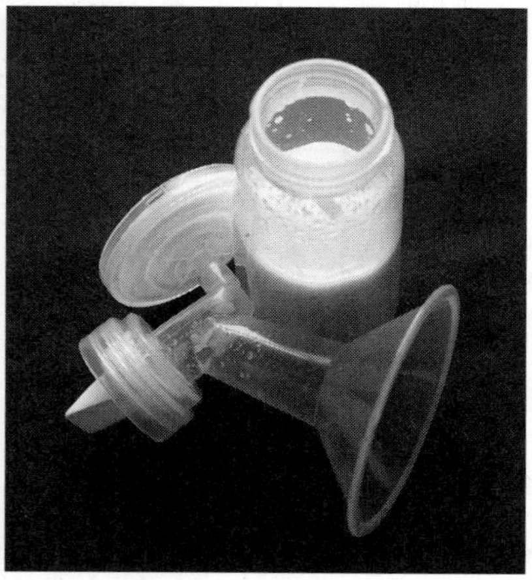

• • •

To make milk faster, suggest nursing strategies that remove milk more fully and more often.

As described in the earlier section "Degree of Mammary Fullness," two different dynamics cause full glands to make milk slower: 1) internal pressure from the accumulated milk, which reduces blood flow and compresses milk-making cells, and 2) higher levels of "feedback inhibitor of lactation," or FIL. As the glands become fuller, the combination of increasing FIL and increasing internal pressure causes milk production to become slower and slower.

But the opposite is also true. Rate of milk production speeds when the glands are more fully drained. On average, babies take 67% of the available milk, which means after feeding, 33% (or a third of the milk) is left in the gland (Kent, 2007). One way to increase the rate of milk production is to drain 90% to 95% of the milk instead of 67%. Suggest experimenting with the following nursing strategies to see which are most effective at boosting production.

Make sure the baby latches deeply and transfers milk effectively. Nursing strategies increase the rate of milk production only if the baby feeds effectively. If needed, weighing baby on a very accurate baby scale (to 2 g) before and after nursing can accurately determine the baby's milk intake (P. P. Meier & Engstrom, 2007; Rankin et al., 2016). If it's possible to express enough milk for a full feed, but the baby does not transfer this much milk during a nursing session, milk production may not be the problem and more nursing will not be the answer. Suggest using the strategies described in Chapter 1 to find an effective feeding position and to be sure the baby latches deeply. Nursing shallowly can reduce the baby's milk intake and drain the glands unevenly, which can slow milk production (Mizuno et al., 2008). Also see Chapters 3 and 8 for conditions that can cause ineffective feeding.

Offer each side more than once at each feed. Each time the baby comes off the first side, suggest offering the other side. If at any point the baby does not stay active (just mouthing the nipple rather than actively sucking and swallowing) or if she falls asleep quickly, suggest using breast compression (see next paragraph) to keep her active longer. If possible and baby is able and willing, encourage the baby to take each side at least twice.

Use breast compression or alternate massage. If the baby stops sucking actively, breast compression or alternate massage can increase milk flow, providing positive reinforcement to keep her feeding actively longer. Compression and massage increases the milk's fat content, one indicator of a more drained gland (Bowles, 2011; Stutte, 1988). For a description of breast compression, see p. 889.

Nurse more times each day. More time spent each day with "drained glands" and less time each day with "full glands" increases the rate of milk production between feeds (Daly et al., 1993). Over time frequent milk removal increases the rate of milk production via other mechanisms (Czank, Henderson, et al., 2007). Over the medium term, more frequent milk removal speeds the metabolic activity of key enzymes used in milk-making, increasing the rate of milk production. Over the long-term, frequent milk removal stimulates the growth and development of more milk-making tissue, increasing the rate of milk production even more.

Help the baby in a light sleep latch. To help increase the number of daily nursing sessions, the baby can be gently guided to latch when drowsy or in a light sleep (also known as "dream feeds"). U.K. research (Colson, DeRooy, & Hawdon, 2003) found that laying sleeping babies tummy down on parents' semi-reclined body triggers inborn feeding behaviors, which can lead to effective nursing, even in late preterm babies.

Avoid soothers and restrict all sucking to nursing. Suggest keeping the baby on the parent's body as much as possible to trigger feeding behaviors and provide all sucking during nursing. Swaddling and soothers, such as pacifiers/dummies and swings, can reduce time spent nursing (Buccini, Perez-Escamilla, Paulino, Araujo, & Venancio, 2017; Nelson, 2017). If supplements are needed and the baby can suck effectively, suggest considering the use of a nursing supplementer to increase mammary stimulation (for details, see p. 897).

• • •

Milk expression can drain glands more fully and speed the rate of milk production.

Consider adding milk expression to the plan if the nursing strategies described above are not enough to reach full milk production, the parent wants the process to go more quickly, and/or the baby nurses ineffectively. Be prepared to discuss expression choices. The first choice when attempting to boost milk production after the first few days (when hand expression is often more effective) is double pumping with a multi-user rental-grade pump. If the family decides to use a pump, talk about pump models, pump fit, and using hands-on techniques to remove more milk (see p. 492). Combining pumping with massage, hand expression, and manual compression was found to remove an average of nearly 50% more milk (Morton et al., 2009).

Offer to help the family formulate a daily plan that will not be too overwhelming and follow up with them in case adjustments to the plan are needed. Encourage them to schedule many of the pumping sessions when others can help with the baby. If no one else is available, encourage them to respond to the baby if she cries during milk expression. Another option is to express milk from the unused side during nursing (Figure 10.4). When they start the plan, if they begin feeling overwhelmed, offer to review and revise the plan to concentrate on those aspects that work best in their situation and eliminate the others. Make sure they know that for every Plan A, there is a Plan B, and a Plan C. Families often need to change what they're doing as they see what works and what doesn't. If the baby is not nursing effectively or will not nurse more often, the following milk-expression strategies may be vital to boosting milk production.

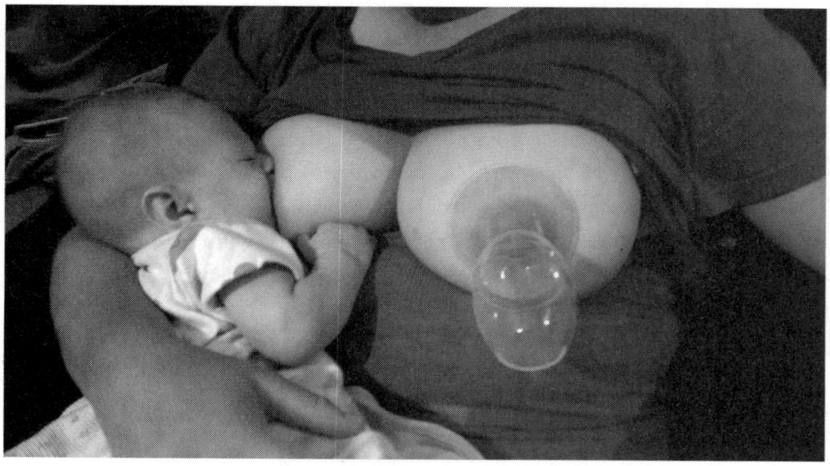

Figure 10.4 If a double-electric pump is unavailable or unmanageable, one simpler way to collect milk is to use a hands-free, all-silicone manual pump like the Haakaa on the unused side during nursing.

But the ultimate goal in most cases is to move away from milk expression to full nursing as soon as possible.

Express milk right after nursing? Milk can be expressed as many times per day as practical to drain the glands more fully and speed milk production. If the baby is very ineffective, to make the daily routine more manageable, it may help to limit the baby to a set period of nursing (perhaps with a nursing supplementer so she doesn't need to be fed again), with a higher priority given to the time spent expressing until the baby becomes more effective. Let the family know that even if at first not much milk is expressed, the main purpose of expressing is to stimulate faster milk production.

Express milk between feeds? Typically, more milk is expressed for supplementation by waiting an hour or more after nursing. This stimulates milk production, too, and usually gives the family of an effective feeder more milk for their efforts than expressing right after a nursing. Let the family decide if they would prefer to keep all feeding-related activities together by expressing right after feeds or express at another time and get more milk.

Intensive pumping. When nursing well, newborns typically go into feeding frenzies during some parts of the day, clustering their nursing sessions close together or even feeding continuously, especially during the evening. Because this is a common pattern babies use to increase milk production, some suggest that using this same type of strategy with pumping might help boost milk production more quickly. No research is yet available to tell us how effective the following strategies are in boosting milk production, but they may help fit in more milk removals.

- ***Power pumping,*** a short-term strategy (popularized by U.S. lactation consultant Catherine Watson Genna), involves putting the pump somewhere the nursing parent passes often and is comfortable sitting or standing (L. Marasco & West, 2020, p. 203). During a several-day period, every time the pump is passed (maybe as often as every 45 to 60 minutes), the nursing parent stops and pumps for 5 to 10 minutes, pumping into the same bottle and using the same pumping pieces without cleaning them for 4 to 6 hours (the length of time milk is considered safe at room temperature). Then the milk is combined and refrigerated and the pump parts cleaned. Because the milk is not refrigerated immediately and the pump pieces are not cleaned after each use, this is appropriate only with healthy term babies.
- ***Cluster pumping,*** a variation from author Stephanie Casemore (Casemore, 2013), involves setting aside an hour (maybe while watching a favorite show, while baby is sleeping, or when help is available) and pumping 10 minutes on and 10 minutes off during this 1-hour period.
- ***Pump like crazy,*** from U.S. lactation consultant Barbara Robertson, in which the nursing parent pumps once every hour for 5 to 10 minutes from 8 am to 9 pm or whatever time period the family chooses (L. Marasco & West, 2020, p. 204).

• • •

Suggest keeping the longest stretch between milk removal no more than 4 to 8 hours.

Because full glands make milk slower, long stretches between nursing and/or milk expressions (usually at night) can slow milk production. Ask the length of the current longest stretch. To avoid giving the message to slow milk production for part of the day, suggest avoiding going longer than 8 hours without either nursing or milk expression (Mohrbacher, 2011). If the baby sleeps longer than 8 hours at night, this means deciding whether to wake the baby to nurse (possibly doing "dream feeds" with baby in a light sleep) or to express milk. For some small-capacity parents, even 8 hours may be long enough to cause milk production to slow. In this case, limit the longest stretch no longer than 4 to 5 hours.

Other Techniques and Strategies to Boost Milk Production

Other techniques and strategies are meant to be used along with the basic dynamics, not as a substitute for them.

The strategies listed in the next point may be helpful if used with the basic milk-removal strategies described in the previous section. They are not meant to be used as an alternative to milk removal.

• • •

A variety of techniques and technologies are used worldwide to boost milk production in lactating families.

Breast massage is used in many cultures to enhance milk production and to prevent problems, such as engorgement and plugged ducts (Bolman, Saju, Oganesyan, Kondrashova, & Witt, 2013). In some Far Eastern countries, breast massage, such as the Oketani method in Japan (Kabir & Tasnim, 2009), is often recommended to nursing families. In China, many families believe that massage is necessary to reach full milk production and an entire profession arose to train women to provide massage to new families. A 2017 Chinese study randomized 80 women after a cesarean delivery into 4 groups (Chu et al., 2017). In 3 groups, breast massage began at 2, 12, or 24 hours respectively and continued 3 times per day for 3 days. The fourth group (the controls) received no massage. The group that started earliest had the highest blood levels of prolactin and reached what the researchers defined as "adequate lactation" the fastest. The blood prolactin levels were higher in all of the massage groups than in the control group, and these differences were statistically significant. After searching Pub Med, Google Scholar, and other databases, a 2015 systematic review (Sadovnikova, 2015) found 10 different massage techniques, some of which were used to boost milk production and some of which were used to alleviate other lactation issues. At this writing, a systematic review is under way to evaluate which techniques are more effective. See p. 879 for details about massage techniques.

Acupuncture and acupressure are practiced worldwide but originate from traditional Chinese medicine. Acupuncture is done by inserting very fine needles into specific areas on the body. Acupressure is done without needles by applying pressure to these areas. See p. 494 in the next chapter for three acupressure points easily reached by parents with normal dexterity.

Chiropractic involves adjusting the bones in the neck and spine to prevent impingement of the nerves, called subluxation. One article (Vallone, 2007) described the experiences of three mothers who had a dramatic improvement in their low milk production after several chiropractic treatments, despite very different circumstances.

Mental imagery and the use of music and audio relaxation techniques. The mind and senses can profoundly affect milk yields during pumping and therefore milk production. The earlier section "Milk Ejection" mentioned the experiences of women with nerve damage between breast and brain who learned to trigger milk ejection with mental imagery alone, even when the physical sensations of nursing were missing (Cowley, 2005, 2014). Several studies found during milk expression that listening to audio recordings of music or using relaxation techniques (Dabas, Joshi, Agarwal, Yadav, & Kachhawa, 2019; Feher, Berger, Johnson, & Wilde, 1989; Keith, Weaver, & Vogel, 2012) reduced anxiety in parents and resulted in higher milk yields. A 2019 Slovenian randomized controlled trial of 64 first-time mothers of term infants (Mohd Shukri et al., 2019) found that those in the group using relaxation therapy intervention had lower stress scores, lower hindmilk cortisol levels, longer sleep duration, and their babies had greater milk intake than the control group.

Kinesio tape is used by some chiropractors and physical and occupational therapists for treating injuries or neurological issues. Unlike athletic tape, its purpose is not to restrict movement but to assist and support movement and stimulate the flow of fluids. The tape's location and direction determine its effects. During lactation, kinesio tape may be used to treat engorgement (see p. 753) and nursing babies with sucking problems as a substitute for hand support of the facial muscles (Marasco & West, 2020, pp. 275-276). A small 2018 U.S. case series followed 11 nursing parents with low milk production (Valdez, Lujan, & Valdez, 2018) who reported an immediate increase in milk output when the kinesio tape was applied to the mammary glands by a trained professional in a fan-like pattern. The tape was left in place for 3 to 5 days, and in some cases, it was reapplied multiple times until milk yields reached the desired level.

Galactogogues

A galactogogue is any substance—drug, herb, food, drink—that speeds milk production.

Galactogogues, or milk-enhancing substances, have been used worldwide through much of human history (Humphrey, 2003; Jacobson, 2007; L. Marasco & West, 2020). Some were passed down by word of mouth from generation to generation. And some—but not all—have been scientifically studied (see next point). They include prescription drugs, botanical and herbal preparations (powders, tablets, capsules, tinctures, and teas), and even some foods and drinks.

If parents are considering using a galactogogue that is not a food or drink, suggest they discuss it with their healthcare provider in light of their health history, as some are contraindicated in some situations (i.e., metoclopramide in a parent with a history of depression). Galactogogues alone are likely to have little effect on milk production. They are most likely to have a small to moderate effect when used in combination with frequent and effective milk removal (Grzeskowiak, Wlodek, & Geddes, 2019). Also, galactogogues are most effective when they treat the underlying cause of low milk production.

> **KEY CONCEPT**
>
> *Galactogogues may provide a small to moderate boost in milk production when chosen well and combined with frequent and effective milk removal.*

• • •

Galactogogues are commonly recommended by healthcare providers and used by nursing families.

A 2016 cross-sectional survey of 82 U.S. healthcare providers (Bazzano et al., 2016) found that more than 70% recommended the use of galactogogues in nursing families with concerns about milk production. The most commonly recommended galactogogue was fenugreek, followed by fennel and milk thistle.

A 2013 Australian survey of 304 mothers who were currently breastfeeding or breastfed during the previous 12 months (Sim, Sherriff, Hattingh, Parsons, & Tee, 2013) found that nearly 60% used an herbal preparation while they were nursing. More than 23% of these mothers used at least one herb to boost milk production. More than 43% considered herbs safer than conventional medications, with more than 70% saying that they purposely avoided taking medications while nursing. The herb most commonly used to boost milk production was fenugreek (used by 18% of the total), following by blessed thistle (6%), fennel (5%), and goat's rue (2%). Only 24% of these mothers told their healthcare providers they were taking herbs.

An Australian qualitative study of 20 mothers who used herbs during breastfeeding (Sim, Hattingh, Sherriff, & Tee, 2014) found that these women chose to use herbal medicines in part because of their concerns about possible adverse effects of conventional medications on their nursing baby. They felt that making their own decision to use herbal preparations enhanced their feelings of autonomy, confidence, and self-efficacy.

• • •

When choosing a galactogogue to speed milk production, consider whether or not it targets the cause of low milk production in that parent.

Just as some antibiotics are more effective with some infections than others, galactogogues are not all equally effective in all cases of low milk production. Encourage any family considering using galactogogues to consult with their healthcare provider. If an herbal or botanical preparation is being considered, consulting with a trained specialist, such as an herbalist, a practitioner of traditional Chinese medicine, or a naturopath would be wise.

In Western countries, the pharmaceutical galactogogues most commonly chosen, metoclopramide and domperidone, boost prolactin blood levels. These drugs do seem to increase milk volumes in some nursing parents (see later point).

In some cases, it may make sense to choose a galactogogue for other reasons. For example, if the nursing parent is anemic, a galactogogue high in iron may help. If a nursing parent has high levels of male hormones (androgens), an antiandrogenic herb may make sense. If diabetes or insulin resistance is a concern, a galactogogue that increases insulin sensitivity may be a good choice. Philip Anderson, a U.S. pharmacist, suggest in one review article (P. O. Anderson, 2017d) that fenugreek—a commonly used plant-based galactogogue—may affect milk production primarily by normalizing insulin levels.

• • •

In most cases, if a galactogogue is going to work, milk production will improve within the first week of use, and it may be used for the short term or long term.

According to U.S. lactation consultants Lisa Marasco and Diana West, if a galactogogue is going to be effective (L. Marasco & West, 2020, p. 210):

> "It typically takes at least 2-5 days to start feeling a difference; if nothing has happened by the end of a week, it likely isn't working for you. Simple situations where either baby or infrequent milk removal caused a drop in supply usually require only short-term use, approximately 1-4 weeks, along with necessary changes. Once full milk production is reestablished, the galactogogue is gradually reduced over 1-2 weeks time. In more difficult cases, a galactogogue may be required indefinitely to sustain a higher level of milk production, though many nursing parents find that they can reduce their dosages after the first 6 months."

• • •

Domperidone and metoclopramide raise blood prolactin levels and may boost milk by a little or a lot.

At this writing, in the U.S., no drugs are officially recognized by the Food and Drug Administration (FDA) for use as galactogogues. However, some drugs designated for other purposes have a side effect of increasing blood prolactin levels. In the U.S., this makes prescribing these drugs to enhance milk-making an "off-label" use. A U.K. double-blinded randomized controlled trial compared milk output and side effects in mothers pumping for babies in the NICU whose milk yields were falling short of their babies' needs (J. Ingram, Taylor, Churchill, Pike, & Greenwood, 2012). One group received domperidone and the other group received metoclopramide, both at 10 mg 3 times per day (30 mg total). Both groups increased milk production by a mean of 31 mL (1 oz.) per 24 hours. The increase in pumping milk yields and the incidence of side effects were roughly comparable in both groups. The differences between these medications were not statistically significant. An online international survey of 1,990 mothers from 25 different countries who took either or both drugs (Hale, Kendall-Tackett, & Cong, 2018) found that the women taking metoclopramide were almost four times more likely to report a side effect compared with those taking domperidone.

Domperidone (Motilium™). This drug is widely used internationally to treat nausea and reflux disease. In Australia it is commonly used to increase milk production. In some countries, a prescription is required. In other countries, such as New Zealand, it can be bought without a prescription. Like metoclopramide (described later in this point), taking domperidone prevents the release of dopamine which increases blood prolactin levels (Hofmeyr, Van Iddekinge, & Blott, 1985). But unlike metoclopramide, domperidone does not cross the blood-brain barrier, so central nervous system side effects are less likely (Hale, 2019). Also, because domperidone has a large molecular weight and high protein-binding, very little passes into mother's milk (Barone, 1999). For these reasons, domperidone is considered compatible with nursing and is rated an L1 (safest) in ***Hale's Medications & Mothers' Milk*** (Hale, 2019). However, due to serious reactions in compromised chemotherapy patients who received high doses of domperidone by IV, in June 2004 the U.S. FDA advised it not be prescribed for nursing mothers. Large-scale studies on domperidone use in Europe and Canada (P. O. Anderson, 2017a) found that women are at a higher risk than men of its more serious side effects and the risk of side effects is higher if the user is obese or has a history of cardiac arrythmias.

KEY CONCEPT

At its recommended doses, domperidone increases milk production significantly in some parents, more modestly in some, and not at all in others..

The Academy of Breastfeeding Medicine (ABM) recommended (Brodribb, 2018) whenever domperidone is being considered that the parent be screened for:

- A history of cardiac arrhythmia, and if there's concern, doing an EKG
- The use of other medications found to increase its effect, such as fluconazole, erythromycin, and macrolide antibiotics

The ABM also recommended using the smallest effective dose for the shortest time possible. In Australia, the typical dosage to increase milk production is 30 to 60 mg per day (Grzeskowiak & Amir, 2015). Two small studies—one in Australia (Wan et al., 2008) and one in Canada (Knoppert et al., 2013)—examined the effects of different doses on safety and milk production. In these studies, the mothers receiving the higher doses produced more milk, but the difference was not statistically significant and none of the babies experienced any side effects. In Canada, a more common dosage (Paul et al., 2015) is 20 to 30 mg taken three to four times daily (a total of 60 to 120 mg).

Domperidone can legally be ordered online from New Zealand pharmacies for personal use without a prescription. Some families order it on their own without medical oversight. Encourage any family to consult with their healthcare provider before taking a medication such as domperidone.

Domperidone increases milk production significantly in some parents, more modestly in some, and not all in others. Most studies on domperidone's effectiveness at increasing milk production (Asztalos et al., 2017; Bazzano et al., 2016; Grzeskowiak, Smithers, Amir, & Grivell, 2018; Haase, Taylor, Mauldin, Johnson, & Wagner, 2016) were done with mothers exclusively expressing milk for preterm babies. In one small Australian study of six mothers (Wan et al., 2008), two of six (one third) had no increase in milk production while taking domperidone, despite an increase in blood prolactin levels. A 2019 meta-analysis combined the data from 239 mothers expressing milk for preterm babies from five randomized controlled trials (Taylor, Logan, Twells, & Newhook, 2019) and found that on average, domperidone increased milk volumes by about 94 mL (3 oz.) per day.

Parents who respond to domperidone usually see an increase in milk production within 48 hours but not usually after 7 days. Typically, it takes 2 to 4 weeks for it to achieve its peak effect (W. Jones & Breward, 2011). A 2019 secondary analysis of a Canadian randomized controlled trial (Asztalos et al., 2019) found the effect on milk production was comparable in those who took domperidone from Days 1 to 14 compared with those who took it from Days 15 to 28. Common side effects include dry mouth, headaches, and abdominal cramps.

Metoclopramide (Reglan™ or Maxeran™). When this drug is effective, taking 10 to 15 mg 3 times per day (30 to 45 mg per day total) usually increases milk production noticeably within a few days, while doses of 15 mg per day do not (Hale, 2019). When given within the first month post-delivery at 10 mg doses three times per day for 7 to 14 days, this drug increased milk production an average of 110% in some mothers with low milk production (Ehrenkranz & Ackerman, 1986; Forinash, Yancey, Barnes, & Myles, 2012; McGuire, 2018). Even among low-producing parents of babies 8- to 12-months old, it was found to increase milk production by 72% (Kauppila et al., 1983).

KEY CONCEPT

Taking metoclopramide during the first 3 days after birth--when prolactin levels are naturally high—does not appear to boost milk production.

However, randomized controlled trials done in the U.S. (Hansen, McAndrew, Harris, & Zimmerman, 2005) and Iran (Sakha & Behbahan, 2008) found that taking metoclopramide during the first 96 hours post-birth, a time when the parent's blood prolactin levels should be naturally high, did not boost milk production. When optimal nursing dynamics are used (early, often, and effective milk removal) milk production in those not taking metoclopramide was comparable to those taking 30 mg of metoclopramide per day.

Because metoclopramide crosses the blood-brain barrier, one side effect is depression, so it is not recommended for parents with a history of depression. The incidence of side effects from metoclopramide (restlessness, irritability, headache, weakness, fatigue, depression) increase when it is taken for longer than a month, which is not recommended (Anfinson, 2002). From the baby's standpoint, this drug is rated an L2 (safer) in ***Hale's Medications and Mothers' Milk***. From the parent's standpoint, one significant concern about this drug is the side effect known as ***tardive dyskinesia***, which is a neurological problem that causes involuntary movements that may become permanent in a small percentage of those who take this medication (Hale et al., 2018).

Weaning gradually from domperidone and metoclopramide. When domperidone or metoclopramide is discontinued, milk production may slow, but not usually to the level it was before it was started. However, this may not be true if low milk production is due to insufficient glandular tissue or other issues unrelated to prolactin levels. To minimize this decrease in milk production, tapering off these drugs gradually by 10 mg per week is recommended (Brodribb, 2018; Hale, 2019).

• • •

Other medications may also boost milk production.

Other medications found to increase milk production include the antipsychotic medications sulpiride and chlorpromazine, recombinant human growth hormone (hGH), and thyrotropin-releasing hormone (TRH), which is given as a nasal spray. These medications, however, are not commonly used to increase milk production because their risks outweigh their benefits.

Metformin (Glucophage™) is another drug that some (L. Marasco & West, 2020, p. 214) suggest may improve milk production by sensitizing insulin receptors in those with insulin resistance, such as parents with diabetes or polycystic ovary syndrome (PCOS). So far, however, research has not confirmed this effect. A 2019 U.S. randomized controlled trial of mothers with low milk production and insulin resistance (L. Nommsen-Rivers et al., 2019) found only 20% of those in the metformin group sustained improved milk production to Day 28 and none of them perceived the metformin as being helpful.

• • •

A variety of plant-based galactogogues are used worldwide to increase milk production.

Throughout human history, many plant-based and herbal preparations have been used to enhance milk production (Humphrey, 2003). But there are some aspects of using plant-based galactogogues that families need to know.

Use with caution. Some botanicals contain the same active ingredients used in prescription medications, which may affect the nursing baby and interact with other herbs or drugs, which is why it's vital to use them with caution. Suggest that any family considering using plant-based galactogogues do so only under the guidance of someone well-versed in their use, such as a certified herbalist, a trained practitioner of traditional Chinese medicine, or a naturopath, so their appropriateness, quality, and potential interactions can be evaluated. At this writing, in the U.S. no regulatory agency monitors herbal preparations for consistency, and their quality can vary widely. A U.S. study found that one in five Ayurvedic herbal products sold in Boston contained dangerous levels of heavy metals, such as mercury and lead (Saper et al., 2004). The website **ConsumerLab.com** provides subscribers with information on the quality of specific brands of herbal preparations.

Different formulations and doses. Herbal preparations are available in many forms, including powders, tablets, capsules, tinctures, and teas. A parent may respond better to one form than another, and different parents may respond better to lower or higher doses. Teas can be especially tricky because the amount of active ingredient increases with longer steeping.

Fenugreek (*Trigonella foenum-graecum*). Fenugreek seed is the most common herbal galactogogue used by Western families (Budzynska, Gardner, Dugoua, Low Dog, & Gardiner, 2012). It was used for generations in Egypt and India and is recommended by lactation books for parents (K. Huggins, 2020). Fenugreek is used in cooking and to add flavor to artificial maple syrup. Doses high enough to boost milk production are usually three capsules three to four times per day or about 6,000 mg per day. It can be taken alone or with other herbal galactogogues or conventional medications. Parents report that it usually takes 24 to 72 hours to notice an increase in milk production, when their sweat and urine begin to smell like maple syrup. Fenugreek is generally recognized as safe (GRAS) by the U.S. FDA (Hale, 2019, p. 291-292).

Research on the efficacy of fenugreek in increasing milk production is mixed. A 2013 U.S. randomized controlled trial compared the effects of fenugreek with a placebo when taken for 3 weeks by 26 mothers pumping for babies born earlier than 31 weeks gestation (Reeder, LeGrand, & O'Connor-Von, 2013). It found no statistically significant differences in milk output between the two groups. But a 2018 meta-analysis that included five studies with 122 women (T. M. Khan, Wu, & Dolzhenko, 2018) found that compared to the placebos, fenugreek was an effective galactogogue.

In animal research (Tahiliani & Kar, 2003), fenugreek in high doses lowered blood level of thyroid hormone T3 in rats. For this reason, it may not be a good choice for those with low thyroid or those at risk of hypothyroidism. The authors of the book ***Making More Milk*** reported (L. Marasco & West, 2020, p. 228):

> "In an online group for adoptive parents inducing lactation, several members reported a drop in milk output when they added fenugreek to their domperidone regime. The common denominator: hypothyroidism."

Another reported adverse effect of fenugreek in humans was suspected GI bleeding in a 30-week preemie after his mother began taking fenugreek, but it was never confirmed as the cause (Hale, 2019, p. 292). As with any other substance, an allergic reaction to fenugreek is possible. One article (Patil, Niphadkar, & Bapat, 1997) describes two cases of allergic reactions to fenugreek. Fenugreek may boost milk production in part because it reduces the effects of insulin resistance (P. O. Anderson, 2017d), so caution is recommended among diabetic nursing parents.

Malunggay (*Moringa oleifera*) rhymes with "balloon guy" and is commonly used as a plant-based galactogogue in the Philippines. Also known as the miracle tree, the drumstick tree, the horseradish tree, and ben oil (benzoil) tree, its leaves, seeds, bark, roots, sap, and flowers are widely used in traditional medicine in the dry topics, where this tree grows. Malunggay leaves can be added to soups or stews, it may be taken in powder form, with 0.5 to 1 teaspoon (5 to 7 g) added to smoothies or taken as a capsule. Unlike many other plant-based galactogogues, research is available on its safety (Stohs & Hartman, 2015) and efficacy, including meta-analyses and systematic reviews (King, Ranguindin, & Dans, 2013). At this writing, there are at least 33 human studies and abstracts published on its use and six randomized placebo-controlled blinded clinical trials (Raguindin, Dans, & King, 2014). No adverse effects were found (Raguindin et al., 2014). Malunggay also qualifies as a "superfood" because it has more iron than spinach, more calcium than milk, more protein than eggs, more potassium than bananas, more vitamin A than carrots, and more vitamin C than oranges.

A Filippino randomized clinical trial (King et al., 2013) found that on Days 4, 5 and 7, the group consuming malunggay produced more milk than the control group, and this difference was statistically significant.

Other herbal galactogogues. A wide variety of herbs are recommended internationally as galactogogues, including blessed thistle, goat's rue, alfalfa, fennel, nettle, and shatavari. Not all herbal galactogogues are considered safe during pregnancy (L. Marasco & West, 2020). For more details, an excellent resource about dosages and quality sources for the plant-based galactogogues mentioned above along with many others is the book ***Making More Milk: The Breastfeeding Guide to Increasing Your Milk Production***, by U.S. lactation consultants Lisa Marasco and Diana West. Some of this information is also available on their website **lowmilksupply.org**.

• • •

Some foods, drinks, and seasonings are recommended in various cultures to enhance milk production.

Many traditional cultures consider foods to be medicinal as well as nutritional, and specific foods are chosen or avoided after birth based on their properties. For example, in the Ayurvedic tradition of eastern India, foods believed to enhance milk-making include pumpkin, sunflower, and sesame seeds, as well as rice pudding with milk and sugar (Jacobson, 2007). In China, foods thought to regulate body warmth and fluids are recommended, such as chicken and seaweed soups, cooked papaya, millet, rice, anise, fennel, dill, cumin, caraway, and ginger.

Grains, such as oatmeal, have a reputation among North American families for speeding milk production, and grain-based drinks are recommended in many cultures. In Mexico, a drink commonly made for nursing parents contains oats or cornmeal simmered in milk. In Europe, coffee-substitutes made from roasted grains, especially barley, are recommended for speeding milk production. For more details, see **mother-food.com**.

Three studies done in Thailand examined the effects of traditionally recommended foods that are considered galactogogues. In a 2014 quasi-experimental study (Thaweekul, Thaweekul, & Sritipsukho, 2014), the 105 mothers who delivered at the hospital during its 1-month period were fed foods that included the locally recommended galactogogues, such as hot basil, lemon basil, sweet basil, banana blossoms, garlic chives, ginger, and pepper. During the following 1-month period, these foods were not served after delivery to its 127 mothers. There were more reports of "breast fullness" at 48 hours in the group that ate the galactogogues (72% versus 57%) and fewer babies in the galactogogue group lost more than 7% of their birth weight (15% versus 24%). In a 2017 nonexperimental Thai study using self-report surveys (Buntuchai, Pavadhgul, Kittipichai, & Satheannoppakao, 2017), the researchers found a statistically significant association between the consumption of galactogogues (banana flower, lemon basil, Thai basil, bottle gourd, and pumpkin) and 24-hour milk intake (calculated by test weights) between 1 and 3 months in its exclusively nursing babies. This study also found an association between the consumption of certain protein foods (egg, tofu, chicken, fish, and shrimp) and greater 24-hour milk intake by the babies. Along the same lines, a previously mentioned Thai randomized controlled trial of 120 poorly nourished mothers of term newborns (Achalapong, 2016) found that during the first days after birth, those supplemented with eggs, milk, or both produced more milk at 48 and 72 hours compared to those fed the regular diet.

• • •

Consuming the placenta after birth is thought by some to improve mood and milk production, but this practice has risks and these claims have not been verified.

In many mammal species, mothers consume their placenta after birth (known as ***placentophagia***), however, this practice was unknown in humans until the 1970s, and its origins are unknown (Young & Benyshek, 2010). Although the placenta is used in traditional Chinese medicine, its use is unrelated to childbirth recovery and nursing. At this writing, this practice is most common among white, married, middle-class women living in the western U.S., 70% to 80% of whom consume dried placenta in capsule form (Selander, Cantor, Young, & Benyshek, 2013) rather than cooked or raw. For a fee, some birth practitioners and companies will steam and dry the placenta after birth and then grind it to a powder for encapsulation (Joseph, Giovinazzo, & Brown, 2016).

Proponents of this practice say it has a wide range of (unproven) benefits, such as providing nutrition, pain relief, improved mood and energy, hormone replacement, and increased milk production (Hayes, 2016). Others questioned why providing the placental hormones that are meant to be low during lactation (estrogen, progesterone) would improve milk production. In fact, a 2019 U.S. randomized, placebo-controlled trial of 27 women (Young et al., 2019) found no difference between the two groups in either blood prolactin levels or newborn weight gain. The U.S. Centers for Disease Control and Prevention (CDC) recommended against this practice due to a case report of a baby who acquired a late-onset *Group B Streptococcus agalactiae* (GBS) infection that was eventually traced to the mother's ingestion of placental capsules (Buser et al., 2017). According to the CDC, no standards exist for safe processing of the placenta for human consumption and the process typically used does not eradicate infectious pathogens.

In addition to reported benefits of placenta consumption after birth, reported adverse effects (Joseph et al., 2016) include bad-tasting burps, headaches, stomach cramps, diarrhea, constipation, pelvic pain, lack of milk, and emotional symptoms.

Strategies for Supplementing that Enhance Milk-Making

If a baby needs to be supplemented, the volume of supplement needed depends on the baby's weight gain.

When a nursing baby needs to be supplemented, assuming the baby is an effective feeder, the goal is to strike a delicate balance between giving the least amount of supplement needed, while actively nursing as much as possible to stimulate faster milk production. Babies need to be well nourished to gain weight and thrive, and also to feed effectively. If a baby with low milk intake becomes weak, this can compromise her ability to nurse. For details on choices of supplement and volume of milk needed by age, see p. 226.

• • •

Discuss the options for feeding method and the advantages of using a nursing supplementer to increase mammary stimulation.

A nursing supplementer, also known as a feeding-tube device, can provide needed supplement while baby nurses, keeping the baby actively feeding longer to stimulate faster milk production. It also avoids the need to spend more time feeding the baby again after nursing. Not all parents are comfortable using nursing supplementers (Borucki, 2005), so discuss the range of options and support the parents in their choice. The decision may depend in part on the level of milk production: close to full milk production, making some milk, or making little or no milk, as well as the baby's ability to nurse effectively. For the pros and cons of each supplemental feeding method, see p. 896.

• • •

If the baby is supplemented by bottle, encourage the family to use techniques and products that reinforce nursing.

Some aspects of using feeding bottles and nipples/teats can work for or against continued nursing. For details on how flow, shape, feeding technique, and other aspects of bottle-feeding can be tailored to encourage nursing, see p. 902-903.

• • •

When it becomes obvious that a parent is unable to fully nourish the baby by nursing alone, this can be emotionally devastating, and the family may need some help in processing this loss. As U.S. lactation consultant Lisa Marasco wrote (L. Marasco, 2005, p. 29):

If exclusive nursing is not possible due to low milk production, provide empathy, support, and a chance to grieve this loss before making decisions.

> "When a primary lactation failure is evident, great sensitivity is needed in guiding the mother through the process of deciding how she wants to proceed. Remember that she is facing a complex situation that does not offer a guarantee of full results, and that she may even have come to us hesitantly, afraid of 'fanaticism' that ignores the emotions and realities of her situation. As much as we want to see her do what it takes to breastfeed her baby, anything that feels like subtle pressure can heap more guilt upon her, resulting in anger and resentment toward us and anyone else who she feels does not appreciate the difficulty and hard work involved.
>
> "An approach that may be helpful is to present information...[about] all of the possible tangible techniques to increase milk supply, but at the same time also emphasizing the relational and nurturing aspects of the nursing relationship so that the milk is not her only focus."

When full nursing is not an option, discuss the possibility of partially nursing with supplements (Thorley, 2005). Depending on how much milk-making tissue is present and the nursing dynamics, the parent may also find—like the parent inducing lactation—that with frequent nursing, milk production may continue to increase over time (K Huggins et al., 2000). Frequent nursing causes more milk-making glandular tissue to grow, so even if parents must continue to supplement with this baby, they may eventually be able to eliminate the supplement after solid foods are started or exclusively nurse later babies (Wilson-Clay & Hoover, 2017, p. 69).

Overabundant Milk Production

U.S. family physician Anne Eglash offers what she calls a "commonsense" definition of overabundant milk production, also known as oversupply, hyperlactation, hyperactive milk ejection reflex, and hypergalactia (Eglash, 2014, p. 423):

Some nursing parents produce much more milk than their baby needs.

> "...the state of producing excessive milk, which leads to discomfort and may compel a nursing mother to express and store milk beyond what the baby is taking, assuming normal infant growth."

Keep in mind that even if the baby is gaining much more weight than average, if the nursing parent and baby are happy and comfortable, their situation does not meet this definition and is not a problem. If, however, either parent or baby suffers from some of the symptoms described in this section, it may make sense to consider taking steps to slow milk production.

• • •

Causes of overabundant milk production may be partly anatomical and partly cultural.

Milk production is best regulated by a baby's appetite. However, some parents are just naturally large milk producers. And in some cultures, the "lactation rules" given to families cause them to manipulate their baby's feeding rhythms or express milk much more often than necessary, which can cause problems with milk production. As U.S pediatrician Christina Smillie wrote (Smillie et al., 2005):

> "...[I]n the absence of a cultural history of easy and ubiquitous breastfeeding, and without an established understanding of the physiology of breastfeeding and lactation, healthcare providers now often pass on to mothers historical recommendations and rules about breastfeeding for which there are no clear physiological rationale. Many of these rules—at least so many minutes on a side, always feed on both sides, always offer the full side—probably date back to those days of 4-hour feeds, and are essentially strategies for maximizing milk production. Thus, as more and more women are breastfeeding in the United States, we are seeing more women who already have plenty of milk trying to breastfeed according to these culturally defined rules...
>
> "Although normal variations in maternal anatomy and physiology and certain infant temperaments can certainly interact to create this clinical picture, more commonly, the initial cause of hyperlactation is cultural misinformation about optimal breastfeeding practices. Moreover, even when there are maternal or infant primary predispositions to rapid milk production, homeostatic mechanisms should normally lead to self-correction. However, cultural ideas about breastfeeding can interfere with these physiological mechanisms."

Another possible cause of overabundant milk production is suggested by two case reports (Powers & Tapia, 2015): a history of long-term use of progestin-only contraceptives. These two women with oversupply described in these case reports exclusively pumped for their babies. The one characteristic both women had in common was a history of long-term use of progestin-only birth control methods. Clearly, more research is needed to confirm this association.

• • •

When milk production occurs outside the context of pregnancy and lactation, known as "galactorrhea," it is usually caused by a health problem or medication.

On occasion, someone who is not pregnant or nursing begins producing milk from both sides. Called ***galactorrhea***, a person with this condition should be referred to a healthcare provider for evaluation (Huang & Molitch, 2012). Because nursing is not involved, this is in an entirely different category from the overabundant milk production described in this section, but some refer to this condition as "overproduction." This may be a sign of elevated prolactin levels caused by a benign pituitary tumor (adenoma), an overactive thyroid (thyroxicosis), or other health problem (Trimeloni & Spencer, 2016). It may occur in people with normal prolactin levels (Huang & Molitch, 2012). It even occurs rarely (in less than 1% of cases) after breast augmentation surgery (Basile & Basile, 2015). Galactorrhea can also be a side effect of some medications, such as tricyclic antidepressants, theophylline, amphetamines, and some contraceptives (Wichman & Cunningham, 2008).

Coping with Too Much Milk

Many nursing parents think that making lots of milk is a plus, not a minus. But there are real drawbacks of oversupply for both parent and baby.

Overabundant milk production can make nursing challenging for the baby.

Difficulty coping with a fast milk flow. With overabundant milk production, milk flow is usually very fast, especially during the first milk ejection (D. K. Prime, Kent, Hepworth, Trengove, & Hartmann, 2012), which depending on the baby may lead to some of the following feeding behaviors (Smillie et al., 2005):

- Pulling back, clamping down, or using biting or chewing mouth movements during nursing to slow milk flow
- Coming on and off during nursing sessions
- Keeping the nipple loosely in her mouth while milk flows in

Some babies fuss during milk ejection, coughing, sputtering, or arching away. Many swallow lots of air when gulping milk, spit up regularly, and pass lots of gas. Although many believe excess gas is due to swallowed air, this is not the case, as air cannot pass from the stomach into the intestines. It is usually caused by a high volume of low-fat milk passing quickly through baby's intestines (see later point). Other common symptoms include unwillingness to nurse while falling asleep and general colicky or fussy behaviors (Douglas & Hill, 2011). If the fussy behavior occurs during feeds, the cause is most likely difficulty coping with fast milk flow. If it occurs after feeds, it may be due to too much low-fat milk. Other possible symptoms include not feeding even when obviously hungry, not taking the second side, and a complete unwillingness to nurse at all (nursing strike, see p. 128).

Some of these symptoms may also occur in the baby with reflux disease and hypersensitivity, intolerance, or allergy.

Symptoms of high-milk-volume feeds may include:

- Very fast weight gain, with some babies exceeding by double, triple, or more the average weight gain of 2 pounds (900 g) per month during the first 3 months
- Fussiness between feeds
- Explosive green, frothy, or watery stools
- Continuous feeding cues even after taking ample milk

Continuous feeding cues. Many of these babies always seem to be ravenous and unsatisfied despite large weight gains, which convinces many families that their problem is not too much milk but too little milk (Smillie et al., 2005). These behaviors can occur during nursing when a baby gets mostly high-sugar, low-fat milk. There may be so much milk in a full, overproducing mammary gland that the baby cannot drain it well enough to reach the fattier hindmilk. Fat triggers the release in a baby's gut of a peptide called cholecystokinin (CCK), which aids in digestion and in regulation of intake, leaving a baby feeling satisfied and relaxed after a full meal. Nursing babies may release more CCK than formula-fed babies (Marchini, Simoni, Bartolini, & Linden, 1993), but a nursing baby taking mostly high-sugar, low-fat milk presumably releases less CCK, leaving her feeling unsatisfied, despite consuming large volumes (Smillie et al., 2005).

Stools that are green, frothy, or watery or contain mucus or blood. The sugar in this high-sugar, low-fat milk is mostly lactose (milk sugar), and if the baby receives enough of it, it may overwhelm her gut, causing watery, frothy, or green stools (Woolridge & Fisher, 1988). Green stools may also be a normal variation or a symptom of the baby's sensitivity to a food or medication she receives directly or indirectly through mother's milk. For more details, see p. 561. Some experts (Smillie et al., 2005) questioned whether the combination of colicky symptoms and mucus or blood in the stools—which are usually associated with allergy—might instead be symptoms of overabundant milk production alone. If so, slowing milk production (see next section) will resolve these symptoms.

• • •

To make milk flow more manageable for the baby, suggest starter nursing positions and other strategies.

Before bringing down an overabundant milk production (see next section), the following strategies may help the baby better cope with the fast milk flow.

- **Nurse in starter or side-lying positions,** which give the baby more control over milk flow (Figure 10.5 and p. 23-29).
- **Do what some call the "milk shake"** (personal communication, Christina Smillie, August 2019) by spending a half a minute or so before nursing massaging each side like warming modeling clay or kneading dough, only gentler. Research on hands-on pumping (Morton, 2012) found that massage and compression dislodge some of the fat sticking to the walls of the alveoli, nearly doubling the milk-fat content, which can keep a baby feeling full longer to help break this "vicious cycle."
- **Nurse more often,** before feeling so full.
- **Nurse when the baby is drowsy or sleepy,** which can mean calmer feeds.
- **Try frequent burping and breaks** so the baby can pace herself.

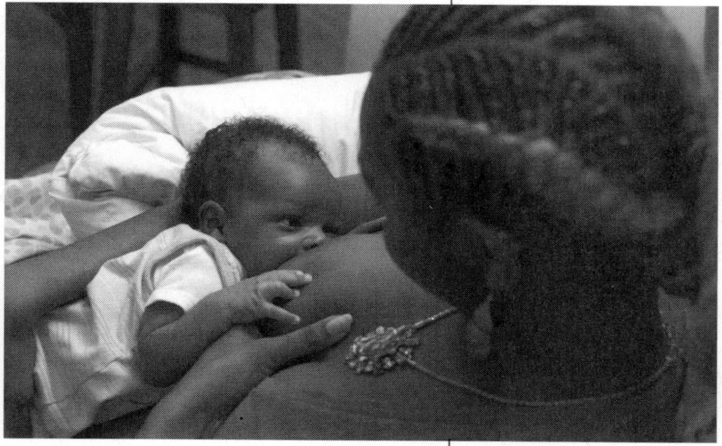

Figure 10.5 In starter positions, the baby's head is above the nipple, making it easier for her to manage milk flowing "uphill." ©2020 Nancy Mohrbacher Solutions, Inc.

Rather than offering the baby a full mammary gland, some recommend expressing the first milk ejection to decrease flow and make nursing more manageable for the baby. The drawback to this strategy is that on average about 45% of the available milk is expressed with the first milk ejection (Kent et al., 2008). So if this is done regularly, it can boost milk production even more, making overproduction worse instead of better. If pumping is necessary for the nursing parent's comfort, suggest pumping slightly less each time until it is no longer necessary. If pumping 3 oz. (89 mL) total, stop pumping after 2.5 oz. (75 mL). After a day or two, cut back more.

• • •

Overabundant milk production can make nursing uncomfortable for the parent and increase the risk of mastitis.

Not all overproducing parents have all the following symptoms of too much milk.

- **Profuse milk leakage** during and between feeds
- **Painful nipples.** When an overwhelmed baby clamps down, chews, or clenches her jaw to slow milk flow, this may cause pinched, injured, or infected nipples (Smillie et al., 2005).
- **Painful mammary glands.** Many overproducing parents experience

milk ejections (especially the first) as painful or "knife-like" (Livingstone, 1996). With fast milk production, mammary fullness and tenderness commonly cause discomfort (Witt, Mason, Burgess, Flocke, & Zyzanski, 2014), with some feeling full even shortly after nursing.

- **Recurring mastitis** of all types (plugged ducts, infections, abscesses) are associated with overabundant milk production (Campbell, 2006; Riordan & Nichols, 1990) due to regularly occurring and prolonged periods of mammary fullness.

Strategies for Making Less Milk

Before slowing milk production, be absolutely sure the behaviors and symptoms are not due to other causes.

The symptoms described in the previous section, such as nipple pain, recurring mastitis, or the baby gulping, coughing, and sputtering during nursing may have other causes, so before taking steps to slow milk production, be sure to rule them out. A baby with an airway abnormality, tongue-tie, or a neurological impairment, for example, might find it difficult to cope with even an average milk flow. And recurring mastitis and painful nursing can occur when a baby latches shallowly or nurses ineffectively for other reasons. Slowing milk production when overproduction is not the cause will not address the real issue and can lead to slow weight gain and low milk production.

Make special note of the baby's weight gain, as in most cases of overabundant milk production, a baby will gain weight at double, triple, or more of the expected early weight gain of 2 pounds (900 g) per month. Although a small percentage of babies shut down or feed poorly with overabundant milk flow, if a baby is gaining in the normal range or below, overabundant milk production may not be the cause of baby's or parent's symptoms. No matter what the underlying cause, if a baby is not gaining more weight than average, slowing milk production is unlikely to help.

• • •

It may be difficult to convince parents to slow their milk production.

Even when during the early months a baby is gaining much more than the average 2 pounds (900 grams) per month and suffering from the symptoms previously described, it is often difficult to convince nursing parents to agree to slow milk production because they may interpret the baby's behaviors as signs of hunger, leading them to believe that their milk production is low, not high, and worry that they don't have enough milk. Parents may also be influenced by cultural messages about how easy it is to "lose their milk." In ***The Breastfeeding Atlas***, U.S. lactation consultants Barbara Wilson-Clay and Kay Hoover suggest using pre- and post-feed test weights to show parents exactly how much milk their baby takes at feeds to provide objective information that links the baby's unhappiness during nursing with too much milk, not too little (Wilson-Clay & Hoover, 2017, p. 86).

• • •

When overabundant milk production is confirmed, suggest strategies to slow production using the dynamic "full glands make milk slower."

As described earlier in this chapter, two different dynamics cause full glands to make milk slower: 1) internal pressure from milk filling the gland, which reduces blood flow and compresses milk-making cells, and 2) higher levels of the substance known as ***feedback inhibitor of lactation***, or FIL, which research (Hernandez et al., 2008; Stull et al., 2007) found is likely to be serotonin in the milk. As the glands become fuller, the combination of increasing FIL and increasing internal pressure cause milk production to become slower and slower. These dynamics can be used to slow milk production in an overproducing parent without limiting the baby's nursing time by using the following strategies.

One side per feed or for 3-hour periods. In some cases of mild-to-moderate overproduction, limiting a baby to one side per feed (returning the baby to that side more than once if needed) may be enough to bring milk production under control. In other cases, offering the same side each time the baby shows feeding cues within a 3-hour time window and alternating sides every 3 hours can resolve the symptoms. During this 3-hour period, if the unused side feels full or uncomfortable, the parent removes (by nursing or expressing) the minimum volume of milk needed to stay comfortable. In cases of moderate-to-severe overproduction, however, other measures are needed.

Full drainage and block feeding. One Dutch article described the "full drainage and block feeding" (FDBF) method and the experiences of four mothers who used it to slow milk production (van Veldhuizen-Staas, 2007). The first step at the beginning of the first treatment day was using an effective breast pump to drain both sides as fully as possible (Berghuijs, 2000), then latching the baby immediately. Any time during the next 3 hours the baby showed feeding cues, the mothers offered the same side. After 3 hours, the mothers began offering the other side at all feeds for the next 3 hours. Depending on the severity of the mother's overproduction, the time blocks were increased to 4, 6, 8, or for one mother, 12 hours. For some mothers, no further use of the pump was needed; for others, draining their breasts fully one or two more times helped.

A more intuitive "modified" block feeding. During her years in practice at her U.S. lactation clinic, pediatrician Christina Smillie saw more than 1,400 overproducing parents and their babies. In response, she developed a variation of block feeding she called "modified block feeding," which she considered less rule-oriented and more supportive of a parent's intuition and the emotional connection with the baby (Smillie et al., 2005). The underlying goal was to help parents avoid focusing on rules and learn to use their own and their baby's comfort as their guide. At this writing, Dr. Smillie said (personal communication, August 2019) that when the strategies recommended on p. 460 are used, modified block feeding is rarely needed, but in extreme cases, she may recommend it.

Smillie described this approach as alternately draining each gland well, and then leaving it full longer than before to slow milk production. Depending on the level of milk production, she recommended for a period of several days to a week the parent use a pump once each day to drain the glands as fully as possible. The purpose of this drainage was to minimize the risk of mastitis and give the baby access to the high-fat milk that encouraged longer intervals between feeds. As in the previous strategy, the parent offered the same side for periods of time, but rather than using the clock to determine when to switch sides, Smillie divided the day into unequal blocks of time based on the family's lifestyle (Table 10.5) and alternated the side used in the morning each day. The purpose of alternating the "morning side" was to avoid uneven stimulation and slow milk production faster. Smillie defined "morning" as the time the parents consider themselves up for the day until lunchtime, "afternoon" as lunchtime to dinnertime, "evening" as dinner time until bedtime, and "night" from bedtime until they're up for the day. These times can vary from day to day. The side listed in each block of time (L=left, R=right) should be favored, with the side in

TABLE 10.5 The More Intuitive Modified Block Feeding to Slow Milk Production

Time	Day 1	Day 2	Day 3	Day 4	Day 5: Done
Morning	L (R)	R (L)	L (R)	R (L)	L (R)
Afternoon	R (L)	L (R)	R (L)	L (R)	R (L)
Evening	L (R)	R (L)	L (R)	R (L)	L (R)
Night	Any	Any	Any	Any	Any

Adapted from (C. Smillie, personal communication, August, 2019)

parentheses used whenever it feels right to the parent or baby. During parents' usual sleeping hours, Smillie encouraged them to do what felt right to them. She also encouraged parents to use this strategy for 5 days only, as she found that when she didn't give a specific end date, some families continued it for weeks and even months. If used long-term, this strategy could become just another rule-based system that could artificially make milk production too high or too low. The goal is for parents to learn to nurse by "feel" by responding to their baby and to avoid external nursing rules, which may cause overproduction.

• • •

If needed, some drugs and/or herbal preparations can be used to slow milk production.

If the methods in the previous point do not resolve the symptoms of overabundant milk production, parents may want to consult with their healthcare provider about using drugs or herbs (sometimes referred to as "anti-galactogogues") to slow milk production.

Herbs to slow milk production. As with galactogogues, it's important when using herbal preparations during lactation to consult with someone knowledgeable in their use, such as an herbalist, a practitioner of traditional Chinese medicine, or a naturopath.

- ***Sage*** (Sativa officinalis). Consulting with a knowledgeable practitioner is especially important when using sage, as its essential oil is toxic, and this form should be avoided. To use sage to slow milk production, steep 1 tablespoon of fresh whole leaf dried herb in one cup (0.25 L) of boiling water for 10 to 15 minutes. Drink 3 to 6 cups per day until milk production has slowed enough that the parent's and baby's symptoms have resolved, then discontinue (Humphrey, 2003). U.S. family physician, Dr. Anne Eglash provided an overview (Eglash, 2014) of different substances that can be used to slow milk production. Regarding sage, if sage extract is used, she suggests taking one dose and waiting 8 to 12 hours to note any side effects (such as nausea, vomiting, dizziness). If there are no side effects, consider taking a stronger dose.
- ***Other herbs.*** Eglash suggested other possible herbs to slow milk production (Eglash, 2014). For example, jasmine flowers and peppermint tea can be applied topically. Jasmine is suspected of reducing prolactin levels. This is also true of parsley, which can be eaten with meals. U.S. pediatrician Christina Smillie (personal communication, August 2019) suggested parents with oversupply use a strong, sugarless mint candy (like Altoids™) by starting with 1 or 2 mints with each nursing or milk expression.

Homeopathic remedies to slow milk production. In her 2014 article on hypergalactia, Eglash listed several homeopathic remedies reported to slow milk production, including Lac caninum 30C, Pulsatilla 30C, and Ricinus communis 30C. Trained homeopathic medicine specialists would choose among these treatments depending on the parent's symptoms. Purchased in pellet form, these remedies are taken 5 pellets under the tongue 2 or 3 times per day until there is a noticeable decrease in milk production.

Medications to slow milk production. Both prescribed and over-the-counter medications can also be used in this way.

- ***Pseudoephedrine*** (Sudafed™). One Australian study of eight lactating women (Aljazaf et al., 2003) found that when compared with a placebo, a single 60-mg dose of this common decongestant reduced milk production by a mean of 24%. U.S. lactation consultant Barbara Wilson-Clay noted in *The Breastfeeding Atlas* that some parents in her practice who took this medication under the guidance of their healthcare providers responded best when they took one 60 mg dose before bedtime and others got better results when this daily dose was spread evenly throughout the day (Wilson-Clay & Hoover, 2017, p. 87). It's important that the original formula be used and not the "PE" version available in many U.S. pharmacies. Due to its effect on milk production, this drug is not usually recommended for nursing parents, but it passes into milk in very low levels (0.4-0.6% of the maternal dose), and no side effects were reported in nursing babies (Hale, 2019, p. 639).
- ***Oral contraceptives containing estrogen.*** For overabundant milk production after 3 weeks post-birth, some physicians prescribe a 4- to 7-day course of low-dose oral contraceptive pills with estrogen and progesterone once per day (Wilson-Clay & Hoover, 2017, p. 87). According to a Cochrane Review (Oladapo & Fawole, 2012), estrogen effectively decreases milk production. Vaginal bleeding may occur after this treatment, and it may disrupt the effects of nursing on fertility.
- ***Cabergoline as a last resort.*** If none of these strategies or treatments help and the parent decides to wean, as a last resort, Eglash prescribed cabergoline, 0.25 twice per day for 1 day (Eglash, 2014). This "dry-up" medication was found to have fewer side effects than bromocriptine (Aydin et al., 2010), a medication used in years past by hospitals. Due to cabergoline's long half-life of 63 to 69 hours, Eglash recommended parents "pump and dump" for 5 days after taking it.

RESOURCES

bit.ly/BA2-Galactogogues—An article about galactogogues suitable for sharing by Dr. Frank Nice.

bit.ly/BA2-LLLITransgender—La Leche League International's webpage on nursing in transgender and non-binary families.

Cassar-Uhl, D. (2014). *Finding Sufficiency: Breastfeeding with Insufficient Glandular Tissue.* Amarillo, TX: Praeclarus Press.

firstdroplets.com—Videos by Dr. Jane Morton for parents of term and preterm babies show how to maximize milk production by learning hand expression before birth and using it after birth.

Humphrey, S. (2003). *The Nursing Mother's Herbal.* Minneapolis, MN: Fairview Press.

lowmilksupply.org—An online resource created by the authors of the book, *Making More Milk,* it includes strategies for boosting low milk production, including galactogogues.

Marasco, L. & West, D. (2020). *Making More Milk: The Breastfeeding Guide to Increasing Your Milk Production,* 2nd ed. New York, NY: McGraw Hill.

MobiMotherhood.org—A website for parents experiencing nursing challenges such as low milk production. MOBI stands for "mothers overcoming breastfeeding issues."

REFERENCES

Achalapong, J. (2016). Effect of egg and milk supplement on breast milk volume at 48 and 72 hours postpartum: A randomized-controlled trial. *Thai Journal of Obstetrics and Gynaecology, 24*(1), 20-25.

Acuna-Muga, J., Ureta-Velasco, N., de la Cruz-Bertolo, J., et al. (2014). Volume of milk obtained in relation to location and circumstances of expression in mothers of very low birth weight infants. *Journal of Human Lactation, 30*(1), 41-46.

Agostoni, C., Marangoni, F., Lammardo, A. M., et al. (2001). Breastfeeding duration, milk fat composition and developmental indices at 1 year of life among breastfed infants. *Prostaglandins, Leukotrienes & Essential Fatty Acids, 64*(2), 105-109.

Aljazaf, K., Hale, T. W., Ilett, K. F., et al. (2003). Pseudoephedrine: Effects on milk production in women and estimation of infant exposure via breastmilk. *British Journal of Clinical Pharmacology, 56*(1), 18-24.

Allen, J. C., Keller, R. P., Archer, P., et al. (1991). Studies in human lactation: Milk composition and daily secretion rates of macronutrients in the first year of lactation. *American Journal of Clinical Nutrition, 54*(1), 69-80.

Anderson, A. M. (2001). Disruption of lactogenesis by retained placental fragments. *Journal of Human Lactation, 17*(2), 142-144.

Anderson, N. K., Beerman, K. A., McGuire, M. A., et al. (2005). Dietary fat type influences total milk fat content in lean women. *Journal of Nutrition, 135*(3), 416-421.

Anderson, P. O. (2017a). Domperidone: The forbidden fruit. *Breastfeeding Medicine, 12,* 258-260.

Anderson, P. O. (2017b). Drugs that suppress lactation, part 1. *Breastfeeding Medicine, 12,* 128-130.

Anderson, P. O. (2017c). Drugs that suppress lactation, part 2. *Breastfeeding Medicine, 12,* 199-201.

Anderson, P. O. (2017d). Herbal use during breastfeeding. *Breastfeeding Medicine, 12*(9), 507-509.

Anfinson, T. J. (2002). Akathisia, panic, agoraphobia, and major depression following brief exposure to metoclopramide. *Psychopharmacology Bulletin, 36*(1), 82-93.

Anjarwati, N., Waluyanti, F. T., & Rachmawati, I. N. (2019). Exclusive breastfeeding for twin babies and its influencing factors: A study in East Java, Indonesia. *Comprehensive Child and Adolescent Nursing, 42*(Supplement 1), 261-266.

Asztalos, E. V., Campbell-Yeo, M., da Silva, O. P., et al. (2017). Enhancing human milk production with domperidone in mothers of preterm infants. *Journal Human Lactation, 33*(1), 181-187.

Asztalos, E. V., Kiss, A., daSilva, O. P., et al. (2019). Role of days postdelivery on breast milk production: A secondary analysis from the EMPOWER trial. *International Breastfeeding Journal, 14,* 21.

Auer, C., & Gromada, K. K. (1998). A case report of breastfeeding quadruplets: Factors perceived as affecting breastfeeding. *Journal of Human Lactation, 14*(2), 135-141.

Aydin, Y., Atis, A., Kaleli, S., et al. (2010). Cabergoline versus bromocriptine for symptomatic treatment of premenstrual mastalgia: A randomised, open-label study. *European Journal of Obstetrics & Gynecology and Reproductive Biology, 150*(2), 203-206.

Barone, J. A. (1999). Domperidone: A peripherally acting dopamine2-receptor antagonist. *Annals of Pharmacotherapy, 33*(4), 429-440.

Bartick, M., & Reyes, C. (2012). Las dos cosas: An analysis of attitudes of latina women on non-exclusive breastfeeding. *Breastfeeding Medicine, 7*(1), 19-24.

Basile, F. V., & Basile, A. R. (2015). Diagnosis and management of galactorrhea after breast augmentation. *Plastic and Reconstructive Surgery. , 135*(5), 1349-1356.

Bazzano, A. N., Littrell, L., Brandt, A., et al. (2016). Health provider experiences with galactagogues to support breastfeeding: A cross-sectional survey. *Journal of Multidisciplinary Healthcare, 9,* 623-630.

Beck, C. T., & Watson, S. (2008). Impact of birth trauma on breast-feeding: A tale of two pathways. *Nursing Research, 57*(4), 228-236.

Berghuijs, S. (2000). Casus. *Nederlandse Verniging van Lactatiekundigen Info*, 31-32.

Berlin, C. M. (2007). "Exclusive" breastfeeding of quadruplets. *Breastfeeding Medicine, 2*(2), 125-126.

Berry, C. A., Thomas, E. C., Piper, K. M., et al. (2007). The histology and cytology of the human mammary gland and breastmilk. In T. W. Hale & P. E. Hartmann (Eds.), *Hale and Hartmann's Textbook of Human Lactation* (pp. 35-47). Amarillo, TX: Hale Publishing.

Bertini, G., Breschi, R., & Dani, C. (2015). Physiological weight loss chart helps to identify high-risk infants who need breastfeeding support. *Acta Paediatrica, 104*(10), 1024-1027.

Betzold, C. M., Hoover, K. L., & Snyder, C. L. (2004). Delayed lactogenesis II: A comparison of four cases. *Journal of Midwifery & Women's Health, 49*(2), 132-137.

Bjelakovic, L., Trajkovic, T., Kocic, G., et al. (2016). The association of prenatal tocolysis and breastfeeding duration. *Breastfeeding Medicine, 11,* 561-563.

Bolman, M., Saju, L., Oganesyan, K., et al. (2013). Recapturing the art of therapeutic breast massage during breastfeeding. *Journal of Human Lactation, 29*(3), 328-331.

Borucki, L. C. (2005). Breastfeeding mothers' experiences using a supplemental feeding tube device: Finding an alternative. *Journal of Human Lactation, 21*(4), 429-438.

Boskabadi, H., & Zakerihamidi, M. (2017). The correlation between frequency and duration of breastfeeding and the severity of neonatal hyperbilirubinemia. *Journal of Maternal-Fetal & Neonatal Medicine, 31*(4), 457-463.

Bosschaart, N., Leproux, A., Abdalsalam, O., et al. (2019). Diffuse optical spectroscopic imaging for the investigation of human lactation physiology: A case study on mammary involution. *Journal of Biomedical Optics, 24*(5), 1-8.

Bowles, B. C. (2011). Breast massage: A "handy" multipurpose tool to promote breastfeeding success. *Clinical Lactation, 2*(4), 21-24.

Bravi, F., Wiens, F., Decarli, A., et al. (2016). Impact of maternal nutrition on breast-milk composition: A systematic review. *American Journal of Clinical Nutrition, 104*(3), 646-662.

Brockway, M., Benzies, K., & Hayden, K. A. (2017). Interventions to improve breastfeeding self-efficacy and resultant breastfeeding rates: A systematic review and meta-analysis. *Journal of Human Lactation, 33*(3), 486-499.

Brodribb, W. (2018). ABM Clinical Protocol #9: Use of galactogogues in initiating or augmenting maternal milk production, second revision 2018. *Breastfeeding Medicine, 13*(5), 307-314.

Buccini, G. D. S., Perez-Escamilla, R., Paulino, L. M., et al. (2017). Pacifier use and interruption of exclusive breastfeeding: Systematic review and meta-analysis. *Maternal and Child Nutrition, 13*(3).

Budzynska, K., Gardner, Z. E., Dugoua, J. J., et al. (2012). Systematic review of breastfeeding and herbs. *Breastfeeding Medicine, 7*(6), 489-503.

Buntuchai, G., Pavadhgul, P., Kittipichai, W., et al. (2017). Traditional galactagogue foods and their connection to human milk volume in Thai breastfeeding mothers. *Journal of Human Lactation, 33*(3), 552-559.

Buser, G. L., Mato, S., Zhang, A. Y., et al. (2017). Late-onset infant Goup B Streptococcus infection associated with maternal consumption of capsules containing dehydrated placenta--Oregon, 2016. *Morbidity and Mortality Weekly Report, 66*(25), 677-678.

Butte, N. F. (2005). Energy requirements of infants. *Public Health Nutrition, 8*(7A), 953-967.

Butte, N. F., Garza, C., Stuff, J. E., et al. (1984). Effect of maternal diet and body composition on lactational performance. *American Journal of Clinical Nutrition, 39*(2), 296-306.

Bystrova, K., Widstrom, A. M., Matthiesen, A. S., et al. (2007). Early lactation performance in primiparous and multiparous women in relation to different maternity home practices. A randomised trial in St. Petersburg. *International Breastfeeding Journal, 2,* 9.

Campbell, S. H. (2006). Recurrent plugged ducts. *Journal of Human Lactation, 22*(3), 340-343.

Casemore, S. (2013). *Exclusively Pumping Breast Milk: A Guide to Providing Expressed Breast Milk for Your Baby,* revised edition. Napanee, Ontario, Canada: Gray Lion Publishing.

Casey, J. R. R., Banks, J., Braniff, K., et al. (2019). The effects of expressing antenatal colostrum in women with diabetes in pregnancy: A retrospective cohort study. *Australian and New Zealand Journal of Obstetrics and Gynaecology.* doi:10.1111/ajo.12966.

Cassar-Uhl, D. (2014). *Finding Sufficiency: Breastfeeding With Insufficient Glandular Tissue.* Amarillo, Texas: Praeclarus Press, LLC.

Cassar-Uhl, D., & Liberatos, P. (2018). Use of shared milk among breastfeeding mothers with lactation insufficiency. *Maternal and Child Nutrition, 14 Supplement 6,* e12594.

Chatterton, R. T., Jr., Hill, P. D., Aldag, J. C., et al. (2000). Relation of plasma oxytocin and prolactin concentrations to milk production in mothers of preterm infants: Influence of stress. *Journal of Clinical Endocrinology and Metabolism, 85*(10), 3661-3668.

Chu, J. Y., Zhang, L., Zhang, Y. J., et al. (2017). [The effect of breast massage at different time in the early period after cesarean section]. *Zhonghua Yu Fang Yi Xue Za Zhi [Chinese Journal of Preventative Medicine], 51*(11), 1038-1040.

Chubukov, A. S., Belentseva, P. N., & Makarov, E. I. (1973). [Effect of vitamin B_{12} on lactation]. *Akushersfvo i Ginekologila (Mosk), 49*(8), 61-62.

Cobo, E. (1993). Characteristics of the spontaneous milk ejecting activity occurring during human lactation. *Journal of Perinatal Medicine, 21*(1), 77-85.

Colson, S., DeRooy, L., & Hawdon, J. (2003). Biological nurturing increases duration of breastfeeding for a vulnerable cohort. *MIDIRS Midwifery Digest, 13*(1), 92-97.

Cowley, K. C. (2005). Psychogenic and pharmacologic induction of the let-down reflex can facilitate breastfeeding by tetraplegic women: A report of 3 cases. *Archives of Physical Medicine and Rehabilitation, 86*(6), 1261-1264.

Cowley, K. C. (2014). Breastfeeding by women with tetraplegia: Some evidence for optimism. *Spinal Cord, 52*(3), 255.

Cox, D. B., Kent, J. C., Casey, T. M., et al. (1999). Breast growth and the urinary excretion of lactose during human pregnancy and early lactation: Endocrine relationships. *Experimental Physiology, 84*(2), 421-434.

Cox, D. B., Owens, R. A., & Hartmann, P. E. (1996). Blood and milk prolactin and the rate of milk synthesis in women. *Experimental Physiology, 81*(6), 1007-1020.

Cregan, M. D., & Hartmann, P. E. (1999). Computerized breast measurement from conception to weaning: Clinical implications. *Journal of Human Lactation, 15*(2), 89-96.

Cromi, A., Serati, M., Candeloro, I., et al. (2015). Assisted reproductive technology and breastfeeding outcomes: A case-control study. *Fertility and Sterility, 103*(1), 89-94.

Crume, T. L., Juhl, A. L., Brooks-Russell, A., et al. (2018). Cannabis use during the perinatal period in a state with legalized recreational and medical marijuana: The association between maternal characteristics, breastfeeding patterns, and neonatal outcomes. *Journal of Pediatrics, 197,* 90-96.

Czank, C., Henderson, J. J., Kent, J. C., et al. (2007). Hormonal control of the lactation cycle. In T. W. Hale & P. E. Hartmann (Eds.), *Hale & Hartmann's Textbook of Human Lactation* (pp. 89-111). Amarillo, TX: Hale Publishing.

Czank, C., Mitoulas, L., & Hartmann, P. E. (2007). Human milk composition-nitrogen and energy content. In T. W. Hale & P. E. Hartmann (Eds.), *Hale & Hartmann's Textbook of Human Lactation* (pp. 75-88). Amarillo, TX: Hale Publishing.

Czosnykowska-Lukacka, M., Krolak-Olejnik, B., & Orczyk-Pawilowicz, M. (2018). Breast milk macronutrient components in prolonged lactation. *Nutrients, 10*(12).

Dabas, S., Joshi, P., Agarwal, R., et al. (2019). Impact of audio assisted relaxation technique on stress, anxiety and milk output among postpartum mothers of hospitalized neonates: A randomized controlled trial. *Journal of Neonatal Nursing, 25*(4), 200-204.

Daly, S. E., & Hartmann, P. E. (1995). Infant demand and milk supply. Part 2: The short-term control of milk synthesis in lactating women. *Journal of Human Lactation, 11*(1), 27-37.

Daly, S. E., Kent, J. C., Owens, R. A., et al. (1996). Frequency and degree of milk removal and the short-term control of human milk synthesis. *Experimental Physiology, 81*(5), 861-875.

Daly, S. E., Owens, R. A., & Hartmann, P. E. (1993). The short-term synthesis and infant-regulated removal of milk in lactating women. *Experimental Physiology, 78*(2), 209-220.

Damato, E. G., Dowling, D. A., Madigan, E. A., et al. (2005). Duration of breastfeeding for mothers of twins. *Journal of Obstetric, Gynecologic & Neonatal Nursing, 34*(2), 201-209.

Damato, E. G., Dowling, D. A., Standing, T. S., et al. (2005). Explanation for cessation of breastfeeding in mothers of twins. *Journal of Human Lactation, 21*(3), 296-304.

DaMota, K., Banuelos, J., Goldbronn, J., et al. (2012). Maternal request for in-hospital supplementation of healthy breastfed infants among low-income women. *Journal of Human Lactation, 28*(4), 476-482.

Dangat, K. D., Kale, A. A., & Joshi, S. R. (2011). Maternal supplementation of omega 3 fatty acids to micronutrient-imbalanced diet improves lactation in rat. *Metabolism, 60*(9), 1318-1324. doi:02.001.

De Carvalho, M. (1983). Effect of frequent breast feeding on early milk production and infant weight gain. *Pediatrics, 72,* 307-311.

De Coopman, J. (1993). Breastfeeding after pituitary resection: Support for a theory of autocrine control of milk supply? *Journal of Human Lactation, 9*(1), 35-40.

Demirci, J., Schmella, M., Glasser, M., et al. (2018). Delayed lactogenesis II and potential utility of antenatal milk expression in women developing late-onset preeclampsia: A case series. *BMC Pregnancy & Childbirth, 18*(1), 68.

Demirci, J. R., Glasser, M., Fichner, J., et al. (2019). "It gave me so much confidence": First-time U.S. mothers' experiences with antenatal milk expression. *Maternal and Child Nutrition,* e12824.

Dennis, C. L. (2003). The breastfeeding self-efficacy scale: Psychometric assessment of the short form. *Journal of Obstetric, Gynecologic & Neonatal Nursing, 32*(6), 734-744.

Dewey, K. G. (2001). Maternal and fetal stress are associated with impaired lactogenesis in humans. *Journal of Nutrition, 131*(11), 3012S-3015S.

Dewey, K. G., Finley, D. A., & Lonnerdal, B. (1984). Breast milk volume and composition during late lactation (7-20 months). *Journal of Pediatric Gastroenterology and Nutrition, 3*(5), 713-720.

Dewey, K. G., Nommsen-Rivers, L. A., Heinig, M. J., et al. (2003). Risk factors for suboptimal infant breastfeeding behavior, delayed onset of lactation, and excess neonatal weight loss. *Pediatrics, 112*(3 Pt 1), 607-619.

Dimitraki, M., Tsikouras, P., Manav, B., et al. (2016). Evaluation of the effect of natural and emotional stress of labor on lactation and breast-feeding. *Archives of Gynecology and Obstetrics, 293*(2), 317-328.

Doucet, S., Soussignan, R., Sagot, P., et al. (2009). The secretion of areolar (Montgomery's) glands from lactating women elicits selective, unconditional responses in neonates. *PLoS One, 4*(10), e7579.

Douglas, P., & Hill, P. (2011). Managing infants who cry excessively in the first few months of life. *British Medical Journal, 343,* d7772.

Du, G. L., Liu, Z. H., Chen, M., et al. (2015). Sheehan's syndrome in Xinjiang: Clinical characteristics and laboratory evaluation of 97 patients. *Hormones (Athens), 14*(4), 660-667.

Dusdieker, L. B., Booth, B. M., Stumbo, P. J., et al. (1985). Effect of supplemental fluids on human milk production. *Journal of Pediatrics, 106*(2), 207-211.

Edge, D. S., & Segatore, M. (1993). Assessment and management of galactorrhea. *Nurse Practitioner, 18*(6), 35-36, 38, 43-34, passim.

Eglash, A. (2014). Treatment of maternal hypergalactia. *Breastfeeding Medicine, 9*(9), 423-425.

Ehrenkranz, R. A., & Ackerman, B. A. (1986). Metoclopramide effect on faltering milk production by mothers of premature infants. *Pediatrics, 78*(4), 614-620.

Engstrom, J. L., Meier, P. P., Jegier, B., et al. (2007). Comparison of milk output from the right and left breasts during simultaneous pumping in mothers of very low birthweight infants. *Breastfeeding Medicine, 2*(2), 83-91.

Erickson, E. N., & Emeis, C. L. (2017). Breastfeeding outcomes after oxytocin use during childbirth: An integrative review. *Journal of Midwifery & Women's Health, 62*(4), 397-417.

Evans, K. C., Evans, R. G., Royal, R., et al. (2003). Effect of caesarean section on breast milk transfer to the normal term newborn over the first week of life. Archives of Disease in Childhood. *Fetal and Neonatal Edition, 88*(5), F380-382.

Everett, M. (1982). Pyridoxine to suppress lactation. *Journal of the Royal College of General Practitioners, 32*(242), 577-578.

FDA. (1994). Bromocriptine indication widthrawn. *FDA Med Bulletin, 24*(2), 2.

Feher, S., Berger, L., Johnson, J., et al. (1989). Increasing breast milk production for premature infants with a relaxation/imagery audiotape. *Pediatrics, 83*(1), 57-60.

Fisher, W., Wang, J., George, N. I., et al. (2016). Dietary iodine sufficiency and moderate insufficiency in the lactating mother and nursing infant: A computational perspective. *PLoS One, 11*(3), e0149300.

Flaherman, V. J., Beiler, J. S., Cabana, M. D., et al. (2016). Relationship of newborn weight loss to milk supply concern and anxiety: The impact on breastfeeding duration. *Maternal and Child Nutrition, 12*(3), 463-472.

Flaherman, V. J., Schaefer, E. W., Kuzniewicz, M. W., et al. (2015). Early weight loss nomograms for exclusively breastfed newborns. *Pediatrics, 135*(1), e16-23.

Follin, C., Link, K., Wiebe, T., et al. (2013). Prolactin insufficiency but normal thyroid hormone levels after cranial radiotherapy in long-term survivors of childhood leukaemia. *Clinical Endocrinology (Oxford), 79*(1), 71-78.

Forinash, A. B., Yancey, A. M., Barnes, K. N., et al. (2012). The use of galactogogues in the breastfeeding mother. *Annals of Pharmacotherapy, 46*(10), 1392-1404.

Freeman, M. E., Kanyicska, B., Lerant, A., et al. (2000). Prolactin: structure, function, and regulation of secretion. *Physiological Reviews, 80*(4), 1523-1631.

French, C. A., Cong, X., & Chung, K. S. (2016). Labor epidural analgesia and breastfeeding: A systematic review. *Journal of Human Lactation, 32*(3), 507-520.

Galante, L., Milan, A. M., Reynolds, C. M., et al. (2018). Sex-specific human milk composition: The role of infant sex in determining early life nutrition. *Nutrients, 10*(9).

Galipeau, R., Dumas, L., & Lepage, M. (2017). Perception of not having enough milk and actual milk production of first-time breastfeeding mothers: Is there a difference? *Breastfeeding Medicine, 12,* 210-217.

Galipeau, R., Goulet, C., & Chagnon, M. (2012). Infant and maternal factors influencing breastmilk sodium among primiparous mothers. *Breastfeeding Medicine, 7,* 290-294.

Garbin, C. P., Deacon, J. P., Rowan, M. K., et al. (2009). Association of nipple piercing with abnormal milk production and breastfeeding. *Journal of the American Medical Association, 301*(24), 2550-2551.

Gardner, H., Kent, J. C., Hartmann, P. E., et al. (2015). Asynchronous milk ejection in human lactating breast: Case series. *Journal of Human Lactation, 31*(2), 254-259.

Gardner, H., Kent, J. C., Lai, C. T., et al. (2015). Milk ejection patterns: An intra- individual comparison of breastfeeding and pumping. *BMC Pregnancy & Childbirth, 15,* 156.

Gay, M. C. L., Koleva, P. T., Slupsky, C. M., et al. (2018). Worldwide variation in human milk metabolome: Indicators of breast physiology and maternal lifestyle? *Nutrients, 10*(9).

Geddes, D. T. (2007a). Gross anatomy of the lactating breast. In T. W. Hale & P. E. Hartmann (Eds.), *Hale & Hartmann's Textbook of Human Lactation* (pp. 19-34). Amarillo, TX: Hale Publishing.

Geddes, D. T. (2007b). Inside the lactating breast: The latest anatomy research. *Journal of Midwifery & Women's Health, 52*(6), 556-563.

Going, J. J., & Moffat, D. F. (2004). Escaping from Flatland: Clinical and biological aspects of human mammary duct anatomy in three dimensions. *Journal of Pathology, 203*(1), 538-544. doi:10.1002/path.1556.

Gokceoglu, E., & Kucukoglu, S. (2017). The relationship between insufficient milk perception and breastfeeding self-efficacy among Turkish mothers. *Global Health Promotion, 24*(4), 53-61.

Grajeda, R., & Perez-Escamilla, R. (2002). Stress during labor and delivery is associated with delayed onset of lactation among urban Guatemalan women. *Journal of Nutrition, 132*(10), 3055-3060.

Gridneva, Z., Tie, W. J., Rea, A., et al. (2018). Human milk casein and whey protein and infant body composition over the first 12 months of lactation. *Nutrients, 10*(9).

Grzeskowiak, L. E., & Amir, L. H. (2015). Pharmacological management of low milk supply with domperidone: Separating fact from fiction. *Medical Journal of Australia, 202*(6), 298.

Grzeskowiak, L. E., Leggett, C., Costi, L., et al. (2018). Impact of serotonin reuptake inhibitor use on breast milk supply in mothers of preterm infants: A retrospective cohort study. *British Journal of Clinical Pharmacology, 84*(6), 1373-1379.

Grzeskowiak, L. E., Smithers, L. G., Amir, L. H., et al. (2018). Domperidone for increasing breast milk volume in mothers expressing breast milk for their preterm infants: A systematic review and meta-analysis. *British Journal of Obstetrics and Gynaecology, 125*(11), 1371-1378.

Grzeskowiak, L. E., Wlodek, M. E., & Geddes, D. T. (2019). What evidence do we have for pharmaceutical galactagogues in the treatment of lactation insufficiency?-A narrative review. *Nutrients, 11*(5).

Haase, B., Taylor, S. N., Mauldin, J., et al. (2016). Domperidone for treatment of low milk supply in breast pump-dependent mothers of hospitalized preterm infants: A clinical protocol. *Journal of Human Lactation, 32*(2), 373-381.

Haastrup, M. B., Pottegard, A., & Damkier, P. (2014). Alcohol and breastfeeding. *Basic & Clinical Pharmacology & Toxicology, 114*(2), 168-173.

Hahn-Holbrook, J., Saxbe, D., Bixby, C., et al. (2019). Human milk as "chrononutrition": Implications for child health and development. *Pediatric Research, 85*(7), 936-942.

Haile, Z. T., Chavan, B. B., Teweldeberhan, A., et al. (2017). Association between gestational weight gain and delayed onset of lactation: The moderating effects of race/ethnicity. *Breastfeeding Medicine, 12,* 79-85.

Hale, T. W. (2019). *Hale's Medications & Mothers' Milk: A Manual of Lactational Pharmacology* (18th ed.). New York, NY: Springer Publishing Company.

Hale, T. W., Kendall-Tackett, K., & KCong, Z. (2018). Domperidone versus metoclopramide: Self-reported side effects in a large sample of breastfeeding mothers who used these medications to increase milk production. *Clinical Lactation, 9*(1), 10-17.

Handlin, L., Jonas, W., Petersson, M., et al. (2009). Effects of sucking and skin-to-skin contact on maternal ACTH and cortisol levels during the second day postpartum-Influence of epidural analgesia and oxytocin in the perinatal period. *Breastfeeding Medicine* (4), 207-220.

Hansen, W. F., McAndrew, S., Harris, K., et al. (2005). Metoclopramide effect on breastfeeding the preterm infant: A randomized trial. *Obstetrics & Gynecology, 105*(2), 383-389.

Hartmann, P. E., & Kulski, J. K. (1978). Changes in the composition of the mammary secretion of women after abrupt termination of breast feeding. *Journal of Physiology, 275,* 1-11.

Hauck, Y. L., Summers, L., White, E., et al. (2008). A qualitative study of Western Australian women's perceptions of using a Snoezelen room for breastfeeding during their postpartum hospital stay. *International Breastfeeding Journal, 3,* 20.

Hayes, E. H. (2016). Consumption of the placenta in the postpartum period. *Journal of Obstetric, Gynecologic & Neonatal Nursing, 45*(1), 78-89.

Heinig, M. J., Nommsen, L. A., Peerson, J. M., et al. (1993). Energy and protein intakes of breast-fed and formula-fed infants during the first year of life and their association with growth velocity: the DARLING Study. *American Journal of Clinical Nutrition, 58*(2), 152-161.

Heise, A. M., & Wiechmann, D. (2018). Letter to the editor: D-MER—An open question. *Clinical Lactation, 9*(3), 104-105.

Heise, A. M., & Wiessinger, D. (2011). Dysphoric milk ejection reflex: A case report. *International Breastfeeding Journal, 6*(1), 6.

Henly, S. J., Anderson, C. M., Avery, M. D., et al. (1995). Anemia and insufficient milk in first-time mothers. *Birth, 22*(2), 86-92.

Hennart, P., Delogne-Desnoeck, J., Vis, H., et al. (1981). Serum levels of prolactin and milk production in women during a lactation period of thirty months. *Clinical Endocrinology, 14*(4), 349-353.

Hernandez, L. L., Stiening, C. M., Wheelock, J. B., et al. (2008). Evaluation of serotonin as a feedback inhibitor of lactation in the bovine. *Journal of Dairy Science, 91*(5), 1834-1844.

Hill, P. D., Aldag, J. C., Chatterton, R. T., et al. (2005). Comparison of milk output between mothers of preterm and term infants: The first 6 weeks after birth. *Journal of Human Lactation, 21*(1), 22-30.

Hill, P. D., Aldag, J. C., Zinaman, M., et al. (2007). Comparison of milk output between breasts in pump-dependent mothers. *Journal of Human Lactation, 23*(4), 333-337.

Hill, P. D., & Humenick, S. S. (1989). Insufficient milk supply. *Image: Journal of Nursing Scholarship, 21*(3), 145-148.

Hillervik-Lindquist, C. (1991). Studies on perceived breast milk insufficiency. A prospective study in a group of Swedish women. *Acta Paediatrica Scandinavica Supplement, 376,* 1-27.

Hilson, J. A., Rasmussen, K. M., & Kjolhede, C. L. (2004). High prepregnant body mass index is associated with poor lactation outcomes among white, rural women independent of psychosocial and demographic correlates. *Journal of Human Lactation, 20*(1), 18-29.

Hofmeyr, G. J., Van Iddekinge, B., & Blott, J. A. (1985). Domperidone: Secretion in breast milk and effect on puerperal prolactin levels. *British Journal of Obstetrics and Gynaecology, 92*(2), 141-144.

Hoover, K. L., Barbalinardo, L. H., & Platia, M. P. (2002). Delayed lactogenesis II secondary to gestational ovarian theca lutein cysts in two normal singleton pregnancies. *Journal of Human Lactation, 18*(3), 264-268.

Houston, M. J., Howie, P. W., & McNeilly, A. S. (1983). Factors affecting the duration of breast feeding: 1. Measurement of breast milk intake in the first week of life. *Early Human Development, 8*(1), 49-54.

Huang, W., & Molitch, M. E. (2012). Evaluation and management of galactorrhea. *American Family Physician, 85*(11), 1073-1080.

Huggins, K. (2020). *The Nursing Mother's Companion* (8th ed.). Boston, MA: Harvard Common Press.

Huggins, K., Petok, E., & Mireles, O. (2000). Markers of lactation insufficiency: A study of 34 mothers. *Current Issues in Clinical Lactation, 25–35.*

Hull, V., Thapa, S., & Pratomo, H. (1990). Breast-feeding in the modern health sector in Indonesia: The mother's perspective. *Social Science & Medicine, 30*(5), 625-633.

Humphrey, S. (2003). *The Nursing Mother's Herbal.* Minneapolis, MN: Fairview Press.

Hurst, N. M., Valentine, C. J., Renfro, L., et al. (1997). Skin-to-skin holding in the neonatal intensive care unit influences maternal milk volume. *Journal of Perinatology, 17*(3), 213-217.

Ingram, J., Taylor, H., Churchill, C., et al. (2012). Metoclopramide or domperidone for increasing maternal breast milk output: A randomised controlled trial. *Archives of Disease in Childhood. Fetal and Neonatal Edition, 97*(4), F241-245.

Ingram, J. C., Woolridge, M. W., Greenwood, R. J., et al. (1999). Maternal predictors of early breast milk output. *Acta Paediatrica, 88*(5), 493-499.

Islam, M. M., Peerson, J. M., Ahmed, T., et al. (2006). Effects of varied energy density of complementary foods on breast-milk intakes and total energy consumption by healthy, breastfed Bangladeshi children. *American Journal of Clinical Nutrition, 83*(4), 851-858.

Jacobson, H. (2007). *Mother Food: A Breastfeeding Diet Guide with Lactogenic Foods and Herbs - Build Milk Supply, Boost Immunity, Lift Depression, Detox, Lose Weight, Optimize a Baby's IQ, and Reduce Colic and Allergies.* Ashland, OR: Rosalind Press.

Jain, D. (2013). A ray of hope for a woman with Sheehan's syndrome. *BMJ Case Reports, 2013.*

Johnston, K., Vowels, M., Carroll, S., et al. (2008). Failure to lactate: A possible late effect of cranial radiation. *Pediatric Blood & Cancer, 50*(3), 721-722.

Jones, E., & Hilton, S. (2009). Correctly fitting breast shields are the key to lactation success for pump dependent mothers following preterm delivery. *Journal of Neonatal Nursing, 15*(1), 14-17.

Jones, W., & Breward, S. (2011). Use of domperidone to enhance lactation: What is the evidence? *Community Practitioner, 84*(6), 35-37.

Joseph, R., Giovinazzo, M., & Brown, M. (2016). A literature review on the practice of placentophagia. *Nursing for Women's Health, 20*(5), 476-483.

Jutte, J., Hohoff, A., Sauerland, C., et al. (2014). In vivo assessment of number of milk duct orifices in lactating women and association with parameters in the mother and the infant. *BMC Pregnancy & Childbirth, 14,* 124.

Kabir, N., & Tasnim, S. (2009). Oketani lactation management: A new method to augment breast milk. *Journal of Bangladesh College of Physicians & Surgeons, 27*(3), 155.

Kair, L. R., & Colaizy, T. T. (2016). When breast milk alone is not enough: Barriers to breastfeeding continuation among overweight and obese mothers. *Journal of Human Lactation, 32*(2), 250-257.

Katzer, D., Pauli, L., Mueller, A., et al. (2016). Melatonin concentrations and antioxidative capacity of human breast milk according to gestational age and the time of day. *Journal of Human Lactation, 32*(4), NP105-NP110.

Kauppila, A., Arvela, P., Koivisto, M., et al. (1983). Metoclopramide and breast feeding: transfer into milk and the newborn. *European Journal of Clinical Pharmacology, 25*(6), 819-823.

Keith, D. R., Weaver, B. S., & Vogel, R. L. (2012). The effect of music-based listening interventions on the volume, fat content, and caloric content of breast milk-produced by mothers of premature and critically ill infants. *Advances in Neonatal Care, 12*(2), 112-119.

Kennedy, K. I. (2010). Fertility, sexuality, and contraception during lactation. In J. Riordan & K. Wambach (Eds.), *Breastfeeding and Human Lactation* (4th ed., pp. 705-736). Boston, MA: Jones and Bartlett.

Kent, J. C. (2007). How breastfeeding works. *Journal of Midwifery & Women's Health, 52*(6), 564-570.

Kent, J. C., Gardner, H., & Geddes, D. T. (2016). Breastmilk production in the first 4 weeks after birth of term infants. *Nutrients, 8*(12).

Kent, J. C., Gardner, H., Lai, C. T., et al. (2018). Hourly breast expression to estimate the rate of synthesis of milk and fat. *Nutrients, 10*(9).

Kent, J. C., Hepworth, A. R., Sherriff, J. L., et al. (2013). Longitudinal changes in breastfeeding patterns from 1 to 6 months of lactation. *Breastfeeding Medicine, 8,* 401-407.

Kent, J. C., Mitoulas, L., Cox, D. B., et al. (1999). Breast volume and milk production during extended lactation in women. *Experimental Physiology, 84*(2), 435-447.

Kent, J. C., Mitoulas, L. R., Cregan, M. D., et al. (2008). Importance of vacuum for breastmilk expression. *Breastfeeding Medicine, 3*(1), 11-19.

Kent, J. C., Mitoulas, L. R., Cregan, M. D., et al. (2006). Volume and frequency of breastfeedings and fat content of breast milk throughout the day. *Pediatrics, 117*(3), e387-395.

Kent, J. C., Ramsay, D. T., Doherty, D., et al. (2003). Response of breasts to different stimulation patterns of an electric breast pump. *Journal of Human Lactation, 19*(2), 179-186; quiz 187-178, 218.

Khan, S., Prime, D. K., Hepworth, A. R., et al. (2013). Investigation of short-term variations in term breast milk composition during repeated breast expression sessions. *Journal of Human Lactation, 29*(2), 196-204.

Khan, T. M., Wu, D. B., & Dolzhenko, A. V. (2018). Effectiveness of fenugreek as a galactagogue: A network meta-analysis. *Phytotherapy Research, 32*(3), 402-412. doi:10.1002/ptr.5972

Kim, B. Y. (2016). Factors that influence early breastfeeding of singletons and twins in Korea: A retrospective study. *International Breastfeeding Journal, 12,* 4.

Kim, S. J., Kim, M., & Kim, M. J. (2014). The affecting factors of breast anthropometry in Korean women. *Breastfeeding Medicine, 9*(2), 73-78.

Kimura, C., & Matsuoka, M. (2007). Changes in breast skin temperature during the course of breastfeeding. *Journal of Human Lactation, 23*(1), 60-69.

King, J. S., Ranguindin, P. F. N., & Dans, L. F. (2013). Moringa oleifera (malunggay) as a galactagogue for breastfeeding mothers: A systematic review and meta-analysis of randomized controlled trials. *Philippine Journal of Pediatrics, 61*(2), 34-42.

Knight, C. H., Peaker, M., & Wilde, C. J. (1998). Local control of mammary development and function. *Reviews of Reproduction, 3*(2), 104-112.

Knoppert, D. C., Page, A., Warren, J., et al. (2013). The effect of two different domperidone doses on maternal milk production. *Journal of Human Lactation, 29*(1), 38-44.

Kolasa, K. M., Firnhaber, G., & Haven, K. (2015). Diet for a healthy lactating woman. *Clinical Obstetrics and Gynecology, 58*(4), 893-901.

Koning, L. (2011). How two lesbian mamas share breastfeeding duties. Retrieved from **offbeathome.com/co-breastfeeding**.

Kunz, C., & Lonnerdal, B. (1992). Re-evaluation of the whey protein/casein ratio of human milk. *Acta Paediatrica, 81*(2), 107-112.

Lamberts, S. W., & Macleod, R. M. (1990). Regulation of prolactin secretion at the level of the lactotroph. *Physiological Reviews, 70*(2), 279-318.

Laway, B. A., Mir, S. A., & Zargar, A. H. (2013). Recovery of prolactin function following spontaneous pregnancy in a woman with Sheehan's syndrome. *Indian Journal of Endocrinology and Metabolism, 17*(Supplement 3), S696-699.

Lawrence, R. A., & Lawrence, R. M. (2016). *Breastfeeding: A Guide for the Medical Profession* (8th ed.). Philadelphia, PA: Elsevier.

Lee, N. (1995). More on pierced nipples. *Journal of Human Lactation, 11*(2), 89.

Lee, S., & Kelleher, S. L. (2016). Biological underpinnings of breastfeeding challenges: The role of genetics, diet, and environment on lactation physiology. American *Journal of Physiology, Endocrinology and Metabolism, 311*(2), E405-422.

Leeners, B., Rath, W., Kuse, S., et al. (2005). Breast-feeding in women with hypertensive disorders in pregnancy. *Journal of Perinatal Medicine, 33*(6), 553-560.

Leung, A. M., Pearce, E. N., & Braverman, L. E. (2011). Iodine nutrition in pregnancy and lactation. *Endocrinology & Metabolism Clinics of North America, 40*(4), 765-777.

Lind, J. N., Perrine, C. G., & Li, R. (2014). Relationship between use of labor pain medications and delayed onset of lactation. *Journal of Human Lactation, 30*(2), 167-173.

Livingstone, V. (1996). Too much of a good thing. Maternal and infant hyperlactation syndromes. *Canadian Family Physician, 42,* 89-99.

Lopez, M. A. C., Rodriguez, J. L. R., & Garcia, M. R. (2013). Physiological and pathological hyperprolactemia: Can we minimize errors in the clinical practice? In G. M. Nagy & B. E. Toth (Eds.), *Prolactin: InTechOpen*.

Lou, Z., Zeng, G., Huang, L., et al. (2014). Maternal reported indicators and causes of insufficient milk supply. *Journal of Human Lactation, 30*(4), 466-473; quiz 511-462.

Love, S. M., & Barsky, S. H. (2004). Anatomy of the nipple and breast ducts revisited. *Cancer, 101*(9), 1947-1957.

MacDonald, T., Noel-Weiss, J., West, D., et al. (2016). Transmasculine individuals' experiences with lactation, chestfeeding, and gender identity: A qualitative study. *BMC Pregnancy & Childbirth, 16,* 106.

Mandel, D., Lubetzky, R., Dollberg, S., et al. (2005). Fat and energy contents of expressed human breast milk in prolonged lactation. *Pediatrics, 116*(3), e432-435.

Mannion, C., & Mansell, D. (2012). Breastfeeding self-efficacy and the use of prescription medication: A pilot study. *Obstetrics and Gynecology International, 2012,* 562704.

Marasco, L. (2005). Polycystic ovary syndrome. *Leaven, 41*(2), 27-29.

Marasco, L. (2006). The impact of thyroid dysfunction on lactation. *Breastfeeding Abstracts, 25*(2), 11-12.

Marasco, L., & West, D. (2020). *Making More Milk: The Breastfeeding Guide to Increasing Your Milk Production* (2nd ed.). New York, NY: McGraw Hill.

Marchini, G., Simoni, M. R., Bartolini, F., et al. (1993). The relationship of plasma cholecystokinin levels to different feeding routines in newborn infants. *Early Human Development, 35*(1), 31-35.

Marshall, A. M., Nommsen-Rivers, L. A., Hernandez, L. L., et al. (2010). Serotonin transport and metabolism in the mammary gland modulates secretory activation and involution. *Journal of Clinical Endocrinology & Metabolism, 95*(2), 837-846.

Mathur, G. P., Chitranshi, S., Mathur, S., et al. (1992). Lactation failure. *Indian Pediatrics, 29*(12), 1541-1544.

Matthiesen, A. S., Ransjo-Arvidson, A. B., Nissen, E., et al. (2001). Postpartum maternal oxytocin release by newborns: Effects of infant hand massage and sucking. *Birth, 28*(1), 13-19.

McGuire, T. M. (2018). Drugs affecting milk supply during lactation. *Australian Prescriber, 41*(1), 7-9.

McLennan, J. D. (2001). Early termination of breast-feeding in periurban Santo Domingo, Dominican Republic: Mothers' community perceptions and personal practices. *Revista Panamericana de Salud Publica, 9*(6), 362-367.

McNeilly, A. S., & McNeilly, J. R. (1978). Spontaneous milk ejection during lactation and its possible relevance to success of breast-feeding. *British Medical Journal, 2*(6135), 466-468.

McNeilly, A. S., Robinson, I. C., Houston, M. J., et al. (1983). Release of oxytocin and prolactin in response to suckling. *British Medical Journal (Clinical Research Ed.), 286*(6361), 257-259.

Mead, L. J., Chuffo, R., Lawlor-Klean, P., et al. (1992). Breastfeeding success with preterm quadruplets. *Journal of Obstetric, Gynecologic, and Neonatal Nursing, 21*(3), 221-227.

Meier, P. (2004). Choosing a correctly-fitted breastshield. *Medela Messenger, 21,* 8-9.

Meier, P. P., & Engstrom, J. L. (2007). Test weighing for term and premature infants is an accurate procedure. *Archives of Disease in Childhood. Fetal and Neonatal Edition, 92*(2), F155-156.

Meier, P. P., Engstrom, J. L., Fleming, B. A., et al. (1996). Estimating milk intake of hospitalized preterm infants who breastfeed. *Journal of Human Lactation, 12*(1), 21-26.

Mennella, J. A., & Pepino, M. Y. (2010). Breastfeeding and prolactin levels in lactating women with a family history of alcoholism. *Pediatrics, 125*(5), e1162-1170.

Michaels, A. M., & Wanner, H. (2013). Breastfeeding twins after mastectomy. *Journal of Human Lactation, 29*(1), 20-22.

Mikami, F. C. F., Francisco, R. P. V., Rodrigues, A., et al. (2018). Breastfeeding twins: Factors related to weaning. *Journal of Human Lactation,* doi:10.1177/0890334418767382.

Miyai, K., Tokushige, T., & Kondo, M. (2008). Suppression of thyroid function during ingestion of seaweed "Kombu" (Laminaria japonoca) in normal Japanese adults. *Endocrine Journal, 55*(6), 1103-1108.

Mizuno, K., Nishida, Y., Mizuno, N., et al. (2008). The important role of deep attachment in the uniform drainage of breast milk from mammary lobe. *Acta Paediatrica, 97*(9), 1200-1204.

Mohd Shukri, N. H., Wells, J., Eaton, S., et al. (2019). Randomized controlled trial investigating the effects of a breastfeeding relaxation intervention on maternal psychological state, breast milk outcomes, and infant behavior and growth. *American Journal of Clinical Nutrition.*

Mohrbacher, N. (1996). Mothers who forgo breastfeeding for pumping. *Ameda/Egnell Circle of Caring, 9*(2), 1-2.

Mohrbacher, N. (2011). The 'Magic Number' and long-term milk production. *Clinical Lactation, 2*(1), 15-18.

Morton, J. (2012). The importance of hands. *Journal of Human Lactation, 28*(3), 276-277.

Morton, J. (2019). Hands-on or hands-off when first milk matters most? *Breastfeeding Medicine, 14*(5), 295-297.

Morton, J., Hall, J. Y., Wong, R. J., et al. (2009). Combining hand techniques with electric pumping increases milk production in mothers of preterm infants. *Journal of Perinatology, 29*(11), 757-764.

Murase, M., Wagner, E. A., C, J. C., et al. (2017). The relation between breast milk sodium to potassium ratio and maternal report of a milk supply concern. *Journal of Pediatrics, 181,* 294-297 e293.

Napierala, M., Mazela, J., Merritt, T. A., et al. (2016). Tobacco smoking and breastfeeding: Effect on the lactation process, breast milk composition and infant development. A critical review. *Environmental Research, 151,* 321-338.

Napierala, M., Merritt, T. A., Mazela, J., et al. (2017). The effect of tobacco smoke on oxytocin concentrations and selected oxidative stress parameters in plasma during pregnancy and post-partum—An experimental model. *Human & Experimental Toxicology, 36*(2), 135-145.

Neifert, M. R., McDonough, S. L., & Neville, M. C. (1981). Failure of lactogenesis associated with placental retention. *American Journal of Obstetrics & Gynecology, 140*(4), 477-478.

Nelson, A. M. (2017). Risks and benefits of swaddling healthy infants: An integrative review. *MCN: American Journal of Maternal/Child Nursing, 42*(4), 216-225.

Neville, M. C., Allen, J. C., Archer, P. C., et al. (1991). Studies in human lactation: Milk volume and nutrient composition during weaning and lactogenesis. *American Journal of Clinical Nutrition, 54*(1), 81-92.

Neville, M. C., Keller, R., Seacat, J., et al. (1988). Studies in human lactation: Milk volumes in lactating women during the onset of lactation and full lactation. *American Journal of Clinical Nutrition, 48*(6), 1375-1386.

Neville, M. C., McFadden, T. B., & Forsyth, I. (2002). Hormonal regulation of mammary differentiation and milk secretion. *Journal of Mammary Gland Biology and Neoplasia, 7*(1), 49-66.

Neville, M. C., & Morton, J. (2001). Physiology and endocrine changes underlying human lactogenesis II. *Journal of Nutrition, 131*(11), 3005S-3008S.

Newton, M., & Newton, N. R. (1948). The let-down reflex in human lactation. *Journal of Pediatrics, 33*(6), 698-704.

Noel, G. L., Suh, H. K., & Frantz, A. G. (1974). Prolactin release during nursing and breast stimulation in postpartum and nonpostpartum subjects. *Journal of Clinical Endocrinology and Metabolism, 38*(3), 413-423.

Nommsen-Rivers, L., Thompson, A., Riddle, S., et al. (2019). Feasibility and acceptability of metformin to augment low milk supply: A pilot randomized controlled trial. *Journal of Human Lactation, 35*(2), 261-271.

Nommsen-Rivers, L. A. (2016). Does insulin explain the relation between maternal obesity and poor lactation outcomes? An overview of the literature. *Advances in Nutrition, 7*(2), 407-414.

Nommsen-Rivers, L. A., Heinig, M. J., Cohen, R. J., et al. (2008). Newborn wet and soiled diaper counts and timing of onset of lactation as indicators of breastfeeding inadequacy. *Journal of Human Lactation, 24*(1), 27-33.

Oladapo, O. T., & Fawole, B. (2012). Treatments for suppression of lactation. *Cochrane Database of Systematic Reviews*(9), CD005937. doi:10.1002/14651858.CD005937.pub3.

Olsen, A. (1940). Nursing under conditions of thirst or excessive ingestion of fluids. *Acta Obstetricia et Gynecologica Scandinavica, 20*(4), 313-343.

Otsuka, K., Dennis, C. L., Tatsuoka, H., et al. (2008). The relationship between breastfeeding self-efficacy and perceived insufficient milk among Japanese mothers. *Journal of Obstetric, Gynecologic & Neonatal Nursing, 37*(5), 546-555.

Pai, V. P., Hernandez, L. L., Stull, M. A., et al. (2015). The type 7 serotonin receptor, 5-HT 7, is essential in the mammary gland for regulation of mammary epithelial structure and function. *BioMed Research International, 2015,* 364746.

Pang, W. W., & Hartmann, P. E. (2007). Initiation of human lactation: secretory differentiation and secretory activation. *Journal of Mammary Gland Biology and Neoplasia, 12*(4), 211-221.

Parker, L. A., Sullivan, S., Krueger, C., et al. (2012). Effect of early breast milk expression on milk volume and timing of lactogenesis stage II among mothers of very low birth weight infants: A pilot study. *Journal of Perinatology, 32*(3), 205-209.

Patil, S. P., Niphadkar, P. V., & Bapat, M. M. (1997). Allergy to fenugreek (Trigonella foenum graecum). *Annals of Allergy, Asthma, and Immunology, 78*(3), 297-300.

Paul, C., Zenut, M., Dorut, A., et al. (2015). Use of domperidone as a galactagogue drug: A systematic review of the benefit-risk ratio. *Journal of Human Lactation, 31*(1), 57-63.

Perrin, M. T., Fogleman, A. D., Newburg, D. S., et al. (2017). A longitudinal study of human milk composition in the second year postpartum: Implications for human milk banking. *Maternal and Child Nutrition, 13*(1).

Pieh-Holder, K. L., Scardo, J. A., & Costello, D. H. (2012). Lactogenesis failure following successful delivery of advanced abdominal pregnancy. *Breastfeeding Medicine, 7*(6), 543-546.

Pisacane, A., & Continisio, P. (2004). Breastfeeding and perceived changes in the appearance of the breasts: A retrospective study. *Acta Paediatrica, 93*(10), 1346-1348.

Powers, D., & Tapia, V. (2015). Hyperlactation associated with oral contraception use: A case report, part 1. *Clinical Lactation, 6*(3), 66-71.

Prentice, A. (1989). Evidence for local feedback control of human milk secretion. *Biochemical Society Transactions, 17,* 489-492.

Prentice, P., Ong, K. K., Schoemaker, M. H., et al. (2016). Breast milk nutrient content and infancy growth. *Acta Paediatrica, 105*(6), 641-647.

Preusting, I., Brumley, J., Odibo, L., et al. (2017). Obesity as a predictor of delayed lactogenesis II. *Journal of Human Lactation, 33*(4), 684-691.

Prime, D. K., Geddes, D. T., & Hartmann, P. E. (2007). Oxytocin: Milk ejection and maternal-infant well-being. In T. W. Hale & P. E. Hartmann (Eds.), *Hale & Hartmann's Textbook of Human Lactation* (pp. 141-155). Amarillo, TX: Hale Publishing.

Prime, D. K., Kent, J. C., Hepworth, A. R., et al. (2012). Dynamics of milk removal during simultaneous breast expression in women. *Breastfeeding Medicine, 7*(2), 100-106.

Raguindin, P. F., Dans, L. F., & King, J. F. (2014). Moringa oleifera as a galactagogue. *Breastfeeding Medicine, 9*(6), 323-324.

Ramsay, D. T., Kent, J. C., Hartmann, R. A., et al. (2005). Anatomy of the lactating human breast redefined with ultrasound imaging. *Journal of Anatomy, 206*(6), 525-534.

Ramsay, D. T., Kent, J. C., Owens, R. A., et al. (2004). Ultrasound imaging of milk ejection in the breast of lactating women. *Pediatrics, 113*(2), 361-367.

Ramsay, D. T., Mitoulas, L. R., Kent, J. C., et al. (2005). The use of ultrasound to characterize milk ejection in women using an electric breast pump. *Journal of Human Lactation, 21*(4), 421-428.

Rankin, M. W., Jimenez, E. Y., Caraco, M., et al. (2016). Validation of test weighing protocol to estimate enteral feeding volumes in preterm infants. *Journal of Pediatrics, 178,* 108-112.

Rasmussen, K. (2007). Association of maternal obesity before conception with poor lactation performance. *Annual Review of Nutrition* (27), 103-121.

Rasmussen, K. M., & Kjolhede, C. L. (2004). Prepregnant overweight and obesity diminish the prolactin response to suckling in the first week postpartum. *Pediatrics, 113*(5), e465-471.

Reeder, C., LeGrand, A., & O'Connor-Von, S. K. (2013). The effect of fenugreek on milk production and prolactin levels in mothers of preterm infants. *Clinical Lactation, 4*(4), 159-165.

Reisman, T., & Goldstein, Z. (2018). Case report: Induced lactation in a transgender woman. *Transgender Health, 3*(1), 24-26.

Reza, S., Rahmani, S., Mohsen, J. Z., et al. (2013). Prevalence and causes of exclusive breastfeeding failure in 6 months after birth in Iranian infants. *Breastfeeding Medicine, 8*(4), 426-427.

Rinker, B., Veneracion, M., & Walsh, C. P. (2008). The effect of breastfeeding on breast aesthetics. *Aesthetic Surgery Journal, 28*(5), 534-537.

Riordan, J. M., & Nichols, F. H. (1990). A descriptive study of lactation mastitis in long-term breastfeeding women. *Journal of Human Lactation, 6*(2), 53-58.

Rioux, F. M., Savoie, N., & Allard, J. (2006). Is there a link between postpartum anemia and discontinuation of breastfeeding? *Canadian Journal of Dietetic Practice and Research, 67*(2), 72-76.

Rossoni, E., Feng, J., Tirozzi, B., et al. (2008). Emergent synchronous bursting of oxytocin neuronal network. *PLoS Computational Biology, 4*(7), e1000123.

Sadovnikova, A. S., I; Koehler, S; Plott, J. (2015). *Systematic review of breast massage techniques around the world in databases and on YouTube.* Paper presented at the Academy of Breastfeeding Medicine 20th Annual International Meeting, Los Angeles.

Saint, L., Maggiore, P., & Hartmann, P. E. (1986). Yield and nutrient content of milk in eight women breast-feeding twins and one woman breast-feeding triplets. *British Journal of Nutrition, 56*(1), 49-58.

Saint, L., Smith, M., & Hartmann, P. E. (1984). The yield and nutrient content of colostrum and milk of women from giving birth to 1 month post-partum. *British Journal of Nutrition, 52*(1), 87-95.

Sakha, K., & Behbahan, A. G. (2008). Training for perfect breastfeeding or metoclopramide: Which one can promote lactation in nursing mothers? *Breastfeeding Medicine, 3*(2), 120-123.

Salahudeen, M. S., Koshy, A. M., & Sen, S. (2013). A study of the factors affecting time to onset of lactogenesis-II after parturition. *Journal of Pharmacy Research, 6*(1), 68-72.

Saper, R. B., Kales, S. N., Paquin, J., et al. (2004). Heavy metal content of ayurvedic herbal medicine products. *Journal of the American Medical Association, 292*(23), 2868-2873.

Sauer, C. W., Boutin, M. A., & Kim, J. H. (2017). Wide variability in caloric density of expressed human milk can lead to major underestimation or overestimation of nutrient content. *Journal of Human Lactation, 33*(2), 341-350.

Schaal, B., Doucet, S., Sagot, P., et al. (2006). Human breast areolae as scent organs: Morphological data and possible involvement in maternal-neonatal coadaptation. *Developmental Psychobiology, 48*(2), 100-110.

Scheplyagina, L. A. (2005). Impact of the mother's zinc deficiency on the woman's and newborn's health status. *Journal of Trace Elements in Medicine and Biology, 19*(1), 29-35.

Selander, J., Cantor, A., Young, S. M., et al. (2013). Human maternal placentophagy: A survey of self-reported motivations and experiences associated with placenta consumption. *Ecology of Food & Nutrition, 52*(2), 93-115.

Serrano-Nascimento, C., Salgueiro, R. B., Vitzel, K. F., et al. (2017). Iodine excess exposure during pregnancy and lactation impairs maternal thyroid function in rats. *Endocrine Connections, 6*(7), 510-521.

Shivaprasad, C. (2011). Sheehan's syndrome: Newer advances. *Indian Journal of Endocrinology and Metabolism, 15 Suppl 3,* S203-207.

Sim, T. F., Hattingh, H. L., Sherriff, J., et al. (2014). Perspectives and attitudes of breastfeeding women using herbal galactagogues during breastfeeding: A qualitative study. *BMC Complementary & Alternative Medicine, 14,* 216.

Sim, T. F., Sherriff, J., Hattingh, H. L., et al. (2013). The use of herbal medicines during breastfeeding: A population-based survey in Western Australia. *BMC Complementary & Alternative Medicine, 13,* 317.

Smillie, C. M., Campbell, S. H., & Iwinski, S. (2005). Hyperlactation: How left-brained 'rules' for breastfeeding can wreak havoc with a natural process. *Newborn and Infant Nursing Reviews, 5*(1), 49-58.

Smith, L. (2021). Postpartum care. In K. Wambach & B. Spencer (Eds.), *Breastfeeding and Human Lactation* (6th ed., pp. 247-280). Burlington, MA: Jones & Bartlett Learning.

Sonnenblick, E. B., Shah, A. D., Goldstein, Z., et al. (2018). Breast imaging of transgender individuals: A review. *Current Radiology Reports, 6*(1), 1.

Sozmen, M. (1992). Effects of early suckling of cesarean-born babies on lactation. *Biology of the Neonate, 62,* 67-68.

Sperling, D., & Robinson, L. (2018). Induced lactation in a transgendered female partner. *Journal of Obstetric, Gynecologic & Neonatal Nursing, 47*(Supplement 3S), S61.

Stohs, S. J., & Hartman, M. J. (2015). Review of the safety and efficacy of Moringa oleifera. *Phytotherapy Research, 29*(6), 796-804.

Strode, M. A., Dewey, K. G., & Lonnerdal, B. (1986). Effects of short-term caloric restriction on lactational performance of well-nourished women. *Acta Paediatrica Scandavica, 75*(2), 222-229.

Stuebe, A. M., Meltzer-Brody, S., Pearson, B., et al. (2015). Maternal neuroendocrine serum levels in exclusively breastfeeding mothers. *Breastfeeding Medicine, 10*(4), 197-202.

Stull, M. A., Pai, V., Vomachka, A. J., et al. (2007). Mammary gland homeostasis employs serotonergic regulation of epithelial tight junctions. *Proceedings of the National Academy of Sciences of the USA., 104*(42), 16708-16713.

Stutte, P. (1988). The effects of breast massage on volume and fat content of human milk. *Genesis, 10*(2), 22-25.

Tahiliani, P., & Kar, A. (2003). Mitigation of thyroxine-induced hyperglycaemia by two plant extracts. *Phytotherapy Research, 17*(3), 294-296.

Taylor, A., Logan, G., Twells, L., et al. (2019). Human milk expression after domperidone treatment in postpartum women: A systematic review and meta-analysis of randomized controlled trials. *Journal of Human Lactation, 35*(3), 501-509.

Thanaboonyawat, I., Chanprapaph, P., Lattalapkul, J., et al. (2013). Pilot study of normal development of nipples during pregnancy. *Journal of Human Lactation, 29*(4), 480-483.

Thaweekul, P., Thaweekul, Y., & Sritipsukho, P. (2014). The efficacy of hospital-based food program as galactogogues in early period of lactation. *Journal of the Medical Association of Thailand, 97*(5), 478-482.

Thayer, Z. M., Agustin Bechayda, S., & Kuzawa, C. W. (2018). Circadian cortisol dynamics across reproductive stages and in relation to breastfeeding in the Philippines. *American Journal of Human Biology, 30*(4), e23115.

Thompson, J. F., Heal, L. J., Roberts, C. L., et al. (2010). Women's breastfeeding experiences following a significant primary postpartum haemorrhage: A multicentre cohort study. *International Breastfeeding Journal, 5,* 5.

Thorley, V. (2005). Breast hypoplasia and breastfeeding: A case history. *Breastfeeding Review, 13*(2), 13-16.

Toppare, M. F., Kitapci, F., Senses, D. A., et al. (1994). Lactational failure--Study of risk factors in Turkish mothers. *Indian Journal of Pediatrics, 61*(3), 269-276.

Torris, C., Thune, I., Emaus, A., et al. (2013). Duration of lactation, maternal metabolic profile, and body composition in the Norwegian EBBA I-study. *Breastfeeding Medicine, 8*(1), 8-15.

Trimeloni, L., & Spencer, J. (2016). Diagnosis and management of breast milk oversupply. *Journal of the American Board of Family Medicine, 29*(1), 139-142.

Ureno, T. L., Berry-Caban, C. S., Adams, A., et al. (2019). Dysphoric milk ejection reflex: A descriptive study. *Breastfeeding Medicine.*

Ureno, T. L., Buchheit, T. L., Hopkinson, S. G., et al. (2018). Dysphoric milk ejection reflex: A case series. *Breastfeeding Medicine, 13*(1), 85-88.

Uvnas-Moberg, K. (2014). *Oxytocin: The Biological Guide to Motherhood.* Amarillo, TX: Praeclarus Press.

Uvnas-Moberg, K., & Kendall-Tackett, K. (2018). The mystery of D-MER: What can hormonal research tell us about dysphoric milk-ejection reflex? *Clinical Lactation, 9*(1), 23-29.

Valdez, J., Lujan, C., & Valdez, M. (2018). Effects of kinesio tape application on breast milk production [abstract]. *Breastfeeding Medicine, 13*(Supplement 2), S-36.

Vallone, S. (2007). The role of subluxation and chiropractic care in hypolactation. *Journal of Clinical Chiropractic Pediatrics, 8*(1-2), 518-524.

van Veldhuizen-Staas, C. G. (2007). Overabundant milk supply: An alternative way to intervene by full drainage and block feeding. *International Breastfeeding Journal, 2,* 11.

VanHouten, J., Dann, P., McGeoch, G., et al. (2004). The calcium-sensing receptor regulates mammary gland parathyroid hormone-related protein production and calcium transport. *Journal of Clinical Investigation, 113*(4), 598-608.

Vazirinejad, R., Darakhshan, S., Esmaeili, A., et al. (2009). The effect of maternal breast variations on neonatal weight gain in the first seven days of life. *International Breastfeeding Journal, 4,* 13.

Wan, E. W., Davey, K., Page-Sharp, M., et al. (2008). Dose-effect study of domperidone as a galactagogue in preterm mothers with insufficient milk supply, and its transfer into milk. *British Journal of Clinical Pharmacology, 66*(2), 283-289.

Watson, C. J. (2006). Involution: Apoptosis and tissue remodelling that convert the mammary gland from milk factory to a quiescent organ. *Breast Cancer Research, 8*(2), 203.

Weisstaub, A. R., Zeni, S., de Portela, M. L., et al. (2006). Influence of maternal dietary calcium levels on milk zinc, calcium and phosphorus contents and milk production in rats. *Journal of Trace Elements in Medicine and Biology, 20*(1), 41-47.

West, D., & Hirsch, E. (2008). *Breastfeeding after Breast and Nipple Procedures.* Amarillo, TX: Hale Publishing.

Wichman, C. L., & Cunningham, J. L. (2008). A case of venlafaxine-induced galactorrhea? *Journal of Clinical Psychopharmacology, 28*(5), 580-581.

Wiffen, J., & Fetherston, C. (2016). Relationships between assisted reproductive technologies and initiation of lactation: Preliminary observations. *Breastfeeding Review, 24*(1), 21-27.

Wilde, C. J., Addey, C. V., Boddy, L. M., et al. (1995). Autocrine regulation of milk secretion by a protein in milk. *Biochemical Journal, 305* (Pt 1), 51-58.

Willis, C. E., & Livingstone, V. (1995). Infant insufficient milk syndrome associated with maternal postpartum hemorrhage. *Journal of Human Lactation, 11*(2), 123-126.

Wilson-Clay, B., & Hoover, K. (2017). *The Breastfeeding Atlas* (6th ed.). Manchaca, TX: LactNews Press.

Wilson, E., Perrin, M. T., Fogleman, A., et al. (2015). The intricacies of induced lactation for same-sex mothers of an adopted child. *Journal of Human Lactation, 31*(1), 64-67.

Witt, A., Mason, M. J., Burgess, K., et al. (2014). A case control study of bacterial species and colony count in milk of breastfeeding women with chronic pain. *Breastfeeding Medicine, 9*(1), 29-34.

Woolridge, M. W., & Fisher, C. (1988). Colic, "overfeeding", and symptoms of lactose malabsorption in the breast-fed baby: A possible artifact of feed management? *Lancet, 2*(8607), 382-384.

Yamada, R., Rasmussen, K. M., & Felice, J. P. (2019). "What is 'enough,' and how do I make it?": A qualitative examination of questions mothers ask on social media about pumping and providing an adequate amount of milk for their infants. *Breastfeeding Medicine, 14*(1), 17-21.

Yamauchi, Y., & Yamanouchi, I. (1990). Breast-feeding frequency during the first 24 hours after birth in full-term neonates. *Pediatrics, 86*(2), 171-175.

Yokoyama, Y., & Ooki, S. (2004). Breast-feeding and bottle-feeding of twins, triplets and higher order multiple births. *Nippon Koshu Eisei Zasshi, 51*(11), 969-974.

Young, S. M., & Benyshek, D. C. (2010). In search of human placentophagy: A cross-cultural survey of human placenta consumption, disposal practices, and cultural beliefs. *Ecology of Food & Nutrition, 49*(6), 467-484.

Young, S. M., Gryder, L. K., Cross, C. L., et al. (2019). Ingestion of steamed and dehydrated placenta capsules does not affect postpartum plasma prolactin levels or neonatal weight gain: Results from a randomized, double-bind, placebo-controlled pilot study. *Journal of Midwifery & Women's Health, 64*(4), 443-450.

Zangen, S., Di Lorenzo, C., Zangen, T., et al. (2001). Rapid maturation of gastric relaxation in newborn infants. *Pediatric Research, 50*(5), 629-632.

Zelazniewicz, A., & Pawlowski, B. (2019). Maternal breast volume in pregnancy and lactation capacity. *American Journal of Physical Anthropology, 168*(1), 180-189.

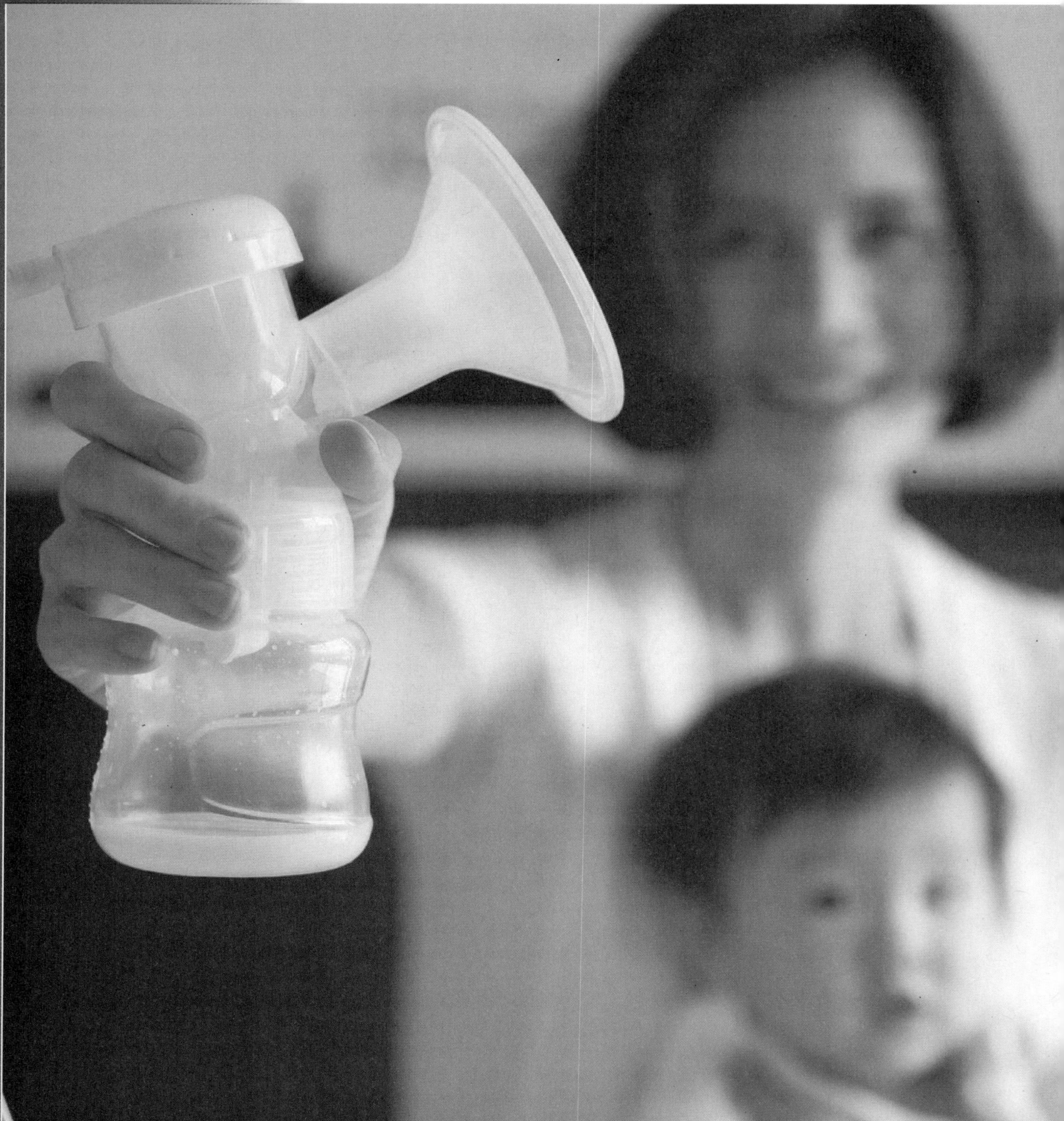

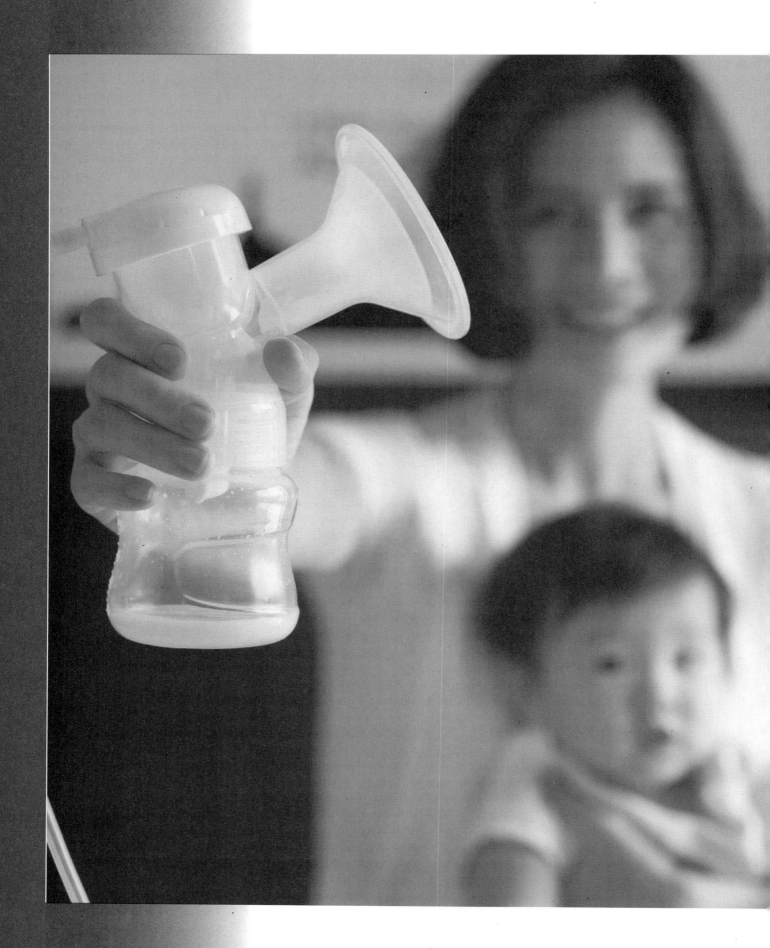

Milk Expression and Storage

11

MILK EXPRESSION BASICS

Why Express Milk?

Some milk expression is associated with reduced early use of formula and longer nursing duration, but regular and exclusive pumping is associated with a shorter nursing duration.

The effect of milk expression on nursing outcomes depends on several factors: the method used, whether it occurs during pregnancy or after birth, and how often milk is expressed: occasionally, regularly, or exclusively.

Hand expression during pregnancy and the first week. Learning to hand-express milk is one of the Baby Friendly Hospital Initiative's "Ten Steps to Successful Breastfeeding." Learning this skill gives nursing parents more control over their comfort and their ability to provide milk for their baby. Research on early hand expression indicates that learning this skill benefits lactation outcomes both early and later.

- ***Hand expression during the last month of pregnancy.*** Australian research on diabetic mothers who expressed and stored colostrum beginning at 36 weeks (Forster et al., 2017) found hand expression was a safe practice if done near the end of an uncomplicated pregnancy. In a 2019 Australian retrospective cohort study (Casey, Banks, Braniff, Buettner, & Heal, 2019), learning to express colostrum during the last month of pregnancy was associated with reduced formula supplementation in the hospital. In a U.S qualitative semi-structured interview study (Demirci, Glasser, Fichner, Caplan, & Himes, 2019), its 19 first-time mothers reported that expressing and storing colostrum during the last month of pregnancy gave them more confidence in their ability to fully nurse their baby.
- ***Hand expression during the hospital stay.*** An Italian study in which the 1,760 study parents often hand-expressed colostrum and spoon-fed it to their newborns (Bertini, Breschi, & Dani, 2015) found that none of these newborns lost more than 10% of birth weight. In a U.S. study (Flaherman, Beiler, Cabana, & Paul, 2016), early excess weight loss was associated with a lack of confidence in milk production and increased odds of weaning before 6 months. A U.S. randomized controlled trial of 68 mothers of newborns 12 to 36 hours old having latching or sucking problems (Flaherman et al., 2012) found that more of those randomized to the hand-expression group (96%) were still nursing at 2 months compared with those in the breast-pump group (73%). The mothers in the hand-expression group were also more comfortable hand expressing in front of others, as compared with those in the pumping group.

Due to these positive effects of hand expression on early nursing, U.S. pediatrician Jane Morton created the website **firstdroplets.com**, which provides videos for parents explaining the advantages of learning hand expression and using it after delivery, even when feeding is going well. The videos also demonstrate how to do hand expression. For families who expect a delay in their milk increase after birth (e.g., parents nursing for the first time or those who are diabetic), hand-expressing and collecting colostrum during pregnancy is one way to avoid the use of formula until milk increase occurs (Cox, 2006; Forster et al., 2017).

> **KEY CONCEPT**
>
> *Learning hand expression during late pregnancy and using it after birth improves confidence and nursing outcomes.*

Pumping a little or a lot. On the other hand, while occasional pumping appears to increase nursing duration (Win, Binns, Zhao, Scott, & Oddy, 2006), frequent regular or exclusive pumping appears to shorten it (Bai, Fong, Lok, Wong, & Tarrant, 2017; Felice, Cassano, & Rasmussen, 2016; Pang et al., 2017; Yourkavitch et al., 2018). Even so, in some countries, plans to pump after delivery are nearly universal in nursing families. One U.S. cross-sectional study of 100 breastfeeding women, who were interviewed in the hospital after delivery (Loewenberg Weisband, Keim, Keder, Geraghty, & Gallo, 2017) found that 98% planned to pump, with 69% intending to start within weeks. Nearly 29% intended to start pumping within the first few days after delivery.

In the U.S., the only developed country without paid parental leave and where many families receive free breast pumps through their health insurance companies, it's easy to assume that many nursing parents plan to pump because they will be returning to work. However, in Australia, where there is a 1-year paid maternity leave for many families, pumping rates are still very high. A 2016 Australian prospective cohort study included 1,003 women after the birth of a healthy term baby at three hospitals in Melbourne (Johns, Amir, McLachlan, & Forster, 2016). At the first interview, 24 to 48 hours after birth, 60% already had a breast pump. At 2 weeks after delivery, 60% had used their pump, with 40% pumping several times each day. By 6 months, 83% owned a pump and 40% pumped at least occasionally. Only 10% of this study population used their pump because they returned to work.

KEY CONCEPT

Compared with direct nursing, many find pumping unpleasant, but for various reasons, it is nearly universal in some countries.

• • •

Parents express milk for many reasons, and their reasons change over time.

In the Australian study described in the previous point (Johns et al., 2016), the main reasons most of the study mothers gave for pumping milk (from most to least common) were: 1) to be able to go out and leave the baby (23%), 2) not enough milk (17%), 3) latching struggles (8.5%), and 4) too much milk (8.5%). Other reasons included to return to work (8.5%), nipple pain (6%), so someone else can feed the baby (5%), father wanted to feed baby (3%), and wanted to measure milk (2%), and to store extra milk (2%).

In the U.S. (Loewenberg Weisband et al., 2017), among those interviewed within a day or two after birth who had already started pumping, the reasons given were: 1) to keep up milk supply when away from baby (73%), 2) to increase milk supply (67%), 3) latching struggles (27%), and 4) to create a freezer stash of milk for return to work (27%). One U.S. longitudinal qualitative study of 20 pumping mothers used in-depth, semi-structured interviews conducted from pregnancy through the end of human-milk feeding (Felice et al., 2017). These mothers described pumping as "time-consuming, costly, and unpleasant" compared with direct nursing but felt it was necessary to meet their feeding goals. Their reasons for pumping changed over time. At first, many pumped because of latching struggles or to establish milk production, while later they pumped for other reasons, such as return to work, to replace nursing sessions after alcohol consumption, or during separations for reasons other than work, so the baby's father could participate, and to create a milk surplus to use after weaning.

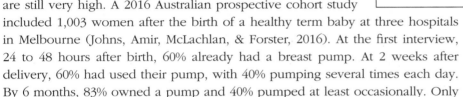

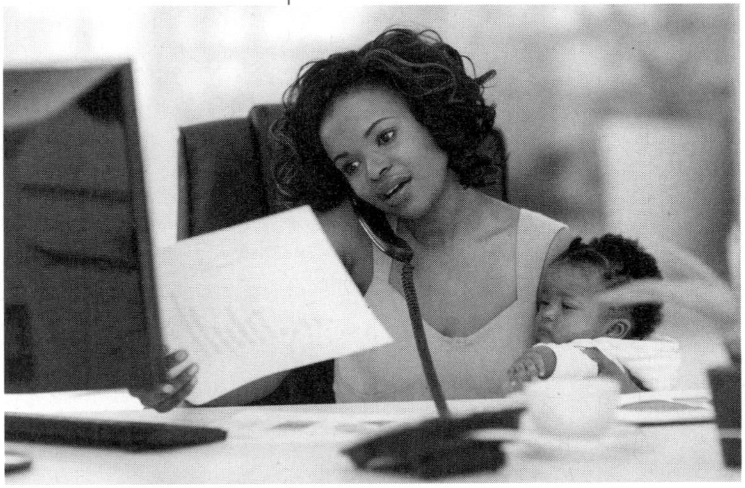

How Much Milk to Expect

To be effective, milk expression usually requires practice and conditioning.

On their first try, few parents express much milk; some only a few drops. Suggest thinking of the first milk expressions as practice sessions and any milk as a bonus. Make sure parents know that whatever method they use, milk expression is a learned skill and with practice more milk will come. The key to effective milk expression is to condition the body to respond with milk ejection to the feel of the expression method. This can be as much psychological as it is physical (see next section). Even if just a few drops are expressed, this is a good sign, and with practice, it's reasonable to expect more milk within a few days.

• • •

When nursing is going well, the milk available to express will increase over the first 5 weeks or so after birth.

As described in the previous chapter, on a baby's first day of life, total milk production averages a little more than 1 ounce (about 37 mL) of colostrum, the first milk (Saint, Smith, & Hartmann, 1984). If nursing goes well, by the time the baby is about 5 weeks old, the average nursing parent will reach peak milk production of 25 to 35 ounces (750 to 1035 mL) per day (Kent, Gardner, & Geddes, 2016; Kent et al., 2013). As milk production sharply increases during the first weeks (Kent et al., 2016), more milk is available for expression.

After about 5 weeks, daily milk production reaches its peak, and then stays relatively stable—within about 2 to 5 ounces (59 to 148 mL)—until the baby starts other foods at about 6 months of age, which causes production to gradually decrease (Islam, Peerson, Ahmed, Dewey, & Brown, 2006). Table 11.1 illustrates how feeding volumes increase as baby grows.

• • •

Other factors affect how much milk parents can express at a session.

In addition to the daily volume of milk produced, other factors affect the volume of milk expressed at a session.

Exclusively nursing? If a nursing baby also receives other foods or drinks, less milk is produced (Islam et al., 2006). Lower milk production means less milk available to express. If baby is not exclusively nursing, the volume of milk expressed will vary depending on how close the parent is to full milk production. For example, if about half of baby's milk intake comes from nursing, expect to express about half the milk that the parent of an exclusively nursing baby the same age would express.

> **KEY CONCEPT**
>
> *Many factors affect milk yields, including whether milk is expressed between regular nursing sessions or whether it replaces a nursing.*

Time elapsed since the last milk removal. Since the last nursing session or milk expression, the longer the parent waits to express milk, the greater the milk yield—to a point. For example, by waiting 2 hours, parents are likely to express more milk than if they expressed after just 1 hour. But if parents regularly wait so long that their mammary glands feel full, over time milk production will slow, which will lead to less milk expressed. On average, if parents whose baby is exclusively nursing express between regular nursing sessions they should expect to express about half a feed. If parents express for a missed feed, it is reasonable to expect to express a full feed. See Table 11.1 for feeding volumes during exclusive nursing by age.

Storage capacity. As explained in the previous chapter (see p. 416) storage capacity is the maximum volume of milk available to the baby when the mammary gland is at its fullest time of the day. Storage capacity varies among parents, from

TABLE 11.1 Average Feeding Volume by Age

Baby's Age	Avg. Milk Intake Per Feed	Avg. Milk Intake Per Day
First week	1-2 oz. (30-59 mL)	10-20 oz. (300-600 mL) after Day 4
Weeks 2 and 3	2-3 oz. (59-89 mL)	15-25 oz. (450-750 mL)
Months 1 to 6	3-4 oz. (89-118 mL)	25-30 oz. (750-887 mL)

Adapted from (Kent et al., 2016; Kent et al., 2013; Kent et al., 2006)

baby to baby in the same parent, and is not necessarily related to mammary size. Parents with a larger storage capacity usually express more milk at a session than those with a small storage capacity.

Time of day. Most parents express more milk in the morning than they do later in the day. This may be in part because babies older than a few weeks tend to feed less often during the night, leading to greater milk accumulation by morning (Kent et al., 2006).

Pump quality, fit, and practice time. When using a breast pump, other factors being equal, in general, multi-user pumps offer more combinations of vacuum and speed (cycle) settings than the pump models available for purchase. More setting combinations allow users to tailor their settings to their body's response. Research on milk yields from seven different pumping patterns (Kent, Ramsay, Doherty, Larsson, & Hartmann, 2003) found that about half of its study mothers responded well to all pumping patterns, but half of them didn't, with some only responding well to one pattern..

Pump fit can also affect milk yields (E. Jones & Hilton, 2009; P. Meier, 2004). A too-small nipple tunnel (the opening the nipple is drawn into during pumping) can compress milk ducts and slow milk flow. Also, fit may change with time and pump use, as nipples expand in size (Wilson-Clay & Hoover, 2017, p. 82). A parent who had a good fit when pumping began may need a larger nipple tunnel with more pumping over time (E. Jones & Hilton, 2009; P. Meier, Motykowski, & Zuleger, 2004). Unlike direct nursing and hand expression, with regular pumping, nipple length and diameter increase in size (Francis & Dickton, 2019). For illustrations of how to get a good pump fit, see p. 907-908.

Because milk ejection is, in part, a conditioned response, practice with a pump can help a parent's body learn to respond faster to its feel (Kent et al., 2003). With practice, the pump will trigger more milk ejections and pump yields will increase.

Emotional state. If a parent feels upset, frustrated, stressed, or angry, this releases adrenaline, which blocks the release of oxytocin and milk ejection (D.K. Prime, Geddes, & Hartmann, 2007). It is not unusual for parents pumping for preterm babies to pump less milk when they receive bad news about their baby's condition (Chatterton et al., 2000). If milk yields go down when a parent experiences negative emotions, suggest taking a break and trying to express later.

> **KEY CONCEPT**
>
> *Anger, frustration, and upset can reduce milk yields.*

Whether hands-on pumping techniques are used. Using the pump alone yields less milk than when massage and compression are also used (Alekseev & Ilyin, 2016; Morton et al., 2009). For details on hands-on pumping techniques, see the later point on p. 492.

• • •

If a baby takes more milk from a bottle than a parent can express at a session, this is not necessarily a sign of low milk production.

Many babies take more milk from a bottle than during a nursing session (Azad et al., 2018; Kramer et al., 2004; Li, Magadia, Fein, & Grummer-Strawn, 2012). Unless pacing techniques are used during bottle-feeding (see p. 902-903), this may be in part because the bottle provides a more consistent milk flow, which can override a baby's appetite control mechanism and cause overfeeding. During nursing, milk flow varies with milk ejection, and babies typically consume less milk during direct nursing. Unless there are other signs of low milk production, taking more milk from the bottle does not necessarily indicate a problem with milk production.

• • •

Most often, milk yields from one side are higher than the other.

Studies that measure pumping milk yields (Engstrom, Meier, Jegier, Motykowski, & Zuleger, 2007; Ramsay, Mitoulas, Kent, Larsson, & Hartmann, 2005) found that there is often a significant difference in milk yields between sides, with only 1 in 4 pumping parents producing the same milk volumes on both sides. If a parent seems concerned because one side yields more milk, first check the pump fit, as one nipple may be larger and need a different size nipple tunnel. However, what matters to the baby is getting enough milk overall, not whether each side yields the same milk volume. Some differences in milk output and production may relate to usage, as some favor one side during nursing. One side, however, may simply be a naturally larger milk producer. One U.S. study of 95 exclusively pumping mothers (Hill, Aldag, Zinaman, & Chatterton, 2007) found that milk output per breast was not necessarily associated with a mother's dominant hand, number of children, or previous breastfeeding experience. If parents are concerned about appearing lopsided, reassure them that both sides will most likely return to their original size after weaning.

Milk Ejection While Expressing

Triggering milk ejections—or let downs—is necessary for effective milk expression.

During nursing and milk expression, most milk leaves the mammary gland only when milk ejections occur. Without them, most milk stays in the gland. A milk ejection occurs when the hormone oxytocin is released into the bloodstream, which causes the muscles around the milk-producing alveoli (the myoepithelial cells) to squeeze and milk ducts to widen, pushing the milk out of the nipple.

Some nursing parents perceive milk ejection as a tingling feeling, pressure, increased thirst, milk leakage, even pain, while others feel nothing (Ramsay, Kent, Owens, & Hartmann, 2004; Ramsay et al., 2005). When a baby nurses, on average, it takes about a minute for a milk ejection to occur (Ramsay et al., 2004). The most reliable indicator of milk ejection during nursing is audible swallowing and during milk expression, visibly faster milk flow.

• • •

While nursing, most parents have multiple milk ejections and should also expect this while expressing milk.

Australian research (Cobo, 1993; Kent et al., 2008) found most nursing parents averaged 3 to 4 milk ejections during a nursing session, with a range of 1 to 17. One Australian study (Ramsay et al., 2004) used ultrasound to observe milk ejections during 166 nursing sessions with 45 mothers and found 88% of its study mothers felt their first milk ejection, but none felt their subsequent milk ejections. In another Australian study of 11 breastfeeding mothers (Ramsay et al., 2005), four of the study mothers felt more than one milk ejection. Since so many nursing parents—even experienced parents—are unaware they have more than one milk ejection, many will not realize they should expect multiple milk ejections while expressing milk.

During both pumping and nursing, parents experience a comparable number of milk ejections. In on Australian study (Ramsay & Hartmann, 2005), multiple milk ejections occurred during 95% of its pump sessions.

• • •

With more milk ejections, more milk is expressed—to a point.

More milk ejections during nursing means more milk consumed by the baby (Ramsay et al., 2004). This is also true about milk yields during expression, but the law of diminishing returns also applies. Australian breast-pump research (Kent et al., 2008) found that when the study mothers set their pumps at their highest comfortable vacuum setting, on average during the first milk ejection they expressed a little less than half of their available milk. "Available milk" is defined as the mammary gland's fullness when expression begins multiplied by that person's storage capacity. If more milk is expressed than the baby takes at his largest feed, available milk during milk expression can exceed 100%.

As the volume of milk in the gland decreases, milk flow slows. Less milk is expressed with each subsequent milk ejection. See Table 11.2 for the average results of 21 breastfeeding mothers using a multi-user double electric breast pump. In this Australian study (Kent et al., 2008), after two milk ejections, about 76% of the available milk was expressed (an average total milk volume of 90 mL, or 3 ounces). With four milk ejections, on average, nursing parents express about 99% of the available milk. After four milk ejections, the volume of milk expressed continued to decrease. The fifth and sixth milk ejections yielded only 7 mL, or about ¼ ounce each.

KEY CONCEPT

Time and practice are needed for the parent's body to become conditioned to the feel of the milk-expression method.

• • •

A parent's body can become conditioned to a specific feel and may need extra help when starting to express or when changing methods.

Milk ejection is in part a conditioned response (Kent et al., 2003). This means that when a parent's body becomes used to a particular feel, if this feel changes, extra help may be needed to trigger milk ejections. This can happen when an exclusively nursing parent starts expressing milk, when switching from one pump to another, when switching from hand expression to a pump, or vice versa.

TABLE 11.2 Average Volume of Milk Expressed During Each Milk Ejection

Milk Ejection	Average Percent of Available Milk Expressed	Average Volume of Milk Expressed
1st	45%	54 mL (1.8 oz.)
2nd	76%	37 mL (1.3 oz.)
3rd	88%	16 mL (0.5 oz.)
4th	99%	13 mL (0.4 oz.)
5th	104%	7 mL (0.2 oz.)
6th	109%	7 mL (0.2 oz.)
7th	111%	2 mL (0.1 oz.)

Adapted from (Kent et al., 2008)

An individual's responsiveness to different feels will also vary. In one Australian study (Kent et al., 2003), 28 mothers tested seven different breast pump cycling and suction patterns. Half responded well to all seven patterns, while the other half responded well only to some patterns or even to just one.

• • •

Whether parents are comfortable in their environment can affect milk ejection.

Changing the environment can sometimes produce higher milk yields. This may be done in several ways.

Express milk in a comfortable, familiar place, perhaps always sitting in the same comfortable chair, with good arm and back support, to allow complete relaxation.

Minimize distractions. Some start by turning off their phone, playing some relaxing music, and/or gathering what they need, such as a drink, a snack, or something to read. If at home with older children, suggest planning ahead for their needs. If away from home, suggest finding a comfortable, private place, where it's possible to relax without worrying about interruptions.

Follow a pre-expression ritual. Preparing to express in the same way each time can be a psychological trigger for relaxation and milk ejection. Possibilities include:

- Wrap a blanket, sweater, or jacket around the shoulders for warmth.
- Use gentle massage, gently tapping, rubbing, or rolling the nipples for stimulation.
- Spend 5 minutes relaxing by using childbirth breathing exercises, guided relaxation techniques, or just sitting quietly, using mental imagery to picture a warm beach or other relaxing setting.

• • •

If needed, massage, compression, and other sensory stimulation may help trigger milk ejections while expressing.

Massage is an essential ingredient of effective hand expression (see next section). With breast pumps, we used to think that just holding the pump parts against the nipples and letting the pump operate was enough to effectively express milk. We know now that pump alone only extracts some of the milk. When compression is either built in to a pump's function (Alekseev & Ilyin, 2016) or the user massages and compresses during the pump session (Morton et al., 2009), this pressure and touch helps trigger milk ejection and boosts milk yields. For details on how to do hands-on pumping techniques, see p. 492.

Any of the sensory pathways, as well as the mind and emotions (Cobo, 1993; Cowley, 2014), can help trigger milk ejections. If at first extra help is needed to trigger milk ejections, in addition to using massage and compression, suggest experimenting with the strategies below to see which work best. This will vary from person to person.

- **Sight:** Look at the baby or a photo or video of the baby.
- **Smell:** Smell the baby's blanket or clothing.
- **Touch:** Apply warmth to the mammary glands using wet or dry heat. Interrupt expressing several times to massage again.
- **Taste:** Sip a favorite warm drink or have a snack to help relax.

- **Hearing:** Listen to a recording of the baby cooing or crying. If the baby is not there, call and check on him, or as a distraction, call someone to chat. Access audio relaxation files, which can reduce stress and improve milk yields (Dabas, Joshi, Agarwal, Yadav, & Kachhawa, 2019; S. Feher, L. Berger, J. Johnson, & J. Wilde, 1989). Listening to music can also improve milk yields and even increase milk fat content (Ak, Lakshmanagowda, G, & Goturu, 2015; Keith, Weaver, & Vogel, 2012).
- **Mind/feelings:** Close the eyes, relax, and imagine the feel of skin-to-skin contact with the baby or imagine the baby nursing. Think loving thoughts about the baby.

Two Canadian articles described several women whose nerve pathways between breast and brain were physically damaged by cervical spinal cord injuries and were able to trigger milk releases with mental imagery alone (Cowley, 2005, 2014).

• • •

If milk ejection while expressing is delayed or inhibited, suggest expressing from one side while the baby nurses on the other side.

Some parents let down their milk easily to hand expression and pumping, while others find it more challenging. For a tiny minority, it may seem impossible. When parents try all of the previous tips and still struggle to express any milk, one nearly sure-fire strategy is for the baby to stimulate milk ejection by nursing while the parent expresses from the other side. An older baby may need little help (Figure 11.1). With a smaller baby, some parents hand-express with their free hand, using pillows to help support the baby's weight at the other side. Others use either a hands-free pump or one that can be operated with one hand. Expressing while the baby nurses can help condition a parent's body to the feel of the expression method, so that with practice milk ejections will happen even when the baby is not nursing.

• • •

If milk ejection is inhibited by stress or upset, suggest taking a break and trying again later.

A parent going through an emotional or physical crisis may find that milk ejection is temporarily affected. In extreme situations, this may affect milk production. If this happens, encourage continued nursing and/or expressing. Assure the family that milk ejection and production will quickly return to normal.

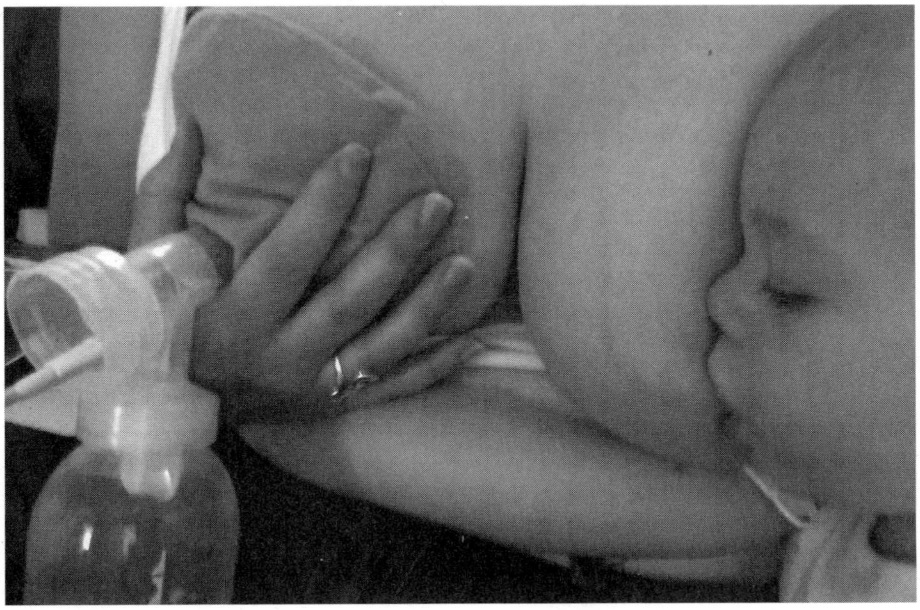

Figure 11.1 When milk ejection during pumping is a challenge, a good starting point is to pump one side while nursing on the other, so the baby can trigger the let-downs

MILK EXPRESSION METHODS

Deciding How to Express Milk

The most popular expression methods vary by decade and locale.

In some areas, such as rural coastal Kenya (Talbert, Tsofa, Mumbo, Berkley, & Mwangome, 2018), the idea of expressing milk and feeding it to the baby is foreign. In some parts of the developing world, however, hand expression is more common than breast pumps because pumps are beyond many families' means and power sources are not readily available (Glynn & Goosen, 2005).

In developed countries, electric breast pumps became more popular in recent years. A study on milk-expression trends in Australia between 1993 and 2003 (Binns, Win, Zhao, & Scott, 2006) noted that 60% of the mothers of term babies used and preferred manual pumps during the first 6 months after birth. However, in a 2016 Australian study of 772 mothers of term babies (Johns et al., 2016), there was a marked rise in the use of electric pumps, with 73% of first-time mothers using an electric pump compared with 55% of mothers with older children. Multiple expression methods were common in this group, as 65% also used a manual pump. More than half of these mothers also hand-expressed milk.

As previously noted, nearly all (98%) of U.S. families expect to get and use a breast pump after birth (Loewenberg Weisband et al., 2017). At this writing, the U.S. Affordable Care Act mandates that health-insurance companies provide families with a free pump. The type of free pump received varies by state, with the majority of states providing double electric pumps (Martin, 2011). Even before the passage of the Affordable Care Act, many U.S. families owned and used more than one type of pump (Labiner-Wolfe, Fein, Shealy, & Wang, 2008).

• • •

Parents' milk-expression needs vary by how often they express.

To better understand the situation of a family choosing an expression method, ask:

- **How often do they plan to express milk?** The parent separated from a hospitalized baby will have very different needs from those planning to express milk for an occasional missed feed. The expression method used is much more important if it needs to substitute for a nursing baby often or exclusively.
- **Are they familiar with any methods and do they have a preference?** If so, discuss the pros and cons of the preferred method in their situation (see next point) and mention other possible appropriate methods, so they can make an informed choice. If they have no preference, offer to describe the choices appropriate in their situation. For details about types of breast pumps, see Table 11.3 on p. 487.

• • •

Discuss hand expression and breast pumps, emphasizing that using them together usually gives the best results.

Rather than an either/or choice, suggest families think of hand expression and breast pumping as complementary. Unless for some reason one of them is not an option or the nursing parent gets significantly better results with hand expression alone, in most cases, using them together produces higher milk yields. For details on how to most effectively combine them with hands-on pumping techniques, see p. 492.

Some of the advantages of learning hand expression include:

- It's free of charge.
- In some parents, the skin-to-skin contact more quickly triggers milk ejection compared to the feel of plastic pump parts against the skin.
- During the first few days post-birth, it may be more effective than a pump in expressing the thick colostrum (Ohyama, Watabe, & Hayasaka, 2010).
- To some parents, it feels more "natural."
- Learning this skill during pregnancy boosts self-confidence in nursing (Demirci et al., 2019).
- It can be used as a back-up method when a pump malfunctions, parts are missing or lost, or its power source is unavailable.
- It's eco-friendly with no solid waste, no special equipment, and requires no electricity or other power sources, so it's ideal in emergencies.
- There are no "fit" issues.
- There is nothing to store or transport.
- Before and after expressing, the only thing that needs to be washed is the parent's hands.

But hand expression also has some drawbacks.

- There is a learning curve.
- It requires physical effort and can become tiring.
- It may take more time than double pumping if hand-expressing one side at a time.
- Hand expression alone may not yield as much milk as a double-electric pump, which can be a problem when establishing milk production with hand expression only (Lussier et al., 2015; T. Slusher et al., 2007; T. M. Slusher et al., 2012).
- Some parents feel uncomfortable with the act and even the idea of hand expressing.

Some advantages of using breast pumps include:

- Automatic pumps do much of the physical work of expressing.
- Double pumps usually express more milk in less time.
- There may be less of a learning curve than with hand expression.
- It may be more comfortable in those with limited hand movement or chronic wrist or hand pain.
- With hands-free double-pumping, it's possible to multi-task while expressing.
- For some, it is more effective than hand expression alone at establishing milk production when a baby is not yet nursing (Lussier et al., 2015; T. Slusher et al., 2007; T. M. Slusher et al., 2012).

Breast pumps also have drawbacks.

- The cost: double electric pumps may be beyond some families' means and some cheaper pumps may be ineffective or painful.
- Pump parts can break, melt, get lost, or be left behind by mistake, rendering the pump nonfunctional.

- Power sources may not always be available.
- The pump's sound may be irritating or draw unwelcome attention.
- The pump parts in contact with the milk need to be washed after each use, and a place to wash pump parts may not always be available.
- Less eco-friendly, as many pumps and their parts end up in landfills.

Hand Expression

Suggest experimenting with finger positions and techniques until hand expression works effectively.

Hand expression can stimulate milk production, provide milk for the baby, and relieve mammary fullness or engorgement. It is a useful skill that every nursing parent should know.

If parents plan to feed the baby the expressed milk, suggest they:

- Find a relaxing setting, such as a private, comfortable area with good body support.
- Wash hands thoroughly with soap and warm water.
- Have on hand a clean collection container, either one with a wide mouth, such as a cup, or during the first days after birth—when milk volumes are small—a clean spoon.

Finger placement: finding the "sweet spot." Effective hand-expression techniques vary from person to person. What's most important is finding the "sweet spot" on the mammary glands for best milk flow. Instructions that recommend finger placement using the areola as a guide can be misleading because of the large variation in areola size. Those with very large areolae may find their sweet spot within their areola and those with small areolae may find their sweet spot well away from it. During the early learning stages, one U.S. online video by pediatrician Jane Morton (**bit.ly/BA2-StanfordHandExpress**) suggests applying small circle band-aids to these sweet spots to make finding them easier the next time. Suggest parents tailor any instructions to their comfort and results.

KEY CONCEPT

Hand expression is a useful skill every nursing parent should have.

Hand-expression instructions vary by instructor (Becker & Roberts, 2009). The following technique is a combination of several, including one from the World Health Organization (WHO, 2009):

1. Before expressing, spend some time gently massaging the glands with hands and fingertips, a soft baby brush, or a warm towel. This video demo shows possible massage techniques, including fingertip tapping: **bit.ly/BA2-BolmanMassage**.
2. Sit up, leaning slightly forward to allow gravity to help with milk flow.
3. At the first expression, to find the sweet spots, start by putting thumb on top of the gland and fingers below about 1.5 inches (4 cm) from the nipple. Apply steady pressure into the gland toward the chest wall a few times. If no milk comes, shift finger and thumb placement farther away or closer to the nipple and compress again a few times. Repeat, moving finger and thumb until slightly firmer tissue is felt and pressure yields more milk. At future hand expressions, skip the "finding" phase and place fingers directly on this area.

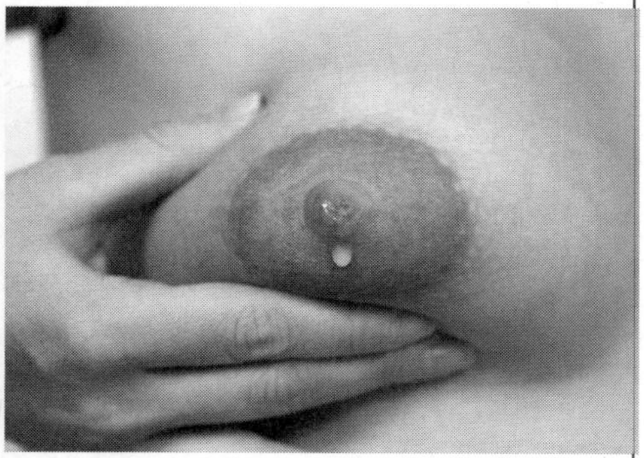

Figure 11.2 Hand expression is more comfortable and effective when the fingers are pushed back toward the chest wall rather than sliding out toward the nipple.

4. Apply steady pressure into the gland toward the chest wall, not toward the nipple. The idea is to put pressure on areas of milk within the gland.
5. As this inward pressure is applied, compress the pads of the thumb and fingers together (pushing in, not pulling out toward the nipple), finding a good rhythm of press-compress-relax, like a baby's sucking pattern.
6. Alternate sides every few minutes (5 or 6 times in total at each expression), rotating finger position, so that all areas of the mammary gland are expressed and feel soft, which usually takes about 20 to 30 minutes.

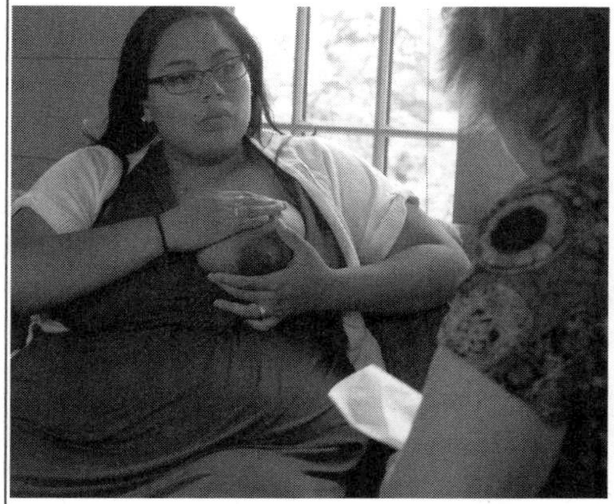

Figure 11.3 After warming her breast, this pregnant mother uses massage to help stimulate milk flow before hand expressing. ©2020 Nancy Mohrbacher Solutions, Inc.

Avoid sliding the fingers along the skin. See a video demonstration of one version of this technique at **bit.ly/BA2-StanfordHandExpress**.

If parents feel pain or discomfort, they may be compressing too hard, sliding their fingers along the skin, or squeezing the nipple itself, which can be both ineffective and painful. Ask them to describe what they are doing to determine what changes will make expression more comfortable.

• • •

With practice, a parent may be able to hand express while the baby nurses or express both sides at the same time.

To hand-express milk while baby is nursing, some use pillows or cushions to support the baby's body, so they have both hands free. Some learn to hand-express milk from both sides simultaneously, with the right hand expressing the right side and the left hand expressing the left side, with collection containers on a stable surface just below nipple level.

• • •

How hand expression during pregnancy is done depends in part on whether or not the milk will be collected and stored.

The first point in this chapter described why learning to express milk during the last month of an uncomplicated pregnancy is safe and recommended. If the pregnancy is low risk enough that the parent's healthcare provider considers it safe to continue having sex (which releases the same hormones as milk expression), then it is also safe to express milk.

Around the 36th or 37th week of pregnancy is a good time to begin. Start by warming the mammary glands. If the milk is not going be collected and stored right away, expressing in the shower may be a good beginning. If collecting the colostrum, expressing after a shower a bath may make the process easier. After warming the glands, use massage (Figure 11. 3) to stimulate the release of the hormone oxytocin, which triggers milk flow. Then follow the steps described in the description of hand expression technique beginning on the previous page. If any pain or discomfort is felt, suggest stopping and evaluating what needs to change. Ideally, hand expression should always be done gently enough to feel comfortable.

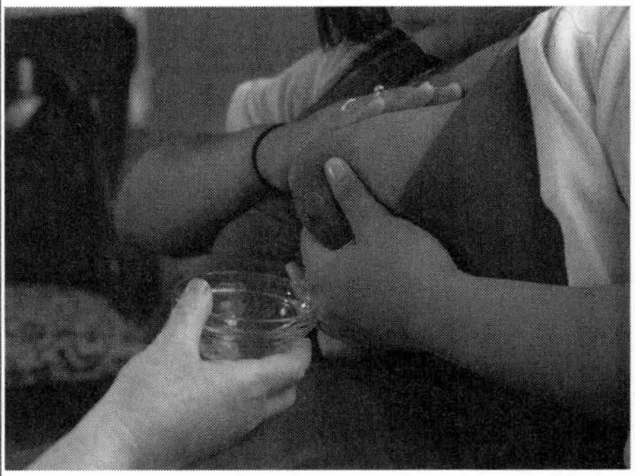

Figure 11.4 Depending on the volume of colostrum expressed, it may be collected in a small cup, vial, or syringe. ©2020 Nancy Mohrbacher Solutions, Inc.

If the plan is to collect and store the expressed colostrum, the drops can be sucked up into a syringe or collected in a small clean cup (Figure 11.4) or vial. Plan to hand-express milk from both sides for about 5 minutes per side. Some parents do this just once each day. Others do it more often, depending on the situation. The collected colostrum can be stored in the refrigerator between collections. If a syringe is used, avoid overfilling it to allow room for expansion during freezing. Once the syringe is full enough, put on the cap and freeze. If the colostrum will be used to supplement the newborn during the first days after birth, plan to freeze it in volumes of no larger than 10 to 20 mL, (0.3 to 0.5 oz.).

The Warm Bottle Method

The warm bottle method is a low-tech way to provide relief to an engorged parent.

A middle ground between hand expression and a pump, the warm bottle method can be ideal for an engorged parent without access to an effective pump who has not mastered hand expression or whose mammary glands are so taut that hand expression is difficult.

• • •

This method uses a glass bottle with a mouth about 2 inches (5 cm) in diameter and requires access to hot water.

Any clean glass bottle with a mouth diameter of at least 2 inches (5 cm) will work. A 1 liter or larger bottle is ideal. To use this method, suggest the parent:

- Slowly fill the bottle with hot water and let it stand for a few minutes.
- Wrap a cloth around the bottle and pour out the hot water.
- Allow the neck of the bottle to cool and then place the mouth over the nipple and areola to form an airtight seal.
- As the bottle cools slowly, gentle suction is created, which draws the nipple into the bottle's neck. The warmth of the bottle and the gentle suction usually triggers a milk ejection, expressing milk.
- When the milk flow slows, break the suction and remove the mammary gland.
- If discomfort is felt break the suction. (Limit the time the bottle is on the gland.)
- Pour out the milk and repeat on the other side.

If the glass bottle and the parent's hands are clean, this milk can be stored or fed. Avoid too-rapid cooling, as it causes more suction, which can lead to discomfort.

Breast Pumps

If parents ask for help in choosing a breast pump, ask about their situation, including how often they plan to pump.

When a pump is only used occasionally, its type, make, and model are not critical for meeting long-term feeding goals. A 2016 Cochrane Review on milk-expression methods (Becker, Smith, & Cooney, 2016) examined 34 randomized controlled trials and found no consistent differences in milk yield among manual and electric pumps. This is encouraging for families in resource-poor areas. This systematic review found that many of the strategies to increase milk yields during expression described beginning on p. 491 may offset the use of a less-effective pump. Its authors noted that (Becker et al., 2016, p. 3):

> "Low-cost measures such as starting to express milk early for an infant unable to breastfeed, relaxation, breast massage, warming of the breasts, hand expression, and lower-cost pumps may be as effective, or more, than large electric pumps for some outcomes."

Most manual pumps require the muscle power of squeezing or pushing a handle to operate (see later point), so if a parent uses it often or exclusively, it could quickly become tiring. This is why for many families planning to pump often or exclusively, manual pumps are not optimal. That said, however, a U.S. randomized controlled trial of low-income U.S. women receiving either a double electric pump or a manual pump when returning to work (Hayes et al., 2008) found no differences in nursing outcomes between the two groups.

TABLE 11.3 Types of Breast Pumps Well Suited for Different Situations

Situation	Manual Pump	Single-User Double Electric Pump	Multi-User Double Electric Pump (rental-grade)
Pumping occasionally (<1 missed feed/day)	X	X	X
Pumping daily (>1 missed feed/day ≥5 days/week)		X	X
Baby not nursing, establishing full milk production			X
Baby not nursing, maintaining full milk production		X	X

Adapted from (Eglash & Malloy, 2015; P. P. Meier, Patel, Hoban & Engstrom, 2016)

• • •

There is no one "best" breast pump.

It is tempting to assume that a pump brand with lots of research to its name must provide the highest milk yields. However, much of the breast-pump research is sponsored by the breast-pump industry, which has a vested interest in presenting its products in the best possible light. Studies that compare pumps often evaluate the previous version of the company's product against its "new-and-improved" version (P. P. Meier, Engstrom, Janes, Jegier, & Loera, 2012; Post, Stam, & Tromp, 2016), which does not compare one brand to others. Or a new feature, like 2-phase pumping (a pump programmed to provide faster then slower pump cycling) is introduced with the claim that it yields "more milk faster," but according to the fine print, this claim is only true when comparing double pumping with single pumping. In other words, this new feature actually pumped the same milk volumes overall as its previous single-phase version. In studies that compare one brand of breast pump to another, research done in NICUs (Burton et al., 2013) and that followed mothers of term babies for 6 months (M. Fewtrell et al., 2019) found the "premium" brands and models no more effective than the others.

When helping families sort through their options, keep in mind that there is no single "best" pump. Nursing parents respond differently to the same pumping patterns (Kent et al., 2003). In most situations there are multiple pump options, all of which may be good choices. See Table 11.3 for suggestions on what basic types of pumps are well suited to which situations.

• • •

Manual pumps are operated in several different ways.

Manual pumps have no motor and rely on the user to generate suction, either with a foot (pedal pumps) or using a hand to squeeze or pull a handle. See the last point in this section for suggestions on what type of pumping rhythm to try with manual pumps.

Since the last edition of this book, a new type of manual pump entered the marketplace that is unlike the others. Made by several different companies and composed entirely of food-grade silicone, the user squeezes the soft container

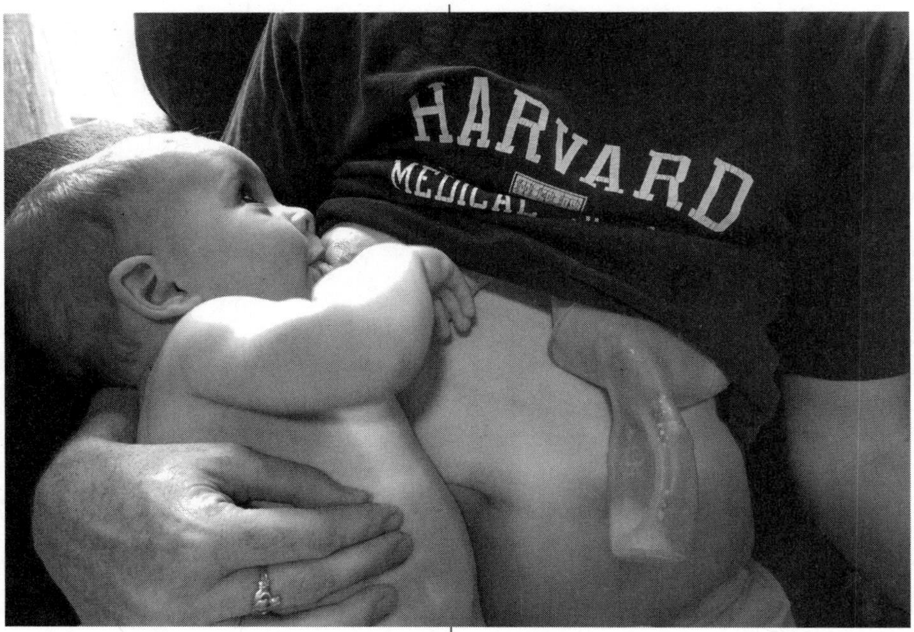

Figure 11.5 All-silicone manual pumps can simplify pumping by collecting milk on one side while baby nurses on the other.

to generate the suction, covers the nipple with the opening, and releases the squeeze, which fixes the pump to that side. Depending on the shape of the mammary gland, the user may be able to leave it there hands-free while its continuous suction draws out the milk. This all-silicone pump can be used to collect milk on one side while baby nurses on the other side (Figure 11.5).

The popularity of this new type of all-silicone manual pump has raised questions.

- Does its regular use during the early weeks contribute to oversupply?
- Is its continuous suction (rather than the suction-and-release action of other manual and electric pumps) less effective at boosting or maintaining milk production?

We don't yet have the answers to these questions, but caution is warranted.

• • •

When a family depends on a pump to regularly or exclusively substitute for a nursing baby, some pump features are important to consider.

When a parent is "pump dependent," or relies on a pump to build or maintain milk production, what features are important?

Multi-user, rental-grade electric pumps. When establishing milk production without a nursing baby, a multi-user pump is usually the first choice, when available (Eglash & Malloy, 2015; P. P. Meier et al., 2016). Due to their high cost, these pumps are usually rented and are designed to be shared by multiple users, who each own their own "milk collection kit," so their milk never comes in contact with the milk of another user. One aspect of these multi-user pumps that makes them especially well-suited to establishing milk production is that most provide more suction and cycles settings than the single-user pumps more commonly purchased. Having more settings allows parents to better customize the pump to their body's response. Although sometimes referred to as "hospital-grade," this term is unrelated to pump effectiveness. It is used by the pump manufacturers to describe whether the pump has a two-pronged or three-pronged plug.

Single-user double electric pumps. When a family purchases a breast pump that will be used often or exclusively, suggest they consider the following basic features:

- **A motor warranty of at least 1 year,** a sign of durability
- **Several "fit" options.** Pumps whose nipple tunnels are made of hard plastic should have at least 3 different nipple-tunnel diameters available separately (see p. 907-908).

- **Separate vacuum (suction) and cycle (speed) controls,** to better customize pump settings to an individual's body response
- **A maximum suction level of at least 250 mm/Hg**

Other pump features that may affect parents' choice include:

- **Power sources.** Do they need their pump to run on batteries as well as electricity?
- **Noise level and quality.** Will they be pumping in a place where noise level or quality could be an issue? Do they find the pump sound tolerable, or is it really irritating?
- **Easy care and cleaning.** How many pump parts need to be cleaned after use? The design of some pumps allows expressed milk or milk particles to enter its tubing, making it necessary to sometimes clean or replace the pump tubing or spend extra time allowing the pump to run after pumping to dry out the tubing. Other pumps are designed with a solid barrier between the milk and the tubing to eliminate this issue.
- **Hands-free option.** Some pumps are designed to be used hands free. Hands-free pumps fall into two main categories: 1) pumps with tubing that connects the milk-collection pieces to the pump motor (some motors are small enough to attach to the user's clothing for greater freedom of movement), or 2) pumps whose motor is part of the milk-collection unit and do not require tubing or bottles, giving the user complete freedom of movement. At this writing, the second type is more expensive and its effectiveness depends in large part on the shape of the user's mammary glands and whether the pump's nipple opening fits well enough to maintain the consistent air seal needed for pump suction. Some pumps can be adapted for hands-free use with special bands or bras.

• • •

If there is less than 20 minutes to pump, consider a double pump; if single-pumping, switch sides often.

Double pumps save time (Becker et al., 2016). Single pumping usually takes about 20 to 30 minutes total, as it's necessary to pump one side at a time. A double pump allows both sides to be pumped at the same time, which can cut expression time in half.

If single-pumping, suggest switching sides when the milk flow slows, usually every 5 to 7 minutes, and expressing from each side several times at each pump session. Because both sides should be well drained using this approach, the milk's fat content should be the same as double-pumping. In some parents, alternating sides more effectively triggers milk ejection (Morton et al., 2009).

• • •

Milk-flow rates during pumping vary greatly among parents but are consistent over time in individuals, which can help determine how many minutes to pump.

Table 11.2 on p. 479 reflects average milk flow rates during pumping, but individuals' expression patterns vary tremendously. A 2012 Australian study of 34 mothers whose milk flow was measured throughout multiple 15-minute pump sessions (D. K. Prime, Kent, Hepworth, Trengove, & Hartmann, 2012) found huge variations in their milk flow. Some pumped 60% of their available milk within the first minute of pumping, while others pumped as much as 20% of their available milk as late as 14 minutes into their pump sesions. The most significant finding was that although milk-flow patterns varied from person to person, they stayed consistent in the same person over time. In fact, a 2017

Australian study by the same team (Gardner et al., 2017) found that these milk-flow patterns were even consistent from the first baby to the second.

Individualizing pumping time. This information revealed how we can help families find their own optimal length of pumping, assuming they are using the pump alone rather than hands-on pumping (see p. 492). To help parents determine the optimal number of minutes they should pump, first suggest they pump several times for about 20 minutes and observe their milk flow. If milk flow ends within the first 5 minutes of pumping, that should be an adequate length of time for them. But if they are still getting considerable milk near the 15-minute mark, a longer pump session would provide better milk removal.

• • •

When using a manual or electric breast pump, adjust the pump's vacuum and cycle options to produce higher milk yields.

Whether the pump is electric with automatic suction-and-release or manual, where users control its suction and cycling with their hands, the following strategies may help pump more milk faster.

Pump cycles (speed). If the baby is nursing and the parent's body is conditioned to the baby's sucking patterns, suggest starting with this approach either by hand or with the pump's cycle settings to mimic the baby's nursing pattern.

- Start at a fast speed to trigger milk ejection more quickly
- At milk ejection—when milk starts flowing faster—decrease the speed to slow to drain the milk faster.
- As the milk flow slows to a trickle, return to a fast speed again to more quickly trigger the next milk ejection
- Repeat until done, using milk flow as a guide.

It is always wise to experiment and use whatever approach produces faster milk flow. Some of the "2-phase" pumps can cycle as fast as 120 cycles per minute (cpm), but Australian research (Ramsay et al., 2006) found that 86% of its study mothers expressed no milk at all at this very fast cycle speed, so suggest minimizing any time spent at that setting. (In some pumps, 120 cpm is the first phase of its "2-phase" pumping.) Before milk ejection, at a pump setting of 120 cpm mothers average only 1 to 2.7 mL of milk (Kent et al., 2008) compared with 10 mL (about one-third ounce) at 60 cpm (Ramsay et al., 2005).

Pump vacuum. Australian research found that milk yields are higher and milk flows faster when pump vacuum is set at the highest comfortable setting during milk ejection (Kent et al., 2008). The highest comfortable vacuum setting varies by person and could be anywhere in the pump's vacuum range. Some had the highest milk yields at an electric pump's lowest vacuum setting.

KEY CONCEPT

Too-high pump suction can inhibit milk ejection, so the goal is to use the highest suction setting that's truly comfortable, which varies greatly among parents.

Encourage parents to experiment with their pump's controls, as individuals respond differently to the same stimuli. For example, one U.S. study (P. P. Meier et al., 2008) found that in those study mothers who were conditioned to pumping at a fixed cycle speed (50 cpm), the time it took for their first milk ejection to occur was delayed by a full minute when they switched to a pump that began at 120 cpm. As parents experiment with their pump's controls, encourage them to use those settings that produce the fastest milk flow.

MILK EXPRESSION STRATEGIES

Boosting Milk Yields

In the days after birth, a relaxed environment, skin-to-skin contact, warm compresses, and reverse pressure softening may boost milk yields.

Expressing thick colostrum after birth, when milk volumes are low, may be challenging for some parents and the healthcare providers who help them. Expressing colostrum within the first hour of delivery usually yields much more milk than if the first expression occurs later (see the later section "Stage 1: The First Few Days" on p. 498). When colostrum is not forthcoming, it may help to keep in mind that milk expression is not like turning on a faucet. As described in the previous section on milk ejection, the release of oxytocin is vital to milk removal. For oxytocin release to occur, parents need to feel emotionally comfortable, so a relaxed environment and patience are important. In addition to the massage that is a normal part of hand-expressing, it may also help to first spend 15 minutes or more in skin-to-skin contact with the baby, which triggers oxytocin release. Warm compresses on the mammary glands also contribute to relaxation and oxytocin release. For some, the use of reverse pressure softening (see p. 885) makes hand-expression of colostrum more effective.

• • •

When milk yields in pump-dependent parents are lower than expected, first review the basics.

Before offering strategies to boost production, first start with these questions:

- **How many times per day do they pump?** Don't focus on the time intervals between sessions (e.g., every 3 hours), as this doesn't give the full picture. Instead, ask the times of each pump session on a typical day and then add them together for the daily total. If this number is less than 8, ask if they would consider adding more pump sessions.
- **About how many minutes long is each pump session?** Are they single- or double-pumping? Are they using hands-on pumping techniques (see next point)? If so, ask them to go over what they are doing at each pump session step by step. They may be missing a step or two, or there may be some ways to increase the effectiveness of their routine.
- **What is the longest stretch between pump sessions?** Stretches longer than about 8 hours cause a slow decrease in milk production for many (Mohrbacher, 2011). If they're not pumping at least once during the night, ask if they would be willing to do so.
- **Which pump(s) are they using?** Which brands and models? Are these pumps effective enough for their situation? If not, is it possible for them to upgrade?
- **When was the pump fit last checked?** Even with a good fit at first, pump fit can change with time and pumping (Francis & Dickton, 2019; P. Meier et al., 2004; Wilson-Clay & Hoover, 2017). For details about checking pump fit, see p. 907-908.
- **How much time do they spend each day in skin-to-skin contact with their baby?** Skin-to-skin contact is associated with higher milk yields (Acuna-Muga et al., 2014; Hurst, Valentine, Renfro, Burns, & Ferlic, 1997).
- **What is their feeding goal?** Parents who plan to pump short term may not want to spend as much time on boosting milk production as those who intend to express long term.

> **KEY CONCEPT**
>
> *Usually, parents who say they pump every 3 hours don't pump 8 times per day. Ask when each pump session occurred in the last 24 hours.*

Ask about health-related factors that affect milk production.

Discuss aspects of the nursing parent's health that might affect milk production, such as taking a medication that affects lactation, a history of breast or chest surgery, or any other health problems. See Box 10.2 on p. 441 for a complete list.

• • •

Hands-on pumping is an effective strategy, which research found increased milk yields by an average of nearly 50%.

Whenever milk yields are critical—pumping for a very tiny preemie, increasing low milk production, returning to work full time away from baby—hands-on pumping techniques can effectively pump more milk. Hands-on pumping was developed by U.S. pediatrician Jane Morton, and her research revealed that for the best results, it is not wise to rely on the pump alone. Using manual techniques (massage, compression, hand expression) with the pump makes a major short-term and long-term difference in milk yields. In Morton's study, 52 mothers pumped exclusively for 8 weeks for very tiny preemies in the NICU (Morton et al., 2009). Those who used hands-on pumping techniques averaged nearly 50% more milk than those who used the pump alone.

In years past, those pumping milk for very preterm babies typically peaked at about 3 to 4 weeks after delivery and then plateaued or declined in milk volumes (Hill, Aldag, Chatterton, & Zinaman, 2005), but thanks to hands-on pumping, the mothers in Morton's study were still seeing an increase in milk production 8 weeks after delivery.

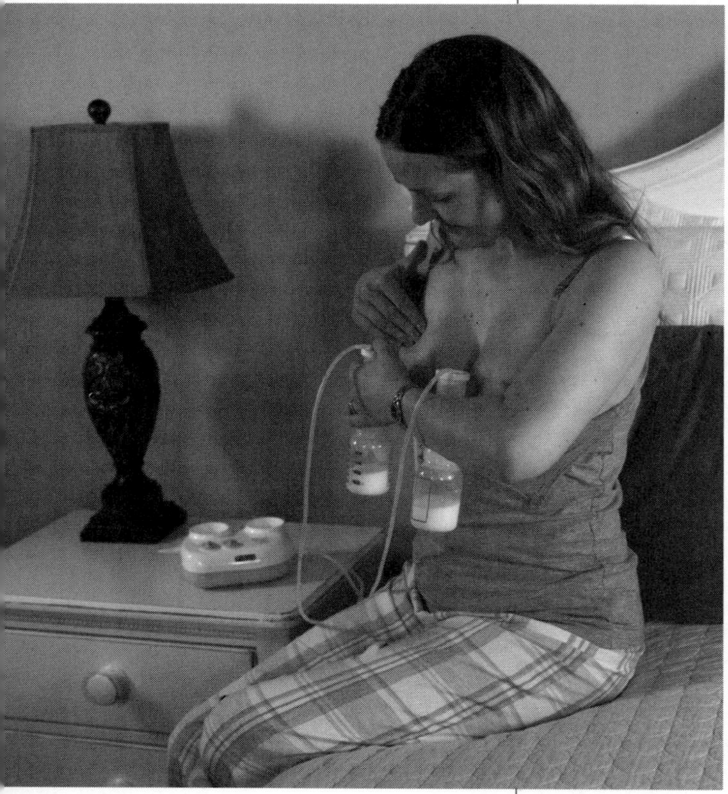

Figure 11.6 This mother shows how to support her double pump kit with one hand and arm while using the other hand to do the compression and massage for hands-on pumping.

To do hands-on pumping, follow the steps below. In the Morton study, a pump session using these techniques took on average 25 minutes. A video demo from Stanford University is suitable for sharing with families at **bit.ly/BA2-HandsOnPumpingDemo**.

1. **Massage** both mammary glands. Allow about a minute or so of massage, which stimulates the hormones that enhance milk flow.
2. **Double pump while compressing and massaging.** This can be done one-handed while using the other hand and arm to support the pump pieces (Figure 11.6) or using a hands-free pumping band or bra to free both hands (shown in the video demo).
3. **Massage again.** After milk flow during double pumping slows to a trickle (after maybe 10 to 15 minutes), take off the pump parts and massage again for a minute or so, taking special care to massage any areas that still feel hard or full.
4. **Finish with either hand expression or single pumping,** whichever is more effective, focusing on one side at a time and going back and forth from side to side, using compression and massage on that side until both sides feel well drained.

Hands-on pumping is most effective when used after milk increase, usually the third or fourth day after birth. For pumping strategies effective before then, see p. 498. To provide the above instructions to families, share this author's post at **bit.ly/BA2-HandsOnPumpNM** which includes links to the Stanford videos.

• • •

A Turkish study of 39 mothers who were exclusively pumping for preterm babies randomized which breast was warmed before pumping (Yigit et al., 2012). A compress was warmed for 1 minute in a microwave set at 180 W and then applied to one breast for 20 minutes, followed by a pump session. This process was repeated twice a day at the same time intervals for 3 days. The researchers found that the warmed breast yielded on average about 40% more than the unwarmed breast.

Applying warmth before pumping increased milk yields by about 40%.

• • •

Research found several audio techniques that increased milk yields during pumping.

Audio-assisted relaxation techniques and music therapy effectively reduced stress and anxiety and increased milk yields and milk fat content.

Guided relaxation techniques. As described earlier in this chapter, a lactating parent's emotions during milk expression can affect milk ejection and therefore milk yields. A 2019 Indian non-blinded randomized controlled trial (Dabas et al., 2019) found that of its 74 mothers of preterm babies, those who used audio-assisted relaxation techniques had reduced stress and anxiety scores and had statistically significant increases in milk output (69 mL versus 54 mL, about a 22% increase). In one U.S. study (S. D. Feher, L. R. Berger, J. D. Johnson, & J. B. Wilde, 1989) its mothers expressed 121% more milk during the second week while listening at times other than pumping to a 20-minute audiotape on relaxation and visual imagery than they did while pumping at other times.

Music therapy also appears to be effective at reducing stress and increasing pumping milk yields. Another Indian study compared the effects of music therapy before and during pump sessions on both milk yields and stress levels (Ak et al., 2015). Each mother of a preterm baby served as her own control, receiving music therapy for 2 pump sessions and pumping for 2 sessions without music. It found that the music therapy was associated with significantly lower stress levels and significantly higher milk volumes.

Comparison of both strategies. A U.S. randomized controlled trial divided the mothers of 162 preterm and critically ill babies into 4 groups and followed them for 14 days (Keith et al., 2012). The control group (D), received standard support and lactation education. The other 3 groups received mp3 players with a video screen and 12 minutes of one of the following:

KEY CONCEPT

Providing exclusively pumping parents with an audio file of guided relaxation and music improved their milk yields.

A. Audio guided relaxation techniques

B. Audio guided relaxation techniques plus lullabies on guitar

C. Audio guided relaxation techniques, lullabies on guitar, and images of their baby

Although there was no statistically significant difference in the number of pump sessions among the 4 groups, the mothers in the control group D produced the smallest volumes of milk. Those in group A, who listened only to the audio relaxation techniques, pumped the highest milk volumes, as well as the milk that was highest in fat content. The differences among the groups were statistically significant.

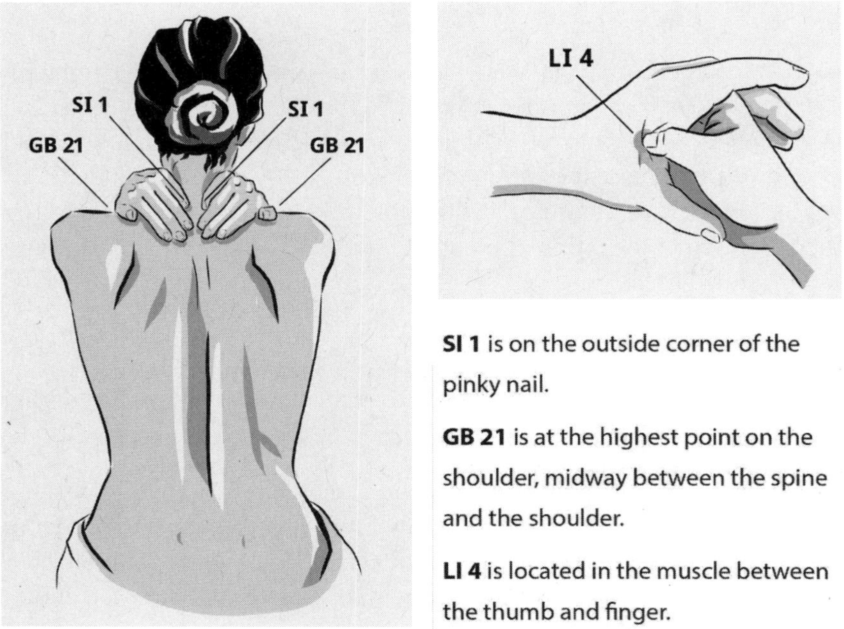

SI 1 is on the outside corner of the pinky nail.

GB 21 is at the highest point on the shoulder, midway between the spine and the shoulder.

LI 4 is located in the muscle between the thumb and finger.

Figure 11.7 The acupressure (acupoints) points found effective at boosting milk production are SI 1 on the outside corner of the pinky nail, GB 21 at the highest point on the shoulder midway between the spine and the shoulder, and LI 4 in the muscle between thumb and finger. ©2020 Julia Eva Bacon, used with permission.

• • •

Acupuncture and acupressure boost pumping milk yields in some.

Acupuncture and acupressure are practiced worldwide but originate from traditional Chinese medicine. Acupuncture is done by inserting very fine needles into specific areas on the body. Acupressure is done without needles by applying pressure to these areas (see p. 881-884). A 2015 Iranian randomized clinical trial on 60 lactating women with low milk production measured the effects of acupressure on pumping milk yields (Esfahani, Berenji-Sooghe, Valiani, & Ehsanpour, 2015). The women in the intervention group were trained to apply on 12 consecutive days bilateral pressure to three acupressure points (SI 1, LI 4, and GB 21, see Figure 11.7) for 2 to 5 minutes three times per day. The control group received routine education. Before the intervention began, milk yields at 1 hour after nursing were comparable in the two groups (10.5 mL in the intervention group and 9.5 mL in the control group). At both 2 and 4 weeks, the acupressure group pumped significantly more milk (33 mL vs. 18 mL and 36 mL vs. 18 mL). These three acupressure points are easily reached by parents with normal dexterity, but this is also something a partner or support person could do.

• • •

Strategies to boost milk production usually boost pumping milk yields.

See the section beginning on p. 442 in the previous chapter for a variety of strategies to boost milk production. These include basic dynamics (like more frequent and effective milk removal) and others, including the use of galactogogues, or milk-enhancing substances. Boosting milk production is an off-label use of drugs like metoclopramide (Reglan™) and domperidone (Motilium™), which contribute to a small-to-moderate increase in some users. For details on these drugs and some commonly used plant-based and galactogogues, see p. 449. It is appropriate for lactation supporters to provide information to parents and their healthcare providers about these options, so they evaluate them in light of the parent's medical history.

Relieving Engorgement

The tissue swelling that comes with engorgement (see p. 748) can make milk expression challenging. Begin with the previous strategies mentioned for triggering milk ejection during expression and those for boosting milk yields in the previous section. In addition, the following strategies may also be helpful.

During engorgement, massage and reverse pressure softening may boost milk yields.

Breast massage. As mentioned previously, various types of breast massage are used worldwide during lactation. Research and clinical practice (Bolman, Saju, Oganesyan, Kondrashova, & Witt, 2013) found some types of massage helpful in relieving engorgement. At about time stamp 2:50, this video demo shows a technique for using olive oil and massage together during engorgement to relieve swelling: **bit.ly/BA2-BolmanMassage**

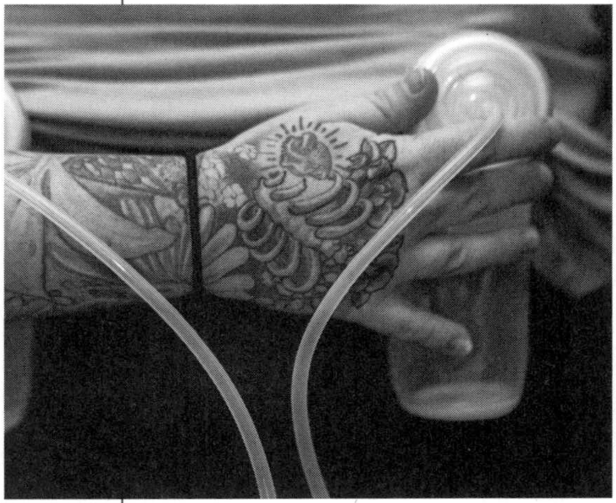

Reverse pressure softening (RPS) is a technique developed by U.S. lactation consultant Jean Cotterman (Cotterman, 2004), which involves using gentle finger and hand pressure to move the tissue swelling of engorgement further back into the mammary gland, making it easier for the baby to latch. When RPS is used before pumping or hand expression, it may help the milk flow more quickly and easily (p. 885).

Storing Milk While Exclusively Nursing

Several approaches can be used to express and store milk while exclusively nursing. Because babies take, on average, less than 70% of the available milk at a feed (Kent, 2007), there will usually be some milk left to express, even right after a nursing. But by waiting a little while, there will be more available milk to express. Most nursing parents express more milk in the morning than later in the day, perhaps because after the newborn period babies tend to have longer stretches between feeds at night (see p. 78).

Expressing both sides about 30 to 60 minutes after a morning nursing usually yields the most milk for storage without affecting nursing.

• • •

If an hour passes between a milk expression and the next nursing, the baby's feeding pattern will not usually be affected. However, if the baby wants to feed sooner, encourage the parent to nurse anyway. Most babies will be patient with the slower milk flow. The baby may simply feed longer, take each side more than once, or want to nurse again sooner than usual.

If the baby wants to nurse soon after expressing both sides, encourage the parent to go ahead and nurse.

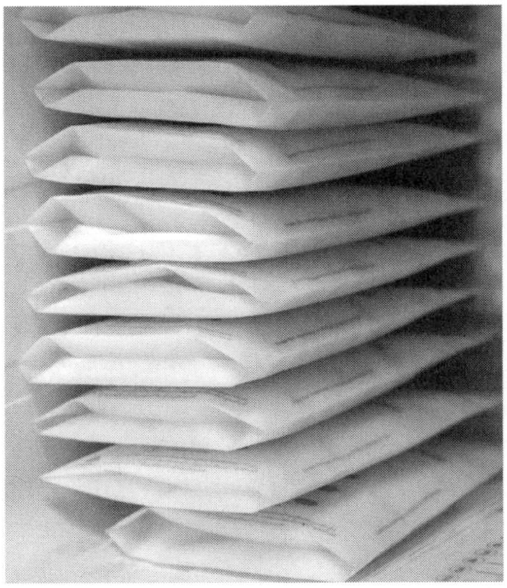

• • •

Some parents feel more comfortable expressing from one side, leaving the other side fuller in case the baby wants to nurse. This can work especially well if the baby usually takes one side at a feed, but this way less milk will be expressed for storage.

Another option is to express milk from one side during or between feeds.

Expressing for Regularly Missed Feeds

Knowing milk-production basics enables parents to keep it steady long term, even when regularly separated from the baby.

Whether nursing parents are regularly away from their baby due to employment, school, or other commitments, they can continue to nurse and maintain milk production. See Chapter 15, "Employment" on p. 656-659 for specific tips for planning daily routines and milk expression strategies to help maintain milk production over the long term.

Exclusive Pumping

When nursing is not an option, exclusive pumping can make it possible for the baby to be partially or exclusively human-milk fed.

Effective milk expression becomes critical when parents want their baby to be exclusively or mostly human-milk fed but they either choose not to nurse directly or their baby cannot nurse due to illness, prematurity, or other reasons. In these situations, milk expression must take the baby's place in establishing milk production. Effective expression is also vital when a parent needs to maintain milk production temporarily, such as during a nursing strike, a separation, or when taking a medication incompatible with nursing. This section describes expression strategies that can help families in different situations meet their feeding goals.

• • •

Exclusive pumping is becoming more common.

U.S. and Australian studies published between 2005 and 2010 (Clemons & Amir, 2010; Geraghty, Khoury, & Kalkwarf, 2005) found that most of those exclusively pumping (about 4% to 5% of nursing families) were parents of preterm babies who had not made the transition to direct nursing. But during the next decade, the percentage of families exclusively pumping rose. A 2017 U.S. prospective study that surveyed 478 mothers (Loewenberg Weisband et al., 2017) found that the percentage of the mothers who exclusively pump was about 7%.

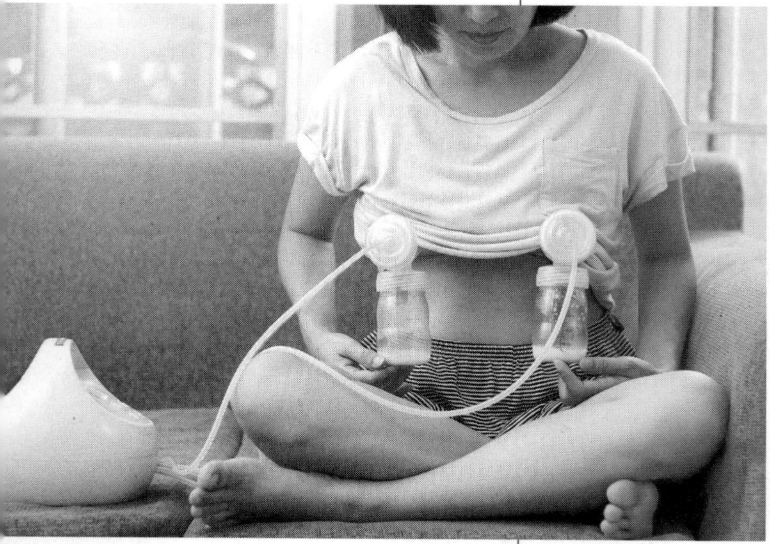

Increases in exclusive pumping appear to be more extreme in Asia. A Hong Kong prospective study that followed the feeding practices of 2,450 mothers for 12 months in 2006 and 2007 and then again in 2011 and 2012 (Bai et al., 2017) found that among the 2006 and 2007 group, about 5% to 8% of those with 3-month-old babies exclusively pumped. By 2011 to 2012, this rose to 18% to 19%. Another 2017 multi-ethnic Asian study (Pang et al., 2017) used data from the 1,247 women in the Growing Up in Singapore Towards healthy Outcomes (GUSTO) birth cohort and found that nearly 17% of its study mothers exclusively pumped.

Exclusive pumping is linked to shorter duration of lactation. All of these studies found that families who exclusively pumped had a shorter duration of human-milk feeding and an earlier introduction of formula compared with those who either mixed-fed or who only directly nursed. This is not surprising, as exclusive pumping is more time consuming than direct nursing. For this reason, it's important to give exclusively pumping families emotional support as they continue doing "triple-duty" (pump, feed, clean) to provide mother's milk to their babies.

• • •

Some parents plan to directly nurse but end up exclusively pumping at birth because their baby was very preterm, very ill, or was unable to nurse effectively for other reasons. In other cases, birth-related emotional or physical trauma can trigger anxiety, which can influence feeding. In one U.K. study on the effect of parenting style on nursing (Brown & Arnott, 2014), 508 U.K. women with babies 0 to 12 months old completed a questionnaire about breastfeeding duration and behaviors. It measured their anxiety levels and their attitudes about routine and nurturing behaviors. The authors noted that the subset of study women who exclusively pumped (7% of the 430 women whose babies were human-milk fed) had the highest anxiety levels and suggested a possible connection between early trauma, anxiety, and exclusive pumping (Brown & Arnott, 2014, p. e83893):

Anxiety may influence some parents' decision to exclusively pump.

> "...a negative birth experience can have a major impact on a new mother. It can increase maternal anxiety for her infant that can last into childhood. Concerns regarding growth and milk supply are especially strong. Here, mothers who expressed breast milk at birth reported the highest levels of anxiety regarding their infant suggesting that early parenting style may be affected by significant experiences surrounding the birth and first year."

Another source of anxiety that leads some families to exclusively pump is a history of childhood sexual abuse. Many with this history find nursing a healing experience, but for others, the act of nursing can raise anxiety levels and trigger flashbacks (Kendall-Tackett, Cong, & Hale, 2013; Klaus, 2010). Although these families start nursing at similar or higher rates than other families, the incidence of nursing problems may be higher (Elfgen, Hagenbuch, Gorres, Block, & Leeners, 2017) and duration of nursing may be shorter (Coles, Anderson, & Loxton, 2016). For more details see p. 840.

• • •

A 2019 U.S. cross-sectional, mixed-methods online survey administered to a convenience sample of 1,215 current or previous exclusively pumping mothers (Jardine, 2019) found that 71% received no information about exclusive pumping before their baby's birth. The 24% who had heard about it before birth reported feeling more knowledgeable about exclusive pumping and experienced less of the negative feelings (frustration, insecurity, depression, rejection, embarrassment, envy, and guilt) than those who were unaware of this option. The author suggested including some information about exclusive pumping during pregnancy.

Exclusive pumping may be a more positive experience when parents learn something about it before their baby's birth.

Establishing Full Milk Production with Pumping

Many parents unexpectedly faced with a pump instead of a nursing baby have strong feelings about their situation. If a baby is born very preterm, see p. 344 for more about this emotional rollercoaster. Many find exclusive pumping exhausting, even degrading, with some feeling "like a cow" (Bujold, Feeley, Axelin, & Cinquino, 2018). Other common feelings are "paradoxical," in other words, pumping feels like both a connection to their baby and a wedge between them. If the baby is ill or very preterm, parents may need to grieve the normal birth and nursing they expected before accepting their situation emotionally.

If parents didn't plan to exclusively pump, most have very mixed feelings about it, especially at first.

• • •

If parents are exclusively pumping or considering it when they could be nursing, offer to help them meet their feeding goals before discussing the advantages of direct nursing.

The most important thing when discussing exclusive pumping with families is to avoid making any assumptions about their feeding goals. Rather than trying to talk them into nursing, a better start is to say: "I can help you. I have the information you need to make this work." When some exclusively pumping parents are told first why they should instead begin direct nursing, they may tune this out and contact someone else.

Exclusive pumping is possible for most families, but once they knows this and know you are willing to help them, it is also important for them to know that exclusive pumping takes much more time and work than direct nursing—often double or triple the time due to the time it takes to pump, feed, and clean equipment. Some parents are unaware of this and may be motivated by this information to nurse instead.

KEY CONCEPT

When parents express the desire to exclusively pump, offer help and support before discussing alternatives.

If the parent considering exclusive pumping is in the midst of nursing struggles, it's important to convey that most nursing problems are fixable. However, in some cases, parents may feel stressed and/or exhausted from working on nursing and may want to take a break from it. If so, convey that even after taking a break, it is possible to return to direct nursing later when they are feeling more relaxed and ready. For details, see the later section on p. 508, "Transitioning to Direct Nursing."

Stage 1: The First Few Days

If the goal is full milk production, due to the unique hormonal dynamics of the first 2 weeks, suggest setting as a goal full production by about 10 days or so.

Full milk production is about 750 to 887 mL (25 to 30 ounces) per baby per day (Spatz, 2021, p. 408). As explained on p. 410 in the previous chapter, during the first 2 weeks after birth, mammary stimulation and milk removal profoundly affect blood levels of prolactin, a hormone involved in milk production. This intense hormonal response is unique to the first 2 weeks, so during this critical time window, parents get the maximum results for their pumping efforts. It is possible to increase milk production later, but it requires much more time and effort. For this reason, a logical goal is to reach full milk production within the first 2 weeks.

Make sure the family knows that the milk production goal of 750 mL per day per baby is about as much milk as the baby will ever need, no matter how big he gets (for details, see p.424-425). In the first 2 weeks after birth, the parent's body is hormonally primed for making milk, and the research-based pumping strategies in this section and the next can help families reach this goal.

• • •

For higher long-term milk yields, suggest starting to pump within the first hour after birth.

An early start to pumping after birth can make a huge difference in milk yields, even 6 weeks later (Figure 11.8). Several U.S. studies of mothers pumping for very-low-birthweight (VLBW) babies (Furman, Minich, & Hack, 2002; L. A. Parker, Sullivan, Krueger, & Mueller, 2015; M. G. Parker et al., 2019) found that delaying the first pump session longer than 6 to 8 hours was associated with lower milk yields and decreased odds of providing any human milk at 7 days and at 40 weeks gestation.

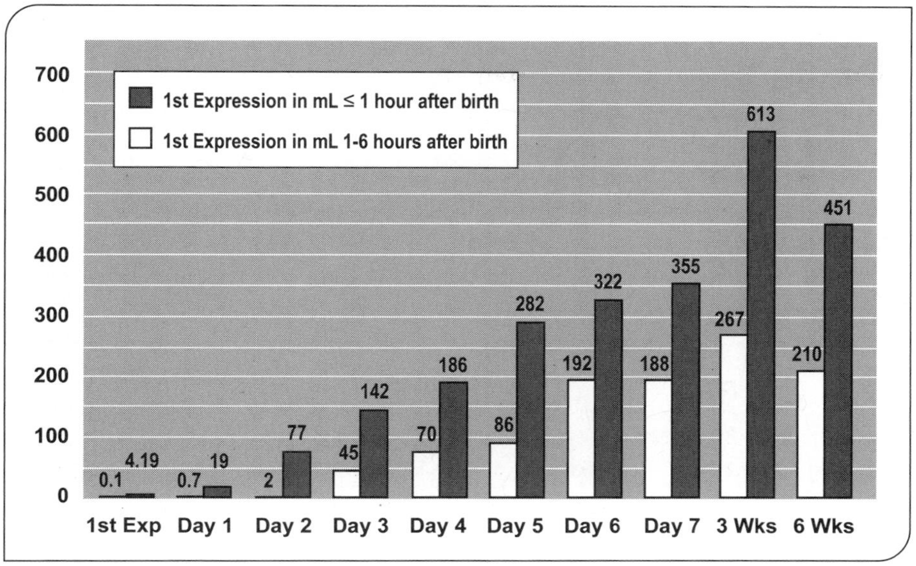

Figure 11.8 This graph illustrates the huge difference in milk production, even at 6 weeks, among those who began pumping within the first hour after birth and those who began 1 to 6 hours after delivery. Adapted from (L.A. Parker et al., 2012).

In 2012, a U.S. randomized controlled trial (L. A. Parker, Sullivan, Krueger, Kelechi, & Mueller, 2012) put 20 mothers pumping for VLBW babies into one of two groups:

1. Pumping began within 1 hour of delivery
2. Pumping began 1 to 6 hours after delivery

Milk yields were measured at different time points during the first 6 weeks (Figure 11.8) and the differences were considerable, even at 6 weeks. The researchers concluded that starting milk expression within the first hour after delivery increases milk volumes and decreases time to milk increase (lactogenesis II) after birth.

• • •

During the first 5 days, at least 5 times per day, suggest the parents follow double pumping with hand expression.

If possible, use an effective double pump. It's easy to understand why double pumping (pumping both sides at once) saves time over single pumping (one side at a time). However, the research is mixed on whether double pumping stimulates higher milk yields than single pumping (Becker et al., 2016). One U.K. randomized controlled trial of 62 mothers pumping exclusively for their preemies (M. S. Fewtrell et al., 2016) found one factor associated with greater milk yields at 10 days was double pumping. In any case, its time-saving aspect may be crucial to making exclusive pumping workable for many families.

The first choice when establishing exclusive pumping is a multi-user rental-grade pump, which is available in most hospitals. (The rationale for this recommendation was explained on p. 486-487.) Once milk production is established, switching to a single-user double electric pump will work well for most. Whatever the family's milk expression options, make sure they are aware of the pumping strategies in this section.

Make sure to get a good pump fit. When a pump's nipple tunnel is too large or too small, this can compromise pump effectiveness and comfort. Another factor associated with higher milk yields on Day 10 in the U.K. study mentioned above (M. S. Fewtrell et al., 2016) was the perceived comfort of the pump. For details on pump fit, see the p. 907-908.

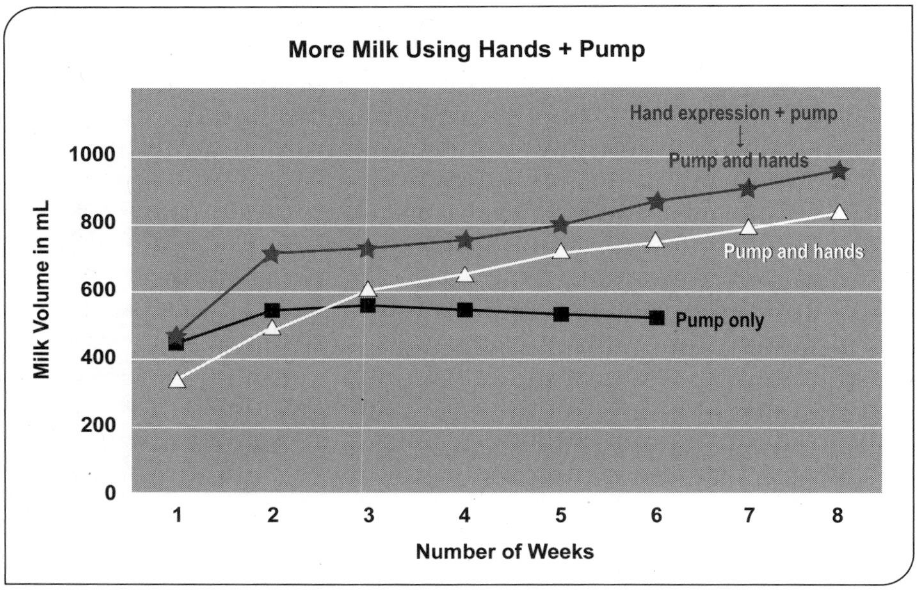

Figure 11.9 Milk yields from 3 groups of mothers pumping for VLBW babies. The black squares used the pump alone, the white triangles began hands-on pumping after milk increase, and the gray stars hand-expressed ≥5 times per day after pumping during the first 5 days and started hands-on pumping after milk increase. ©2020 Jane Morton, used with permission.

Follow double pumping with hand expression. As described in the first point of this chapter, learning hand expression during the last month of an uncomplicated pregnancy is recommended for all families. This skill is valuable to parents who are exclusively pumping in two ways. First, if a pump is not provided within the first hour after delivery, they can start hand-expressing. Second, if a pump is available within the first hour, research (Morton et al., 2009) indicates that for the first 5 days, following pump sessions with hand expression—expressing into the pump's nipple tunnel—at least 5 times per day resulted in much higher milk yields even 8 weeks later (Figure 11.9).

• • •

During the first few days, plan to pump at least 8 to 10 times daily for about 15 minutes and expect very little milk.

Expect small milk volumes. Because small volumes of milk are produced during the early days, some suggest thinking of these early pump sessions as "putting in their order" for more milk later. Some parents express nothing, some express drops of milk, others as much as a teaspoon (5 mL). Most do not express much more than this at first. However, each time milk is removed and the mammary glands stimulated, it signals the body to increase the rate of milk production. Make sure the family knows that the colostrum, or first milk, is concentrated nourishment and immunities, providing the baby with protection from illness and infection, and that no amount is too small to save for the baby.

Pump at least 8 times per day. As with nursing, establishing full milk production by pumping and hand expressing requires that milk be removed early, often, and effectively. In general—but especially during the first 2 weeks—the earlier, more often, and more fully the milk is expressed, the more milk will be produced (M. S. Fewtrell et al., 2016; Morton et al., 2009). To stimulate full milk production, parents exclusively pumping should plan to express milk at least as often as a baby would be nursing, no less than 8 to 10 times each day. As a visual reminder, some suggest each morning the pumping parent place ten candies or other snacks by their pump to help remind them to meet this goal (Wilson-Clay & Hoover, 2017).

In a study of 52 mothers pumping for VLBW babies (Morton et al., 2009), U.S. pediatrician Jane Morton found that falling below 7 pump sessions per day during the first 2 weeks significantly decreased the likelihood of reaching full milk production. A U.K. study of 62 mothers exclusively pumping for preemies (M. S. Fewtrell et al., 2016) found an association between number of pump sessions and milk volumes at 10 days.

Families are sometimes told not to worry about expressing milk in the beginning because they can always increase their milk production later when the baby is nursing. But following this well-meaning advice can seriously undermine their ability to meet their long-term feeding goals. Later, after the hormones of childbirth are at lower levels, increasing milk production is usually more difficult.

• • •

Until full production is reached, suggest going no longer than 5 to 6 hours at most between pump sessions, or pumping at least once during the night.

As explained in the previous chapter, when the mammary glands become full of milk, two dynamics signal the body to slow the rate of milk production:

1. The accumulation of a substance in the milk called "feedback inhibitor of lactation" (FIL for short) (Prentice, 1989), which appears to be serotonin (L. L. Hernandez et al., 2008)
2. Internal pressure from fullness

Many newborns take, on average, one long 4- to 5-hour sleep stretch per day, which may or may not be at night. When the mammary glands stay full longer than that, the "full glands make milk slower" dynamic may slow milk production (Kent, Prime, & Garbin, 2012). Pumping more often takes advantage of the "drained glands make milk faster" dynamic to more quickly move toward full production. For this reason, suggest pumping at least once during the night until full milk production is reached.

• • •

Skin-to-skin contact and pumping near baby increase milk yields. If the baby is in the NICU, suggest asking about pumping at baby's bedside.

A classic U.S. study (Hurst et al., 1997) found that even 1 hour of skin-to-skin contact per day is enough to increase pumping milk yields. A more recent Spanish study (Acuna-Muga et al., 2014) found that its 26 mothers pumped the most milk right after skin-to-skin contact with their baby. Pumping at their baby's bedside also yielded more milk than when they pumped in another room at the hospital or at home.

From a practical standpoint, if parents of ill or preterm babies are limited to pumping away from their baby, pumping is often delayed in order to talk to their baby's healthcare provider or because the pumping room is unavailable. Making it easier to pump more often is one good reason to encourage parents to pump at their baby's bedside (Spatz, 2021). Another good reason is the message it sends families about the importance of pumping. The sensory stimulation of looking at and touching the baby may also be one reason for the higher milk yields at baby's bedside. If this option is not offered, suggest the family request it.

Stage 2: From Milk Increase to Full Production

During the first 2 weeks post-birth, expressing at least 8 times per day is vital to reaching full milk production.

During the critical first 2 weeks after delivery, with every nursing or pump session, blood prolactin levels (a hormone vital to milk production) rise significantly. Higher blood prolactin levels activate or ***upregulate*** prolactin receptors in the mammary gland that determine milk production. A classic U.S. study (De Carvalho, Robertson, Friedman, & Klaus, 1983) concluded that the number of prolactin receptors upregulated during these early weeks may influence the peak level of milk production for that baby. Most families find that trying to increase milk production after the first 2 weeks takes more time and work, due to normal changes in hormonal levels (p. 410).

• • •

When milk increase occurs, usually around Day 3 or 4, suggest using the hands-on pumping techniques at all pump sessions.

Because "drained glands make milk faster," removing more milk at pump sessions increases rate of milk production so the family will reach full milk production faster (Morton et al., 2009). Encourage families to use the hands-on pumping techniques described on p. 492 (video demo at: **bit.ly/BA2-HandsOnPumpingDemo**) at as many pump sessions per day as possible. The research on this method (Morton et al., 2009) found that the mothers who used it averaged nearly 50% higher milk yields with nearly double the milk fat content (Morton et al., 2012) as compared with those who used the pump alone without incorporating these techniques. Compared with those who used the pump alone, whose milk yields peaked at 3 to 4 weeks and then plateaued or declined, those using hands-on pumping saw their milk yields continue to increase through the entire 8 weeks of the study.

• • •

Rather than trying to pump at regular time intervals, suggest focusing each day on the total number of pump sessions.

Some healthcare providers suggest families pump at specific time intervals (e.g., every 3 hours). However, for many, this makes pumping more challenging because life often interferes. Medical appointments, visitors, and other distractions can often postpone regular pump sessions and decrease the total number of daily milk removals.

Keep the focus on the daily total. Because the number of pump sessions per day is more important than the intervals between them, suggest instead that parents focus on the daily goal of 8 to 10 pump sessions and pump whenever it is most convenient, trying to avoid stretches longer than 5 or 6 hours or so until full milk production is reached. Typically, nursing babies do not feed at regular time intervals (Benson, 2001), so there is nothing magical about pumping by the clock. Vastly more important to meeting long-term milk production goals is the total number of milk removals per day (M. S. Fewtrell et al., 2016; Morton et al., 2009). By keeping the focus there, many families find it easier to fit in the recommended number of daily pump sessions and reach full production more quickly. On some days, it might be easier to pump every hour for part of the day followed by a longer 4-hour stretch, and this is fine. This pumping pattern is actually closer to how a baby nurses.

KEY CONCEPT

Encourage parents to cluster pump sessions closer together at convenient times to fit in more sessions.

• • •

If parents plan to provide pumped milk on a short-term basis, help them tailor their pumping routine to their goals.

Some families have no intention of nursing their baby but due to illness or prematurity decide to pump their milk after delivery on a short-term basis while baby is especially vulnerable. In this case, less intensive pumping efforts and reaching a lower level of milk production could be the focus, rather than stimulating full milk production. If a family's goal is to express milk short-term, encourage the nursing parent to do so at whatever level of milk expression will meet the baby's short-term needs and that the parent finds acceptable. Let the family know that with gradual weaning they can discontinue pumping whenever desired without pain.

TABLE 11.4 Pumping Strategies for Achieving Full Milk Production by Stage

	Stage 1: Birth (Start ≤ 1 Hour) to Milk Increase (Day 3 or 4)	Stage 2: Milk Increase (Day 3 or 4) to Full Production	Stage 3: At Full Production
Number of daily pump sessions	8-10, followed by hand expression ≥ 5/day	8-10, using hands-on pumping techniques	6-7
Pumping duration	15 minutes/side	≥ 20-30 minutes	≥ 10-15 minutes/side
Longest stretch between pump sessions	≤ 5-6 hours	≤ 5-6 hours	≤ 8 hours

Adapted from (Morton et al., 2009)

• • •

If parents are pumping for more than one baby, it will probably take longer to reach full milk production.

Parents of twins, triplets, and higher-order multiples will obviously need much more milk than families who delivered a single baby. To reach full milk production for multiples, suggest continuing using hands-on pumping techniques and continued night-time pumping of the Stage 2 recommendations until milk production reaches 750 mL (25 ounces) per baby per day. Then proceed to Stage 3.

• • •

If full milk production is not reached by Day 10, consider possible reasons.

See the later section on p. 506, "Troubleshooting Falling Milk Yields."

• • •

Research on the use of oxytocin during pumping is mixed.

Studies on oxytocin tablets and nasal sprays have not found their use produces higher milk yields (D.K. Prime et al., 2007). One U.K. randomized controlled trial (M. S. Fewtrell, Loh, Blake, Ridout, & Hawdon, 2006) found no benefit to using oxytocin nasal spray 3 to 5 minutes before pumping during the first 5 days of life. Although the 21 mothers using the oxytocin spray pumped more milk at first, by the fifth day, there were no differences between those who used the oxytocin spray and the 21 mothers who used the placebo nasal spray.

Stage 3: At Full Milk Production

Once full milk production is reached, suggest decreasing the number and length of pump sessions while monitoring daily milk yield at least once a week.

When 750 mL (25 ounces) of milk per day per baby is reached, this means enough prolactin receptors were upregulated to allow for experimentation with the pumping routine without putting milk production at long-term risk. In this situation, even if production dips, it should be possible to quickly bring it back up again, as long as it doesn't stay low for longer than 2 or 3 weeks.

Decrease milk expressions to 6 to 7 times per day. The number of pump sessions needed each day to maintain production will vary among parents, depending on storage capacity (see next section). Encourage the parent to start by experimenting within the parameters in Table 11.4. In most cases, 6 to 7 pump sessions per day are necessary to maintain long-term milk production. However, some with a very small storage capacity may notice a decrease at 7 daily sessions. If this happens, this means more pump sessions are needed to maintain milk production.

Decrease pumping time to 10 to 15 minutes. For most parents, this is long enough. If milk production slows, it may be necessary to pump longer. See p. 489-490 for a research-based strategy for helping parents tailor their length of milk expression to their own milk flow.

• • •

Suggest trying to sleep for 8 hours at night without pumping.

When it's time to try sleeping through the night without pumping, suggest starting by pumping as the last thing before going to sleep at night and the first thing upon awakening in the morning. What happens will provide clues to storage capacity. In general, those with a larger storage capacity can do this without too much discomfort or painful fullness. For their first morning expression, they may express 300 mL (10 ounces) or more. Those with a smaller storage capacity, on the other hand, may awaken before morning with discomfort, yet be unable to express more than 150 mL (5 ounces) or so (Mohrbacher, 2011).

Maintaining Full Milk Production

In some cases, previously nursing parents need to exclusively pump to maintain an already established milk production.

Examples of situations when exclusive pumping is needed to help maintain milk production in those who already have established milk production include:

- Nursing strikes
- Temporary interruption of nursing because they are taking an incompatible drug or need to have a diagnostic test using radioactive compounds.
- Hospitalization (either of parent or baby), which involves separation.
- Separation from the baby during a business or personal trip.

Temporary interruptions of nursing for any reason can be both emotionally and physically stressful for nursing couples. If it is abrupt, the stress is compounded. The parent may feel stressed about pumping and worry about how the baby will react to the change or the absence. Other worries may include concerns about mastitis and maintaining milk production. The family may need emotional support during this time and a listening ear.

In situations like these, the baby may find it stressful to change feeding methods (for options, see p. 986) and/or to be introduced to new foods. If the nursing couple is not usually separated, this will add to their stress. If so, encourage the parent to ask the baby's caregiver to give him lots of cuddling and holding to help make up for the separation and the loss of nursing.

The 'Magic Number' and Other Basics

In light of individual differences, giving all parents the same guidelines for maintaining milk production is not helpful.

Some older studies drew conclusions about the average number of minutes and daily pump sessions needed to maintain milk production (de Carvalho, Anderson, Glangreco, & Pittard, 1985). One U.S. study of 32 mothers of preterm babies born at 28 to 30 weeks gestation (Hopkinson, Schanler, & Garza, 1988) concluded that to maintain milk production, mothers needed to express at least five times per day for a total of more than 100 minutes. However, this study was done before storage capacity (see next point) was understood. With a greater understanding of the impact of individual differences, recommending that all parents express for the same number of minutes and number of daily pump sessions no longer makes sense. A pumping plan needs to be tailored to each individual, based on their storage capacity and other individual characteristics.

• • •

The number of daily pump sessions needed to maintain production will vary by storage capacity and other factors.

Whether nursing or pumping, the basic dynamics of milk production remain the same:

- **Drained glands make milk faster.** When mammary glands are drained often and well, this sends the signal to the body to make milk faster.
- **Full glands make milk slower.** The accumulation of feedback inhibitor of lactation (FIL) and the internal pressure of mammary fullness both send signals to the body to slow milk-making (Prentice, 1989). The more milk that fills the gland, the slower it is produced.

Storage capacity. How long it takes for the glands to become full depends on this variable, which refers to the maximum volume of milk available to the baby when the gland is at its fullest time of day. Mammary size is determined mostly by the amount of fatty tissue, so storage capacity is unrelated to size (Daly, Owens, & Hartmann, 1993).

Large-capacity parents can comfortably store more milk without feeling full and, therefore, need to pump less often to maintain production. They also tend to express more milk each time. Small-capacity parents feel full faster and need to express more often for the same daily milk yield. Parents at both ends of the storage-capacity spectrum can make ample milk, but the number of daily pump sessions needed to maintain production can vary greatly.

To use storage capacity as a guide, suggest parents note feelings of fullness, ideally never allowing themselves to get too full or stay that way too long without expressing milk. When the glands get and stay too full, this puts them at risk for both slowed milk production and mastitis (see p. 415).

Determining their "magic number." Depending on storage capacity, each parent has a specific number of daily pump sessions needed to maintain milk production over the long term. This is their "magic number" (Mohrbacher, 2011). (For more, see p. 657). If parents are exclusively pumping, they can estimate their magic number by reaching full production and then experimenting. For most, the magic number will be somewhere between 5 and 7 pump sessions per day. For those with a very small storage capacity, it may be more; if very large, it may be less. However, some large-capacity parents who cut back to fewer than 5 daily pump sessions report that production stays steady for a month or two, then declines precipitously (Mohrbacher, 1996). Parents will know they have found their magic number when their milk production stays steady without dropping.

KEY CONCEPT

The "magic number" is the number of daily milk removals needed to maintain full milk production.

The length of each pump session. This factor can affect the magic number because increasing the length of pumping ("drained glands make milk faster") can sometimes offset fewer daily milk expressions. In the U.S. study on hands-on pumping (Morton et al., 2009), the authors noted that after the first 2 weeks, its study mothers were able to decrease the number of pump sessions to 6 or 7 and yet with the fuller milk removal of hands-on pumping, they were still seeing an increase in milk production until the study ended at 8 weeks.

The longest stretch between pump sessions. Because full glands make milk slower, very long stretches between pump sessions may slow milk production. Parents with a large storage capacity sometimes push the envelope and go as long as 10 to 12 hours as their longest daily stretch. Be sure to ask any parent with milk production issues about this variable. In some cases, a flagging milk production can be boosted simply by decreasing the longest stretch.

• • •

When a parent who is exclusively pumping reaches full milk production, it may be okay to switch to a single-user double electric pump that is smaller and more portable.

With the necessary prolactin receptors upregulated and a full milk production of at least 750 mL (25 ounces) per day per baby, it is usually possible to maintain milk production with a smaller, more portable double electric pump. There are a wide range of automatic double pumps available for sale, some that include carry bags with insulated milk-cooling areas. When changing pumps, milk ejection may be temporarily affected due to the new feel. If so, see p. 480-481 for strategies that may help shorten the adjustment period.

• • •

Suggest recording the 24-hour milk yield at least once a week, so if it decreases, a quick response is possible.

Keeping an eye on the 24-hour milk yield is important, because the faster nursing parents respond to a drop in milk production, the sooner they'll rebound. If they take steps to increase milk production within a week or two, it is usually fairly easy to recover from a drop, but if they wait to take action for 3 or 4 weeks or longer, some glandular tissue may involute—or revert to its prepregnancy condition. Once some involution occurs, it may be difficult to bring milk yields up. For milk-boosting strategies, see p. 442.

Troubleshooting Falling Milk Yields

When pumping milk yields unexpectedly drop, first review the basics.

Before suggesting strategies to boost faltering milk yields, start by reviewing the basics.

- **How many times per day are they pumping?** Don't focus on the time intervals between pump sessions (e.g., every 3 hours), as this does not give a complete picture. Instead, ask about the time of each pump session on a typical day and then add the sessions together for the daily total. How close is this to their magic number (see previous section)?
- **About how many minutes is each pump session?** Has this changed recently? Are they single or double pumping? Hands-on pumping?
- **What is the longest stretch between pump sessions?** Stretches longer than about 8 hours will cause milk production to decrease slowly or quickly for many.
- **Which pump(s) are they using?** Which brand and model? Is this a good choice for their situation? If not, can they upgrade?
- **When was the pump fit last checked?** Even with a good fit at first, pump fit can change with time and pumping (Francis & Dickton, 2019; P. Meier et al., 2004; Wilson-Clay & Hoover, 2017). For details about checking fit, see p. 907-908.

- **How much daily skin-to-skin contact with their baby do they have?** Skin-to-skin contact is associated with higher milk yields (Acuna-Muga et al., 2014; Hurst et al., 1997).
- **What is their feeding goal?** Parents who plan to pump short term may not want to spend as much time on milk removal as those who intend to express long term.

• • •

Ask about health-related factors that may affect milk production.

Discuss aspects of the nursing parent's health that might affect milk production, such as taking a medication that affects lactation, a history of breast or chest surgery, thyroid problems, or any other health or physical issues that can affect milk production. See Box 10.2 on p. 441 for a more complete list.

• • •

Discuss possible strategies to boost milk production.

Discuss options for boosting milk yields and determine which are acceptable to them.

- **Use hands-on pumping techniques.** Even if they say they are doing hands-on pumping, ask them to describe step-by-step what they are doing when they pump to see if they might be missing a step or two or whether they could improve on their routine in any way.
- **Pump more times per day.** Their number of pump sessions may have dropped below their magic number, when milk production decreases (Mohrbacher, 2011). In this case, more than 8 expressions per day will increase milk production in most. (For small-capacity parents, this number may be higher.) Going from 6 to 7 pump sessions per day is unlikely to boost yields. The sessions don't have to be at regular intervals. It's okay to pump every hour during the part of the day that the pumping parent has help. See p. 447 for some strategies for increasing pumping intensity short term.
- **Decrease the length of the longest stretch.** If at night they are going 8 hours or longer without pumping, ask if they could fit in one pump session at night. Or ask if they could pump closer to their bedtime or sooner in the morning.
- **Consider other options to boost milk production.** See the section in the previous chapter starting on p. 442 for strategies for boosting milk production, including the use of galactogogues, or milk-enhancing substances. Boosting milk yields is an off-label use of drugs like metoclopramide (Reglan™) and domperidone (Motilium™), which cause a moderate increase in milk yields in some users. For details on these drugs and some commonly used plant-based and herbal galactogogues, see p. 449.

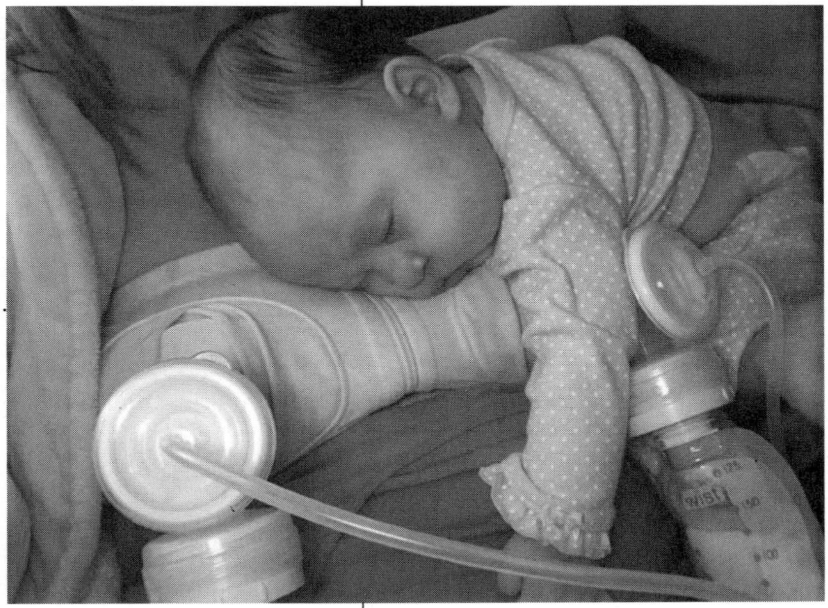

After Reaching Full Production, What's Next?

After reaching full milk production, be sure parents know their options.

Parents who achieve full milk production may wonder where to go from there. Pumping for a non-nursing baby brings many rewards. Parents say it feels great to see their baby grow and thrive on their milk, and it sets their mind at ease to know they're giving their baby the best (Bower, Burnette, Lewis, Wright, & Kavanagh, 2017; Ikonen, Paavilainen, & Kaunonen, 2015). Mother's milk is recommended for at least a baby's first year (AAP, 2012). But even motivated families find it difficult to make exclusive pumping work long-term because it takes much more time and effort than direct nursing.

> **KEY CONCEPT**
>
> *Transitioning to direct nursing is possible no matter how long the parent was expressing.*

Be sure the family knows that in addition to continuing with exclusive pumping, they have other options as well. Transitioning their baby to direct nursing is one—no matter how long they've been pumping. Make sure they know, too, that if they decide instead to wean from pumping, there are ways to do it that are comfortable and safe.

Transitioning to Direct Nursing

At any age, most babies can make the transition to nursing.

As described in the first chapter, babies are hardwired to nurse. Adoptive nursing in Australia involves transitioning 6- to 12-month-old babies to nursing because adoptions are not allowed there before this age (Gribble, 2005a). The instinctive feeding behaviors babies use to find the nipple, latch, and nurse were observed even in babies older than 1 year (Gribble, 2005b; Smillie, 2017).

Suggest parents think of this transition as a learning process that requires time and patience. Parents may sometimes feel awkward, anxious, or frustrated. Encourage them to consider their first attempts as "getting acquainted" sessions and enjoy the cuddling as they keep trying.

• • •

During this transition, keep all interactions on the parent's body pleasant and happy.

Never let nursing attempts become a battle. While near the nipple, give the baby lots of skin-to-skin and eye contact. Smile, talk, and enjoy each other. If the baby wants to move away, allow him to do so and come back to it at another time. If the baby fusses or cries, encourage the parent to stop and comfort him, so the baby does not associate the parent's body with frustration or unhappiness.

• • •

The starter positions are a good way to begin.

These positions (Figure 11.10 shows one example) make the most of babies' innate feeding behaviors. For details, see p. 23-29.

• • •

If the baby doesn't latch at first, suggest trying while he's in a light sleep or drowsy state.

Inborn feeding behaviors continue to be triggered while baby's in a light sleep (Colson, 2003, 2019). The parent will know the baby is in a light sleep when some body part moves (eyes moving under eyelids, mouth moving, etc.). To reduce latching struggles, a sleeping baby can be placed on the parent's semi-reclined body. Some babies latch more easily when drowsy or in a light sleep because their instinctive behaviors are triggered without conscious awareness of previous negative experiences.

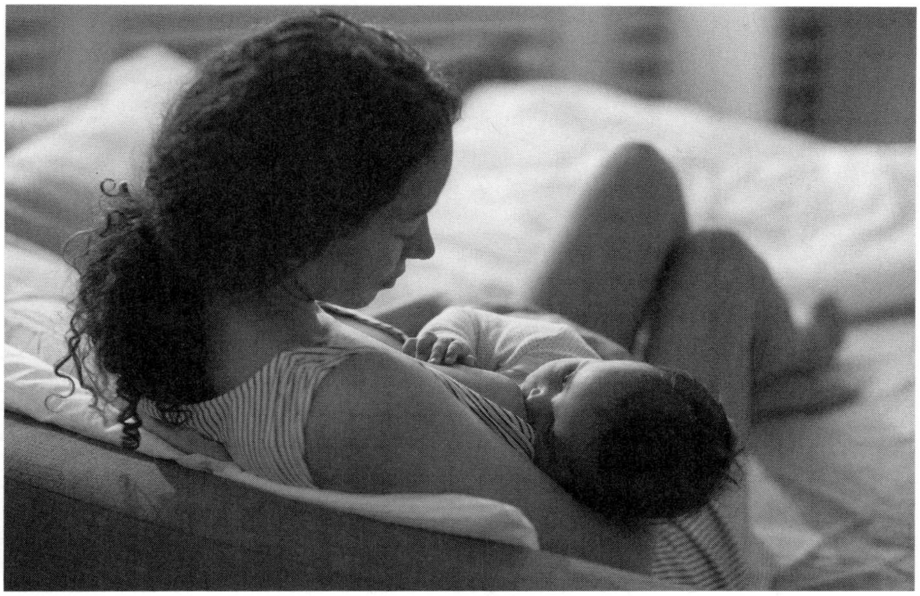

Figure 11.10 One example of a starter position that may make the transition to nursing easier because it triggers baby's inborn feeding behaviors.

• • •

Other strategies and tools may also help babies transition to nursing more easily.

It may also help to approach this transition the same way as a nursing strike. See p. 129 in Chapter 3, "Latching and Nursing Struggles" for an overview of parent and baby issues that can affect the act of nursing and the section "Strategies to Achieve Settled Nursing" on p. 129 for specific tips and tools. See also p. 680 in Chapter 16, "Relacation, Induced Lactation, and Emergencies."

• • •

It may take time for the baby to latch easily and nurse well.

Parents often feel discouraged if their baby does not take to nursing quickly. Assure them that the early nursing sessions are the most challenging and that with time and practice, it will get easier.

• • •

If the parents are anxious about not knowing how much milk their baby takes during nursing, explain how to gauge milk intake.

One emotional barrier that prevents many families from transitioning from exclusive pumping to direct nursing is their worry about accurately gauging their baby's milk intake. This may be especially difficult with babies born preterm or ill. Following familiar routines that were instrumental in keeping their baby alive and healthy in the NICU can feel comforting. On an emotional level, direct nursing may feel risky, even after the baby is no longer at risk and could nurse effectively and well. Explain that nursing is a normal behavior (like walking and talking) that babies are hardwired to do and that by helping their baby learn to nurse, they are not only making their feeding routines easier and less time-consuming, learning to nurse contributes to their baby's growth and development.

Regarding gauging milk intake, share expected weight gains and less reliable signs, such as diaper output and behavior after feeding. In addition to arranging for regular weight checks during the transition, encourage them to take note of their baby's diaper output and post-feeding behavior before transitioning to nursing, so that they will be more aware of what to look for afterward.

If, in spite of this information, the parents are still very anxious about not knowing how much milk the baby consumes while nursing, suggest for the first week arranging for a weight check with the baby's healthcare provider every day or every few days. If the family has the means and an accurate baby scale (to 2 g) is available for rent, suggest considering a 1-week rental, to do daily weight checks at home. This may help set their minds at ease during this transition. These scales are often available where breast pumps are rented.

Weaning from Exclusive Pumping

Like any other weaning, it is more comfortable and less risky to wean from pumping gradually.

If a parent decides to wean from pumping, rather than transitioning the baby to nursing, there are several possible approaches that can be used individually or in combination to make it more gradual and comfortable.

If at any time during weaning the mammary glands feel very full, encourage parents to pump to comfort without doing a full pumping. Remaining too full for too long increases the risk of pain and mastitis. With this in mind, possible approaches include:

- **Eliminate one daily pump session every 3 days or so,** leaving for last the first morning and last evening pump sessions. This gives milk production time to adjust downward before dropping another pumping. When a pump session is dropped, adjust the timing so all sessions are about the same time interval apart. Repeat until fully weaned from pumping.
- **Gradually increase the intervals between pump sessions.** For example, if the previous routine was to pump every 3 hours during the day, delay to 4 to 5 hours, and wait 3 days or so to increase the time intervals again. Repeat until the parent no longer feels the need to pump.
- **Keep the number of pump sessions per day the same, but stop sooner.** For example, if parents were pumping 120 mL (4 ounces) at each session, stop pumping after 90 mL (3 ounces). Give their body 3 days or so to adjust and repeat until they no longer feel the need to pump.

• • •

While weaning from pumping, pumping to comfort as needed is in parents' best interest.

Whether parents choose one of the methods in the previous point or combine several of them, pumping to comfort as needed will not prolong the process. It will simply make it more comfortable and prevent painful fullness from developing into mastitis. The goal is a gradual weaning with a minimum of risk and discomfort.

Another weaning strategy sometimes recommended when there is already a blocked duct, or a hardened area in the mammary gland, is to fully drain that side and then go for longer and longer stretches without pumping. Encourage parents to use whichever of these strategies works best for them.

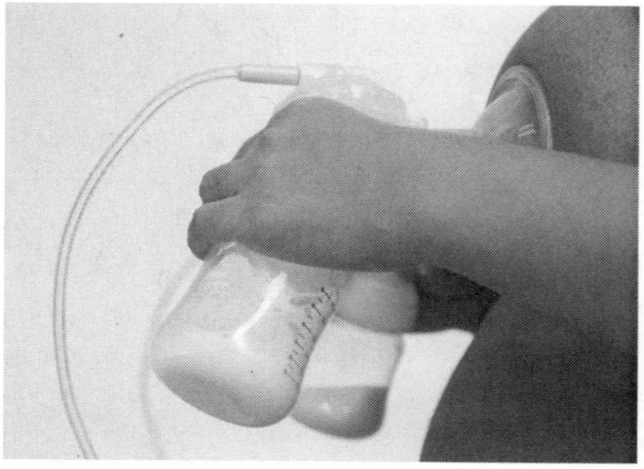

MILK STORAGE AND HANDLING

Milk Storage Guidelines

For Full-Term, Healthy Babies

The live cells in freshly expressed human milk kill bacteria, keeping milk fresh longer. Two Spanish studies found that when freshly expressed human milk is refrigerated, its bacteria-killing properties stay active for the first few days, but begin to decline after 72 hours (Martinez-Costa et al., 2007; Silvestre, Lopez, March, Plaza, & Martinez-Costa, 2006). The authors of the Academy of Breastfeeding Medicine (ABM) milk-storage guidelines (Eglash, Simon, & Academy of Breastfeeding, 2017) noted that the safety of milk storage at room temperature depends upon how clean the storage conditions are and how warm the room temperature. After reviewing the studies, its authors concluded that at the temperature range of 50° F to 85° F (10° C to 29° C), 4 hours should be safe. If the conditions are very clean, it may be safe to store freshly expressed human milk for up to 6 to 8 hours at room temperature.

Freshly expressed human milk takes longer to spoil at room temperature than pasteurized cow's milk because its bioactive cells kill bacteria.

• • •

One U.S. study, which attempted to more closely replicate the conditions parents face daily, found that milk stored at slightly below room temperature (60º F/15º C) was safe to use for up to 24 hours (Hamosh, Ellis, Pollock, Henderson, & Hamosh, 1996).

Fresh milk can be safely stored in an insulated cooler bag with frozen ice packs for up to 24 hours.

• • •

Some of the first studies of refrigerated milk were limited to 24 hours (Pittard, Anderson, Cerutti, & Boxerbaum, 1985). Later research extended the study period to 5 days and found that bacterial counts continued to be low during this entire time (Sosa & Barness, 1987). A Belgian study (Pardou, Serruys, Mascart-Lemone, Dramaix, & Vis, 1994) found that even after 8 days of refrigeration, some batches of milk actually had bacterial levels lower than when the milk was first expressed. These researchers concluded that milk used within 8 days should be refrigerated, rather than frozen, because the antimicrobial qualities of human milk are better preserved by refrigeration.

Storage guidelines for refrigerated human milk changed over the years as studies examined it for longer periods of time.

There is more to milk-storage guidelines than bacterial count. If the milk's bacterial count (one gauge of milk spoilage) is the only factor considered, the 8-day guideline for refrigerated milk makes sense. But when milk is refrigerated longer than 72 hours, other changes occur, such as a decrease in vitamin C levels and antioxidant properties (Buss, McGill, Darlow, & Winterbourn, 2001; Hanna et al., 2004). For this reason, some recommend using refrigerated milk within a shorter time, such as 4 or 5 days (Eglash et al., 2017; F. Jones, 2019). If a baby is ill or preterm, shorter guidelines may also be used (see later section "For the Hospitalized Baby").

> **KEY CONCEPT**
> *Guidelines for refrigerated milk vary by whether the main concern is spoilage or nutrient loss.*

Milk placement matters. The best area to store refrigerated milk is in the back of the refrigerator and away from the door, where there is greater temperature fluctuation.

Consider the situation. It is always better to use expressed milk sooner rather than later, but if the parents of a young baby find an 8-day-old container of expressed milk in the back of the refrigerator, they should consider their situation. The authors of the ABM guidelines noted that if the milk was stored under very clean conditions, it's okay to feed a healthy term baby milk that was refrigerated for 5 to 8 days. If the length of storage time makes the milk questionable, ask if the family has more expressed milk available. If so, it may be wise to discard the older milk. But if the only other option is to give infant formula, using the stored milk is most likely the better choice. When in doubt, suggest smelling the expressed milk. Spoiled milk usually smells sour.

• • •

Storage guidelines for frozen milk vary by organization and in some by type of freezer.

According to the author of the Human Milk Banking Association of North America (HMBANA) guidelines, any freezer that's cold enough to keep ice cream solidly frozen is cold enough to freeze human milk (F. Jones, 2019). HMBANA's milk-storage guidelines for healthy term babies include a range of acceptable options for frozen milk:

- Ideal: ≤3 months
- Optimal: ≤6 months
- Acceptable: Up to 12 months in a deep freeze

The ABM guidelines (Eglash et al., 2017) noted that although milk frozen at 0° F (-18° C) is safe indefinitely from bacterial contamination, some components—like fat, protein, carbohydrates, and vitamin C—decrease over time.

Milk placement and the volume stored matters. Suggest the parents store the milk in the back of the freezer away from the door due to fluctuating temperatures. If stored in a refrigerator/freezer, suggest putting the milk on a rack or shelf away from the freezer walls to avoid warming during the automatic defrost cycle (Eglash et al., 2017). Before freezing, suggest filling the container no more than about three-quarters full to allow for the normal expansion of the milk during freezing and to tighten bottle caps after the milk is completely frozen to allow displaced air to escape.

• • •

It is normal for the smell of refrigerated or frozen expressed milk to change over time.

The composition of human milk changes during storage (Garcia-Lara et al., 2012). Although the bacterial levels of refrigerated milk decrease during the first 48 to 72 hours (Martinez-Costa et al., 2007; Silvestre et al., 2006) and stay stable while it is frozen, as with other foods, the enzymes in milk, such as lipase, continue to function (USDA, 2013). Lipase breaks down milk fat into free fatty acids, which increases the acidity of the milk (Vazquez-Roman et al., 2016) and sometimes produces a soapy or rancid smell and/or flavor (Hung, Hsu, Su, & Chang, 2018). Some parents notice this change in smell after a short time in the refrigerator or freezer. In other cases, it takes a longer time for the stored milk to develop this smell (Mohrbacher, 2014). Freezing slows but does not stop the lipase from breaking down the fat in the milk (Berkow et al., 1984; Bitman, Wood, Mehta, Hamosh, & Hamosh, 1983). In fact, the authors of the ABM's Clinical Protocol #8 on human milk storage and handling wrote that this breakdown of the milk may be beneficial (Eglash et al., 2017, p. 393), because it "has antimicrobial effects preventing the growth of microorganisms in thawed refrigerated milk (Handa et al., 2014)."

The baby's reaction and the milk's safety. As long as the milk-storage guidelines are followed, the guidelines from both the ABM and HMBANA deem it safe to feed babies expressed milk that develops a soapy or rancid smell or flavor during storage (Eglash et al., 2017; F. Jones, 2019). According to the guidelines from the ABM, there is no evidence that this change in smell or taste causes babies to reject this milk. The authors of the ABM's clinical protocol also pointed out that many foods adults eat–such as eggs, cheese, and fish—contain the free fatty acids that cause a similar smell but this smell does not necessarily reflect the taste of these foods.

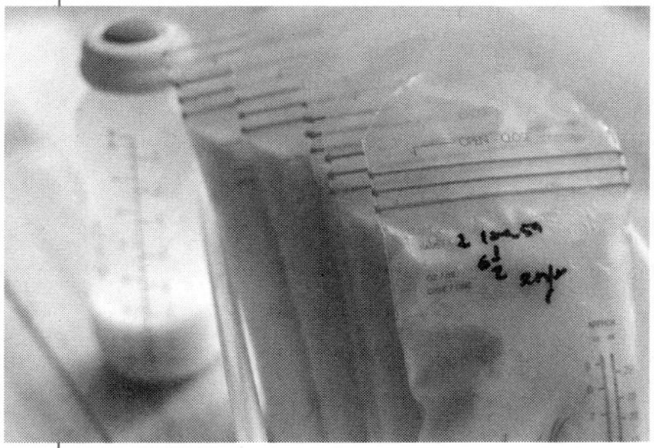

What to do when a baby refuses to drink smelly milk. Most babies accept milk that smells soapy or rancid, but there are exceptions. When this happens, what should parents do? One 2014 article (Mohrbacher, 2014) described the experiences of families who found different solutions. First, suggest experimenting to determine the length of storage time needed for the milk to acquire the smell or taste. In some cases, it may happen weeks after freezing. In this case, providing milk expressed before that time, either refrigerated milk or milk frozen for shorter periods, may solve the problem. For some families, though, even a short refrigeration is long enough for this change in smell or taste to occur. As one parent wrote (Mohrbacher, 2014, pp. 5-6):

> "I developed a system where I used that day's fresh milk for the next day's daycare supply. On Friday, I would collect the milk and scald it....Come Sunday night, I would place those bags in the fridge to prepare for Monday at daycare. I felt very fortunate that I only had to do this on Friday."

To scald or not to scald? In addition to using milk before it acquires the soapy or rancid smell, it is also possible in many cases to prevent the smell from occurring. If the family can't use the milk quickly enough, HMBANA's guidelines mentioned scalding the milk before cooling and storing it as another option (F. Jones, 2019). To scald expressed milk, put the freshly expressed milk in a pan on the stove and heat it to about 180° F (82° C) or until bubbles form around the edges but it is not yet boiling. After that temperature is reached, cool the milk quickly and either refrigerate or freeze it. Scalding prevents this change in smell by deactivating the enzyme lipase in the milk. (Scalding will not help if the milk has already acquired this smell or flavor.) Of course, heating expressed milk is not usually recommended, because it destroys some of its bioactive immune factors. For this reason, the ABM does not recommend scalding. But for some families, scalding may be the only way their expressed milk can be used.

Using milk that already smells soapy or rancid. Even if a baby refuses stored milk that smells soapy or rancid, discarding the milk is not the only option.

- ***Mix it with fresher milk that has not yet acquired the smell or taste.*** Families report (Mohrbacher, 2014) that different ratios of fresh or refrigerated milk to smelly milk are acceptable to different babies. Some may accept milk that is 50:50 fresh to smelly milk. If so, try increasing the ratio of smelly milk until the upper limit is reached. Others accept mixtures that are 60:40, 70:30, or 80:20. Whatever the ratio, this strategy allows the stored milk to be used.
- ***Donate it to a milk bank.*** In the 2019 HMBANA guidelines (F. Jones, 2019), its author stated that if a milk donor meets its criteria, this milk can be pooled with other donor milk and used by sick and preterm infants. Make sure the family knows that this milk could be a lifesaver for another baby.

TABLE 11.5 Mature Milk Storage Times for Healthy Term Babies at Home

Milk Storage/ Handling	Deep Freeze (0°F/-18°C)	Refrigerator/ Freezer (0°F/-18°C)	Refrigerator (39°F/4°C)	Room Temperature (50°F-85°F/ 10°C-29°C)
Fresh	Optimal: ≤ 6 mo. Okay: ≤ 12 mo.	Ideal: ≤ 3 mo. Okay: ≤ 6 mo.	Ideal: 4 days Okay if very clean conditions: 5-8 days	Ideal: ≤ 4 hours Okay if very clean conditions: 6-8 hours
Frozen, thawed in fridge	Do not refreeze	Do not refreeze	≤ 24 hours	≤ 4 hours
Thawed, warmed, not fed	Do not refreeze	Do not refreeze	≤ 4 hours	Until feed ends
Fed	Discard	Discard	Discard	Until feed ends

Adapted from (CDC, 2019; Eglash et al., 2017; F. Jones, 2019)

• • •

Milk that collects in breast shells, or "drip milk," should be discarded.

Milk that collects in breast shells was found in one study (Lucas, Gibbs, & Baum, 1978) to contain half the fat of actively expressed milk. It was also found to contain higher levels of common skin bacteria (Gessler, Bischoff, Wiegand, Essers, & Bossart, 2004), probably due to prolonged skin contact. For these reasons, current HMBANA guidelines (F. Jones, 2019) recommend discarding "drip milk" rather than storing it or feeding it to the baby.

• • •

Current guidelines either provide no recommendation about refreezing thawed milk or recommend against it. Partially defrosted milk should be considered on a case-by-case basis.

A power outage is the most likely situation in which the safety of refreezing thawed or partially thawed milk is an issue. The authors of the ABM guidelines wrote (Eglash et al., 2017, p. 392):

> "There is little information on refreezing thawed human milk. Bacterial growth and loss of antibacterial activity in thawed milk will vary depending on the technique of milk thawing, duration of the thaw, and the amount of bacteria in the milk at the time of expression. At this time no recommendations can be made on the refreezing of thawed human milk."

The HMBANA guidelines recommended against refreezing thawed human milk (F. Jones, 2019). When milk is only partially thawed, these guidelines suggested being flexible and basing the final decision on the answers to these questions:

- Was the milk raw or pasteurized before freezing? Raw milk will likely retain more antibacterial properties.
- For how long and at what temperature was it frozen? Milk frozen at a lower temperature for a shorter time is likely to be safer.
- About how much of the container is thawed? The lower the percentage of thawed to frozen milk, the better.
- Can the milk be refrigerated and used within the storage guidelines? Using the thawed milk quickly is preferable.

- What is the baby's gestational age and health? The older and healthier the baby, the less likelihood there is that feeding the refrozen milk later will be a problem.

• • •

Recommendations vary on how long milk leftover after a feed can be safely used.

When a baby takes milk from a bottle or a cup, the milk mixes with his saliva, introducing more bacteria into the milk. In the ABM Clinical Protocol #8 (Eglash et al., 2017), its authors noted that there is insufficient research on which to base recommendations for this situation, but it suggested that it seems reasonable to discard any remaining milk within 1 to 2 hours after the feed.

In the HMBANA guidelines (F. Jones, 2019), on the other hand, its author suggested that it is safe to put any leftover milk into the refrigerator for up to 4 hours. After that time, it should be discarded.

In a 2018 article (Fogleman et al., 2018), U.S. researchers summarized the results of two small pilot studies that examined the bacterial and immunological characteristics of unused and leftover milk from 12 mothers, some of which was freshly expressed and some of which was previously frozen. The researchers examined these batches during 6 days of refrigeration at 6° C. They concluded that these characteristics were stable throughout the 6 days in all of the milk samples and encouraged more research to be done before guidelines are revised.

• • •

Each batch of milk should be labeled with the date and in some cases the baby's name and the time it was expressed.

Including the day, month, and year on the milk-storage container will allow the milk to be used in the order it was expressed. If the milk will be given in a group setting, such as a hospital or daycare facility, the baby's name should also be written on each container. If the milk will be fed to a preterm baby or donated to a milk bank, labeling the container with the time of day it was expressed may also be important.

• • •

To avoid waste, store milk in volumes no larger than the baby might take at a feed.

For the baby older than about 1 month, suggest parents start by freezing their milk in 2- to 4-ounce (60-118 mL) quantities, which is about how much the average baby takes during nursing (Kent et al., 2013). Small volumes thaw and warm faster, and less milk will be discarded if the baby does not take it all. If the baby wants more milk, it can always be added. While sorting out how much milk is right for their baby, suggest parents store some smaller 1- to 2-ounce (30-59 mL) volumes to provide a little extra if needed.

• • •

On average, nursing babies take much less milk per day than babies bottle-fed formula.

Although there is a large range of normal milk intakes among nursing babies (Kent et al., 2013; Kent et al., 2006), on average, the exclusively nursing baby takes less milk per day than the baby who is bottle-fed formula. One U.S. study found that at 4 months of age, nursing babies consumed on average 25% fewer calories than formula-fed babies of the same age, even though their weight gains were comparable (Butte, Garza, Smith, & Nichols, 1984). Another U.S. study found that at 6 months nursing babies, on average, consume 23% less milk than their formula-feeding counterparts (Heinig, Nommsen, Peerson, Lonnerdal, & Dewey, 1993). This could be important information for parents gauging their baby's milk needs by their neighbor's formula-fed baby. (For more details on the reasons for this difference, see p. 192-194.

• • •

Milk expressed at different sessions can be combined and labeled with the date of the oldest milk.

When batches of expressed milk are combined, the milk should be dated according to the oldest milk. For example, if refrigerated milk from May 10 is combined with milk expressed and cooled on May 11, the combined batch should be dated May 10. To reduce the risk of contamination, HMBANA recommends limiting the number of times milk is added to a container and to start a new container every 24 hours (F. Jones, 2019).

Both the ABM and HMBANA recommend cooling freshly expressed milk before adding it to refrigerated milk. Fresh milk can be added to frozen milk, as long as there is less fresh milk than frozen milk, and it is first cooled for about an hour, so it does not thaw the top layer.

• • •

For the baby whose milk intake is largely or exclusively expressed milk, suggest the family make their first priority feeding fresh milk, second refrigerated milk, and third frozen milk.

If a baby who directly nurses is fed expressed milk occasionally, frozen milk is fine. But in families where expressed milk comprises a large percentage of the baby's milk intake, encourage parents not to cycle all of their expressed milk through the freezer before feeding it to the baby. Because freezing deactivates some of the bioactive factors in human milk (Raoof, Adamkin, Radmacher, & Telang, 2016; Rollo, Radmacher, Turcu, Myers, & Adamkin, 2014; Takci et al., 2012), it's better to prioritize feeding fresh milk first, refrigerated milk second, and frozen milk third, when the others are not available. The sooner the baby receives the milk after it is expressed, the fewer nutrients and bioactive factors will be lost and the closer it will be to the milk received during direct nursing.

• • •

There is no evidence that milk stored during a candida infection should be discarded.

Parents sometimes feel anxious about using milk frozen when they had thrush. A Brazilian study found low levels of live yeast in human milk that was previously frozen and thawed (Rosa, Novak, de Almeida, Medonca-Hagler, & Hagler, 1990) and concluded that freezing milk may not kill yeast. However, the researchers acknowledge the possibility that the milk became contaminated with live yeast during its handling. There is currently no evidence to indicate that milk expressed and stored during a nipple candida infection or thrush in baby's mouth can cause a recurrence. In the ABM Clinical Protocol #8, its authors wrote (Eglash et al., 2017, p. 393):

> "If a mother has breast or nipple pain from a bacterial or yeast infection, there is no evidence that her stored expressed milk needs to be discarded."

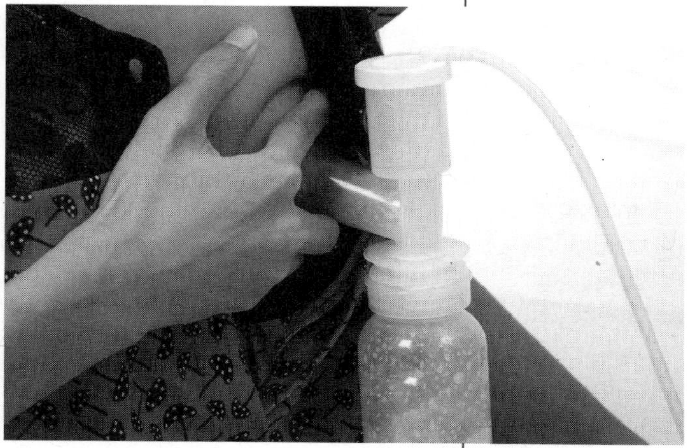

If parents are concerned, an alternative to discarding stored milk is to use it while parent and baby are being treated for thrush. If that's not possible, another alternative is to warm the expressed milk to temperatures that kill yeast. Milk banks heat milk to 63 degrees C (144.5 degrees F) for 30 minutes, which will kill bacteria and yeast. One reference (L. Amir & Hoover, 2002) states that candida dies within minutes at a temperature of 122 degrees F (60 degrees C). Of course, if the milk is heated, cool it to between room temperature and body temperature before feeding it.

For Hospitalized Babies

Parents of a preterm or sick baby need to ask about milk-storage guidelines at their baby's hospital. In many institutions, sterile storage containers are provided and special labeling processes followed (P. P. Meier, Johnson, Patel, & Rossman, 2017). The hospital may also specify how much milk to put in each container and provide storage times for fresh, refrigerated, and frozen milk that differ from those for healthy term babies and home use. For sick or preterm babies, HMBANA recommends expressed milk be refrigerated immediately, rather than allowing it to stay at room temperature (F. Jones, 2019). Milk storage guidelines also differ if fortifier is added to the milk. Human milk is not sterile, and bacteriologic screening is not usually recommended because there are currently no generally agreed-upon acceptable levels of bacteria in the milk (F. Jones, 2019).

Suggest the parents of a hospitalized baby ask the hospital staff for their milk storage guidelines, which vary by institution.

Preterm and sick babies are at greater risk for serious and even life-threatening health problems, so stricter hygiene precautions are needed. Simple steps like handwashing before expressing milk can be critical in preventing contamination of the milk (Novak, Da Silva, Hagler, & Figueiredo, 2000). For more details, see p. 372 for the section "Milk Handling and Safety" in Chapter 9, "The Preterm Baby."

KEY CONCEPT

Shorter storage times and stricter hygiene may be recommended when storing milk for ill or preterm babies.

• • •

In previous years, to decrease the risk of milk contamination, part of routine hygiene recommendations for parents of vulnerable babies included washing the nipple before milk expression and discarding the first drops of milk. However, research (Pittard, Geddes, Brown, Mintz, & Hulsey, 1991) found no difference in milk contamination when these procedures were followed, so they are no longer recommended (F. Jones, 2019). Normal hygiene is considered sufficient.

Cleaning the nipples before expressing and discarding the first few drops of milk are no longer recommended.

Handling and Preparing Milk

For milk expressed for healthy term babies, washing, rinsing, and drying storage containers, along with good handwashing are considered sufficient to prevent milk contamination (F. Jones, 2019; Pittard et al., 1991). Regular sterilization or sanitization of milk storage containers or pump parts is not currently recommended, because no benefits to these extra procedures were found. Other precautions may be recommended when expressing milk for sick or hospitalized babies.

Before storing milk, any reusable storage container should be washed in hot, soapy water, rinsed well, and air dried.

• • •

Layers. Because most parents are familiar with the appearance of homogenized cow's milk, some worry when their expressed milk separates into milk and cream. Reassure them this separation is normal in any milk that is not homogenized. Before the milk is fed to the baby, suggest first swirling it gently to mix the layers.

Expressed milk separates into layers over time and its color may vary.

Colors. Usually human milk appears either bluish, yellowish, or even brownish in color. However, consuming some foods, food dyes, and medications, can change the color of the milk to pink (Quinn, Ailsworth, Matthews, Kellams, & Shirley, 2018) or pink-orange (orange soda or gelatins), green (algae, kelp, multivitamins or green drinks) (Naor, Fridman, Kouadio, Merlob, & Linder,

2019; Yazgan, Demirdoven, Yazgan, Toraman, & Gurel, 2012), and even black (minocycline) (Anderson, 2018). Frozen milk may take on a yellowish color, which is not a sign of spoilage.

• • •

Suggest thawing frozen milk gently and gradually, keeping heat low.

Freezing and heating human milk reduces some of its immune properties that kill bacteria, making it more vulnerable to contamination (J. Hernandez, Lemons, Lemons, & Todd, 1979). When thawing or warming milk, keep heat low, using one of the following methods (Eglash et al., 2017):

- Thaw it in the refrigerator overnight, which results in less fat loss than thawing in warm water (Thatrimontrichai, Janjindamai, & Puwanant, 2012). Once thawed, milk can be refrigerated for up to 24 hours.
- Hold the container under warm running water for a few minutes.
- Hold the container in water that has been previously heated on the stove to ideally no more than body temperature (98° F/37° C). If the water cools and the milk is not yet thawed, remove the container of milk and reheat the water. Do not heat the milk on the stove burner directly.
- Thaw in a waterless warming device.

According to HMBANA guidelines (F. Jones, 2019), another option is to thaw milk at room temperature, making sure that once it is completely thawed, it is immediately refrigerated.

If using water to thaw or warm milk, tilt or hold the container, so the water cannot seep under the lid. Thawed milk should not be kept at room temperature. It should be either fed immediately or refrigerated.

• • •

Expressed milk can be fed cold or it can be warmed to between room and body temperature.

Healthy term and older babies often willingly drink chilled milk directly from the refrigerator, which the HMBANA guidelines considers the safest choice (F. Jones, 2019). But some term babies prefer their milk warmed, and warming is important for preterm babies, as cold milk may lower body temperature.

To warm milk before feeding, allow about 20 minutes (Eglash et al., 2017) and hold the container under lukewarm running water or hold it in a pan of lukewarm water that has been previously heated to no more than about body temperature (98° F/37° C) on the stove. Too much heat during warming can cause potentially dangerous hot spots in the milk (Bransburg-Zabary, Virozub, & Mimouni, 2015), and it deactivates the milk's bioactive proteins and decreases its fat content (Eglash et al., 2017).

KEY CONCEPT

Discourage families from warming expressed milk in a microwave.

• • •

A microwave should not be used to thaw or warm human milk.

Despite the fact that 12% of U.S. parents use microwaves to thaw or warm expressed milk (Labiner-Wolfe & Fein, 2013), this practice is not recommended and should be discouraged. Warming human milk in a microwave reduces bacterial levels (Ben-Shoshan, Mandel, Lubetzky, Dollberg, & Mimouni, 2016), but it also reduces much of its anti-infective factors, such as IgA (Quan et al., 1992; Sigman, Burke, Swarner, & Shavlik, 1989). Also, microwaves heat liquids unevenly (Ovesen, Jakobsen, Leth, & Reinholdt, 1996), so even if the milk is swirled or shaken afterwards, hot spots remain that can burn the baby's throat.

• • •

In the U.S., according to the Centers for U.S. Disease Control and Prevention (CDC, 2018) and the Occupational Safety and Health Administration (OSHA) (Clark, 1992), human milk is not considered a biohazardous material, so rubber gloves are not needed when human milk is handled or fed, nor is a separate refrigerator required. At workplaces and at child care facilities, human milk can be stored along with other foods in a common refrigerator and no special precautions are needed (Eglash et al., 2017). If it's discarded, human milk can also be safely poured down the drain.

Human milk is not a biohazardous substance, so no gloves or other special precautions are needed when handling it. It can be safely poured down the drain when discarded.

Storage Containers

With the exception of the containers described in the next point, the best choice for storing expressed milk is composed of food-grade material and has a tight-fitting, solid lid (rather than one with a nipple/teat). If the baby gets most of his nourishment from direct nursing and only occasionally receives expressed milk, the type of storage container is not a major concern (F. Jones, 2019). But when a baby receives most of his nourishment from expressed milk, the storage container should be chosen carefully.

Glass and most solid plastic containers with solid, tight-fitting lids are recommended for both hospital and home use.

With all types of storage containers—glass, hard plastic, and bags—milk components are affected, especially fat (Chang, Chen, & Lin, 2012). Percentage of milk fat is significantly lower in stored milk and its total protein and carbohydrate concentrations are higher. After reviewing the research, the authors of the ABM Clinical Protocol #8 (Eglash et al., 2017) concluded the effects of glass and polypropylene plastic containers on stored milk were similar in terms of:

- How much fat stuck to the sides of the containers (Garza, Johnson, Harrist, & Nichols, 1982)
- Concentrations of IgA
- Number of viable white blood cells (Goldblum, Garza, Johnson, Harrist, & Nichols, 1981)

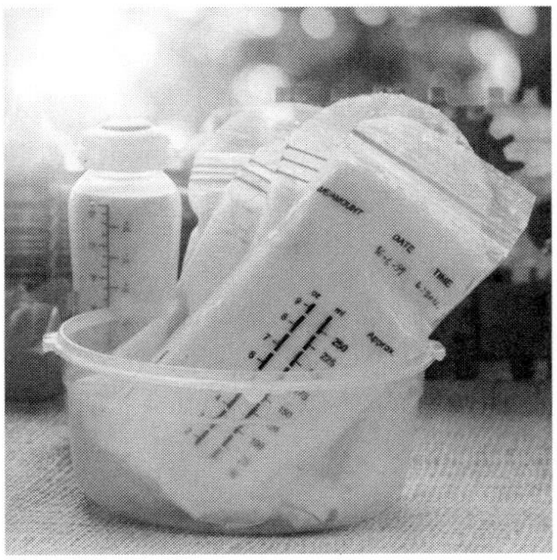

But the effects of polyethylene milk storage bags on the expressed milk were different. There was a significant 60% drop in the milk's IgA concentrations (Goldblum et al., 1981), as well as a marked drop in the milk's bacteria-fighting capability when compared with milk stored in Pyrex tempered glass containers (Takci et al., 2012).

• • •

Specimen cups are used to collect urine or other body fluids but should not be used to store expressed milk because they may contain potentially harmful chemicals that could be absorbed into the milk (Blouin, Coulombe, & Rhainds, 2014).

Avoid storing expressed milk in specimen cups and containers made from polycarbonate plastic and stainless steel.

Polycarbonate bottles containing BPA or BPS. These hard-plastic bottles contain the chemicals bisphenol-A (BPA) or bisphenol-S (BPS) and are also not recommended for storing expressed milk because under certain conditions these chemicals, which are estrogen disruptors, could leach into the milk and potentially affect the baby (vom Saal & Hughes, 2005).

Stainless steel containers are not recommended by HMBANA for storing expressed milk (F. Jones, 2019) because studies found the milk in these containers had fewer live cells and the components were less bioactive when compared with milk stored in polyethylene bags (Manohar, Williamson, & Koppikar, 1997) or glass (Williamson & Murti, 1996).

• • •

Milk storage bags can be used to store expressed milk for home use.

For many parents, polyethylene milk storage bags have practical advantages. They take up less storage space than hard-sided containers and can be attached directly to breast pump attachments in place of a bottle, reducing the need to transfer milk and the risk of contamination. Because they are not reused, there is less to wash. However, this makes them less eco-friendly than reusable containers.

Types of milk bags. Some types of milk bags are sturdier than others. Storing expressed milk in plastic sandwich bags, for example, is not recommended because they are thin and tear easily (F. Jones, 2019). Some bags called "disposable bottle liners" are made primarily as part of a commercial feeding system rather than intended for milk storage. These feeding bags tend to be thinner and more prone to splitting. If this type of bag is used to store milk, suggest the parents safeguard the milk by first inserting the bag of milk inside another bag before sealing and storing it.

Why home use only? Milk storage bags are not usually recommended for hospitalized babies because they are not airtight like hard-sided containers, and there is a greater risk of leaking. In HMBANA's 2019 guidelines, its author noted that when a parent is supplying limited volumes of milk to a preterm baby, it's vital that the milk retain as many milk components as possible (F. Jones, 2019). As described in an earlier point, the 60% decrease in milk antibodies that occurred when milk was stored in milk bags (Goldblum et al., 1981) is significant, and a loss that an at-risk newborn cannot afford.

Best practices when storing milk in bags. HMBANA's guidelines suggest these strategies for families using milk storage bags (F. Jones, 2019):

- Leave space for milk expansion when freezing milk.
- Close the bag tightly.
- Lie the bags flat during freezing.
- After the milk is frozen, insert the bags into a disposable freezer bag and seal it or into a bin with a lid for extra protection.

Reducing the Risks of Milk Sharing

Lactation supporters can help milk-sharing families reduce risk.

One major change since the last edition of this book is the rise of vast milk-sharing networks created by families to fill their need for human milk. A 2018 U.S. study that included both a qualitative survey and a national sample (O'Sullivan, Geraghty, & Rasmussen, 2018) found that 17% of its U.S. sample either provided or received human milk from other families through these milk-sharing networks, despite recommendations against milk sharing from the U.S. Food and Drug Administration. (USFDA, 2018). The grass-roots growth of milk sharing reflects a widespread belief among parents in the importance of human milk to their babies.

BOX 11.1 Four Pillars of Safe Milk Sharing

1. Informed Choice	2. Donor Screening	3. Safe Handling	4. Home Pasteurization
• Explore all infant and child feeding options, including their risks and benefits	• Identify the health, lifestyle, and social factors incompatible with milk sharing • Foster clear, honest communication between milk-sharing families • Screen for HIV, HTLV, hepatitis B and C, syphilis, and rubella	• Check mammary glands and skin regularly for lesions and sores • Follow guidelines for handling, storing, transporting, and shipping human milk	• Learn techniques for heat-treating shared milk at home to reduce infection risk • Make an informed choice based on donor criteria between using raw or heat-treated milk

Adapted from (Walker & Armstrong, 2012); also see **eatsonfeets.org/#FourPillars**

Milk sharing is usually done without guidance from healthcare providers or lactation supporters. Two U.S. authors (McCloskey & Karandikar, 2018) examined the challenges milk-sharing parents face and described an approach to working with families that facilitates an open discussion about the pros and cons of milk sharing with a focus on promoting safety and reducing risk. Parents often reach out to other families through the websites and social-media pages of organizations like Eats on Feets and Human Milk 4 Human Babies without seeking professional counsel. But when given the opportunity, we can provide information that can help families reduce risks associated with milk sharing.

In 2012, Eats on Feets' founder Shell Walker published its "four pillars of breast milk sharing" (Walker & Armstrong, 2012), which is available on its website **eatsonfeets.org/#fourPillars**. See Box 11.1 for a summary.

All lactation supporters should be familiar with these recommendations to understand what information many families receive about milk sharing. In addition to sharing this information with families who don't have it, there are other ways lactation supporters can help families reduce the risks of milk sharing.

Make current milk storage and handling guidelines available. A 2017 internet survey of 321 milk-sharing families (Reyes-Foster, Carter, & Hinojosa, 2017) found that the vast majority used safe practices. Even so, it may be helpful to provide the latest milk storage and handling guidelines listed in this chapter

Recommend families avoid milk for sale. According to a 2015 online survey of 392 milk-sharing families (Reyes-Foster, Carter, & Hinojosa, 2015), 95% of milk donors and recipients meet in person in their local communities. Only 5% of those surveyed shipped their milk to other locations or received shipped milk. Also, the vast majority of milk sharing is done without financial compensation. Yet a highly publicized U.S. study (Keim, McNamara, Kwiek, & Geraghty, 2015) focused on online milk sales. This research team bought milk online that was shipped to them for analysis. Of the 102 milk samples received, none of them contained any of the drugs of abuse they were looking for. Unlike the usual milk-sharing experience, in which donors and recipients meet locally and form a relationship, the researchers asked the milk donors to ship the milk any way they wanted, without regard for milk safety. Some of these batches took up to 5 days to arrive. Not surprisingly, these batches had very high levels of bacterial contamination. Another interesting finding about this milk for sale (Keim, Kulkarni, et al., 2015) was that it contained about 10% cow's milk, which was likely added to the human milk to increase its volume and therefore the price paid.

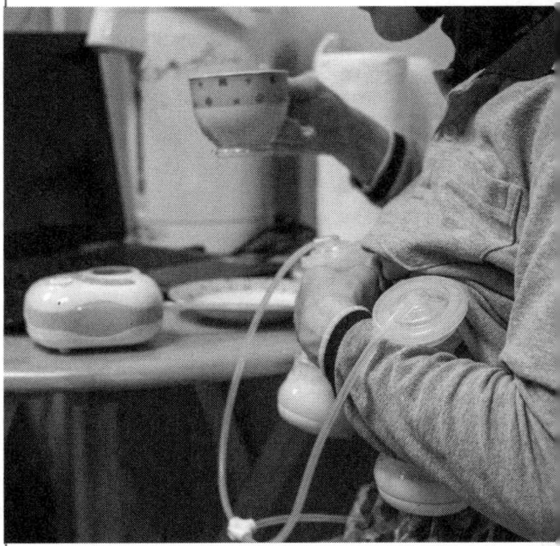

RESOURCES

bit.ly/BA2-BolmanMassage—A 4.5-minute video showing some of the techniques described in the article Bolman, M., Saju, L, Oganesyan, K., et al. (2013). Recapturing the art of therapeutic breast massage during breastfeeding. Journal of Human Lactation, 28(3):328-331.

bit.ly/BA2-HandsOnPumpingDemo—A 9.5 minute video demonstrating by Dr. Jane Morton of hands-on pumping techniques, which incorporates manual expression and massage.

bit.ly/BA2-HandsOnPumpNM—Blog post summary from this author about how to do hands-on pumping with links to the Stanford videos.

bit.ly/BA2-PumpingPretermHandout—"Pumping Milk for Your Preterm Baby" (English and Spanish) by Kay Hoover and Barbara Wilson-Clay. A 4-page booklet with full-color photos, a weekly pumping log, and low-literacy text with instructions for those exclusively pumping from birth.

bit.ly/BA2-StanfordHandExpress—A 7.5 minute video by Dr. Jane Morton demonstrating the manual expression technique used at Stanford University Hospital.

REFERENCES

AAP. (2012). Breastfeeding and the use of human milk. *Pediatrics, 129*(3), e827-e841.

Acuna-Muga, J., Ureta-Velasco, N., de la Cruz-Bertolo, J., et al. (2014). Volume of milk obtained in relation to location and circumstances of expression in mothers of very low birth weight infants. *Journal of Human Lactation, 30*(1), 41-46.

Ak, J., Lakshmanagowda, P. B., G, C. M. P., et al. (2015). Impact of music therapy on breast milk secretion in mothers of premature newborns. *Journal of Clinical and Diagnostic Research, 9*(4), CC04-06.

Alekseev, N. P., & Ilyin, V. I. (2016). The mechanics of breast pumping: Compression stimuli increased milk ejection. *Breastfeeding Medicine, 11,* 370-375.

Amir, L., & Hoover, K. (2002). Candidiasis and breastfeeding. In (Vol. 6). Schaumburg, IL: La Leche League International.

Anderson, P. O. (2018). Unusual milk colors. *Breastfeeding Medicine, 13*(3), 172-173.

Azad, M. B., Vehling, L., Chan, D., et al. (2018). Infant feeding and weight gain: Separating breast milk from breastfeeding and formula from food. *Pediatrics, 142*(4).

Bai, D. L., Fong, D. Y., Lok, K. Y., et al. (2017). Practices, predictors and consequences of expressed breast-milk feeding in healthy full-term infants. *Public Health Nutrition, 20*(3), 492-503.

Becker, G. E., & Roberts, T. (2009). Do we agree? Using a Delphi technique to develop consensus on skills of hand expression. *Journal of Human Lactation, 25*(2), 220-225.

Becker, G. E., Smith, H. A., & Cooney, F. (2016). Methods of milk expression for lactating women. *Cochrane Database of Systematic Reviews, 9,* CD006170. doi:10.1002/14651858.CD006170.pub5

Ben-Shoshan, M., Mandel, D., Lubetzky, R., et al. (2016). Eradication of cytomegalovirus from human milk by microwave irradiation: A pilot study. *Breastfeeding Medicine, 11,* 186-187.

Benson, S. (2001). What is normal? A study of normal breastfeeding dyads during the first sixty hours of life. *Breastfeeding Review, 9*(1), 27-32.

Berkow, S. E., Freed, L. M., Hamosh, M., et al. (1984). Lipases and lipids in human milk: Effect of freeze-thawing and storage. *Pediatric Research, 18*(12), 1257-1262.

Bertini, G., Breschi, R., & Dani, C. (2015). Physiological weight loss chart helps to identify high-risk infants who need breastfeeding support. *Acta Paediatrica, 104*(10), 1024-1027.

Binns, C. W., Win, N. N., Zhao, Y., et al. (2006). Trends in the expression of breastmilk 1993-2003. *Breastfeeding Review, 14*(3), 5-9.

Bitman, J., Wood, D. L., Mehta, N. R., et al. (1983). Lipolysis of triglycerides of human milk during storage at low temperatures: A note of caution. *Journal of Pediatric Gastroenterology and Nutrition, 2*(3), 521-524.

Blouin, M., Coulombe, M., & Rhainds, M. (2014). Specimen plastic containers used to store expressed breast milk in neonatal care units: A case of precautionary principle. *Canadian Journal of Public Health, 105*(3), e218-220.

Bolman, M., Saju, L., Oganesyan, K., et al. (2013). Recapturing the art of therapeutic breast massage during breastfeeding. *Journal of Human Lactation, 29*(3), 328-331.

Bower, K., Burnette, T., Lewis, D., et al. (2017). "I had one job and that was to make milk." *Journal of Human Lactation, 33*(1), 188-194.

Bransburg-Zabary, S., Virozub, A., & Mimouni, F. B. (2015). Human milk warming temperatures using a simulation of currently available storage and warming methods. *PLoS One, 10*(6), e0128806.

Brown, A., & Arnott, B. (2014). Breastfeeding duration and early parenting behaviour: The importance of an infant-led, responsive style. *PLoS One, 9*(2), e83893.

Bujold, M., Feeley, N., Axelin, A., et al. (2018). Expressing human milk in the NICU: Coping mechanisms and challenges shape the complex experience of closeness and separation. *Advances in Neonatal Care, 18*(1), 38-48.

Burton, P., Kennedy, K., Ahluwalia, J. S., et al. (2013). Randomized trial comparing the effectiveness of 2 electric breast pumps in the NICU. *Journal of Human Lactation, 29*(3), 412-419.

Buss, I. H., McGill, F., Darlow, B. A., et al. (2001). Vitamin C is reduced in human milk after storage. *Acta Paediatrica, 90*(7), 813-815.

Butte, N. F., Garza, C., Smith, E. O., et al. (1984). Human milk intake and growth in exclusively breast-fed infants. *Journal of Pediatrics, 104*(2), 187-195.

Casey, J. R. R., Banks, J., Braniff, K., et al. (2019). The effects of expressing antenatal colostrum in women with diabetes in pregnancy: A retrospective cohort study. *Australian and New Zealand Journal of Obstetrics and Gynaecology.* doi:10.1111/ajo.12966.

CDC. (2018, 1/24/2018). Are special precautions needed while handling breast milk? Retrieved from **cdc.gov/breastfeeding/faq/#handling-breast-milk**.

CDC. (2019, June 2019). Storage and preparation of breast milk. Retrieved from **cdc.gov/breastfeeding/pdf/preparation-of-breast-milk_H.pdf**.

Chang, Y. C., Chen, C. H., & Lin, M. C. (2012). The macronutrients in human milk change after storage in various containers. *Pediatrics and Neonatology, 53*(3), 205-209.

Chatterton, R. T., Jr., Hill, P. D., Aldag, J. C., et al. (2000). Relation of plasma oxytocin and prolactin concentrations to milk production in mothers of preterm infants: Influence of stress. *Journal of Clinical Endocrinology and Metabolism, 85*(10), 3661-3668.

Clark, R. A. (1992). Breast milk does not constitute occupational exposure as defined by standard. Retrieved from **osha.gov/pls/oshaweb/owadisp.show_document?p_table=INTERPRETATIONS&p_id=20952**.

Clemons, S. N., & Amir, L. H. (2010). Breastfeeding women's experience of expressing: A descriptive study. *Journal of Human Lactation, 26*(3), 258-265.

Cobo, E. (1993). Characteristics of the spontaneous milk ejecting activity occurring during human lactation. *Journal of Perinatal Medicine, 21*(1), 77-85.

Coles, J., Anderson, A., & Loxton, D. (2016). Breastfeeding duration after childhood sexual abuse: An Australian cohort study. *Journal of Human Lactation, 32*(3), NP28-35.

Colson, S. (2003). Biological nurturing increases duration of breastfeeding for a vulnerable cohort. *MIDRIS Midwifery Digest, 13*(1), 92-97.

Colson, S. (2019). *Biological Nurturing: Instinctual Breastfeeding* (2nd ed.). Amarillo, TX: Praeclarus Press.

Cotterman, K. J. (2004). Reverse pressure softening: A simple tool to prepare areola for easier latching during engorgement. *Journal of Human Lactation, 20*(2), 227-237.

Cowley, K. C. (2005). Psychogenic and pharmacologic induction of the let-down reflex can facilitate breastfeeding by tetraplegic women: A report of 3 cases. *Archives of Physical Medicine and Rehabilitation, 86*(6), 1261-1264.

Cowley, K. C. (2014). Breastfeeding by women with tetraplegia: Some evidence for optimism. *Spinal Cord, 52*(3), 255.

Cox, S. (2006). Expressing and storing colostrum antenatally for use in the newborn period. *Breastfeeding Review, 14*(3), 5-8.

Dabas, S., Joshi, P., Agarwal, R., et al. (2019). Impact of audio assisted relaxation technique on stress, anxiety and milk output among postpartum mothers of hospitalized neonates: A randomized controlled trial. *Journal of Neonatal Nursing, 25*(4), 200-204.

Daly, S. E., Owens, R. A., & Hartmann, P. E. (1993). The short-term synthesis and infant-regulated removal of milk in lactating women. *Experimental Physiology, 78*(2), 209-220.

de Carvalho, M., Anderson, D. M., Glangreco, A., et al. (1985). Frequency of milk expression and milk production by mothers of nonnursing premature neonates. *American Journal of Diseases of Children, 139,* 483-485.

De Carvalho, M., Robertson, S., Friedman, A., et al. (1983). Effect of frequent breast-feeding on early milk production and infant weight gain. *Pediatrics, 72*(3), 307-311.

Demirci, J. R., Glasser, M., Fichner, J., et al. (2019). "It gave me so much confidence": First-time U.S. mothers' experiences with antenatal milk expression. *Maternal and Child Nutrition,* e12824. doi:10.1111/mcn.12824.

Eglash, A., & Malloy, M. L. (2015). Breastmilk expression and breast pump technology. *Clinical Obstetrics and Gynecology, 58*(4), 855-867.

Eglash, A., Simon, L., & Academy of Breastfeeding, M. (2017). ABM Clinical Protocol #8: Human milk storage information for home use for full-term infants, revised 2017. *Breastfeeding Medicine, 12*(7), 390-395.

Elfgen, C., Hagenbuch, N., Gorres, G., et al. (2017). Breastfeeding in women having experienced childhood sexual abuse. *Journal of Human Lactation, 33*(1), 119-127.

Engstrom, J. L., Meier, P. P., Jegier, B., et al. (2007). Comparison of milk output from the right and left breasts during simultaneous pumping in mothers of very low birthweight infants. *Breastfeeding Medicine, 2*(2), 83-91.

Esfahani, M. S., Berenji-Sooghe, S., Valiani, M., et al. (2015). Effect of acupressure on milk volume of breastfeeding mothers referring to selected health care centers in Tehran. *Iranian Journal of Nursing and Midwifery Research, 20*(1), 7.

Feher, S. D., Berger, L. R., Johnson, J. D., et al. (1989). Increasing breast milk production for premature infants with a relaxation/imagery audiotape. *Pediatrics, 83*(1), 57-60.

Felice, J. P., Cassano, P. A., & Rasmussen, K. M. (2016). Pumping human milk in the early postpartum period: Its impact on long-term practices for feeding at the breast and exclusively feeding human milk in a longitudinal survey cohort. *American Journal of Clinical Nutrition, 103*(5), 1267-1277.

Felice, J. P., Geraghty, S. R., Quaglieri, C. W., et al. (2017). "Breastfeeding" without baby: A longitudinal, qualitative investigation of how mothers perceive, feel about, and practice human milk expression. *Maternal and Child Nutrition, 13*(3).

Fewtrell, M., Kennedy, K., Lukoyanova, O., et al. (2019). Short-term efficacy of two breast pumps and impact on breastfeeding outcomes at 6 months in exclusively breastfeeding mothers: A randomised trial. *Maternal and Child Nutrition, 15*(3), e12779.

Fewtrell, M. S., Kennedy, K., Ahluwalia, J. S., et al. (2016). Predictors of expressed breast milk volume in mothers expressing milk for their preterm infant. *Archives of Disease in Childhood. Fetal and Neonatal Edition, 101*(6), F502-F506.

Fewtrell, M. S., Loh, K. L., Blake, A., et al. (2006). Randomised, double blind trial of oxytocin nasal spray in mothers expressing breast milk for preterm infants. *Archives of Disease in Childhood. Fetal and Neonatal Edition, 91*(3), F169-174.

Flaherman, V. J., Beiler, J. S., Cabana, M. D., et al. (2016). Relationship of newborn weight loss to milk supply concern and anxiety: The impact on breastfeeding duration. *Maternal and Child Nutrition, 12*(3), 463-472.

Flaherman, V. J., Gay, B., Scott, C., et al. (2012). Randomised trial comparing hand expression with breast pumping for mothers of term newborns feeding poorly. *Archives of Disease in Childhood. Fetal and Neonatal Edition, 97*(1), F18-23.

Fogleman, A. D., Meng, T., Osborne, J., et al. (2018). Storage of unfed and leftover mothers' own milk. *Breastfeeding Medicine, 13*(1), 42-49.

Forster, D. A., Moorhead, A. M., Jacobs, S. E., et al. (2017). Advising women with diabetes in pregnancy to express breastmilk in late pregnancy (Diabetes and Antenatal Milk Expressing [DAME]): A multicentre, unblinded, randomised controlled trial. *Lancet, 389*(10085), 2204-2213.

Francis, J., & Dickton, D. (2019). Physical analysis of the breast after direct breastfeeding compared with hand or pump expression: A randomized clinical trial. *Breastfeeding Medicine. 14*(10), 705-711.

Furman, L., Minich, N., & Hack, M. (2002). Correlates of lactation in mothers of very low birth weight infants. *Pediatrics, 109*(4), e57.

Garcia-Lara, N. R., Escuder-Vieco, D., Garcia-Algar, O., et al. (2012). Effect of freezing time on macronutrients and energy content of breastmilk. *Breastfeeding Medicine, 7,* 295-301.

Gardner, H., Kent, J. C., Prime, D. K., et al. (2017). Milk ejection patterns remain consistent during the first and second lactations. *American Journal of Human Biology, 29*(3).

Garza, C., Johnson, C. A., Harrist, R., et al. (1982). Effects of methods of collection and storage on nutrients in human milk. *Early Human Development, 6*(3), 295-303.

Geraghty, S. R., Khoury, J. C., & Kalkwarf, H. J. (2005). Human milk pumping rates of mothers of singletons and mothers of multiples. *Journal of Human Lactation, 21*(4), 413-420.

Gessler, P., Bischoff, G. A., Wiegand, D., et al. (2004). Cytomegalovirus-associated necrotizing enterocolitis in a preterm twin after breastfeeding. *Journal of Perinatology, 24*(2), 124-126.

Glynn, L., & Goosen, L. (2005). Manual expression of breast milk. *Journal of Human Lactation, 21*(2), 184-185.

Goldblum, R. M., Garza, C., Johnson, C. A., et al. (1981). Human milk banking I: Effects of container upon immunologic factors in mature milk. *Nutrition Research, 1*(449-459).

Gribble, K. D. (2005a). Adoptive breastfeeding. *Breastfeeding Review, 13*(3), 6.

Gribble, K. D. (2005b). Post-institutionalized adopted children who seek breastfeeding from their new mothers. *Journal of Prenatal & Perinatal Psychology & Health, 19*(3), 217-235.

Hamosh, M., Ellis, L. A., Pollock, D. R., et al. (1996). Breastfeeding and the working mother: Effect of time and temperature of short-term storage on proteolysis, lipolysis, and bacterial growth in milk. *Pediatrics, 97*(4), 492-498.

Handa, D., Ahrabi, A. F., Codipilly, C. N., et al. (2014). Do thawing and warming affect the integrity of human milk? *Journal of Perinatology, 34*(11), 863-866.

Hanna, N., Ahmed, K., Anwar, M., et al. (2004). Effect of storage on breast milk antioxidant activity. *Archives of Disease in Childhood. Fetal and Neonatal Edition, 89*(6), F518-520.

Hayes, D. K., Prince, C. B., Espinueva, V., et al. (2008). Comparison of manual and electric breast pumps among WIC women returning to work or school in Hawaii. *Breastfeeding Medicine, 3*(1), 3-10.

Heinig, M. J., Nommsen, L. A., Peerson, J. M., et al. (1993). Energy and protein intakes of breast-fed and formula-fed infants during the first year of life and their association with growth velocity: The DARLING Study. *American Journal of Clinical Nutrition, 58*(2), 152-161.

Hernandez, J., Lemons, P., Lemons, J., et al. (1979). Effect of storage processes on the bacterial growth-inhibiting activity of human breast milk. *Pediatrics, 63*(4), 597-601.

Hernandez, L. L., Stiening, C. M., Wheelock, J. B., et al. (2008). Evaluation of serotonin as a feedback inhibitor of lactation in the bovine. *Journal of Dairy Science, 91*(5), 1834-1844.

Hill, P. D., Aldag, J. C., Chatterton, R. T., et al. (2005). Comparison of milk output between mothers of preterm and term infants: The first 6 weeks after birth. *Journal of Human Lactation, 21*(1), 22-30.

Hill, P. D., Aldag, J. C., Zinaman, M., et al. (2007). Comparison of milk output between breasts in pump-dependent mothers. *Journal of Human Lactation, 23*(4), 333-337.

Hopkinson, J. M., Schanler, R. J., & Garza, C. (1988). Milk production by mothers of premature infants. *Pediatrics, 81*(6), 815-820.

Hung, H. Y., Hsu, Y. Y., Su, P. F., et al. (2018). Variations in the rancid-flavor compounds of human breastmilk under general frozen-storage conditions. *BMC Pediatrics, 18*(1), 94.

Hurst, N. M., Valentine, C. J., Renfro, L., et al. (1997). Skin-to-skin holding in the neonatal intensive care unit influences maternal milk volume. *Journal of Perinatology, 17*(3), 213-217.

Ikonen, R., Paavilainen, E., & Kaunonen, M. (2015). Preterm infants' mothers' experiences with milk expression and breastfeeding: An integrative review. *Advances in Neonatal Care, 15*(6), 394-406.

Islam, M. M., Peerson, J. M., Ahmed, T., et al. (2006). Effects of varied energy density of complementary foods on breast-milk intakes and total energy consumption by healthy, breastfed Bangladeshi children. *American Journal of Clinical Nutrition, 83*(4), 851-858.

Jardine, F. M. (2019). Breastfeeding without nursing: "If only I'd known more about exclusively pumping before giving birth". *Journal of Human Lactation, 35*(2), 272-283.

Johns, H. M., Amir, L. H., McLachlan, H. L., et al. (2016). Breast pump use amongst mothers of healthy term infants in Melbourne, Australia: A prospective cohort study. *Midwifery, 33,* 82-89.

Jones, E., & Hilton, S. (2009). Correctly fitting breast shields are the key to lactation success for pump dependent mothers following preterm delivery. *Journal of Neonatal Nursing, 15*(1), 14-17.

Jones, F. (2019). *Best Practice for Expressing, Storing, and Handling Human Milk in Hospitals, Homes, and Child Care Settings* (4th ed.). Fort Worth, TX: Human Milk Banking Association of North America.

Keim, S. A., Kulkarni, M. M., McNamara, K., et al. (2015). Cow's milk contamination of human milk purchased via the internet. *Pediatrics, 135*(5), e1157-1162.

Keim, S. A., McNamara, K., Kwiek, J. J., et al. (2015). Drugs of abuse in human milk purchased via the internet. *Breastfeeding Medicine, 10*(9), 416-418.

Keith, D. R., Weaver, B. S., & Vogel, R. L. (2012). The effect of music-based listening interventions on the volume, fat content, and caloric content of breast milk-produced by mothers of premature and critically ill infants. *Advances in Neonatal Care, 12*(2), 112-119.

Kendall-Tackett, K., Cong, Z., & Hale, T. W. (2013). Depression, sleep quality, and maternal well-being in postpartum women with a history of sexual assault: A comparison of breastfeeding, mixed-feeding, and formula-feeding mothers. *Breastfeeding Medicine, 8*(1), 16-22.

Kent, J. C. (2007). How breastfeeding works. *Journal of Midwifery & Women's Health, 52*(6), 564-570.

Kent, J. C., Gardner, H., & Geddes, D. T. (2016). Breastmilk production in the first 4 weeks after birth of term infants. *Nutrients, 8*(12).

Kent, J. C., Hepworth, A. R., Sherriff, J. L., et al. (2013). Longitudinal changes in breastfeeding patterns from 1 to 6 months of lactation. *Breastfeeding Medicine, 8,* 401-407.

Kent, J. C., Mitoulas, L. R., Cregan, M. D., et al. (2008). Importance of vacuum for breastmilk expression. *Breastfeeding Medicine, 3*(1), 11-19.

Kent, J. C., Mitoulas, L. R., Cregan, M. D., et al. (2006). Volume and frequency of breastfeedings and fat content of breast milk throughout the day. *Pediatrics, 117*(3), e387-395.

Kent, J. C., Prime, D. K., & Garbin, C. P. (2012). Principles for maintaining or increasing breast milk production. *Journal of Obstetric, Gynecologic & Neonatal Nursing, 41*(1), 114-121.

Kent, J. C., Ramsay, D. T., Doherty, D., et al. (2003). Response of breasts to different stimulation patterns of an electric breast pump. *Journal of Human Lactation, 19*(2), 179-186; quiz 187-178, 218.

Klaus, P. (2010). The impact of childhood sexual abuse on childbearing and breastfeeding: The role of maternity caregivers. *Breastfeeding Medicine, 5*(4), 141-145.

Kramer, M. S., Guo, T., Platt, R. W., et al. (2004). Feeding effects on growth during infancy. *Journal of Pediatrics, 145*(5), 600-605.

Labiner-Wolfe, J., & Fein, S. B. (2013). How US mothers store and handle their expressed breast milk. *Journal of Human Lactation, 29*(1), 54-58.

Labiner-Wolfe, J., Fein, S. B., Shealy, K. R., et al. (2008). Prevalence of breast milk expression and associated factors. *Pediatrics, 122 Suppl 2,* S63-68.

Lawrence, R. A., & Lawrence, R. M. (2016). *Breastfeeding: A Guide for the Medical Profession* (8th ed.). Philadelphia, PA: Elsevier.

Li, R., Magadia, J., Fein, S. B., et al. (2012). Risk of bottle-feeding for rapid weight gain during the first year of life. *Archives of Pediatric & Adolescent Medicine, 166*(5), 431-436.

Loewenberg Weisband, Y., Keim, S. A., Keder, L. M., et al. (2017). Early breast milk pumping intentions among postpartum women. *Breastfeeding Medicine, 12,* 28-32.

Lucas, A., Gibbs, J. A., & Baum, J. D. (1978). The biology of human drip breast milk. *Early Human Development, 2*(4), 351-361.

Lussier, M. M., Brownell, E. A., Proulx, T. A., et al. (2015). Daily breastmilk volume in mothers of very low birth weight neonates: A repeated-measures randomized trial of hand expression versus electric breast pump expression. *Breastfeeding Medicine, 10*(6), 312-317.

Manohar, A. A., Williamson, M., & Koppikar, G. V. (1997). Effect of storage of colostrum in various containers. *Indian Pediatrics, 34*(4), 293-295.

Martin, K. (2011). A time and place to pump: What lactation consultants need to know about the new federal protections for employed breastfeeding mothers. *Clinical Lactation, 2*(2), 20-21.

Martinez-Costa, C., Silvestre, M. D., Lopez, M. C., et al. (2007). Effects of refrigeration on the bactericidal activity of human milk: A preliminary study. *Journal of Pediatric Gastroenterology and Nutrition, 45*(2), 275-277.

McCloskey, R. J., & Karandikar, S. (2018). A liberation health approach to examining challenges and facilitators of peer-to-peer human milk sharing. *Journal of Human Lactation, 34*(3), 438-447.

Meier, P. (2004). Choosing a correctly-fitted breastshield. *Medela Messenger, 21,* 8-9.

Meier, P., Motykowski, J. E., & Zuleger, J. L. (2004). Choosing a correctly-fitted breastshield for milk expression. *Medela Messenger, 21,* 8-9.

Meier, P. P., Engstrom, J. L., Hurst, N. M., et al. (2008). A comparison of the efficiency, efficacy, comfort, and convenience of two hospital-grade electric breast pumps for mothers of very low birthweight infants. *Breastfeeding Medicine, 3*(3), 141-150.

Meier, P. P., Engstrom, J. L., Janes, J. E., et al. (2012). Breast pump suction patterns that mimic the human infant during breastfeeding: greater milk output in less time spent pumping for breast pump-dependent mothers with premature infants. *Journal of Perinatology, 32*(2), 103-110.

Meier, P. P., Johnson, T. J., Patel, A. L., et al. (2017). Evidence-based methods that promote human milk feeding of preterm infants: An expert review. *Clinical Perinatology, 44*(1), 1-22.

Meier, P. P., Patel, A. L., Hoban, R., et al. (2016). Which breast pump for which mother: An evidence-based approach to individualizing breast pump technology. *Journal of Perinatology, 36*(7), 493-499.

Mohrbacher, N. (1996). Mothers who forgo breastfeeding for pumping. *Ameda/Egnell Circle of Caring, 9*(2), 1-2.

Mohrbacher, N. (2011). The 'magic number' and long-term milk production. *Clinical Lactation, 2*(1), 15-18.

Mohrbacher, N. (2014). When stored milk smells soapy or rancid. *Breastfeeding Today, 26*(12), 4-6.

Morton, J., Hall, J. Y., Wong, R. J., et al. (2009). Combining hand techniques with electric pumping increases milk production in mothers of preterm infants. *Journal of Perinatology, 29*(11), 757-764.

Morton, J., Wong, R. J., Hall, J. Y., et al. (2012). Combining hand techniques with electric pumping increases the caloric content of milk in mothers of preterm infants. *Journal of Perinatology, 32*(10), 791-796.

Naor, N., Fridman, E., Kouadio, F., et al. (2019). Green breast milk following ingestion of blue-green algae: A case report. *Breastfeeding Medicine, 14*(3), 203-204.

Novak, F. R., Da Silva, A. V., Hagler, A. N., et al. (2000). Contamination of expressed human breast milk with an epidemic multiresistant Staphylococcus aureus clone. *Journal of Medical Microbiology, 49*(12), 1109-1117.

O'Sullivan, E. J., Geraghty, S. R., & Rasmussen, K. M. (2018). Awareness and prevalence of human milk sharing and selling in the United States. *Maternal and Child Nutrition, 14 Supplement 6,* e12567.

Ohyama, M., Watabe, H., & Hayasaka, Y. (2010). Manual expression and electric breast pumping in the first 48 h after delivery. *Pediatrics International, 52*(1), 39-43.

Ovesen, L., Jakobsen, J., Leth, T., et al. (1996). The effect of microwave heating on vitamins B1 and E, and linoleic and linolenic acids, and immunoglobulins in human milk. *International Journal of Food Science and Nutrition, 47*(5), 427-436.

Pang, W. W., Bernard, J. Y., Thavamani, G., et al. (2017). Direct vs. expressed breast milk feeding: Relation to duration of breastfeeding. *Nutrients, 9*(6).

Pardou, A., Serruys, E., Mascart-Lemone, F., et al. (1994). Human milk banking: Influence of storage processes and of bacterial contamination on some milk constituents. *Biology of the Neonate, 65*(5), 302-309.

Parker, L. A., Sullivan, S., Krueger, C., et al. (2012). Effect of early breast milk expression on milk volume and timing of lactogenesis stage II among mothers of very low birth weight infants: A pilot study. *Journal of Perinatology, 32*(3), 205-209.

Parker, L. A., Sullivan, S., Krueger, C., et al. (2015). Association of timing of initiation of breastmilk expression on milk volume and timing of lactogenesis stage II among mothers of very low-birth-weight infants. *Breastfeeding Medicine, 10*(2), 84-91.

Parker, M. G., Melvin, P., Graham, D. A., et al. (2019). Timing of first milk expression to maximize breastfeeding continuation among mothers of very low-birth-weight infants. *Obstetrics & Gynecology, 133*(6), 1208-1215.

Pittard, W. B., 3rd, Anderson, D. M., Cerutti, E. R., et al. (1985). Bacteriostatic qualities of human milk. *Journal of Pediatrics, 107*(2), 240-243.

Pittard, W. B., 3rd, Geddes, K. M., Brown, S., et al. (1991). Bacterial contamination of human milk: Container type and method of expression. *American Journal of Perinatology, 8*(1), 25-27.

Post, E. D., Stam, G., & Tromp, E. (2016). Milk production after preterm, late preterm and term delivery; effects of different breast pump suction patterns. *Journal of Perinatology, 36*(1), 47-51.

Prentice, A. (1989). Evidence for local feedback control of human milk secretion. *Biochemical Society Transactions, 17,* 489-492.

Prime, D. K., Geddes, D. T., & Hartmann, P. E. (2007). Oxytocin: Milk ejection and maternal-infant well-being. In T. W. Hale & P. E. Hartmann (Eds.), *Hale & Hartmann's Textbook of Human Lactation* (pp. 141-155). Amarillo, TX: Hale Publishing.

Prime, D. K., Kent, J. C., Hepworth, A. R., et al. (2012). Dynamics of milk removal during simultaneous breast expression in women. *Breastfeeding Medicine, 7*(2), 100-106.

Quan, R., Yang, C., Rubinstein, S., et al. (1992). Effects of microwave radiation on anti-infective factors in human milk. *Pediatrics, 89*(4 Pt 1), 667-669.

Quinn, L., Ailsworth, M., Matthews, E., et al. (2018). Serratia marcescens colonization causing pink breast milk and pink diapers: A case report and literature review. *Breastfeeding Medicine, 13*(5), 388-394.

Ramsay, D. T., & Hartmann, P. E. (2005). Milk removal from the breast. *Breastfeeding Review, 13*(1), 5-7.

Ramsay, D. T., Kent, J. C., Owens, R. A., et al. (2004). Ultrasound imaging of milk ejection in the breast of lactating women. *Pediatrics, 113*(2), 361-367.

Ramsay, D. T., Mitoulas, L. R., Kent, J. C., et al. (2006). Milk flow rates can be used to identify and investigate milk ejection in women expressing breast milk using an electric breast pump. *Breastfeeding Medicine, 1*(1), 14-23.

Ramsay, D. T., Mitoulas, L. R., Kent, J. C., et al. (2005). The use of ultrasound to characterize milk ejection in women using an electric breast pump. *Journal of Human Lactation, 21*(4), 421-428.

Raoof, N. A., Adamkin, D. H., Radmacher, P. G., et al. (2016). Comparison of lactoferrin activity in fresh and stored human milk. *Journal of Perinatology, 36*(3), 207-209.

Reyes-Foster, B. M., Carter, S. K., & Hinojosa, M. S. (2015). Milk sharing in practice: A descriptive analysis of peer breastmilk sharing. *Breastfeeding Medicine, 10*(5), 263-269.

Reyes-Foster, B. M., Carter, S. K., & Hinojosa, M. S. (2017). Human milk hand storage practices among peer milk-sharing mothers. *Journal of Human Lactation, 33*(1), 173-180.

Rollo, D. E., Radmacher, P. G., Turcu, R. M., et al. (2014). Stability of lactoferrin in stored human milk. *Journal of Perinatology, 34*(4), 284-286.

Rosa, C. A., Novak, F. R., de Almeida, J. A., et al. (1990). Yeasts from human milk collected in Rio de Janeiro, Brazil. *Revista de Microbiologia, 21*(4), 361-363.

Saint, L., Smith, M., & Hartmann, P. E. (1984). The yield and nutrient content of colostrum and milk of women from giving birth to 1 month post-partum. *British Journal of Nutrition, 52*(1), 87-95.

Sigman, M., Burke, K. I., Swarner, O. W., et al. (1989). Effects of microwaving human milk: Changes in IgA content and bacterial count. *Journal of the American Dietetic Association, 89*(5), 690-692.

Silvestre, D., Lopez, M. C., March, L., et al. (2006). Bactericidal activity of human milk: Stability during storage. *British Journal of Biomedical Science, 63*(2), 59-62.

Slusher, T., Slusher, I. L., Biomdo, M., et al. (2007). Electric breast pump use increases maternal milk volume in African nurseries. *Journal of Tropical Pediatrics, 53*(2), 125-130.

Slusher, T. M., Slusher, I. L., Keating, E. M., et al. (2012). Comparison of maternal milk (breastmilk) expression methods in an African nursery. *Breastfeeding Medicine, 7*(2), 107-111.

Smillie, C. M. (2017). How infants learn to feed: A neurobehavioral model. In C. W. Genna (Ed.), *Supporting Sucking Skills in Breastfeeding Infants* (3rd ed., pp. 89-111). Burlington, MA: Jones & Bartlett Learning.

Sosa, R., & Barness, L. (1987). Bacterial growth in refrigerated human milk. *American Journal of Diseases of Children, 141*(1), 111-112.

Spatz, D. L. (2021). The use of human milk and breastfeeding in the neonatal intensive care unit. In K. Wambach & B. Spencer (Eds.), *Breastfeeding and Human Lactation* (6th ed., pp. 397-441). Burlington, MA: Jones & Bartlett Learning.

Takci, S., Gulmez, D., Yigit, S., et al. (2012). Effects of freezing on the bactericidal activity of human milk. *Journal of Pediatric Gastroenterology and Nutrition, 55*(2), 146-149.

Talbert, A. W., Tsofa, B., Mumbo, E., et al. (2018). Knowledge of, and attitudes to giving expressed breastmilk to infants in rural coastal Kenya; focus group discussions of first time mothers and their advisers. *International Breastfeeding Journal, 13,* 16.

Thatrimontrichai, A., Janjindamai, W., & Puwanant, M. (2012). Fat loss in thawed breast milk: Comparison between refrigerator and warm water. *Indian Pediatrics, 49*(11), 877-880.

USDA. (2013, 6/15/13). Freezing and food safety. Retrieved from **https://www.fsis.usda.gov/wps/portal/fsis/topics/food-safety-education/get-answers/food-safety-fact-sheets/safe-food-handling/freezing-and-food-safety/CT_Index**.

USFDA. (2018, 3/22/18). Use of donor human milk. Retrieved from **https://www.fda.gov/science-research/pediatrics/use-donor-human-milk**.

Vazquez-Roman, S., Escuder-Vieco, D., Garcia-Lara, N. R., et al. (2016). Impact of freezing time on dornic acidity in three types of milk: Raw donor milk, mother's own milk, and pasteurized donor milk. *Breastfeeding Medicine, 11*(2), 91-93.

vom Saal, F. S., & Hughes, C. (2005). An extensive new literature concerning low-dose effects of bisphenol A shows the need for a new risk assessment. *Environmental Health Perspectives, 113*(8), 926-933.

Walker, S., & Armstrong, M. (2012). The four pillars of safe breast milk sharing. *Midwifery Today International Midwife*(101), 34-37.

WHO. (2009). Infant and young child feeding: Model Chapter for textbooks for medical students and allied health professionals. *Geneva, Switzerland: World Health Organization.*

Williamson, M. T., & Murti, P. K. (1996). Effects of storage, time, temperature, and composition of containers on biologic components of human milk. *Journal of Human Lactation, 12*(1), 31-35.

Wilson-Clay, B., & Hoover, K. (2017). *The Breastfeeding Atlas* (6th ed.). Manchaca, TX: LactNews Press.

Win, N. N., Binns, C. W., Zhao, Y., et al. (2006). Breastfeeding duration in mothers who express breast milk: A cohort study. *International Breastfeeding Journal, 1,* 28.

Yazgan, H., Demirdoven, M., Yazgan, Z., et al. (2012). A mother with green breastmilk due to multivitamin and mineral intake: A case report. *Breastfeeding Medicine, 7,* 310-312.

Yigit, F., Cigdem, Z., Temizsoy, E., et al. (2012). Does warming the breasts affect the amount of breastmilk production? *Breastfeeding Medicine, 7*(6), 487-488.

Yourkavitch, J., Rasmussen, K. M., Pence, B. W., et al. (2018). Early, regular breast-milk pumping may lead to early breast-milk feeding cessation. *Public Health Nutrition, 21*(9), 1726-1736.

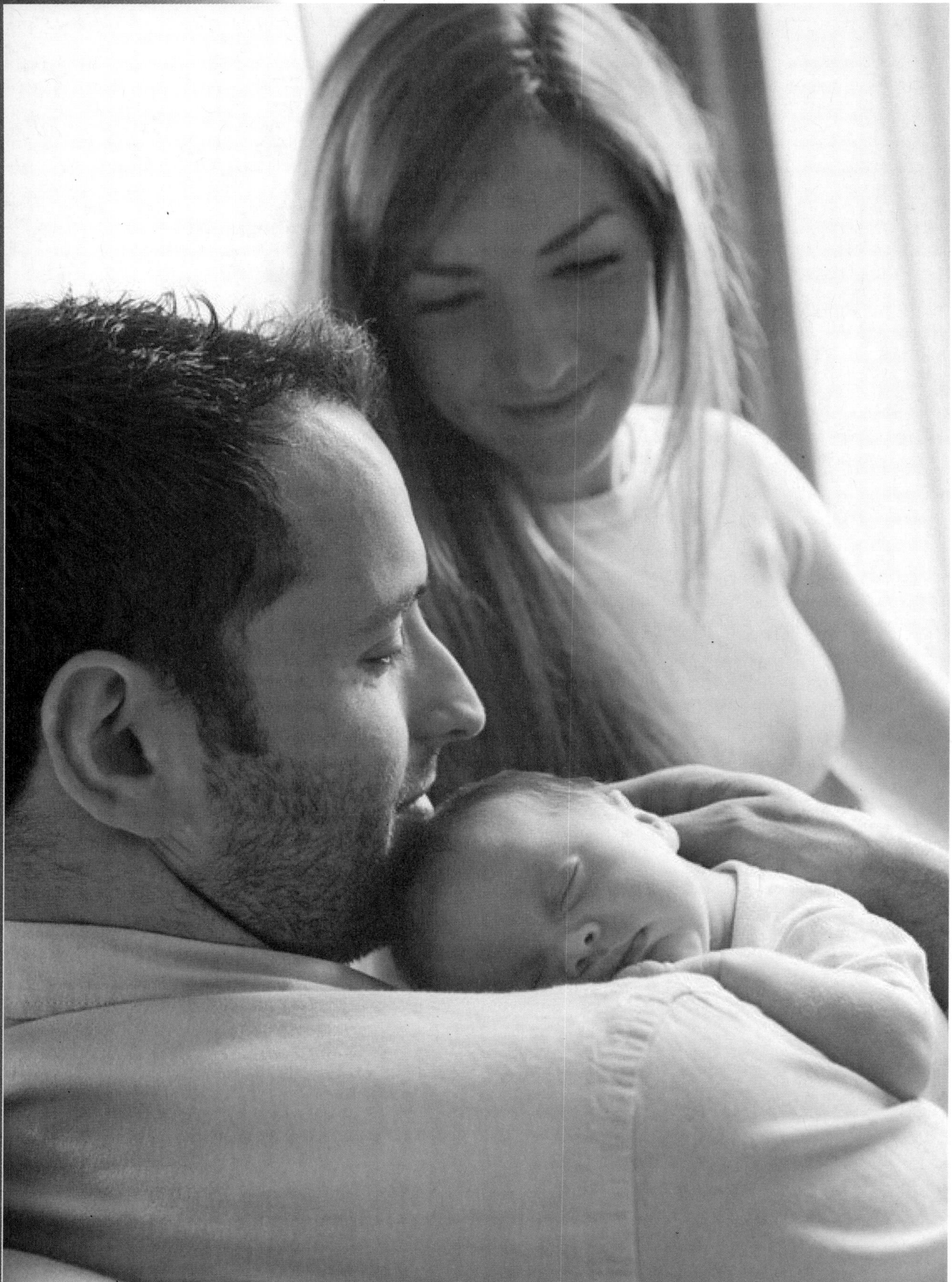

Sex, Fertility, and Contraception

12

NURSING AND SEXUALITY

Changes in Sexual Desire and a Couple's Relationship

During the early months after birth, many nursing parents feel less sexual desire than they did before they began lactating.

After a baby's birth, there are many dynamics that can decrease nursing parents' sexual desire and create tension in their relationship with their partner.

- The often-unexpected time and energy it takes to care for a newborn—nonstop days and sleepless nights, which can cause extreme fatigue and mood swings
- The intense emotional focus on feelings of love and oneness with the baby, often to the exclusion of others
- Changing feelings about their relationship, i.e., some have trouble seeing their partner as both parent and lover
- Little uninterrupted "couple time"
- Feelings of being "touched out" during round-the-clock nursing, making the nursing parent less responsive to the partner's touch
- Birth-related physical or emotional issues, such as discomfort from episiotomy stitches or grief from a disappointing or traumatic birth
- Baby-related challenges, such as health problems or colic
- Hormonal shifts that can contribute to mood swings
- Fears of pregnancy or worries about contraception

KEY CONCEPT

Many nursing parents feel less sexual desire and are less sexually active for several months after birth.

One U.K. cross-sectional study of 484 mothers' sexual experiences during the first 6 months post-delivery (Barrett et al., 2000) found that 67% had sex less often than before pregnancy, and only 5% had sex more often. Comparing sex before and after birth, 38% described it as "less good," 47% "about the same," and 10% "improved."

• • •

If nursing parents feel less interested in sex, encourage them to talk about it with their partner.

When sex becomes a lower priority for long periods, the partner may feel hurt and confused. The birth of a baby is one of the most stressful times for a couple, and during times of change, couples need to communicate openly. When vague feelings of unhappiness surface, it is time to talk. The partner may need reassurance that the lack of sexual desire is not a personal rejection, but a common response to caring for a young baby. Nursing parents may feel better knowing that their partner will not insist on something they are not comfortable giving. Suggest they tell their partner they are willing to work with them to find other ways acceptable to them both that strengthen and deepen their relationship.

• • •

Some nursing parents report heightened sexual responsiveness after birth.

For some, the deep feelings of inner peace that can come with nursing spill over into their sexual relationship with their partner. The warmth and tenderness that caring for an infant stimulates sometimes enhances sexual desire and creates a deeper sexual bond between nursing parents and their partners. One mother said, "There's something about nursing a baby that gives you an all's-right-with-the-world feeling. I feel so loving toward my whole family, not just toward my baby. Sex just seems to be a natural expression of this good feeling" (Kenny, 1973, p. 220).

Some couples find the rounded curves of pregnancy and lactation sexually attractive. Some have fewer worries about pregnancy at these times, allowing for freer sexual expression.

• • •

Research is mixed on the effects of nursing on interest in sex after birth.

In the mid-20th century, sex-research pioneers Masters and Johnson found that breastfeeding mothers were more comfortable with their sexuality and more anxious to resume sexual relations with their partners than formula-feeding mothers (Masters & Johnson, 2010). But many social, cultural, and psychological factors affect the expression of an individual's sexuality.

It is not surprising that research on sexual behavior is mixed, and conclusions vary by country and culture.

- **Germany:** A longitudinal cohort study of 315 women (Wallwiener et al., 2017) found that at 4 months, exclusively breastfeeding mothers were much more likely to be sexually inactive than those who were formula or mixed feeding.
- **Canada:** A study of 316 women found that breastfeeding was associated with a longer delay in resuming sex after birth (Rowland, Foxcroft, Hopman, & Patel, 2005).
- **Uganda:** The timing of resumption of sex after birth was affected in part by tribal customs (Alum, Kizza, Osingada, Katende, & Kaye, 2015).
- **Philippines and Bangladesh:** Breastfeeding mothers were less interested in sex after childbirth than those who didn't breastfeed (Islam & Khan, 1993).
- **Iran:** A survey of 200 women (Malakoti, Zamanzadeh, Maleki, & Farshbaf Khalili, 2013) found that breastfeeding women were less interested in resuming sex between 3 and 6 months after birth than their formula-feeding counterparts.
- **Kuwait:** Breastfeeding mothers were more sexually active than those who formula-fed (al Bustan, el Tomi, Faiwalla, & Manav, 1995).
- **Ireland:** At 6 and 12 months, breastfeeding was associated (along with other factors) with a loss of interest in sex. This loss of interest was also associated with dissatisfaction with their body (O'Malley, Higgins, Begley, Daly, & Smith, 2018).

Research from the U.S. and U.K. is mixed. Some studies found no differences in sexual activity after childbirth among breastfeeding and formula-feeding women (Grudzinskas & Atkinson, 1984; Robson, Brant, & Kumar, 1981). However, a more recent U.S. study (Yee, Kaimal, Nakagawa, Houston, & Kuppermann, 2013) found exclusive breastfeeding was associated with less sexual activity as compared to women who mixed fed or exclusively formula-fed. Some suggest breastfeeding may be a "swing factor," sometimes enhancing sexual desire and sometimes an obstacle to its expression.

A U.S. study that examined the sexual feelings and activity of the nursing parent's partner (van Anders, Hipp, & Kane Low, 2013) found that its 114 partners (95 men, 18 women, and 1 unspecified) found that—unlike some earlier studies—

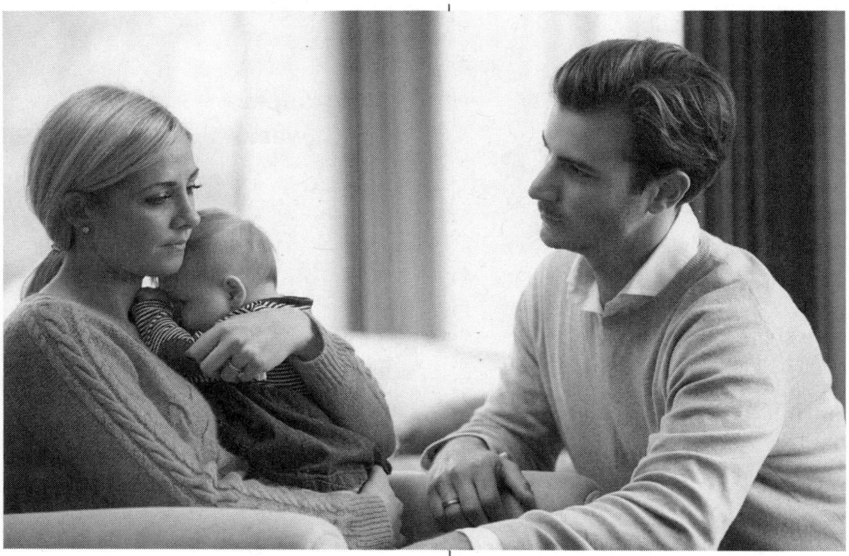

breastfeeding and intensity of breastfeeding did not seem to affect this group's sexual feelings and behavior.

Two fascinating U.S. studies found that exposure to breastfeeding mothers can affect other women's sexuality. In these studies (Jacob et al., 2004; Spencer et al., 2004), non-pregnant, non-lactating women smelled a breastfeeding mother's scent (via pads worn on the breastfeeding mother's breast or armpit), which affected them hormonally by either increasing their sexual desire for their partner or regulating their menstrual cycles. If they didn't have a partner, it increased their sexual fantasies.

• • •

After the birth of a baby, it can be challenging to find a time and a place to make love and fit "couple time" into a routine.

Some have reported an almost psychic link between nursing parents and their babies that makes them so closely attuned to each other that the baby wakes up whenever the nursing parent feels strong emotions, including sexual arousal. Fortunately, this type of "radar" is usually short-lived, occurring only while the baby is small. As the baby matures and becomes less dependent, the intensity of the nursing relationship may diminish.

Time spent together as a couple, whether or not it involves sex, is vital. After the birth of a baby, changes often happen quickly. Ideally, adult partners should support each other as they adjust to their new life as a family. Especially while sex is at a premium, their relationship will more likely stay strong if they make it a priority to be intimate in other ways. If nursing and baby care leave the parent feeling "touched out," for example, suggest finding other ways to be romantic, such as sharing a favorite meal served by candlelight.

In the early period after birth, one way the partner can show real caring and love is by pitching in and taking care of household chores—perhaps the best foreplay. Most nursing parents find it overwhelming to keep up with their usual chores while caring for a tiny baby. If the partner takes over the chores, the nursing parent may find it easier to relax and be more open to sex. Sometimes it may be necessary to explain to the partner what needs to be done, as the partner may be oblivious to the chores usually handled by someone else. Suggest being openly appreciative of the partner's efforts to make their life easier—whether it's by doing household chores or by being patient when the baby consumes most of the available time and energy.

Although some couples think they need to arrange for time away from the baby for "couple time," this is not a requirement. Many nursing parents are more comfortable and relaxed when their baby is near and schedule their couple time at home or take their baby along when they go out with their partner.

• • •

A good relationship may lead to better support for nursing.

One Brazilian study of 153 families (Falceto, Giugliani, & Fernandes, 2004) found that the quality of a couple's relationship was not associated with nursing duration, but that a good relationship between the couple was associated with good support for nursing from the partner.

Nursing and Sex: The Practical Details

In many parts of the world, birthing parents are advised by their healthcare providers to wait until the 6-week checkup before resuming vaginal sex. However, many start earlier. In a Canadian study of 149 women (Rowland et al., 2005), nearly 39% of those nursing resumed sex before their 6-week checkup. In some studies, how quickly parents resume sex after birth depended in part on the type of birth and the degree of perineal damage. An Israeli prospective study (Lurie et al., 2013) found that women who delivered vaginally without an episiotomy or tear resumed sex at on average about 4.5 weeks after birth. Those who delivered by cesarean or had an episiotomy or tear resumed sex on average 2 to 3 weeks later.

Most couples resume sex by 8 to 10 weeks after delivery.

How soon after birth parents resume sex, however, varies around the world. In a large Australian multicenter study (McDonald & Brown, 2013), only 15% of women began having vaginal sex by 4 weeks and only 41% by 6 weeks. By 2 months this rose to 65%, and by 3 months, it had increased to 78%. As in the previous Israeli study, those who had an episiotomy, tear, or cesarean delivery resumed sex later than those who didn't. A 2015 systematic review (Andreucci et al., 2015) had similar findings. When women experienced 3rd or 4th degree tears during birth or had any other traumatic birth experience, they were likely to resume sex later than those who didn't have these experiences.

In some studies, no connection was found between type of delivery and resumption of sex. In the U.S., 150 first-time mothers were followed during pregnancy and for 6 months after delivery (Connolly, Thorp, & Pahel, 2005). By 6 weeks, 57% resumed sex. By 12 weeks, this had risen to 82%, and by 24 weeks, 90%. No association was found between type of delivery or episiotomy and when they resumed sex. Another U.S. study (Yee et al., 2013) found that only about 61% of couples had resumed sex by 8 to 10 weeks after birth.

• • •

At birth, levels of estrogen fall. For this reason, in the first weeks after birth, lactating parents have lower estrogen levels than they do at other times, and low estrogen levels can cause vaginal dryness. But lactation extends this period of low estrogen for at least 6 months, and sometimes for the entire duration of lactation (Lawrence & Lawrence, 2016, p. 706). A U.S. study of 244 women during the first 6 weeks after birth (Agarwal, Kim, Korst, & Hughes, 2015) compared symptoms of vaginal dryness in those who breastfed and bottle-fed (Table 12.1). Some of these study women were using hormonal contraception, which could affect the results. But even in the first 6 weeks—before many women resume sexual relations—noticeably more breastfeeding women reported vaginal dryness than bottle-feeding women.

Low estrogen levels during lactation may cause vaginal dryness, which is easily remedied with lubricants.

TABLE 12.1 Incidence of Vaginal Dryness in Women After Birth by Feeding Method

	Post-Delivery		3 Weeks After Birth		6 Weeks After Birth	
	Breast	Bottle	Breast	Bottle	Breast	Bottle
Vaginal Dryness	1%	3%	13%	4%	18%	2%

Adapted from (Agarwal et al., 2015)

In addition to causing vaginal dryness in some women, low estrogen levels during breastfeeding may also cause vaginal tightness and tenderness. A 2001 U.S. retrospective study found an association between breastfeeding and painful intercourse (Signorello, Harlow, Chekos, & Repke, 2001). Breastfeeding women were 4 times as likely to report painful intercourse as those who didn't breastfeed. A 2018 Irish prospective longitudinal cohort study of 832 first-time mothers (O'Malley et al., 2018) found at 6 months, breastfeeding was associated with vaginal dryness.

If a nursing parent finds intercourse painful or uncomfortable, more foreplay may help. If that is not enough, suggest using a water-based lubricant, such as K-Y jelly. Another option is prescribed estrogen-based creams or suppositories, which research found can be helpful with no apparent effect on lactation (Wisniewski & Wilkinson, 1991).

• • •

During lactation, milk leakage may occur while having sex.

The hormonal changes during lovemaking stimulate a milk ejection in some nursing parents. If either partner considers this an issue, suggest feeding the baby or expressing milk before making love to reduce milk flow. Once the milk is flowing, it can be stopped by applying gentle pressure to the nipples. A towel on hand to catch leaked milk may also help.

Fondling and lovemaking do not need to be restricted during lactation. The mammary glands should not be considered "off limits," unless the nursing parent wants them to be. Some enjoy the presence of milk during lovemaking.

• • •

Some cultures prohibit sexual relations during lactation or until the child reaches a certain age or developmental milestone.

In her classic 1983 book, *A Practical Guide to Breastfeeding*, Jan Riordan, EdD wrote: "Pressures and problems of sexual relations while lactating are as ancient as woman herself. Physicians during the 17th century recommended breastfeeding, but insisted that sexual relations during lactation would spoil the milk and endanger the life of the child" (Riordan, 1983, pp. 338-339). Because human milk substitutes led to higher rates of infant death, wet nurses became popular, allowing mothers to stop breastfeeding to meet their husbands' sexual needs without compromising their babies' health.

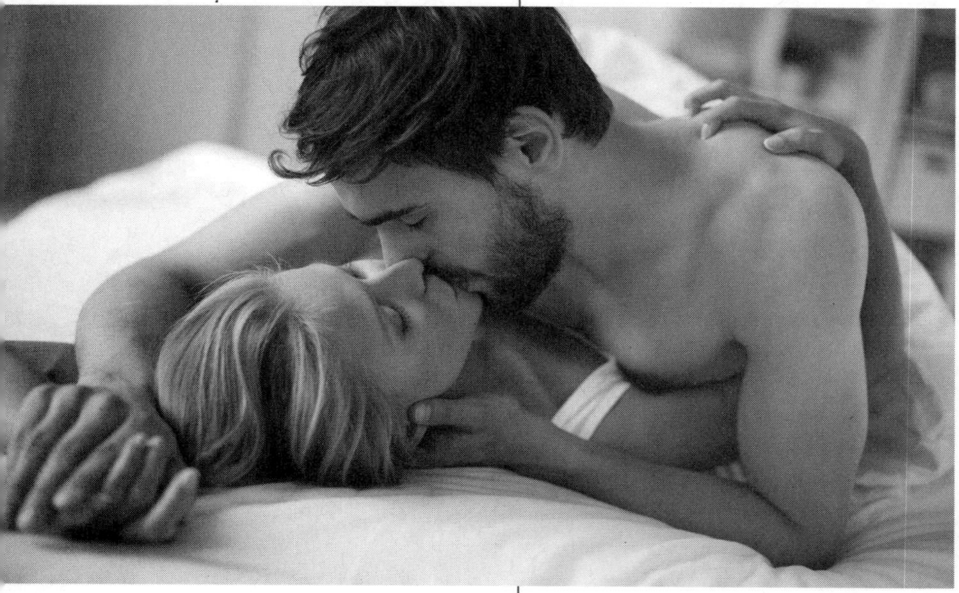

Due to the high value placed on child-spacing, some cultures insist on complete abstinence from sex for a specific period of time—from a few weeks to a year or even longer. In some places, resumption of sexual relations is determined by a developmental milestone, such as the eruption of the baby's teeth or the beginning of crawling or walking (Ford & Beach, 1950). Nigeria is one country where a long period of abstinence after birth is considered the cultural norm. However, studies done in two different regions of Nigeria found that most couples resume sex within 6 to 12 weeks after delivery (Adanikin, Awoleke, Adeyiolu, Alao, & Adanikin, 2015; Anzaku & Mikah, 2014).

NURSING, FERTILITY, AND CONTRACEPTION

The Effects of Nursing on Fertility

Nursing delays the return of fertility after birth.

The hormones released in the nursing parent during feeds interact with many body processes to prolong the period of infertility after birth. One study from Argentina found that breastfeeding affects the development of the egg (ovum) within the ovary (Velasquez, Trigo, Creus, Campo, & Croxatto, 2006).

However, the child-spacing effect of nursing in a large population depends in part on the feeding rhythm common in that culture, as well as duration of nursing and the use of other contraceptives. In cultures where nursing exclusively and intensively is common, the effect on fertility is greater. In cultures that encourage longer intervals between feeds, feeding schedules, or mix nursing with formula use, the effect on fertility is less (M. H. Labbok, 2015). One study demonstrated the profound effect of cultural practices on fertility by analyzing the number of pregnancies prevented by nursing in different countries (Becker, Rutstein, & Labbok, 2003). According to the researchers' calculations, if no parent nursed in Brazil, this would increase the number of births per year by only 1% to 4%, whereas no nursing in Uganda would increase the number of births annually by 50%.

> **KEY CONCEPT**
>
> *The child-spacing effect of nursing in a large population depends in part on the feeding rhythm common in that culture.*

In some traditional societies, nursing alone is responsible for a typical child-spacing of several years. For example, in the !Kung tribe of Botswana, despite the absence of sexual taboos during nursing, births were spaced an average of 44 months apart (Konner & Worthman, 1980). The !Kung children were given free access to nursing and might feed briefly several times per hour around the clock for the first years of life. At this end of the spectrum, exclusive and intensive nursing followed by a gradual introduction of solid foods and continued nursing day and night was reported to delay ovulation for up to 4 years (McNeilly, 2001).

This birth-spacing effect of nursing is nature's way of making sure birthing parents can give the baby their full attention and their body has a chance to recover from pregnancy and childbirth (Haig, 2014). In both developing and industrialized nations, adequate spacing can be crucial to the survival of both birthing parent and child. An analysis of research done in 17 countries concluded that a spacing of at least 36 to 59 months is optimal for the health outcomes of both birthing parent and child in developing countries (Rutstein, 2005). In the U.S., studies indicated that spacing of at least 28 months reduces maternity-related risks significantly (Klerman, Cliver, & Goldenberg, 1998; Zhu, Rolfs, Nangle, & Horan, 1999).

Before the Menses Resume

A baby's nursing rhythm plays a major role in the return to fertility.

The time between birth and the first nursing is one of the first aspects of the nursing rhythm associated with fertility, with a shorter time between birth and the first feed associated with a longer delay in the return of menses (WHO, 1998b).

The World Health Organization did a prospective study of more than 4,000 breastfeeding women in seven countries and found that 7 of the 10 factors significantly associated with the delay in menstruation after birth involved babies' breastfeeding rhythms (WHO, 1998a, 1998b). But there's more about nursing that affects fertility than just the hormones released from active sucking. One Chilean study of 99 mother/baby pairs found that sucking activity and length were not associated with a delay in the return of menses, but time at the breast in non-sucking pauses was (Prieto, Cardenas, & Croxatto, 1999). So, sensory aspects of nursing other than sucking may also affect the return to fertility.

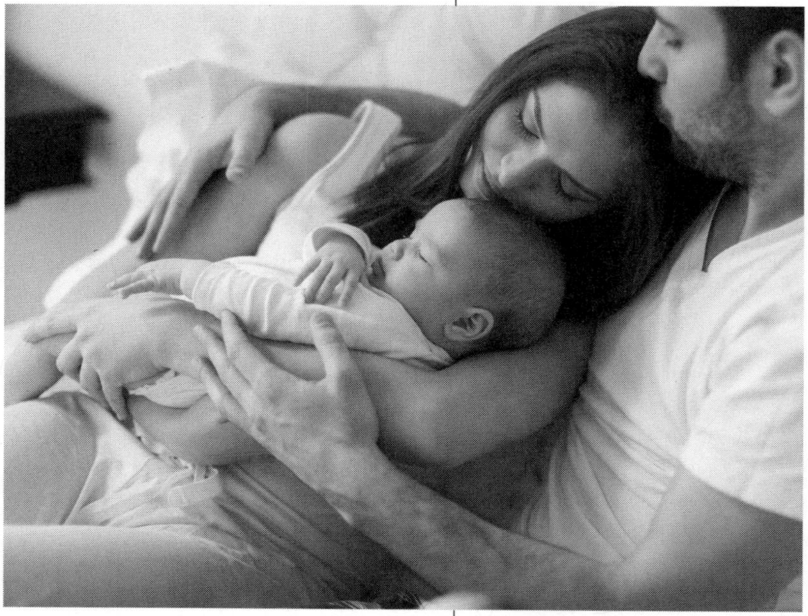

Nursing rhythms vary tremendously from place to place. Research has not yet pinpointed exactly how many times and how long a baby needs to nurse each day to suppress fertility because a "nursing session" means something so different to different families. Western families, for example, may consider a nursing session a lengthy, ritualized activity, which may involve changing the baby's diaper/nappy, preparing a drink, settling into a certain chair, and then spending a long while feeding. In contrast, in a developing country, it may be common practice to keep the baby on the parent's body, nursing at the slightest cue for just a few minutes 15 to 20 times each day. These two babies may get about the same amount of milk in 24 hours, but the immense differences in their nursing rhythms make it difficult to quantify the nursing needed to delay fertility.

Generally speaking, nursing exclusively and often day and night—with no long stretches between feeds—produces a longer period of infertility after birth than scheduled or supplemented nursing. This is because the baby's time nursing affects a lactating parent's hormonal balance. One randomized 2-month intervention trial with 141 low-income mothers in Honduras found that in the group that began feeding their babies supplemental food at 4 months, 20% more were menstruating at 6 months compared with the mothers who exclusively breastfed between 4 and 6 months (Dewey, Cohen, Rivera, Canahuati, & Brown, 1997). When parents begin to give their baby other foods, this decreases the amount of time spent nursing and alters the nursing parent's hormonal balance. A Chilean study found that ovulation before the first menstrual period occurred more often in women who supplemented their baby by bottle (Diaz et al., 1991).

KEY CONCEPT

Nursing rhythms have a profound effect on both fertility and the return of menses.

Depending on nursing parents' individual body chemistry (see next point), they will eventually reach a "tipping point" when their hormonal levels change enough to permit menstruation and ovulation (M. Labbok, Valdes, & Aravena, 2002). For details on how nursing can be used reliably to space babies, see "Lactational Amenorrhea Method (LAM)" in the next section.

• • •

A nursing parent's body chemistry also plays a major role in when fertility returns.

Population studies reveal how nursing rhythms affect the return to fertility in large groups, but averages do not always apply to individuals. Because we do not yet fully understand all of the hormonal interactions and body processes involved in how nursing suppresses fertility, it is impossible to accurately predict when an individual parent will return to fertility (McNeilly, 2001).

Differences in body chemistry explain in part why return to fertility can vary so widely among nursing parents whose babies have similar feeding rhythms and sucking stimulation. It also explains in part why some parents who exclusively nurse day and night resume their menses within 8 weeks of giving birth while others resume their menses at 12 months, 24 months, or longer, even when their baby has long stretches of sleep or receives regular supplements.

A parent's body chemistry does not usually change from one pregnancy to the next, which explains why research found that the single most significant predictor of when menstruation will resume after birth is the parent's experience after a previous pregnancy (WHO, 1998b). However, if the feeding rhythm varies greatly from one baby to the next, the return to fertility is likely to vary (M. Labbok et al., 2002).

• • •

The nursing parent's nutritional status appears to have little effect on the return of fertility.

Some studies led researchers to believe that nursing parents with more fat stores and better nutrition began menstruating earlier than those with less fat stores and poorer nutrition, but these studies did not control for nursing frequency or supplementation of the baby (Frisch, 1988; Prema, Naidu, Neelakumari, & Ramalakshmi, 1981). Research on breastfeeding mothers that controlled for these factors concluded that fat stores and nutritional status have little effect on the return of menses and fertility (Kurz, Habicht, Rasmussen, & Schwager, 1993; Wasalathanthri & Tennekoon, 2001).

A small U.S. study (Domer et al., 2015) examined the effects of percentage of body fat on length of time to first ovulation after birth. Among these well-nourished U.S. women, the researchers found no association between body composition and duration of infertility. In the women who lost a greater percentage of their body fat during the early weeks after delivery, ovulation tended to return earlier, but this association was not statistically significant.

• • •

During the first 6 months of nursing, if menstruation occurs, it usually precedes ovulation.

Nursing increases the likelihood that the first menstruation will be anovulatory (not preceded by ovulation), especially if menstruation starts during the baby's first 6 months of life. Because pregnancy is impossible without ovulation, some refer to this as the "warning" period. In those who nurse exclusively and intensively, there may be up to three menstrual cycles before conception can occur (M. H. Labbok, 2007).

The longer the menses are delayed by nursing, the more likely it is that ovulation will occur before the first menstruation. In one Australian study, mothers whose babies were older than 1 year were more than 2.5 times more likely to ovulate before their first menstrual period than mothers whose babies were younger than 3 months (Lewis, Brown, Renfree, & Short, 1991). According to one Indian study, the younger the baby when the mother's menses returned, the more anovulatory cycles the mother was likely to have (Singh, Suchindran, & Singh, 1993). In this study, after 9 months post-birth, though, no differences in fertility were associated with continuing to breastfeed. The effect of nursing on fertility as children mature will depend in large part on the amount of time they spend nursing, which is much more variable in older children.

• • •

Milk expression does not appear to affect fertility in the same way as nursing.

The body's hormonal response to milk expression may not be the same as nursing, so suggest families do not equate milk expression with nursing in terms of its effect on fertility (Valdes, Labbok, Pugin, & Perez, 2000). See the later section "Lactational Amenorrhea Method" for research on milk expression and its effects on fertility in employed parents.

• • •

How solid foods are started and their effect on nursing rhythms can affect when menstruation and fertility return.

Once solid foods are started, the way they're given can affect whether the nursing parent's menses return quickly or whether the period of natural infertility is prolonged. To delay the return of the menses as long as possible, three studies (Cooney, Nyirabukeye, Labbok, Hoser, & Ballard, 1996; Kazi, Kennedy, Visness, & Khan, 1995; Kennedy, 2002) found a nursing parent can:

- Nurse first, before offering solid foods.
- Introduce solid foods gradually.
- Continue nursing often day and night, going no longer than 4 hours without nursing during the day and 6 hours at night.

If a family wants to speed the return of the menses, suggest they give solids before nursing, introduce lots of solid foods quickly, and increase the intervals between feeds.

• • •

As a baby nurses less often, the chances of ovulating before menstruating increase.

Some changes that can alter a nursing parent's hormonal balance and increase the odds of ovulating before the first post-birth menstruation include:

- Starting solid foods or significantly increasing other foods (fluids or solids)
- Longer intervals between feeds at night
- Decreasing nursing frequency
- Decreasing total time nursing
- Weaning from nursing

Be sure the family knows that any changes that decrease nursing frequency increase the possibility of ovulation and pregnancy.

• • •

If a nursing parent's goal is to become fertile before the menses return naturally, one option is to cut back on nursing.

The intensity of nursing needed to suppress fertility will vary from person to person, depending on body chemistry. If a nursing parent wants fertility to return sooner than it would return naturally, suggest gradually increasing the intervals between feeds and/or giving the baby more of other foods. One expert suggests that because the hormonal response to nursing is greater at night, one effective way to begin is by limiting night feeds (M. H. Labbok, 2008). When mammary stimulation decreases enough to cross an individual's hormonal threshold, fertility will return. Most nursing parents become fertile without having to wean completely, but there are exceptions (see next point).

Hormonal medical treatments were used to speed nursing parents' return to fertility, but the research on their safety and efficacy is still preliminary. At this writing, decreasing nursing is the recommended approach (Kauffman, 2007).

• • •

For some unusually sensitive individuals who previously nursed exclusively and intensively, even token nursing can be enough to prevent pregnancy (Gray et al., 1990). In these rare cases, even after regular menstruation begins, pregnancy may not occur. In this situation, encourage the family to weigh the risks to the current baby of weaning with the benefits of returning to fertility. Once a baby weans completely, fertility usually returns within about 30 days (Kauffman, 2007).

Rarely, it may be impossible to become pregnant until the baby is completely weaned from nursing.

After the Menses Resume

Light bleeding or spotting is the first indication of the return to fertility (M. H. Labbok, 2008). One U.S. study (Campbell & Gray, 1993) found that ovulation was nearly 10 times more likely to precede "regular" or "heavy" bleeding, as opposed to "spotting" or "light" bleeding. If the family's goal is not to conceive again soon, make sure they know that bleeding increases the chances of getting pregnant.

If more than 8 weeks after birth, vaginal bleeding lasts for 2 days or more or if bleeding occurs that is like a menses, assume pregnancy is possible.

• • •

Even after a nursing parent begins menstruating again, for a while, nursing reduces the chances of conceiving. One Chilean study (Diaz et al., 1992) found that when mothers breastfed intensively day and night, each month of breastfeeding after menstruation resumed reduced their chances of conceiving by an average of more than 7%. This is because, in many cases, the hormones of nursing cause a deficient egg and follicle and a deficient luteal phase, and the hormonal levels in the second half of the menstrual cycle are too low to maintain a pregnancy. One 2015 Tanzanian study of families that included 315 children (Mattison, Wander, & Hinde, 2015) found that breastfeeding for more than 2 years was associated with longer birth intervals.

Continuing to nurse after the menses resume reduces the chances of conceiving and maintaining a pregnancy.

• • •

Sometimes a sudden increase in a baby's nursing (such as during an illness) or milk expression can cause regular menstruation to temporarily stop. The amount of extra stimulation needed to suppress menstruation will vary from person to person. If this happens, suggest parents assume they are fertile and pregnancy is possible.

After menstruation resumes, an increase in nursing or milk expression may suppress it again, but, assume fertility has returned.

Nursing and Contraception

A family planning method that is popular and effective in one culture may be unacceptable in another (Chertok & Zimmerman, 2007). Before discussing options, ask what types of contraception the couple is considering and which methods they would not find acceptable. Other information that might rule in or rule out some methods include (Berens & Labbok, 2015):

- The family's financial resources, healthcare options, and locally available methods
- Their nursing rhythm and the baby's age (LAM and hormonal methods)
- The nursing parent's age (hormonal methods)

Cultural and religious values, as well as other factors, will affect the family planning choices each couple finds acceptable.

- The partner's opinion
- Their childbearing goals (temporary or permanent methods)
- Any health issues (temporary or permanent methods, hormonal methods)

Non-Hormonal Methods

Non-hormonal methods of contraception are the first choice for nursing families since they have no negative impact on nursing.

The Lactational Amenorrhea Method (LAM)—see next section—has the advantage of improving nursing outcomes. At the very least, however, all of the non-hormonal methods have no effect on nursing, because there is nothing to pass into the milk, affect milk production, or alter milk composition. Be sure that those who are fully nursing a baby younger than 6 months are aware of LAM, as it is a reliable interim option while the family considers other longer-term alternatives.

Lactational Amenorrhea Method (LAM)

If a family is fully nursing, the baby is less than 6 months old, and the menses have not resumed, the protection from pregnancy is about the same as that provided by birth-control pills.

Many families are confused about the effects of nursing on fertility. One 2018 Turkish study (Ozsoy, Aksu, Akdolun Balkaya, & Demirsoy Horta, 2018) found that 4 out of 5 mothers surveyed believed that breastfeeding was not effective as contraception. However, it can be effective under the right circumstances. The Lactational Amenorrhea Method, or LAM, is a temporary family planning method that does not require abstinence and was found in research conducted worldwide to be at least 98% reliable during the first 6 months after delivery (Berens & Labbok, 2015; M. H. Labbok, 2015). This method consists of nursing rhythms (see next point) that provide families with more than just a prolonged period of natural infertility. Because LAM also promotes optimal nursing, it leads to better health outcomes for the family, saves money that would otherwise be spent on supplements and contraceptives, and gives nursing parents control over their fertility. LAM is also acceptable to virtually all religious groups.

Some reasons families give for choosing LAM over other methods are:

1. They want a break from using a device or taking a prescribed medication.
2. They want more time before deciding on a long-term or permanent method of contraception.
3. They prefer a natural method of child-spacing.

LAM's effectiveness is independent of a family's education, religion, country of origin, and available nursing support.

LAM has its roots in a meeting of two dozen researchers held in August 1988 in Bellagio, Italy, whose combined opinion is referred to as the Bellagio Consensus. After evaluating the research on nursing and fertility from developed and developing countries, these researchers came to a better understanding of how an individual could use the natural delay in menses as a method of contraception. This led to the development in 1990 of the algorithm (see next point) that became known as LAM at the Institute for Reproductive Health in Georgetown University in Washington DC (*Guidelines: Breastfeeding, family planning, and the Lactational Amenorrhea Method--LAM,* 1994).

KEY CONCEPT

Lactational Amenorrhea Method (LAM) is an effective form of contraception that was studied worldwide.

• • •

To practice LAM, the answer to three specific questions must be "no."

Nursing parents are taught LAM by asking them these three questions:

1. Have your menses returned? (Defined as 2 consecutive days of bleeding after 8 weeks post-delivery or a vaginal bleed considered to be a menses.)
2. Are you supplementing regularly or allowing long periods without nursing either day or night?
3. Is your baby more than 6 months old?

When the answer is "no" to all three questions, there is a less than a 2% chance of pregnancy (M. H. Labbok et al., 1994). It's also important to keep asking these same questions regularly. When the answer to any of these questions is "yes," to avoid pregnancy, the family should begin using another method of contraception.

• • •

To better research and understand LAM, nursing patterns needed to be defined.

The key to suppression of fertility through nursing is to nurse frequently day and night. To make it easier for families and healthcare providers to understand the impact of feeding on fertility, researchers defined nursing patterns by dividing the three main categories—full, partial, and token breastfeeding—into six subcategories:

KEY CONCEPT

The key to suppressing fertility while lactating is nursing often day and night.

Full breastfeeding

- ***Exclusive breastfeeding***—Baby receives only mother's milk and no other liquids or solids.
- ***Almost exclusive breastfeeding***—Along with breastfeeding, baby receives no more than two mouthfuls daily of other foods, drinks, and/or vitamins/minerals.

Partial breastfeeding

- ***High partial breastfeeding***—Breastfeeding is the vast majority of feeds.
- ***Medium partial breastfeeding***—About half of all feeds are at the breast.
- ***Low partial breastfeeding***—The vast majority of daily feeds are not at the breast.

Token breastfeeding

- ***Occasional breastfeeding***—The baby feeds minimally, occasionally, or irregularly, not necessarily daily at the breast.

Since these definitions of nursing patterns were created, organizations have created various versions of them, which are not identical. An international consensus on these definitions is needed (M. H. Labbok & Starling, 2012).

Families can rely on LAM with confidence when they nurse exclusively or almost exclusively (the patterns in the "full breastfeeding" category), at least until the menses return, the nursing pattern changes, or the baby turns 6 months old. Research indicates that high partial breastfeeding—with supplements comprising no more than 5% to 15% of a baby's feeds—can also effectively suppress fertility, especially if baby nurses first before receiving the supplements. However, if the supplementation increases or the baby begins going longer without nursing day or night, risk of becoming fertile increases (Gray et al., 1990). Medium partial breastfeeding delays return of fertility for some but is not a reliable method to prevent pregnancy. Low partial and token breastfeeding have little effect on fertility.

• • •

Even if parents do not have a clear understanding of how LAM works, if they are exclusively nursing, pregnancy rates appear to be comparable to those supported in using LAM.

Although families using LAM have a slightly higher frequency of nursing, compared to families who simply exclusively nurse (M. H. Labbok, 2015), an analysis of 75 surveys conducted in 45 developing countries (Fabic & Choi, 2013) found that only 26% of women who described themselves as LAM users were correctly practicing it. However, a 2015 Cochrane Review (Van der Wijden & Manion, 2015) compared nursing families who were informed and supported in using LAM and families who exclusively nursed (no supplements given) but did not receive instruction and support on LAM. It found no clear differences in pregnancy rates between these two groups.

• • •

After 6 months, some studies found LAM effective under certain conditions.

LAM was originally limited to 6 months, because this is when introduction of other foods is recommended. But several studies found that if the menses have not returned, solids are given after the baby nurses, and there are no gaps in nursing longer than 4 hours during the day and 6 hours at night, very few pregnancies occur (Cooney et al., 1996; Kazi et al., 1995). In one study done in Rwanda (Cooney et al., 1996), where return of menses occurs on average 12 months after birth, use of a modified LAM was extended from 6 to 9 months with no reported pregnancies. In this extended version of LAM, mothers were also asked the question: "Are you fully or nearly fully breastfeeding your baby during the first 6 months?" and if the baby was between 7 and 9 months, "Are you breastfeeding before giving other foods, so that the baby's hunger is satisfied first with breast milk, and then with other foods?"

• • •

LAM appears to be slightly less effective in employed mothers expressing milk.

One Chilean study (Valdes et al., 2000) found LAM to be about 95% effective in preventing pregnancy in women who hand-expressed their milk at work, as compared with the 98% or more effectiveness found in other studies among those practicing LAM who were not separated from their babies. In the study of employed mothers, nearly half of the 170 mothers provided their milk exclusively for 6 months, despite their separation from their babies, and half of these women (28.2% of the total) were still not menstruating at 6 months.

Other Natural Methods

Other natural methods involve abstaining from sex during fertile times.

The Academy of Breastfeeding Medicine 2015 Clinical Protocol #13 on contraception during nursing (Berens & Labbok, 2015) lists four methods of "fertility awareness" natural family planning:

- Billings ovulation method (OM)
- Creighton model
- Symptothermal method
- Marquette method.

Any of these natural family planning methods can be used by a nursing family even before the menses have returned. These methods all involve observing some combination of cervical mucus, temperature, and/or hormonal monitoring, which determines fertile times. The couples using these methods then abstain from intercourse when they are fertile. A study on the efficacy of the Marquette method during the first year after birth (Bouchard, Fehring, & Schneider, 2013) found it to be 98% effective when used correctly.

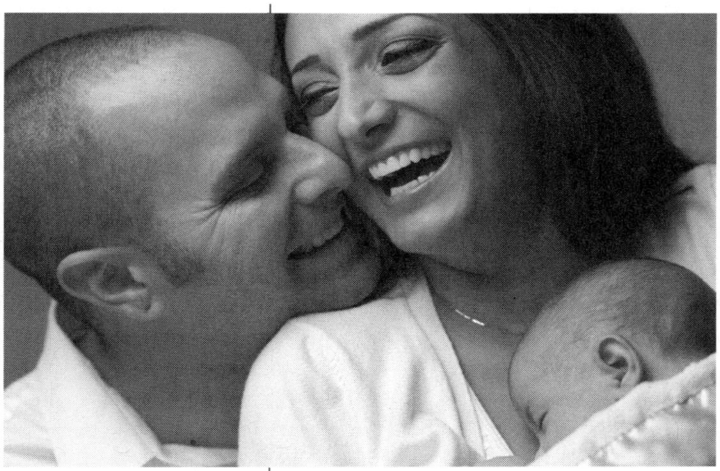

Barrier Methods and Spermicides

Condoms, diaphragms, and other barriers can be used alone or with other methods.

For the nursing family, barrier methods, such as condoms, diaphragms, contraceptive sponges, and cervical caps, have advantages over other contraceptive methods. They do not affect nursing, they are easily available in most places, some provide protection from sexually transmitted diseases, they are relatively inexpensive, and they can be used along with other methods. For example, if the family is using a natural family planning method to determine fertile times (see previous section), barrier methods can be used only during periods of fertility, rather than abstaining from intercourse. When used correctly, condoms and diaphragms are generally considered to be very effective in preventing pregnancy (Berens & Labbok, 2015).

Barrier methods also have some disadvantages. Unless lubricated condoms are used, they can cause irritation due to vaginal dryness from low estrogen levels during nursing. In this case, lubricant or spermicides can be used with them. Diaphragms and cervical caps require a physical exam for refitting after giving birth and whenever its user's weight varies by more than 10 lbs. (4.5 kg). Allergic reactions can occur in response to the materials used to make these devices. Some also consider them inconvenient and feel they limit spontaneous sex.

KEY CONCEPT

Barrier methods of contraception have no impact on nursing.

• • •

Spermicides used alone or with a barrier method do not affect nursing.

Spermicides can reduce the transmission of some infections and provide welcome lubrication during early nursing (Berens & Labbok, 2015). However, some brands may cause irritation in sensitive people.

Non-Hormonal IUDs

Non-hormonal IUDs reliably prevent pregnancy and are compatible with nursing.

An intrauterine device (IUD) is one form of contraception that is inserted into the uterus and left in place long-term. It works by altering its user's hormonal state to prevent fertilization or implantation of a fertilized egg. Highly effective at preventing pregnancy, a non-hormonal IUD does not affect milk production, milk composition, or the nursing baby (Berens & Labbok, 2015).

• • •

To reduce risk of expulsion, IUDs should be inserted at least 3 days after birth.

According to a systematic review of the literature (Berry-Bibee et al., 2016), there is a higher risk that an IUD will be involuntarily expelled from the uterus if it is inserted within the first 3 days following birth rather than after 3 days. No

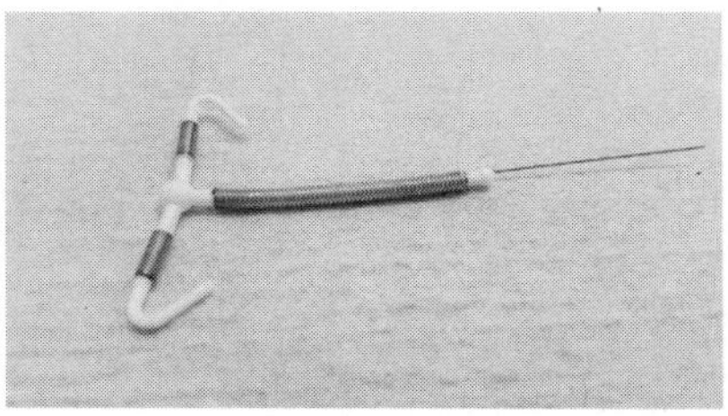

difference in expulsion risk was found between those who nursed and those who didn't. This same review concluded that perforation of the uterus and infections associated with insertion of an IUD are rare events. The risk of perforation may be higher among nursing parents, but the risk of infection does not appear to be higher in nursing versus non-nursing parents.

Surgical Sterilization

Vasectomy and tubal ligation effectively prevent pregnancy, but surgery on the nursing parent may cause an interruption of nursing.

Both of these surgeries involve physically blocking the pathway between sperm and egg. Surgical sterilization should be considered permanent, as reversal cannot be guaranteed. Fewer risks are associated with a vasectomy, which may be done as an office procedure. Surgery on a male partner has no effect on nursing.

When nursing parents have a tubal ligation, however, they face the risks associated with any surgery, and if performed shortly after birth, there likely will be a temporary interruption of nursing during the vulnerable early weeks after birth. Also, the pain from the surgery may make nursing uncomfortable afterwards. Suggest families planning a tubal ligation after birth allow enough time between birth and the surgery to express milk for any missed feeds.

KEY CONCEPT

Tubal ligation surgery does not affect nursing, but nursing parent and baby will be apart and should plan for this.

• • •

A full or partial hysterectomy will not affect nursing or milk production.

The removal of the uterus and/or ovaries will not affect milk production, which is regulated by hormones secreted from the hypothalamus and pituitary glands. However, when nursing parents undergo any surgery, they will likely need help in maintaining nursing during the hospital stay. For details, see p. 859-861 in Chapter 19.

Hormonal Methods

Controversy exists about whether hormonal contraceptive methods affect milk production in some users.

One concern about the use in nursing families of contraceptives containing progestin and/or estrogen is their possible effect on milk production, especially if they are started during the early weeks after birth (Hale, 2019, pp. 178-180). A 2015 Cochrane Review (Lopez et al., 2015) examined studies comparing breastfeeding outcomes in three different groups of women, those who used:

- Non-hormonal contraceptive methods
- Progestin-only methods
- Combined oral contraceptive methods, which include estrogen (see next section)

These scientists concluded that the results were inconsistent across 11 trials. Two of 8 trials noted less breastfeeding among women using hormonal birth control. One of these 2 studies included a combined oral contraceptive pill containing both estrogen and progestin. In the other study, women used a hormonal IUD. The authors of the Cochrane Review wrote that it was difficult to come to definitive conclusions because "the evidence was limited for any particular hormonal method."

The World Health Organization's 2015 publication "Medical Eligibility Criteria for Contraceptive Use" (WHO, 2015) recommended that nursing families avoid using progestin-only contraception during the first 6 weeks after birth. It also recommended nursing families avoid using combined hormonal contraceptives containing both progestin and estrogen during the first 6 months after birth.

Because the current research is not strong enough to make evidence-based recommendations, in its 2015 Clinical Protocol #13 (Berens & Labbok, 2015), the Academy of Breastfeeding Medicine (ABM) suggested informing families that hormonal contraceptive methods may decrease milk production, especially during the early weeks when it is initially being established. The ABM also suggested hormonal methods be discouraged in families where these situations are present:

- Low milk production with this child or a history of lactation failure
- History of breast or chest surgery
- Twins, triplets, or higher-order multiples
- Preterm birth (when milk production is already at risk)
- When health is compromised in the nursing parent or baby

For nursing families, the World Health Organization also recommended hormonal methods be considered after non-hormonal methods due to milk-production concerns.

The U.S. Centers for Disease Control and Prevention (CDC), however, provides different recommendations for nursing families about hormonal contraceptives. In its published guidelines, "U.S. Medical Eligibility for Contraceptive Use" (CDC, 2016), the CDC rates progestin-only contraceptives for nursing families—even during the early weeks—in category 2, which is defined as "the advantages of using the method generally outweigh the theoretical or proven risks." For more details, see the next section.

• • •

Children who were exposed to estrogen and/or progesterone through human milk have been followed for 17 years, with no harmful effects found. However, some professionals still have concerns.

In the book *Hale's Medications and Mothers' Milk*, hormonal methods of contraception containing progestin and/or estrogen, are rated as an L3. This category is considered compatible with nursing, but less research on nursing families is available than categories L1 and L2 (Hale, 2019, pp. 178-180). Several cases of breast enlargement (gynecomastia) were reported in babies whose nursing parents were using hormonal contraception, but this side effect is extremely rare.

When nursing parents use combined oral contraceptives containing both progestin and estrogen (see later section), the amount of estrogen their babies receive is similar to what they would receive from the naturally occurring estrogen in mother's milk. Studies have followed health outcomes in the children of parents who used progestin-only methods for up to 17 years (Pardthaisong, Yenchit, & Gray, 1992) and found no short- or long-term negative effects. A 2016 systematic review of the safety of progesterone-releasing vaginal rings (Carr, Gaffield, Dragoman, & Phillips, 2016) found no negative health effects on nursing babies. Another 2016 systematic review that looked at the effects of the whole range of progestin-only contraceptives (Phillips et al., 2016) had similar findings. However, some experts still have concerns. In her 2015 overview of sexuality, contraception, and lactation, the late U.S. physician and international expert on sexuality and contraception during lactation, Miriam Labbok wrote (M. H. Labbok, 2015):

> "…these studies have been inadequately designed to determine whether a risk of either serious or subtle long-term effects exists. Animal data suggest there is an effect of progestogen on the developing brain; whether similar effects occur after progestogen exposure in humans is unclear."

Progestin-Only Methods

Progestin-only hormonal methods, which include a variety of options, are considered by most to be compatible with nursing, but they are not considered the first choice for nursing families, especially during the early weeks.

Progestin-only methods prevent pregnancy by thickening cervical mucus, making sperm penetration more difficult, blocking ovulation, and thinning the uterine lining. However, since the onset of lactation occurs due to the rapid fall in natural progesterone levels after the delivery of the placenta, the use of methods that include progestin—a synthetic progesterone—in the early weeks has the potential to disrupt lactation. While studies have not yet identified any problems with these methods in large groups of women when initiated after 6 weeks post-birth (Phillips et al., 2016), there are anecdotal reports of insufficient milk after these methods were started (Stuebe, Bryant, Lewis, & Muddana, 2016).

It's helpful for families to know that there are differences among the following types of progestin-only methods that may make one a better choice than another.

- **Progestin-only minipill** is most effective when taken at about the same time each day. It is slightly less effective (and less forgiving of missed pills) than the combined pill containing progesterone and estrogen. Irregular bleeding, a commonly reported side effect of the minipill, is less likely while nursing (Berens & Labbok, 2015).
- **Progestin-only IUD** works like a non-hormonal IUD with the addition of small amounts of progestin released into its user's system over time. Depending on the model used, these devices may be effective for up to 12 years after insertion. They provide just slightly better pregnancy prevention than non-hormonal IUDs (0.2% of those using hormonal IUDs become pregnant versus 0.8% of those using non-hormonal IUDs). A 2009 study found that insertion of hormonal IUDs immediately after birth resulted in a shorter duration and less exclusive nursing (Chen, Creinin, Reeves, & Schwarz, 2009). In another study, though, these differences in outcomes were not evident (Turok et al., 2017). Immediate insertion after birth also increases the risk that the IUD will be involuntarily expelled from the uterus (Turok et al., 2017).
- **Progestin-releasing vaginal ring** is inserted in the vagina and removed for a week every 21 days (Kestelyn et al., 2018; Phillips et al., 2016).
- **Progestin-only injectable** (i.e. Depo-Provera or DPMA) is injected every 3 months. Since it is not reversible, care should be taken in its use during lactation. About 6% of women worldwide reportedly use injectables (Jacobstein & Polis, 2014).
- **Progestin-only implant** (i.e. Norplant or Implanon) is inserted under the skin and prevents pregnancy for up to 5 years. Some implants, such as Nesterone or Elcometrine, deliver an orally inactive progesterone that baby cannot absorb, making it a better choice for nursing parents (Diaz, 2002). Progestin-only implants are reportedly used by only about 1% of women worldwide (Jacobstein & Polis, 2014).

Timed-released methods (often referred to as long-acting reversible contraception or LARC) are often recommended in low-income populations. They provide highly effective and continuous protection from pregnancy over a long period of time independent of human error. One noteworthy difference among these methods is that the amount of hormone available to the baby through the milk is less with pills, implants and progestin-only IUDs and more with injectables, such as Depo-Provera (DPMA) (Sober & Schreiber, 2014).

• • •

Controversy exists about how soon after birth nursing parents should start using progestin-only methods. The World Health Organization recommends delaying these methods until nursing has been well established for at least 6 weeks (WHO, 2015).

Some recommend nursing parents start progestin-only methods no earlier than 6 weeks postpartum. Others consider it acceptable to start using them earlier.

The American College of Obstetricians and Gynecologists (ACOG) based its recommendations on the "U.S. Medical Eligibility Criteria" guidelines from the U.S. Centers for Disease Control and Prevention (CDC), which considers starting these methods immediately after birth compatible with nursing (ACOG, 2016; CDC, 2016). The CDC's criteria put progestin-only contraception in its category 2, which means the benefits of using these methods at this time are generally believed to outweigh the risks.

KEY CONCEPT

The World Health Organization (WHO) recommends delaying the use of progestin-only methods for 6 weeks after birth.

Some healthcare providers recommend nursing parents start progestin-only methods at birth, especially if providers consider them at high risk of pregnancy before their first post-delivery checkup (Bennett & Mannel, 2018). A 2014 U.S. study (Brownell et al., 2014) found that nearly three-quarters of the low-income mothers who received progestin-only injectables (Depo-Provera or DPMA) during their hospital stay had not planned before birth to use that method of contraception. When considering contraception soon after birth, it is important to keep in mind that when nursing is exclusive or nearly exclusive, the risk of pregnancy in the first 6 to 12 weeks approaches zero, leading to overlap of protection and the possible risk of a negative impact on lactation.

Effects of progestin on milk production. One concern about early use of progestin-only methods is their potential effect on the hormonal balance needed to establish milk production. In the first days after birth, the biological trigger for the rapid increase in milk production (called lactogenesis II or secretory activation) is the sharp drop in progesterone that naturally occurs after the delivery of the placenta. If nursing parents receive an injection of progestin (a synthetic progesterone) right after delivery, this might alter their hormonal state enough to undermine milk production.

One 1984 three-center study done in Hungary and Thailand found a 12% decrease in milk volume among mothers taking the progestin-only minipill (the mothers using non-hormonal methods had a 6% decrease) (Tankeyoon et al., 1984). However, some studies reported that mothers using progestin-only methods had slightly better milk volumes and longer duration of breastfeeding than mothers using non-hormonal methods (Halderman & Nelson, 2002; Koetsawang, 1987; Sinchai et al., 1995).

During the past decades, more studies were conducted on the use of progestin-only methods during the first 6 weeks after birth. Early studies (Halderman &

Nelson, 2002; Hannon et al., 1997) did not use reliable techniques to determine differences in milk production among its study participants. A 2012 systematic review (Brownell et al., 2012) examined all clinical trials, randomized clinical trials, and comparative studies that reviewed the effects of Depo-Provera (or DPMA) on nursing during the first 6 weeks. Its authors concluded that at that time all of the available evidence was weak and provided an inadequate basis on which to determine a cause-and-effect relationship between early DPMA use and poor nursing outcomes.

In a 2014 U.S. study of 183 low-income women who delivered in one of four New York hospitals (Dozier, Nelson, Brownell, Howard, & Lawrence, 2014), nearly 63% of the 127 women who used Depo-Provera received it in the hospital immediately after birth. To gauge the effects of Depo-Provera on milk production, these researchers examined the percentage of women who weaned their babies early. After analyzing the relationship between early administration of Depo-Provera and breastfeeding cessation, the study authors concluded that if the Depo-Provera had an effect on lactation, it was most likely minimal.

Two studies compared early introduction (1 to 3 days after birth) with late introduction (after 6 weeks) of progestin-only methods. One Brazilian study compared early insertion of a progestin-releasing implant with the late injection of Depo-Provera (DPMA) (Brito et al., 2009). A U.S. study compared the early insertion of a progestin-releasing implant with insertions of the same contraceptive after 6 weeks. Both studies had similar results. Overall duration of exclusive breastfeeding was comparable in its two groups and any differences were not statistically significant. In the Brazilian study, babies in the early introduction group had a trend toward greater weight gain. In the U.S. study, there was no difference between the early and late groups in the number of women experiencing lactation failure.

KEY CONCEPT

Hormonal contraceptives may negatively affect milk production.

A 2014 Indian prospective study randomized 150 women into a group that received a progestin-releasing injectable before hospital discharge (between 2 and 10 days after birth) and compared their lactation experience with a group of 100 women who received no hormonal contraception (Singhal, Sarda, Gupta, & Goel, 2014). At 3 weeks, 3 months, and 6 months, the babies' gains in weight and height were comparable in the two groups. In the group that received the progestin-releasing injectable, 100% of the women were satisfied with their milk production, compared with 95% in the control group who received no hormonal contraception.

In a 2015 Brazilian study (Braga et al., 2015), 24 women had a progestin-releasing implant inserted within 48 hours of birth. The researches gave the study mothers oral doses of deuterium so they could calculate the volume of milk intake in the newborns by measuring the deuterium ingested by the babies. The researchers concluded that the median volume of milk intake on the first day of the study and Day 29 was similar in both groups.

A 2017 Brazilian study followed for 12 months two groups, each comprised of 50 women, who were randomized into either early (less than 48 hours after birth) and late (after 6 weeks) insertion of a progestin-releasing implant (Carmo, Braga, Ferriani, Quintana, & Vieira, 2017). No difference in the babies' growth (weight, height, head circumference) between the two groups was found at 14, 40, 90, 180, 270, and 360 days.

Although these studies found no milk-production issues with early initiation of progestin-only methods, when considering the timing of starting these methods, suggest the family and their healthcare provider factor in the period of natural infertility nursing provides while the baby is primarily nursed. (See the previous section on LAM.)

Effects of progestin on the baby. In addition to any concerns about milk production, some experts have concerns that the young baby may have difficulty metabolizing progestin during the newborn period (M. H. Labbok, 2015). However, the majority of experts consider these methods compatible with nursing. One U.S. expert wrote that progestin-only methods, "...do not appear to have clinically relevant effects on the infant's health" (Hale, 2019, p. 179). The exposure to progestin in the infant is not clinically relevant in part because it is not easily absorbed by the baby's gut (Shaaban, 1991). As of this writing, the children of nursing parents who used progestin-only methods were followed for up to 17 years, with no long-term effects found on growth or development, including sexual development (Nilsson et al., 1986; Pardthaisong et al., 1992).

• • •

There are anecdotal reports of nursing parents who experienced a drop in milk production after starting progestin-only methods.

Individual case reports of nursing parents who had a decrease in milk production after starting progestin-only methods are one reason these methods are not recommended by the World Health Organization during the first 6 weeks after birth (WHO, 2015). As explained in the previous point, however, research on large numbers of nursing parents does not confirm this effect. It may be helpful to share with families that individual differences in body chemistry and response can produce different reactions (Stuebe et al., 2016). For this reason, if a family decides to use a progestin-only method, it might be best to choose one that can be quickly discontinued, such as the minipill, rather than one that cannot quickly be reversed, such as Depo-Provera. That way if there is a noticeable decrease in milk production, they can discontinue it.

Methods Containing Estrogen

Contraceptive methods containing estrogen are not recommended until the baby is older, some say at least 6 months old.

Contraceptives containing estrogen are considered the last choice for nursing parents, because the amount of estrogen in earlier versions of combined oral contraceptives decreased milk production and lactation duration. A Cochrane Review on methods for suppressing lactation after birth (Oladapo & Fawole, 2012) included 11 trials that involved 4 different estrogen preparations, all of which were found to be effective in suppressing lactation.

The most common estrogen-containing contraceptive method is the combined oral contraceptive pill, which is taken daily and contains both estrogen and progestin. Other methods that combine estrogen and progestin include:

- Transdermal patch (replaced weekly)
- Combined vaginal ring (replaced monthly)

Like Depo-Provera (DPMA), described in the previous section, these above two methods give continuous highly effective protection from pregnancy and as long as they stay in place are immune to human error.

Combined hormonal methods are not recommended for users over 35 who smoke and those with clotting problems, estrogen-dependent cancers, or severe migraines (CDC, 2016; Hale, 2019).

The U.S. Centers for Disease Control and Prevention (CDC) categorized these methods differently depending on when they are started after birth (CDC, 2016):

- **Birth to 3 weeks:** Category 4, "an unacceptable health risk"
- **3 to 6 weeks:** Category 3, "the theoretical or proven risks usually outweigh the advantages"
- **After 6 weeks:** Category 2: "the advantages of using the method generally outweigh the theoretical or proven risks"

Concerns first arose about the use of combined oral contraceptives by nursing parents in the 1980s, when higher-estrogen pills taken during the first weeks post-delivery were found to decrease milk production between 20% and 40% (Koetsawang, 1987; WHO, 1988). When combined oral contraceptives with lower-dose estrogen were started after full milk production was established, they had less effect on both nursing duration and milk production. However, some of the studies included in a 2015 Cochrane Review (Lopez et al., 2015) found lower milk production among some of those using combined methods. A 2018 study that used the data from the large U.S. Infant Feeding Practices Study II (Goulding, Wouk, & Stuebe, 2018) included 1,349 U.S. mothers who both planned to breastfeed for at least 4 months and used contraception. The researchers found that those who used progestin-only methods were more likely to meet their nursing goals and those who used combined methods were least likely to meet their nursing goals. Women using non-hormonal methods fell in the middle.

KEY CONCEPT

The World Health Organization recommends delaying the use of contraceptives containing estrogen for the first 6 months.

Due to the documented risks of these combined methods, the World Health Organization recommended that nursing parents avoid combined methods until the baby is at least 6 months old, when the introduction of solid foods can offset any decrease in milk production (WHO, 2015).

• • •

Nursing babies whose parents uses combined oral contraceptives receive no more estrogen than they would receive during nursing.

Both estrogen and progestin are considered compatible with nursing. One U.S. author wrote that estrogen-containing methods "...secreted into milk in minute quantities and do not appear to have clinically relevant effects on the infant's health. Studies of these products in breastfeeding women have found typical [relative infant doses] to be less than 1%" (Hale, 2019, p. 179). Hormonal contraceptives have been used by nursing parents for several decades, and no short- or long-term effects of estrogen on nursing babies have been reported.

• • •

Previous concerns about changes in milk composition with combined contraceptives appear to be unfounded.

Although some early studies noted slight changes in milk composition in mothers using hormonal contraception, later studies found no cause for concern (Dorea & Miazaki, 1999; Dorea & Myazaki, 1998). The changes observed were within the normal variations in milk composition from feed to feed and day to day.

• • •

If a nursing parent uses a method containing estrogen, suggest continued nursing while monitoring the baby's weight gain.

A nursing parent using a contraceptive method containing estrogen should watch for any signs of decreased milk production. Suggest scheduling regular checkups with the baby's healthcare provider to monitor her weight gain, the most reliable gauge of adequate milk intake.

Emergency Contraception

There are different types of emergency contraceptives, and they are all compatible with lactation.

Emergency contraception is used to prevent pregnancy after unprotected sex. It is most effective if it is used within 72 hours of intercourse, but it may be given up to 120 hours afterwards. Emergency options include (Shen, Che, Showell, Chen, & Cheng, 2017):

- Insertion of a copper IUD
- Combined oral contraceptives containing both estrogen and progestin
- High doses of progestin, such as levonorgestrel (LNG), which is used in many of the previously described progestin-only contraceptive methods

As an emergency contraceptive, LNG is usually given in two 0.75 mg doses 12 hours apart. Studies have examined its use in women. One 2007 Chilean study measured breastfeeding mothers' blood and milk levels of LNG after receiving a single 1.5 mg dose (Gainer et al., 2007). The estimated infant exposure to this drug during the first 8 hours, when the levels were highest, was 1.0 µg, and during the first 24 hours was 1.6 µg, which the Academy of Breastfeeding Medicine considered minimal and compatible with continued breastfeeding (Berens & Labbok, 2015). In a 2013 Israeli prospective, observational cohort study, researchers compared 71 breastfeeding women who received the 1.5 mg dose of LNG with a control group of 72 breastfeeding women who were taking an antiprogesterone drug (Polakow-Farkash et al., 2013). Infant adverse effects were rare in both groups, and the authors concluded there was no need to interrupt nursing.

REFERENCES

ACOG. (2016). Committee Opinion Number 670 (2016): Immediate postpartum long-acting reversible contraception. Retrieved from **acog.org/Clinical-Guidance-and-Publications/Committee-Opinions/Committee-on-Obstetric-Practice/Immediate-Postpartum-Long-Acting-Reversible-Contraception**.

Adanikin, A. I., Awoleke, J. O., Adeyiolu, A., et al. (2015). Resumption of intercourse after childbirth in southwest Nigeria. *European Journal of Contraception & Reproductive Health Care, 20*(4), 241-248.

Agarwal, S. K., Kim, J., Korst, L. M., et al. (2015). Application of the estrogen threshold hypothesis to the physiologic hypoestrogenemia of lactation. *Breastfeeding Medicine, 10*(2), 77-83.

al Bustan, M. A., el Tomi, N. F., Faiwalla, M. F., et al. (1995). Maternal sexuality during pregnancy and after childbirth in Muslim Kuwaiti women. *Archives of Sexual Behavior, 24*(2), 207-215.

Alum, A. C., Kizza, I. B., Osingada, C. P., et al. (2015). Factors associated with early resumption of sexual intercourse among postnatal women in Uganda. *Reproductive Health, 12,* 107.

Andreucci, C. B., Bussadori, J. C., Pacagnella, R. C., et al. (2015). Sexual life and dysfunction after maternal morbidity: A systematic review. *BMC Pregnancy & Childbirth, 15,* 307.

Anzaku, A., & Mikah, S. (2014). Postpartum resumption of sexual activity, sexual morbidity and use of modern contraceptives among Nigerian women in Jos. *Annals of Medical and Health Science Resesarch, 4*(2), 210-216.

Barrett, G., Pendry, E., Peacock, J., et al. (2000). Women's sexual health after childbirth. *British Journal of Obstetrics and Gynaecology, 107*(2), 186-195.

Becker, S., Rutstein, S., & Labbok, M. H. (2003). Estimation of births averted due to breast-feeding and increases in levels of contraception needed to substitute for breast-feeding. *Journal of Biosocial Science, 35*(4), 559-574.

Bennett, C. J., & Mannel, R. (2018). Walking the medicaid policy tightrope between long-acting reversible contraception and lactation. *Journal of Human Lactation, 34*(3), 433-437.

Berens, P., & Labbok, M. (2015). ABM Clinical Protocol #13: Contraception during breastfeeding, revised 2015. *Breastfeeding Medicine, 10*(1), 3-12.

Berry-Bibee, E. N., Tepper, N. K., Jatlaoui, T. C., et al. (2016). The safety of intrauterine devices in breastfeeding women: A systematic review. *Contraception, 94*(6), 725-738.

Bouchard, T., Fehring, R. J., & Schneider, M. (2013). Efficacy of a new postpartum transition protocol for avoiding pregnancy. *Journal of the American Board of Family Medicine, 26*(1), 35-44.

Braga, G. C., Ferriolli, E., Quintana, S. M., et al. (2015). Immediate postpartum initiation of etonogestrel-releasing implant: A randomized controlled trial on breastfeeding impact. *Contraception, 92*(6), 536-542.

Brito, M. B., Ferriani, R. A., Quintana, S. M., et al. (2009). Safety of the etonogestrel-releasing implant during the immediate postpartum period: A pilot study. *Contraception, 80*(6), 519-526.

Brownell, E. A., Fernandez, I. D., Howard, C. R., et al. (2012). A systematic review of early postpartum medroxyprogesterone receipt and early breastfeeding cessation: Evaluating the methodological rigor of the evidence. *Breastfeeding Medicine, 7*(1), 10-18.

Brownell, E. A., Lussier, M. M., Dozier, A. M., et al. (2014). The discordance between planned use and actual receipt of immediate postpartum depot medroxyprogesterone among low-income women. *Breastfeeding Medicine, 9*(6), 290-293.

Campbell, O. M., & Gray, R. H. (1993). Characteristics and determinants of postpartum ovarian function in women in the United States. *American Journal of Obstetrics & Gynecology, 169*(1), 55-60.

Carmo, L., Braga, G. C., Ferriani, R. A., et al. (2017). Timing of etonogestrel-releasing implants and growth of breastfed infants: A randomized controlled trial. *Obstetrics & Gynecology, 130*(1), 100-107.

Carr, S. L., Gaffield, M. E., Dragoman, M. V., et al. (2016). Safety of the progesterone-releasing vaginal ring (PVR) among lactating women: A systematic review. *Contraception, 94*(3), 253-261.

CDC. (2016). U.S. medical eligibility criteria for contraceptive use, 2016. *Morbidity and Mortality Weekly Report, 65*(3), 1-104.

Chen, B. A., Creinin, M. D., Reeves, M. F., et al. (2009). Breastfeeding continuation among women using the levonorgestrel-releasing intrauterine device after vaginal delivery. *Contraception, 80,* 204.

Chertok, I. R., & Zimmerman, D. R. (2007). Contraceptive considerations for breastfeeding women within Jewish law. *International Breastfeeding Journal, 2,* 1.

Connolly, A., Thorp, J., & Pahel, L. (2005). Effects of pregnancy and childbirth on postpartum sexual function: A longitudinal prospective study. *International Urogynecology Journal and Pelvic Floor Dysfunction, 16*(4), 263-267.

Cooney, K. A., Nyirabukeye, T., Labbok, M. H., et al. (1996). An assessment of the nine-month lactational amenorrhea method (MAMA-9) in Rwanda. *Studies in Family Planning, 27*(3), 102-171.

Dewey, K. G., Cohen, R. J., Rivera, L. L., et al. (1997). Effects of age at introduction of complementary foods to breast-fed infants on duration of lactational amenorrhea in Honduran women. *American Journal of Clinical Nutrition, 65*(5), 1403-1409.

Diaz, S. (2002). Contraceptive implants and lactation. *Contraception, 65*(1), 39-46.

Diaz, S., Aravena, R., Cardenas, H., et al. (1991). Contraceptive efficacy of lactational amenorrhea in urban Chilean women. *Contraception, 43*(4), 335-352.

Diaz, S., Cardenas, H., Brandeis, A., et al. (1992). Relative contributions of anovulation and luteal phase defect to the reduced pregnancy rate of breastfeeding women. *Fertility and Sterility, 58*(3), 498-503.

Domer, M. C., Beerman, K. A., Ahmadzadeh, A., et al. (2015). Loss of body fat and associated decrease in leptin in early lactation are related to shorter duration of postpartum anovulation in healthy US women. *Journal of Human Lactation, 31*(2), 282-293.

Dorea, J. G., & Miazaki, E. S. (1999). The effects of oral contraceptive use on iron and copper concentrations in breast milk. *Fertility and Sterility, 72*(2), 297-301.

Dorea, J. G., & Myazaki, E. (1998). Calcium and phosphorus in milk of Brazilian mothers using oral contraceptives. *Journal of the American College of Nutrition, 17*(6), 642-646.

Dozier, A. M., Nelson, A., Brownell, E. A., et al. (2014). Patterns of postpartum depot medroxyprogesterone administration among low-income mothers. *Journal of Women's Health (Larchmont), 23*(3), 224-230.

Fabic, M. S., & Choi, Y. (2013). Assessing the quality of data regarding use of the lactational amenorrhea method. *Studies in Family Planning, 44*(2), 205-221.

Falceto, O. G., Giugliani, E. R., & Fernandes, C. L. (2004). Couples' relationships and breastfeeding: Is there an association? *Journal of Human Lactation, 20(*1), 46-55.

Ford, C., & Beach, F. (1950). *Patterns of Sexual Behavior.* New York: Harper & Row

Frisch, R. E. (1988). Fatness and fertility. *Scientific American, 258*(3), 88-95.

Gainer, E., Massai, R., Lillo, S., et al. (2007). Levonorgestrel pharmacokinetics in plasma and milk of lactating women who take 1.5 mg for emergency contraception. *Human Reproduction, 22*(6), 1578-1584.

Goulding, A. N., Wouk, K., & Stuebe, A. M. (2018). Contraception and breastfeeding at 4 months postpartum among women intending to breastfeed. *Breastfeeding Medicine, 13*(1), 75-80.

Gray, R. H., Campbell, O. M., Apelo, R., et al. (1990). Risk of ovulation during lactation. *Lancet, 335*(8680), 25-29.

Grudzinskas, J. G., & Atkinson, L. (1984). Sexual function during the puerperium. *Archives of Sexual Behavior, 13*(1), 85-91.

Guidelines: Breastfeeding, family planning, and the Lactational Amenorrhea Method—LAM. (1994). Washington, DC: Institute for Reproductive Health, Georgetown University.

Haig, D. (2014). Troubled sleep: Night waking, breastfeeding and parent-offspring conflict. *Evolutionary Medicine and Public Health, 2014*(1), 32-39.

Halderman, L. D., & Nelson, A. L. (2002). Impact of early postpartum administration of progestin-only hormonal contraceptives compared with nonhormonal contraceptives on short-term breast-feeding patterns. *American Journal of Obstetrics & Gynecology, 186*(6), 1250-1256; discussion 1256-1258.

Hale, T. W. (2019). *Hale's Medications & Mothers' Milk: A Manual of Lactational Pharmacology* (18th ed.). New York, NY: Springer Publishing Company.

Hannon, P. R., Duggan, A. K., Serwint, J. R., et al. (1997). The influence of medroxyprogesterone on the duration of breast-feeding in mothers in an urban community. *Archives of Pediatrics & Adolescent Medicine, 151*(5), 490-496.

Islam, M. M., & Khan, H. T. A. (1993). Pattern of coital frequency in rural Bangladesh. *Journal of Family Welfare, 39,* 38-43.

Jacob, S., Spencer, N. A., Bullivant, S. B., et al. (2004). Effects of breastfeeding chemosignals on the human menstrual cycle. *Human Reproduction, 19*(2), 422-429.

Jacobstein, R., & Polis, C. B. (2014). Progestin-only contraception: Injectables and implants. *Best Practice & Research: Clinical Obstetrics & Gynaecology, 28*(6), 795-806.

Kauffman, R. P. (2007). Reproductive bioenergetics, infertility, and ovulation induction in the lactating female. In T. W. Hale & P. F. Hartmann (Eds.), *Hale & Hartmann's Textbok of Human Lactation* (pp. 319-342). Amarillo, TX: Hale Publishing.

Kazi, A., Kennedy, K. I., Visness, C. M., et al. (1995). Effectiveness of the lactational amenorrhea method in Pakistan. *Fertility and Sterility, 64*(4), 717-723.

Kennedy, K. I. (2002). Efficacy and effectiveness of LAM. *Advances in Experimental Medicine and Biology, 503,* 207-216.

Kenny, J. A. (1973). Sexuality of pregnant and breastfeeding women. *Archives of Sexual Behavior, 2(*3), 215-229.

Kestelyn, E., Van Nuil, J. I., Umulisa, M. M., et al. (2018). High acceptability of a contraceptive vaginal ring among women in Kigali, Rwanda. *PLoS One, 13*(6), e0199096.

Klerman, L. V., Cliver, S. P., & Goldenberg, R. L. (1998). The impact of short interpregnancy intervals on pregnancy outcomes in a low-income population. *American Journal of Public Health, 88*(8), 1182-1185.

Koetsawang, S. (1987). The effects of contraceptive methods on the quality and quantity of breastmilk. *International Journal of Gynaecology and Obstetrics, 25*(suppl), 115-128.

Konner, M., & Worthman, C. (1980). Nursing frequency, gonadal function, and birth spacing among !Kung hunter-gatherers. *Science, 207*(4432), 788-791.

Kurz, K. M., Habicht, J. P., Rasmussen, K. M., et al. (1993). Effects of maternal nutritional status and maternal energy supplementation on length of postpartum amenorrhea among Guatemalan women. *American Journal of Clinical Nutrition, 58*(5), 636-642.

Labbok, M., Valdes, V., & Aravena, R. (2002). Determinants of menses return in lactating women. In M. K. Davis, C. Isaacs, L. A. Hanson, & A. L. Wright (Eds.), *Advances in Experimental Medicine and Biology: Integrating Population Outcomes, Biological Mechanisms and Research Methods in the Study of Human Milk and Lactation* (pp. 285-287). New York: Kluwer Academic Plenum Publishers.

Labbok, M. H. (2007). Breastfeeding, birth spacing, and family planning. In T. W. Hale & P. F. Hartmann (Eds.), *Hale & Hartmann's Textbook of Human Lactation* (pp. 305-318). Amarillo, TX: Hale Publishing.

Labbok, M. H. (2008). Breastfeeding, fertility, and family planning. *Global Library of Women's Medicine.* Retrieved from **http://www.glowm.com/section_view/item/396**

Labbok, M. H. (2015). Postpartum sexuality and the Lactational Amenorrhea Method for contraception. *Clinical Obstetrics and Gynecology, 58*(4), 915-927.

Labbok, M. H., Perez, A., Valdes, V., et al. (1994). The Lactational Amenorrhea Method (LAM): A postpartum introductory family planning method with policy and program implications. *Advances in Contraception, 10(*2), 93-109.

Labbok, M. H., & Starling, A. (2012). Definitions of breastfeeding: Call for the development and use of consistent definitions in research and peer-reviewed literature. *Breastfeeding Medicine, 7*(6), 397-402.

Lawrence, R. A., & Lawrence, R. M. (2016). *Breastfeeding: A Guide for the Medical Profession* (8th ed.). Philadelphia, PA: Elsevier.

Lewis, P. R., Brown, J. B., Renfree, M. B., et al. (1991). The resumption of ovulation and menstruation in a well-nourished population of women breastfeeding for an extended period of time. *Fertility and Sterility, 55*(3), 529-536.

Lopez, L. M., Grey, T. W., Stuebe, A. M., et al. (2015). Combined hormonal versus nonhormonal versus progestin-only contraception in lactation. *Cochrane Database of Systematic Reviews*(3), CD003988. doi:10.1002/14651858.CD003988.pub2.

Lurie, S., Aizenberg, M., Sulema, V., et al. (2013). Sexual function after childbirth by the mode of delivery: A prospective study. *Archives of Gynecology and Obstetrics, 288*(4), 785-792.

Malakoti, J., Zamanzadeh, V., Maleki, A., et al. (2013). Sexual function in breastfeeding women in family health centers of Tabriz, Iran, 2012. *Journal of Caring Sciences, 2*(2), 141-146.

Masters, W., & Johnson, V. (2010). *Human Sexual Response.* Bronx, NY: Ishi Press.

Mattison, S. M., Wander, K., & Hinde, K. (2015). Breastfeeding over two years is associated with longer birth intervals, but not measures of growth or health, among children in Kilimanjaro, TZ. *American Journal of Human Biology, 27*(6), 807-815.

McDonald, E. A., & Brown, S. J. (2013). Does method of birth make a difference to when women resume sex after childbirth? *British Journal of Obstetrics and Gynaecology, 120*(7), 823-830.

McNeilly, A. S. (2001). Neuroendocrine changes and fertility in breast-feeding women. *Progress in Brain Research, 133,* 207-214.

Nilsson, S., Mellbin, T., Hofvander, Y., et al. (1986). Long-term follow-up of children breast-fed by mothers using oral contraceptives. *Contraception, 34*(5), 443-457.

O'Malley, D., Higgins, A., Begley, C., et al. (2018). Prevalence of and risk factors associated with sexual health issues in primiparous women at 6 and 12 months postpartum; A longitudinal prospective cohort study (the MAMMI study). *BMC Pregnancy Childbirth, 18*(1), 196.

Oladapo, O. T., & Fawole, B. (2012). Treatments for suppression of lactation. *Cochrane Database of Systematic Reviews*(9), CD005937. doi:10.1002/14651858.CD005937.pub3

Ozsoy, S., Aksu, H., Akdolun Balkaya, N., et al. (2018). Knowledge and opinions of postpartum mothers about the Lactational Amenorrhea Method: The Turkish experience. *Breastfeeding Medicine, 13*(1), 70-74.

Pardthaisong, T., Yenchit, C., & Gray, R. (1992). The long-term growth and development of children exposed to Depo-Provera during pregnancy or lactation. *Contraception, 45*(4), 313-324.

Phillips, S. J., Tepper, N. K., Kapp, N., et al. (2016). Progestogen-only contraceptive use among breastfeeding women: A systematic review. *Contraception, 94*(3), 226-252.

Polakow-Farkash, S., Gilad, O., Merlob, P., et al. (2013). Levonorgestrel used for emergency contraception during lactation-a prospective observational cohort study on maternal and infant safety. *Journal of Maternal-Fetal & Neonatal Medicine, 26*(3), 219-221.

Prema, K., Naidu, A. N., Neelakumari, S., et al. (1981). Nutrition--fertility interaction in lactating women of low income groups. *British Journal of Nutrition, 45*(3), 461-467.

Prieto, C. R., Cardenas, H., & Croxatto, H. B. (1999). Variability of breast sucking, associated milk transfer and the duration of lactational amenorrhoea. *Journal of Reproduction and Fertility, 115*(2), 193-200.

Riordan, J. (1983). *A Practical Guide to Breastfeeding.* St. Louis, MO: The C.V. Mosby Company.

Robson, K. M., Brant, H. A., & Kumar, R. (1981). Maternal sexuality during first pregnancy and after childbirth. *British Journal of Obstetrics and Gynaecology, 88*(9), 882-889.

Rowland, M., Foxcroft, L., Hopman, W. M., et al. (2005). Breastfeeding and sexuality immediately post partum. *Canadian Family Physician, 51,* 1366-1367.

Rutstein, S. O. (2005). Effects of preceding birth intervals on neonatal, infant and under-five years mortality and nutritional status in developing countries: Evidence from the demographic and health surveys. *International Journal of Gynaecology and Obstetrics, 89 Suppl 1,* S7-24.

Shaaban, M. M. (1991). Contraception with progestogens and progesterone during lactation. *Journal of Steroid Biochemistry and Molecular Biology, 40*(4-6), 705-710.

Shen, J., Che, Y., Showell, E., et al. (2017). Interventions for emergency contraception. *Cochrane Database of Systematic Reviews, 8,* CD001324. doi:10.1002/14651858.CD001324.pub5.

Signorello, L. B., Harlow, B. L., Chekos, A. K., et al. (2001). Postpartum sexual functioning and its relationship to perineal trauma: A retrospective cohort study of primiparous women. *American Journal of Obstetrics & Gynecology, 184*(5), 881-888; discussion 888-890.

Sinchai, W., Sethavanich, S., Asavapiriyanont, S., et al. (1995). Effects of a progestogen-only pill (Exluton) and an intrauterine device (Multiload Cu250) on breastfeeding. *Advances in Contraception, 11*(2), 143-155.

Singh, K. K., Suchindran, C. M., & Singh, K. (1993). Effects of breast feeding after resumption of menstruation on waiting time to next conception. *Human Biology, 65(1*), 71-86.

Singhal, S., Sarda, N., Gupta, S., et al. (2014). Impact of injectable progestogen contraception in early puerperium on lactation and infant health. *Journal of Clinical and Diagnostic Ressearch, 8*(3), 69-72.

Sober, S., & Schreiber, C. A. (2014). Postpartum contraception. *Clinical Obstetrics and Gynecology, 57*(4), 763-776.

Spencer, N. A., McClintock, M. K., Sellergren, S. A., et al. (2004). Social chemosignals from breastfeeding women increase sexual motivation. *Hormones and Behavior, 46*(3), 362-370.

Stuebe, A. M., Bryant, A. G., Lewis, R., et al. (2016). Association of etonogestrel-releasing contraceptive implant with reduced weight gain in an exclusively breastfed infant: Report and literature review. *Breastfeeding Medicine, 11,* 203-206.

Tankeyoon, M., Dusitsin, N., Chalapati, S., et al. (1984). Effects of hormonal contraceptives on milk volume and infant growth. WHO Special Programme of Research, Development and Research Training in Human Reproduction Task force on oral contraceptives. *Contraception, 30*(6), 505-522.

Turok, D. K., Leeman, L., Sanders, J. N., et al. (2017). Immediate postpartum levonorgestrel intrauterine device insertion and breast-feeding outcomes: A noninferiority randomized controlled trial. *American Journal of Obstetrics & Gynecology, 217*(6), 665 e661-665 e668.

Valdes, V., Labbok, M. H., Pugin, E., et al. (2000). The efficacy of the Lactational Amenorrhea Method (LAM) among working women. *Contraception, 62*(5), 217-219.

van Anders, S. M., Hipp, L. E., & Kane Low, L. (2013). Exploring co-parent experiences of sexuality in the first 3 months after birth. *Journal of Sexual Medicine, 10*(8), 1988-1999.

Van der Wijden, C., & Manion, C. (2015). Lactational amenorrhoea method for family planning. *Cochrane Database of Systematic Reviews*(10), CD001329. doi:10.1002/14651858.CD001329.pub2.

Velasquez, E. V., Trigo, R. V., Creus, S., et al. (2006). Pituitary-ovarian axis during lactational amenorrhoea. I. Longitudinal assessment of follicular growth, gonadotrophins, sex steroids and inhibin levels before and after recovery of menstrual cyclicity. *Human Reproduction, 21*(4), 909-915.

Wallwiener, S., Muller, M., Doster, A., et al. (2017). Sexual activity and sexual dysfunction of women in the perinatal period: A longitudinal study. *Archives of Gynecology and Obstetrics, 295*(4), 873-883.

Wasalathanthri, S., & Tennekoon, K. H. (2001). Lactational amenorrhea/anovulation and some of their determinants: A comparison of well-nourished and undernourished women. *Fertility and Sterility, 76(2*), 317-325.

WHO. (1988). Effects of hormonal contraceptives on breast milk composition and infant growth. *Studies in Family Planning, 19,* 36-69.

WHO. (1998a). The World Health Organization multinational study of breast-feeding and lactational amenorrhea. I. Description of infant feeding patterns and of the return of menses. World Health Organization Task Force on Methods for the Natural Regulation of Fertility. *Fertility and Sterility, 70*(3), 448-460.

WHO. (1998b). The World Health Organization multinational study of breast-feeding and lactational amenorrhea. II. Factors associated with the length of amenorrhea. World Health Organization Task Force on Methods for the Natural Regulation of Fertility. *Fertility and Sterility, 70*(3), 461-471.

WHO. (2015). *Medical Eligibility Criteria for Contraceptive Use.* Geneva, Switzerland: World Health Organization.

Wisniewski, P. M., & Wilkinson, E. J. (1991). Postpartum vaginal atrophy. *American Journal of Obstetrics and Gynecology, 165*(4 Pt 2), 1249-1254.

Yee, L. M., Kaimal, A. J., Nakagawa, S., et al. (2013). Predictors of postpartum sexual activity and function in a diverse population of women. *Journal of Midwifery & Women's Health, 58*(6), 654-661.

Zhu, B. P., Rolfs, R. T., Nangle, B. E., et al. (1999). Effect of the interval between pregnancies on perinatal outcomes. *New England Journal of Medicine, 340*(8), 589-594.

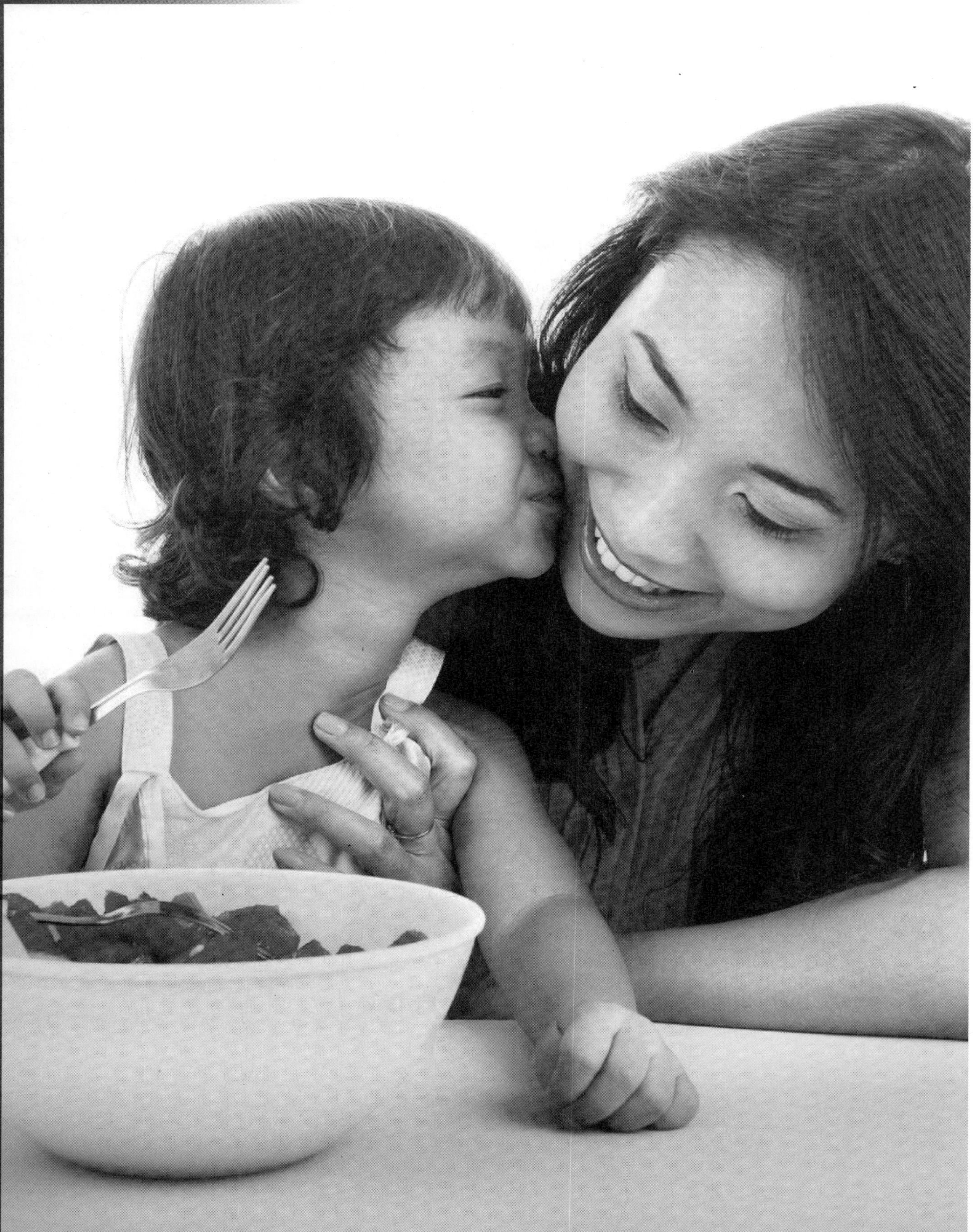

Nutrition, Exercise, and Lifestyle Issues

13

NUTRITION FOR NURSING PARENTS

Nutrition Basics

When talking to parents, keep nutrition information simple.

The same basic nutritional guidelines recommended for nursing parents also apply to the rest of the family. Suggest parents focus on eating a nutrient-dense diet, choosing fresh foods in as close to their natural state as possible. Fresh fruits and vegetables, whole-grain breads and cereals, and foods rich in calcium and protein are all good choices. The specific foods chosen from these categories vary by personal preferences, culture, climate, and family finances.

KEY CONCEPT

Nutrition-dense foods—fruits, vegetables, whole grains, and foods rich in calcium and protein—are good choices for nursing parents.

Keep diet information simple. If families consider the nutritional recommendations during lactation complicated, this may convince them not to nurse. According to one medical lactation textbook: "...[O]ne barrier to breastfeeding for some women is the 'diet rules' they see as being too hard to follow or too restrictive" (Lawrence & Lawrence, 2016, p. 285).

• • •

Suggest busy parents keep nutritious foods on hand that don't require much preparation.

The biggest challenge for many nursing families is finding the time for food shopping and preparation. But many foods are both nutritious and easy to eat as snacks or quick meals, such as cheese and crackers, yogurt, nuts, whole-grain bread, sprouts, sliced tomatoes, fresh fruits, whole or sliced raw vegetables, and hard-boiled eggs. Some parents find smaller, more frequent meals easier to manage than three larger meals. Suggest parents notice if they feel better after a healthy snack and drink whenever they nurse, rather than preparing larger meals. Some dietetic professionals recommend frozen and canned fruits and vegetables when fresh foods are not available, to reduce preparation time and make it easier for the family to eat more of these healthy foods

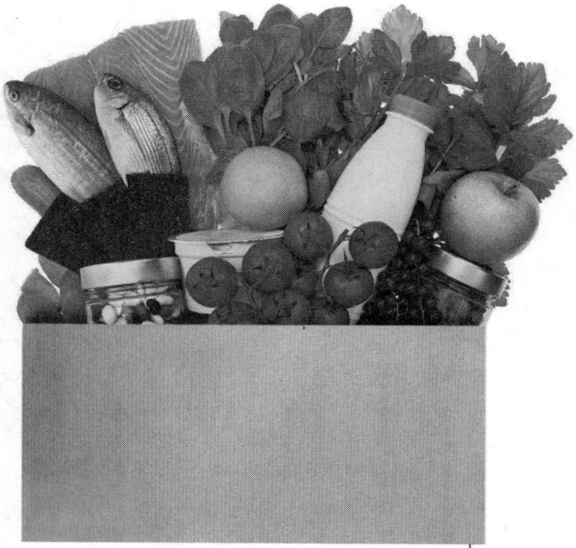

Other ways to simplify meal preparation include planning meals 7 days at a time to cut down on trips to buy food and washing and cutting vegetables in large batches for snacking or adding to a salad or a main dish. Suggest when cooking to make double batches of main dishes and freeze half for quick meals on hectic days. Another strategy is to use a slow cooker to start dinner in the morning that will be ready during the hectic early evening hours. If others ask how they can help, suggest asking for meals. For some families, take-out/take-away meals may also be an option.

• • •

To keep it simple, suggest nursing parents "eat to hunger" rather than counting calories.

Milk production is estimated to use about 500 calories per day (IOM, 2005), with some of this energy coming from body stores acquired during pregnancy. There is no need for an average-weight parent to keep careful track of daily caloric intake. A simpler strategy is just to "eat to hunger," which means using appetite as a guide. Most parents feel hungrier while nursing, so encourage them to trust their appetite and choose nutritious foods because they provide more energy and increase resistance to illness. If a parent is overweight when giving birth, limiting sweetened drinks and high-fat snack foods can help bring weight down during lactation (see later section on weight loss).

• • •

Even when food is scarce, most nursing parents make ample milk, but when low milk production is an issue, focus on lactation-critical nutrients.

A perfect diet isn't necessary. A nursing parent's diet is only one source of the energy and nutrients needed to make milk. Energy and most nutrients can also be drawn from the body stores laid down during pregnancy (Hopkinson, 2007). Even mildly malnourished nursing parents in developing countries produce plenty of good quality milk for their babies. In one study from Gambia, a developing country where food supplies were limited, when researchers gave breastfeeding mothers nutritional supplements, their babies did not gain more weight than the babies of women whose diets were not supplemented (Prentice et al., 1983). A meta-analysis that examined research from around the globe found that only when famine or near-famine conditions last weeks or more does milk production or milk quality suffer (Prentice, Goldberg, & Prentice, 1994). One Dutch study found that even in famine conditions, among previously well-nourished women with good body stores, milk production may be only slightly affected (C. Smith, 1947).

Activity levels also affect nutritional needs. During the first 4 to 5 weeks after birth, most nursing parents are less physically active than they are at other times in their lives (Butte & King, 2005). This reduces their need for calories.

When low milk production is an issue and the usual strategies aren't helping (see p. 442), take a closer look at the nursing parent's diet. In this situation, U.S. lactation consultants Lisa Marasco and Diana West (Marasco & West, 2019) suggest focusing on the lactation-critical nutrients that research (S. Lee & Kelleher, 2016) found may affect milk production.

- **Protein** intake recommended during lactation is 65 g to 100 g per day. A Thai randomized controlled trial of 120 poorly nourished mothers of term newborns (Achalapong, 2016) found that during the first days after birth, those supplemented with high-protein foods—in this case, eggs, milk, or both—produced more milk at 48 and 72 hours compared to those fed the regular diet.
- **Vitamin B_{12}** deficiency is possible in vegan families, some vegetarians, those with a history of weight-loss surgery (see later section), and anyone with a digestion or absorption problem like Crohn's disease.
- **Calcium** may aid in prolactin release, which is vital to milk production. Recommended daily intake of calcium during lactation is 1000 mg (Kolasa, Firnhaber, & Haven, 2015).
- **Iron.** Anemia (usually caused by low iron levels) is a risk factor for low milk production (Mathur, Chitranshi, Mathur, Singh, & Bhalla, 1992; Rioux, Savoie, & Allard, 2006) and delayed milk increase after birth (Salahudeen, Koshy, & Sen, 2013).
- **Zinc** is involved in several body functions related to milk production (S. Lee & Kelleher, 2016). During pregnancy it plays a role in the development of glandular tissue. After birth, it assists in milk increase and keeping the milk-making cells working. After weaning, it aids the process of involution.
- **Iodine** is essential to normal thyroid function, which is critical to making milk (Leung, Pearce, & Braverman, 2011). During pregnancy and lactation, the daily iodine requirement is 250 to 290 µg/L, and many fall short (Fisher, Wang, George, Gearhart, & McLanahan, 2016).

Too much iodine, however, can also reduce thyroid function (Miyai, Tokushige, & Kondo, 2008; Serrano-Nascimento et al., 2017).

- **Omega-3 fatty acids and healthy fats** in the nursing parent's diet increases their content in the milk but can also increase the milk's total fat content in lean women (N. K. Anderson et al., 2005)..
- **Fiber.** A Norwegian study (Torris et al., 2013) found an association in mothers on a low-fiber diet with a shorter duration of nursing.

For more details about lactation-critical nutrients, see p. 412.

• • •

When nursing parents go on a fast, be sure they know that any changes in the baby's nursing patterns or behavior are temporary.

Parents may fast (go without food and/or drink) for an extended period of time. Common reasons for fasting include weight loss and religious beliefs or practices. When nursing parents fast, it may impact their energy level and their baby's behavior. Ethiopian researchers interviewed and conducted focus groups with 199 Muslim and orthodox Christian families and their caregivers (Bazzano, Potts, & Mulugeta, 2018). In line with their religious beliefs, these women fasted even when pregnant and lactating. The only possible exception was the immediate post-birth period. While they fasted, some reported that their milk production was lower and nursing was difficult. But they continued because they felt it was their duty. Another larger Ethiopian study (Desalegn, Lambert, Riedel, Negese, & Biesalski, 2018) examined the effects of extensive fasting (200 days per year) required in the Orthodox Tewahedo religion. After evaluating the nutritional status of its 572 study women, they found that during the longer Lent fasting times, more than half were malnourished, which could negatively affect the health of both breastfeeding mothers and babies, as well as milk production. Israeli research (D. R. Zimmerman et al., 2009) examined both milk composition and babies' behavior during the 24-hour fast of Yom Kippur in 48 breastfeeding women with babies between 1 and 6 months old. After mothers abstained from all food and drink for 24 hours, their milk was higher in sodium, calcium, and protein and lower in phosphorus and lactose. During the fast, some mothers thought their babies wanted to breastfeed more often or seemed fussier than usual. The researchers suggested reassuring parents in this situation that any change in feeding pattern or behavior is temporary and will return to normal after the fast, as long as the mother nurses whenever the baby shows feeding cues.

• • •

The fatty-acids profile of mother's milk varies by the type of fats in the nursing parent's diet.

The overall amount of fat, protein, and milk sugar (lactose) in human milk is not affected by diet (Aumeistere et al., 2019), but the proportion of various types of fatty acids in milk varies by the parent's diet (Miliku et al., 2019). For example, eating more unsaturated fats (found mainly in fish, nuts, seeds and plant oils) produces milk higher in unsaturated fats than a diet higher in animal products. Parents who eat more fish or take fish oil or cod liver oil supplements produce milk richer in DHA (Aumeistere, Ciprovica, Zavadska, & Volkovs, 2018; Olafsdottir, Thorsdottir, Wagner, & Elmadfa, 2006). A 2018 Spanish study (Barreiro, Regal, Lopez-Racamonde, Cepeda, & Fente, 2018) found that among mothers with a diet rich in fish, even after 1 year of lactation, their milk was a good source of healthy fats. For greater intake of long-chain polyunsaturated fatty acids (like DHA and ARA) and carotenoids like beta-carotene (found in red, yellow and orange fruits and vegetables), see next point.

• • •

Greater intake by the baby of long-chain polyunsaturated fatty acids like DHA and ARA (also known as omega-3 fatty acids) and carotenoids (nutrients such as beta-carotene found in red, yellow and orange fruits and vegetables) is associated with better infant psychomotor development (Zielinska, Hamulka, Grabowicz-Chadrzynska, et al., 2019).

Increasing the number of colorful fruits and vegetables in the nursing parent's diet each day benefits both parent and baby.

Carotenoids are present in formula in only trace amounts. Their level in human milk depends largely on the nursing parent's diet (Zielinska, Hamulka, & Wesolowska, 2019). As one U.S. randomized trial (Essa et al., 2018) found, however, eating more colorful fruits and vegetables has the potential to benefit more than just the baby. The consumption of more fruits and vegetable each day in the intervention group also reduced the type of inflammation in the mammary tissue linked to breast cancer.

• • •

Nursing parents who are vitamin deficient may make milk lower in some vitamins.

A perfect diet is not necessary to make high-quality milk. But a nursing parent without good body stores and an inadequate diet who is chronically malnourished or becomes vitamin deficient due to poor nutrient absorption from illness or weight-loss surgery may be at risk of producing milk that is lower in some vitamins. These include vitamins A, D, B_1, B_2, B_6, and B_{12} (Allen, Donohue, & Dror, 2018; Hopkinson, 2007). In this case, an improved diet or vitamin supplements would bring milk vitamin levels back to normal (see the section "Supplements: Vitamin, Minerals, Omega-3s, Probiotics").

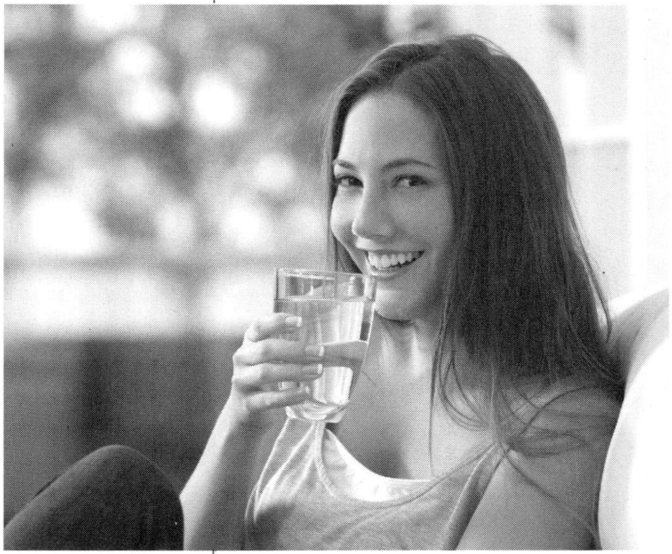

Some scientists note that our current estimates of adequate nutritional intake for both babies and nursing parents are based on very limited data (Allen et al., 2018). They say multicenter studies are needed to refine our understanding of basic nutritional needs during lactation. A 2017 systematic review examined the results of 59 observational and 43 interventional studies on maternal diet and milk composition (Keikha, Bahreynian, Saleki, & Kelishadi, 2017) and found that increased intake of fat-soluble vitamins (A, D, E, and K) resulted in higher levels in the milk, as well as vitamins B_1 and C.

Fluids

Suggest nursing parents "drink to thirst."

By "drinking to thirst," nursing parents should receive all the fluids they need (USDA, 2015). During lactation, most parents feel thirstier more often, so they may find themselves drinking more fluids than before. Encourage them to take a drink at the first sign of thirst, rather than waiting until they feel parched. If parents notice they are feeling thirsty while the baby nurses, suggest routinely having a drink handy when they get ready to feed.

While water is always a good choice, other fluids, such as fruit and vegetable juices, milk, and soups can satisfy thirst and provide needed nutrients. Avoid high-sugar drinks or those sweetened with sugar substitutes, like sodas (USDA, 2015).

• • •

Contrary to popular belief, drinking more fluids is not associated with increased milk production.

When parents express worry about milk production, the first advice they often receive is to drink more fluids. Although severe dehydration could potentially reduce milk production, even mild dehydration does not. A classic 1940 study examined the effect on milk production of reducing nursing mothers' daily fluid intake by 1 liter (Olsen, 1940), with no change found in their milk production. One U.S. study (Dusdieker, Booth, Stumbo, & Eichenberger, 1985) found that when mothers drank 25% more fluids than when they "drank to thirst," there was no statistically significant difference in milk production. In fact, during the "more fluids" period, the mothers produced slightly less milk.

• • •

Nursing parents will know if they are drinking enough fluids by their stools and the color of their urine.

Pale yellow urine indicates nursing parents are most likely drinking enough fluids. Constipation (hard, dry stools) and darker, more concentrated urine with a stronger smell are signs that they need to drink more (Lawrence & Lawrence, 2016). When constipated, nursing parents may be able to avoid the need for commercial laxatives by drinking more liquids and eating more fresh and dried fruits (prunes and pear especially) and increasing their consumption of fiber, such as raw vegetables and whole grains.

• • •

It is not necessary for nursing parents to "drink milk to make milk."

Cow's milk is not consumed by older children and adults in many parts of the world because most people worldwide are lactose intolerant later in life. After dairy farming became widespread among northern European peoples, these cultures developed a tolerance for cow's milk in adulthood.

Drinking cow's milk is not essential during lactation. Milk is one possible source of protein and calcium, but if nursing parents do not like milk or if the baby is sensitive to milk in their diet, there are other sources of these nutrients. Because yogurt and cheeses are processed, some parents and babies who are sensitive to straight cow's milk can tolerate them. Other excellent sources of calcium are foods fortified with calcium like soy milk, rice milk, almond milk, tofu, and orange juice. Good sources of calcium that require eating larger amounts include bok choy, Chinese mustard greens, sesame seeds, kale, white beans, Brazil nuts, and broccoli (Hopkinson, 2007).

Supplements: Vitamins, Minerals, Omega-3s, Probiotics

Well-nourished nursing parents with healthy vitamin D levels may not need vitamin or mineral supplements.

While supplements may benefit malnourished parents, those on a restricted diet (see next point), or those with a history of weight-loss surgery (see later section), the best way for well-nourished nursing parents to get the nutrients they need is through a balanced and healthy diet. One exception is vitamin D (see next point).

• • •

Undernourished or nutrient-deficient nursing parents will benefit from supplements.

Parents whose sunlight exposure is limited, are chronically undernourished, have a history of weight-loss surgery, or on a very restricted diet may eventually develop vitamin or mineral deficiencies that can lead to a decrease in the levels of some nutrients in the milk, such as iodine, choline, A, D, B_1, B_2, B_6, or B_{12}, which may affect their nursing baby's health (Allen, 2012; Allen et al., 2018; Stoutjesdijk, Schaafsma, Dijck-Brouwer, & Muskiet, 2018). Those at risk include nursing parents on vegan diets, those with intestinal parasites, and those with a history of weight-loss surgery (see later section). Also at risk are those with Crohn's disease and other malabsorption disorders. In this case, vitamin-and-mineral supplements may be important.

Vitamin D. Due to lifestyle changes, depletion of the ozone layer, and warnings about sun exposure, the percentage of birthing parents and children suffering from vitamin D deficiency is high worldwide, especially in non-tropical latitudes. Vitamin D is actually a hormone precursor made by the body when the skin is exposed to the ultraviolet rays of the sun. Only about 10% to 20% of our vitamin D intake is meant to come from the food we eat (Papadimitriou, 2017; C. L. Wagner, Taylor, & Hollis, 2008). When nursing parents are vitamin D deficient, vitamin D supplements can both restore their own vitamin D levels and increase the amount in the milk, which assures healthy vitamin D levels in the baby. For more details, see p. 296.

KEY CONCEPT

Some vitamin and mineral deficiencies may affect levels in mother's milk.

Vitamin B_{12}. Vegan nursing parents consume no animal products, so to safeguard their health and their baby's health, vitamin B_{12} supplements are necessary. See p. 568 for details. The same may be true for nursing parents with a history of weight-loss surgery (see p. 580) or any other health condition that interferes with nutrient absorption.

Iron. If a nursing parent becomes iron-deficient or anemic, iron supplements can help bring iron levels up to normal. However, iron levels in milk are not affected by the nursing parent's blood iron levels, and taking iron supplements will not affect the level of iron in the milk (Lawrence & Lawrence, 2016, p. 304).

• • •

Taking mega-doses of some fat-soluble vitamins is not recommended, as this may be harmful to both nursing parent and baby.

Water-soluble vitamins, which include vitamin C and the B-complex vitamins (thiamin [B_1], riboflavin [B_2], niacin [B_3], pantothenic acid [B_5], pyridoxine [B_6], biotin [B_7], folic acid or folate [B_9], and cobalamin [B_{12}]) are flushed through a nursing parent's system daily and do not accumulate. So if a nursing parent is taking higher-than-recommended doses of these vitamins to treat a health problem (such as B_2 for migraine, B_6 for neuritis, C for the common cold), this should not affect nursing (Sauberan, 2019).

Fat-soluble vitamins, which are stored in fat and tissue, include vitamins A, D, E, and K and should not be taken in mega-doses unless the nursing parent is deficient and being treated to bring blood levels up to normal. Vitamin A is secreted into human milk and is stored in the liver. Doses of more than 5,000 IUs of vitamin A per day are not recommended for adults (Hale, 2019, p. 783).

Vitamin D is also a fat-soluble vitamin, but it behaves more like a hormone because it is made in our bodies during skin exposure to the sun. Due to the rise in vitamin D deficiency worldwide, larger-than-recommended doses may be beneficial to many nursing parents and babies. For details, see p. 295.

• • •

If nursing parents consume few omega-3 fatty acids in their diet, a supplement may be beneficial.

As described in a previous point, the total amount of fat in human milk usually stays stable independent of diet. But diet plays a major role in the proportion of different types of fats in the milk. In babies, greater intake of long-chain polyunsaturated fatty acids like DHA and ARA (also known as omega-3 fatty acids) and carotenoids (nutrients such as beta-carotene found in red, yellow and orange fruits and vegetables) is associated with better psychomotor development (Zielinska, Hamulka, Grabowicz-Chadrzynska, et al., 2019).

In areas where fish consumption is common (one serving of oily fish per week), recommended levels of DHA and other omega-3 fatty acids are found in mother's milk (Aumeistere et al., 2018; Tian et al., 2019). However, if a parent's diet is low in omega-3s, regularly taking an omega-3 supplement may benefit the nursing baby, although long-term studies have not yet confirmed this. Omega-3 supplements increase levels of DHA in milk (Cimatti et al., 2018). See also p. 837 on taking omega-3 supplements as a treatment for postpartum depression.

• • •

The research on the benefits of probiotics for nursing parents is mixed.

Will taking probiotics during pregnancy and lactation improve baby's health by decreasing incidence of allergy and gastrointestinal problems (Baldassarre et al., 2018)? According to some studies, yes (Rautava, 2018), according to other studies, no (Cabana et al., 2017; Mantaring et al., 2018). However, Spanish research (see p. 763) found that taking probiotics during pregnancy and lactation may prevent and/or treat mastitis in nursing parents. More research is needed.

Foods to Eat or Avoid

There are no specific foods that should be consumed or avoided during lactation.

Nursing parents with healthy eating habits do not usually need to change their diet during lactation. They don't have to drink cow's milk or eat any other specific foods, and no specific foods should be avoided by every lactating parent. Although exceptions exist, most nursing parents can eat anything they like in moderation—including chocolate, garlic, and spicy foods—without any effect on their baby.

• • •

When nursing parents eat foods with different flavors, this gives the baby a preview of the tastes he'll experience later from solid foods at the family table.

During pregnancy and lactation, all mammal young are exposed to the flavors of the foods their mothers eat through amniotic fluid (Lipchock, Reed, & Mennella, 2011) and their mother's milk. This helps babies recognize safe foods when they are ready to expand their diet to non-milk foods (Mennella, Reiter, & Daniels, 2016).

Several studies found that when nursing parents eat a food regularly during pregnancy and lactation, their babies are more likely to accept its flavor later as a solid food. In one U.S. study (Mennella, Jagnow, & Beauchamp, 2001), mothers drank either carrot juice or water 4 days per week for 3 weeks during pregnancy. When carrots were introduced as a solid food, the babies' enjoyment of them was rated higher by the mothers who drank the carrot juice than by the mothers who drank the water.

KEY CONCEPT

Nursing parents do not need to eat or avoid any specific foods or drinks.

In another U.S. randomized controlled trial (Mennella, Daniels, & Reiter, 2017), lactating mothers began drinking vegetable, beet, celery, and carrot juices for 1 or 3 months, beginning at different time periods after birth. Researchers found that when mothers drank the vegetable juices starting at 2 weeks post-delivery, this had a much greater effect on their babies' acceptance of carrot-flavored baby cereal at 6 months than if they started drinking the juices at 6 or 10 weeks post-delivery. One month of juice-drinking after birth had a greater effect on baby's acceptance of that flavor than 3 months of juice drinking.

A Danish study found that some food flavor compounds appeared in mother's milk within 1 to 2 hours after ingestion (Hausner, Bredie, Molgaard, Petersen, & Moller, 2008). In one U.S. study (Mennella & Beauchamp, 1991a), an hour or two after breastfeeding the mothers swallowed concentrated capsules of garlic extract, and their milk acquired a distinct garlicky smell, but the babies who were fed this garlicky milk did not refuse it or act fussy. Instead, they drank more milk than usual. A 2019 French study (S. Wagner et al., 2019) found that babies weaned between 8 and 12 months were attracted to the odors of green vegetables, cheese, and fish when their mothers ate these foods during pregnancy and lactation.

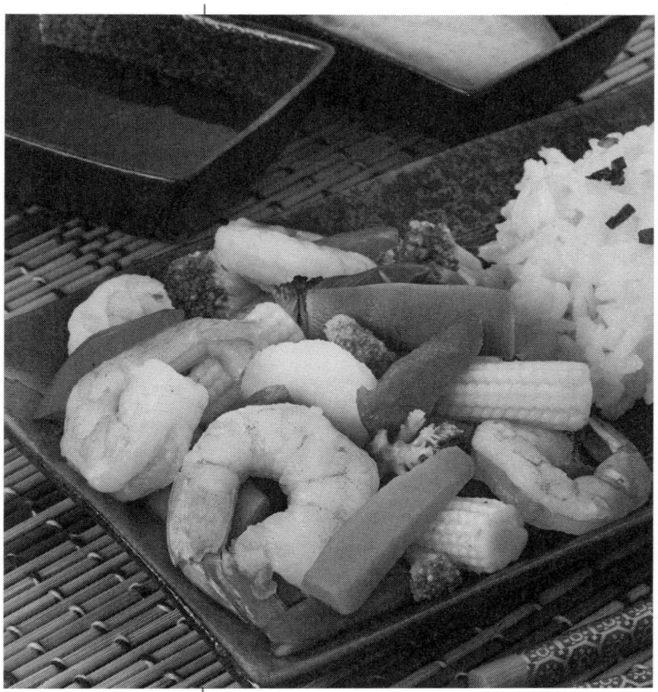

Food preferences acquired during nursing appear to last for years. One 2019 U.S. prospective cohort study followed 1,396 mothers and children (Beckerman, Slade, & Ventura, 2019) and found that even at 6 years of age, the children of the mothers who consumed more vegetables and breastfed longer ate more vegetables independent of their sociodemographics and availability of fruits and vegetables.

Is Baby Reacting to Something in the Parent's Diet?

When a baby is fretful or gassy, many nursing parents wrongly assume something they ate is the cause.

Fussiness and gassiness are normal during the newborn period and are unlikely to be a reaction to something in the parent's diet. During the first year, only about 5% of nursing babies react to a food their parent consumes, with cow's milk being the most common offending food in Western countries (Kvenshagen, Halvorsen, & Jacobsen, 2008).

Most nursing parents can eat any food they like in moderation without any effect on their baby. Yet many nursing parents are told to avoid specific foods, which vary from culture to culture. For example, Chinese and Southeast Asian mothers are advised to avoid cold liquids because they are not good for mother or baby (Lauwers & Swisher, 2015). Some Hispanic women are cautioned to avoid pork, chili peppers, and tomatoes, while some African-American mothers are warned to avoid onions. In Australia, cabbage, chocolates, spicy foods, peas, onions, and cauliflower are thought to cause colic, gas, diarrhea, and rashes in the nursing baby (Wambach & Spencer, 2021, p. 753).

As described in the previous section, nursing babies usually benefit when their parents eat a varied diet because the flavors from the foods parents eat enter the milk (Mastorakou, Ruark, Weenen, Stahl, & Stieger, 2019), providing babies with a preview of the tastes they'll experience at the family table when they are older (Mennella et al., 2017).

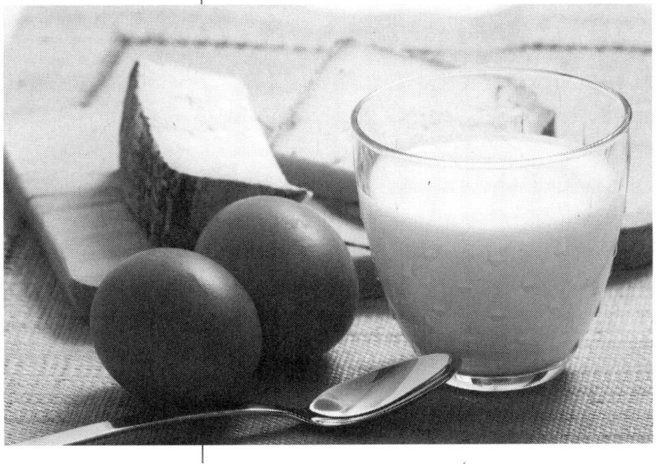

Even when a baby does react to a food in the parent's diet, the specific food that causes a reaction will vary from baby to baby. For this reason, telling all nursing parents to avoid the same foods will do no good. Plus perceived "diet rules" dissuade some parents from nursing (Gabriel, Gabriel, & Lawrence, 1986).

• • •

Before assuming the baby is reacting to something in the parent's diet, ask if the baby has been fed anything other than human milk.

When a baby fusses, some parents assume it was something they ate, even if the baby is also consuming formula or other foods. Because the percentage of nursing babies who react to foods their parents eat is small (see previous point), it is far more likely a baby will react to a food he is given directly, such as formula or solids, rather than to a food in his parent's diet. Ask if:

- The baby is fed teas or other remedies for colic or crying
- Other adults or children might be feeding the baby something other than mother's milk
- The baby gets supplemental feeds from the other parent or a caregiver

• • •

Ask if the parent or baby is taking any medications, vitamins, or supplements and whether the reaction started after they were introduced.

On average only about 1% of a medication passes into the milk (Hale, 2019), but a very sensitive baby may still have a reaction. If the baby's reaction started after the parent began taking a drug, vitamins, or other supplements, this will provide a clue. If a drug or supplement may be a contributing cause, suggest the parent ask the healthcare provider for an alternative.

• • •

Ask how many caffeinated drinks the nursing parent consumes daily.

Very little caffeine (about 1.5% of the maternal dose) passes into the milk. But it takes much longer for caffeine to clear a young baby's system as compared with an older baby. For more details, see the next section.

• • •

A reaction to a food in the parent's diet is more likely if there is a family history of allergy and the baby has physical symptoms.

Although a baby affected by a food his lactating parent eats is an exception to the rule, it can happen. Symptoms of food hypersensitivity, intolerance, or allergy include:

- Skin reactions: eczema, dermatitis, hives, rash, dry skin
- Gastrointestinal reactions: vomiting, diarrhea, pain, blood or mucus in stools (ABM, 2011)
- Respiratory reactions: congestion, runny nose, wheezing, coughing

When a baby has a reaction like these, there is likely to be a family history of allergy. If one parent has allergies, the baby has a 20% to 40% risk of being allergic, and if both parents have allergies, the baby's risk increases to 50% to 80% (Ferreira & Seidman, 2007).

• • •

A reaction to a food in the parent's diet is more likely if there is a family history of allergy and the baby has physical symptoms.

If a baby seems to react acutely to something in the parent's diet, ask whether a new food was consumed recently, especially one that is either strong or spicy, or if a large quantity of one food was consumed. If too much of one food is the issue, eating it in more moderate amounts may be enough to resolve the reaction.

Case reports (Cooper & Cooper, 1996) document two Swiss breastfed babies who developed a rash within 1 hour after their mothers ate a dish with red pepper, with the rash disappearing within 12 to 48 hours. Based on many years of clinical experience, U.S. physicians Ruth and Robert Lawrence (Lawrence & Lawrence, 2016, p. 315) wrote that typically a baby's reaction to a food eaten by the parent resolves within 24 hours

• • •

Dairy is the most common allergen to affect nursing babies via the milk in Western countries. In China, the most common food is egg. Here's some of what we know.

The most common food to cause a reaction in babies through mother's milk in Western countries is dairy, followed by other protein foods.

Incidence of cow-milk protein allergy in nursing babies. During the first year, about 5% of nursing babies react to cow-milk protein through the milk, with the most common reactions being pain behavior and gastrointestinal and respiratory symptoms (Kvenshagen et al., 2008).

Early formula supplements sensitize babies. Although a baby can be sensitized to allergy in the womb (Szepfalusi et al., 2000), it happens more commonly after birth. Research found that exposure to cow-milk protein via early formula supplements increases the risk that a baby may develop cow-milk-protein allergy (CMPA). In one Danish study of 1,749 newborns followed for their first year of life (Host, Husby, & Osterballe, 1988), only 0.5% (9) of the exclusively breastfed babies reacted to cow's milk in their mothers' diet, and all of these babies were given infant formula during their first days of life in the hospital, in some cases without the mothers' knowledge. The younger the baby when cow's milk is introduced, the more likely it is to sensitize a baby to allergy.

A 2019 Irish retrospective study compared the feeding histories of 55 children diagnosed later with CMPA with 55 age- and sex-matched children tolerant of cow's milk (Kelly, DunnGalvin, Murphy, & J, 2019). During the first 24 hours, some of the study babies were exclusively breastfed, some were exclusively formula fed, and some (nearly 46% of the breastfed babies) were breastfed with formula supplements. Using logistical regression, they found that the only factor that significantly predicted the development of CMPA was formula supplementation during the first 24 hours. These early formula supplements had a 74% diagnostic accuracy. The breastfed babies fed formula during their first 24 hours were ***7 times more likely to develop CMPA*** than the babies exclusively breastfed during their first day. This study also had a prospective arm that examined the reasons 179 nursing newborns received formula on their first day of life in the hospital. The authors wrote (Kelly et al., 2019):

> "Breastfed babies are still being put at significantly increased risk of CMPA by receiving supplemental formula in the first 24 hours of life, despite the major predictors of supplementation being subjective and remediable in other ways. Mothers and healthcare providers should be better educated on the benefits of exclusive breastfeeding and resourced adequately to avoid unnecessary formula supplementation to reduce the risk of development of CMPA.".

Cow-milk protein in the nursing parent's diet enters the milk. When a nursing baby develops CMPA, he may react to the cow-milk protein in mother's milk. In a Finnish study (Sorva, Makinen-Kiljunen, & Juntunen-Backman, 1994), one group of study mothers consumed dairy and the researchers detected a cow's milk antibody (the protein beta-lactoglobulin) in the mothers' milk within 1 to 2 hours after consumption. A U.S. study (Clyne & Kulczycki, 1991) reported that the level of IgG (another cow's milk protein) was higher in the milk of mothers of colicky babies as compared with the milk of other mothers. In this study, the level of this cow's milk protein was even higher in the milk of the mothers with colicky babies than the level in infant formula (up to 8.5 µg/mL versus up to 6.4 µg/mL).

KEY CONCEPT

Nursing newborns fed formula during their first 24 hours were 16 times more likely to develop cow-milk-protein allergy than those exclusively nursed.

In another U.S. study (Jakobsson & Lindberg, 1983), 35 of 66 mothers of colicky babies reported a decrease in their babies' colicky behavior when they eliminated milk and milk products from their diets. The behaviors reappeared twice when the mothers ate dairy as a challenge.

• • •

When parents eliminate a food that they were eating regularly, it may take weeks for it to clear fully from their system.

Eliminating a food for a day or two will usually resolve a baby's acute reaction to a new food. But if the baby reacts to a food the nursing parent was eating often, it may take longer for it to clear and for the baby's symptoms to resolve fully. Also, symptoms like congestion, eczema, wheezing, and crying often start gradually, so it may take time before the connection between the parent's diet and the baby's reaction becomes obvious.

Expected response to elimination diets. When parents go on a dairy-free diet, for example, some babies respond within a few days, but it often takes 2 to 3 weeks for the cow-milk protein to clear fully from their system and the baby's reaction to resolve completely. A 2017 Thai study of 19 lactating mothers, 4 of whom had babies with CMPA (Matangkasombut et al., 2017), began with the mothers avoiding all dairy for 1 week. Then they consumed one dose of cow's milk before going back on the elimination diet again. For the next 7 days, the researchers measured their milk levels of the cow-milk protein beta-lactoglobulin. In the hours after they consumed the cow's milk, the mothers' milk level of this protein rose from 0.58 ng/L to a peak of 1.23 ng/L. Milk levels were still significantly elevated at 3 and 7 days, and these differences were statistically significant. The level of the cow-milk protein was the same in the mothers whose babies had CMPA and the mothers of the healthy babies. During this challenge, 3 of the 4 babies with CMPA developed symptoms, such as rash or congestion.

Dairy elimination and bone health. Some nursing parents worry that their bone health may be at risk when they reduce their calcium intake by eliminating dairy. A Finnish study (Holmberg-Marttila et al., 2001) examined the effect on bone mineral density of eliminating cow's milk from a breastfeeding mother's diet and concluded that elimination of dairy for a few months was not associated with greater-than-normal loss of bone mineral density. If nursing parents or their healthcare providers are concerned, one option is to take calcium supplements while avoiding dairy.

Other foods to eliminate. If eliminating dairy and all foods containing cow-milk protein does not improve the baby's symptoms, in Clinical Protocol #24 (ABM, 2011) from the Academy of Breastfeeding Medicine (ABM), its authors suggested eliminating the following food one by one:

- Eggs
- Corn
- Soy
- Citrus fruits
- Nuts
- Peanuts
- Wheat

If the baby's symptoms continue and other causes were ruled out (see next point), another option is for the nursing parent to go on a low-allergen diet consisting of lamb, rice, squash, and pears (ABM, 2011). If parents plan to make any major changes in their diet, suggest eliminating no more than one or two foods at a time, so they can more easily pinpoint the cause. Also suggest getting skilled help from a registered dietitian in evaluating their diet.

• • •

If a baby's stools contain blood and/or mucus and eliminating dairy does not resolve it, rule out other causes. In most cases, it will clear in time with continued nursing.

In one study of babies with blood in the stool (Pumberger, Pomberger, & Geissler, 2001), the blood disappeared after the nursing parents eliminated dairy from their diet, but this symptom is not always caused by allergy or hypersensitivity.

Other causes of blood in the stool. In fact, in a 2019 U.S. prospective longitudinal study (Lazare, Brand, Fazzari, Noor, & Daum, 2019), one group of 19 exclusively breastfeeding mothers whose babies had blood in their stools followed a dairy-and-soy elimination diet and then did a challenge with these foods at 3-week intervals. In spite of the elimination diets, every one of these 19 babies continued to test positive for blood in the stool. A Finnish study of 40 babies between 1 and 6 months old with bloody stools (Arvola et al., 2006) found after dairy elimination diets and dairy challenges that only 18% had cow-milk-protein allergy. The researchers found evidence in 20% of the babies that indicated a virus may have triggered the bleeding. They concluded that "rectal bleeding in infants is generally a benign and self-limiting disorder" (Arvola et al., 2006, p. e761). They recommended elimination diets whenever a baby has bloody stools, since this resolved the symptoms of some babies, but they noted that in the vast majority of cases, this symptom was not an indicator of a serious health problem.

Other possible causes of blood in the stool, such as an anal fissure, were listed in a 2017 overview article on this topic (Pai & Fox, 2017). Among possible infectious and inflammatory conditions that might cause bloody stools, it included infant cow-milk-protein allergy, antibiotic use (which can cause gut damage), gastrointestinal infection, and a family history of inflammatory bowel disease.

If the baby's healthcare provider recommends suspending nursing during a trial of hypoallergenic formula, suggest the family discuss the possibility of continuing to nurse and share the ABM's Clinical Protocol #24, which is free and downloadable in multiple languages at **bfmed.org/protocols**.

A 2014 Israeli historical prospective comparative study of 77 babies who had an incident of rectal bleeding (Reiter, Morag, Mazkereth, Strauss, & Maayan-Metzger, 2014) concluded that an incident of rectal bleeding in the newborn period does not increase the risk of developing hypersensitivities or food allergies during childhood.

• • •

If an elimination diet identifies an offending food, it is usually possible for the nursing parent to eat this food again within 6 months or so.

Suggest nursing parents try adding a small amount of any offending food back into their diet as an experiment when the baby is 9 to 12 months old. Although children's allergic reactions to some foods are lifelong, a reaction to cow's milk is usually outgrown, often by 1 year (Ferreira & Seidman, 2007). See p. 138 for recommendations on when and how to introduce offending foods into the diet of a baby who has a skin rash or other symptoms of allergy.

Caffeine, Chocolate, and Herbal Teas

Moderate caffeine intake by the nursing parent is not a problem for most babies.

Very little caffeine (about 1.5% of the maternal dose) passes into a mother's milk (Berlin, Denson, Daniel, & Ward, 1984). But it takes much longer for caffeine to clear a young baby's system as compared with an older baby. The half-life of caffeine is about 96 hours in a newborn, 14 hours in a 3- to 5-month-old baby, 2.6 hours in a baby older than 6 months, and 5 hours in an adult (Hale, 2019, p. 99). U.S. studies (Nehlig, 1994; Ryu, 1985a, 1985b) found that most parents need to drink more than 5 cups of coffee per day before their nursing baby is affected.

KEY CONCEPT

Most babies are not affected by moderate consumption of coffee, tea, chocolate, or herbal tea by the nursing parent.

How much caffeine is okay while nursing? One cup of coffee—depending on type and preparation—usually contains about 100 mg to 150 mg of caffeine. A 2018 Swiss systematic review (McCreedy, Bird, Brown, Shaw-Stewart, & Chen, 2018) was unable to draw conclusions about caffeine intake during lactation because the evidence is so limited. But after reviewing the literature, the European Food Safety Authority (EFSA, 2015) concluded that a daily intake of 2 cups of coffee (200 mg of caffeine) "does not give rise to safety concerns" for the nursing baby. Other experts say that 2 to 3 cups of coffee (300 mg or less of caffeine) per day might be a safe level (P. O. Anderson, 2018c), with the caution that lower levels of caffeine consumption are advised for parents of preterm babies and newborns.

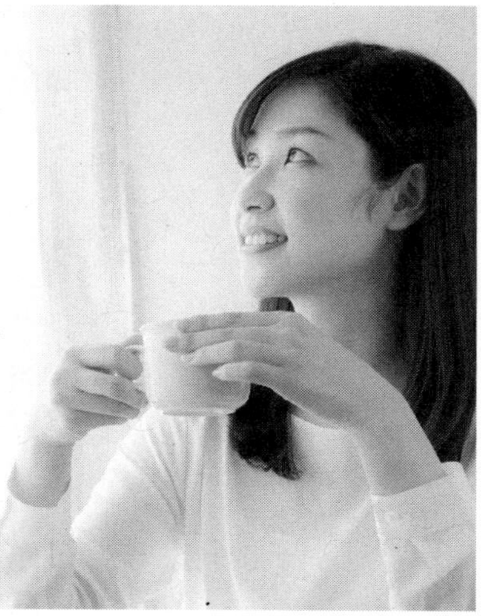

A 2012 Brazilian prospective cohort study examined at 3 months post-birth the effect of breastfeeding mothers' coffee consumption on the sleep patterns of their 885 babies (Santos, Matijasevich, & Domingues, 2012). Whether the mothers consumed more or less than 300 mg of caffeine per day, the researchers found no differences in the babies' sleep patterns.

• • •

If parents are worried their baby is reacting to caffeine, ask how much caffeine they are consuming from all sources.

Sources of caffeine include coffee, iced and hot teas, colas, other caffeine-containing soft drinks (be sure to ask about serving size), and any over-the-counter caffeine-containing drugs, such as some pain relievers, cold remedies, and diuretics.

If parents consume 750 mg of caffeine or more per day—the amount of caffeine in five 5-oz (150 mL) cups of coffee—and the baby seems irritable, fussy, and doesn't sleep long, suggest substituting caffeine-free beverages for 2 to 3 weeks and see if the baby's behavior changes. Eliminating caffeine suddenly may cause headaches, so it may be best to taper down gradually. If caffeine is causing the reaction, within 2 weeks of eliminating caffeine, the parent should notice a difference (P. O. Anderson, 2018c). .

• • •

In addition to the possible effects on a nursing baby's behavior, there are other drawbacks to consuming too much caffeine while nursing.

Higher levels of caffeine consumption by a nursing parent may have other drawbacks besides an irritable baby. Research found an association between caffeine consumption and mammary pain that occurs around menstruation (Ader, South-Paul, Adera, & Deuster, 2001; Eren et al., 2016). Consuming more than 450 mg per day of caffeine was also associated with lower iron levels in human milk (Hale, 2019; Munoz, Lonnerdal, Keen, & Dewey, 1988).

• • •

Chocolate contains a substance similar to caffeine, but in much smaller amounts.

Chocolate contains theobromine, which is similar to caffeine and can produce the same effect if consumed in large amounts (Berlin & Daniel, 1981). Although the theobromine in chocolate is similar to caffeine, there is much less theobromine in chocolate than caffeine in coffee. A small cup of brewed drip coffee contains about 100 mg to 150 mg of caffeine, while a cup of decaffeinated coffee contains about 3 mg of caffeine, and 1 ounce of milk chocolate contains about 6 mg of theobromine, as well as a small amount of caffeine.

Moderate consumption of chocolate does not usually cause a reaction in nursing babies, but large amounts of chocolate can. In one case report (P. O. Anderson, 2018c), a mother who did not drink coffee consumed about 250 g of cocoa per day. By 12 hours after birth, her baby was irritable, jittery, and cried inconsolably, which persisted for days. After tapering down her chocolate intake over a 10-day period, her baby's symptoms subsided.

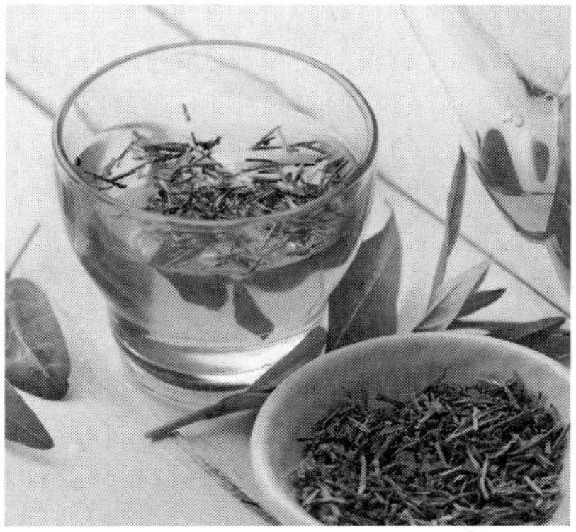

• • •

Herbs can act like drugs, and some herbal teas may affect nursing.

Many of today's modern medications come from the herbs used in teas and home remedies. Like drugs, herbs can act as stimulants or tranquilizers and can also affect other body processes. Licorice, for example, can increase blood pressure, so it should be avoided by those with hypertension (Humphrey, 2003, p. 42). Before consuming an herb, it is important to learn about its use.

Some herbs can affect nursing. For example, in significant amounts sage, peppermint, and parsley may reduce milk production (Humphrey, 2003; Marasco & West, 2020). While major brands of herbal teas are safe for nursing parents, teas marketed as "private" brands or teas brewed from individual herbs should be used with caution.

• • •

Suggest parents prepare herbal teas as directed and drink them in moderation.

If parents are concerned about their herbal-tea consumption, mention that the strength of a tea depends on its preparation. The longer the tea leaves are steeped, the stronger the tea. By decreasing the steeping time, parents can decrease the tea's potency.

During lactation, suggest parents strive for moderation in all foods and drinks so that reactions in their baby are less likely to occur. A parent who drinks a few cups of herbal tea each day is unlikely to have a problem. But reactions are more likely if parents drink a quart (.946 liter) or more of tea each day, or if the tea is potent or contains active ingredients.

Bone Health

During lactation, some of the calcium in the milk comes from the nursing parent's bones, which is borrowed during nursing and replaced after weaning.

During lactation, the nursing parent's body draws some of the calcium needed in the milk from the parent's bones, causing a temporary decrease in bone mineral density. Ultimately, though, bone strength is regained. A 2019 overview article (B. A. Ryan & Kovacs, 2019) explained how this process of bone loss and bone gain works in the body, based on the findings of human and animal studies. After weaning, a reversal of the bone-loss process occurs to create an increase in bone formation. By 6 to 12 months after weaning, the bone mineral density of the spine and hips has returned to their prepregnancy values (Kovacs, 2016). Two large prospective studies, one American and one Canadian (Cooke-Hubley et al., 2019; Crandall et al., 2017), found that neither lactation nor number of births affects the parent's risk of low bone density or fractures.

KEY CONCEPT

The greater a parent's lifetime nursing duration, the greater the bone strength later in life.

The main predictor of bone loss later in life appears to be low calcium intake from childhood to early adulthood (Cross, Hillman, Allen, Krause, & Vieira, 1995).

Long-term nursing and bone health. Longer lifetime nursing is associated with improved health outcomes for nursing parents, including a lower risk of hypertension, Type 2 diabetes, and breast and ovarian cancers (Chowdhury et al., 2015; Rameez et al., 2019). A 2012 U.K. study that measured body composition, bone area, bone mineral content and bone density in 145 women (Wiklund et al., 2012) looked at the impact of long-term nursing on bone density. It found that 16 to 20 years after the birth of the last child, a lifetime nursing duration of 33 or more months was associated with significantly better bone strength in the hip and tibia. The researchers attributed the improved bone strength to the hormonal changes that occur during nursing.

• • •

Calcium intake from food or supplements during lactation is not the primary source of the calcium in human milk.

Most of the calcium needed for milk production does not come from dietary calcium intake (Kent, Arthur, Mitoulas, & Hartmann, 2009). Instead, it comes from a combination of calcium drawn from nursing parents' bones (Kovacs, 2016) and a decrease in the calcium excreted in their urine (King, 2001).

For nursing parents eating a varied and nutritious diet, taking calcium supplements is probably unnecessary. In fact, consuming too much calcium increases the risk of kidney stones and urinary tract infections (Sorensen, 2014). However, if a parent's diet is low in calcium, suggest consuming more calcium-rich foods. Good sources of calcium include low-fat dairy products (milk, yogurt, cheese, ice cream), dark green, leafy vegetables (broccoli, collard greens, bok choy), canned sardines and salmon with bones, tofu, almonds, corn tortillas, and foods fortified with calcium (some orange juices, cereals, breads). In lactating women on low-calcium diets, increasing consumption of calcium-rich foods was associated with less bone loss during pregnancy and nursing (O'Brien et al., 2006).

Vegetarian and Vegan Families

Ask vegetarian parents to describe what foods they eat and what specific foods they avoid.

Vegetarian diets cover a wide range of possibilities. Some vegetarians avoid red meat but eat poultry, seafood, milk products, and eggs. Ovo-lacto-vegetarians avoid all red meat, seafood, and poultry (flesh foods) but eat milk products and eggs. Lacto-vegetarians avoid flesh foods and eggs but eat milk products. Ovo-vegetarians avoid flesh foods and milk products, but eat eggs. All of these diets include some form of animal products.

Vegan diets, on the other hand, include no animal products, the only dietary source of vitamin B_{12}. To avoid a vitamin B_{12} deficiency, vegan nursing parents (and those who consume very little animal protein) need to take steps to make sure they receive vitamin B_{12}, either from foods enriched with vitamin B_{12} or by taking regular vitamin B_{12} supplements (see next point).

• • •

Research (Weder, Hoffmann, Becker, Alexy, & Keller, 2019) found that children raised on a vegan diet can grow and gain weight normally, but because the sole dietary source of vitamin B_{12} is animal products, vegan diets—which include no animal products—must be supplemented to avoid putting both nursing parent and nursing baby at risk of developing a vitamin B_{12} deficiency (Baroni et al., 2018). This deficiency in nursing parents leads to milk low in vitamin B_{12}, which increases risk of deficiency in their nursing baby. Systematic reviews and studies on vitamin B_{12} levels in the milk of meat-eating, vegetarian, and vegan mothers (Dror & Allen, 2018; Pawlak et al., 2018) indicate that there is still much to learn, but the science is clear that a vitamin B_{12} deficiency during infancy can lead to lifelong health and development issues in exclusively nursing babies.

Vegan families consume no animal products, so finding a reliable source of vitamin B_{12} is vital to preventing vitamin B_{12} deficiency in both nursing parents and nursing babies.

Symptoms of vitamin B_{12} deficiency in the baby often develop before symptoms in the nursing parent, appearing within the first few months of life or going unrecognized until later (Roschitz et al., 2005). Early symptoms often include irritability and lack of interest in feeding, which can lead to slow weight gain, failure to thrive, and eventually neurological problems (El & Celikkaya, 2019). Other common symptoms include fatigue, pale skin, a lack of eye contact, vomiting, diarrhea or constipation, a slowing or reversal of normal development (losing the ability to sit up) (Weiss, Fogelman, & Bennett, 2004). Low muscle tone (hypotonia) is another possible symptom. The nursing parent may have no symptoms, but blood or milk testing can detect this deficiency.

KEY CONCEPT

Nursing parents on vegan diets need to eat foods enriched with vitamin B_{12} or take supplements.

Treating a vitamin B_{12} deficiency. If a vitamin B_{12} deficiency is caught early, any neurological problems may be reversed when treated with vitamin B_{12} supplements (Casella, Valente, de Navarro, & Kok, 2005); if not caught early, they may be irreversible.

Avoiding a vitamin B_{12} deficiency. One way a vegan parent can safeguard the baby's long-term health and development is to take vitamin B_{12} supplements or eat foods fortified with vitamin B_{12} (Baroni et al., 2018). A 2019 overview article on diet during pregnancy and lactation (Sebastiani et al., 2019) recommended that vegan parents who are not taking a vitamin B_{12} supplement eat 4 servings each day of a vitamin B_{12} fortified food. In the developing world, providing vitamin B_{12} supplements during pregnancy and early lactation not only improved blood and milk vitamin B_{12} levels, it also improved weight gain, most likely due in part to improved feeding ability in the vitamin B_{12} sufficient babies (A. D. Smith, 2018).

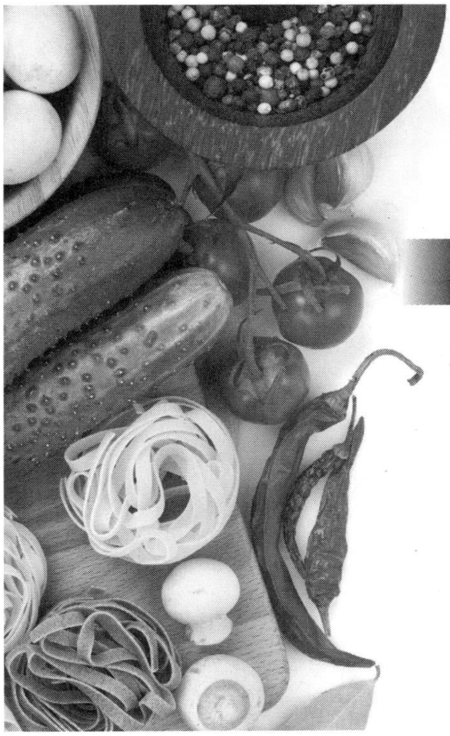

• • •

A U.S. cross-sectional study of 74 lactating mothers (M. T. Perrin, Pawlak, Dean, Christis, & Friend, 2018) analyzed their milk samples and found—as described on p. 427—that although the overall fat content of the milk was comparable, the types of fats found in the milk samples varied by diet. Due to low seafood consumption among all three groups, the milk levels of the omega-3 fatty acid DHA were low. The milk of the vegan mothers was higher in unsaturated fats and other omega-3 fatty acids and lower in saturated fats, and trans fats. The milk from vegan parents also had a lower ratio of omega-6 fatty acids to omega-3s compared with the vegetarian and meat-eaters. All of the differences are considered normal variations in human milk composition.

The types of fat in human milk vary among meat-eaters, vegetarians, and vegans.

Weight and Weight Loss

Weight Loss after Birth and Dieting

Many—but not all—nursing parents lose weight gradually during the first 6 months after birth.

During the early weeks after birth, nursing parents are usually less active than during pregnancy. But because some of the fat reserves laid down during pregnancy are mobilized for milk production, weight loss is normal during this period. The U.S. Institute of Medicine estimates that nursing parents who "eat to hunger" lose on average about 0.8 kg (1.6 pounds) per month during the first 6 months of lactation (IOM, 2005). These are averages, and some parents gain weight during lactation. One U.S. study of 24 mothers compared those exclusively breastfeeding with those doing mixed feeds and concluded that exclusive nursing promotes greater weight loss than combining nursing and formula feeds (Hatsu, McDougald, & Anderson, 2008). A 2019 U.S. study of 370 women who exclusively breastfed their babies for at least 1 month (Tahir et al., 2019) also found that breastfeeding intensity affected weight loss, with the study women who exclusively nursed for 3 to 6 months losing more weight than those who exclusively nursed for a shorter time.

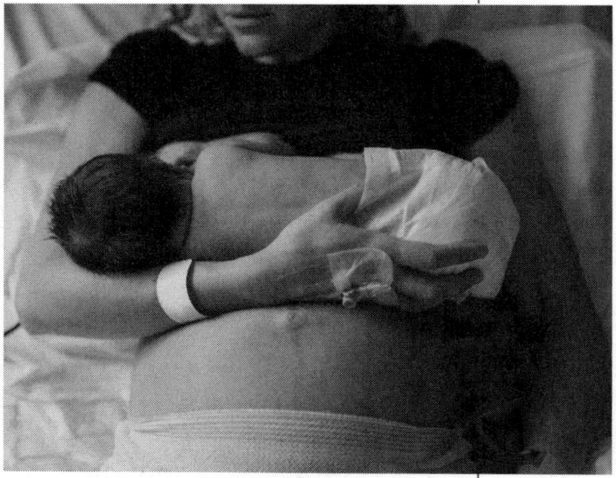

As one 2017 U.K. survey of 182 mothers (Schalla, Witcomb, & Haycraft, 2017) found, the idea that nursing takes off the weight is an effective motivator that convinces many new parents to give nursing a try. Overall, however, the research on nursing and weight loss is mixed, in part because studies do not always use the same definition of nursing or measure weight change at the same time points. One U.S. systematic review of 37 prospective studies and 8 retrospective studies (Neville, McKinley, Holmes, Spence, & Woodside, 2014) noted that the majority of studies found no association between nursing and weight or changes in body composition, although the findings depended in part on the time points that the weights were measured and the intensity of nursing. Its authors found that among the 5 studies that were considered of the highest quality, four of these studies found a positive association between nursing and weight change.

After 6 months, weight tends to become more stable unless the parent eats fewer calories and begins exercising regularly.

• • •

If nursing parents want to lose weight faster, suggest avoiding extreme weight loss programs while eating less and exercising more.

After giving birth, parents are vulnerable to retaining some of the weight gained during pregnancy. There are good reasons to take steps to return to prepregnancy weight other than concerns about attractiveness. Research (Rooney, Schauberger, & Mathiason, 2005) found an association between retaining weight more than 6 months after birth and obesity later in life.

When parents choose to eat less to lose weight, encourage them to eat nutrient-dense foods and consider a vitamin-and-mineral supplement. Although a minimum of 1800 calories per day is usually recommended during lactation, one study found that eating as little as 1500 calories per day during the first 6 months of nursing did not affect milk production or composition in previously well-nourished mothers (Strode, Dewey, & Lonnerdal, 1986). But even if milk production is not affected, eating poorly can compromise a parent's health and energy by depleting reserves. Encourage parents to eat a healthy diet for their own sake to increase their resistance to illness and energy.

One U.S. study found that when breastfeeding mothers lowered their calorie intake by 25%, they safely lost about 1 pound (0.45 kg) per week without affecting their baby's growth (Dusdieker, Hemingway, & Stumbo, 1994). Another U.S. study found that when 40 overweight women cut 500 calories from their daily diet and added a 45-minute exercise routine 4 days a week, those in the diet-and-exercise group lost more weight than those in the control group, while the average weight gain of the babies in both groups stayed the same (Lovelady, Garner, Moreno, & Williams, 2000).

To promote faster weight loss, suggest parents begin by increasing their activity level and eliminating 100 calories per day from their diet. If they want to do more, suggest they plan to eat at least 1800 calories per day in nutrient-dense foods.

• • •

Extremely low carb diets are not recommended during lactation.

Popular low-carbohydrate diets such as the Paleo, Ketogenic, and Atkins diets work by reducing carbohydrate intake to such a low level that the body goes into ***ketosis***, when fats are burned for fuel instead of carbohydrates. While this metabolic change does not seem to be harmful in non-lactating individuals, at this writing, there are more than 12 case reports of lactating women who were hospitalized with the life-threatening condition known as ***ketoacidosis*** (in which blood pH decreases to a dangerous level) as a result of going on a diet with adequate calories but extremely low in carbohydrates (Al Alawi & Falhammar, 2018; Nnodum, Oduah, Albert, & Pettus, 2019). Hospitalization and medical treatment, which included providing needed carbohydrates, resolved the condition within a few days and in most cases nursing continued.

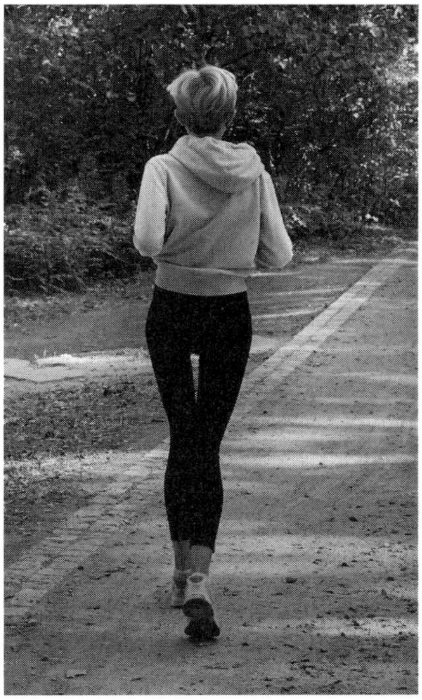

Nearly 100 years ago, dairy science identified this condition—known as "bovine ketosis" or "lactation ketoacidosis"—in milk cows who were unable to consume enough calories to offset the metabolic needs of milk-making (Stinson, 1929).

If parents want to try a low-carb diet, suggest they consider a moderate version that includes some carbohydrates, such as the maintenance phase of the South Beach diet. Suggest they also discuss diet options with a nutrition professional, such as a registered dietitian, so they can choose the diet most compatible with their health history.

Underweight and Eating Disorders

Underweight nursing parents and those with an eating disorder are at risk for vitamin deficiencies, which can affect milk composition.

Nursing parents who are undernourished run the risk of depleting their nutritional stores to provide the nutrients the baby needs. Until their body stores are gone, the milk composition will remain normal. One Italian study of 1,272 women found that being underweight before pregnancy was not associated with lower initiation or duration of breastfeeding (Giovannini, Radaelli, Banderali, & Riva, 2007).

However, even if nursing parents are not vitamin deficient, depleting their body stores may leave them with less energy and a lower resistance to illness. If they become chronically malnourished and vitamin deficient their milk levels of some vitamins, including vitamin A, D, B_6, and B_{12}, may fall below normal. With extreme malnutrition lasting for weeks, milk production may eventually decrease (C. Smith, 1947). For details, see the previous sections "Nutrition Basics" and "Supplements: Vitamins, Minerals, Omega-3s, Probiotics." When nursing parents are malnourished, the most cost- and resource-effective strategy is to supplement them rather than the baby.

• • •

Eating disorders may affect birth outcomes and growth in exclusively nursing babies.

An eating disorder is defined as abnormal eating habits that negatively affect a person's physical or mental health. One example is ***anorexia nervosa***, which involves trouble maintaining a healthy weight for height due to extreme limitation of food intake and/or compulsive exercising. Those who are anorexic often have a distorted body image, thinking they are overweight when they are actually very thin. Those with ***bulimia nervosa***, another example, may eat excessively (binge) and then induce vomiting (purge), with accompanying feelings of guilt or shame.

Unhealthy eating habits before or during pregnancy were found to contribute to problems with birth and baby's growth. U.S. researchers used the data from the large Norwegian Mother and Child Cohort Study, which included more than 50,000 families, to examine the effects of eating disorders and birth outcomes (Watson et al., 2017). In those with active eating disorders during pregnancy, outcomes differed.

- Anorexia nervosa—64% greater risk of babies shorter in length at birth
- Bulimia nervosa and other binging disorders—Increased incidence of pregnancy complications, such as high blood pressure, diabetes, and pre-eclampsia
- All eating disorders—More delivery complications (prolonged labor, cesarean birth, induction of labor)

A healthy weight gain during pregnancy, however, offset these risks.

Regarding lactation, in Norway, 98% of the families in this large study nursed their babies, providing much data on eating disorders and exclusive nursing (E. M. Perrin et al., 2015). Although the mothers with eating disorders successfully breastfed their babies, the growth of these babies differed from other babies. During the first 2 months of life, these babies had slower weight-for-length growth, although still within the normal range. The researchers had several theories about why this might be true. They noted that many of these mothers resumed their unhealthy eating habits after birth, which may have affected their milk production. However, another study (Micali, Simonoff, & Treasure, 2009) found that women with eating disorders were more likely to have early nursing problems, which is another possible reason. Although these babies had slower weight-for-length growth during the first 2 months, after 4 months, they had faster weight-for-length growth than other babies.

A 2015 U.K. study that looked at symptoms and behavior patterns during pregnancy and afterward among women with an active eating disorder or a history of eating disorders (Easter et al., 2015). It confirmed what many other studies found: pregnancy and the early months after birth are a time when many women with active eating disorders experience less depression and anxiety. However, in those with a history of an eating disorder, these symptoms worsened during pregnancy.

• • •

Some parents with eating disorders embrace nursing; others reject it.

Although nursing is nearly universal at birth in Norway (see previous point), that is not the case everywhere. A 2018 meta-ethnographic study (Fogarty, Elmir, Hay, & Schmied, 2018) synthesized the findings of 12 studies that examined the challenges faced during and after pregnancy by women with eating disorders.

Many described their experiences as like a "tug of war" between two competing forces: their baby's needs and the fierce pull of their eating disorder. Despite their struggles, some developed healthier eating habits during pregnancy and even grew to love their new shape. However, once their babies were born, the mothers saw breastfeeding in two opposite ways. Some considered nursing a welcome way to lose more weight more quickly and embraced it. As one mother said (Stapleton, Fielder, & Kirkham, 2008, p. 111):

> "I think it was partly about me behaving selfishly. It was knowing (breastfeeding) brought your figure back more quickly so I kept putting off weaning him because I know the weight was still dropping off me."

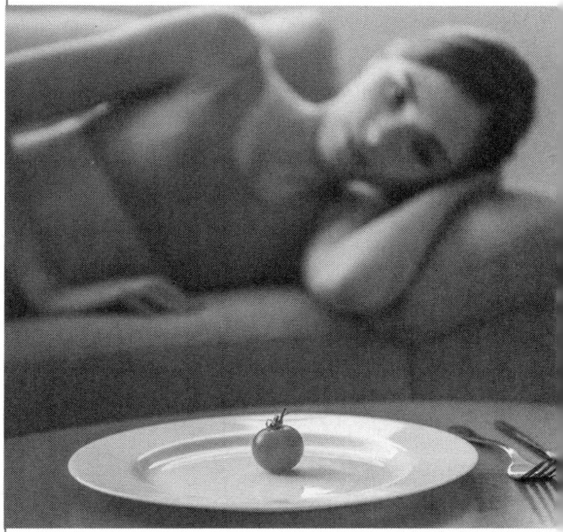

But other mothers considered breastfeeding a barrier to resuming their previous eating-disorder behaviors. As one mother said (L. Little & Lowkes, 2000, p. 303):

> "As soon as I could walk after I had her, I started doing exercises again… I just wanted to get the fat off. I was going to the gym 2 or 3 hours a day in the morning at 3:30 [am] until 5:30 [am] or 2 [am] until 5. Just to get the fat off. I didn't even attempt to breastfeed; I was so focused on losing the weight."

A U.K. interview study recruited 16 women who had eating disorders since adolescence (Stapleton et al., 2008). Most of them (11 of 16) began breastfeeding after birth, and some described feeling "desperate" to nurse because it affirmed that they were good mothers and because they felt they could eat foods they would not otherwise eat for fear of gaining weight. Feeling pride in their body's ability to nourish their infants helped to soften some mothers' negative body image. A minority (5 of 16) rejected breastfeeding because they believed it was incompatible with their restrictive eating, bingeing/purging behaviors, and/or intense exercise regimens. They also felt that their emotional need to get back to these behaviors quickly after birth outweighed the importance of breastfeeding.

Nine of the 16 mothers did not share their eating disorder with their healthcare providers. Those who did worried that knowing about their eating disorder might make their healthcare provider more likely to criticize them or keep a closer eye on them. The researchers noted that pregnancy and the early post-delivery period provides a window of opportunity for those with eating disorders to change their self-image and adopt healthier behaviors.

• • •

A 2019 U.K. prospective observational longitudinal study followed 99 mothers from pregnancy through 1 year after birth, 46 healthy controls, 38 with a current eating disorder, and 25 with a history of an eating disorder (Martini, Taborelli, Schmidt, Treasure, & Micali, 2019). The researchers found that mothers with a current or past eating disorder were more likely to express concern about their children overeating and becoming overweight. They were also less aware than the healthy controls of their child's signs of hunger and fullness.

Parents with a current or past eating disorder may be more likely to nurse on a schedule and be less aware of their baby's hunger and satiety cues.

An older study that compared the infant-feeding patterns of 16 mothers with eating disorders with 20 healthy controls (Evans & le Grange, 1995) found that although the two groups breastfed for a similar length of time (7.6 months in the eating disorder group and 7.0 months in the control group), their approaches to nursing were very different. Ten of the 13 mothers in the eating disorder group who nursed their babies fed them on a rigid feeding schedule, whereas only 2 of the 18 mothers in the healthy control group nursed by the clock. The researchers noted that using a rigid feeding schedule—which was recommended by healthcare providers—led to confusion and anxiety in the mothers with an eating disorder. When the babies showed hunger cues outside the recommended feeding times, some expressed guilt because they interpreted their baby's behavior as signs of an infant eating disorder that arose from their own conflicts with food or as signs of their own inability to meet their child's needs. The mothers in the eating disorder group were 4 times more likely to rate their baby as a fussy eater compared with the controls.

Obesity

Excess body fat releases hormones that may disrupt development of the mammary glands during puberty and pregnancy and alter the body's response to sucking during lactation.

A high body mass index (BMI) may be the result of poor diet and lack of exercise. Or it may be a side effect of medications taken for health problems or metabolic disorders such as low thyroid (hypothyroidism) and polycystic ovary syndrome. According to the World Health Organization (WHO, 2018), in 2016 39% of the world's population 18 years and older were overweight and 13% were obese. Due to the obesity epidemic, the physical effects of excess body fat on metabolic health is a major research focus. Most studies use the World Health Organization's definitions of overweight and obesity (Table 13.1).

Obesity, metabolic health, and milk production. Animal and human studies provide clues to some of the effects of obesity on metabolic health and possibly milk production. One way excess body fat affects metabolism is by releasing estrogen, which may disrupt body functions. Estrogen can also inhibit milk production (Oladapo & Fawole, 2012). Body fat behaves like an immune system organ by releasing the hormones that trigger metabolic syndrome, a constellation of conditions such as insulin resistance, high blood pressure, high blood sugar, fat around the middle and abnormal blood cholesterol and triglycerides. Metabolic syndrome increases risk of heart disease, stroke and diabetes. The poor metabolic health that occurs as a result may also affect lactation (Nommsen-Rivers LA; Thompson, 2017).

Effects on mammary development. Normal mammary growth during puberty requires the formation of fat pads where milk ducts will grow. But excess body fat during puberty (and during pregnancy) can negatively affect mammary development. Obese mice who developed large fat pads during puberty grew abnormal milk ducts and fewer of the muscles around the milk-making cells that cause milk ejection (Kamikawa et al., 2009). Losing weight was found to reverse some of these changes in mice (Chamberlin, D'Amato, & Arendt, 2017).

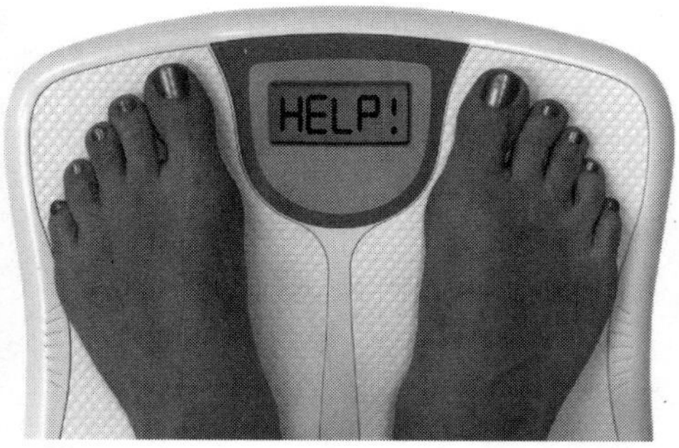

TABLE 13.1 WHO Body Mass Index (BMI) Classifications

Weight	Body Mass Index (BMI)
Obese	> 30
Overweight	25-30
Normal weight	18.5-25
Underweight	< 18.5

Adapted from (WHO, 2018)

Delay in milk increase after birth. Several U.S. studies found an association between prepregnancy obesity and a delay in milk increase after birth (secretory activation or lactogenesis II) (Chapman & Perez-Escamilla, 1999; Dewey, Nommsen-Rivers, Heinig, & Cohen, 2003; Hilson, Rasmussen, & Kjolhede, 2004; Matias, Dewey, Quesenberry, & Gunderson, 2014; Preusting, Brumley, Odibo, Spatz, & Louis, 2017; Turcksin, Bel, Galjaard, & Devlieger, 2014). The most recent (Preusting et al., 2017) was a prospective observational cohort study of 216 women. In the group with a BMI of 30 or less, 46% experienced a delay in milk increase (after 72 hours), while the group with a BMI of more than 30, nearly 58% experienced a delay. A greater weight gain during pregnancy had this same effect.

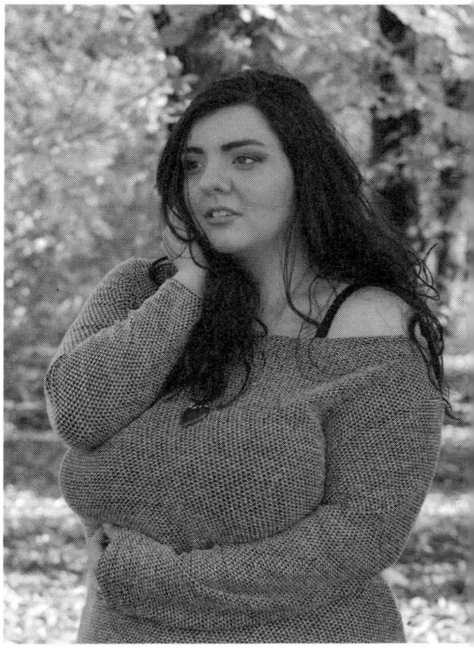

However, this delay in milk increase after birth among parents with high BMIs may not be entirely related to the physical effects of excess body fat on hormonal levels. Other research (Bystrova et al., 2007; Kair & Colaizy, 2016a; Kugyelka, Rasmussen, & Frongillo, 2004) found that overweight and obese women were less likely to nurse their newborns within the first 2 hours after birth, which is also associated with a delay in milk increase.

Decreased prolactin response to baby's sucking. A 2013 Swedish study found that after birth, when prolactin levels in normal-weight and obese mothers were tested (Follin et al., 2013), the levels were comparable. But during the first week, the prolactin surges that occur during nursing were lower in the women with high BMIs, which the researchers thought may make long-term milk production more challenging to maintain. An older U.S. study measured mothers' blood prolactin levels after birth (Rasmussen & Kjolhede, 2004) and found the prolactin response to baby's sucking was lower among overweight and obese mothers on Day 2, but not on Day 7.

Other potential obesity-related hormonal changes. In studies on rats (Buonfiglio et al., 2016), obesity was associated with prolactin resistance, which occurs when prolactin receptors do not respond normally to the appropriate level of prolactin in the blood. Insulin resistance and diabetes in obese parents may also affect milk production (for more details, see p. 843) (Nommsen-Rivers, 2016). Some obese parents also have higher levels of androgens (male hormones) that may affect mammary development and milk production (Carlsen, Jacobsen, & Romundstad, 2006).

KEY CONCEPT

Obese parents are at greater risk of not nursing and early weaning, but this may only be due in part to physical factors.

Obesity-related medical conditions. Overweight and obese parents are also more likely to suffer from medical conditions that may affect early nursing, such as diabetes, which has been linked to later milk increase, and polycystic ovary syndrome (PCOS) (Arthur, Smith, & Hartmann, 1989; Neubauer et al., 1993). For details, see p. 843 and 852 in Chapter 19.

• • •

Concerns about milk production are universal among nursing parents everywhere. This can make it difficult to determine what percentage of families actually experience low milk production versus what is termed "perceived insufficient milk," meaning that the worry is real but the milk production is normal (see p. 420). In one 2016 U.S. study (Kair & Colaizy, 2016b), more than 19,000 mothers were surveyed. Of the 19% who were obese and 23% who were overweight, "insufficient milk" was the most common reason they gave for discontinuing nursing. In this study, 44% of the obese mothers and 42% of

Newborns of obese nursing parents are more likely to receive formula supplements during their hospital stay than newborns of normal-weight parents.

the overweight mothers gave this reason, as compared with 41% of the normal-weight mothers. However, the researchers had no data on the babies' weight gain or any other objective measure of whether these families had a real or "perceived" case of insufficient milk.

Another study, however, examined the need for supplementation more objectively. A 2019 U.S. secondary analysis of data collected after birth in a Baby-Friendly hospital (Colling, Ward, Beck, & Nommsen-Rivers, 2019) compared the number of babies of obese mothers who received medically indicated formula supplements with the babies of normal-weight mothers. Rates of exclusive breastfeeding were 70% among the obese mothers compared with 84% in the non-obese mothers. After adjusting for the medical conditions that sometimes accompany obesity, the researchers concluded that the risk of receiving medically indicated formula supplements in the hospital after birth was much higher among the babies of the obese mothers. The authors (Colling et al., 2019, p. 236) wrote:

> "In a setting with high obesity prevalence and strong support for exclusive breastfeeding, obesity accounted for 36% of medically indicated formula and 21% of the elective formula use."

• • •

The psychological, emotional, and social aspects of obesity affect nursing outcomes, too.

Nursing is a complex behavior with physical, psychological, emotional, and social aspects. Unrelated to any physical effects of obesity on milk production and hormonal responsiveness, obesity before and during pregnancy is associated with a decreased likelihood of ***any*** nursing at all after birth. Obese parents are also less likely to exclusively nurse and more likely to nurse for a shorter time. A 2019 systematic review and meta-analysis that included 30 cohort studies (Huang, Ouyang, & Redding, 2019) concluded that when parents are obese before pregnancy, they are less likely to begin nursing after birth and more likely to stop early. The authors of a 2018 systematic review and meta-analysis that included 28 studies (Flores, Mielke, Wendt, Nunes, & Bertoldi, 2018) also concluded that obesity before pregnancy and excess weight gain during pregnancy were associated with less exclusive nursing.

In addition to the physical factors described in the previous point, other factors can have a profound effect on nursing in obese parents. As the U.S. authors of the book *Making More Milk* (Marasco & West, 2020, p. 154) wrote:

> "Beyond the physical factors are the more intangible but equally important psychosocial issues of low self-esteem, shaming, and discrimination. Parents with a high BMI are not always comfortable with exposing their bodies and may not want to nurse in front of others, even at home. They are more likely to be harassed and therefore less likely to breastfeed in public, reducing nursing and milk removal opportunities that can contribute to less milk over time."

One barrier: nursing around others. Nursing parents with high BMIs report that their reluctance to nurse in front of others was one major barrier to meeting their feeding goals. This was true whether they were "in public" or in their own homes (Massov, 2015). A 2018 U.S. qualitative study that compared the perceptions of normal-weight and obese mothers (McKenzie, Rasmussen, & Garner, 2018) concluded that a major barrier to nursing among obese mothers was the problem of nursing "around others" rather than just nursing in public. They felt nursing was both socially and physically awkward for them and that because of their larger body size, it was much more difficult to minimize their body exposure and nurse discreetly.

In the article summarizing her interviews with obese nursing mothers, Kay Hoover shared strategies they developed to deal with this issue. For more coverage, some wore a tank top with holes cut in the nipple area under their shirt. One said, "It took a long time to feel comfortable enough with myself to be able to breastfeed in public. I finally decided that breastfeeding was best for my baby, so 'tough' if they have a problem seeing my fat rolls" (Hoover, 2008, p. 6).

Cultural beliefs play a role, too. For example, in areas where virtually all families nurse, obese parents begin nursing at the same rate as normal-weight parents. However, even in areas where nursing at birth is virtually universal, overweight and obese parents stop nursing earlier. One Australian study of 1,803 women found that overweight and obese women were more likely to wean their babies by 6 months than normal-weight women (Oddy et al., 2006). In Denmark, where 98% of families nurse, one study of 37,459 Danish women (J. L. Baker, Michaelsen, Sorensen, & Rasmussen, 2007) found that the greater the prepregnant BMI, the earlier breastfeeding stopped. A 2018 U.S. study using a sample of obese Hispanic mothers from a randomized controlled trial (Shin et al., 2018) found that the greater their acculturation to U.S. customs and values, the less nursing they did at 1 month after delivery.

KEY CONCEPT

In cultures that shame the obese or discriminate against them, parents with a high BMI have poorer nursing outcomes.

How a culture views weight and obesity can affect nursing behaviors. In most Western cultures, for example, obesity is considered a negative, which is why body exposure during nursing is so difficult for these families. In one French study (Mok et al., 2008), the main reason given by obese women for deciding not to nurse was "decency." In cultures that view obesity negatively, when compared to normal-weight parents, obese parents are more likely to have body-image dissatisfaction and to suffer from postpartum depression. A 2014 systematic review and meta-analysis that included 62 studies and more than 540,000 women (Molyneaux, Poston, Ashurst-Williams, & Howard, 2014) concluded that overweight and obese women were more likely than normal-weight women to experience depression and anxiety, as well as eating disorders. Negative body image as an independent factor is also associated with lower nursing rates (Bigman, Wilkinson, Homedes, & Perez, 2018).

Yet in some cultures, there is no link between weight and nursing rates. One example is the Cree women in northern Quebec, Canada, where overweight and obesity are common (Vallianatos et al., 2006). If a culture does not consider obesity a negative, its nursing parents may be less likely to feel embarrassed or self-conscious about exposing their bodies around others.

• • •

Are obese nursing families more likely than normal-weight families to have latching problems after birth? A 2019 Israeli prospective observational study of 109 mothers of term babies (Mangel, Mimouni, Mandel, Mordechaev, & Marom, 2019) divided them into four groups by prepregnancy BMI. The researchers found that the higher the BMI, the larger the breasts. Nipple diameter, nipple length and areola diameter correlated significantly with breast size, too. Surprisingly, the percentage of mothers who had latching difficulties during the newborn period was about the same in all four groups: 15.5%. Even so, the higher the BMI, the lower the likelihood of breastfeeding at 6 months among the study families.

After birth, even with larger mammary glands and larger nipples, obesity does not necessarily lead to more latching struggles than in normal-weight families.

A 2018 Australian secondary analysis followed 477 overweight and obese mothers for the first 4 months after delivery and found that the number and type of nursing problems was the same across the weight ranges. The researchers (Mallan, Daniels, Byrne, & de Jersey, 2018, p. 1) wrote: "Overall, it does not appear that overweight women are more likely to experience a range of specific breastfeeding problems in the first months compared to non-overweight women."

• • •

After birth, many overweight and obese parents receive a lower quality of lactation care than other parents.

Cultural discrimination may play a role in the lower quality of care obese and overweight parents receive after birth. According to a U.S. 2016 study that used data from the CDC Pregnancy Risk Assessment Monitoring System (PRAMS) from three states (Kair, et al, 2016a) found that during the hospital stay, mothers who had high prepregnancy BMIs were less likely than normal-weight mothers to:

- Breastfeed during the first hour after birth
- Be exposed to pro-breastfeeding hospital practices
- Receive information about breastfeeding from a staff member
- Be given a telephone number for breastfeeding help after discharge
- Be told the importance of nursing on cue

A 2014 qualitative study that conducted in-depth interviews with 34 healthcare providers (Garner, Ratcliff, Devine, Thornburg, & Rasmussen, 2014) found that these clinicians considered helping obese parents with nursing more physically challenging and time-consuming than helping normal-weight families. They also believed that obese parents were more likely to have nursing problems. One factor that may affect the perception that helping obese families nurse is more difficult is the 2016 study (Chapman, Doughty, Mullin, & Perez-Escamilla, 2016) that found the usual lactation assessment tools (such as the LATCH tool) are not as reliable with overweight and obese families as they are with normal-weight families.

What can be done to provide a better quality of care for these families? In a 2018 Swedish qualitative semi-structured interview study of 11 obese mothers, one mother described the huge improvement that occurred in her care between her first and second child (Claesson, Larsson, Steen, & Alehagen, 2018, p. 7):

> "When I was there with my first child, they often talked about my obesity and it was written 27 times that I was very overweight. This time they looked into my eyes and saw me as I was. Nobody focused on what I looked like. It is important that you receive the same information regardless of your weight."

• • •

Using some strategies during pregnancy and after birth may make it easier for overweight and obese parents to meet their nursing goals.

Like all families, overweight and obese families benefit from receiving practical help and support for nursing.

During pregnancy, suggest the following strategies to promote a healthy weight, a better birth, and a clear understanding of nursing dynamics and milk production.

- Nutritional counseling to keep pregnancy weight gain in the recommended range by putting the focus on consuming nutrient-rich foods and avoiding non-nutritious choices, such as soda and candy (Jevitt, Hernandez, & Groer, 2007).

- Learn the basics of how milk production works (Kaymaz & Yildirim, 2016).
- During the last month of pregnancy, learn and practice hand expression, which is demonstrated on the website **firstdroplets.com.**
- Arrange for a labor support person and learn non-drug pain management techniques to help reduce the odds of a cesarean delivery.

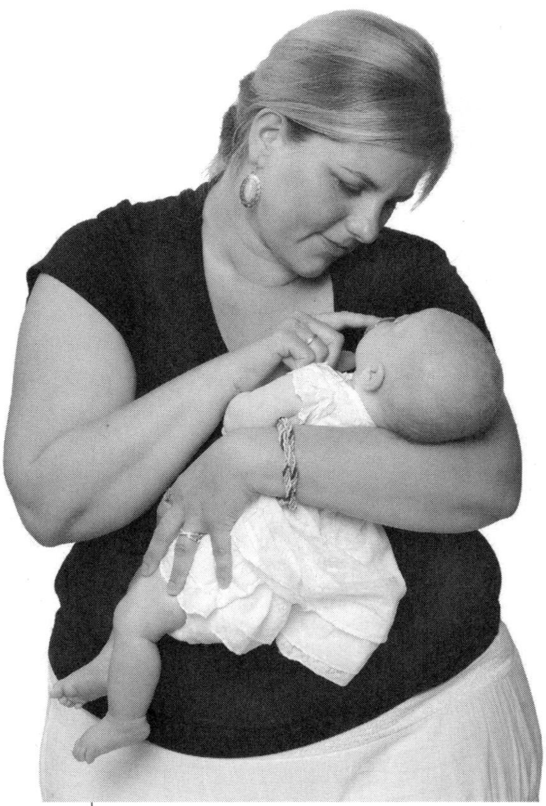

After birth, emphasize nursing early, often, and effectively to promote healthy milk production

- Plan to keep the newborn in skin-to-skin contact during the first 1 to 2 hours and nurse as soon as possible, ideally within the first 2 hours after birth.
- Limit separation and encourage the nursing couple to share lots of skin-to-skin and body contact and frequent feeds, ideally at least 8 to 12 feeds per 24 hours.
- During the first few days, several times each day after nursing, express extra colostrum into a spoon to feed the baby some "dessert" to stimulate milk production and prevent excess weight loss (see **firstdroplets.com** (Morton, 2019).

Finding a comfortable feeding position was one of the practical challenges U.S. lactation consultant Kay Hoover, M.Ed., IBCLC reported after interviewing several obese breastfeeding mothers (Hoover, 2008). Getting comfortable is vital for frequent nursing. If nursing is uncomfortable, parents may be a tempted to postpone it, which may affect early milk production. Some of the mothers with high BMIs Hoover interviewed expressed their fear of suffocating their baby with their large, heavy breasts. Hoover suggested using positions that do not rest a heavy gland on the baby's chest. See p. 23-29 in Chapter 1 for starter positions that provide alternatives to the sometimes-challenging upright positions.

Inflammation of the mammary folds. Another challenge some of the mothers Hoover interviewed also experienced was inflammation of the breast skin folds, sometimes caused by clothing friction, which involved itching, burning, and pain. Called "intertrigo," this can be prevented or treated with daily cleaning and drying of the skin folds.

Keep nursing. Once parents with high BMIs get through the first month of nursing, it usually becomes more manageable. A 2015 study used the data from the U.S. Infant Feeding Practices Study II and compared nursing outcomes among 115 normal-weight mothers and 580 obese mothers (O'Sullivan, Perrine, & Rasmussen, 2015). Its authors concluded that by 2 months after delivery obesity had no effect on nursing rates. But during the first month, many obese families did not nurse exclusively due to concerns about insufficient milk. The researchers concluded that extra lactation support would benefit obese parents.

Targeted efforts may be needed to provide this extra support, since obese nursing parents are perceived by healthcare providers as having more lactation difficulties and being more time consuming and physically challenging to help (Garner et al., 2014). Also, they are less likely to receive lactation information and help in the hospital (Kair & Colaizy, 2016a), and less likely to ask for help with nursing from others when it's needed (Mok et al., 2008).

• • •

A nursing parent with a high BMI may have an unrealistic view of the baby's weight, which may affect nursing outcomes.

When parents have ongoing weight issues of their own, this commonly leads to concerns (founded or unfounded) about their child's weight. A 2019 U.S. prospective quantitative, self-report online survey received responses from 206 women with high BMIs who gave birth within the previous 6 months (E. Zimmerman, Rodgers, O'Flynn, & Bourdeau, 2019). The researchers found that the higher the mothers' BMI, the greater the negative association with exclusive nursing at 6 months. They attributed the nursing issues to body dissatisfaction, the mothers' own disordered eating habits, concerns about their child's weight, as well as low breastfeeding self-efficacy.

An unhealthy relationship with food sometimes leads to poor nursing choices. A Japanese study of 1,496 women found that many mothers had unrealistic views of their baby's weight (Yakura, 1997). Many (23% to 58%) rated their normal-weight babies as obese, especially among those who dieted during adolescence. These mothers used both appropriate (frequent exercise) and inappropriate strategies to try to prevent future obesity in their children. Inappropriate strategies included reducing the frequency of nursing, diluting formula, and not allowing snacking between meals.

It may be helpful for the family to know that exclusive nursing appears to be protective of obesity for the children of obese parents (Patel et al., 2018).

Weight-Loss Surgery

Many parents with a history of weight-loss surgery need to take vitamin and mineral supplements to avoid deficiencies.

Weight-loss surgery (sometimes called metabolic and bariatric surgery, or MBS) is usually considered by those with a body mass index (BMI) of greater than 40 and for some can be life-saving. Its purpose is to improve metabolic health, which may happen even before the expected dramatic weight loss (Vidal, Corcelles, Jimenez, Flores, & Lacy, 2017).

Types of procedures. These procedures limit the amount of food the digestive system can hold by either reducing the stomach volume with bands (gastric band surgery), surgically removing most of the stomach (sleeve gastrectomy), or reducing stomach size and bypassing part of the small intestine (gastric bypass surgery). After the surgery, weight loss averages 25% to 35% of original body weight by 18 months.

Their effects on nutrient absorption. These surgeries affect the body's ability to absorb nutrients from food, with some procedures having a greater effect than others. For example, after the Roux-en-Y type of gastric bypass surgery (where food completely bypasses part of the small intestine) about 25% of patients develop protein deficiencies. But after adjustable gastric band surgery, only 2% develop this deficiency (Handzlik-Orlik, Holecki, Orlik, Wylezol, & Dulawa, 2015). (Table 13.2 shows the risk of specific nutrient deficiencies after gastric bypass surgery.) This is why it is so important for nursing parents with a history of weight-loss surgery to take any recommended nutritional supplements. For information on the current recommendations, go to **bit.ly/BA2-NutritionBariatric** (Parrott et al., 2017). These guidelines also recommend regular blood tests post-surgery to monitor for nutritional deficiencies.

KEY CONCEPT

Vitamin deficiencies are common after some types of weight-loss surgery.

TABLE 13.2 Risk of Nutrient Deficiencies after Gastric Bypass Surgery

Deficiency	Gastric Bypass Surgery Risk Factor
Protein	≤ 25%
Iron	≤ 50% (at 4 years)
Vitamin A	10% (at 4 years)
Vitamin B_1	18%
Vitamin B_6	17%
Vitamin B_9 (folate)	22% (at 2 years)
Vitamin B_{12}	33% - 37% (at 3 years)

Adapted from (Handzlik-Orlik et al., 2015)

A vitamin B_{12} deficiency in a nursing parent puts the exclusively nursing baby at risk for neurological and other health issues (see p. 569). Several cases of vitamin B_{12} deficiencies were reported among nursing babies whose mothers had a history of weight-loss surgery (Celiker & Chawla, 2009; Grange & Finlay, 1994; Wardinsky et al., 1995). Due to this and other possible nutritional deficiencies, suggest nursing parents ask their healthcare provider to monitor their nutritional status regularly during pregnancy and lactation. It may also be wise to monitor the nutritional status of their nursing baby (McGuire, 2018).

• • •

Milk composition appears to be the same among those with a history of weight-loss surgery as those without this history.

Is milk composition different in lactating parents with a history of weight-loss surgery? Two studies compared milk composition in samples of colostrum (Jans, Matthys, Lannoo, Van der Schueren, & Devlieger, 2015) and mature milk (Jans et al., 2018) in lactating women with and without a history of weight-loss surgery and found no significant differences.

• • •

Encourage nursing families to learn the basics of milk production, take regular supplements as directed, and monitor their own health and their baby's weight and health.

At this writing, little research is available about nursing after weight-loss surgery. Although the currently published studies do not show much exclusive nursing among these families, they do not include enough information to gauge whether the rarity of exclusive nursing is due to the effects of weight-loss surgery on milk production or other common issues that undermine nursing.

One small retrospective chart review of 24 women with a history of weight-loss surgery who said they wanted to breastfeed (Caplinger et al., 2015) found that one baby of the 24 exclusively breastfed. Formula supplements were started on average on Day 5. At 2 weeks, the average infant weight gain was low. Reasons for the supplementation were not provided, so it's not obvious if the supplements were medically indicated. Another study (Gascoin et al., 2017) found that rates of breastfeeding were low among women with a history of gastric bypass surgery compared with controls (22% versus 51%), which the researchers attributed to the fact that obese women breastfeed at a lower rate than normal-weight women. However, in a 2018 Brazilian study (Gimenes et al., 2018), 3 of the 13 children exclusively breastfed for their first 6 months and the rest (10 of the 13) partially breastfed. The researchers found the children who exclusively breastfed had healthier weight and blood-sugar levels than those who received formula.

For parents with a history of weight-loss surgery, some basic recommendations (McGuire, 2018) include:

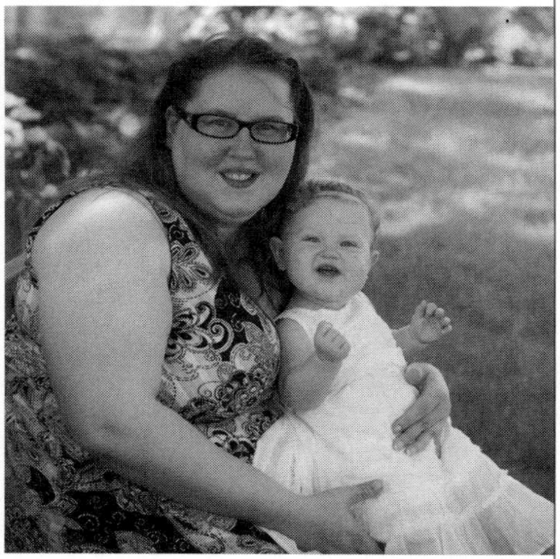

- Share their history with the baby's healthcare provider.
- Follow the guidelines for nutritional supplementation
- Arrange for the nursing parent to have regular blood tests to rule out nutritional deficiencies.
- If exclusively nursing, monitor baby's weight gain at regular checkups and be aware of the signs to check the baby for nutrient deficiencies.

A 2019 U.K. consensus statement (Shawe et al., 2019) recommended breastfeeding for parents with a history of weight-loss surgery along with regular monitoring of the nursing parent for nutritional deficiencies. A consensus statement by the Austrian Society of Gynaecology and Obstetrics (Stopp, Falcone, Feichtinger, & Gobl, 2018) concluded that there are no contraindications for breastfeeding after weight-loss surgery.

EXERCISE

Moderate exercise benefits the nursing parent in many ways.

Moderate exercise improves cardiovascular fitness, blood lipid profiles, and insulin response (Lovelady, Fuller, Geigerman, Hunter, & Kinsella, 2004; Lovelady, Hunter, & Geigerman, 2003; Lovelady, Nommsen-Rivers, McCrory, & Dewey, 1995). A regular resistance exercise program beginning after 4 weeks post-delivery was also found to slow the temporary loss of bone density that occurs during lactation (Colleran, Hiatt, Wideman, & Lovelady, 2019).

KEY CONCEPT

Exercise has a positive effect on physical and emotional well-being.

Exercise also has emotional benefits. One U.S. prospective, randomized, controlled trial of 202 adults (Blumenthal et al., 2007) found that exercise can alleviate depression as effectively as anti-depressant medications. An Australian qualitative study of six breastfeeding mothers enrolled in a formal exercise program (Rich, Currie, & McMahon, 2004) reported some of the benefits the mothers enjoyed:

- A greater feeling of well-being
- Improved body image and easier weight control
- Enhanced relationships with others, including their baby

Some considered exercise a great stress-reliever that made them less frazzled when their baby was unsettled. Some expressed concern when they began exercising that the exercise might cause decreased milk production, but over time this did not turn out to be an issue. A U.S. study of 156 adults (Babyak et al., 2000) found that exercise provided significant therapeutic benefit to those with major depression.

• • •

Moderate exercise is compatible with lactation.

U.S. studies (Dewey, Lovelady, Nommsen-Rivers, McCrory, & Lonnerdal, 1994; Lovelady, Lonnerdal, & Dewey, 1990) found no effect of exercise on milk production. Even when nursing parents both exercise and eat less to lose weight, milk production appears unaffected (Lovelady, 2004). Also, no significant differences in milk composition were found after moderate exercise (Carey, Quinn, & Goodwin, 1997; Larson-Meyer, 2002; McCrory, 2000).

A 2012 meta-analysis of randomized controlled trials examined the effects of exercise on the babies' weight gain and growth and concluded that (Daley et al., 2012, p. 108) "mothers can exercise and breastfeed without detriment to the growth of their infants." The authors of an Australian study of 587 mothers interviewed them seven times from birth to 12 months post-birth (Su, Zhao, Binns, Scott, & Oddy, 2007) and found that exercise did not affect nursing outcomes at usual exercise levels.

A 2019 Iranian study of 28 lactating women (Tartibian, 2019) found that the milk of the mothers engaged in regular and moderate aerobic exercise had slightly higher concentrations of IgA compared with the milk of the control mothers. The researchers concluded that exercise was not a contraindication to lactation.

• • •

Exercising to exhaustion increases levels of lactic acid in the milk, but there is no need to postpone nursing.

In one U.S. study (Wallace, Inbar, & Ernsthausen, 1992), researchers analyzed mothers' milk before and after extreme exercise and compared their babies' acceptance of the before-exercise milk with the milk expressed after exercise. After exercise, the mothers' milk was higher in lactic acid, and the babies—who were fed the milk by medicine dropper—were judged by the authors to be less accepting of the after-exercise milk. Oddly, the researchers did not consider the impact of the medicine-dropper feeding method (which was new to the babies) on the babies' reactions. This study was widely publicized, along with its recommendations that parents nurse their babies before exercising or provide expressed milk for feeding afterwards and avoid nursing for as long as 90 minutes after exercise. In a later study that attempted to replicate this using familiar bottles to feed the babies the post-exercise, high-lactic-acid milk (Wright, Quinn, & Carey, 2002), researchers found that even after maximal exercise, there was no difference in the babies' acceptance of the pre-and post-exercise milk. In a review of the literature, U.S researchers concluded that (Dewey & McCrory, 1994, p. 450S) "altered acceptance of breastmilk due to higher lactic acid concentrations post-exercise is not likely to be a problem in most cases."

• • •

When nursing parents are ready to start exercising after birth, suggest they first talk to their healthcare provider and then start gradually.

In a review of the literature (Larson-Meyer, 2002), one author suggested that during the first 6 weeks after birth, before nursing parents start exercising, to first discuss it with their healthcare provider and then start slowly and gradually, being alert to their comfort. If the exercise feels good, it's probably all right. But if the parent feels very tired, dehydrated, or if anything hurts, it's better to stop. If bright red vaginal bleeding occurs after exercise that is greater in volume than during a menstrual cycle, suggest seeing a healthcare provider.

• • •

It may be easier for a new parent to exercise more often if the baby is included.

Lack of time can make exercising difficult to fit into daily routines. One U.S. study used focus groups to understand what would motivate low-income mothers to eat well, exercise, and achieve a healthy weight after birth (MacMillan Uribe & Olson, 2019). They found that appealing to the mothers' health was not as motivating as focusing on the baby and the mother-baby interaction. For this reason, it may be more effective to suggest ways parents can combine exercise with other activities they do with the baby. For example, walking with the baby in a stroller, pram, sling, or a baby carrier provides both exercise and a change of scene. If the weather is bad, suggest walking inside an enclosed shopping mall or gym. There are also special strollers designed for running or jogging with a baby. Exercise videos can be watched and followed at home. Some exercise books for new mothers feature routines that include the baby. In one Australian study, its mothers reported that exercise became more fun when their baby was included (Rich et al., 2004).

• • •

Little specific information is available to guide elite athletes during lactation.

Few studies are available on managing lactation and professional athletic careers. A 2016 Canadian semi-structured interview study (Giles, Phillipps, Darroch, & McGettigan-Dumas, 2016) described the lactation experiences of 14 elite distance runners who breastfed while training and competing in professional athletic events. Despite the challenges they experienced, they nursed their babies longer than the general population at that time. They described several challenges they encountered.

- **Conflicting demands.** Pumping milk was often their solution to the conflicting demands of meeting the baby's need for milk while carving out the time needed to train and compete.
- **Limited access to relevant lactation information.** As one study mother said (Giles et al., 2016, p. 630): "The whole lactic acid thing was a concern. I actually just went online to see if there was anything [about it] and there was nothing." After trying to get the information needed from the internet, peers, and health professionals, some turned to other elite athletes to find out how they managed and followed their example.
- **Concerns about the baby's health.** This challenge mainly revolved around how best to balance nursing duration with their need to train for events. These mothers described their very careful consideration of when to wean, factoring in their child's needs as well as their own.

A 2018 British evidence summary from an expert group meeting offered some specific suggestions for lactating athletes (Bo et al., 2018, p. 4):

> "Elite athletes who exercise intensively may lose too much weight and should compensate with higher energy intake. Athletes may find exercise more comfortable after breastfeeding. Breastfeeding athletes may also find a fitted bra with features of greater breast elevation more comfortable than a standard encapsulation sport bra."

GROOMING: HAIR CARE, TANNING, AND PIERCINGS

No evidence exists that nursing parents' use of hair-care products will affect their nursing baby.

Some chemicals in hair-care products, such as hair dyes and permanents, may be absorbed through the user's skin, but even so, there is no report of a nursing baby being affected. If a parent's scalp is healthy and intact, less will be absorbed than if the skin on the scalp is scratched or abraded.

• • •

Ultraviolet light is used in tanning beds to create a tan. Parents are also exposed to ultraviolet light when outdoors and exposed to the sun.

No evidence exists that parents' use of a tanning bed will affect their nursing baby.

• • •

Over the years, nipple piercing has become more common (Sadove & Clayman, 2008). One U.K. study of more than 10,000 people aged 16 and older (Bone, Ncube, Nichols, & Noah, 2008) found that 10% (1,934) had body piercings other than the earlobe. Of these, 9% (143) had nipple piercings, with twice as many men as women and most were between 16 and 24 years old.

Some parents with pierced nipples have successfully nursed, but some have experienced feeding problems related to their piercing.

Several reported examples exist of mothers successfully breastfeeding with pierced nipples, obviously removing any jewelry when nursing (Wilson-Clay & Hoover, 2017, p. 75). One report describes a mother who removed the ring from one of her nipples after birth and breastfed from one breast only (N. Lee, 1995). For a review of possible breastfeeding problems associated with nipple piercing and questions to ask a parent with pierced nipples, see p. 742.

SUBSTANCE USE DURING LACTATION

Alcohol

Specific recommendations on alcohol consumption and nursing vary worldwide. Since the last edition of this book, research has called into question the previous recommendation that drinking alcohol in moderation is compatible with nursing (see later point).

How much alcohol consumption is compatible with nursing is controversial and varies by country and organization.

The authors of the 2012 policy statement on breastfeeding by the American Academy of Pediatrics (AAP) Committee on Breastfeeding (AAP, 2012, p. e833) wrote:

> "Alcohol…may blunt prolactin response to suckling and negatively affects infant motor development. Thus, ingestion of alcoholic beverages should be minimized and limited to an occasional intake but no more than 0.5 g alcohol per kg body weight, which for a 60 kg [132 lb.] mother is approximately 2 oz. liquor, 8 oz. wine, or 2 beers. Nursing should take place 2 hours or longer after the alcohol intake to minimize its concentration in the ingested milk."

> **KEY CONCEPT**
> *A small amount of alcohol is acceptable for the nursing parent.*

In the AAP's 2013 article about the transfer of drugs and therapeutics into human milk (Sachs & Committee On, 2013, p. e800), its authors gave as reasons for concern about alcohol consumption during lactation "impaired motor development or postnatal growth, decreased milk consumption, sleep disturbances."

In *Hale's Medications and Mothers' Milk*, its author wrote (Hale, 2019, p. 276): "… mothers who ingest alcohol in moderate amounts can generally return to breastfeeding as soon as they feel neurologically normal. A good rule is 2 hours for each drink. Chronic or heavy consumers of alcohol should not breastfeed."

Some take an even stricter stance on alcohol consumption during lactation. After reviewing the literature, a 2002 Canadian article (Koren, 2002) concluded that there is no known safe amount of alcohol in human milk and recommended that lactation supporters help families determine the amount of time to refrain from nursing after any amount of drinking to be sure no alcohol is present in the milk. An Australian systematic review of the literature (Giglia, Binns, & Alfonso, 2006) concluded with the following recommendations for nursing parents: No alcohol in the first month. After the first month, limit alcohol intake to one to two standard drinks per day and drink them just after breastfeeding to limit the amount of alcohol the baby receives. If a mother wants to drink more than this, express milk before drinking and consider skipping one nursing session.

• • •

The percentage of nursing parents who consume alcohol varies widely around the world.

Yet drinking alcohol while nursing is common in many countries. The following studies found that the percentage of nursing parents who consume alcohol varied by country.

- U.S.: 36% (Breslow, Falk, Fein, & Grummer-Strawn, 2007)
- Canada: 20% (Popova, Lange, & Rehm, 2013)
- Australia: 32% to 71% (Arora et al., 2017; Wilson et al., 2017); those consuming >2 drinks/day were nearly twice as likely to stop nursing by 6 mo. as those who drank less (Giglia & Binns, 2008).
- Brazil: 12% (Nascimento et al., 2013)
- Germany: 20.5% (Logan et al., 2016)
- Nepal: 43% (Aryal et al., 2016)

• • •

Some parents may nurse longer if they receive stricter guidelines about alcohol consumption during nursing as compared with feeling unsure about a more liberal phrasing.

Some worry that telling new parents not to drink alcohol or to severely restrict its use during lactation may convince many not to nurse at all or to cut nursing short. What is the best approach? Well-known lactation advocate and researcher Ted Greiner conducted a survey of female university students in South Korea as a first step in determining how three possible messages affected their feelings about nursing (Greiner, 2019b). The three messages were:

1. Breastfeeding is compatible with moderate but not heavy drinking of alcohol.
2. You can use alcohol while breastfeeding, but only on rare occasions and only 1 to 2 drinks at a time. Too much alcohol can harm the breastfeeding process. After each drink, you should wait 2 hours before breastfeeding to keep the child from being affected.
3. You should never use alcohol while you are breastfeeding.

Most of the young women surveyed were not yet mothers and 90% currently consumed alcohol, 79% said they would avoid alcohol while nursing, and 12% said they would reduce it. The last two statements, which were more strictly worded were associated with more young women planning to breastfeed and for a longer time. Regarding the first statement, the authors (Greiner, 2019b, p. 33) wrote:

> "The more moderately worded message was more complex and required a specific set of activities….[It] left it up to the mother to define

what moderate vs. heavy drinking would be. This may have made any that did want to drink while breastfeeding feel so insecure that they decided it would be safer to reduce how much they breastfed or not to breast feed at all."

• • •

In a nursing parent, milk alcohol levels are roughly equal to blood alcohol levels, because alcohol passes very easily both into and out of the milk (Chien, Liu, Huang, Hsu, & Chao, 2005; Mennella & Beauchamp, 1991c). This means that there's no benefit to "pumping and dumping," as it will not hasten the removal of the alcohol from the milk (Koren, 2002). The alcohol just naturally passes back into the bloodstream as blood alcohol levels drop. Another factor that influences blood alcohol concentration is the nursing parent's weight, as after one drink, lighter adults have higher blood alcohol concentrations than heavier adults (Greiner, 2019a). The amount of alcohol that reaches the nursing baby also depends upon whether or not milk is expressed before drinking (see next point).

The alcohol in one drink clears the body quickly—no need to pump and dump—so a nursing parent can reduce baby's exposure by waiting 2 to 3 hours to nurse.

Alcohol with or without food. After one alcoholic drink without food, nursing parents' blood alcohol levels peak at about 20 to 40 minutes after the drink (Chien et al., 2005; Mennella & Beauchamp, 1991c). If they have a drink with a meal, their peak blood alcohol levels occur about 60 to 90 minutes later (Lawton, 1985). It takes a 120-pound woman 2 to 3 hours to completely eliminate from her body the alcohol in one regular serving of beer or wine (P. O. Anderson, 2018a).

Calculating the clearance time of more than one drink. However, the more alcohol adults drink, the longer it takes for it to clear their body. Canadian researchers (Ho, Collantes, Kapur, Moretti, & Koren, 2001) created a chart using average alcohol elimination time and factoring in the nursing parent's weight, time since drinking began, and number of drinks. Using this information, this chart calculates the time needed for alcohol to clear a nursing parent's body. View this chart at **bit.ly/BA2-AlcoholCalculator**.

The Health Council of the Netherlands provides nursing parents with a simpler calculation. If they have a standard drink (10g of alcohol), they avoid nursing for 3 hours; if more than one drink, multiply the 3-hour period by the number of drinks (HealthCounciloftheNetherlands, 2005).

Baby's alcohol exposure. It is estimated that babies receive about 5% to 6% of the lactating parent's dose of alcohol through the milk (Haastrup, Pottegard, & Damkier, 2014). Because a newborn's liver is immature, it is likely that the younger baby eliminates alcohol from his system more slowly than an older baby, so more caution is warranted during the newborn period (Marek & Kraft, 2014).

• • •

One U.S. study (Pepino & Mennella, 2008) found that along with eating a meal before drinking, nursing or expressing milk before drinking alcohol reduced alcohol availability in the nursing parent's body. These effects added to one another, so if nursing parents both ate a meal (reducing alcohol availability by 38%) and expressed milk within the hour before drinking, this reduced the total availability of alcohol in their system by 58%.

Both eating a meal and expressing milk before drinking decrease alcohol availability in a nursing parent's system.

The researchers suggested that the change in metabolism triggered by nursing or milk expression may exist to speed nutrient processing to more efficiently meet the increased energy demands of lactation.

• • •

Alcohol disrupts a nursing parent's hormonal balance and decreases the volume of milk the baby takes at a nursing session.

Some cultural folklore considers beer to have special properties to relax a nursing parent and enhance milk flow and production. When studies found that beer increased mothers' prolactin levels (Carlson, Wasser, & Reidelberger, 1985; De Rosa, Corsello, Ruffilli, Della Casa, & Pasargiklian, 1981; Koletzko & Lehner, 2000), this was thought to validate this belief. However, a body of research led by U.S. scientist Julie Mennella found that far from enhancing milk flow, when mothers drank alcohol, their babies breastfed more often, but consumed 20% to 27% less milk (Mennella, 1998, 2001; Mennella & Beauchamp, 1993). Although babies took less milk for the first 4 hours after their mothers drank alcohol, they compensated by feeding more often and by taking more milk 8 to 16 hours after this exposure (Mennella, 2001).

In one of these studies (Mennella & Beauchamp, 1991b), a noticeable change in the odor of the mothers' milk paralleled the changes in alcohol concentration in the milk. In an effort to determine if the change in the milk's flavor caused this decrease in milk intake, babies were fed bottles of expressed milk, one set of bottles with alcohol flavor added and another set without (Mennella, 1997). The babies took significantly more of the alcohol-flavored milk than the plain milk, so the researchers concluded that the babies did not take less from the breast because they rejected the milk's alcohol flavor.

One mechanism that may contribute to the babies' reduced milk intake during nursing was later found to be hormonal. U.S. researchers (Cobo, 1973; Mennella, Pepino, & Teff, 2005) found that while mothers' blood prolactin levels increased after drinking alcohol—mirroring the findings of earlier research—their oxytocin levels significantly decreased, which could inhibit milk ejection. The researchers concluded that while alcohol may relax nursing parents, it disrupts the hormonal balance needed for let-down, reducing the availability of milk to the baby.

Later research by this same U.S. team (Mennella & Pepino, 2008) found that a nursing parent's prolactin response to alcohol varied depending on whether their blood alcohol levels were increasing or decreasing. If parents pumped while blood alcohol increased, their prolactin levels increased, but if they pumped while their blood alcohol levels decreased, their prolactin response was delayed. A nursing parent's body responses to sucking are complex and alcohol's effects on these dynamics are not yet fully understood.

• • •

Exposure to alcohol in mother's milk leads to babies sleeping less.

According to some folklore, babies sleep better after their nursing parent drinks alcohol, but one U.S. study (Mennella & Gerrish, 1998) found that alcohol produced the opposite effect. Although the babies who were fed their mother's expressed milk with alcohol added fell asleep sooner, they slept for a significantly shorter time during the 3.5 hours after receiving the spiked expressed milk than they did when they were fed plain mother's milk. When non-alcoholic vanilla-flavored milk was tried instead of the alcohol-flavored milk, no differences in sleep patterns were found. The researchers (Mennella & Garcia-Gomez, 2001) concluded that the alcohol changed the babies' sleep-wake patterns, resulting in less sleep overall. When the time of the study was extended to 24 hours, the researchers found that the babies initially spent less time in active sleep, which they compensated for by spending more time in active sleep in the 20.5 hours after the initial alcohol exposure.

• • •

Drinking large amounts of alcohol or drinking regularly over time, may harm the nursing baby.

What studies called into question previous recommendations about alcohol and lactation? A population-based study used data from research on fetal alcohol syndrome (FASD) in South Africa to examine the association between FASD and drinking during pregnancy and nursing (May et al., 2016). After controlling for exposure during pregnancy, it found evidence that in this population—also affected by malnutrition and poverty—alcohol use during nursing (as compared with only drinking during pregnancy) was associated with a greater incidence of the physical features of FASD. Children exposed to alcohol in mother's milk were six times more likely to have a FASD diagnosis at age 7 years as compared with children not exposed during nursing. These mothers nursed on average 21 months and reported regular weekend binge drinking involving more than four drinks per occasion. The children of the mothers who avoided alcohol during pregnancy and drank only during breastfeeding were smaller and had lower verbal IQ scores than the children whose mothers did not drink.

A 2018 Australian study used the data from several large population studies (Gibson & Porter, 2018) and found an association between alcohol consumption during breastfeeding and a reduction in abstract reasoning in the exposed children at ages 6 and 7 years. This study had methodological issues (Genna, 2019), which was also true of other older studies with similar findings. A U.S. study (R. E. Little, Anderson, Ervin, Worthington-Roberts, & Clarren, 1989) found that when mothers who breastfed for at least 3 months regularly consumed two or more alcoholic drinks per day, their babies scored slightly lower on motor development at 1 year. Mental development was similar in both groups. However, babies in the "breastfed" group included babies who received up to 16 ounces (480 mL) per day of cow's milk or formula. When researchers attempted to replicate this study and extend it to 18 months (R. E. Little, Northstone, & Golding, 2002), no such association was found.

Tobacco

If parents smoke cigarettes, encourage them to nurse and to quit smoking. If they can't quit completely, suggest while lactating they smoke as little as possible.

In the U.S., about 11% of pregnant women smoke cigarettes, with this percentage higher in Europe (Cohen et al., 2018). Of those who quit smoking during pregnancy, 50% to 80% relapse within the first 6 months after birth. Although many parents who smoke consider formula-feeding "safer" than nursing (see next point), the opposite is true. When parents who smoke do not nurse, it increases the baby's risk of developing infections, respiratory illness, respiratory allergy, asthma, and sudden infant death syndrome (Du, Ellert, Lampert, Mensink, & Schlaud, 2012; Guedes & Souza, 2009; Karmaus et al., 2008; Ladomenou, Kafatos, & Galanakis, 2009). One U.S. case-control study (Klonoff-Cohen et al., 1995) examined the relationship between sudden infant death syndrome (SIDS) and smoking and found that while "overall breastfeeding was protective for SIDS…this effect was evident only among nonsmokers." In other words, smoking negated nursing's protective effect and babies of smoking parents had a rate of SIDS equal to nonsmoking bottle-feeding parents.

In addition to the lack of bioactive factors such as antibodies in formula, there may be other reasons for these differences in health outcomes. One U.S. study (Ogbuanu, Karmaus, Arshad, Kurukulaaratchy, & Ewart, 2009) found an association between not breastfeeding and reduced lung function at age 10 years. In 2019, this same finding was replicated in 6- to 9-year-old Austrian children (Moshammer & Hutter, 2019). A Turkish study (Yilmaz et al., 2009) found that when mothers smoked cigarettes but did not breastfeed, their 6-month-old babies had lower blood levels of the antioxidants vitamins A, C, and E. The blood levels of these vitamins were not lower, however, in the babies whose smoking mothers breastfed.

No matter how a baby is fed, exposure to secondhand or passive smoking can be harmful (see last point in the section), but nursing can offset some of the negative health outcomes associated with passive smoking (Y. Q. Liu et al., 2016; B. F. Moore et al., 2017; Nafstad, Jaakkola, Hagen, Botten, & Kongerud, 1996). One Greek study of 240 babies found an increased incidence of the lower respiratory infection bronchiolitis in families who smoked, except when babies were breastfed (Chatzimichael et al., 2007). Another Greek study (Ladomenou et al., 2009) also found an increased incidence of all types of infections during the first year of life in babies whose households included a nonsmoking nursing parent but at least one person who smoked.

Smoking during pregnancy is associated with lower birth weight, greater risk of preterm birth, and other health risks to parent and baby (Einarson & Riordan, 2009). This can be a strong motivator for many nursing parents to quit before birth (Giglia et al., 2006; O'Campo, Faden, Brown, & Gielen, 1992). The more cigarettes smoked, the greater the chance the baby may be affected. Nicotine withdrawal symptoms in newborns were documented in one U.S. study that compared exposed and unexposed babies after birth (Stroud et al., 2009).

If parents can't or won't stop smoking, see the later point on strategies to minimize baby's exposure to nicotine (Vagnarelli et al., 2006).

• • •

Parents who smoke are less likely to nurse, and those who do nurse are more likely to wean earlier, but physical effects of smoking may only be partly responsible for these differences.

While there may be some physical causes for the differences in nursing rates among smokers and nonsmokers, parents' intent to nurse and their decision to start nursing after birth are likely unrelated to any physical effects of smoking. Research (Cohen et al., 2018) confirms that smoking parents are less likely to both plan to nurse during pregnancy and initiate nursing after birth. Shorter duration of nursing was also found in households where other smokers live, even if the nursing parent is a nonsmoker (Lok, Wang, Chan, & Tarrant, 2018). A 2019 systematic review examined the results of eight prospective cohort studies and performed a meta-analysis on two studies that included 1,382 women (Suzuki et al., 2019) and concluded that the odds of discontinuing nursing before 6 months was significantly higher in those exposed to secondhand smoke during pregnancy.

Physical effects of smoking on lactation. When considering why smokers wean earlier than nonsmokers, the physical effects of smoking must be weighed. For example, does nicotine affect a parent's hormonal levels, milk production, and/or milk composition? At this writing, the answer seems to be yes. The authors of a 2016 review of the literature on how smoking affects the lactation process (Napierala, Mazela, Merritt, & Florek, 2016) concluded that nicotine (both in smokers and those exposed to secondhand smoke) may reduce levels in nursing parents of both oxytocin and prolactin (Napierala et al., 2017) and may reduce the fat levels in milk by as much as 20% (Andersen et al., 1982; Baheiraei et al., 2014).

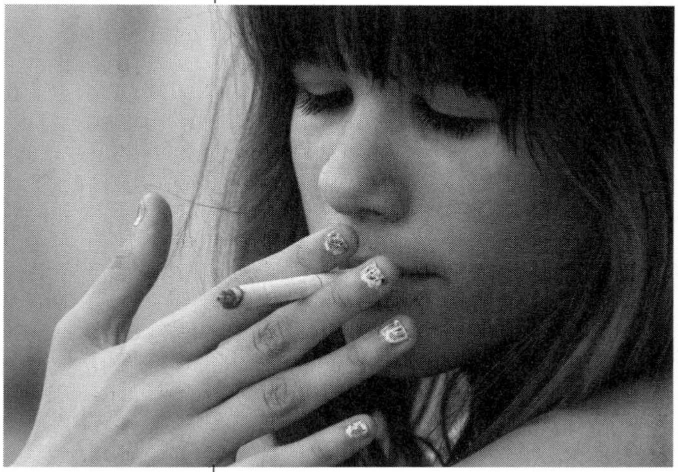

But some findings are puzzling. Although some suggest that smoking reduces milk production, evidence points in the opposite direction. A 2016 U.S. population-based study examined weight gains among babies of nonsmokers, light smokers (1-19 cigarettes/day), and heavy smokers (20+ per day) (Shenassa, Wen, & Braid, 2016) and found that among babies born at average weight, smoking did not significantly affect weight gain. But in the babies born small-for-gestational age (SGA), there was a marginally significant ***greater*** weight gain among the babies whose nursing parents smoked.

Effects of smoking during pregnancy on newborn sucking. Whether or not nicotine directly affects milk production, if nicotine exposure during pregnancy decreases babies' sucking ability at birth, that could certainly cause lower milk production during the critical first 2 weeks of nursing. Studies done on male mice pups found that exposure to cigarette smoke during pregnancy and lactation appeared to cause brain inflammation and an imbalance of free radicals and antioxidants (oxidative stress) (Chan et al., 2016). A 2019 Italian study examined the nursing and neurological scores of 70 newborns, half of whom were born to smoking and half to nonsmoking parents (Bertini, Elia, Lori, & Dani, 2019). At discharge, the babies of the smoking parents had significantly lower scores on the LATCH nursing assessment tool and significantly poorer neurological evaluations. A Turkish study (Memis & Yalcin, 2019) found an association between higher levels of chemical pollutants associated with smoking in mother's milk and an increased rate of feeding problems after birth. As mentioned in the previous point, withdrawal symptoms were documented after birth in babies exposed to smoking during pregnancy (Stroud et al., 2009), which could also affect babies' suck and feeding effectiveness.

Other possible causes of shorter nursing duration among smokers. Some research provides clues to the social and psychological factors at work. For example, one older study that examined the infant-feeding decisions of 4,000 women in the U.S. south in the 1960s (Underwood, Hester, Laffitte, & Gregg, 1965) found a trend that heavier smokers were more likely to nurse. This study was done at a time when women with more education and income were less likely to nurse and poorer, less educated women (who are also more likely to be smokers) were more likely to nurse. In this study, 58% of those smoking more than one pack of cigarettes per day initiated breastfeeding compared with 46% of the nonsmokers. At this writing, the opposite is true: more educated and higher-income parents are more likely to nurse and less-educated and lower-income parents are less likely to nurse. Some researchers (Tanda, Chertok, Haile, & Chavan, 2018) describe how challenging it is to separate the effects of the parents' socioeconomic status from their decision to smoke and to nurse.

In a Canadian study (Ratner, Johnson, & Bottorff, 1999), researchers surveyed 228 mothers and found that earlier weaning in smoking mothers had less to do with the physical effects of smoking and more to do with mothers' anxiety about how smoking affected their milk and their baby. They concluded that most smoking women wean to formula earlier because they think it is safer.

A 2009 U.S. survey of 204 mothers (Lucero et al., 2009) confirmed that despite the recommendations that smoking mothers nurse for better health outcomes, 80% of its mothers believed that breastfeeding women should not smoke at all. Only 25% of the study mothers who were current smokers considered it acceptable for a breastfeeding mother to smoke even one cigarette per day, and only 2% thought it was acceptable for breastfeeding mothers to use nicotine replacement therapies to help them quit smoking (see next point). Another qualitative U.S. study of 44 low-income women (Goldade, Nichter, Adrian, Tesler, & Muramoto, 2008) found these women thought smoking while breastfeeding could harm their baby and that smoking made their milk toxic and addictive. They reported being unable to stop smoking and received little encouragement to nurse.

KEY CONCEPT

Most healthcare providers and smoking parents mistakenly believe it is not safe for smokers to nurse.

What about those who advise families about nursing and smoking? The American Academy of Pediatrics' 2012 policy statement on breastfeeding tells pediatricians that although smoking should be strongly discouraged for health reasons (AAP, 2012, p. e833), "Maternal smoking is not an absolute contraindication to breastfeeding…." Yet a descriptive study of 209 U.S. pediatricians (Lucero et al., 2009) found that less than half recommended that smoking parents breastfeed. Most were likely to recommend formula feeding and were unsure about the safety of nicotine replacement therapies for nursing parents.

In light of these findings, it is not surprising that at both 10 weeks and 6 months more than twice as many nonsmoking parents are nursing (Jedrychowski et al., 2008; J. Liu, Rosenberg, & Sandoval, 2006). More education about smoking and nursing is obviously needed among both families and healthcare providers.

• • •

Nicotine-replacement products used to quit smoking are compatible with nursing.

Nicotine replacement products provide blood nicotine levels high enough to prevent or reduce withdrawal symptoms but without the "buzz" of cigarettes. They are also missing the tars, carbon monoxide, and lung irritants that come with smoking. According to a 2018 Cochrane Review article (Hartmann-Boyce, Chepkin, Ye, Bullen, & Lancaster, 2018), use of these products increases the chances of successfully quitting smoking by 50% to 60%, regardless of whether they're used in a study or at home. These products come in a variety of forms.

Nicotine gums, lozenges, tablets, inhalers, and nasal sprays are used intermittently over the course of the day, so blood and milk nicotine levels rise and fall. When using these products, suggest the same strategy recommended for the smoking parent (see next point): use them after nursing and if possible wait 2 to 3 hours before the next nursing, when nicotine levels in blood and milk are lower (Hale, 2019, p. 551-552). If a baby wants to nurse before that time, though, suggest the parent go ahead. Nicotine gums were found to produce blood levels averaging only 30% to 60% of those produced by smoking (Schatz, 1998). Nicotine blood levels from nicotine inhalers are only about 12% (Hale, 2019, p. 551-552). On average, when used as recommended, one of these replacement products would provide about as much nicotine per day as less than one pack of cigarettes (Schatz, 1998).

Transdermal nicotine patches provide a steady level of nicotine in the user's blood and milk, which if used correctly, should be lower than smoking. Suggest parents remove the patch at bedtime for lower nicotine levels at night (Schatz, 1998). One Australian study of 15 breastfeeding mothers found that while their babies' milk intake remained stable while they used the patch, the babies received 70% less nicotine and its metabolite cotinine than while smoking. These researchers (Ilett et al., 2003, p. 516) wrote: "Undertaking maternal smoking cessation with the nicotine patch is, therefore, a safer option than continued smoking."

E-cigarettes, also known as Electronic Nicotine Delivery Systems (ENDS), are used by some to quit smoking. They look like a regular cigarette, are battery-powered, and are designed to mimic the experience of smoking without exposing the user or those in the environment to the harmful compounds released while smoking cigarettes. Sometimes referred to as "vaping," according to Hale (Hale, 2019, p. 552), more research is needed, but the amount of nicotine delivered by e-cigarettes is likely minimal and comparable to a nicotine inhaler. However, the dose of nicotine will depend on how many times per day it is used.

• • •

If a nursing parent continues to smoke, suggest strategies to minimize the baby's exposure to nicotine and secondhand smoke.

Nicotine and cotinine (a byproduct of nicotine breakdown) are concentrated in human milk. U.K. research (Luck & Nau, 1984, 1985) found that on average nicotine levels were three times higher in nursing parents' milk than in their blood. One Canadian study (Becker et al., 1999) comparing urine cotinine levels in smokers' nursing and formula-fed babies found five times more cotinine in the urine of smokers' nursing babies than in those who did not nurse. Cotinine inhaled from passive smoking was associated with increased incidence of respiratory problems, but cotinine in mother's milk was not. To reduce a nursing baby's exposure to nicotine, suggest these strategies.

Smoke fewer cigarettes per day. While quitting is ideal, if parents won't or can't quit, to decrease the baby's exposure to nicotine, suggest cutting back on the number of cigarettes they smoke per day. It may motivate parents to cut back to know about several studies (Canivet, Ostergren, Jakobsson, Dejin-Karlsson, & Hagander, 2008; Reijneveld, Lanting, Crone, & Van Wouwe, 2005; Shenassa & Brown, 2004) that found a link between smoking and increased incidence of colic, even in formula-feeding families.

Smoke after nursing. The half-life of nicotine—the amount of time it takes for half the nicotine to be eliminated from the body— is 95 minutes (Steldinger, Luck, & Nau, 1988). After smoking a cigarette, a nursing parent's blood and milk nicotine levels first rise and then fall over time. One Swedish study (Dahlstrom, Lundell, Curvall, & Thapper, 1990) found that smoking right before nursing caused a 10-fold increase in the amount of nicotine the baby received. Smoking after nursing—ideally waiting 2 to 3 hours before the next nursing—allows the milk nicotine levels to fall significantly before the baby nurses again. However, if the baby wants to nurse sooner, nursing is better than giving formula (Myr, 2004). Another incentive to smoke after nursing comes from a U.S. study of 15 mothers and babies (Mennella, Yourshaw, & Morgan, 2007), which found that the babies spent significantly less time sleeping when the mothers smoked right before breastfeeding.

KEY CONCEPT

Smokers have many ways to reduce their nursing baby's exposure to nicotine and secondhand smoke.

Smoke outside or in a separate room. No matter how a baby is fed, breathing cigarette smoke (passive smoking) poses health risks for everyone in the family. One German study (Bajanowski et al., 2008) found that nicotine levels in the hair and in spinal and heart fluids in formula-fed babies who died of SIDS were five times higher than in the babies who were nursed, leading the researchers to conclude that passive smoking may be more important to health than exposure to nicotine derivatives through nursing. Exposure to passive smoking was found to increase the incidence of infections in non-nursing babies, but nursing provides some protection against infection (Ladomenou et al., 2009). Encourage parents to create smoke-free zones anywhere their baby spends a lot of time (home, car).

Cannabis

Cannabis—which may be used for medical or recreational purposes—affects its users via the body's endocannabinoid system.

Since the last edition of this book, cannabis was legalized for medical and recreational use in Canada and in many U.S. states, although at this writing it is still illegal under U.S. federal law. Because in the past cannabis was illegal in most areas, research on its short- and long-term effects, especially during pregnancy and lactation, is scarce and conflicting.

Cannabis use after legalization. A significant number of families use cannabis, and its use is likely to increase with legalization, even before we have a clear understanding of its effects. Parents who use cannabis often believe that because it is natural, it is less harmful than alcohol. In one U.K. study (D. G. Moore et al., 2010), cannabis was the only illegal drug pregnant women continued to use until birth. A U.S. cross-sectional study of 3.207 respondents from the Colorado Pregnancy Risk Assessment Monitoring System (Crume et al., 2018) found that the self-reported statewide prevalence of cannabis use during pregnancy was about 6% and during lactation 5%. Cannabis use during pregnancy was associated with a 50% increased risk of low birth weight, but there was no association with small-for-gestational-age, preterm birth, or NICU admission after birth. Cannabis use may be greater among different socioeconomic groups. In another article about Colorado cannabis use (Wang, 2017), participants of the state's low-income food subsidy program (WIC) in its largest county (more than 26% of the state's WIC participants) were surveyed. Of the 4% overall who reported using cannabis, 36% used it during pregnancy and 18% while nursing.

Cannabis products. The term cannabis includes different product types made from the *Cannabis sativa* or hemp plant, its cousin, *Cannabis indica*, or a hybrid of the two, which include

- Marijuana—From its dried leaves, stems, and flower buds
- Hashish—From the resin in its flower buds,
- Oils—By extracting cannabidiol (CBD) from the plant and diluting it with a carrier oil like coconut oil or hemp-seed oil

Delta-9-tetrahydrocannabinol (THC) is the psychoactive ingredient in cannabis that causes its users to feel "high." The cannabis products available today contain much higher levels of THC than the cannabis decades ago. Today's products have been genetically engineered so that rather than the 1% level of THC that was common in the 1960s and 1970s, it is as high as 30%. New forms of cannabis are available, such as the hard, amber-colored solid made from its resin and used for "dabbing," which involves heating it with vape pens or other specialty devices and inhaling it for a more intense high.

CBD oils do not have the psychoactive effect of other cannabis products because their THC levels are so low. Some reported benefits of using CBD oils are reduced pain, anxiety, and depression. Reported side effects of CBD oils include fatigue, diarrhea, and changes in weight and appetite. CBD oils are not currently approved for use by the U.S. Food and Drug Administration, and like other plant-derived herbal products, their labels may not accurately reflect their content. Typically, CBD oils contain a larger number of the more than 400 existing cannabinoid substances than other cannabis products. At this writing, no research is available on the short- or long-term effects of CBD oil on lactation or on the baby during pregnancy or nursing. Synthetic THC and CBD products are now available for treating pain and the nausea of chemotherapy. These products may be available as a transdermal patch or a topical cream.

The endocannabinoid system is responsible for the physical effects of cannabis products on the human body. This system includes a network of cannabinoid receptors and endocannabinoid molecules, which are also a normal ingredient of human milk. This system is believed to play a role in mood, coordination and movement, appetite, weight regulation, brain aging (Bilkei-Gorzo, 2012), and neural development before and after birth, including infant sucking. When researchers blocked the CB1 receptors (one of the body's two cannabinoid receptors) in mouse newborns, the baby mice were unable to suck and extract milk (Mechoulam, Berry, Avraham, Di Marzo, & Fride, 2006). In a later study, U.S. scientists analyzed human-milk samples and identified endocannabinoids and related compounds that may play a role in establishing babies' sucking response after birth (Gaitan, Wood, Zhang, Makriyannis, & Lammi-Keefe, 2018). In babies who suffered brain damage during birth, cannabis (without the THC) was used successfully to treat them due to its effects on this endocannabinoid system (Fernandez-Lopez, Lizasoain, Moro, & Martinez-Orgado, 2013).

• • •

Recent research gives new insight into how THC is absorbed by lactating parents and enters milk.

The THC in cannabis passes into the milk, stays in the body for weeks, and in regular users, may accumulate.

THC absorption when smoked and eaten. When cannabis is smoked, more THC is absorbed than when it is eaten. According to Hale (Hale, 2019, p. 105), in occasional cannabis users, about 10% to 14% of the THC is absorbed by the body, while in regular users, between 23% and 27% is absorbed. When cannabis is eaten, the absorption is lower: 4% to 12%.

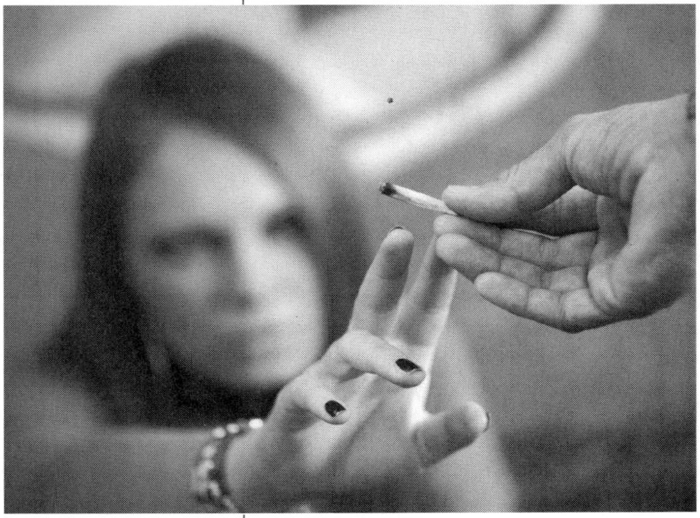

Positive urine screens and child protective services. Once THC is absorbed by the body, it enters the fatty tissues and is stored there for weeks. This means that urine screens done even several weeks after the last use will be positive for cannabis. Parents need to know this because if they use cannabis during pregnancy and they give birth within a few weeks of their last use, they may test positive for THC. Even in places where cannabis is legal for medical and recreational use, a positive urine screen may require the staff in some birthing facilities to contact child protective services for an evaluation.

THC passes into mother's milk. Until 2018, the only evidence available about THC transfer into milk was from case reports. Two 2018 prospective experimental studies provided more information on how THC passes into the milk and how long it stays there. In one small U.S. study of 8 women (seven occasional cannabis users and one regular user) (T. Baker et al., 2018), the study women were asked to abstain from cannabis use for 24 hours. Then they were given doses of cannabis to smoke that were carefully measured by a Colorado dispensary. Milk samples were taken just before exposure and at 1 hour, 2 hours and 4 hours after exposure. The researchers analyzed the milk and found that the peak level of THC occurred at 1 hour after exposure, and the relative infant dose of THC was 2.5% of the mothers' dose. A second 2018 U.S. study (Bertrand, Hanan, Honerkamp-Smith, Best, & Chambers, 2018) took milk samples from 50 cannabis-using lactating women, two thirds of whom were nursing a child younger than 1 year. THC (as well as other cannabinoid compounds) was found in 63% of the milk samples and was detected in the milk for up to 6 days after the last cannabis use. Although on average, the doses of THC the infants ingested via the milk were relatively low, the researchers noted that there was great variability in the milk THC concentrations, so some of the babies were exposed to daily doses of cannabinoids close to a typical adult dose.

KEY CONCEPT

THC reached its peak level 1 hour after cannabis was smoked and was detected in the milk for up to 6 days.

Earlier case reports found that in heavy cannabis users, the level of THC in milk and blood were up to 8 times higher than the levels in occasional users (Perez-Reyes & Wall, 1982). Although the half-life of cannabis is 25 to 57 hours, when it is used regularly, THC is stored in body fat, increasing its half-life up to 4 days (Djulus, Moretti, & Koren, 2005). After a nursing parent uses cannabis, THC can be detected in the baby's urine for up to 3 weeks. Exposure to secondhand cannabis smoke increases the amount of THC the baby receives.

Effects of cannabis on the nursing baby. The most significant concern many experts have about cannabis use during pregnancy and nursing is the possible effect of THC on the baby's rapidly developing brain. THC is quickly absorbed by both the milk and the brain. One article (Tortoriello et al., 2014) used mouse models to describe how repeated cannabis exposure can disrupt neurological development, with the potential to cause permanent neurobehavioral and cognitive impairment. An older study that examined the effects of cannabis exposure in nursing babies during the first month of life (Astley & Little, 1990) found that the exposed babies were more likely to have decreased motor development at 1 year as compared with the babies who were not exposed.

Effects of cannabis on lactation. Human studies found that after cannabis use, prolactin levels in nursing mothers were significantly lower compared with those not exposed (Mendelson, Mello, & Ellingboe, 1985; Ranganathan et al., 2009). A 2017 review article (Mourh & Rowe, 2017) summarized the findings of seven animal studies in which the exposed lactating animals had lower prolactin and oxytocin levels, and their babies did less sucking in comparison to those not exposed. These findings mean that cannabis use may affect the nursing parent's hormonal response to sucking and the baby's ability to suck, which both have the potential to reduce milk removal and milk production.

• • •

Because research is scant and conflicting, recommendations about cannabis use during nursing vary.

Because so little research is available on the short- and long-term effects of cannabis on the user, the nursing baby, and the process of lactation (see previous point), recommendations about cannabis use during nursing vary widely. For example, two systematic reviews came to opposite conclusions. One (Ordean, 2014) concluded that the effects of cannabis during lactation are unclear, so nursing parents should be told about the health advantages of nursing as well as the possible harmful effects of cannabis use. The other systematic review (Seabrook, Biden, & Campbell, 2017) concluded that medical cannabis should not be given to nursing parents due to the risks associated with poor neurobehavioral outcomes and that nursing parents should be advised to reduce or stop using cannabis.

What should lactation specialists tell pregnant and nursing parents about cannabis use? The central messages provided by many of the major health organizations (Reece-Stremtan & Marinelli, 2015; S. A. Ryan et al., 2018) are similar—with a few exceptions—to the recommendations given to cigarette smokers.

- There's a lot we don't know about the effects of cannabis on the baby's developing brain, and just because cannabis is legal in some areas and "natural," that does not mean it is safe to use during pregnancy and lactation.
- After giving birth, if a urine screen for cannabis is positive—which can happen even several weeks after the last use—child protective services may be contacted.
- Keep the baby away from any contact with secondhand cannabis smoke.
- If cannabis is recommended for medical reasons, talk to a healthcare provider about possible alternative treatments, and if none exist, weigh the risks and benefits of continuing to nurse while using cannabis.
- If at all possible, stop using cannabis during pregnancy and while nursing. If stopping cannabis use altogether is not an option, reduce as much as possible its use while nursing.

Clinical Protocol #21 from the Academy of Breastfeeding Medicine described its recommendations about cannabis use while nursing this way (Reece-Stremtan & Marinelli, 2015, p. 137):

> "Information regarding long-term effects of marijuana use by the breastfeeding mother on the infant remains insufficient to recommend complete abstention from breastfeeding initiation or continuation based on the scientific evidence at this time...."

Here's how the clinical report of the American Academy of Pediatrics (S. A. Ryan et al., 2018, p. 11) expressed it:

> "Present data are insufficient to assess the effects of exposure of infants to maternal marijuana use during breastfeeding. As a result, maternal marijuana use while breastfeeding is discouraged. Because the potential risk of infant exposure to marijuana metabolites are unknown, women should be informed of the potential risk of exposure during lactation and encouraged to abstain from using any marijuana products while breastfeeding."

Opioids, NAS, and Treatments

Over the last decade, the use of opioids—both legal and illegal—skyrocketed.

The term ***opioid*** was once used to distinguish opiates (drugs derived from opium) from the drugs made synthetically that attach to the opiate receptors in the body. Now, though, "opioid" is an umbrella term used to define the entire family of opiates, both natural opiates and their synthetic versions.

Prescription opioids are some of the most commonly used narcotic pain relievers. They include codeine, morphine, oxycodone, fentanyl, and hydrocodone. Morphine is often given for pain relief after a cesarean delivery because due to its short half-life—1.5 to 2 hours—it leaves the body quickly, which is an advantage in nursing parents. After an oral dose, morphine reaches its peak level in only about 30 minutes (Hale, 2019, p. 528-529).

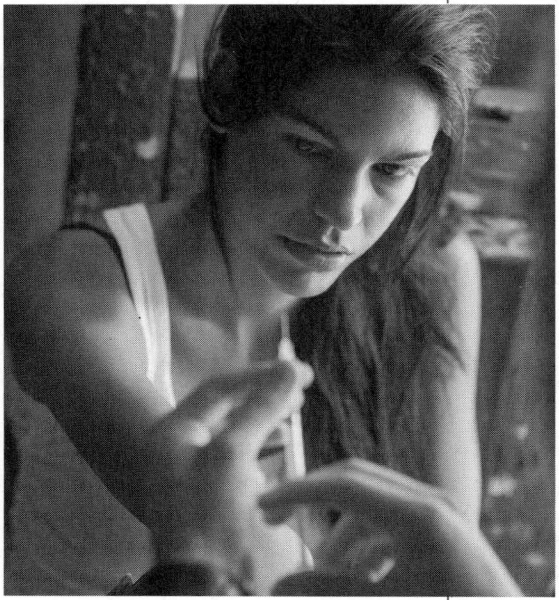

The opioid epidemic. In the U.S. during the past decade, opioid drugs, which can be an appropriate choice when taken short term, were overprescribed for longer periods, which led to rising drug dependence (called ***opioid use disorder***). Between 1999 and 2014, the number of parents starting prenatal care with opioid use disorder increased 333% (Clark, 2019). This led to many more infants going through opioid withdrawal after birth (see next point). This epidemic also included increasing rates of opioid overdose deaths, which the U.S. National Institute on Drug Abuse (NIDA, 2019) called a national crisis. Because regular use of opioids can be expensive, many of those with a dependence on opioids seek illegal sources of these drugs, especially when their tolerance for the drug rises and they need to increase their dosage to produce the same effect.

Heroin, a highly addictive opioid, is not used for medical treatment in the U.S. Some who develop opioid use disorder switch to heroin because it costs much less than prescribed opioids. A retrospective analysis of heroin use in the U.S. (Cicero, Ellis, Surratt, & Kurtz, 2014) concluded that heroin is no longer a drug primarily associated with poverty in the inner cities. Its use has become more widespread. Heroin users who want to get sober may enroll in programs that provide legal drugs like methadone and buprenorphine, to help them kick the habit (see the last section in this chapter).

• • •

Most babies born to opioid-dependent parents experience withdrawal, a stressful process that nursing can help moderate.

Neonatal abstinence syndrome, or ***NAS***, is the withdrawal process that occurs when a baby is born to a parent regularly using opioids, including opioid-substitute drugs like methadone and buprenorphine to treat opioid dependence. According to one study (Winkelman, Villapiano, Kozhimannil, Davis, & Patrick, 2018), the U.S. incidence of NAS increased five-fold between 2004 and 2014.

NAS incidence and symptoms. NAS occurs in between 55% to 94% of opioid exposed newborns (Hudak et al., 2012). Its symptoms occur in the areas of the body where the opiate receptors are located, such as the central nervous system and the digestive tract. Neurological symptoms include a high-pitched cry, tremors, high muscle tone, hyperactive reflexes, temperature instability, fast breathing, and even seizures. Digestive symptoms include vomiting, diarrhea, poor weight gain, and poor feeding, which may include uncoordinated sucking that may contribute to nursing challenges (Howard et al., 2018).

Nursing eases NAS. Newborns with NAS who nurse or receive expressed human milk have better outcomes than those exclusively formula-fed. In two large studies, babies who nursed or received any expressed milk had shorter hospital stays. A 2016 U.S. retrospective study of 3,725 babies with NAS (Short, Gannon, & Abatemarco, 2016) compared those who were nursed with those who were formula-fed. The average hospital stay was nearly 10% shorter (10 days versus 12 days) in the nursing group. A 2019 retrospective cohort study analyzed data collected prospectively on 1,738 babies born with NAS and divided them into two groups: those who received any human milk and those who received none (Favara et al., 2019). They found that the group who received any human milk needed drug therapy for a shorter time and had a shorter hospital stay compared with babies exclusively formula-fed. In a 2019 systematic review of eight studies that evaluated the effects of feeding method on babies born with NAS (McQueen, Taylor, & Murphy-Oikonen, 2019, p. 1), its authors wrote:

> "...for newborns exposed to methadone, breastfeeding was associated with decreased incidence and duration of pharmacologic treatment, shorter hospital length of stay, and decreased severity of NAS....Women who are stable on opioid substitution treatment should be provided with appropriate education and support to breastfeed."

Rooming-in and NAS. Rooming-in during the hospital stay also leads to better NAS outcomes. A 2017 literature review (Grossman, Seashore, & Holmes, 2017) described studies from Canada and Germany that found babies with NAS who stayed in their parent's room after birth had shorter hospital stays, too. A 2016 U.S. study (Holmes et al., 2016) also found that rooming-in decreased the length of hospital stay in babies with NAS (12 versus 17 days), as well as decreasing their need for drug therapy (27% versus 46%), and substantially lowering their healthcare costs ($5,000 versus $11,000 USD)..

Other non-drug treatments. Before drug therapy is used to treat a baby's NAS symptoms, ideally non-drug treatments are tried first. Both skin-to-skin contact and nursing are considered non-pharmacologic treatments for NAS, in addition to swaddling and a quiet environment.

• • •

When a person develops an opioid dependence, drug therapy involves regular use of a drug that acts on the opiate receptors in the body, such as methadone and buprenorphine. Drug therapy may be used long-term, and may even be lifelong. The goal of drug therapy is to block the euphoria that comes with opioid use while relieving the craving and suppressing withdrawal symptoms. Rather than simply treating the symptoms, some opioid treatment programs also provide counseling and behavioral therapy to treat the underlying mental-health issues that lead to drug dependence. Sometimes referred to as ***medication-assisted treatment***, or MAT, receiving both drug therapy and counseling is most likely to help those who are drug dependent turn their lives around. Keep in mind that most drug dependence is a form of self-medication in those with untreated trauma and other mental-health issues who are struggling to cope (see previous section).

The medications used to treat adults for opioid dependence are compatible with nursing, but without good-quality lactation help and support, nursing rates are low in these families.

The most common drugs used to treat opioid use disorder are methadone and buprenorphine, and both are rated using Hale's lactation risk categories (Hale, 2019) as L2 drugs, meaning available research on their use during lactation indicates they are compatible with nursing.

Methadone. Studies examined the effects of methadone in both blood and milk on the nursing baby for up to 6 months (Bogen et al., 2011; Jansson, Choo, Velez, Lowe, & Huestis, 2008). The authors of the American Academy of Pediatrics clinical report on neonatal drug withdrawal (Hudak et al., 2012, p. e548) wrote:

> "...there is no clear reason to discourage breastfeeding in mothers who adhere to methadone or buprenorphine maintenance treatment."

Buprenorphine. Both short-term and long-term studies (Gower et al., 2014; Ilett et al., 2012; Jansson et al., 2016) found low concentrations of this drug in mother's milk in parents on long-term drug therapy. Sustained-release pellets of this drug are available that provide a low daily dose over weeks. But the buprenorphine patch produces higher blood levels for up to 7 days, and there is no data on its potential effects on the nursing baby (Hale, 2019, p. 92).

Nursing during treatment for opioid use disorder. . Nursing initiation and duration vary greatly among birthing parents in treatment for opioid-use disorder, depending on the model of care, whether consistent lactation advice is given, and how much lactation support is available. For example, one U.S. retrospective chart review of 276 mothers and babies with NAS (Wachman, Byun, & Philipp, 2010) found that while 68% were eligible to nurse (see Table 13.3 on p. 604), only 24% initiated nursing, with 60% of these stopping within 1 week. Another U.S. retrospective chart review had a completely different outcome. After its 85 mothers gave birth to babies with NAS (O'Connor, Collett, Alto, & O'Brien, 2013), 76% initiated nursing, with 66% still nursing 6 to 8 weeks later.

KEY CONCEPT

More opioid-dependent families nurse longer when they received integrated care that addressed medical, social, and psychological needs.

Why did so many more mothers nurse longer in the second study? The answer can be found in a 2019 systematic review of four studies on nursing during opioid treatment (Doerzbacher & Chang, 2019). Its authors concluded that the interventions that effectively increased nursing initiation and duration were "embedded within alternative models of care." In other words, their basic approach to caring for these families increased the level of help and support they received for nursing. For example, comprehensive prenatal care insured that the families received information about nursing and encouragement to nurse even before their baby was born. Rooming-in kept families together during the hospital stay. Social services provided opioid-dependent parents with counseling, as well as appropriate drug therapy. As the authors of this systematic review (Doerzbacher & Chang, 2019, p. 1163) wrote:

> "Each model is comprehensive, addressing the medical, social, and psychological needs of the mother and newborn and providing obstetrical care and substance use treatment with an integrated transdisciplinary approach. Each model incorporates strategies to build and maintain maternal strengths and capabilities while fostering the integrity of the mother/infant dyad. Each care setting was staffed by healthcare professionals who were committed to providing holistic, supportive, and trauma-informed care that is sensitive to the unique needs of these women."

Along the same lines, a 2018 U.S. retrospective cohort study (Schiff et al., 2018) examined the factors that affected whether or not these families decided to nurse and for those who started nursing, the factors that kept them going over time. Like the previous systematic review, the authors found that the most important factors were prenatal education, the availability of specialized programs for opioid-dependent parents, and staff perceptions. Because many of these factors were not fully in place in the hospital where this study was conducted, the nursing initiation rate was 50% and by hospital discharge, only 33% of these families were nursing. Its authors recommended that hospitals implement guidelines to create integrated programs and provide staff training to ensure consistent messages, making this a normal part of the care they provide.

BOX 13.1 Some Reliable Sources on Substance Use During Lactation

LactMed (U.S.)
Part of the National Library of Medicine's Toxicology Data Network (TOXNET)
Access its electronic database at: **bit.ly/BA2-LactMed**

e-Lactancia.org (Europe, in English and Spanish)
Created by APILAM (Association for the Promotion of and Cultural and Scientific Research into Breastfeeding), a European organization of health professionals

Infant Risk Center (U.S.)
infantrisk.com
Experts available by phone Monday through Friday at 806-352-2519

Adapted from Hale, T. W. (2019). Hale's Medications & Mothers' Milk: A Manual of Lactational Pharmacology (18th ed.). New York, NY: Springer Publishing Company.

The experience of nursing during opioid-substitute therapy. Studies using focus groups and semi-structured interviews provide insights into the barriers faced by opioid-dependent parents before and after birth. Lack of support and misinformation from healthcare providers was cited as a major barrier to nursing in one U.S. interview study (Demirci, Bogen, & Klionsky, 2015). In another U.S. qualitative study (McGlothen, Cleveland, & Gill, 2018), a mother described how confusing it was to have the lactation consultant tell her that her opioid-substitute therapy was compatible with breastfeeding while other healthcare providers told her she shouldn't breastfeed while on methadone. These study mothers also described how important it was to them to do the best for their baby and how much they valued support from both healthcare providers and their peers.

In another U.S. qualitative study (Howard et al., 2018), the 25 mothers all roomed-in with their newborns. Nearly three quarters (72%) breastfed, with 40% continuing until hospital discharge. Among their newborns, 36% required drug treatment for NAS. They described the hospital environment as both a source of support and tension as they struggled to make their own decisions about their baby's care. They also described feeling a stigma, both from within themselves and from those around them that negatively affected their self-confidence as mothers. Some described the effects their history of abuse and trauma had on their decision not to nurse, as well as their attachment to their baby. Some described how having a baby contributed to their resiliency and gave them a greater sense of purpose in life.

Methamphetamines

Methamphetamine is contraindicated during nursing, and its use can quickly lead to dependence.

Methamphetamine, or meth, is a stimulant drug that affects the central nervous system and is highly addictive. It is used in many forms: a powder, a pill, or as crystal meth, which looks like glass fragments or rocks. It can be smoked, snorted, injected, or ingested orally or anally. According to Hale (Hale, 2019), its lactation risk category is L5, which means its use is so hazardous to the nursing baby that nursing is contraindicated.

Pump and dump for at least 100 hours after use. According to Hale's lactation risk categories (Hale, 2019, p. 488-489), meth is considered an L5, meaning it is considered so hazardous to the nursing baby that its use is contraindicated

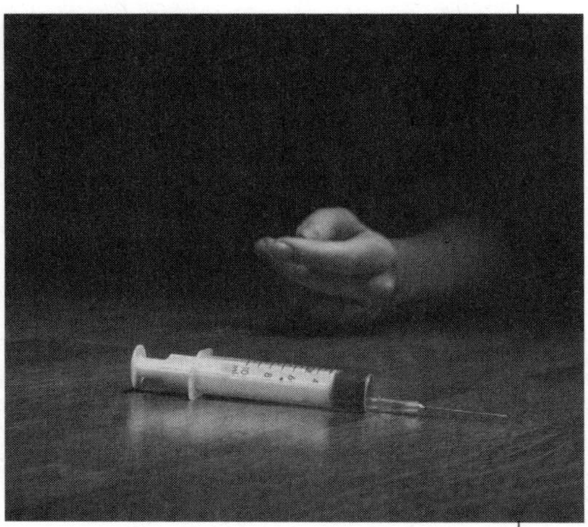

during lactation. After one dose of methamphetamine, the recommendation is to pump and dump for at least 100 hours. This is how long a 2016 study found it took for meth to be undetectable in the milk of users (Chomchai, Chomchai, & Kitsommart, 2016). In *Hale's Medications & Mothers' Milk* (Hale, 2019, pp. 488-489), its author noted that another way to minimize a nursing baby's exposure to meth is to wait to resume nursing until the parent's urine screen is negative, which according to the testing in the Chomchai study, was an additional 30 to 75 hours, depending on the dose. See Table 13.3 on p. 604 for guidelines on whether a nursing parent who is using meth or has a history of meth use should be supported to continue nursing, carefully evaluated, or discouraged from nursing. If parents use meth regularly, assume they lack the good judgment needed to avoid nursing while under the influence and encourage them to seek treatment.

Cocaine

After using cocaine, a nursing parent should pump and dump for at least 24 hours, as its use contraindicated during nursing.

Like meth, cocaine is a central nervous system stimulant that can be smoked, snorted, or injected. With repeated uses, tolerance can develop. Cocaine passes into milk in significant amounts and can cause cocaine intoxication in the nursing baby. Reported symptoms in the baby include irritability, vomiting, dilated pupils, tremors, and increased heart and respiratory rates (Cressman et al., 2012).

Pump and dump for at least 24 hours after use. Although the effects of cocaine on the nursing parent can fade within 20 to 30 minutes, cocaine is metabolized slowly and was found in adults' urine for up to 7 days and even longer in babies' urine (Hale, 2019, p. 170-172). In one case report (Chasnoff, Lewis, & Squires, 1987), cocaine was found in mother's milk for as long as 36 hours. Because illicit drugs are rarely pure, cocaine may also contain other drugs that may be harmful to the nursing baby. Like methamphetamines, according to Hale's lactation risk categories (Hale, 2019), cocaine is an L5, which means this drug is considered so hazardous to the nursing baby that its use is contraindicated during lactation. After one dose of cocaine, the recommendation (Hale, 2019) is that nursing parents pump and dump for at least 24 hours before nursing again. See Table 13.3 on p. 604 for guidelines on when nursing parents who use illegal drugs should be encouraged to nurse, carefully evaluated, or discouraged from nursing.

Topical cocaine can also be hazardous to babies. In one case report (P. O. Anderson, 2018b; Chaney, Franke, & Wadlington, 1988), a mother applied cocaine to her nipples to relieve soreness. Three hours later, she nursed the baby with a nipple shield and the baby developed convulsions and breathing problems.

Hallucinogenic Drugs

Hallucinogenic drugs, such as angel dust, ecstasy, and LSD, are contraindicated during nursing.

Significant amounts of PCP (angel dust), gamma hydroxybutyric acid (ecstasy), and LSD (acid) pass easily through the blood-brain barrier, which make them very likely to transfer quickly into human milk (Hale, 2019). According to Hale's lactation risk categories (Hale, 2019), these drugs are rated an L5, which means they are considered so hazardous to the nursing baby that their use is contraindicated during lactation. The book *Hale's Medications & Mothers' Milk* (2019) provides specific information on these drugs:

- **PCP** (half-life of 24 to 51 hours)—Because it is stored in fatty tissue, PCP can be detected in the user's urine for 14 to 30 days. One mother who took PCP 41 days before she began lactating still had measurable milk levels of PCP after her baby was born (P. O. Anderson, 2018b; Kaufman, Petrucha, Pitts, & Weekes, 1983).
- **Ecstasy** (half-life of 20 to 60 minutes)—Depending on dose, recommend after use the lactating parent pump and dump for at least 12 to 24 hours.
- **LSD** (half-life of 3 hours)—This very potent drug crosses the blood-brain barrier and may cause hallucinations in the baby. LSD can be found in the parent's urine for 34 to 120 hours.

Nursing and the Use of Illegal Substances

Some parents with a history of illegal substance use can be supported to nurse.

In most cases, untreated mental-health issues lead to regular use of illegal substances as a type of self-medication. Termed ***substance use disorder*** (SUD), an Australian study (Staiger, Thomas, Ricciardelli, & McCabe, 2011) found that 76% of those diagnosed with SUD suffered from depressive disorders and 25% had four or more different mental-health diagnoses. Illegal substance use can occur in any family, but it is more likely in those who are poor, unemployed, lack safe housing, transportation, and social support, and those with a history of trauma. Using illegal substances during pregnancy is a cause for concern because it increases risk for birth defects, fetal growth restrictions, preterm birth, impaired neurological development, and after birth, signs of toxicity or withdrawal (Hudak et al., 2012).

In families with a history of illegal drug use, nursing may be risky. The most common concern in this situation is whether the nursing baby will be exposed to dangerous substances through the milk. When parents use illegal drugs, use of multiple drugs is the norm, in part because illegal drugs are often cut with other substances. Because psychiatric disorders are so common in these families, the nursing parent may also be taking psychiatric medications. Infection, such as HIV (see p. 824) and hepatitis B and C (see p. 817) are also more common in illegal drug users. The nursing baby may also face dangers from risky behaviors. Yet in spite of the risks, the authors of Clinical Protocol #21 from the Academy of Breastfeeding Medicine (ABM) (Reece-Stremtan & Marinelli, 2015, p. 135) wrote:

> "...drug-exposed infants, who are at high risk for an array of medical, psychological, and developmental issues, as well as their mothers, stand to benefit significantly from breastfeeding."

There is little available research on the use of illegal drugs during lactation. This picture is complicated even more by the fact that it can be difficult to separate a baby's exposure to a drug during pregnancy from exposure through the milk.

Unfortunately, the decision to nurse a baby after birth does not decrease the likelihood that a previous illegal drug user will use again. For that reason, the ABM's Clinical Protocol #21 described specific topics to discuss with families who have a history of illegal drug use to determine if nursing should be

TABLE 13.3 Nursing Considerations in Those with a History of Illegal Substance Use

	Support Nursing (All)	Carefully Evaluate	Discourage Nursing (Any)
Started prenatal care	Soon after pregnancy is confirmed	≥2nd trimester	No prenatal care and no plans for pediatric care
Permission to discuss treatment with counselor	Yes, counselor confirms sobriety maintenance	Yes, counselor confirms sobriety	No, won't give consent
Treatment plans	Continuing treatment	Plans to enter treatment	None, not willing to enter treatment
Attained sobriety	As an outpatient	As an inpatient	No, + urine screen, behavior indicates active drug use, chronic alcohol use
Last substance use	≥90 days before birth	30-90 days before birth	Relapsed ≤30 days before birth
Any psychiatric medications	If yes, compatible with nursing	If yes, compatible with nursing	Incompatible with nursing
Other nursing contraindications	No	No	Yes
Medication or treatment	On stable maintenance	Starting maintenance	Not yet

Adapted from (Reece-Stremtan & Marinelli, 2015)

considered (Table 13.3). It is difficult for any lactation supporter to imagine discouraging a family from nursing. But in situations where the nursing parent is using dangerous substances that could harm the baby, the risks of nursing may outweigh all of its positives.

• • •

When nursing parents are under the influence of illegal drugs, no matter how the baby is fed, their ability to provide adequate care is impaired.

Even if nursing parents formula-feed or withhold nursing for the recommended length of time after drug use, they have a responsibility to keep the baby safe. While on drugs, recommend making arrangements for the baby to be cared for by someone sober, as drug use at the very least puts the baby at risk for inadequate care. In most parts of the world, healthcare providers—including lactation specialists—are considered mandated reporters, meaning if they believe a baby is at risk, they are obligated to notify either the baby's primary healthcare provider or child protective services.

RESOURCES

bfmed.org/protocols—Free and downloadable, fully referenced protocols available in multiple languages, suitable for sharing with healthcare providers:

- #21: Guidelines for breastfeeding and substance use or substance use disorder
- #24: Allergic proctocolitis in the exclusively breastfed infant
- #29: Iron, zinc, and vitamin D supplementation during breastfeeding

bit.ly/BA2-AlcoholCalculator—From Canadian scientists, created for parents and professionals to determine—based on parent weight and number of alcoholic drinks—the length of time needed for alcohol to completely clear the milk

Hale, T. W. (2019). *Hale's Medications & Mothers' Milk: A Manual of Lactational Pharmacology* (18th ed.). New York, NY: Springer Publishing Company.

REFERENCES

AAP. (2012). Breastfeeding and the use of human milk. *Pediatrics, 129*(3), e827-e841.

ABM. (2011). ABM Clinical Protocol #24: Allergic proctocolitis in the exclusively breastfed infant. *Breastfeeding Medicine, 6*(6), 435-440.

Achalapong, J. (2016). Effect of egg and milk supplement on breast milk volume at 48 and 72 hours postpartum: A randomized-controlled trial. *Thai Journal of Obstetrics and Gynaecology, 24*(1), 20-25.

Ader, D. N., South-Paul, J., Adera, T., et al. (2001). Cyclical mastalgia: Prevalence and associated health and behavioral factors. *Journal of Psychosomatic Obstetrics & Gynaecology, 22*(2), 71-76.

Al Alawi, A. M., & Falhammar, H. (2018). Lactation ketoacidosis: Case presentation and literature review. *BMJ Case Reports, 2018*. doi:10.1136/bcr-2017-223494

Allen, L. H. (2012). B vitamins in breast milk: Relative importance of maternal status and intake, and effects on infant status and function. *Advances in Nutrition, 3*(3), 362-369.

Allen, L. H., Donohue, J. A., & Dror, D. K. (2018). Limitations of the evidence base used to set recommended nutrient intakes for infants and lactating women. *Advances in Nutrition, 9*(supplement 1), 295S-312S.

Andersen, A. N., Lund-Andersen, C., Larsen, J. F., et al. (1982). Suppressed prolactin but normal neurophysin levels in cigarette smoking breast-feeding women. *Clinical Endocrinology (Oxford), 17*(4), 363-368.

Anderson, N. K., Beerman, K. A., McGuire, M. A., et al. (2005). Dietary fat type influences total milk fat content in lean women. *Journal of Nutrition, 135*(3), 416-421.

Anderson, P. O. (2018a). Alcohol use during breastfeeding. *Breastfeeding Medicine, 13*(5), 315-317.

Anderson, P. O. (2018b). Drugs of abuse during breastfeeding. *Breastfeeding Medicine, 13*(6), 405-407.

Anderson, P. O. (2018c). Potentially toxic foods while breastfeeding: Garlic, caffeine, mushrooms, and more. *Breastfeeding Medicine*. doi:10.1089/bfm.2018.0192

Arora, A., Manohar, N., Hayen, A., et al. (2017). Determinants of breastfeeding initiation among mothers in Sydney, Australia: Findings from a birth cohort study. *International Breastfeeding Journal, 12*, 39.

Arthur, P. G., Smith, M., & Hartmann, P. E. (1989). Milk lactose, citrate, and glucose as markers of lactogenesis in normal and diabetic women. *Journal of Pediatric Gastroenterology and Nutrition, 9*(4), 488-496.

Arvola, T., Ruuska, T., Keranen, J., et al. (2006). Rectal bleeding in infancy: Clinical, allergological, and microbiological examination. *Pediatrics, 117*(4), e760-768.

Aryal, K. K., Thapa, N., Mehata, S., et al. (2016). Alcohol consumption during pregnancy and postpartum period and its predictors in Sindhupalchowk District, Nepal. *Journal of Nepal Health Research Council, 14*(34), 143-153.

Astley, S. J., & Little, R. E. (1990). Maternal marijuana use during lactation and infant development at one year. *Neurotoxicology and Teratology, 12*(2), 161-168.

Aumeistere, L., Ciprovica, I., Zavadska, D., et al. (2019). Impact of maternal diet on human milk composition among lactating women in Latvia. *Medicina (Kaunas), 55*(5).

Aumeistere, L., Ciprovica, I., Zavadska, D., et al. (2018). Fish intake reflects on DHA level in breast milk among lactating women in Latvia. *International Breastfeeding Journal, 13*, 33.

Babyak, M., Blumenthal, J. A., Herman, S., et al. (2000). Exercise treatment for major depression: Maintenance of therapeutic benefit at 10 months. *Psychosomatic Medicine, 62*(5), 633-638.

Baheiraei, A., Shamsi, A., Khaghani, S., et al. (2014). The effects of maternal passive smoking on maternal milk lipid. *Acta Medica Iranica, 52*(4), 280-285.

Bajanowski, T., Brinkmann, B., Mitchell, E. A., et al. (2008). Nicotine and cotinine in infants dying from sudden infant death syndrome. *International Journal of Legal Medicine, 122*(1), 23-28.

Baker, J. L., Michaelsen, K. F., Sorensen, T. I., et al. (2007). High prepregnant body mass index is associated with early termination of full and any breastfeeding in Danish women. *American Journal of Clinical Nutrition, 86*(2), 404-411.

Baker, T., Datta, P., Rewers-Felkins, K., et al. (2018). Transfer of inhaled cannabis Into human breast milk. *Obstetrics & Gynecology, 131*(5), 783-788.

Baldassarre, M. E., Palladino, V., Amoruso, A., et al. (2018). Rationale of probiotic supplementation during pregnancy and neonatal period. *Nutrients, 10*(11).

Baroni, L., Goggi, S., Battaglino, R., et al. (2018). Vegan nutrition for mothers and children: Practical tools for healthcare providers. *Nutrients, 11*(1).

Barreiro, R., Regal, P., Lopez-Racamonde, O., et al. (2018). Comparison of the fatty acid profile of Spanish infant formulas and Galician women breast milk. *Journal of Physiology and Biochemistry, 74*(1), 127-138.

Bazzano, A. N., Potts, K. S., & Mulugeta, A. (2018). How do pregnant and lactating women, and young children, experience religious food restriction at the community level? A qualitative study of fasting traditions and feeding behaviors in four regions of Ethiopia. *PLoS One, 13*(12), e0208408.

Becker, A. B., Manfreda, J., Ferguson, A. C., et al. (1999). Breast-feeding and environmental tobacco smoke exposure. *Archives of Pediatrics and Adolescent Medicine, 153*(7), 689-691.

Beckerman, J. P., Slade, E., & Ventura, A. K. (2019). Maternal diet during lactation and breast-feeding practices have synergistic association with child diet at 6 years. *Public Health Nutrition, 1-9*.

Berlin, C. M., Jr., & Daniel, C. H. (1981). Excretion of theobromine in human milk and saliva. *Pediatric Research, 15*, 492.

Berlin, C. M., Jr., Denson, H. M., Daniel, C. H., et al. (1984). Disposition of dietary caffeine in milk, saliva, and plasma of lactating women. *Pediatrics, 73*(1), 59-63.

Bertini, G., Elia, S., Lori, S., et al. (2019). Abnormal neurological soft signs in babies born to smoking mothers were associated with lower breastfeeding for first three months. *Acta Paediatrica, 108*(7), 1256-1261.

Bertrand, K. A., Hanan, N. J., Honerkamp-Smith, G., et al. (2018). Marijuana use by breastfeeding mothers and cannabinoid concentrations in breast milk. *Pediatrics, 142*(3).

Bigman, G., Wilkinson, A. V., Homedes, N., et al. (2018). Body image dissatisfaction, obesity and their associations with breastfeeding in Mexican women, a cross-sectional study. *Maternal and Child Health Journal, 22*(12), 1815-1825.

Bilkei-Gorzo, A. (2012). The endocannabinoid system in normal and pathological brain ageing. *Philosophical Transactions of the Royal Society B: Biological Sciences (London), 367*(1607), 3326-3341.

Blumenthal, J. A., Babyak, M. A., Doraiswamy, P. M., et al. (2007). Exercise and pharmacotherapy in the treatment of major depressive disorder. *Psychosomatic Medicine, 69*(7), 587-596.

Bo, K., Artal, R., Barakat, R., et al. (2018). Exercise and pregnancy in recreational and elite athletes: 2016/2017 evidence summary from the IOC expert group meeting, Lausanne. Part 5. Recommendations for health professionals and active women. *British Journal of Sports Medicine, 52*(17), 1080-1085.

Bogen, D. L., Perel, J. M., Helsel, J. C., et al. (2011). Estimated infant exposure to enantiomer-specific methadone levels in breastmilk. *Breastfeeding Medicine, 6*(6), 377-384.

Bone, A., Ncube, F., Nichols, T., et al. (2008). Body piercing in England: A survey of piercing at sites other than earlobe. *British Medical Journal, 336*(7658), 1426-1428.

Breslow, R. A., Falk, D. E., Fein, S. B., et al. (2007). Alcohol consumption among breastfeeding women. *Breastfeeding Medicine, 2*(3), 152-157.

Buonfiglio, D. C., Ramos-Lobo, A. M., Freitas, V. M., et al. (2016). Obesity impairs lactation performance in mice by inducing prolactin resistance. *Scientific Reports, 6*, 22421.

Butte, N. F., & King, J. C. (2005). Energy requirements during pregnancy and lactation. *Public Health Nutrition, 8*(7A), 1010-1027.

Bystrova, K., Widstrom, A. M., Matthiesen, A. S., et al. (2007). Early lactation performance in primiparous and multiparous women in relation to different maternity home practices. A randomised trial in St. Petersburg. *International Breastfeeding Journal, 2*, 9.

Cabana, M. D., McKean, M., Caughey, A. B., et al. (2017). Early probiotic supplementation for eczema and asthma prevention: A randomized controlled trial. *Pediatrics, 140*(3).

Canivet, C. A., Ostergren, P. O., Jakobsson, I. L., et al. (2008). Infantile colic, maternal smoking and infant feeding at 5 weeks of age. *Scandanavian Journal of Public Health, 36*(3), 284-291.

Caplinger, P., Cooney, A. T., Bledsoe, C., et al. (2015). Breastfeeding outcomes following bariatric surgery. *Clinical Lactation, 6*(4), 144-152.

Carey, G. B., Quinn, T. J., & Goodwin, S. E. (1997). Breast milk composition after exercise of different intensities. *Journal of Human Lactation, 13*(2), 115-120.

Carlsen, S. M., Jacobsen, G., & Romundstad, P. (2006). Maternal testosterone levels during pregnancy are associated with offspring size at birth. *European Journal of Endocrinology, 155*(2), 365-370.

Carlson, H. E., Wasser, H. L., & Reidelberger, R. D. (1985). Beer-induced prolactin secretion: A clinical and laboratory study of the role of salsolinol. *Journal of Clinical Endocrinology and Metabolism, 60*(4), 673-677.

Casella, E. B., Valente, M., de Navarro, J. M., et al. (2005). Vitamin B12 deficiency in infancy as a cause of developmental regression. *Brain & Development, 27*(8), 592-594.

Celiker, M. Y., & Chawla, A. (2009). Congenital B12 deficiency following maternal gastric bypass. *Journal of Perinatology, 29*(9), 640-642.

Chamberlin, T., D'Amato, J. V., & Arendt, L. M. (2017). Obesity reversibly depletes the basal cell population and enhances mammary epithelial cell estrogen receptor alpha expression and progenitor activity. *Breast Cancer Research, 19*(1), 128.

Chan, Y. L., Saad, S., Pollock, C., et al. (2016). Impact of maternal cigarette smoke exposure on brain inflammation and oxidative stress in male mice offspring. *Scientific Reports, 6,* 25881.

Chaney, N. E., Franke, J., & Wadlington, W. B. (1988). Cocaine convulsions in a breast-feeding baby. *Journal of Pediatrics, 112*(1), 134-135.

Chapman, D. J., Doughty, K., Mullin, E. M., et al. (2016). Reliability of lactation assessment tools applied to overweight and obese women. *Journal of Human Lactation, 32*(2), 269-276.

Chapman, D. J., & Perez-Escamilla, R. (1999). Identification of risk factors for delayed onset of lactation. *Journal of the American Dietetic Association, 99*(4), 450-454; quiz 455-456.

Chasnoff, I. J., Lewis, D. E., & Squires, L. (1987). Cocaine intoxication in a breast-fed infant. *Pediatrics, 80*(6), 836-838.

Chatzimichael, A., Tsalkidis, A., Cassimos, D., et al. (2007). The role of breastfeeding and passive smoking on the development of severe bronchiolitis in infants. *Minerva Pediatrica, 59*(3), 199-206.

Chien, Y. C., Liu, J. F., Huang, Y. J., et al. (2005). Alcohol levels in Chinese lactating mothers after consumption of alcoholic diet during postpartum "doing-the-month" ritual. *Alcohol, 37*(3), 143-150.

Chomchai, C., Chomchai, S., & Kitsommart, R. (2016). Transfer of methamphetamine (MA) into breast milk and urine of postpartum women who smoked MA tablets during pregnancy: Implications for initiation of breastfeeding. *Journal of Human Lactation, 32*(2), 333-339.

Chowdhury, R., Sinha, B., Sankar, M. J., et al. (2015). Breastfeeding and maternal health outcomes: A systematic review and meta-analysis. *Acta Paediatrica, 104*(467), 96-113.

Cicero, T. J., Ellis, M. S., Surratt, H. L., et al. (2014). The changing face of heroin use in the United States: A retrospective analysis of the past 50 years. *JAMA Psychiatry, 71*(7), 821-826.

Cimatti, A. G., Martini, S., Munarini, A., et al. (2018). Maternal supplementation with krill oil during breastfeeding and long-chain polyunsaturated fatty acids (LCPUFAs) composition of human milk: A feasibility study. *Frontiers in Pediatrics, 6,* 407.

Claesson, I. M., Larsson, L., Steen, L., et al. (2018). "You just need to leave the room when you breastfeed" Breastfeeding experiences among obese women in Sweden - A qualitative study. *BMC Pregnancy & Childbirth, 18*(1), 39.

Clark, R. R. S. (2019). Breastfeeding in women on opioid maintenance therapy: A review of policy and practice. *Journal of Midwifery & Women's Health, 64*(5), 545-558.

Clyne, P. S., & Kulczycki, A., Jr. (1991). Human breast milk contains bovine IgG. Relationship to infant colic? *Pediatrics, 87*(4), 439-444.

Cobo, E. (1973). Effect of different doses of ethanol on the milk-ejecting reflex in lactating women. *American Journal of Obstetrics & Gynecology, 115*(6), 817-821.

Cohen, S. S., Alexander, D. D., Krebs, N. F., et al. (2018). Factors associated with breastfeeding initiation and continuation: A meta-analysis. *Journal of Pediatrics, 203,* 190-196 e121.

Colleran, H. L., Hiatt, A., Wideman, L., et al. (2019). The effect of an exercise intervention during early lactation on bone mineral density during the first year postpartum. *Journal of Physical Activity & Health, 16*(3), 197-204.

Colling, K., Ward, L., Beck, A., et al. (2019). Contribution of maternal obesity to medically indicated and elective formula supplementation in a baby-friendly hospital. *Breastfeeding Medicine, 14*(4), 236-242.

Cooke-Hubley, S., Gao, Z., Mugford, G., et al. (2019). Parity and lactation are not associated with incident fragility fractures or radiographic vertebral fractures over 16 years of follow-up: Canadian Multicentre Osteoporosis Study (CaMos). *Archives of Osteoporosis, 14*(1), 49.

Cooper, R. L., & Cooper, M. M. (1996). Red pepper-induced dermatitis in breast-fed infants. *Dermatology, 193*(1), 61-62.

Crandall, C. J., Liu, J., Cauley, J., et al. (2017). Associations of parity, breastfeeding, and fractures in the Women's Health Observational Study. *Obstetrics & Gynecology, 130*(1), 171-180.

Cressman, A. M., Koren, G., Pupco, A., et al. (2012). Maternal cocaine use during breastfeeding. *Canadian Family Physician, 58*(11), 1218-1219.

Cross, N. A., Hillman, L. S., Allen, S. H., et al. (1995). Calcium homeostasis and bone metabolism during pregnancy, lactation, and postweaning: A longitudinal study. *American Journal of Clinical Nutrition, 61*(3), 514-523.

Crume, T. L., Juhl, A. L., Brooks-Russell, A., et al. (2018). Cannabis use during the perinatal period in a state with legalized recreational and medical marijuana: The association between maternal characteristics, breastfeeding patterns, and neonatal outcomes. *Journal of Pediatrics, 197,* 90-96.

Dahlstrom, A., Lundell, B., Curvall, M., et al. (1990). Nicotine and cotinine concentrations in the nursing mother and her infant. *Acta Paediatrica Scandanavica, 79*(2), 142-147.

Daley, A. J., Thomas, A., Cooper, H., et al. (2012). Maternal exercise and growth in breastfed infants: A meta-analysis of randomized controlled trials. *Pediatrics, 130*(1), 108-114.

De Rosa, G., Corsello, S. M., Ruffilli, M. P., et al. (1981). Prolactin secretion after beer. *Lancet, 2*(8252), 934.

Demirci, J. R., Bogen, D. L., & Klionsky, Y. (2015). Breastfeeding and methadone therapy: The maternal experience. *Substance Abuse, 36*(2), 203-208.

Desalegn, B. B., Lambert, C., Riedel, S., et al. (2018). Ethiopian orthodox fasting and lactating mothers: Longitudinal study on dietary pattern and nutritional status in rural Tigray, Ethiopia. *International Journal of Environmental Research and Public Health, 15*(8).

Dewey, K. G., Lovelady, C. A., Nommsen-Rivers, L. A., et al. (1994). A randomized study of the effects of aerobic exercise by lactating women on breast-milk volume and composition. *New England Journal of Medicine, 330*(7), 449-453.

Dewey, K. G., & McCrory, M. A. (1994). Effects of dieting and physical activity on pregnancy and lactation. *American Journal of Clinical Nutrition, 59*(2 Suppl), 446S-452S; discussion 452S-453S.

Dewey, K. G., Nommsen-Rivers, L. A., Heinig, M. J., et al. (2003). Risk factors for suboptimal infant breastfeeding behavior, delayed onset of lactation, and excess neonatal weight loss. *Pediatrics, 112*(3 Pt 1), 607-619.

Djulus, J., Moretti, M., & Koren, G. (2005). Marijuana use and breastfeeding. *Canadian Family Physician, 51,* 349-350.

Doerzbacher, M., & Chang, Y. P. (2019). Supporting breastfeeding for women on opioid maintenance therapy: A systematic review. *Journal of Perinatology, 39*(9), 1159-1164.

Dror, D. K., & Allen, L. H. (2018). Vitamin B-12 in human milk: A systematic review. *Advances in Nutrition, 9*(supplement_1), 358S-366S.

Du, Y., Ellert, U., Lampert, T., et al. (2012). Association of breastfeeding and exposure to maternal smoking during pregnancy with children's general health status later in childhood. *Breastfeeding Medicine, 7*(6), 504-513.

Dusdieker, L. B., Booth, B. M., Stumbo, P. J., et al. (1985). Effect of supplemental fluids on human milk production. *Journal of Pediatrics, 106*(2), 207-211.

Dusdieker, L. B., Hemingway, D. L., & Stumbo, P. J. (1994). Is milk production impaired by dieting during lactation? *American Journal of Clinical Nutrition, 59*(4), 833-840.

Easter, A., Solmi, F., Bye, A., et al. (2015). Antenatal and postnatal psychopathology among women with current and past eating disorders: Longitudinal patterns. *European Eating Disorder Review, 23*(1), 19-27.

EFSA. (2015). Scientific opinion on the safety of caffeine. *European Food Safety Authority Journal, 13*(5), 4102.

Einarson, A., & Riordan, S. (2009). Smoking in pregnancy and lactation: A review of risks and cessation strategies. *European Journal of Clinical Pharmacology, 65*(4), 325-330.

El, C., & Celikkaya, M. E. (2019). Infants with vitamin B12 deficiency-related neurological dysfunction and the effect of maternal nutrition. *Annals of Medical Research, 26*(1), 63-67.

Eren, T., Aslan, A., Ozemir, I. A., et al. (2016). Factors affecting mastalgia. *Breast Care (Basel), 11*(3), 188-193.

Essa, A. R., Browne, E. P., Punska, E. C., et al. (2018). Dietary intervention to increase fruit and vegetable consumption in breastfeeding women: A pilot randomized trial measuring inflammatory markers in breast milk. *Journal of the Academy of Nutrition and Dietetics, 118*(12), 2287-2295.

Evans, J., & le Grange, D. (1995). Body size and parenting in eating disorders: A comparative study of the attitudes of mothers towards their children. *International Journal of Eating Disorders, 18*(1), 39-48.

Favara, M. T., Carola, D., Jensen, E., et al. (2019). Maternal breast milk feeding and length of treatment in infants with neonatal abstinence syndrome. *Journal of Perinatology, 39*(6), 876-882.

Fernandez-Lopez, D., Lizasoain, I., Moro, M. A., et al. (2013). Cannabinoids: Well-suited candidates for the treatment of perinatal brain injury. *Brain Science, 3*(3), 1043-1059.

Ferreira, C. T., & Seidman, E. (2007). Food allergy: A practical update from the gastroenterological viewpoint. *Jornal de Pediatria (Rio J), 83*(1), 7-20.

Fisher, W., Wang, J., George, N. I., et al. (2016). Dietary iodine sufficiency and moderate insufficiency in the lactating mother and nursing infant: A computational perspective. *PLoS One, 11*(3), e0149300.

Flores, T. R., Mielke, G. I., Wendt, A., et al. (2018). Prepregnancy weight excess and cessation of exclusive breastfeeding: A systematic review and meta-analysis. *European Journal of Clinical Nutrition, 72*(4), 480-488.

Fogarty, S., Elmir, R., Hay, P., et al. (2018). The experience of women with an eating disorder in the perinatal period: A meta-ethnographic study. *BMC Pregnancy & Childbirth, 18*(1), 121.

Follin, C., Link, K., Wiebe, T., et al. (2013). Prolactin insufficiency but normal thyroid hormone levels after cranial radiotherapy in long-term survivors of childhood leukaemia. *Clinical Endocrinology (Oxford), 79*(1), 71-78.

Gabriel, A., Gabriel, K. R., & Lawrence, R. A. (1986). Cultural values and biomedical knowledge: Choices in infant feeding. Analysis of a survey. *Social Science and Medicine, 23*(5), 501-509.

Gaitan, A. V., Wood, J. T., Zhang, F., et al. (2018). Endocannabinoid metabolome characterization of transitional and mature human milk. *Nutrients, 10*(9).

Garner, C. D., Ratcliff, S. L., Devine, C. M., et al. (2014). Health professionals' experiences providing breastfeeding-related care for obese women. *Breastfeeding Medicine, 9*(10), 503-509.

Gascoin, G., Gerard, M., Salle, A., et al. (2017). Risk of low birth weight and micronutrient deficiencies in neonates from mothers after gastric bypass: A case control study. *Surgery for Obesity and Related Diseases, 13*(8), 1384-1391.

Genna, C. W. (2019). Alcohol use during lactation and offspring outcomes. *Clinical Lactation, 10*(2), 81-86.

Gibson, L., & Porter, M. (2018). Drinking or smoking while breastfeeding and later cognition in children. *Pediatrics, 142*(2).

Giglia, R. C., & Binns, C. W. (2008). Alcohol, pregnancy and breastfeeding; A comparison of the 1995 and 2001 National Health Survey data. *Breastfeeding Review, 16*(1), 17-24.

Giglia, R. C., Binns, C. W., & Alfonso, H. S. (2006). Which women stop smoking during pregnancy and the effect on breastfeeding duration. *BMC Public Health, 6,* 195.

Giles, A. R., Phillipps, B., Darroch, F. E., et al. (2016). Elite distance runners and breastfeeding. *Journal of Human Lactation, 32*(4), 627-632.

Gimenes, J. C., Nicoletti, C. F., de Souza Pinhel, M. A., et al. (2018). Nutritional status of children from women with previously bariatric surgery. *Obesity Surgery, 28*(4), 990-995.

Giovannini, M., Radaelli, G., Banderali, G., et al. (2007). Low prepregnant body mass index and breastfeeding practices. *Journal of Human Lactation, 23*(1), 44-51.

Goldade, K., Nichter, M., Adrian, S., et al. (2008). Breastfeeding and smoking among low-income women: Results of a longitudinal qualitative study. *Birth, 35*(3), 230-240.

Gower, S., Bartu, A., Ilett, K. F., et al. (2014). The wellbeing of infants exposed to buprenorphine via breast milk at 4 weeks of age. *Journal of Human Lactation, 30*(2), 217-223.

Grange, D. K., & Finlay, J. L. (1994). Nutritional vitamin B12 deficiency in a breastfed infant following maternal gastric bypass. *Pediatric Hematology and Oncology, 11*(3), 311-318.

Greiner, T. (2019a). Alcohol and breastfeeding, a review of the issues. *World Nutrition, 10*(1), 63-88.

Greiner, T. (2019b). Effect of differently worded messages about alcohol on intent to breastfeed among university women in South Korea: A survey. *World Nutrition, 10*(2), 22-39.

Grossman, M., Seashore, C., & Holmes, A. V. (2017). Neonatal abstinence syndrome management: A review of recent evidence. *Reviews on Recent Clinical Trials, 12*(4), 226-232.

Guedes, H. T., & Souza, L. S. (2009). Exposure to maternal smoking in the first year of life interferes in breast-feeding protective effect against the onset of respiratory allergy from birth to 5 yr. *Pediatric Allergy and Immunology, 20*(1), 30-34.

Haastrup, M. B., Pottegard, A., & Damkier, P. (2014). Alcohol and breastfeeding. *Basic & Clinical Pharmacology & Toxicology, 114*(2), 168-173.

Hale, T. W. (2019). *Hale's Medications & Mothers' Milk: A Manual of Lactational Pharmacology* (18th ed.). New York, NY: Springer Publishing Company.

Handzlik-Orlik, G., Holecki, M., Orlik, B., et al. (2015). Nutrition management of the post-bariatric surgery patient. *Nutrition in Clinical Practice, 30*(3), 383-392.

Hartmann-Boyce, J., Chepkin, S. C., Ye, W., et al. (2018). Nicotine replacement therapy versus control for smoking cessation. *Cochrane Database of Systematic Reviews, 5,* CD000146. doi:10.1002/14651858.CD000146.pub5

Hatsu, I. E., McDougald, D. M., & Anderson, A. K. (2008). Effect of infant feeding on maternal body composition. *International Breastfeeding Journal, 3,* 18.

Hausner, H., Bredie, W. L., Molgaard, C., et al. (2008). Differential transfer of dietary flavour compounds into human breast milk. *Physiology & Behavior, 95*(1-2), 118-124.

HealthCounciloftheNetherlands. (2005). *Risks of Alcohol Consumption Related to Conception, Pregnancy and Breastfeeding.* (2004/22). Hague, The Netherlands: Health Council of the Netherlands Retrieved from **https://www.researchgate.net/publication/46690960_Risks_of_Alcohol_Consumption_Related_to_Conception_Pregnancy_and_Breastfeeding**.

Hilson, J. A., Rasmussen, K. M., & Kjolhede, C. L. (2004). High prepregnant body mass index is associated with poor lactation outcomes among white, rural women independent of psychosocial and demographic correlates. *Journal of Human Lactation, 20*(1), 18-29.

Ho, E., Collantes, A., Kapur, B. M., et al. (2001). Alcohol and breast feeding: Calculation of time to zero level in milk. *Biology of the Neonate, 80*(3), 219-222.

Holmberg-Marttila, D., Sievanen, H., Sarkkinen, E., et al. (2001). Do combined elimination diet and prolonged breastfeeding of an atopic infant jeopardise maternal bone health? *Clinical and Experimental Allergy, 31*(1), 88-94.

Holmes, A. V., Atwood, E. C., Whalen, B., et al. (2016). Rooming-in to treat neonatal abstinence syndrome: Improved family-centered care at lower cost. *Pediatrics, 137*(6).

Hoover, K. L. (2008). Maternal obesity: Problems of breastfeeding with large breasts. *Women's Health Report,* pp. 6,10.

Hopkinson, J. (2007). Nutrition in lactation. In T. W. Hale & P. Hartmann (Eds.), *Hale & Hartmann's Textbook of Human Lactation* (pp. 381-382). Amarillo, TX: Hale Publishing.

Host, A., Husby, S., & Osterballe, O. (1988). A prospective study of cow's milk allergy in exclusively breast-fed infants. Incidence, pathogenetic role of early inadvertent exposure to cow's milk formula, and characterization of bovine milk protein in human milk. *Acta Paediatrica Scandanavica, 77*(5), 663-670.

Howard, M. B., Wachman, E., Levesque, E. M., et al. (2018). The joys and frustrations of breastfeeding and rooming-in among mothers with opioid use disorder: A qualitative study. *Hospital Pediatrics, 8*(12), 761-768.

Huang, Y., Ouyang, Y. Q., & Redding, S. R. (2019). Maternal prepregnancy body mass index, gestational weight gain, and cessation of breastfeeding: A systematic review and meta-analysis. *Breastfeeding Medicine, 14*(6), 366-374.

Hudak, M. L., Tan, R. C.; Committee On, D., et al. (2012). Neonatal drug withdrawal. *Pediatrics, 129*(2), e540-560.

Humphrey, S. (2003). *The Nursing Mother's Herbal.* Minneapolis, MN: Fairview Press.

Ilett, K. F., Hackett, L. P., Gower, S., et al. (2012). Estimated dose exposure of the neonate to buprenorphine and its metabolite norbuprenorphine via breastmilk during maternal buprenorphine substitution treatment. *Breastfeeding Medicine, 7,* 269-274.

Ilett, K. F., Hale, T. W., Page-Sharp, M., et al. (2003). Use of nicotine patches in breastfeeding mothers: Transfer of nicotine and cotinine into human milk. *Clinical Pharmacology & Therapeutics, 74*(6), 516-524.

IOM. (2005). *Dietary reference intakes for energy, carbohydrates, fiber, fat, fatty acids, cholesterol, protein, and amino acids.* Washington, DC: National Academy Press.

Jakobsson, I., & Lindberg, T. (1983). Cow's milk proteins cause infantile colic in breast-fed infants: A double-blind crossover study. *Pediatrics, 71*(2), 268-271.

Jans, G., Devlieger, R., De Preter, V., et al. (2018). Bariatric surgery does not appear to affect women's breast-milk composition. *Journal of Nutrition, 148*(7), 1096-1102.

Jans, G., Matthys, C., Lannoo, M., et al. (2015). Breast milk macronutrient composition after bariatric surgery. *Obesity Surgery, 25*(5), 938-941.

Jansson, L. M., Choo, R., Velez, M. L., et al. (2008). Methadone maintenance and long-term lactation. *Breastfeeding Medicine, 3*(1), 34-37.

Jansson, L. M., Spencer, N., McConnell, K., et al. (2016). Maternal buprenorphine maintenance and lactation. *Journal of Human Lactation, 32*(4), 675-681.

Jedrychowski, W., Perera, F., Mroz, E., et al. (2008). Prenatal exposure to passive smoking and duration of breastfeeding in nonsmoking women: Krakow inner city prospective cohort study. *Archives of Gynecology and Obstetrics, 278*(5), 411-417.

Jevitt, C., Hernandez, I., & Groer, M. (2007). Lactation complicated by overweight and obesity: Supporting the Mother and Newborn. *Journal of Midwifery and Women's Health, 52*(6), 606-613.

Kair, L. R., & Colaizy, T. T. (2016a). Obese mothers have lower odds of experiencing pro-breastfeeding hospital practices than mothers of normal weight: CDC Pregnancy Risk Assessment Monitoring System (PRAMS), 2004-2008. *Maternal and Child Health Journal, 20*(3), 593-601.

Kair, L. R., & Colaizy, T. T. (2016b). When breast milk alone is not enough: Barriers to breastfeeding continuation among overweight and obese mothers. *Journal of Human Lactation, 32*(2), 250-257.

Kamikawa, A., Ichii, O., Yamaji, D., et al. (2009). Diet-induced obesity disrupts ductal development in the mammary glands of nonpregnant mice. *Developmental Dynamics, 238*(5), 1092-1099.

Karmaus, W., Dobai, A. L., Ogbuanu, I., et al. (2008). Long-term effects of breastfeeding, maternal smoking during pregnancy, and recurrent lower respiratory tract infections on asthma in children. *Journal of Asthma, 45*(8), 688-695.

Kaufman, K. R., Petrucha, R. A., Pitts, F. N., Jr., et al. (1983). PCP in amniotic fluid and breast milk: Case report. *Journal of Clinical Psychiatry, 44*(7), 269-270.

Kaymaz, N., & Yildirim, S. (2016). Comment on the article "When breast milk alone is not enough: Barriers to breastfeeding continuation among overweight and obese mothers." *Journal of Human Lactation, 32*(3), 574.

Keikha, M., Bahreynian, M., Saleki, M., et al. (2017). Macro- and micronutrients of human milk composition: Are they related to maternal diet? A comprehensive systematic review. *Breastfeeding Medicine, 12*(9), 517-527.

Kelly, E., DunnGalvin, G., Murphy, B. P., et al. (2019). Formula supplementation remains a risk for cow's milk allergy in breast-fed infants. *Pediatric Allergy and Immunology.* doi:10.1111/pai.13108

Kent, J. C., Arthur, P. G., Mitoulas, L. R., et al. (2009). Why calcium in breastmilk is independent of maternal dietary calcium and vitamin D. *Breastfeeding Review, 17*(2), 5-11.

King, J. C. (2001). Effect of reproduction on the bioavailability of calcium, zinc and selenium. *Journal of Nutrition, 131*(4 Suppl), 1355S-1358S.

Klonoff-Cohen, H. S., Edelstein, S. L., Lefkowitz, E. S., et al. (1995). The effect of passive smoking and tobacco exposure through breast milk on sudden infant death syndrome. *Journal of the American Medical Association, 273*(10), 795-798.

Kolasa, K. M., Firnhaber, G., & Haven, K. (2015). Diet for a healthy lactating woman. *Clinical Obstetrics and Gynecology, 58*(4), 893-901.

Koletzko, B., & Lehner, F. (2000). Beer and breastfeeding. *Advances in Experimental Medicine and Biology, 478,* 23-28.

Koren, G. (2002). Drinking alcohol while breastfeeding. Will it harm my baby? *Canadian Family Physician, 48,* 39-41.

Kovacs, C. S. (2016). Maternal mineral and bone metabolism during pregnancy, lactation, and post-weaning recovery. *Physiological Reviews, 96*(2), 449-547.

Kugyelka, J. G., Rasmussen, K. M., & Frongillo, E. A. (2004). Maternal obesity is negatively associated with breastfeeding success among Hispanic but not Black women. *Journal of Nutrition, 134*(7), 1746-1753.

Kvenshagen, B., Halvorsen, R., & Jacobsen, M. (2008). Adverse reactions to milk in infants. *Acta Paediatrica, 97*(2), 196-200.

Ladomenou, F., Kafatos, A., & Galanakis, E. (2009). Environmental tobacco smoke exposure as a risk factor for infections in infancy. *Acta Paediatrica, 98*(7), 1137-1141.

Larson-Meyer, D. E. (2002). Effect of postpartum exercise on mothers and their offspring: A review of the literature. *Obesity Research, 10*(8), 841-853.

Lauwers, J., & Swisher, A. (2015). Special counseling circumstances. In *Counseling the Nursing Mother* (6th ed., pp. 475-491). Burlington, MA: Jones & Bartlett Learning.

Lawrence, R. A., & Lawrence, R. M. (2016). *Breastfeeding: A Guide for the Medical Profession* (8th ed.). Philadelphia, PA: Elsevier.

Lawton, M. E. (1985). Alcohol in breast milk. *Australian and New Zealand Journal of Obstetrics and Gynaecology, 25*(1), 71-73.

Lazare, F. B., Brand, D. A., Fazzari, M. J., et al. (2019). Maternal dairy consumption and hematochezia in exclusively breastfed infants. *Journal of Human Lactation.* doi:10.1177/089033441983.

Lee, N. (1995). More on pierced nipples. *Journal of Human Lactation, 11*(2), 89.

Lee, S., & Kelleher, S. L. (2016). Biological underpinnings of breastfeeding challenges: The role of genetics, diet, and environment on lactation physiology. *American Journal of Physiology-Endocrinology and Metabolism, 311*(2), E405-422.

Leung, A. M., Pearce, E. N., & Braverman, L. E. (2011). Iodine nutrition in pregnancy and lactation. *Endocrinology & Metabolism Clinics of North America, 40*(4), 765-777.

Lipchock, S. V., Reed, D. R., & Mennella, J. A. (2011). The gustatory and olfactory systems during infancy: Implications for development of feeding behaviors in the high-risk neonate. *Clinical Perinatology, 38*(4), 627-641.

Little, L., & Lowkes, E. (2000). Critical issues in the care of pregnant women with eating disorders and the impact on their children. *Journal of Midwifery & Women's Health, 45*(4), 301-307.

Little, R. E., Anderson, K. W., Ervin, C. H., et al. (1989). Maternal alcohol use during breast-feeding and infant mental and motor development at one year. *New England Journal of Medicine, 321*(7), 425-430.

Little, R. E., Northstone, K., & Golding, J. (2002). Alcohol, breastfeeding, and development at 18 months. *Pediatrics, 109*(5), E72-72.

Liu, J., Rosenberg, K. D., & Sandoval, A. P. (2006). Breastfeeding duration and perinatal cigarette smoking in a population-based cohort. *American Journal of Public Health, 96*(2), 309-314.

Liu, Y. Q., Qian, Z., Wang, J., et al. (2016). Breastfeeding modifies the effects of environment tobacco smoke exposure on respiratory diseases and symptoms in Chinese children: The Seven Northeast Cities Study. *Indoor Air, 26*(4), 614-622.

Logan, C., Zittel, T., Striebel, S., et al. (2016). Changing societal and lifestyle factors and breastfeeding patterns over time. *Pediatrics, 137*(5).

Lok, K. Y. W., Wang, M. P., Chan, V. H. S., et al. (2018). Effect of secondary cigarette smoke from household members on breastfeeding duration: A prospective cohort study. *Breastfeeding Medicine, 13*(6), 412-417.

Lovelady, C. A. (2004). The impact of energy restriction and exercise in lactating women. *Advances in Experimental Medicine and Biology, 554,* 115-120.

Lovelady, C. A., Fuller, C. J., Geigerman, C. M., et al. (2004). Immune status of physically active women during lactation. *Medicine & Science in Sports & Exercise, 36*(6), 1001-1007.

Lovelady, C. A., Garner, K. E., Moreno, K. L., et al. (2000). The effect of weight loss in overweight, lactating women on the growth of their infants. *New England Journal of Medicine, 342*(7), 449-453.

Lovelady, C. A., Hunter, C. P., & Geigerman, C. (2003). Effect of exercise on immunologic factors in breast milk. *Pediatrics, 111*(2), E148-152.

Lovelady, C. A., Lonnerdal, B., & Dewey, K. G. (1990). Lactation performance of exercising women. *American Journal of Clinical Nutrition, 52*(1), 103-109.

Lovelady, C. A., Nommsen-Rivers, L. A., McCrory, M. A., et al. (1995). Effects of exercise on plasma lipids and metabolism of lactating women. *Medicine & Science in Sports & Exercise, 27*(1), 22-28.

Lucero, C. A., Moss, D. R., Davies, E. D., et al. (2009). An examination of attitudes, knowledge, and clinical practices among Pennsylvania pediatricians regarding breastfeeding and smoking. *Breastfeeding Medicine, 4*(2), 83-89.

Luck, W., & Nau, H. (1984). Nicotine and cotinine concentrations in serum and milk of nursing smokers. *British Journal of Clinical Pharmacology, 18*(1), 9-15.

Luck, W., & Nau, H. (1985). Nicotine and cotinine concentrations in serum and urine of infants exposed via passive smoking or milk from smoking mothers. *Journal of Pediatrics, 107*(5), 816-820.

MacMillan Uribe, A. L., & Olson, B. H. (2019). Exploring healthy eating and exercise behaviors among low-income breastfeeding mothers. *Journal of Human Lactation, 35*(1), 59-70.

Mallan, K. M., Daniels, L. A., Byrne, R., et al. (2018). Comparing barriers to breastfeeding success in the first month for non-overweight and overweight women. *BMC Pregnancy & Childbirth, 18*(1), 461.

Mangel, L., Mimouni, F. B., Mandel, D., et al. (2019). Breastfeeding difficulties, breastfeeding duration, maternal body mass index, and breast anatomy: Are they related? *Breastfeeding Medicine, 14*(5), 342-346.

Mantaring, J., Benyacoub, J., Destura, R., et al. (2018). Effect of maternal supplement beverage with and without probiotics during pregnancy and lactation on maternal and infant health: A randomized controlled trial in the Philippines. *BMC Pregnancy & Childbirth, 18*(1), 193.

Marasco, L., & West, D. (2020). *Making More Milk: The Breastfeeding Guide to Increasing Your Milk Production* (2nd ed.). New York, NY: McGraw Hill.

Marek, E., & Kraft, W. K. (2014). Ethanol pharmacokinetics in neonates and infants. *Current Therapeutic Research, Clinical and Experimental, 76,* 90-97.

Martini, M. G., Taborelli, E., Schmidt, U., et al. (2019). Infant feeding behaviours and attitudes to feeding amongst mothers with eating disorders: A longitudinal study. *European Eating Disorders Review, 27*(2), 137-146.

Massov, L. (2015). Clinically overweight and obese mothers and low rates of breastfeeding: Exploring women's perspectives. *New Zealand College of Midwives Journal*(51), 23-29.

Mastorakou, D., Ruark, A., Weenen, H., et al. (2019). Sensory characteristics of human milk: Association between mothers' diet and milk for bitter taste. *Journal of Dairy Science, 102*(2), 1116-1130.

Matangkasombut, P., Padungpak, S., Thaloengsok, S., et al. (2017). Detection of beta-lactoglobulin in human breast-milk 7 days after cow milk ingestion. *Paediatrics and International Child Health, 37*(3), 199-203.

Mathur, G. P., Chitranshi, S., Mathur, S., et al. (1992). Lactation failure. *Indian Pediatrics, 29*(12), 1541-1544.

Matias, S. L., Dewey, K. G., Quesenberry, C. P., Jr., et al. (2014). Maternal prepregnancy obesity and insulin treatment during pregnancy are independently associated with delayed lactogenesis in women with recent gestational diabetes mellitus. *American Journal of Clinical Nutrition, 99*(1), 115-121.

May, P. A., Hasken, J. M., Blankenship, J., et al. (2016). Breastfeeding and maternal alcohol use: Prevalence and effects on child outcomes and fetal alcohol spectrum disorders. *Reproductive Toxicology, 63,* 13-21.

McCreedy, A., Bird, S., Brown, L. J., et al. (2018). Effects of maternal caffeine consumption on the breastfed child: A systematic review. *Swiss Medical Weekly, 148,* w14665.

McCrory, M. A. (2000). Aerobic exercise during lactation: Safe, healthful, and compatible. *Journal of Human Lactation, 16*(2), 95-98.

McGlothen, K. S., Cleveland, L. M., & Gill, S. L. (2018). "I'm doing the best that I can for her": Infant-feeding decisions of nothers receiving medication-assisted treatment for an opioid use disorder. *Journal of Human Lactation, 34*(3), 535-542.

McGuire, E. (2018). Nutritional consequences of bariatric surgery for pregnancy and breastfeeding. *Breastfeeding Review, 26*(3), 19-26.

McKenzie, S. A., Rasmussen, K. M., & Garner, C. D. (2018). Experiences and perspectives about breastfeeding in "public": A qualitative exploration among normal-weight and obese mothers. *Journal of Human Lactation, 34*(4), 760-767.

McQueen, K., Taylor, C., & Murphy-Oikonen, J. (2019). Systematic review of newborn feeding method and outcomes related to neonatal abstinence syndrome. *Journal of Obstetric, Gynecologic & Neonatal Nursing, 48*(4), 398-407.

Mechoulam, R., Berry, E. M., Avraham, Y., et al. (2006). Endocannabinoids, feeding and suckling--From our perspective. *International Journal of Obesity (London), 30 Supplement 1,* S24-28.

Memis, E. Y., & Yalcin, S. S. (2019). Human milk mycotoxin contamination: Smoking exposure and breastfeeding problems. *Journal of Maternal-Fetal & Neonatal Medicine,* 1-10.

Mendelson, J. H., Mello, N. K., & Ellingboe, J. (1985). Acute effects of marihuana smoking on prolactin levels in human females. *Journal of Pharmacology and Experimental Therapeutics, 232*(1), 220-222.

Mennella, J. A. (1997). Infants' suckling responses to the flavor of alcohol in mothers' milk. *Alcoholism: Clinical and Experimental Research, 21*(4), 581-585.

Mennella, J. A. (1998). Short-term effects of maternal alcohol consumption on lactational performance. *Alcoholism, Clinical and Experimental Research, 22*(7), 1389-1392.

Mennella, J. A. (2001). Regulation of milk intake after exposure to alcohol in mothers' milk. *Alcoholism, Clinical and Experimental Research, 25*(4), 590-593.

Mennella, J. A., & Beauchamp, G. K. (1991a). Maternal diet alters the sensory qualities of human milk and the nursling's behavior. *Pediatrics, 88*(4), 737-744.

Mennella, J. A., & Beauchamp, G. K. (1991b). The transfer of alcohol to human milk. Effects on flavor and the infant's behavior. *New England Journal of Medicine, 325*(14), 981-985.

Mennella, J. A., & Beauchamp, G. K. (1991c). The transfer of alcohol to human milk. Effects on flavor and the infant's behavior. *New England Journal of Medicine, 325*(14), 981-985.

Mennella, J. A., & Beauchamp, G. K. (1993). Beer, breast feeding and folklore. *Developmental Psychobiology, 26,* 459-466.

Mennella, J. A., Daniels, L. M., & Reiter, A. R. (2017). Learning to like vegetables during breastfeeding: A randomized clinical trial of lactating mothers and infants. *American Journal of Clinical Nutrition, 106*(1), 67-76.

Mennella, J. A., & Garcia-Gomez, P. L. (2001). Sleep disturbances after acute exposure to alcohol in mothers' milk. *Alcohol, 25*(3), 153-158.

Mennella, J. A., & Gerrish, C. J. (1998). Effects of exposure to alcohol in mother's milk on infant sleep. *Pediatrics, 101*(5), E2.

Mennella, J. A., Jagnow, C. P., & Beauchamp, G. K. (2001). Prenatal and postnatal flavor learning by human infants. *Pediatrics, 107*(6), E88.

Mennella, J. A., & Pepino, M. Y. (2008). Biphasic effects of moderate drinking on prolactin during lactation. *Alcoholism: Clinical and Experimental Research, 32*(11), 1899-1908.

Mennella, J. A., Pepino, M. Y., & Teff, K. L. (2005). Acute alcohol consumption disrupts the hormonal milieu of lactating women. *Journal of Clinical Endocrinology & Metabolism, 90*(4), 1979-1985.

Mennella, J. A., Reiter, A. R., & Daniels, L. M. (2016). Vegetable and fruit acceptance during infancy: Impact of ontogeny, genetics, and early experiences. *Advances in Nutrition, 7*(1), 211S-219S.

Mennella, J. A., Yourshaw, L. M., & Morgan, L. K. (2007). Breastfeeding and smoking: Short-term effects on infant feeding and sleep. *Pediatrics, 120*(3), 497-502.

Micali, N., Simonoff, E., & Treasure, J. (2009). Infant feeding and weight in the first year of life in babies of women with eating disorders. *Journal of Pediatrics, 154*(1), 55-60.e51.

Miliku, K., Duan, Q. L., Moraes, T. J., et al. (2019). Human milk fatty acid composition is associated with dietary, genetic, sociodemographic, and environmental factors in the CHILD Cohort Study. *American Journal of Clinical Nutrition.* doi:10.1093/ajcn/nqz229

Miyai, K., Tokushige, T., & Kondo, M. (2008). Suppression of thyroid function during ingestion of seaweed "Kombu" (Laminaria japonoca) in normal Japanese adults. *Endocrine Journal, 55*(6), 1103-1108.

Mok, E., Multon, C., Piguel, L., et al. (2008). Decreased full breastfeeding, altered practices, perceptions, and infant weight change of prepregnant obese women: A need for extra support. *Pediatrics, 121*(5), e1319-1324.

Molyneaux, E., Poston, L., Ashurst-Williams, S., et al. (2014). Obesity and mental disorders during pregnancy and postpartum: A systematic review and meta-analysis. *Obstetrics & Gynecology, 123*(4), 857-867.

Moore, B. F., Sauder, K. A., Starling, A. P., et al. (2017). Exposure to secondhand smoke, exclusive breastfeeding and infant adiposity at age 5 months in the Healthy Start study. *Pediatric Obesity, 12 Supplement 1,* 111-119.

Moore, D. G., Turner, J. D., Parrott, A. C., et al. (2010). During pregnancy, recreational drug-using women stop taking ecstasy (3,4-methylenedioxy-N-methyl-amphetamine) and reduce alcohol consumption, but continue to smoke tobacco and cannabis: Initial findings from the Development and Infancy Study. *Journal of Psychopharmacology, 24*(9), 1403-1410.

Morton, J. (2019). Hands-on or hands-off when first milk matters most? *Breastfeeding Medicine, 14*(5), 295-297.

Moshammer, H., & Hutter, H. P. (2019). Breast-feeding protects children from adverse effects of environmental tobacco smoke. *International Journal of Environmental Research and Public Health, 16*(3).

Mourh, J., & Rowe, H. (2017). Marijuana and breastfeeding: Applicability of the current literature to clinical practice. *Breastfeeding Medicine, 12*(10), 582-596.

Munoz, L. M., Lonnerdal, B., Keen, C. L., et al. (1988). Coffee consumption as a factor in iron deficiency anemia among pregnant women and their infants in Costa Rica. *American Journal of Clinical Nutrition, 48*(3), 645-651.

Myr, R. (2004). Promoting, protecting, and supporting breastfeeding in a community with a high rate of tobacco use. *Journal of Human Lactation, 20*(4), 415-416.

Nafstad, P., Jaakkola, J. J., Hagen, J. A., et al. (1996). Breastfeeding, maternal smoking and lower respiratory tract infections. *European Respiratory Journal, 9*(12), 2623-2629.

Napierala, M., Mazela, J., Merritt, T. A., et al. (2016). Tobacco smoking and breastfeeding: Effect on the lactation process, breast milk composition and infant development. A critical review. *Environmental Research, 151,* 321-338.

Napierala, M., Merritt, T. A., Mazela, J., et al. (2017). The effect of tobacco smoke on oxytocin concentrations and selected oxidative stress parameters in plasma during pregnancy and post-partum — an experimental model. *Human & Experimental Toxicology, 36*(2), 135-145.

Nascimento, A. L., de Souza, A. F., de Amorim, A. C., et al. (2013). Alcohol intake in lactating women assisted in a University Hospital. *Revista Paulista de Pediatria, 31*(2), 198-204.

Nehlig, A., Debry, G. (1994). Consequences on the newborn of chronic maternal consumption of coffee during gestation and lactation: A review. *Journal of the American College of Nutrition, 13*(1), 6-21.

Neubauer, S. H., Ferris, A. M., Chase, C. G., et al. (1993). Delayed lactogenesis in women with insulin-dependent diabetes mellitus. *American Journal of Clinical Nutrition, 58*(1), 54-60.

Neville, C. E., McKinley, M. C., Holmes, V. A., et al. (2014). The relationship between breastfeeding and postpartum weight change--A systematic review and critical evaluation. *International Journal of Obesity (London), 38*(4), 577-590.

NIDA. (2019, January 2019). Opioid overdose crisis. Retrieved from **www.drugabuse.gov/drugs-abuse/opioids/opioid-overdose-crisis**

Nnodum, B. N., Oduah, E., Albert, D., et al. (2019). Ketogenic diet-induced severe ketoacidosis in a lactating woman: A case report and review of the literature. *Case Reports in Nephrology, 2019,* 1214208.

Nommsen-Rivers, L. A. (2016). Does insulin explain the relation between maternal obesity and poor lactation outcomes? An overview of the literature. *Advances in Nutrition, 7*(2), 407-414.

Nommsen-Rivers LA; Thompson, A. W., L; Wagner, E; Woo, J; . (2017). Metabolic syndrome severity score identifies persistently low milk output. *Breastfeeding Medicine, 12*((Supplement 1)), S-22.

O'Brien, K. O., Donangelo, C. M., Zapata, C. L., et al. (2006). Bone calcium turnover during pregnancy and lactation in women with low calcium diets is associated with calcium intake and circulating insulin-like growth factor 1 concentrations. *American Journal of Clinical Nutrition, 83*(2), 317-323.

O'Campo, P., Faden, R. R., Brown, H., et al. (1992). The impact of pregnancy on women's prenatal and postpartum smoking behavior. *American Journal of Preventive Medicine, 8*(1), 8-13.

O'Connor, A. B., Collett, A., Alto, W. A., et al. (2013). Breastfeeding rates and the relationship between breastfeeding and neonatal abstinence syndrome in women maintained on buprenorphine during pregnancy. *Journal of Midwifery & Women's Health, 58*(4), 383-388.

O'Sullivan, E. J., Perrine, C. G., & Rasmussen, K. M. (2015). Early breastfeeding problems mediate the negative association between maternal obesity and exclusive breastfeeding at 1 and 2 months postpartum. *Journal of Nutrition, 145*(10), 2369-2378.

Oddy, W. H., Li, J., Landsborough, L., et al. (2006). The association of maternal overweight and obesity with breastfeeding duration. *Journal of Pediatrics, 149*(2), 185-191.

Ogbuanu, I. U., Karmaus, W., Arshad, S. H., et al. (2009). Effect of breastfeeding duration on lung function at age 10 years: A prospective birth cohort study. *Thorax, 64*(1), 62-66.

Oladapo, O. T., & Fawole, B. (2012). Treatments for suppression of lactation. *Cochrane Database of Systematic Reviews*(9), CD005937. doi:10.1002/14651858.CD005937.pub3

Olafsdottir, A. S., Thorsdottir, I., Wagner, K. H., et al. (2006). Polyunsaturated fatty acids in the diet and breast milk of lactating Icelandic women with traditional fish and cod liver oil consumption. *Annals of Nutrition and Metabolism, 50*(3), 270-276.

Olsen, A. (1940). Nursing under conditions of thirst or excessive ingestion of fluids. *Acta Obstetricia et Gynecologica Scandinavica, 20*(4), 313-343.

Ordean, A. (2014). Marijuana exposure during lactation: Is it safe? *International Journal of Pediatric Research,* e1-e6.

Pai, A. K., & Fox, V. L. (2017). Gastrointestinal bleeding and management. *Pediatric Clinics of North America, 64*(3), 543-561.

Papadimitriou, D. T. (2017). The big vitamin D mistake. *Journal of Preventive Medicine & Public Health, 50*(4), 278-281.

Parrott, J., Frank, L., Rabena, R., et al. (2017). American Society for Metabolic and Bariatric Surgery integrated health nutritional guidelines for the surgical weight loss patient 2016 update: Micronutrients. *Surgery for Obesity and Related Diseases, 13*(5), 727-741.

Patel, N., Dalrymple, K. V., Briley, A. L., et al. (2018). Mode of infant feeding, eating behaviour and anthropometry in infants at 6-months of age born to obese women - A secondary analysis of the UPBEAT trial. *BMC Pregnancy & Childbirth, 18*(1), 355.

Pawlak, R., Vos, P., Shahab-Ferdows, S., et al. (2018). Vitamin B-12 content in breast milk of vegan, vegetarian, and nonvegetarian lactating women in the United States. *American Journal of Clinical Nutrition, 108*(3), 525-531.

Pepino, M. Y., & Mennella, J. A. (2008). Effects of breast pumping on the pharmacokinetics and pharmacodynamics of ethanol during lactation. *Clinical Pharmacology & Therapeutics, 84*(6), 710-714.

Perez-Reyes, M., & Wall, M. E. (1982). Presence of delta9-tetrahydrocannabinol in human milk. *New England Journal of Medicine, 307*(13), 819-820.

Perrin, E. M., Von Holle, A., Zerwas, S., et al. (2015). Weight-for-length trajectories in the first year of life in children of mothers with eating disorders in a large Norwegian Cohort. *International Journal of Eating Disorders, 48*(4), 406-414.

Perrin, M. T., Pawlak, R., Dean, L. L., et al. (2018). A cross-sectional study of fatty acids and brain-derived neurotrophic factor (BDNF) in human milk from lactating women following vegan, vegetarian, and omnivore diets. *European Journal of Nutrition.* doi:10.1007/s00394-018-1793-z

Popova, S., Lange, S., & Rehm, J. (2013). Twenty percent of breastfeeding women in Canada consume alcohol. *Journal of Obstetrics and Gynaecology Canada, 35*(8), 695-696.

Prentice, A. M., Goldberg, G. R., & Prentice, A. (1994). Body mass index and lactation performance. *European Journal of Clinical Nutrition, 48 Suppl 3,* S78-86; discussion S86-79.

Prentice, A. M., Roberts, S. B., Prentice, A., et al. (1983). Dietary supplementation of lactating Gambian women. I. Effect on breast-milk volume and quality. *Human Nutrition. Clinical Nutrition, 37*(1), 53-64.

Preusting, I., Brumley, J., Odibo, L., et al. (2017). Obesity as a predictor of delayed lactogenesis II. *Journal of Human Lactation, 33*(4), 684-691.

Pumberger, W., Pomberger, G., & Geissler, W. (2001). Proctocolitis in breast fed infants: A contribution to differential diagnosis of haematochezia in early childhood. *Postgraduate Medical Journal, 77*(906), 252-254.

Rameez, R. M., Sadana, D., Kaur, S., et al. (2019). Association of maternal lactation with diabetes and hypertension: A systematic review and meta-analysis. *JAMA Network Open, 2*(10), e1913401.

Ranganathan, M., Braley, G., Pittman, B., et al. (2009). The effects of cannabinoids on serum cortisol and prolactin in humans. *Psychopharmacology (Berlin), 203*(4), 737-744.

Rasmussen, K. M., & Kjolhede, C. L. (2004). Prepregnant overweight and obesity diminish the prolactin response to suckling in the first week postpartum. *Pediatrics, 113*(5), e465-471.

Ratner, P. A., Johnson, J. L., & Bottorff, J. L. (1999). Smoking relapse and early weaning among postpartum women: Is there an association? *Birth, 26*(2), 76-82.

Rautava, S. (2018). Probiotic intervention through the pregnant and breastfeeding mother to reduce disease risk in the child. *Breastfeeding Medicine, 13*(S1), S14-S15.

Reece-Stremtan, S., & Marinelli, K. A. (2015). ABM Clinical Protocol #21: Guidelines for breastfeeding and substance use or substance use disorder, revised 2015. *Breastfeeding Medicine, 10*(3), 135-141.

Reijneveld, S. A., Lanting, C. I., Crone, M. R., et al. (2005). Exposure to tobacco smoke and infant crying. *Acta Paediatrica, 94*(2), 217-221.

Reiter, O., Morag, I., Mazkereth, R., et al. (2014). Neonatal isolated rectal bleeding and the risk of hypersensitivity syndromes. *Journal of Perinatology, 34*(1), 39-42.

Rich, M., Currie, J., & McMahon, C. (2004). Physical exercise and the lactating woman: A qualitative pilot study of mothers' perceptions and experiences. *Breastfeeding Review, 12*(2), 11-17.

Rioux, F. M., Savoie, N., & Allard, J. (2006). Is there a link between postpartum anemia and discontinuation of breastfeeding? *Canadian Journal of Dietetic Practice and Research, 67*(2), 72-76.

Rooney, B. L., Schauberger, C. W., & Mathiason, M. A. (2005). Impact of perinatal weight change on long-term obesity and obesity-related illnesses. *Obstetrics & Gynecology, 106*(6), 1349-1356.

Roschitz, B., Plecko, B., Huemer, M., et al. (2005). Nutritional infantile vitamin B12 deficiency: Pathobiochemical considerations in seven patients. *Archives of Disease in Childhood. Fetal and Neonatal Edition, 90*(3), F281-282.

Ryan, B. A., & Kovacs, C. S. (2019). The puzzle of lactational bone physiology: Osteocytes masquerade as osteoclasts and osteoblasts. *Journal of Clinical Investigation, 130,* 3041-3044.

Ryan, S. A., Ammerman, S. D., O'Connor, M. E., et al. (2018). Marijuana use during pregnancy and breastfeeding: Implications for neonatal and childhood outcomes. *Pediatrics, 142*(3).

Ryu, J. E. (1985a). Caffeine in human milk and in serum of breast-fed infants. *Developmental Pharmacology and Therapeutics, 8*(6), 329-337.

Ryu, J. E. (1985b). Effect of maternal caffeine consumption on heart rate and sleep time of breast-fed infants. *Developmental Pharmacology and Therapeutics, 8*(6), 355-363.

Sachs, H. C., & Committee On, D. (2013). The transfer of drugs and therapeutics into human breast milk: An update on selected topics. *Pediatrics, 132*(3), e796-809.

Sadove, R., & Clayman, M. A. (2008). Surgical procedure for reversal of nipple piercing. *Aesthetic Plastic Surgery, 32*(3), 563-565. doi:10.1007/s00266-008-9140-z

Salahudeen, M. S., Koshy, A. M., & Sen, S. (2013). A study of the factors affecting time to onset of lactogenesis-II after parturition. *Journal of Pharmacy Research, 6*(1), 68-72.

Santos, I. S., Matijasevich, A., & Domingues, M. R. (2012). Maternal caffeine consumption and infant nighttime waking: Prospective cohort study. *Pediatrics, 129*(5), 860-868.

Sauberan, J. B. (2019). High-dose vitamins. *Breastfeeding Medicine, 14*(5), 287-289.

Schalla, S. C., Witcomb, G. L., & Haycraft, E. (2017). Body shape and weight loss as motivators for breastfeeding initiation and continuation. *International Journal of Environmental Research and Public Health, 14*(7).

Schatz, B. S. (1998). Nicotine replacement products: Implications for the breastfeeding mother. *Journal of Human Lactation, 14*(2), 161-163.

Schiff, D. M., Wachman, E. M., Philipp, B., et al. (2018). Examination of hospital, maternal, and infant characteristics associated with breastfeeding initiation and continuation among opioid-exposed mother-infant dyads. *Breastfeeding Medicine, 13*(4), 266-274.

Seabrook, J. A., Biden, C. R., & Campbell, E. E. (2017). Does the risk of exposure to marijuana outweight the benefits of breastfeeding: A systematic review. *Canadian Journal of Midwifery Research and Practice, 16*(2), 349-350.

Sebastiani, G., Herranz Barbero, A., Borras-Novell, C., et al. (2019). The effects of vegetarian and vegan diet during pregnancy on the health of mothers and offspring. *Nutrients, 11*(3).

Serrano-Nascimento, C., Salgueiro, R. B., Vitzel, K. F., et al. (2017). Iodine excess exposure during pregnancy and lactation impairs maternal thyroid function in rats. *Endocrine Connections, 6*(7), 510-521.

Shawe, J., Ceulemans, D., Akhter, Z., et al. (2019). Pregnancy after bariatric surgery: Consensus recommendations for periconception, antenatal and postnatal care. *Obesity Reviews, 20*(11), 1507-1522.

Shenassa, E. D., & Brown, M. J. (2004). Maternal smoking and infantile gastrointestinal dysregulation: The case of colic. *Pediatrics, 114*(4), e497-505.

Shenassa, E. D., Wen, X., & Braid, S. (2016). Exposure to tobacco metabolites via breast milk and infant weight gain: A population-based study. *Journal of Human Lactation, 32*(3), 462-471.

Shin, C. N., Reifsnider, E., McClain, D., et al. (2018). Acculturation, cultural values, and breastfeeding in overweight or obese, low-income, Hispanic women at 1 month postpartum. *Journal of Human Lactation, 34*(2), 358-364.

Short, V. L., Gannon, M., & Abatemarco, D. J. (2016). The association between breastfeeding and length of hospital stay among infants diagnosed with neonatal abstinence syndrome: A population-based study of in-hospital births. *Breastfeeding Medicine, 11*(7), 343-349.

Smith, A. D. (2018). Maternal and infant vitamin B12 status and development. *Pediatric Research, 84*(5), 591-592.

Smith, C. (1947). Effects of maternal undernutrition upon newborn infants in Holland (1944-1945). *Journal of Pediatrics, 30,* 229-243.

Sorensen, M. D. (2014). Calcium intake and urinary stone disease. *Translational Andrology and Urology, 3*(3), 235-240.

Sorva, R., Makinen-Kiljunen, S., & Juntunen-Backman, K. (1994). Beta-lactoglobulin secretion in human milk varies widely after cow's milk ingestion in mothers of infants with cow's milk allergy. *Journal of Allergy and Clinical Immunology, 93*(4), 787-792.

Staiger, P. K., Thomas, A. C., Ricciardelli, L. A., et al. (2011). Identifying depression and anxiety disorders in people presenting for substance use treatment. *Medical Journal of Australia, 195*(3), S60-63.

Stapleton, H., Fielder, A., & Kirkham, M. (2008). Breast or bottle? Eating disordered childbearing women and infant-feeding decisions. *Maternal and Child Nutrition, 4*(2), 106-120.

Steldinger, R., Luck, W., & Nau, H. (1988). Half lives of nicotine in milk of smoking mothers: Implications for nursing. *Journal of Perinatal Medicine, 16*(3), 261-262.

Stinson, O. (1929). So-called post-parturient dyspepsia of bovines and its specific treatment. *Veterinary Record, 9,* 115-119.

Stopp, T., Falcone, V., Feichtinger, M., et al. (2018). Fertility, pregnancy and lactation after bariatric surgery—A consensus statement from the OEGGG. *Geburtshilfe Frauenheilkd, 78*(12), 1207-1211.

Stoutjesdijk, E., Schaafsma, A., Dijck-Brouwer, D. A. J., et al. (2018). Iodine status during pregnancy and lactation: A pilot study in the Netherlands. *Netherlands Journal of Medicine, 76*(5), 210-217.

Strode, M. A., Dewey, K. G., & Lonnerdal, B. (1986). Effects of short-term caloric restriction on lactational performance of well-nourished women. *Acta Paediatrica Scandanavica, 75*(2), 222-229.

Stroud, L. R., Paster, R. L., Papandonatos, G. D., et al. (2009). Maternal smoking during pregnancy and newborn neurobehavior: Effects at 10 to 27 days. *Journal of Pediatrics, 154*(1), 10-16.

Su, D., Zhao, Y., Binns, C., et al. (2007). Breast-feeding mothers can exercise: Results of a cohort study. *Public Health Nutrition, 10*(10), 1089-1093.

Suzuki, D., Wariki, W. M. V., Suto, M., et al. (2019). Secondhand smoke exposure during pregnancy and mothers' subsequent breastfeeding outcomes: A systematic review and meta-analysis. *Scientific Reports, 9*(1), 8535.

Szepfalusi, Z., Loibichler, C., Pichler, J., et al. (2000). Direct evidence for transplacental allergen transfer. *Pediatric Research, 48*(3), 404-407.

Tahir, M. J., Haapala, J. L., Foster, L. P., et al. (2019). Association of full breastfeeding duration with postpartum weight retention in a cohort of predominantly breastfeeding women. *Nutrients, 11*(4).

Tanda, R., Chertok, I. R. A., Haile, Z. T., et al. (2018). Factors that modify the association of maternal postpartum smoking and exclusive breastfeeding rates. *Breastfeeding Medicine, 13*(9), 614-621.

Tartibian, B. (2019). The effect of moderate intensity aerobic exercise on breast milk IgA concentrations. *Approaches in Sport Sciences, 1*(1), 15-30.

Tian, H. M., Wu, Y. X., Lin, Y. Q., et al. (2019). Dietary patterns affect maternal macronutrient intake levels and the fatty acid profile of breast milk in lactating Chinese mothers. *Nutrition, 58,* 83-88.

Torris, C., Thune, I., Emaus, A., et al. (2013). Duration of lactation, maternal metabolic profile, and body composition in the Norwegian EBBA I-study. *Breastfeeding Medicine, 8*(1), 8-15.

Tortoriello, G., Morris, C. V., Alpar, A., et al. (2014). Miswiring the brain: Delta9-tetrahydrocannabinol disrupts cortical development by inducing an SCG10/stathmin-2 degradation pathway. *EMBO Journal, 33*(7), 668-685.

Turcksin, R., Bel, S., Galjaard, S., et al. (2014). Maternal obesity and breastfeeding intention, initiation, intensity and duration: A systematic review. *Maternal and Child Nutrition, 10*(2), 166-183.

Underwood, P., Hester, L. L., Laffitte, T., Jr., et al. (1965). The Relationship of Smoking to the Outcome of Pregnancy. *American Journal of Obstetrics and Gynecology, 91,* 270-276.

USDA. (2015). *U.S. Dietary Guidelines for Americans* (8th ed.). Washington, DC: U.S. Department of Agriculture.

Vagnarelli, F., Amarri, S., Scaravelli, G., et al. (2006). TDM grand rounds: Neonatal nicotine withdrawal syndrome in an infant prenatally and postnatally exposed to heavy cigarette smoke. *Therapeutic Drug Monitoring, 28*(5), 585-588.

Vallianatos, H., Brennand, E. A., Raine, K., et al. (2006). Beliefs and practices of First Nation women about weight gain during pregnancy and lactation: Implications for women's health. *Canadian Journal of Nursing Research, 38*(1), 102-119.

Vidal, J., Corcelles, R., Jimenez, A., et al. (2017). Metabolic and bariatric surgery for obesity. *Gastroenterology, 152*(7), 1780-1790.

Wachman, E. M., Byun, J., & Philipp, B. L. (2010). Breastfeeding rates among mothers of infants with neonatal abstinence syndrome. *Breastfeeding Medicine, 5*(4), 159-164.

Wagner, C. L., Taylor, S. N., & Hollis, B. W. (2008). Does vitamin D make the world go 'round'? *Breastfeeding Medicine, 3*(4), 239-250.

Wagner, S., Issanchou, S., Chabanet, C., et al. (2019). Weanling infants prefer the odors of green vegetables, cheese, and fish when their mothers consumed these foods during pregnancy and/or lactation. *Chemical Senses, 44*(4), 257-265.

Wallace, J. P., Inbar, G., & Ernsthausen, K. (1992). Infant acceptance of postexercise breast milk. *Pediatrics, 89*(6 Pt 2), 1245-1247.

Wambach, K., & Spencer, B. (2021). The cultural context of breastfeeding. In K. Wambach & B. Spencer (Eds.), *Breastfeeding and Human Lactation* (6th ed., pp. 739-758). Burlington, MA: Jones & Bartlett Learning.

Wang, G. S. (2017). Pediatric concerns due to expanded cannabis use: Unintended consequences of legalization. *Journal of Medical Toxicology, 13*(1), 99-105.

Wardinsky, T. D., Montes, R. G., Friederich, R. L., et al. (1995). Vitamin B12 deficiency associated with low breast-milk vitamin B12 concentration in an infant following maternal gastric bypass surgery. *Archives of Pediatrics and Adolescent Medicine, 149*(11), 1281-1284.

Watson, H. J., Zerwas, S., Torgersen, L., et al. (2017). Maternal eating disorders and perinatal outcomes: A three-generation study in the Norwegian Mother and Child Cohort Study. *Journal of Abnormal Psychology, 126*(5), 552-564.

Weder, S., Hoffmann, M., Becker, K., et al. (2019). Energy, macronutrient intake, and anthropometrics of vegetarian, vegan, and omnivorous children (1(-)3 years) in Germany (VeChi Diet Study). *Nutrients, 11*(4).

Weiss, R., Fogelman, Y., & Bennett, M. (2004). Severe vitamin B12 deficiency in an infant associated with a maternal deficiency and a strict vegetarian diet. *Journal of Pediatric Hematology/Oncology, 26*(4), 270-271.

WHO. (2018). Obesity and overweight. Retrieved from **https://www.who.int/en/news-room/fact-sheets/detail/obesity-and-overweight**

Wiklund, P. K., Xu, L., Wang, Q., et al. (2012). Lactation is associated with greater maternal bone size and bone strength later in life. *Osteoporosis International, 23*(7), 1939-1945.

Wilson-Clay, B., & Hoover, K. (2017). *The Breastfeeding Atlas* (6th ed.). Manchaca, TX: LactNews Press.

Wilson, J., Tay, R. Y., McCormack, C., et al. (2017). Alcohol consumption by breastfeeding mothers: Frequency, correlates and infant outcomes. *Drug and Alcohol Review, 36*(5), 667-676.

Winkelman, T. N. A., Villapiano, N., Kozhimannil, K. B., et al. (2018). Incidence and costs of neonatal abstinence syndrome among infants with Medicaid: 2004-2014. *Pediatrics, 141*(4).

Wright, K. S., Quinn, T. J., & Carey, G. B. (2002). Infant acceptance of breast milk after maternal exercise. *Pediatrics, 109*(4), 585-589.

Yakura, N. (1997). Mothers' body perception biased to obesity and its effects on nursing behaviors. *Yonago Acta Medica, 40,* 127-145.

Yilmaz, G., Isik Agras, P., Hizli, S., et al. (2009). The effect of passive smoking and breast feeding on serum antioxidant vitamin (A, C, E) levels in infants. *Acta Paediatrica, 98*(3), 531-536.

Zielinska, M. A., Hamulka, J., Grabowicz-Chadrzynska, I., et al. (2019). Association between breastmilk LC PUFA, carotenoids and psychomotor development of exclusively breastfed infants. *International Journal of Environmental Research and Public Health, 16*(7).

Zielinska, M. A., Hamulka, J., & Wesolowska, A. (2019). Carotenoid content in breastmilk in the 3rd and 6th month of lactation and its associations with maternal dietary intake and anthropometric characteristics. *Nutrients, 11*(1).

Zimmerman, D. R., Goldstein, L., Lahat, E., et al. (2009). Effect of a 24+ hour fast on breast milk composition. *Journal of Human Lactation, 25*(2), 194-198.

Zimmerman, E., Rodgers, R. F., O'Flynn, J., et al. (2019). Weight-related concerns as barriers to exclusive breastfeeding at 6 months. *Journal of Human Lactation, 35*(2), 284-291.

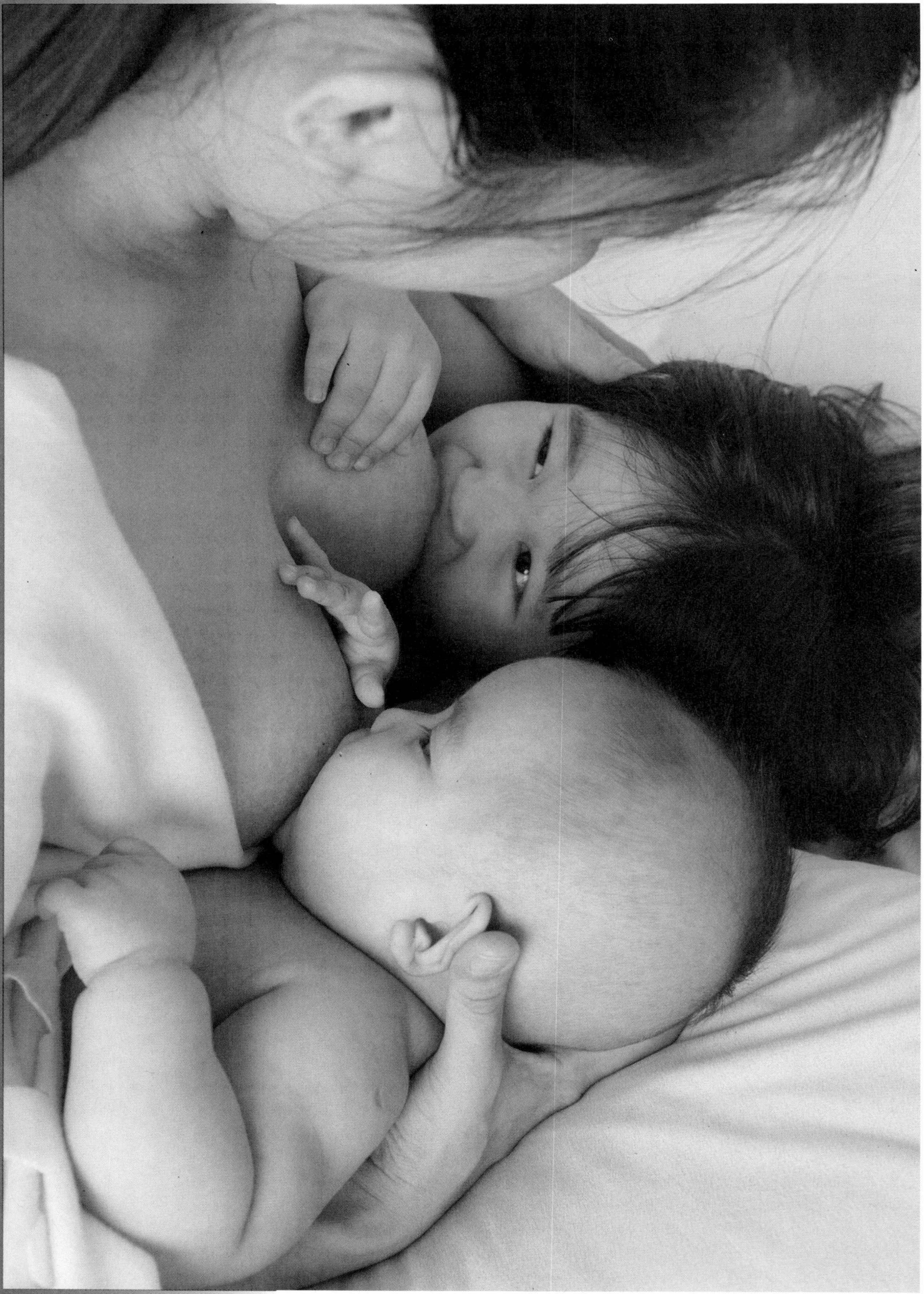

14

Pregnancy and Tandem Nursing

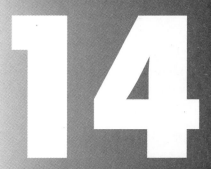

NURSING DURING PREGNANCY

Mixed feelings are common when nursing during pregnancy.

Nursing during a pregnancy and/or continuing to nurse both siblings after birth, known as tandem nursing, is not something most families plan. These practices are considered unusual or even unacceptable by many cultures. A nursing parent may feel pressure from friends and family to wean due to fears that nursing will cause a miscarriage or be too stressful for the nursing parent, but if the child is still avidly nursing, there may also be pressure to continue.

Start by helping the family separate their own feelings from the feelings and opinions of others. Discuss their circumstances and perception of their child's needs. Factors that may influence their decision include:

- The child's age and her physical and emotional need to nurse
- Any nursing-related discomforts, such as nipple pain
- Previous nursing experiences
- Pregnancy-related health issues, such as uterine pain or bleeding, a history of preterm birth, or weight loss during pregnancy
- The partner's feelings about nursing during pregnancy and tandem nursing

If nursing parents seem unsure about their feelings and there are no health issues affecting the situation, suggest postponing a decision and take nursing one day at a time.

• • •

Due to changes in the milk and other factors, most children wean during pregnancy.

In two U.S. studies of women who became pregnant while breastfeeding (Moscone & Moore, 1993; Newton & Theotokatos, 1979), most children (57% and 69%) weaned before their sibling was born. Some reasons pregnancy often leads to weaning include:

- **Changes in the milk.** Most children weaned during the second trimester, when mature milk changes to low-volume, different-tasting colostrum.
- **Nipple pain**, a common side effect of the hormonal changes of pregnancy, which leads many parents to nurse less often and to shorten feeding times.
- **The child's readiness to wean** independent of the pregnancy.

It is not possible to predict whether a child will wean during a pregnancy based on age alone, unless she is younger than 12 months. Although on a physical level, babies need human milk (or a recommended substitute) before 12 months, some do wean (or go on a "nursing strike") at younger ages, which can sometimes be devastating to a nursing parent.

Before 1 year, a child has a biological need for mother's milk, so she will not yet be developmentally ready to wean. But children mature at different rates, so after 1 year, age alone will not be an accurate predictor of weaning readiness. Also, some children wean during pregnancy, and then resume nursing after the baby is born.

• • •

If the nursing parent decides to wean or wants to determine if the child is ready to wean, suggest gentle weaning strategies.

Trying some weaning strategies, such as "don't offer, don't refuse," substitution, and others, can help an unsure parent better gauge if the child is developmentally ready to wean from nursing. For a description of these strategies, see p. 172 in Chapter 5.

Give any parent who's decided to wean support and acceptance. Assure the nursing parent that there are many ways, such as cuddling and focused attention, to meet the child's need for love and acceptance. Also, be sure the family knows that even if the child weans during pregnancy, this is no guarantee the child won't want to nurse after the baby is born. If this happens and the nursing parent does not want the child to nurse, suggest offering her a taste of expressed milk in a spoon or cup. The family may also appreciate receiving reassurance that they can meet the older sibling's needs in other ways.

• • •

If the plan is to keep nursing, suggest being flexible as changes occur.

Although continued nursing can help meet a child's needs during a stressful and tiring time, encourage parents to avoid assumptions about how nursing will go. Emotions and physical comfort during pregnancy can be unpredictable. An open mind and flexibility to changing needs are keys to making nursing during pregnancy a positive experience.

Concerns About the Unborn Baby

If the birthing parent is well-nourished and the older sibling is eating other foods, nursing during pregnancy should not put the pregnancy at risk.

To gain the recommended weight during pregnancy, encourage the birthing parent to rest as needed and eat nutrient-dense foods. Consuming more calories and taking a vitamin/mineral supplement during pregnancy will make meeting nutrient and weight-gain goals easier.

In one U.S. study (Moscone & Moore, 1993), the newborns of 57 mothers who breastfed during pregnancy were healthy at birth and born at the expected weights. Another study of 253 rural Guatemalan women (Merchant, Martorell, & Haas, 1990) compared mothers who weaned 6 months before conceiving with mothers who breastfed into the second and third trimester of pregnancy and found no significant differences in the babies' birth weights. Although the growth of the baby in utero was not affected, this second study noted that the mothers who breastfed during pregnancy showed evidence of reduced maternal fat stores despite consuming more of the nutritional supplements provided than the other mothers. However, these were clinically malnourished or undernourished mothers, and this issue would not apply to birthing parents living in Western countries on adequate diets.

> **KEY CONCEPT**
>
> *Nursing during pregnancy appears to pose no risk to the fetus if the mother is healthy and well-nourished, the pregnancy is low risk, and the older sibling is eating other foods.*

A 2014 Turkish study of 165 pregnant women (Ayrim, Gunduz, Akcal, & Kafali, 2014) found no significant difference in neonatal weight or Apgar scores between the group that overlapped breastfeeding and pregnancy and the group that did not. There were also no differences between these groups in terms of "morning sickness" (hyperemesis gravidarum), incidence of miscarriage, preeclampsia, or preterm labor and birth. However, in the group in which pregnancy and lactation overlapped, the women gained less weight during pregnancy and had lower maternal hemoglobin levels. But these differences had no effect on pregnancy outcomes.

A 2013 Iraqi study of 495 pregnant women (Albadran, 2013) found no difference in birth weight between the group in which lactation overlapped during pregnancy and the group in which the older child weaned before pregnancy.

One factor that appears to significantly affect miscarriage rates is whether or not the older sibling is exclusively nursing during the pregnancy or is also consuming other foods. A 2019 Hungarian study (Molitoris, 2019) analyzed data from more than 10,000 pregnancies over a 13-year period and found that among those exclusively nursing the older sibling, miscarriage rates were 35% as compared with 14% in families where the older nursing sibling also consumed other foods and 15% in those who did not nurse. Because exclusive nursing delays the return of fertility (see p. 533 in Chapter 12), the vast majority of pregnancies are likely to occur after the baby starts solid foods. But for a small minority of families, this information may be vital.

• • •

Clinically malnourished birth parents may need nutritional supplements during pregnancy.

See the later section, "The Nursing Parent's Nutrition, Health, and Comfort."

Effects on the Pregnancy

Uterine contractions occurring during nursing are similar to those occurring during sexual relations.

Many medical studies have been published during the past decade on nursing during pregnancy and none have found any indication of an increased risk of adverse pregnancy outcomes. A 2017 systematic review (Lopez-Fernandez, Barrios, Goberna-Tricas, & Gomez-Benito, 2017), which included 19 studies (6,315 participants, 2,073 cases and 4,242 controls) concluded that nursing during pregnancy does not affect the way pregnancy ends or birth weight. Individual studies found that rates of preterm birth, miscarriage, and low birth weight were similar between groups of women who breastfed during pregnancy and those who did not (Albadran, 2013; Ishii, 2009; Madarshahian & Hassanabadi, 2012).

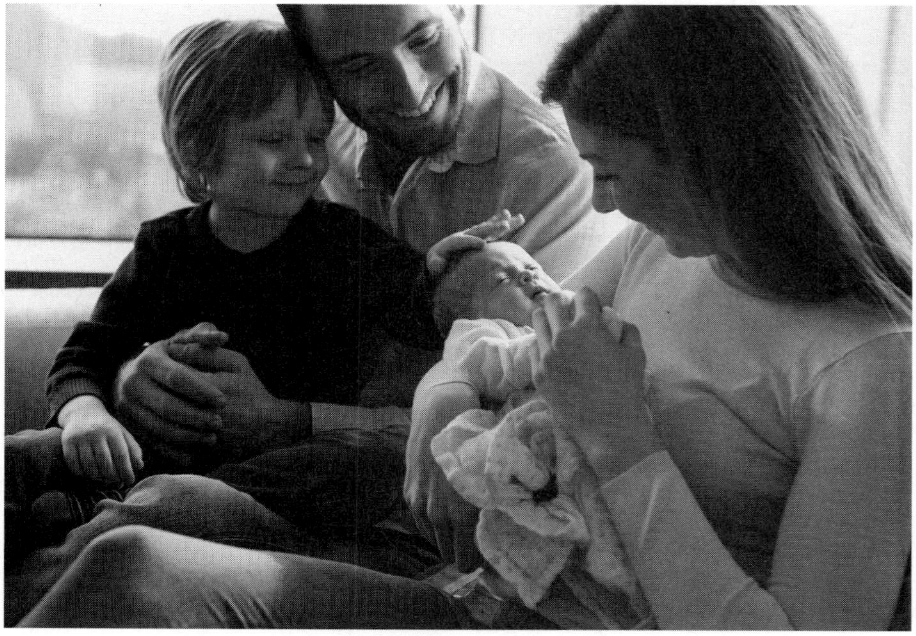

The uterine contractions experienced during nursing are caused by the release of the hormone oxytocin from nipple stimulation and are a normal part of pregnancy. Uterine contractions also occur during sexual activity. Unless the couple has been asked to avoid sexual relations during a high-risk pregnancy due to concerns about potential preterm labor, nursing should not be contraindicated.

Some experience stronger or more frequent contractions in later pregnancy. In one U.S. retrospective study (Moscone & Moore, 1993), 53 of the 57 mothers who breastfed during pregnancy felt no breastfeeding-related contractions and the four who did gave birth to healthy full-term babies.

• • •

After reviewing the literature on the effects of nursing on pregnancy, some health organizations do not support routinely discouraging nursing during pregnancy.

Some healthcare providers advise families to wean during pregnancy "just in case," but support for nursing during pregnancy is increasing. After a review of the literature, the Italian Society of Perinatal Medicine Working Group on Breastfeeding (Cetin et al., 2014) wrote:

> "We found no evidence indicating that healthy women are at higher risk of miscarriage or preterm delivery if they breastfeed while pregnant. No evidence indicates that the pregnancy–breastfeeding overlap might cause intrauterine growth restriction, particularly in women from developed countries. ... In conclusion, currently available data do not support routine discouragement of breastfeeding during pregnancy."

In its 2017 position statement (AAFP, 2017), the American Academy of Family Physicians wrote:

> "Breastfeeding during a subsequent pregnancy is not unusual. If the pregnancy is normal and the mother is healthy, breastfeeding during pregnancy is the woman's personal decision. If the child is younger than 2 years, the child is at increased risk of illness if weaned."

• • •

Weaning may be suggested during a high-risk pregnancy.

There are no specific guidelines on which pregnancy complications are an indication for weaning, and pregnancy caregivers vary widely in their recommendations. Weaning may be suggested if a family is expecting twins, triplets, or more, if uterine pain or bleeding occurs, if there is a history of or symptoms develop of preterm labor, or if there is a less-than-appropriate weight gain during pregnancy. If the nursing parent is uncomfortable with any recommendations, encourage getting a second opinion from a breastfeeding-friendly caregiver.

The Nursing Parent's Nutrition, Health, and Comfort

It is important to stay well-nourished while nursing during pregnancy.

"Eat to hunger" and "drink to thirst" are the basic nutritional recommendations for nursing parents. Nursing during pregnancy increases the usual nutritional requirements (Smith, 2021). Suggest that the nursing and pregnant parent expect to feel hungrier and thirstier than before the pregnancy and to increase food and drink intake accordingly. Staying well-nourished will promote healthy weight gains for parents and children. See p. 554 in Chapter 13 for more specific suggestions for eating nutrient-dense foods.

• • •

If the family is malnourished, there is an increased risk of pregnancy and birth issues, as well as weight gain issues.

Those who are malnourished have few fat stores and may be vitamin deficient. Being malnourished may affect weight gain during pregnancy, the birth weight of the unborn baby, the newborn's weight gain while nursing, and the weight gain of the nursing older sibling. In this situation, the best strategy is to provide nutritional supplements to the pregnant, nursing parent to counteract the malnourishment and improve nutritional status.

One study of 253 Guatemalan women (Merchant et al., 1990) found no significant difference in babies' birth weight when mothers who weaned the older sibling more than 6 months before conception were compared with mothers who breastfed into the second or third trimester of pregnancy. Even though these mothers were consuming nutritional supplements, the birth weights of the newborns tended to be lower the later in pregnancy they weaned the older sibling.

Another study (Siega-Riz & Adair, 1993) found that malnourished Filipino women who breastfed during pregnancy had a poorer weight gain when compared with women who weaned before pregnancy. A study of 113 children in Bhutan (Bohler & Bergstrom, 1996) found that the children who weaned during their mothers' pregnancy had a reduced growth rate during the last months before weaning, when compared with children of the same age who had weaned or continued breastfeeding but whose mothers were not pregnant. A Peruvian study of 133 pregnant women living in poverty (Marquis, Penny, Diaz, & Marin, 2002) found that an overlap between pregnancy and breastfeeding correlated with lower weight gains in the first month of the new baby's life.

A 2015 study of 540 malnourished Egyptian mothers (Shaaban et al., 2015) found that, compared with the group that weaned before becoming pregnant, those who breastfed during pregnancy had an increased incidence of maternal anemia, fetal growth restriction, prolonged labor, cesarean delivery, and low birth weight infants.

A 2015 study of Peruvian women of marginal nutrition status (Pareja, Marquis, Penny, & Dixon, 2015) found no association between breastfeeding during late pregnancy and the birth of small-for-gestational-age (SGA) babies.

• • •

Continued nursing may make pregnancy-related fatigue easier to manage.

Continued nursing during pregnancy may make it easier to convince the nursing baby or toddler to lie down and nurse when it's time to rest. Sometimes well-meaning supporters suggest weaning because they think this will make life easier for the nursing parent. However, in some cases, nursing may be a far easier way to have some restful moments than alternatives to nursing would be if a child was weaned.

• • •

Nausea in early pregnancy may make nursing more challenging.

Managing an active child can be difficult when nausea strikes. For some, nursing does not increase feelings of nausea but holding a squirming child does. For others, increased nausea occurs during nursing, whether or not their child is active. This may be due in part to an increased body awareness during nursing. One strategy that may help is sharing frequent small meals with the child to reduce both nausea and the child's hunger, one motivation to nurse. Another strategy is limiting nursing to a shorter time, such as the length of a favorite song. During pregnancy, as well as afterward, some families find that setting limits on nursing with the older child—such as night weaning--is a workable alternative to complete weaning. For details, see p. 174-175 in Chapter 5.

Whenever there is discomfort of any kind associated with nursing, it is also kind to communicate to the child that this discomfort is not the child's fault and to also avoid blaming the unborn baby.

• • •

A growing abdomen can make nursing increasingly awkward.

In late pregnancy, a disappearing lap and a large abdomen may make it difficult for the child to easily reach the nipple. If so, suggest lying down and trying other positions. An older toddler can be incredibly creative and may nurse leaning over her reclining parent's side or if the parent is sitting upright, over a shoulder. Most toddlers who are motivated to nurse will find a way.

• • •

Most find the changing hormones of pregnancy cause sore or tender nipples and breasts or chests.

Some nursing parents experience nipple and breast or chest tenderness, even before the first menstrual period is missed. Others have no discomfort at all or notice it only late in pregnancy. The duration of nipple and breast/chest soreness is also individual. Of the 39% of the women who reported nipple soreness in one U.S. study (Moscone & Moore, 1993), most experienced it primarily during the first trimester. In another U.S. study (Newton & Theotokatos, 1979), 74% of the mothers reported their nipple soreness lasted for nearly the entire pregnancy, resolving only after their baby's birth.

Nipple and breast or chest pain convinces some to wean during pregnancy. Those who continue nursing learn to cope with the soreness in different ways. To make the soreness more manageable, suggest trying these strategies:

- Vary nursing positions, making sure the child gets a deep latch, with the nipple as far back in her mouth as possible.
- Use childbirth breathing techniques while nursing.
- Ask the child to try to be gentler or limit nursing to a shorter time, assuring the child that the pain is not her fault.
- Hand-express until the milk ejection occurs, as pain decreases when milk is flowing.

• • •

During pregnancy, many feel restless, irritable, or have other strong negative feelings while nursing.

During pregnancy, some experience a feeling of restlessness or irritation with the older child while nursing. Some refer to this as an "antsy" feeling. Two U.S. studies (Moscone & Moore, 1993; Newton & Theotokatos, 1979) found that between 22% and 57% of their pregnant breastfeeding mothers experienced this restlessness or irritation.

If these feelings occur, suggest using distraction during nursing, such as focusing on a smartphone, tablet, or book. Visualization is another kind of distraction that some families find helpful. This might involve thinking about what they value most about nursing and imagining seeing the glowing love flowing from parent to child (Shapiro, 2017, p. 16).

Sarah Shapiro, U.S. lactation consultant and author of the book *Tandem Nursing: A Pocket Guide*, reports that some of the families she has helped found that taking orally 250 mg to 500 mg of magnesium supplements per day during pregnancy helped alleviate these feelings (Shapiro, personal communication, 2018).

Some report developing strong negative feelings termed "nursing aversion" (Yate, 2017) but continued to nurse in spite of these feelings. Feelings of guilt, shame, and confusion may accompany a nursing aversion. Knowing they are not alone in these feelings can be tremendously reassuring and can alleviate this additional suffering. Many online groups offer mutual support for those experiencing nursing aversion.

The Child's Need for Milk

About midway through pregnancy, milk production decreases as milk turns to colostrum.

The hormones that maintain a pregnancy, such as estrogen and progesterone, also cause milk production to decrease. Between 60% and 65% of those who continue nursing during pregnancy report a significant decrease in milk during the fourth or fifth month (Moscone & Moore, 1993; Newton & Theotokatos, 1979). Some nursing babies and toddlers respond to this decrease in milk by nursing less or weaning. Some suddenly begin eating and drinking more other foods and beverages. The change in the milk's taste as it turns from mature milk to colostrum convinces some children to wean. The nursing child who is old enough to talk will often comment on the change in flavor. Some children who wean want to resume nursing after the baby is born. Others continue to nurse during the pregnancy despite these changes.

• • •

If the nursing child is younger than 1 year or is older but is not yet eating much solid food, suggest monitoring her weight gain to make sure she continues to be well-nourished.

For the baby younger than 1 year, the natural pregnancy-related decrease in milk production could compromise her nutritional needs. Suggest the family keep track of the baby's weight gain and if needed, provide appropriate supplements. This may mean more solid foods, donor milk, and/or infant formula. Suggest talking with the baby's healthcare provider for recommendations.

• • •

The older nursing child will not deprive the newborn of colostrum by nursing during pregnancy.

As the milk changes to colostrum in preparation for the birth, reassure the family that the nursing child will not "use up" all the colostrum. No matter how often or long she nurses, colostrum will still be available after birth for the newborn.

• • •

The increased hormones in the milk are compatible with nursing the older child

The hormones that maintain a pregnancy are found in mother's milk, but they are not harmful to the nursing child. The small amount of these hormones the child receives will decrease as milk production decreases. The baby in utero is exposed at a much higher level to the hormones produced by pregnancy than the nursing child.

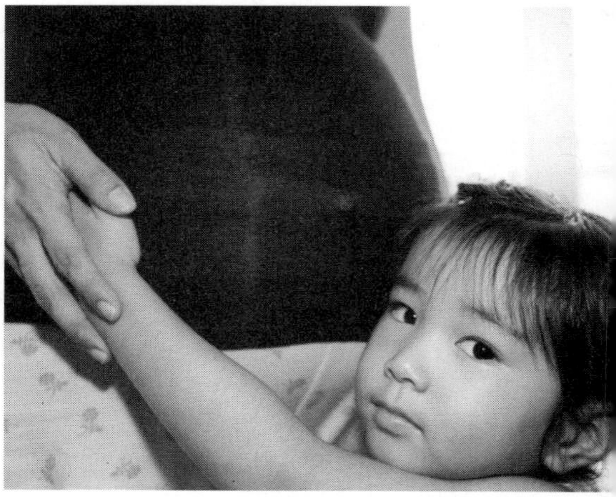

TANDEM NURSING

"Tandem nursing" and "co-nursing" are different.

Some families nurse throughout a pregnancy and then continue to nurse both children after the new baby is born, which is known as tandem nursing. Another definition of tandem nursing is "nursing siblings who are not twins." A different term, "co-nursing," is used to describe adult partners who both nurse one or more children. For more details, see p. 688 in Chapter 16, "Relactation, Induced Lactation, and Emergencies."

• • •

Tandem nursing may happen by design or by default and can be both joyful and stressful.

Families who decide not to actively wean during pregnancy may do so in happy anticipation of nursing the older child and the newborn together. Others continue to nurse for their child's sake without thinking much about tandem nursing. Others approach tandem nursing with concern or even dread. No matter what the feelings during pregnancy, suggest avoiding preconceived ideas about tandem nursing and take it one day at a time.

Planning During Pregnancy

If the older sibling is old enough to understand, suggest preparing her for tandem nursing by discussing the newborn's needs.

If the older sibling is at least 2 or 3 years old, she can begin to learn to wait. One way to help prepare the older child is to talk to her about how her parents responded to her needs as a baby. Also talk about how becoming a "big sister" or "big brother" means helping to take care of the newborn baby by talking to her, touching her gently, and letting her nurse, since milk will be her only food.

It may also be good to talk about how being a "big sister" or "big brother" can sometimes be hard because babies' needs are urgent and sometimes this means waiting. But let the older child know that she will have her needs met, too. It's best to frame challenges in a way that doesn't "blame" the baby. For example, say, "I'm tired and need to rest" rather than "Being pregnant makes me tired, and I need to rest." Some families talk about having lots of love for everyone and how love expands when a new baby arrives (much like milk production increases to meet the needs of both children!), rather than describing a growing family as if there is a fixed amount of love that must now be shared, so everyone gets a little less when a new baby arrives.

• • •

Suggest minimizing any separation from the older sibling at birth, freeze meals, and arrange for household help.

Encourage the family to plan a birth that takes into account the older sibling's need for closeness and minimizes separation. Unnecessary separation can make this stressful adjustment more difficult.

Preparing and freezing meals before the baby is born will help make mealtimes simpler during the baby's early weeks. Household help can also make this time easier. A partner may take a major role, but if other family members or friends offer help, be sure they understand their role in taking care of the house and helping with the older child, allowing the parents to focus on the newborn.

The Practical Details

During the first few days, suggest making it a priority to nurse the newborn often.

The colostrum, or first milk, is a concentrated liquid with the nutrients and antibodies the newborn needs. If the children nurse together, there is no reason to limit the older child's access to nursing. But if the plan is to nurse each child separately, it's important to make it a priority to nurse the newborn often (a minimum of 8 feeds each day) during the first few days after birth. If this becomes challenging, suggest the partner or other helpers give the older sibling focused attention or, if appropriate, take her on special outings. This is a very short time that may even be shorter when two children are nursing, as more nursing can stimulate the milk production to increase sooner than usual. Encourage the family to use their own best judgment on managing early feeds.

• • •

The older sibling may ask to nurse more often in the early weeks, which may cause her stools to change.

When the older sibling sees the newborn nursing, this may temporarily increase her interest in it. In addition to a source of nourishment, nursing for the older sibling is also a source of comfort and closeness. When she feels anxious or threatened by the new baby, she may turn to nursing for reassurance that she is still loved. When she notices her parents' growing attachment to the baby, she may feel the need to reestablish her own relationship by nursing and seeking attention in other ways.

Colostrum and transitional milk can have a laxative effect on the older child, resulting in looser, more frequent stools. This should subside once the transitional milk is replaced by mature milk, which usually occurs about 2 weeks after birth.

• • •

Tandem nursing can help minimize engorgement and ensure abundant milk production.

If the nursing parent is separated from the newborn and/or older sibling, engorgement can still occur. But if it does and the older sibling is willing to nurse, this can help reduce and relieve engorgement as the milk increases. Some older siblings refuse to nurse until the nursing parent's breast or chest is softer, while others are thrilled by the new abundance of milk.

• • •

Normal hygiene is usually enough while tandem nursing, even in case of illness.

The tandem-nursing parent doesn't have to use special hygiene. Regular baths or showers, clean clothes, and reasonable cleanliness are enough. The Montgomery glands near the nipples secrete an anti-bacterial fluid and babies are born with an immunity to most household (and sibling) bacteria, which is enhanced by the antibodies in the milk.

If one sibling has a cold or another common illness, it is not necessary to limit each child to one side, because the children have already been exposed to the bacterium or virus that caused the illness by the time symptoms appear. When an illness becomes obvious, the siblings have already shared the nipples for several days. One exception might be thrush, a fungal infection that can be passed between nursing parents and babies, or any other serious or highly contagious illness. In this case, it may make sense to consider limiting each child to one side until the illness passes.

• • •

Suggest the nursing parent make sure to eat well, drink enough fluids, and get enough rest while tandem nursing.

Just like nursing parents of twins, those who tandem nurse are likely to be hungrier and thirstier than when they nurse just one baby. See p. 554 in Chapter 13 for ideas for nutritious snacks. Encourage the family to plan to have on hand easy, nutritious meals and snacks to eat every few hours and to drink to thirst. Pale urine is a sign of adequate fluid intake. When urine is dark in color, or if constipation develops, these are signs to drink more fluids.

Encourage the family to accept all offers of household help from family and friends or if necessary hire household help. If hiring help is not within their means, suggest asking if a teenager in the neighborhood would be willing to come after school to play with older children and help with household chores.

• • •

The nursing parent is the best one to decide how to manage the children's nursing.

Each nursing parent should feel free to manage the practicalities of tandem nursing in the way that works best within their own family dynamics. While the newborn has a greater physical need for the milk, tandem nursing is easier for some if they are flexible about who nurses first, on which side, and for how long (Gromada, 1992).

The newborn's needs. Some worry about whether the baby is getting the milk she needs when she and the older sibling share nursing. For this reason, the nursing parent may feel strongly about restricting the older sibling's nursing to specific times or only after the baby has finished. If this arrangement works well for the older sibling, it is fine. But if not, reassure the family that most of those who tandem nurse find that because their milk is produced by supply and demand, they have plenty of milk for both children no matter when they nurse. While it may be best to give the newborn first priority to nurse during the early days, switching from one side to the other—or using different feeding positions—is good for the baby, as it promotes healthy eye development. If anyone is worried about baby's milk intake, suggest monitoring baby's weight gain.

The older sibling's needs. How the older sibling feels about sharing nursing and any nursing restrictions will depend on her age and temperament. Some older children can handle restricting nursing to certain times and places; others find being asked to wait even for a few minutes unbearable. Some regress after their sibling's birth and want to nurse like a newborn again. Also, the same child may react differently at different times. Encourage trying different approaches—such as nursing the children together, varying who nurses when throughout the day, or giving the older child consistent nursing times—until the family finds what works best for them. When making these decisions, the nursing parent's feelings are as important as the children's.

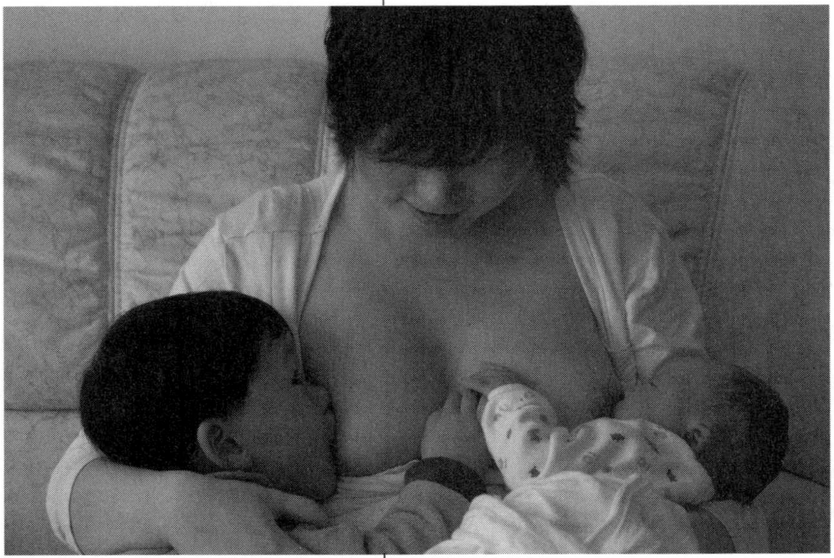

©2019 Melanie Ham, used with permission

For comfort, the nursing parent may want to encourage some consistency in the older sibling's nursing, so that she doesn't nurse all day one day and not at all the next. Removing milk irregularly may increase the risk of mastitis.

The nursing parent's needs. Discuss how the nursing parent is feeling about tandem nursing and ways to balance these feelings with the needs of the children. For example, some feel better about tandem nursing if they nurse both children together, which can cut down on total time spent nursing. Others become restless or irritable when the children nurse together and enjoy tandem nursing more if the children nurse separately. Some feel most comfortable allowing the baby and older child to nurse on cue because there's less conflict. Others feel better about restricting the older sibling's nursing to set times and places. Brainstorm with the family to find practical ways to make tandem nursing subjectively better for them. Let them know, too, that what's really important is finding a routine that works for them rather than any opinions or judgments expressed by those outside the family about what they should do or how tandem nursing should work.

> **KEY CONCEPT**
>
> *Encourage tandem nursing parents to find the nursing arrangements that work best for them.*

If tandem nursing feels overwhelming or unpleasant, encourage the nursing parent to find gradual and positive ways to reduce the number of feeds or wean the older child. (For specific suggestions, see p. 172 in Chapter 5.

• • •

Bedtimes can be a challenge when more than one child nurses to sleep.

Each tandem-nursing family finds its own ways to best navigate bedtimes. In some families, the nursing parent finds a way to nurse both children at once, perhaps in a side-lying position with the younger baby lying on her side facing the parent and the older child leaning over the parent's shoulder. Or perhaps the nursing parent gets into a semi-reclined position and with some pillows for support cradles two children along each side.

In other families, when a partner or support person is available, the nursing parent may nurse one child to sleep while the other adult gives focused attention to the other child. If a partner or support person is not available, it may be possible for the older child to have a special, quiet activity that she is willing to do while the nursing parent lies down with her sibling. Encourage each family to use their creativity to develop a bedtime routine that works for them.

• • •

Help from the partner and use of a baby carrier can make it easier to meet both children's needs.

Using a baby sling or carrier can make it easier to keep the baby close while still having a hand free for the older sibling. If the baby can nurse in the carrier, this makes it easier to give the older child attention while the baby feeds. It may also make it easier for the nursing parent to take the older sibling to outside activities and may distract the older sibling from noticing every time the baby nurses, which may reduce the older sibling's desire to nurse some of the time.

The more active a role a partner can play, if there is one in the family, the better. By spending a lot of time with the older sibling, entertaining her and introducing her to fun activities, this decreases the pressure on the nursing parent to provide for both children's needs. Other family members and friends can also help in this way.

• • •

Tandem nursing while away from home can sometimes be challenging.

One way to reduce requests to nurse while out is to nurse both children before leaving home and offer snacks and drinks to the older sibling while away. Nursing baby in a carrier or sling, as mentioned in the previous point, can also help. For more suggestions on managing nursing while away from home with an older child, see p. 174 in Chapter 5. If it's necessary to nurse both children while out, wearing clothing that permits discreet nursing and using a coverup like a blanket or poncho can make this easier.

Emotional Adjustments

Continuing to nurse after the new baby is born may help ease the emotional adjustment of the older child.

In its 2017 position paper on breastfeeding, the American Academy of Family Physicians addressed both the physical concerns about nursing during pregnancy and the positive emotional benefits for the older child from continuing to nurse after the new baby is born (AAFP, 2017). Regarding the emotional benefits, this paper states, "Breastfeeding the nursing child during pregnancy and after delivery of the next child (tandem nursing) may help provide a smooth transition psychologically for the older child."

• • •

Nursing parents react differently to tandem nursing.

Some nursing parents feel positively about tandem nursing; others do not. Because emotions can vary among individuals and from day to day, do not assume that one person's experience will be the same as another's or that an individual's feelings will remain the same over time.

Many nursing parents decide to tandem nurse because they are focused on the older sibling's needs. It is only natural to focus on the child a parent knows so intimately rather than on the unborn baby, who is still a stranger. However, after birth, many feelings shift dramatically. The hormones of birth and nursing—especially when the experiences with the newborn are positive—enhance parents' natural infatuation with the newborn. All of a sudden, the older child looks so big, and feelings of resentment may arise about taking time away from the newborn to nurse the older child. In one qualitative study of mothers from five European countries, as well as the U.S. and Australia (Watkinson, Murray, & Simpson, 2016), some mothers described what the authors termed "embodied emotions" during breastfeeding, "intense sensations incongruent with the mothers' view of themselves." These included feeling an urgent need to make their child stop nursing or violent urges that passed quickly. In a 2018 overview article on breastfeeding aversion and agitation, one Australian mother shared her intense experience during tandem nursing. Her strong negative emotions—which were often triggered by fatigue while her partner was on business trips—resolved only after she weaned the older sibling (McGuire, 2018). This article also noted that some of the symptoms nursing parents sometimes feel when nursing during pregnancy—such as feelings of skin crawling and toe-curling sensations—may also occur during tandem nursing.

> **KEY CONCEPT**
>
> *Emotional reactions to tandem nursing vary widely among nursing parents.*

Not everyone experiences such a dramatic shift in feelings. But if it happens and the original decision to tandem nurse was made for the sake of the older sibling, this may lead to feelings of guilt and alarm. Assure the family that these opposing feelings—first protective of the older child, then resentful of her demands—are common when a new baby joins the family.

Let the family know that sometimes these same negative feelings can arise even if the older sibling is not nursing. But when nursing is part of this dynamic, negative feelings often become focused there. Having these feelings does not mean a parent will never again enjoy nursing the older child. If there are mood swings, be sure to mention that it is common for life with a new baby to feel like an emotional roller coaster ride. In time, these strong feelings will diminish and a clearer perspective will prevail.

• • •

If the feelings associated with tandem nursing are uncomfortable, suggest possible adjustments.

While nursing a newborn and older child at the same time, some parents become restless or irritable. Some describe their experience as a "creepy-crawly feeling" or have the urge to push their older child off, which is sometimes referred to as "nursing agitation" or a "nursing aversion" (Flower, 2019; Shapiro, 2017). Those who have this experience may worry that there's something wrong with them, so letting them know it is common enough to have earned a name may help them understand that this reaction is not a reflection of their true feelings about their older child. Some feel this way even when the older sibling nurses alone. An older child's teeth and gums may cause friction on the nipple and areola, leading many to describe the "roughness" they feel when their older child sucks in comparison to the gentle suck of their newborn. Some don't notice these differences; others, however, find them disturbing. Some experience the sensations from the older child's sucking as erotic.

Assure the nursing parent that all of these feelings are common and if they are disturbing or uncomfortable, it's time to make adjustments. One author reports that some parents find that taking magnesium supplements (250 mg to 500 mg orally per day) helps reduce these feelings of agitation or aversion (personal communication, S. Shapiro, 2018). But there are many more options. For example, it may help reduce the sensations by varying the older child's feeding positions or nursing the children separately rather than together. Some find they can better handle these feelings by reducing their older child's time nursing, keeping each feed short but not eliminating or postponing them. Others nurse less often by distracting their older child with other activities, postponing feeds, or offering substitutions, such as snacks or drinks before the older child asks to nurse.

When a nursing parent is consistently unhappy with tandem nursing, suggest using weaning strategies to reduce the number of nursing sessions per day. Sometimes nursing fewer times each day—a partial weaning and/or night weaning—is enough so that the parent feels more positively about tandem nursing.

• • •

If the nursing parent feels "touched out," suggest arranging for a little alone time each day.

"Touched out" means feeling an intense need for some personal space after an overabundance of cuddling, holding, and nursing. Between the children's needs and the partner's need for physical intimacy, the nursing parent may sometimes want some time alone to take a few deep breaths, a walk, or any other activity that feels rejuvenating.

Assure the family that these feelings are common. Although the assumption may be that tandem nursing is the cause of these feelings, even if the older child was not nursing, she would still seek closeness and comfort. Suggest arranging for a few minutes alone each day, perhaps to take a bath or shower alone or a short stroll. Even a little "alone time" can go a long way toward elevating the mood.

It helps if tandem-nursing families have a positive attitude and a sense of humor. When those cannot be mustered, it may help to talk to someone who will listen sympathetically, the partner, a friend, other parents who have tandem nursed, or others who are supportive of nursing.

• • •

Even when a family starts tandem nursing with a positive attitude, the nursing parent may discover that it's just not working out. If the adjustments mentioned previously have been tried and the nursing parent still feels uncomfortable or unhappy, for gradual and gentle weaning strategies for the older child, see p. 172 in Chapter 5.

If the decision is made to wean the older child, discuss gradual, gentle weaning strategies.

RESOURCES

Bumgarner, N. (2000). *Mothering Your Nursing Toddler.* Rev. ed. Schaumburg, Illinois: La Leche League International.

Flower, H. (2019). *Adventures in Tandem Nursing,* 2nd edition. Scotts Valley, CA: CreateSpace Independent Publishing.

Shapiro, S. (2017). *Tandem Nursing: A Pocket Guide.* Chatham, NY: First Food Breastfeeding Support.

REFERENCES

AAFP. (2017). Family physicians supporting breastfeeding position paper. Retrieved from **aafp.org/about/policies/all/breastfeeding-support.html**.

Albadran, M. M. (2013). Effect of breastfeeding during pregnancy on the occurrence of miscarriage and preterm labour. *Iraqi Journal of Medical Sciences, 11*(3), 285-289.

Ayrim, A., Gunduz, S., Akcal, B., et al. (2014). Breastfeeding throughout pregnancy in Turkish women. *Breastfeeding Medicine, 9*(3), 157-160.

Bohler, E., & Bergstrom, S. (1996). Child growth during weaning depends on whether mother is pregnant again. *Journal of Tropical Pediatrics, 42*(2), 104-109.

Cetin, I., Assandro, P., Massari, M., et al. (2014). Breastfeeding during pregnancy: Position paper of the Italian Society of Perinatal Medicine and the Task Force on Breastfeeding, Ministry of Health, Italy. *Journal of Human Lactation, 30*(1), 20-27.

Flower, H. (2019). *Adventures in Tandem Nursing* (2nd ed.). St. Petersburg, FL: Flower Press.

Gromada, K. K. (1992). Breastfeeding more than one: multiples and tandem breastfeeding. *NAACOG's Clinical Issues in Perinatal and Women's Health Nursing, 3*(4), 656-666.

Ishii, H. (2009). Does breastfeeding induce spontaneous abortion? *Journal of Obstetrics and Gynaecology, 35*(5), 864-868.

Lopez-Fernandez, G., Barrios, M., Goberna-Tricas, J., et al. (2017). Breastfeeding during pregnancy: A systematic review. *Women and Birth, 30*(6), e292-e300.

Madarshahian, F., & Hassanabadi, M. (2012). A comparative study of breastfeeding during pregnancy: Impact on maternal and newborn outcomes. *Journal of Nursing Research, 20*(1), 74-80.

Marquis, G. S., Penny, M. E., Diaz, J. M., et al. (2002). Postpartum consequences of an overlap of breastfeeding and pregnancy: Reduced breast milk intake and growth during early infancy. *Pediatrics, 109*(4), e56.

McGuire, E. (2018). Breastfeeding aversion and agitation. *Breastfeeding Review, 26*(2), 37-40.

Merchant, K., Martorell, R., & Haas, J. (1990). Maternal and fetal responses to the stresses of lactation concurrent with pregnancy and of short recuperative intervals. *American Journal of Clinical Nutrition, 52*(2), 280-288.

Molitoris, J. (2019). Breast-feeding during pregnancy and the risk of miscarriage. *Perspectives on Sexual and Reproductive Health, 51*(3), 153-163.

Moscone, S. R., & Moore, M. J. (1993). Breastfeeding during pregnancy. *Journal of Human Lactation, 9*(2), 83-88.

Newton, N., & Theotokatos, M. (1979). Breastfeeding during pregnancy in 503 women: Does a psychobiological weaning mechanism exist in humans? *Emotion & Reproduction, 20B,* 845-849.

Pareja, R. G., Marquis, G. S., Penny, M. E., et al. (2015). A case-control study to examine the association between breastfeeding during late pregnancy and risk of a small-for-gestational-age birth in Lima, Peru. *Maternal and Child Nutrition, 11*(2), 190-201.

Shaaban, O. M., Abbas, A. M., Abdel Hafiz, H. A., et al. (2015). Effect of pregnancy-lactation overlap on the current pregnancy outcome in women with substandard nutrition: A prospective cohort study. *Facts, Views & Visions in ObGyn, 7*(4), 213-221.

Shapiro, S. (2017). *Tandem Nursing: A Pocket Guide.* Chatham, New York: CreateSpace Indepdendent Publishing Platform.

Siega-Riz, A. M., & Adair, L. S. (1993). Biological determinants of pregnancy weight gain in a Filipino population. *American Journal of Clinical Nutrition, 57*(3), 365-372.

Smith, L. (2021). Postpartum care. In K. Wambach & B. Spencer (Eds.), *Breastfeeding and Human Lactation* (6th ed., pp. 247-280). Burlington, MA: Jones and Bartlett Learning.

Watkinson, M., Murray, C., & Simpson, J. (2016). Maternal experiences of embodied emotional sensations during breast feeding: An interpretative phenomenological analysis. *Midwifery, 36,* 53-60.

Yate, Z. M. (2017). A qualitative study on negative emotions triggered by breastfeeding; Describing the phenomenon of breastfeeding/nursing aversion and agitation in breastfeeding mothers. *Iran Journal of Nursing and Midwifery Research, 22*(6), 449-454.

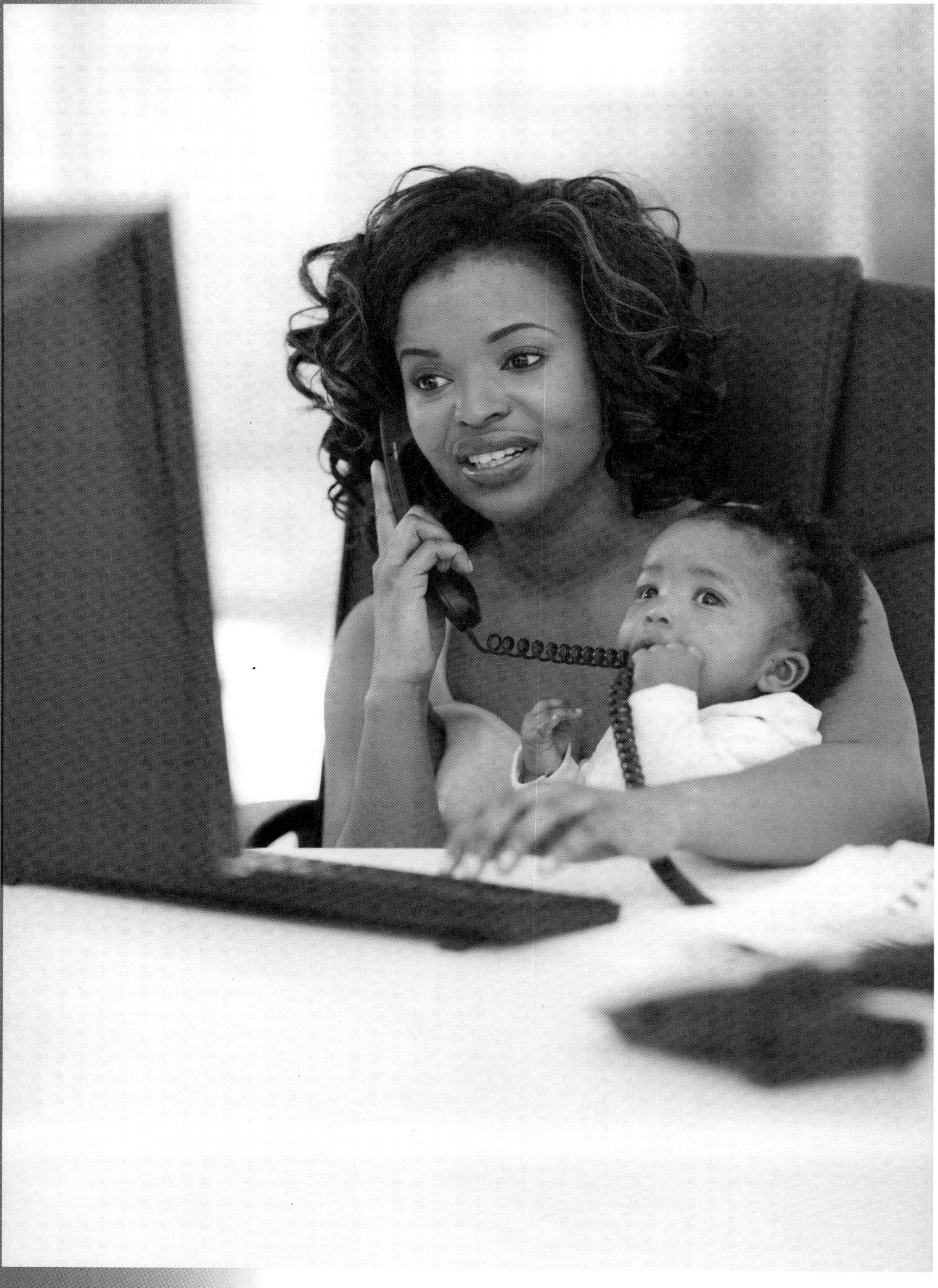

Employment

15

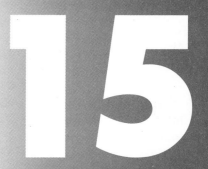

LENGTH OF MATERNITY LEAVE AND NURSING

In whichever country a family lives, length of maternity leave can vary greatly.

Always ask about length of parental leave rather than making assumptions. Even in countries with generous paid maternity leave, not all parents qualify or take the allotted time off. Business owners, for example, may take no break at all. If parents are not at their jobs long enough or did not work enough hours per week to qualify, paid maternity leave may not be an option. At the other end of the spectrum, even in a country like the U.S., where paid leave is primarily dependent on employment agreements rather than government programs, some parents negotiate very generous paid time off after childbirth.

• • •

Whatever the length of maternity leave, nursing parents planning to work part time are more likely to exclusively nurse and to nurse longer than those planning to return to work full time.

A U.S. study analyzed the results of a national survey of 1,573 women (Attanasio, Kozhimannil, McGovern, Gjerdingen, & Johnson, 2013). It found that those women who worked full time during pregnancy and planned to work full time and breastfeed exclusively after birth were at increased risk—even during their baby's first week—of not fulfilling their intention to breastfeed exclusively. The researchers concluded that parents in this situation would benefit from more supportive workplace policies.

Another U.S. study based on a national survey of 2,348 women (Mirkovic, Perrine, Scanlon, & Grummer-Strawn, 2014) found that mothers planning to return to work within 12 weeks of birth and those planning to work full time were less likely to intend to exclusively breastfeed.

A U.S. study found that parents working part time breastfed for about the same length of time as those who were unemployed (Ogbuanu, Glover, Probst, Hussey, & Liu, 2011). The effects of work on nursing rates vary around the world.

- In the U.K., mothers employed part time or self-employed were more likely to breastfeed for at least 4 months as compared with those employed full time (Hawkins, Griffiths, Dezateux, & Law, 2007). U.K. women who worked part time during evening shifts were 70% more likely to begin breastfeeding than unemployed mothers (Zilanawala, 2017).
- In Australia, mothers returning to full-time work before 12 months were less likely to be fully breastfeeding at 6 months or breastfeeding at all at 12 months (Scott, Binns, Oddy, & Graham, 2006). Whether worksite lactation support exists makes a difference, too. In a 2017 study of employees of Australia National University, 24% of the responders agreed or strongly agreed with the statement: "I would have returned to work sooner if worksite was supportive of breastfeeding" (Smith, Javanparast, & Craig, 2017).
- In Taiwan, only about 11% of the women who returned to work for 8- to 12-hour days were breastfeeding at 3 months as compared with the national breastfeeding average of 17% at 3 months (Chen, Wu, & Chie, 2006). Longer workdays and less flexible break times were associated with earlier weaning.

- In New Zealand, at 4 months 39% of the mothers who returned to work full time were breastfeeding as compared with 57% of the women who stayed home (McLeod, Pullon, & Cookson, 2002).
- In Singapore, at 6 months only 20% of the mothers working full-time were breastfeeding as compared with 31% of the mothers at home (Ong, Yap, Li, & Choo, 2005).

One U.S. study noted—not surprisingly—that as daily work hours increase, the number of breastfeeds decreases (Roe, Whittington, Fein, & Teisl, 1999).

• • •

Nursing considerations vary greatly, depending on baby's age when the nursing parent returns to work, whether the work is full time or part time, and whether it's possible to arrange to nurse during work hours.

In general, the older the baby when the nursing parent returns to work, the easier it is to continue nursing long term. This section describes what parents need to know about going back to work full time or part time during six different time windows and the nursing considerations unique to each one, from birth through the first year and beyond.

Birth to 5 Weeks

The most challenging period to return to work is from birth to 5 weeks.

During the first 5 weeks after delivery, birthing parents and babies are most physically vulnerable, babies are most unsettled, and milk production is not yet fully established, which makes returning to work most challenging. Even so, by knowing the basics and planning ahead, families can meet their feeding goals. But if it is an option to either work from home and nurse for even some feeds or delay the return to work for a while longer, encourage the family to seriously consider this.

• • •

If the baby is fed by others during work hours, discuss volume of milk needed and expected feeding patterns.

Feeding volumes. The volume of milk baby needs during the workday will increase significantly between birth and 5 weeks. During this time, baby's stomach grows quickly and the need for milk increases. After the milk increases on the third or fourth day, for the rest of that first week, a full-term newborn's stomach holds comfortably only about 1 oz. (30 mL) of milk (Bergman, 2013). If a bottle is used for some feedings, it's important to avoid overfeeding by using paced bottle-feeding techniques (see p. 902-903 for details).

By the end of the first week, nursing babies consume on average about 1.5 oz. (45 mL) per feed. By the second and third weeks, feeding volumes are usually up to on average 2 to 3 oz. (60 to 90 mL). By the fourth week, on average, a maximum feeding volume is 3 to 4 oz. (90 to 120 mL). This is about how much baby will need per feed until baby is ready for solids at around 6 months.

Feeding patterns. From birth to 5 weeks, most babies are incapable of adjusting well to any sort of feeding schedule. Let the family know that health organizations recommend newborns be fed ***on cue***, meaning whenever baby shows signs that they are hungry, like rooting, hand-to-mouth, and fussing (AAP, 2012; WHO, 2018). It's also helpful for parents to be aware that between 2 and 14 weeks, most babies are fussy for part of the day, even if they are well fed.

Nursing babies usually consume less milk more often than formula-fed babies. Breastfed newborns average 8 to 12 feeds per day. Formula-fed babies average

6 to 8 feeds per day (Sievers, Oldigs, Santer, & Schaub, 2002). Suggest the caregiver encourage small, frequent feeds, as large feeds less often put babies at higher risk of overweight and obesity later (Azad, et al., 2018; Li, Magadia, Fein, & Grummer-Strawn, 2012). For details, see p. 192-193.

• • •

To reach the desired level of milk production after the return to work, the best strategies will depend on the family's goals and whether others will feed the baby during a full-time or part-time workday.

To stimulate an ample milk production during the early weeks, most babies feed intensively, clustering their feeds close together during some parts of the day. Milk production reaches its peak at about 5 weeks (Hill, Aldag, Chatterton, & Zinaman, 2005; Kent, Gardner, & Geddes, 2016). If the nursing parent is not with the baby for these newborn feeding clusters, the decisions on how to handle this will depend on the family's goals and how many hours each day others feed baby.

If the family's goal is to provide human milk exclusively for their baby, they need to understand how milk production works. The key dynamic is how many times each day the milk is removed well, either by feeding or milk expression. A good goal between birth and 5 weeks, when milk production is increasing, is 10 or more milk removals per day. On average, by about 5 weeks, babies consume between 25 and 30 oz. (750 to 887 mL) of milk per day, which is just about the largest daily milk volume baby will ever need. If milk production reaches 25 oz. to 30 oz. (750 to 887 mL) per day during the first 5 weeks, then all that's needed is to keep it steady, which requires less time and effort (see the later section on the magic number).

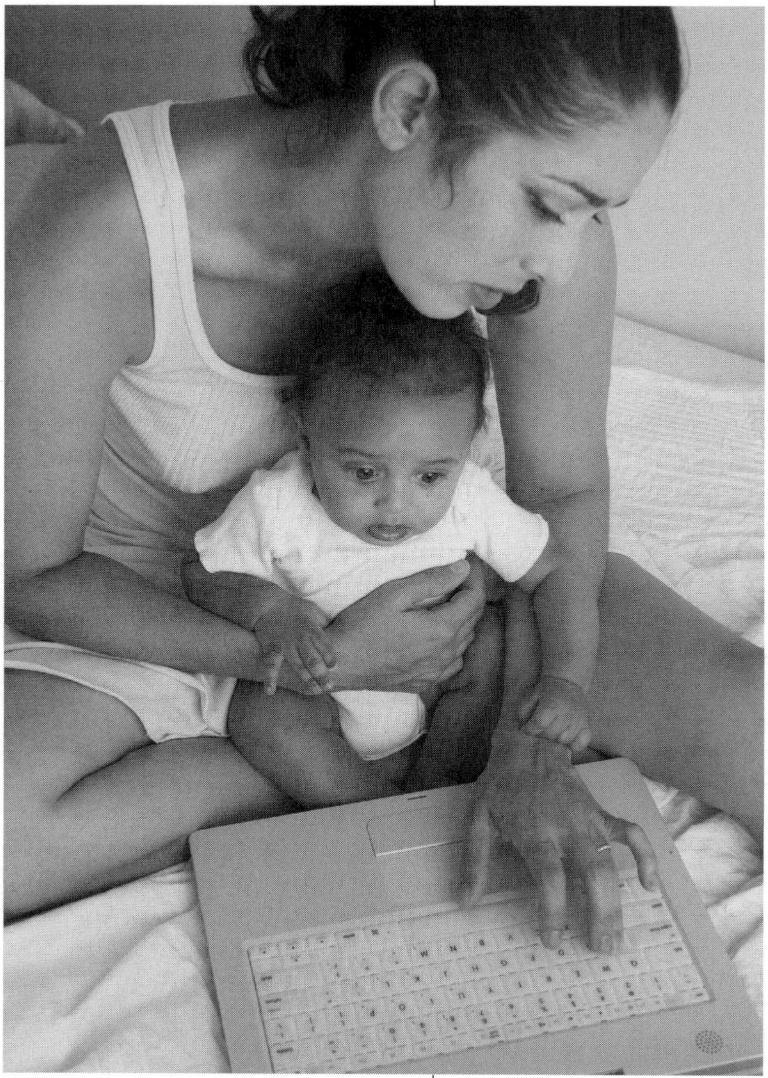

Full-time work. In this situation, each family decides how to best fit in the 10 milk removals per day needed to increase milk production during this time window. Some might find it easier to feed nine times while at home and express milk once during their workday. Others might find more expressions at work easier. The milk removals don't need to be at evenly spaced time intervals. Expressing or nursing every hour works, too. At this stage, a gap of up to 5 to 6 hours once per day will not usually slow milk production. Most important is the total number of daily milk removals and how well the milk is removed.

If feeding mother's milk exclusively is not the family's goal, donor milk or infant formula can be used as a substitute for as many feeds as needed, and the baby can nurse when they are together.

Part-time work. From birth to 5 weeks, just like at other stages, working fewer hours per week provides more flexibility. The need to express milk at work will depend on the work schedule and whether the parent has access to the baby during the workday. If there's a stretch no longer than about 6 hours (including travel time) between feeds, it may work well to nurse baby before leaving for work, then feed next just after they're reunited, fitting in the rest of the 10 daily milk removals while the family is together. An alternative to expressing at work—even if the goal is to leave only mother's milk for baby—is to express after some feeds at home to store extra milk for workdays.

If the part-time work schedule involves working a few very long days (8 to 12 hours or more), expressing milk at work may be needed to stay comfortable and to avoid slowing milk production.

• • •

When returning to work between birth and 5 weeks, suggest going slow, as there may be physical discomforts and emotional challenges.

When returning to work at or before 5 weeks, suggest making self-care a top priority. At 5 weeks, the birth parent is still physically recovering from delivery, which can take months for full recovery. In one U.S. study of women at 5 weeks postpartum (McGovern et al., 2006), breastfeeding mothers reported an average of six childbirth-related physical symptoms such as back pain, headaches, and fatigue. Those who delivered by cesarean had more health problems at 5 weeks than those who delivered vaginally. Another U.S. study interviewed 661 women at 11 weeks after childbirth (Grice et al., 2007) and found that women who returned to work at 5 weeks had much lower mental-health scores at 11 weeks than those still on leave at 11 weeks.

6 Weeks to 3 Months

Most birthing parents who return to work between 6 weeks and 3 months are still recovering from childbirth, and at this age, babies are often fussy in the evenings.

For many U.S. families, return to work occurs during this time window. This is also true for families living in countries that provide 3 months of paid maternity leave.

At this stage, many birthing parents have not yet fully recovered from childbirth. In one U.S. study (McGovern et al., 2007), at 11 weeks, the study women reported an average of four childbirth-related symptoms, such as pain and fatigue. Another U.S. study (Chatterji & Markowitz, 2012) found that women who had less than 12 weeks of maternity leave were at greater risk for depression.

Another challenge during this time window is that evening fussiness in babies usually reaches its peak at around 6 weeks. In many families, this is right around the time that parents get home from work. By 12 to 14 weeks, though, this fussiness usually subsides.

• • •

After 5 weeks, if baby is exclusively nursing and gaining weight well, full milk production is established, and maintaining milk production requires less effort.

If baby is exclusively nursed and is gaining weight well, this indicates full milk production. Many parents are surprised to learn that nursing babies' milk intake stays remarkably stable between 5 weeks and 6 months of age, varying only by about 2 to 4 oz. (60 to 120 mL) per day (Kent et al., 2013).

Be sure to tell the family that they don't have to worry about their baby needing significantly more milk later as he grows. All that's needed is to maintain the current level of milk production. If the goal is for the baby to receive only mother's milk until 6 months, this means focusing on keeping milk production stable. At 6 months, the baby's need for milk decreases when solid foods are started.

• • •

Whether work is full time or part time, maintaining milk production will be determined by how many times each 24-hour day milk is removed well from the mammary glands.

Maintaining milk production for employed parents involves making sure the number of daily milk removals never drops below their magic number (see the later section for details).

Full-time work. If the family's goal is to exclusively provide mother's milk during the workday, before returning to work full time (more than 32 hours per week), near the end of parental leave, count how many times each 24-hour period baby nursed. This number, which varies among individuals, gives a general idea of how many milk removals (feeds plus milk expressions) are needed each day to keep milk production stable over the long term. These milk removals do not have to be at regularly spaced time intervals, such as every 2 or 3 hours. The time between milk removals can vary during the day.

Suggest the family think about the best way to keep the number of daily milk removals steady after the return to work. Plan how many times each day to express milk or how to gain access to the baby for nursing during the workday. Each family can customize their routine.

If the family's goal is not to provide exclusive mother's milk feeds, they can leave donor milk or infant formula as a substitute for as many feeds as needed and nurse when together.

Part-time work. As babies grow and mature, they become more adaptable. Work options that give parents more flexibility between 6 and 12 weeks will make it much easier for families to adjust. The work schedule and family goals will determine whether it's necessary to express milk at work. If the workday is 6 hours or less, it may not be necessary to express milk at work. If workdays are longer, expressing milk may be necessary to stay comfortable and avoid slowing milk production.

4 to 5 Months

Maternity leave of 12 weeks or longer is associated with longer duration of nursing.

In one U.S. study (Ogbuanu, Glover, Probst, Liu, & Hussey, 2011), women who started back to work after 12 weeks were more likely to breastfeed longer than those who returned to work sooner. Why? After 3 months, milk production is well established, and maintaining milk levels is easier than increasing it. Household stress levels may be lower, because baby has outgrown the evening fussy periods that are so common in younger babies. In the U.S. in particular, women whose maternity leave is 3 months or longer may also have more flexible and supportive working conditions, making continued breastfeeding easier (Skafida, 2012).

• • •

From 4 to 5 months of age, whether work is full time or part time, baby's need for milk continues to stay stable.

At this age, an average 24-hour milk intake for an exclusively nursing baby is about 25 to 30 oz. (750 to 887 mL). However, the volume of milk consumed daily is much greater among formula-fed babies this age (Kramer et al., 2004), so caution families not to gauge their nursing baby's need for milk by what a formula-fed baby consumes. For details, see p. 192-193.

As previously explained, when nursing is going well, milk production reaches its peak at about 5 weeks (Hill et al., 2005; Kent et al., 2016). At 4 to 5 months, maintaining milk production is all that's needed. When baby starts solid foods at around 6 months, the need for milk decreases. Just like during the previous time windows, the key dynamic is the number of daily milk removals (feeds plus milk expressions). For more details, see the later section about the magic number.

Full-time work. At 4 to 5 months, assuming a work week of 32 hours or more, start by counting the number of hours baby will be fed by others to calculate how many times per workday to express milk. With full-time work, suggest expressing milk at least every 3 hours or so. If it's possible to have access to baby for feeding even once during the workday, that is better than expression alone.

If the family's plan is not to provide mother's milk for all missed feeds, suggest donor milk or formula as a substitute, nursing when they are together.

Part-time work. Again, more flexibility makes it easier for families to meet their feeding goals.

6 to 8 Months

Solid foods are usually started during this time window, which gradually decreases the volume of milk baby needs, and many babies learn to drink from cups.

Starting solid foods is recommended at around 6 months (AAP, 2012; WHO, 2018). For more details, see Chapter 4, "Solid Foods." Although solids are started at this age, most babies are just learning this new way of eating and are not yet consuming very much. This means human milk (or donor milk or infant formula as substitutes) will still be baby's main food. At this age, in 24 hours an average breastfeeding baby still consumes about 25 to 30 oz. (750 to 887 mL) of milk.

At 6 to 8 months, many babies learn to drink from a cup, so if the return to work happens during this time window, it may not be necessary for baby to feed from a bottle. An average nursing baby this age takes about 3 to 4 oz. (89 to 118 mL) per feed. If a bottle is used, be sure the family shares with baby's caregiver paced bottle-feeding techniques, which slows feedings so baby feels full with less milk. For details, see p. 902-903.

Make sure the family also knows it is normal if the volume of milk expressed starts to decrease slightly as baby begins taking more solid foods. But there may not be a noticeable difference in feeding patterns when the family is together.

Full-time work. At 6 to 8 months, if the baby is receiving only mother's milk and solids and the family wants this to continue, start by expressing milk at work at least every 3 hours or so. Depending on feeding goals, another option is to provide donor milk or infant formula for as many feedings as needed and nurse when together.

Part-time work. Flexibility is a plus. If workdays are short, it may not be necessary to express milk at work. It's possible to express and store milk at home and save it for workdays. If many feedings are missed over long workdays, it may be necessary to express milk at work to stay comfortable.

9 to 11 Months

Between 9 and 11 months, nursing babies gradually need less milk than when they were younger, which they can drink by cup.

At 9 to 11 months, babies still need milk, but because babies are also eating more solid food, they need less milk now than when they were younger. Until babies reach 1 year, health experts recommend continuing to provide mother's milk or a substitute such as donor milk or infant formula (AAP, 2012; WHO, 2018).

By about 9 months of age, most babies are now drinking well from a cup, making feeding bottles optional. If the return to work happens during this time window, bottle-feeding may be completely unnecessary. Many babies this age transition directly from nursing to a cup.

During the 9- to 11-month time window, milk production continues to slowly decrease as babies consume more solid foods. Assure families who notice that less milk is expressed at work that this is a normal part of a baby's transition from a milk-only diet to one that includes solid foods. To stay comfortable at work and to keep milk production where it needs to be, suggest keeping an eye on the total number of milk removals (nursing sessions plus milk expressions) each day. To troubleshoot milk production, see the later section on the magic number. A U.S. study that followed mothers participating in a worksite lactation program (Ortiz, McGilligan, & Kelly, 2004) found that after 9 months, many women who started work when their babies were younger begin phasing out pumping during this time window while continuing to nurse at home.

Full-time work. If others feed baby for 32 or more hours per week, the need to express milk for a 9-to-11-month-old baby, will depend on the level of milk production and family's goals. If the goal is for baby to receive only mother's milk and solids, suggest starting by expressing milk at work about every 3 hours. Depending on the family's goals, donor milk or infant formula can be provided, and nursing can continue when they are together.

Part-time work. If others feed the baby for no longer than 6-hour stretches, it may be possible to nurse just before the work shift and again after they are reunited. To provide milk during the workday, milk can be expressed at home and stored for workdays. If workdays are long, milk expression at work may be necessary to stay comfortable and maintain milk production.

1 Year or Older

For most families, returning to work when the baby is 1 year or older makes continued nursing easier, because little—if any—milk expression is required.

From a lactation perspective, there are many advantages to returning to work after babies turn 1 year. At this stage, babies can simply nurse when they are with their families and during the workday other foods and drinks can be provided. At 1 year, if nursing is not an option during the workday, babies can eat solid foods and whatever drinks the family chooses.

At 1 year, babies are old enough to drink cow's milk from the store, as well as water and other milks, which they can easily drink by cup. Families are no longer limited to providing expressed milk, donor milk, or infant formula during the workday. Some families decide to continue providing expressed milk after 1 year, but it's now just one of many choices.

Because milk production slows gradually during baby's second 6 months, depending on the length of the workday, it may or may not be necessary at first to express milk for the sake of comfort. If uncomfortable fullness develops on the first day back at work, suggest expressing just enough milk to stay comfortable. As long as milk expression is kept just "to comfort," it will likely only be necessary for just a short time as milk production adjusts.

At 1 year, whether the work is full time or part time, nursing and milk production usually require little thought or planning. An exception is work involving overnight shifts or work travel away from baby. In these situations, suggest making sure the nursing parent has whatever equipment—if any—is needed to express milk to comfort while away from baby.

PRIORITIES DURING MATERNITY LEAVE

Baby Time

During the early weeks after birth, suggest making it a priority to nurse long and often to ensure ample long-term milk production.

No matter how long or short the parental leave, suggest the family think of the time at home with their baby after birth as a time of closeness and togetherness. It is also a time to think about their feeding goals and plan for the future. Many of the choices they make during the first month after birth will lay the foundation for their time at work.

One of the most important things to do while on leave is to nurse long and often. This will help set milk production at the level needed to meet long term feeding goals. At every nursing session, the hormone prolactin is released. During the first 2 weeks after birth, each nursing raises the level of prolactin in the blood to higher levels than will occur later. More prolactin in the blood—especially during the first 2 weeks after birth—upregulates the prolactin receptors in the body. The more prolactin receptors upregulated during this critical period, the greater the potential milk production for that baby (De Carvalho, 1983). For details about the vital role of early and frequent nursing to the "lactation curve," and its effect on long-term milk production, see p. 425.

• • •

Ask if there is family support and access to lactation help if needed.

A U.S. qualitative study (Pounds, Fisher, Barnes-Josiah, Coleman, & Lefebvre, 2017) concluded that a key component of employed parents' ability to meet feeding goals is to have both support and lactation help during the early weeks after birth. The study mothers described how overwhelmed they felt after birth and how important the help and support of family was to their ability to continue breastfeeding. Researchers also noted that having access to help with latching issues and other common problems was key to exclusive breastfeeding.

• • •

Suggest waiting until returning to work before adopting the work schedule.

Some families wonder if their baby would adapt more easily to their work routine if they mimic their work schedule at home. That is not usually a good idea. If nursing is going well, milk production is best set by the baby. During maternity leave, limiting nursing to certain times or feeding at predetermined intervals is likely to slow milk production and ultimately undermine a family's ability to meet their long-term feeding goals.

Let the family know that a baby's ability to adapt increases with age. Before birth, a baby receives constant nourishment through the umbilical cord. During the early weeks, the baby learns to adjust to intermittent feeds and this period is less stressful for the baby (and the whole family) if baby is fed on cue, which is recommended to set healthy milk production (AAP, 2012; Chantry, Eglash, & Labbok, 2015; WHO, 2018).

• • •

In the week or two before going back to work, suggest parents note how many times each day the baby nurses to get an idea of their magic number.

Nursing parents differ in their storage capacity, the maximum volume of milk available at their fullest time of the day (for details, see p. 416). This individual difference affects the number of milk removals per day needed to keep milk production stable after going back to work. One way to roughly gauge a person's storage capacity is during the week or two before returning to work, count how many times each 24-hour day the baby nurses. This gives a general idea of how many milk removals per day (nursing sessions plus milk expressions) will be needed to keep milk production steady over the long term. This is sometimes called the magic number. See the later section, "Keeping Milk Production Stable: The 'Magic Number'."

Milk Expression Options and Logistics

Choosing a Method

Hand expression and breast pumps are most effective when used together.

For details, see Chapter 11, p. 482-483.

• • •

To help a family choose a breast pump, ask how many hours per week others will feed the baby.

When a breast pump plays a major role in maintaining milk production, choosing an effective pump can make the difference between meeting or not meeting the family's feeding goals. Many effective pumps are available today, but painful and ineffective pumps still exist, so it's important to choose carefully. The best choice will depend on parents' means and their situation.

For example, in the following situation, the breast pump will likely play a major role in milk production:

- Others feed the baby 32 or more hours per week.
- Baby is younger than 6 months old.
- Family's long-term goal is to provide only expressed milk for missed feeds.

In this case, suggest the family look for a pump with the following features:

- The warranty on the pump motor is at least 1 year (indicates quality and durability)
- Double-pumping capability (user can pump both sides at the same time, a huge time saver)

- At least three different nipple tunnel diameters are available (in pumps where hard plastic covers the nipples)
- Separate controls for vacuum/suction and cycling/speed rather than a single control dial (allows users to customize the pump's settings to their body's response)

See Table 11.3 on p. 487 for a chart that recommends certain categories of pumps (single-user, multi-user, manual) for specific situations. See also p. 487-488 for other pump features that employed nursing parents may want to consider.

In the following situation, the breast pump may play a lesser role in maintaining milk production:

- Others feed the baby less than 32 hours per week.
- In addition to expressed milk, for missed feedings, the family plans to provide donor milk or formula and/or solid foods.

In this case, a pump recommended for "occasional use" might suffice. This might include single pumps (which pump one side at a time) and manual pumps, which require muscle power to operate.

When to Express and How Much to Store

For those returning to work before 1 year with a goal of providing only expressed milk for missed feeds, suggest allowing 3 or 4 weeks to practice milk expression and to store some milk.

Expressing milk is a learned skill. Most nursing parents find—no matter what method they use—that with practice they can express more milk more easily. Milk ejection is triggered in part by the feel of the baby nursing and is a conditioned response. Expressing milk has a different feel than nursing, so it can take some time for the body to respond to this new feel in the same way as it does during nursing (Kent, Ramsay, Doherty, Larsson, & Hartmann, 2003). Allowing a few weeks to practice can help families get comfortable with their expression method, so they can go through this "conditioning phase" at home rather than at work, where there will likely be a more intense need to express quickly and effectively.

Another advantage of starting to express about a month before returning to work is that it allows enough time to store a reserve of milk. If parental leave is at least 8 weeks long, suggest waiting to begin expressing until after milk production reaches its peak, around 4 to 5 weeks after birth (Hill et al., 2005; Kent et al., 2016). With some practice, an expression session in the morning about an hour after nursing usually yields on average about half a feed, or about 1.5 to 2 oz. (45 to 58 mL).

During the first few expressions, while their body adjusts to the new feel of the expression method, most parents express very little milk. After expressing for 4 weeks, a reasonable expectation is to freeze about 14 feeds (half a feed each day for 28 days) as a back-up when it's time to go back to work.

A reserve of frozen milk is an especially good idea for those employed full-time who plan to provide their milk exclusively for a young baby. Once back at work, they can usually expect to express enough milk each day to feed the baby the next day. But it is always good to have some extra milk as a hedge against the unexpected, such as spilled milk or milk left out accidentally.

Different families have different comfort levels with the volume of milk they want to store before returning to work. Some feel anxious if they have less than a full week's worth of feeds. Others are happy to go back with just enough milk to cover their first day.

• • •

During maternity leave, there are several ways to express and store milk—if needed—without interfering with nursing.

One way to store milk without missing feeds is to store whatever milk a parent expresses to stay comfortable during the early weeks. Many feel the need to "express to comfort" when they feel full and their baby is unwilling to nurse. "Expressing to comfort" means expressing just enough milk to relieve any fullness without stimulating more milk production. Any milk expressed can be frozen and combined with other batches expressed later (see p. 516).

Another way to store milk during this time is to schedule a daily milk expression. To avoid upsetting or shortchanging the baby, suggest nursing parents do their best to allow at least an hour between an expression and the next feed. On average, babies only take about 67% of the milk in the breast, (Kent, 2007), so there is usually milk left to express after a feed. To get the most milk at an expression, suggest parents:

- Try expressing in the morning, when most express more milk.
- Express 30 to 60 minutes after a feed and at least an hour before a feed.
- Use hands-on pumping techniques (for details, see p. 492).

If the baby wants to nurse right after a milk expression, go ahead. Most babies are patient and do not mind feeding longer to get the milk they need. Suggest encouraging the baby to go back and forth from side to side several times until done. Remind the family that milk production is continuous, so even if only a few minutes have passed since they finished expressing, there will be some milk there for the baby. Lactating glands are never empty. They are constantly making more milk.

Another option is to express milk from one side while the baby nurses on the other side. Inexpensive, all-silicone breast pumps can make collecting milk from the unused side especially easy. This pump is made entirely of food-grade silicone. To attach it to the unused side, simply squeeze it, center it on the nipple, and release, allowing its gentle, continuous suction to draw milk from the other side while baby nurses. See it in action in the photo on p. 488.

• • •

Unless maternity leave is shorter than 8 weeks, it may not be good investment of time to do much pumping and storing during the first month after birth.

Many employed parents seem to be in a hurry to start expressing milk as soon as baby is born. But that's not always a good investment of their time. On a baby's first day of life, on average, milk production is only about 1 ounce (30 mL) of colostrum, the first milk. When nursing is going well, by the time the baby is about 40 days old, milk production reaches its peak of, on average, 25 to 30 ounces (750 to 887 mL) of milk per day. Milk production increases dramatically during the first weeks, making more milk available for expression over time. Once it reaches its peak at about 5 weeks, milk production stays relatively stable until about 6 months. Table 15.1 illustrates the increase in milk intake at feedings during baby's first month (Kent et al., 2016).

TABLE 15.1 Average Milk Intake by Age

Baby's Age	Ave. Milk Per Feeding	Ave. Milk Per Day
First week	1-2 oz. (30-59 mL)	10-20 oz. (296-591 mL) after Day 4
Weeks 2 and 3	2-3 oz. (59-89 mL)	15-25 oz. (443-750 mL)
Months 1 to 6	3-4 oz. (89-118 mL)	25-30 oz. (750-887 mL)

Adapted from (Kent et al., 2016; Kent et al., 2013)

The volume of milk expressed will also depend on several factors, such as:

- Whether the baby is exclusively nursing, and if not, how much other milks or solids he receives each day
- How much time has passed since the last milk removal
- The time of day
- Parents' emotional state
- Pump quality and fit
- How much practice they've had with the milk-expression method

See p. 487 and 907 for details on pump choices and fit. Because milk ejection, or let-down, is partly a conditioned response, practice with a method can help the expresser's body learn to respond to its feel with more milk ejections, which results in more milk. For more details, see p. 476.

• • •

To avoid waste, suggest storing no more milk in a container than the baby will consume at one feed.

At this writing, milk-storage guidelines recommend that after milk has been warmed and fed, any leftover milk should be discarded within 1 to 2 hours after feeding (Eglash, Simon, & Academy of Breastfeeding, 2017). Average milk intake at a nursing is 3 oz. to 4 oz. (88 to 118 mL), but every baby is different. One Australian study (Kent et al., 2013) found the amount of milk 1- to 6-month-old babies took at a nursing session ranged from very little to about 6 oz. (172 mL). Before parents know how much expressed milk their baby will take, suggest storing some of the expressed milk in 1 to 2 oz. (30 to 59 mL) volumes in case the baby wants just a little more. More milk can always be safely added to the feed. Smaller volumes also have the advantage of warming faster. Also suggest they learn the basics of handling and storing milk. For more details, see p. 511.

Planning Ahead for Work

One aspect of planning for work is deciding whether or not to express milk during the workday, and if not, how to prepare.

If the baby is younger than 1 year, there are several advantages to expressing milk at work:

- Greater comfort and less leaking
- Decreased risk of mastitis
- Easier maintenance of milk production
- Possibly avoiding the cost and health risks of human-milk substitutes

If the nursing parent is not planning to express milk at work, it is important to discuss other options. For example, although it is rare, some individuals with a very large storage capacity (for details, see p. 416) may comfortably go for an 8-hour workday without expressing milk. In unusual cases, large-capacity parents have expressed enough milk at home to meet their baby's need for milk during their work hours. Parents of older babies on solid foods may also be able to get through a workday without expressing, because their milk production is already reduced. But most exclusively nursing parents will find that before the workday is over, they may have painful mammary fullness, which increases the risk of mastitis. Most of those who regularly go 8 hours or more without expressing milk also experience a rapid reduction in milk production. Expressing milk even once during the workday significantly increases comfort and helps maintain milk production overall.

Before discussing options, ask first if the workday will be longer than the baby's longest stretch between feeds at home (usually at night). If the parent is already going this length of time without a problem, it may not be necessary to make any changes.

Partial weaning. If the time at work is much longer than the current longest stretch at home and nursing or expressing milk during the workday is not part of the plan, another possibility is a ***partial weaning***. This is a way to reduce milk production gradually to make it possible to be away from the baby for long stretches without uncomfortable fullness or pain yet still have some milk for feeds at home.

There are different approaches to a partial weaning. One involves first noting the usual feeding times during the workday hours. Then about a week or two before returning to work suggest picking one feed during that time and instead feed a substitute, avoiding the first morning feed when most nursing parents feel full already. Before choosing a substitute for human milk, suggest talking to the baby's healthcare provider for recommendations. Continue to feed this food at about the same time every day. After eliminating that nursing, suggest waiting at least 2 to 3 days before dropping another feed. If uncomfortable fullness develops, suggest expressing just enough milk to feel comfortable and no more. This will cause milk production to slow gradually without pain or risk of mastitis. The partial weaning is complete when the parent feels comfortable without nursing for the time period equal to the entire workday.

Another approach to a partial weaning is to continue to nurse at all feeds while at home and offer the supplements in between. When the baby regularly takes as much supplement as he would take during the workday, the partial weaning is complete.

• • •

If the parent is planning to express milk at work, suggest making sure a private area will be available and, if needed, an electrical outlet.

Before returning to work, suggest asking if the workplace provides a lactation room and/or breast pumps for employees. At this writing in the U.S., free breast pumps are available through many insurance companies (USBC, 2010). If there is no specific area for expressing milk, suggest asking about a private office, empty conference room, storage room, or lounge. Where space is tight, a privacy screen can create a private area. As a last resort—although far from ideal—a car or a restroom/toilet can be used.

For those planning to hand express, a place to wash their hands, privacy, a comfortable chair, and a milk collection container are all that's needed. If using a breast pump, suggest asking if there's an electrical outlet available. If not, some quality breast pumps can be powered by rechargeable batteries.

• • •

The time needed for milk expression at work will depend in part on the expression method.

When calculating the time needed to express milk at work, the total time will depend in part on the expression method used.

- **One side at a time.** Plan for each expression to take between 20 and 30 minutes, plus clean-up and travel to and from the private area.
- **Both sides at once.** Plan for each expression to take at least 10 to 15 minutes, plus clean-up and travel to and from the private area.

To reduce clean-up time, one option is to buy enough extra pump parts for all pump sessions at work, which can be washed at home after work.

• • •

Many parents can fit milk expression into their usual breaks and mealtimes.

The number of pump sessions needed during the workday to maintain milk production depends upon several factors:

- Whether or not the baby is exclusively human-milk fed
- The number of hours per day others feed the baby
- Storage capacity

As a starting point, to calculate how many times the parent of a fully mother's-milk-fed baby younger than 6 months old should plan to express milk at work, suggest dividing by three the number of hours others will feed the baby, including travel time:

- 12 hours, 4 expressions ($12 \div 3 = 4$)
- 9 hours, 3 expressions ($9 \div 3 = 3$)

After following this routine at work for a week or two, adjust as needed. For more details, see the later section, "Daily Routines and Milk Production."

• • •

Most nursing parents working full-time with young babies express milk two to three times per day and spend less than an hour total at work expressing milk.

A U.S. study of 283 mothers working full-time for companies with a workplace lactation program (Slusser, Lange, Dickson, Hawkes, & Cohen, 2004) tracked how many times each day they expressed milk at work and the time they spent at each session. During the period their babies were between 3 and 6 months old, the mothers expressed milk at work on average 2.2 times per day and 85% spent an hour or less on milk expression. By 6 months, the mothers expressed milk on average 1.9 times per day, with 95% spending an hour or less on expression at work.

• • •

Most parents stop expressing milk by their baby's first birthday.

As a baby eats more solid foods, he needs less milk. As his need for milk decreases, so does the need to express milk. As explained in the first section of this chapter, most babies 1 year or older can drink other milks from a cup. By that time, most nursing parents have stopped expressing milk at work, even though they may continue to nurse at home. In one U.S. study of 332 women working for 5 companies that participated in a corporate lactation program (Ortiz et al., 2004), mothers stopped expressing milk at work when their babies were a mean age of 9 months old. The age at which the largest number of mothers stopped expressing milk was 12 months.

• • •

Suggest thinking about where to store expressed milk at work.

Depending on the room temperature at the worksite and the length of the workday, it may or may not be necessary to cool expressed milk. See p. 514 for milk storage times at different temperature ranges. The season and local climate will affect whether or not the milk needs to be cooled while traveling from work to home. As long as the milk storage guidelines are followed, any milk stored at room temperature can be refrigerated and/or frozen later.

If it's necessary to cool the milk, there are several options:

- Pump bag cooler compartment cooled with reusable freezer packs
- Separate cooler bag cooled with freezer packs
- A private or shared refrigerator

To avoid the risk of milk loss or contamination, many prefer storing their milk in a private rather than shared space.

• • •

Human milk is not a biohazardous material and no special precautions are needed at work or at child-care facilities.

According to the U.S. Centers for Disease Control and Prevention (CDC, 2018) and the U.S. Occupational Safety and Health Administration (OSHA) (Clark, 1992), no special precautions, such as rubber gloves or separate storage, are required for handling mother's milk, either in the workplace or at child-care facilities. Contact with expressed milk is not considered an occupational exposure. This means that simple hand washing and cleaning up of spills is all that's needed (Nommsen-Rivers, 1997).

Milk Volumes Needed

The volume of milk the baby will need during the workday can be calculated based on how many hours others feed him.

Another issue that requires planning is how much milk to leave for the baby. The family will quickly learn how much milk baby actually consumes once back at work. But some guidance may be helpful beforehand. On average, nursing babies take about 25 oz. (750 mL) of milk each day (24-hour period), but babies differ. To calculate the volume of milk a baby will need during work hours, add a little extra milk to account for big eaters and use 30 oz. (887 mL) per 24 hours as a benchmark. Then divide this amount by the portion of the day that others feed the baby. For example:

- **6 hours** (one-quarter of a 24-hour day) one-quarter of 30 oz. (887 mL) is 7.5 oz. (252 mL)
- **8 hours** (one-third of a 24-hour day) one-third of 30 oz. (887 mL is 10 oz. (296 mL)
- **12 hours** (half of a 24-hour day) half of 30 oz. (887 mL) is 15 oz. (444 mL).

Most parents working full time are away from their babies for 8 to 12 hours per day, so most of these babies will need between 10 and 15 oz. (296 to 444 mL) of milk. This assumes that the baby nurses often while at home. If the baby feeds very little while at home or if the baby sleeps for very long stretches at night without feeding, the baby will need more milk during work hours. For example, a baby who sleeps 8 hours at night will need the full 30 oz. (887 mL) during the remaining 16 hours left in the day.

As described in the first section of this chapter, between 1 and 6 months, nursing babies need about the same volume of milk per day. After solids are started, the volume of milk needed gradually decreases.

Introducing Another Feeding Method

If others feed the baby during the workday, the family may want help in choosing a feeding method.

Safe and effective alternative feeding methods vary around the world. In the developed world—high-resource countries like Canada, the U.S., Europe, Australia, and New Zealand—most babies between birth and 6 to 9 months are fed by infant feeding bottles. In parts of the developing world where water is not always safe, small straight-sided cups or spoons are often used to feed young babies, because they can be cleaned more easily and are less susceptible to bacterial growth. See p. 894 for details on a variety of alternative feeding methods.

• • •

If the baby will be fed by bottle during the workday, suggest if possible waiting until the baby is at least 3 to 4 weeks old to begin bottle feeding.

Most lactation specialists recommend delaying bottle feeds until at least 3 to 4 weeks of age to allow babies the time to first master nursing. However, if the nursing parent is returning to work within the first month after birth, it may be necessary in some cases to introduce bottles earlier. On the other hand, if the nursing parent is returning to work after 6 months, learning to feed from a bottle may be unnecessary, as many babies this age can transition directly to a cup.

Even if a family chooses to bottle-feed after the return to work, it is not always necessary to introduce the bottle during maternity leave. Some families delay bottles until the return to work and arrange for the caregiver to introduce bottles then. But many parents find that it sets their minds at ease to introduce the bottle earlier, so that they know their baby will accept it.

Many parents are told to start the bottle as early as possible to "get the baby used to it." Some are warned not to wait too long or the baby won't take it. At this writing, although many have strong opinions, there is no reliable evidence to guide us.

• • •

Suggest the parents try different types of bottle nipples/teats and choose the slowest-flow nipple the baby accepts.

Adults are encouraged to eat slowly to activate our "appetite control mechanism," so that we feel full with less food. The same dynamic is true for babies. A baby is more likely to take more milk with a fast-flow bottle, which can lead to overfeeding (Li et al., 2012). A baby using a slow-flow nipple/teat is more likely to feel full after less milk, minimizing the volume of milk needed during the workday.

Because babies' mouths are different shapes, one type of bottle and nipple will not be the best choice for all babies. U.S. lactation specialists Amy Peterson and Mindy Harmer suggest in their book, *Balancing Breast and Bottle* that families start with a teat that widens gradually from base to tip (see p. 901-902 for an illustration), rather than one that widens abruptly (Peterson & Harmer, 2010, p. 53). U.S. lactation consultants Barbara Wilson-Clay and Kay Hoover write in *The Breastfeeding Atlas* (Wilson-Clay & Hoover, 2017, pp. 123-124):

> "...[We] find that an experimental approach is best. Some infants require a narrow-based teat due to poor lip tone and inability to seal to a wide base. Some infants will gag if the teat is too long. Other infants seem not to respond if the teat is too short and insufficient proprioceptive stimulation is provided along the tongue."

Suggest the family try several types and styles of nipples/teats and see which the baby accepts.

• • •

We have no credible evidence on whether it is better for the nursing parent to introduce a bottle to a younger baby or for someone else to introduce it.

When the nursing parent of a younger baby returns to work, in many cases, the best person to introduce a bottle is the baby's caregiver, since the bottle will be a part of their relationship. Bottle-feeding may go more smoothly if the caregiver has the chance to have a few visits and get to know the baby first.

Some, however, believe that it's easiest for nursing parents to introduce the bottle, since they are the person baby knows best. In their book *Balancing Breast and Bottle,* U.S. lactation specialists Amy Peterson and Mindy Harmer wrote (Peterson & Harmer, 2010, p. 52):

> "You, the mother, are the one who is intimately acquainted with your baby's suck. You know what your baby's lips look like when he feeds, how widely he naturally latches on your breast, and how long your let-downs last."

• • •

If a baby is reluctant to take a bottle, there are many strategies to try and, if needed, other ways to feed the baby.

The following strategies may help a reluctant baby accept a bottle. Suggest the family ask the caregiver to experiment to see what works best.

- **Have someone other than nursing parent offer the bottle.** Some babies will not accept a bottle from the nursing parent or from someone else if the nursing parent is within earshot or in the building.
- **Offer the bottle before baby is too hungry.** Babies tend to accept something new more easily if they are feeling calm rather than ravenous.
- **Offer short trials with the bottle at first.** If the baby resists, don't keep at it until baby is screaming. Let the baby play with it and put it away if the baby begins to seem unhappy.
- **Try different feeding positions.** Many babies like to be snuggled close when given a bottle and look into the feeder's eyes, but some babies will not take a bottle when held in their usual nursing position. Try instead to hold baby facing forward, with his back against the caregiver's chest or propped on raised legs, or try the bottle when baby is sitting in an infant seat.
- **Wrap the baby in an item of the nursing parent's clothing** with the parent's scent on it.

- **Warm the bottle nipple/teat to body temperature** by running warm water over it before offering it. Try dipping it in warm mother's milk. If baby is teething, try a nipple that has been chilled in the refrigerator.
- **Tap baby's lips with the bottle nipple,** wait until baby opens, and allow baby to draw the nipple into his mouth rather than pushing it in.
- **Move rhythmically when offering the bottle** to calm baby by walking, rocking, or swaying.
- **Experiment with different types of bottles and nipples/teats.**
- **Try offering the bottle while baby is drowsy or in a light sleep.**
- **If baby is older, give him a bottle to play with** for a few days before attempting a feeding.
- **Give some milk by spoon first** and then offer the bottle or let baby suck on a finger and slip in the bottle along the side as he sucks.

If none of these suggestions work, babies can be fed other ways, with a cup, spoon, or eyedropper. One father discovered by experimenting that his 3-month-old baby, who would not accept a bottle while his mother was a work, would gladly consume by spoon a partially-frozen human-milk "slushie"(Walker, 2011).

• • •

If a baby takes more from a bottle than the volume expressed for a missed feed, this is not necessarily a sign of low milk production.

If a nursing parent is concerned because the baby takes more milk from the bottle than they can express at one sitting, explain that this is likely due to the different flow rates of nursing and bottle. Unless paced-feeding techniques are used (see p. 902-903 for details), the bottle flows consistently. During nursing, however, there is an ebb and flow of milk as milk ejections occur. Due to this natural ebb and flow, a nursing baby may feel full with less milk, whereas the faster, more consistent flow of the bottle may override a baby's "appetite control mechanism" and cause overfeeding (Azad, et al., 2018; Li et al., 2012). Taking more milk from the bottle than is expressed at a session is not a reliable indicator of low milk production. Rather, it is more likely a reflection of these differences in feeding methods (see p. 192-193).

JOB OPTIONS AND CHILD CARE

The first section in this chapter covered the effects of full time and part time work on nursing. This section will review other job options and child-care decisions that can affect feeding outcomes.

Work Schedules and Settings

Suggest the nursing parent look into the possibility of flexible work options.

Although some parents have little flexibility in their jobs, some may discover more options than they expect. The following are possible flexible work arrangements to consider:

- Part time—Working fewer hours per week
- Job-sharing—Sharing one position with another person or parent

- Phase back—Gradually increasing work hours from part time to full time
- Flex-time—Adjusting work hours to baby's routine
- Compressed work week—Working the same hours in fewer days
- Telecommuting—Working from home some or all workdays
- On-site day care—Going to baby for feeds as needed

In one U.S. study (Grice, McGovern, & Alexander, 2008), researchers surveyed 522 women who returned to work within the 6 months after childbirth. Not surprisingly, there was much less perceived spillover of home issues to work when the women had good support from family and friends. Flexible work hours (including the ability to take work home or work some shifts from home) were associated with greater spillover of home issues to work, but job flexibility was perceived as a positive by the women. Also, not surprisingly, the women in professional jobs had greater work flexibility than the women in clerical jobs or those who did manual labor. A later study done by the same U.S. research team (Grice, McGovern, Alexander, Ukestad, & Hellerstedt, 2011) found an association between job and home spillover and decreased mental and physical health, which they concluded may be an unintended consequence of job flexibility.

KEY CONCEPT

Continued nursing is easier in some types of jobs than others.

• • •

Ask for details about the work setting, as some workplaces make continued nursing easier than others.

Continued nursing is easier in some types of jobs than others. A 2018 U.S. study of 1,002 women (Snyder et al., 2018) found significant differences in workplace lactation support among different employment types. Parents with professional or management positions were more likely to get either direct or informal lactation support at their return to work. The least amount of lactation support was provided to lactating employees in the service, production, and transportation industries.

Research found some jobs to be especially challenging, including military (Bales, Washburn, & Bales, 2012; Stevens & Janke, 2003), security guard (Dunn, Zavela, Cline, & Cost, 2004), jobs with 12-hour rotating shifts (Witters-Green, 2003), and physicians during residency (Arthur, Saenz, & Replogle, 2003; Cantu, Gowen, Tang, & Mitchell, 2018).

A 2016 study conducted with 225 mothers in Ghana found that only 9% of those working in formal work settings exclusively breastfed for 6 months because those workplaces did not allow them to bring their babies with them and provided no space or time for milk expression. However, women working in more informal work settings, such as weaving, dressmaking, food and beverage services, and farming, kept their babies with them at work and 91% exclusively breastfed during their babies' first 6 months.

Employer Solutions is a U.S. government video database that features short videos of employers in a wide variety of industries explaining the worksite accommodations they made to support lactation for their employees and why this is an excellent return on investment. This website (**bit.ly/BA2-Employer**) is organized by industry and by the specific accommodations that support nursing in the workplace.

• • •

If the work schedule or setting is inflexible, explore the possibility of reverse cycle nursing.

Reverse cycle nursing means most feeds take place while the nursing parent is home and the baby takes his longest sleep stretch during the workday. Work hours may be scheduled during the baby's naturally occurring longest sleep period. Or the baby may choose to change his feeding rhythm so that he is awake and feeding more often when the nursing parent is home. Some families make nursing work with challenging work schedules or settings by using this approach. If the baby falls into this pattern naturally or the work shift is scheduled around the baby, it can take much of the pressure off to express much milk. However, nursing frequently all night can be exhausting for the nursing parent, and it may not be easy to change a baby's sleep pattern to achieve this.

• • •

In some situations, a note from the parent's or baby's healthcare provider may convince the employer to be more supportive.

U.S. attorney, Jessica Lee, an advocate for families in the workplace, summarized why a note from a doctor can make a big difference in securing pumping or nursing accommodations for lactating employees (Lee, 2017, p. 471):

> "Effective notes, even brief ones, can serve to educate the employer about breastfeeding and pumping, and shift their attitude. In addition to shifting attitudes, notes for breastfeeding workers can be critical for mothers whose only legal entitlement to accommodations is that colleagues with other medical conditions receive accommodations. Often, employer policies require some form of medical certification for their workers to get the changes they need. This may apply to even the most basic accommodations, such as regular break time or allowing a retail worker to keep a bottle of water at her side. In these cases, a doctor's note will shift the conversation from one wherein the worker is asking for a 'favor' to one herein she is asserting a legal right."

According to Lee, the most effective notes contain the following points:

- Explanation about why human milk and regular milk expression are important
- A clear explanation of why the accommodations are necessary for the patient's own health, in addition to the baby's health
- The specific requirements that the patient needs to be able to pump, including the frequency and duration of the required breaks (for example, if the baby is a newborn, 30 minutes of break time every 3 hours)
- A sanitary, private space that is not a bathroom or toilet

If the employee or the baby has a medical condition or impairment, it's key to mention any special needs that entitle them to extra accommodations or protection. For more information, see the website: **bit.ly/BA2-BFAccomm**.

Worksite Lactation Support

Worksite lactation support increases initiation, duration, and exclusivity of nursing.

A 2017 systematic review evaluated workplace lactation interventions in the U.S. (Kim, Shin, & Donovan, 2018), which included providing a breast pump for 1 year, return-to-work consultations with lactation specialists, and telephone support. The authors concluded that these interventions increased breastfeeding initiation, duration, and exclusivity, with better outcomes associated with more available services. A. U.S. study of more than 2,400 mothers (Kozhimannil, Jou, Gjerdingen, & McGovern, 2016) found after controlling for sociodemographic and birth-related factors that women with sufficient break time to express milk at work were 2.6 times more likely to breastfeed exclusively than those who didn't have sufficient break time to express milk and 3 times more likely to be breastfeeding at 6 months. Each month they had both sufficient break time and a private place to express milk, the women were 3.8 times as likely to continue breastfeeding exclusively. Those with a private space but no break time breastfed for 1.36 months longer than those with no break time or private space.

KEY CONCEPT

Nursing even once during the workday reduces the number of pump sessions needed.

In the Academy of Breastfeeding Medicine's 2013 Position Statement, "Breastfeeding Support for Mothers in Workplace Employment or Educational Settings" (Marinelli, Moren, Taylor, & Academy of Breastfeeding Medicine, 2013), interventions proven effective at increasing breastfeeding duration among working families are described:

- Keeping baby and nursing parent together when nursing is being established
- Provision of a longer, ideally paid parental leave after birth
- Workplace accommodations, such as lactation breaks, flexible work hours, access to part-time work when baby is young, infant on site or in close proximity to the workplace
- Employer resources, such as a physical space that is private and clean for nursing or milk expression, education about benefits to employers of supporting nursing
- Legal and public-health policy considerations that promote positive workplace breastfeeding policies

The 2012 Cochrane Review on interventions in the workplace to support breastfeeding (Abdulwadud & Snow, 2012) concluded that if employed nursing families do not receive the worksite support they need, they may not be able to maintain breastfeeding.

A 2017 systematic review that examined 22 articles about worksite lactation support programs in 10 different countries (Dinour & Szaro, 2017) concluded that "maintaining breastfeeding while working is not only possible but also more likely when employers provide the supports that women need to do so. Although some employers may have more extensive breastfeeding support policies and practices than others, all employers can implement a breastfeeding support program that fits their company's budget and resources."

A 2018 U.S. study of a worksite support program in rural Minnesota (Jantzer, Anderson, & Kuehl, 2018) reiterated what many other researchers concluded, that providing a time and place for either nursing or milk expression in the workday can improve job satisfaction as well as helping employed families meet their feeding goals.

• • •

When talking to the boss, encourage the parent to focus on the benefits to the employer of providing worksite lactation support.

Many are reluctant to discuss lactation support at work. Some parents worry that asking for a time and place to nurse or express milk will be seen as requesting special favors. Some feel awkward because nursing feels so personal and they are concerned that it may be perceived as unprofessional to discuss it. Both the employee and employer stand to gain, but most employers are unaware of the benefits to them (Dunn et al., 2004; Soomro, Shaikh, Saheer, & Bijarani, 2016). If parents have information about how nursing will benefit the employer financially, they may feel more comfortable about discussing their needs. An excellent online resource is the U.S. government website that includes the Business Case for Breastfeeding (Garvin et al., 2013). Share this link as a starting point for families who would like more information about the financial benefits to employers of supporting lactation in the workplace: **bit.ly/BA2-BusinessCase**.

For example, the website cited above noted that in employee families who don't breastfeed, companies experience:

- Significantly higher healthcare expenses
- Twice as many 1-day absences due to illness
- Lower employee retention rates after birth (national average: 59%, in companies with worksite lactation support: 94%)

• • •

In some parts of the world, employers may be required by law to provide a time and place for nursing or milk expression.

Before the employee talks to the boss, suggest checking national and state or provincial laws. In the U.S., federal law requires that employers provide all hourly employees with a reasonable amount of break time and a secure, private place to express and store milk (Martin, 2011; Raju, 2014). For details, download the U.S. Breastfeeding Committee publication at this link: **bit.ly/BA2-USBC**.

When discussing lactation laws, however, encourage the family to bring up this subject carefully so the employer does not see it as a veiled threat. Most U.S. worksite breastfeeding laws carry no penalty if not followed. Suggest keeping the main focus on how the company will benefit. In some areas, "Breastfeeding Friendly Employer" awards are offered through local health departments, which may provide positive incentives for local employers.

• • •

In the U.S., more worksite lactation support programs are available to office workers in large companies.

According to a 2017 survey, 42% of U.S. businesses provide lactation support for at least some employees (SHRM, 2017). Research found that lactation support was most likely to be available in large companies as compared with medium with 99 to 499 employees and small companies with 1-99 employees (Snyder et al., 2018).

• • •

Common barriers to worksite lactation support can often be overcome with creative thinking and an open mind.

Barriers to worksite lactation support, such as the following, can usually be overcome (Dinour & Szaro, 2017).

Time away from work duties. If there is a concern about the time spent expressing milk at work, explain that many can express their milk during regular breaks and mealtimes. If this is not enough time, they can ask to make up for time needed by coming in early or leaving later. The employee can also emphasize that the need to express at work is temporary, as most stop expressing by 12 months.

Discomfort with breastfeeding. It may help to choose words carefully. For example, it may help to use the word "lactation" instead of "breastfeeding." Avoid promotional materials with photos of breasts or breastfeeding. Get permission from other parents in the workplace to share their stories so the employer can more clearly see the need.

Resistance from other employees. This can be avoided by including others in the planning process or by providing staff training. To create a greater sense of fairness, some companies offer lactation education and equipment to the partners of employees as well as the nursing employees themselves. Share the financial benefits to the company as a whole (see **bit.ly/BA2-BusinessCase**) and any specifics that might be appropriate.

Lack of available space. If a nursing employee doesn't have a private office, the space needed to nurse or express milk can be as small as 4 feet by 5 feet (1.5 by 2 meters), such as a modified storage room. Suggest the parent brainstorm with the employer about existing areas that could be used. For example, rather than a separate room, a privacy screen could be used in the manager's office to create a private area for nursing or milk expression.

• • •

Even without an official worksite lactation program, companies can still offer benefits and services that support nursing.

In one survey of 157 U.S. businesses, only 28% provided specific lactation support services, yet many offered benefits that promoted lactation, such as (Dunn et al., 2004):

- Maternity leave of 3 months or longer (85%)
- Flex-time, job sharing, or part-time employment options (72%)
- Refrigerator for storage of expressed milk (71%)
- Breaks for expressing milk or nursing (62%)

Access to Baby During the Workday

In some work settings, bringing baby to work or going to the baby for feeds is an option during their workday.

Some companies either allow the baby to stay in the work area or on-site child care is provided. A survey of 157 U.S. companies in Colorado reported that 9% of the companies provided on-site child care (Dunn et al., 2004).

Even if it is not possible to have the baby at work, the nursing parent may be able to go to the baby for some or all feeds by choosing a caregiver near work rather than home. Even one nursing during the workday reduces the time spent expressing milk and the amount of expressed milk the baby needs. Choosing a caregiver near work rather than home also reduces the travel time away from the baby, thereby reducing the need to express milk.

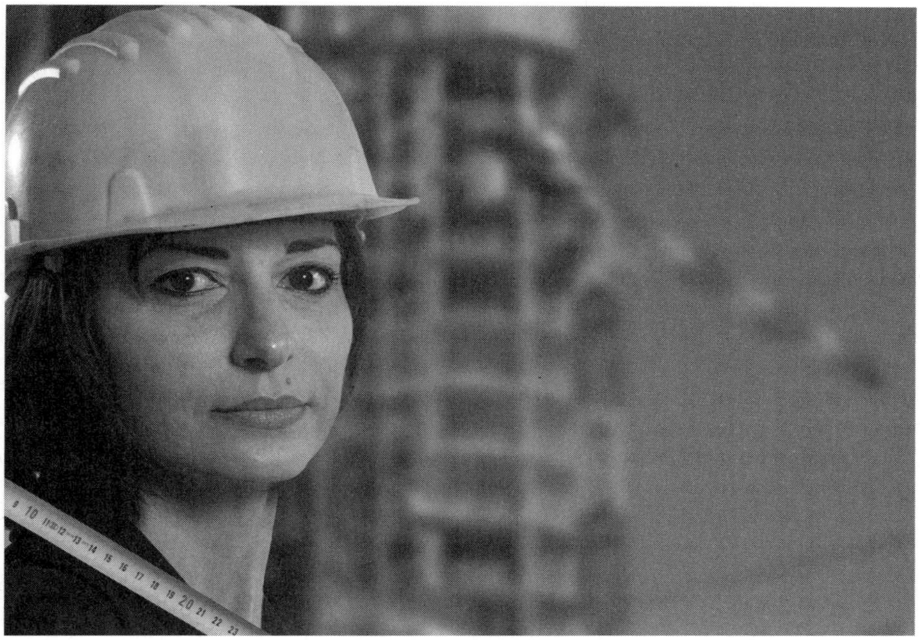

RETURNING TO WORK

In many families, the nursing parent's return to work is a major transition. This section describes ways to make this transition easier and strategies for meeting feeding goals.

Easing the Transition

One way to make the transition back to work easier is to plan to work fewer days and/or fewer hours, even if only for a short time.

To make the first week back at work easier and less stressful, suggest the nursing parent consider starting back to work near the end of the work week, such as on a Thursday or Friday, working shorter hours, or starting back to work part time. A more gradual return to the work schedule may make the transition easier for the whole family.

• • •

If appropriate, suggest wearing work clothes that make it easy to nurse or express milk.

During lactation, the following wardrobe suggestions may make it easier to nurse or express milk at work:

- Have breast pads on hand and an extra top available in case of milk leakage
- Wear two-piece outfits so that nursing or milk expression is possible without having to fully undress
- Wear patterned tops rather than solid colors to better camouflage leaks or spilled milk
- Have a jacket or sweater handy for use as a cover-up if needed

• • •

Encourage the family to accept all offers of help, especially during the most vulnerable first 2 months back at work.

According to one U.S. study (Kimbro, 2006), during the first 2 months back at work, continued lactation is at greatest risk. In this study, employed mothers were 2.2 times more likely to stop breastfeeding than those not yet back at work. Let the family know that if they can keep nursing going for two more months, their odds of continuing are about the same as in families where the nursing parent is not employed. Knowing this may motivate families to proactively take steps to reduce stress during the first months at work.

• • •

Returning to work is a major adjustment for many.

Some of the many adjustments are described by those who participated in one U.S. study (Nichols & Roux, 2004) in which women returned to work on average 11 weeks after giving birth. These mothers:

- Found it difficult to leave their babies
- Had conflicting demands on their time and energy
- Felt overloaded with work-family strains
- Had challenges with child care and financial demands
- Were sleep deprived and experienced mood changes

Although the negatives outweighed the positives, the positives reported included learning to ask for and receive help, their enjoyment of motherhood, the realignment of their priorities and lifestyle to better reflect their new family dynamics, and the satisfaction they derived from their work.

• • •

Encourage the family to seek support from other families who have experience with working and nursing.

There is no substitute for being in contact with others who have been there. Nursing is always easier with emotional support and current information. For some families, coworkers are an important source of ongoing lactation support (Rojjanasrirat, 2004).

If there are no experienced families at work, suggest getting in touch with local in-person or online peer support groups. One U.S. study found that employed parents who attended a support meeting within the first 6 weeks after birth were three times more likely to nurse longer than 6 months and meet their own lactation goals as compared with those who didn't attend a meeting (Chezem & Friesen, 1999). Another U.S. study found that attending a worksite lactation support group at a U.S. public health clinic was one of four significant predictors of breastfeeding duration for a group of mostly Latina mothers (Whaley, Meehan, Lange, Slusser, & Jenks, 2002).

Strategies to Minimize Milk Needed and Avoid Waste

If the baby is younger than 1 year, the volume of milk needed during the workday depends in part on the family's daily routine.

If the baby is younger than 1 year, the following strategies can help keep milk expression to a minimum:

- **Plan to nurse at least twice before leaving the baby with the caregiver.** Nurse once when the nursing parent awakens and again just before leaving baby with the caregiver.

- **Nurse as soon as the nursing parent arrives at the caregiver's after work.** If the baby seems hungry just before the parent arrives, suggest the caregiver feed as little milk as possible so the baby will want to nurse when the parent gets there.
- **Nurse often at home, day and night.** As mentioned earlier, the baby needs a set amount of milk per 24-hour day. The fewer times baby nurses while they're together, the more milk he will need during the workday.
- **Choose a caregiver close to work rather than home to reduce travel time** and therefore time apart.
- **If possible, arrange to nurse baby at least once during the workday.** If the caregiver is nearby, the nursing parent may be able to go to baby or have baby brought to the workplace for a feed.

Depending on the length of the workday, many of these strategies can cut the volume of milk needed during the workday significantly.

• • •

The volume of milk stored and the nipple/teat flow can affect how much milk is discarded and how much baby needs to feel full.

To minimize the volume of expressed milk the baby needs during the workday, suggest the family:

- **Store expressed milk in the smallest volumes baby may take.** The average volume consumed during a nursing is 3 to 4 oz. (88 to 118 mL), but every baby is different. Once the nursing parent is back at work and knows how much the baby usually takes at a feed, the family will know how much milk to store. Suggest also storing some 1- to 2-ounce. (30 to 59 mL) batches to avoid waste in case the baby wants just a little more milk at some feeds.
- **If a young baby is fed by bottle, choose a slow-flow nipple and use paced bottle-feeding techniques.** This allows the baby's "appetite control mechanism" to be triggered earlier so the baby feels full with less milk. Nipple/teat package information is not always an accurate indicator of flow. Suggest experimenting with several brands to see which seems to offer the slowest flow. See p. 902-903 for details on how to do paced bottle-feeding.

Keeping Milk Production Stable: The 'Magic Number'

One way to keep milk production stable long term is to maintain the same number of milk removals per day before and after returning to work (the magic number).

To keep milk production steady as the months go by, suggest that nursing parents continue to remove the milk well the same number of times each day after returning to work as they did near the end of maternity leave. Think of this number of daily milk removals as their ***magic number*** (Mohrbacher, 2011).

An individual's storage capacity will affect how many milk removals per day are needed to keep milk production steady over the long term. A basic dynamic of milk production is drained glands make milk faster and full glands make milk slower. When individuals have a large storage capacity, it takes a longer time for milk to accumulate before they begin to feel full. Many large-capacity parents maintain their milk production on fewer milk removals per day and express more milk at each session than those with a larger capacity. Those with a small storage capacity feel full faster and must remove the milk more often to express the same volume of milk. Both large- and small-capacity parents can make plenty of milk for their babies overall, but their magic number (the number of milk removals needed to keep milk production stable) can vary greatly. Learn more about the magic number at **bit.ly/BA2-MagicNumber**.

In Western cultures, due to the prevalence of bottle-feeding and bottle-feeding norms, over time and as baby grows, many parents believe their nursing babies (like bottle-feeding babies) should nurse fewer and fewer times each day. However, fewer feeds per day is not typical of nursing babies, and this can cause milk production to drop. When the total number of daily milk removals (nursing sessions plus milk expressions) drops below an individual's magic number, (determined in large part by storage capacity), milk production slows (Kent, 2007). For more details, see p. 416.

KEY CONCEPT

A nursing parent's magic number is the number of milk removals (feeds plus milk expressions) per day needed to maintain milk production long term.

Once back at work, suggest making a note at least once per week of how many times each day the milk is removed by either nursing or milk expression. As babies begin sleeping longer at night, the number of daily milk removals can drop below the magic number.

It is not unusual for parents to keep their number of milk expressions at work steady but over time nurse fewer and fewer times per day at home. When milk production decreases, be sure to ask about the 24-hour total number of milk removals, which includes feeds at home and at work, as well as milk expressions at home and at work.. Ask how this daily total number of milk removals compares to what it was during maternity leave. Increasing the daily number of milk removals is often all that's needed to boost decreasing milk production.

• • •

To keep milk production stable over the long term, suggest limiting the longest stretch between milk removals to 8 hours or less.

Because drained glands make milk faster and full glands make milk slower, long stretches between feeds at night can slow milk production. When milk-production issues develop, ask the length of the longest stretch. To avoid going so long between milk removals that a signal is sent to slow milk production, suggest trying to avoid going more than 8 hours without either nursing or expressing milk. For example, if the baby sleeps 10 to 12 hours at night, to keep milk production stable, options include doing a "dream feed" (nurse during light sleep without baby completely waking) or expressing milk. For some small-capacity parents, even 8 hours may be long enough to cause a decrease in milk production. For more details, see p. 416.

• • •

If a job requires travel, keep milk production steady by using the magic number as a guide.

If a nursing parent travels for work without the baby, suggest using the magic number to determine the daily number of milk expressions needed. While on the road, depending on the length of time away, the expressed milk can be cooled, frozen, or discarded. If using a breast pump, suggest bringing extra pump parts and, if needed, extra batteries. There are many creative solutions for storing milk while traveling. Some find ways to freeze the milk and ship it back home on dry ice. Some companies cover the cost of shipping milk as an employee benefit (SHRM, 2017). If the trip is less than a week long, it may be possible to keep the milk refrigerated and carry it back in an insulated bag with cooler packs. For air travel in the U.S., the Transportation Security Administration (TSA) allows an unlimited volume of mother's milk to be hand carried on an aircraft, even when parents travel without the baby.

• • •

When the baby starts eating solid foods, expect milk production to gradually decrease.

Because solid foods take the place of mother's milk in a baby's diet (Islam, Peerson, Ahmed, Dewey, & Brown, 2006), as baby takes more solids, he takes less milk. This is normal, and milk production naturally adjusts downward as baby takes more other foods and less milk. This is important to keep in mind when families report they are expressing less milk at work than they did before. If the baby started solid foods, this may be a normal change. If baby's weight gain is in the normal range, it may not be necessary to increase milk production.

Problem-Solving

If the volume of milk expressed is less milk than the baby consumes during the workday or it has decreased, get more information before offering suggestions.

If a parent says: "My baby is taking more milk than I express at work," or "I used to express more milk at work, but now I'm expressing less," don't assume that milk production is the problem. First rule out other possibilities. To get to the root of the issue, ask:

- The baby's age and how long it's been since the parent's return to work.
- Is the baby fully mother's milk fed? If not, how much and what other foods does baby take?
- What is their total time apart on workdays, including travel time?
- How much milk (and any other foods) does baby take during the workday?
- What is the daily routine, including all nursings, expressions, and other feeds?
- How many milk removals per day were average near the end of parental leave and now?
- What is the longest stretch between milk removals (usually at night)?

Example: Expressing less milk at work than the baby takes

Baby girl 10 weeks old. Mother returned to work 2 weeks ago. Mother and baby are apart 8 hours per day 5 days a week. Baby fully mother's milk fed and taking 20 oz. (591 mL) per day from caregiver. Daily milk removals during maternity leave: 8; now: 5. Daily routine:

- One nursing at home in the morning
- Two milk expressions at work (expressing 12 oz. [355 mL] total)
- Two nursing sessions at home in the evening
- Baby sleeps 8 hours at night, the longest stretch

Baby is fed four 5-oz. (147 mL) bottles by the caregiver.

- One bottle fed at arrival
- Two more bottles fed over the course of the day
- One more bottle fed just before mother arrives to take baby home

Conclusions: The mother is expressing the expected volume of milk. Eight hours apart is one-third of a 24-hour day. Using 30 oz. (887 mL) per day as a benchmark, she should expect to express about one-third of this or about 10 oz. (296 mL). She is expressing 12 oz. (355 mL).

She has two issues: her daily routine and dropping below her magic number. Two simple changes in daily routine could cut in half the amount of expressed milk she needs each day, from 20 oz. (592 mL) to 10 oz. (296 mL).

1. Instead of feeding the baby a bottle of expressed milk upon arrival at the caregiver's, she could nurse before leaving for work.
2. Before picking up the baby at the end of the day, she could ask the caregiver to hold off her baby with very little milk and then nurse when she arrives.

Although her rate of milk production has not yet decreased, she has only been back at work for 2 weeks. She is at risk of slowed milk production, since her daily milk removals recently fell from 8 to 5. Depending on her storage capacity, this may or may not be an issue for her. Make the mother aware of this so that she knows what adjustments to make to increase her rate of milk production if needed.

• • •

There are several reasons a baby may take more milk than expected from the caregiver.

When a baby takes much more milk from the caregiver than expected, it can add tremendous stress to a family's life. To determine the reason, do some detective work.

Compare the baby's milk intake with what's expected. When the workday is between 8 and 12 hours, young babies usually take, on average, 10 to 15 oz. (296 to 444 mL). If the baby consumes the expected volumes, move on to other possible issues. If the baby is consuming much more than expected, try to find out why, starting with a discussion about the family's daily routine. Would it help to nurse more when they are together?

Compare the volume of expressed milk at work with what's expected. For example, if others are feeding the baby for 8 to 12 hours on workdays, how close is the volume expressed to the expected 10 to 15 oz. (296 to 446 mL) of milk)? If the volume of expressed milk is in the expected range, milk production is likely not the problem. If it is low, focus on milk production.

Ask about the feeding method. Is the caregiver using a slow-flow nipple/teat? Is the caregiver using paced bottle-feeding techniques? For details, see p. 902-903.

Other possible issues.

- How much milk is being discarded during the workday? Perhaps the milk needs to be provided in smaller batches.

- Could the caregiver be overfeeding the baby? Some caregivers use overfeeding as a way to keep babies content longer. Another symptom of overfeeding is disinterest in nursing at home. If a baby is gaining well but is feeding very little at home, it may be due to overfeeding during the workday.

• • •

If milk production is low, try to find out why so that strategies to boost milk production address the root cause.

If low milk production is suspected, be sure to consider:

- The peak milk production—Has the baby ever been exclusively nursed? If not, full milk production may not have been established.
- Has the number of daily milk removals dropped below the magic number?
- What is the longest stretch between milk removals—Is it longer than 8 hours?
- Method of milk expression—Is the volume of milk expressed in the expected range? If not, consider pump fit and other strategies for improving its effectiveness. (For details, see p. 442 and 907-908.) If not, is it possible to try another expression method?

Example: Expressing half of what the baby needs during the workday

Baby boy 6 months old. Mother returned to work 4 months ago. Mother and baby are apart 8 hours per day 5 days a week. Baby mostly mother's milk fed. Some formula supplements were needed off and on. Total volume of milk mother expresses at work: 6 oz. (180 mL). Baby needs 12 oz. (355 mL) per workday. Mother's feeding goal is exclusive breastfeeding (plus solids) for at least 1 year. Magic number during maternity leave: 8 to 10; now: 5. Her daily routine:

- One nursing session at home before work
- Two milk expressions at work (expressing 6 oz. [177 ml] total)
- Two nursing sessions at home in the evening
- Baby began sleeping 10 to 12 hours at night—the longest stretch—at about 2 months

Baby is fed three 4-oz. (147 mL) bottles by the caregiver.

Conclusions: The combination of the 10- to 12-hour sleep stretch at night and the drop in the daily milk removals below the magic number—from 9 to 5—most likely explains this mother's difficulty in maintaining her milk production. She said that when her baby started sleeping so long at night, at first she got up to express her milk once during the night and that helped her store enough milk for her workday. She started dropping daily nursing sessions when her friends told her that a baby that age did not need so many feeds each day. After a better understanding of the dynamics working against her, this mother decided to nurse more at home and to get up once during the night to express her milk.

• • •

When an increase in milk production is needed, be prepared to offer several approaches to consider and encourage quick action.

Because nursing parents differ, one approach to increasing milk production will not appeal to everyone. See p. 442 in Chapter 10, "Making Milk" for a range of strategies to suggest. Also, when milk production slows, the sooner action is taken to increase it, the more quickly results are likely to occur. The longer a family waits to take action, the more difficult it can be to boost milk production.

RESOURCES

bit.ly/BA2-ABMWorkplace—Academy of Breastfeeding Medicine Breastfeeding Support for Mothers in Workplace Employment or Educational Settings: Summary Statement.

bit.ly/BA2-BFEurope—EU Project on Promotion of Breastfeeding in Europe. Protection, Promotion and Support of Breastfeeding in Europe: A Blueprint for Action (2004).

bit.ly/BA2-BusinessCase—U.S. Business Case for Breastfeeding (2010).

bit.ly/BA2-ILOWork—International Labour Office, Conditions of Work and Employment Programme. Maternity at Work: A Review of National Legislation (2010).

bit.ly/BA2-MaternityCountry—World Alliance for Breastfeeding Action. Status of Maternity Protection by Country (2011).

bit.ly/BA2-SurgeonGen—U.S. Surgeon General's Call to Action (2011).

Marasco, L. & West, D. (2020). *Making More Milk: The Breastfeeding Guide to Increasing Your Milk Production, 2nd ed.* New York, NY: McGraw Hill.

Mohrbacher, N. (2014). *Working and Breastfeeding Made Simple.* Amarillo TX: Praeclarus Press.

REFERENCES

AP. (2012). Breastfeeding and the use of human milk. *Pediatrics, 129*(3), e827-e841.

Abdulwadud, O. A., & Snow, M. E. (2012). Interventions in the workplace to support breastfeeding for women in employment. *Cochrane Database of Systematic Reviews, 10,* CD006177.

Arthur, C. R., Saenz, R. B., & Replogle, W. H. (2003). The employment-related breastfeeding decisions of physician mothers. *Journal of the Mississippi State Medical Association, 44*(12), 383-387.

Attanasio, L., Kozhimannil, K. B., McGovern, P., et al. (2013). The impact of prenatal employment on breastfeeding intentions and breastfeeding status at 1 week postpartum. *Journal of Human Lactation, 29*(4), 620-628.

Azad, M. B., Vehling, L., Chan, D., et al. (2018). Infant feeding and weight gain: Separating breast milk from breastfeeding and formula from food. *Pediatrics, 142*(4).

Bales, K., Washburn, J., & Bales, J. (2012). Breastfeeding rates and factors related to cessation in a military population. *Breastfeeding Medicine, 7*(6), 436-441.

Bergman, N. J. (2013). Neonatal stomach volume and physiology suggest feeding at 1-h intervals. *Acta Paediatrica, 102*(8), 773-777.

Cantu, R. M., Gowen, M. S., Tang, X., et al. (2018). Barriers to breastfeeding in female physicians. *Breastfeeding Medicine, 13*(5), 341-345.

CDC. (2018, 1/24/2018). Are special precautions needed while handling breast milk? Retrieved from **cdc.gov/breastfeeding/faq/#handling-breast-milk**.

Chantry, C. J., Eglash, A., & Labbok, M. (2015). ABM position on breastfeeding-revised 2015. *Breastfeeding Medicine, 10*(9), 407-411.

Chatterji, P., & Markowitz, S. (2012). Family leave after childbirth and the mental health of new mothers. *The Journal of Mental Health Policy and Economics, 15*(2), 61-76.

Chen, Y. C., Wu, Y. C., & Chie, W. C. (2006). Effects of work-related factors on the breastfeeding behavior of working mothers in a Taiwanese semiconductor manufacturer: A cross-sectional survey. *BMC Public Health, 6,* 160.

Chezem, J., & Friesen, C. (1999). Attendance at breast-feeding support meetings: Relationship to demographic characteristics and duration of lactation in women planning postpartum employment. *Journal of the American Dietetic Association, 99*(1), 83-85.

Clark, R. A. (1992). Breast milk does not constitute occupational exposure as defined by standard. Retrieved from **osha.gov/pls/oshaweb/owadisp.show_document?p_table=INTERPRETATIONS&p_id=20952**.

De Carvalho, M. (1983). Effect of frequent breast feeding on early milk production and infant weight gain. *Pediatrics, 72,* 307-311.

Dinour, L. M., & Szaro, J. M. (2017). Employer-based programs to support breastfeeding among working mothers: A systematic review. *Breastfeeding Medicine, 12,* 131-141.

Dunn, B. F., Zavela, K. J., Cline, A. D., et al. (2004). Breastfeeding practices in Colorado businesses. *Journal of Human Lactation, 20*(2), 170-177.

Eglash, A., Simon, L., & Academy of Breastfeeding, M. (2017). ABM Clinical Protocol #8: Human milk storage information for home use for full-term infants, revised 2017. *Breastfeeding Medicine, 12*(7), 390-395.

Garvin, C. C., Sriraman, N. K., Paulson, A., et al. (2013). The business case for breastfeeding: A successful regional implementation, evaluation, and follow-up. *Breastfeeding Medicine, 8*(4), 413-417.

Grice, M. M., Feda, D., McGovern, P., et al. (2007). Giving birth and returning to work: The impact of work-family conflict on women's health after childbirth. *Annals of Epidemiology, 17*(10), 791-798.

Grice, M. M., McGovern, P. M., & Alexander, B. H. (2008). Flexible work arrangements and work-family conflict after childbirth. *Occupational Medicine (Lond), 58*(7), 468-474.

Grice, M. M., McGovern, P. M., Alexander, B. H., et al. (2011). Balancing work and family after childbirth: A longitudinal analysis. *Women's Health Issues, 21*(1), 19-27.

Hawkins, S. S., Griffiths, L. J., Dezateux, C., et al. (2007). The impact of maternal employment on breast-feeding duration in the UK Millennium Cohort Study. *Public Health Nutrition, 10*(9), 891-896.

Hill, P. D., Aldag, J. C., Chatterton, R. T., et al. (2005). Comparison of milk output between mothers of preterm and term infants: The first 6 weeks after birth. *Journal of Human Lactation, 21*(1), 22-30.

Islam, M. M., Peerson, J. M., Ahmed, T., et al. (2006). Effects of varied energy density of complementary foods on breast-milk intakes and total energy consumption by healthy, breastfed Bangladeshi children. *American Journal of Clinical Nutrition, 83*(4), 851-858.

Jantzer, A. M., Anderson, J., & Kuehl, R. A. (2018). Breastfeeding support in the workplace: The relationships among breastfeeding support, work-life balance, and job satisfaction. *Journal of Human Lactation, 34(*2), 379-385.

Kent, J. C. (2007). How breastfeeding works. *Journal of Midwifery & Women's Health, 52*(6), 564-570.

Kent, J. C., Gardner, H., & Geddes, D. T. (2016). Breastmilk production in the first 4 weeks after birth of term infants. *Nutrients, 8*(12).

Kent, J. C., Hepworth, A. R., Sherriff, J. L., et al. (2013). Longitudinal changes in breastfeeding patterns from 1 to 6 months of lactation. *Breastfeeding Medicine, 8,* 401-407.

Kent, J. C., Ramsay, D. T., Doherty, D., et al. (2003). Response of breasts to different stimulation patterns of an electric breast pump. *Journal of Human Lactation, 19*(2), 179-186; quiz 187-178, 218.

Kim, J. H., Shin, J. C., & Donovan, S. M. (2018). Effectiveness of workplace lactation interventions on breastfeeding outcomes in the United States: An updated systematic review. *Journal of Human Lactation,* 890334418765464.

Kimbro, R. T. (2006). On-the-job moms: Work and breastfeeding initiation and duration for a sample of low-income women. *Maternal and Child Health Journal, 10*(1), 19-26.

Kozhimannil, K. B., Jou, J., Gjerdingen, D. K., et al. (2016). Access to workplace accommodations to support breastfeeding after passage of the Affordable Care Act. *Women's Health Issues, 26*(1), 6-13.

Kramer, M. S., Guo, T., Platt, R. W., et al. (2004). Feeding effects on growth during infancy. *Journal of Pediatrics, 145*(5), 600-605.

Lee, J. (2017). Supporting breastfeeding moms at work: How a doctor's note can make the difference. *Breastfeeding Medicine, 12*(8), 470-472.

Li, R., Magadia, J., Fein, S. B., et al. (2012). Risk of bottle-feeding for rapid weight gain during the first year of life. *Archives of Pediatric & Adolescent Medicine, 166*(5), 431-436.

Marinelli, K. A., Moren, K., Taylor, J. S., et al. (2013). Breastfeeding support for mothers in workplace employment or educational settings: Summary statement. *Breastfeeding Medicine, 8*(1), 137-142.

Martin, K. (2011). A time and place to pump: What lactation consultants need to know about the new federal protections for employed breastfeeding mothers. *Clinical Lactation, 2*(2), 20-21.

McGovern, P., Dowd, B., Gjerdingen, D., et al. (2007). Mothers' health and work-related factors at 11 weeks postpartum. *The Annals of Family Medicine, 5*(6), 519-527.

McGovern, P., Dowd, B., Gjerdingen, D., et al. (2006). Postpartum health of employed mothers 5 weeks after childbirth. *The Annals of Family Medicine, 4*(2), 159-167.

McLeod, D., Pullon, S., & Cookson, T. (2002). Factors influencing continuation of breastfeeding in a cohort of women. *Journal of Human Lactation, 18*(4), 335-343.

Mirkovic, K. R., Perrine, C. G., Scanlon, K. S., et al. (2014). Maternity leave duration and full-time/part-time work status are associated with US mothers' ability to meet breastfeeding intentions. *Journal of Human Lactation, 30*(4), 416-419.

Mohrbacher, N. (2011). The 'Magic Number' and long-term milk production. *Clinical Lactation, 2*(1), 15-18.

Nichols, M. R., & Roux, G. M. (2004). Maternal perspectives on postpartum return to the workplace. *Journal of Obstetric, Gynecologic, & Neonatal Nursing, 33*(4), 463-471.

Nommsen-Rivers, L. (1997). Universal precautions are not needed for health care workers handling breast milk. *Journal of Human Lactation, 13*(4), 267-268.

Ogbuanu, C., Glover, S., Probst, J., et al. (2011). Balancing work and family: Effect of employment characteristics on breastfeeding. *Journal of Human Lactaction, 27*(3), 225-238; quiz 293-225.

Ogbuanu, C., Glover, S., Probst, J., et al. (2011). The effect of maternity leave length and time of return to work on breastfeeding. *Pediatrics, 127*(6), e1414-1427.

Ong, G., Yap, M., Li, F. L., et al. (2005). Impact of working status on breastfeeding in Singapore: Evidence from the National Breastfeeding Survey 2001. *European Journal of Public Health, 15*(4), 424-430.

Ortiz, J., McGilligan, K., & Kelly, P. (2004). Duration of breast milk expression among working mothers enrolled in an employer-sponsored lactation program. *Pediatric Nursing, 30*(2), 111-119.

Peterson, A., & Harmer, M. (2010). *Balancing Breast and Bottle: Reaching Your Breastfeeding Goals.* Amarillo, TX: Hale Publishing.

Pounds, L., Fisher, C. M., Barnes-Josiah, D., et al. (2017). The role of early maternal support in balancing full-time work and infant exclusive breastfeeding: A qualitative study. *Breastfeeding Medicine, 12,* 33-38.

Raju, T. N. (2014). Reasonable break time for nursing mothers: A provision enacted through the Affordable Care Act. *Pediatrics, 134*(3), 423-424.

Roe, B., Whittington, L. A., Fein, S. B., et al. (1999). Is there competition between breastfeeding and maternal employment? *Demography, 36*(2), 157-171.

Rojjanasrirat, W. (2004). Working women's breastfeeding experiences. *MCN American Journal of Maternal and Child Nursing, 29*(4), 222-227; quiz 228-229.

Scott, J. A., Binns, C. W., Oddy, W. H., et al. (2006). Predictors of breastfeeding duration: Evidence from a cohort study. *Pediatrics, 117*(4), e646-655.

SHRM. (2017). *2017 Employee Benefits: Remaining Competitive in a Challenging Talent Marketplace.* Alexandria, VA: Socieity for Human Resource Management.

Sievers, E., Oldigs, H. D., Santer, R., et al. (2002). Feeding patterns in breast-fed and formula-fed infants. *Annals of Nutrition and Metabolism, 46*(6), 243-248.

Skafida, V. (2012). Juggling work and motherhood: The impact of employment and maternity leave on breastfeeding duration: A survival analysis on Growing Up in Scotland data. *Maternal and Child Health Journal, 16*(2), 519-527.

Slusser, W. M., Lange, L., Dickson, V., et al. (2004). Breast milk expression in the workplace: A look at frequency and time. *Journal of Human Lactation, 20*(2), 164-169.

Smith, J., Javanparast, S., & Craig, L. (2017). Bringing babies and breasts into workplaces: Support for breastfeeding mothers in workplaces and childcare services at the Australian National University. *Breastfeeding Review, 25*(1), 45-56.

Snyder, K., Hansen, K., Brown, S., et al. (2018). Workplace breastfeeding support varies by employment type: The service workplace disadvantage. *Breastfeeding Medicine, 13*(1), 23-27.

Soomro, J. A., Shaikh, Z. N., Saheer, T. B., et al. (2016). Employers' perspective of workplace breastfeeding support in Karachi, Pakistan: A cross-sectional study. *International Breastfeeding Journal, 11*(1), 24.

Stevens, K. V., & Janke, J. (2003). Breastfeeding experiences of active duty military women. *Military Medicine, 168*(5), 380-384.

USBC. (2010). *Workplace Accommodations to Support and Protect Breastfeeding.* Washington, D.C.: U.S. Breastfeeding Committee.

Walker, M. (2011). Clinics in Human Lactation #8: *Breastfeeding and Employment: Making It Work.* Amarillo, TX: Hale Publishing.

Whaley, S. E., Meehan, K., Lange, L., et al. (2002). Predictors of breastfeeding duration for employees of the Special Supplemental Nutrition Program for Women, Infants, and Children (WIC). *Journal of the American Dietetic Association, 102*(9), 1290-1293.

WHO. (2018). Infant and young child feeding. Retrieved from **who.int/mediacentre/factsheets/fs342/en/index.html**.

Wilson-Clay, B., & Hoover, K. (2017). *The Breastfeeding Atlas* (6th ed.). Manchaca, TX: LactNews Press.

Witters-Green, R. (2003). Increasing breastfeeding rates in working mothers. *Families, Sytems & Health, 21,* 415-434.

Zilanawala, A. (2017). Maternal nonstandard work schedules and breastfeeding behaviors. *Maternal and Child Health Journal, 21*(6), 1308-1317.

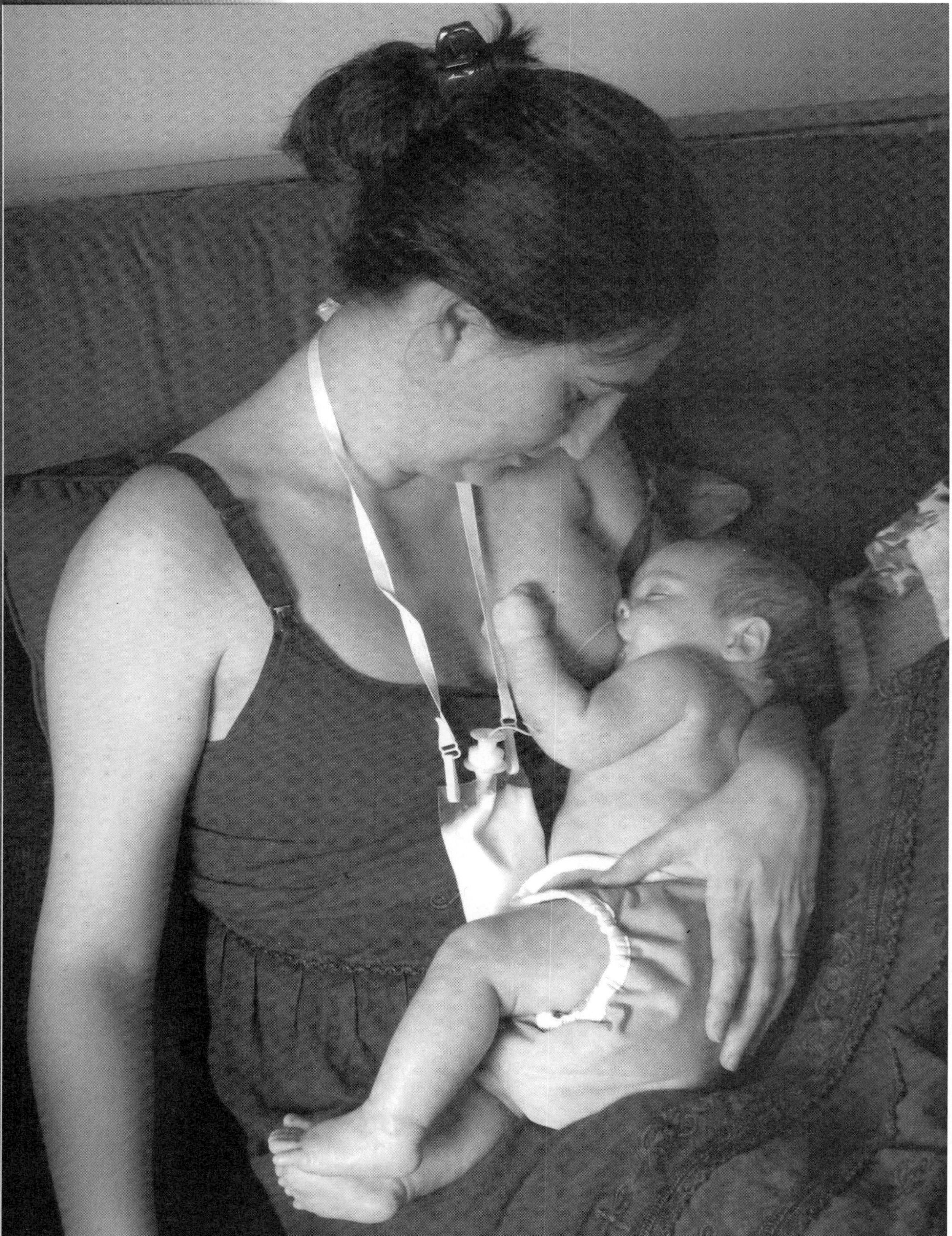

Relactation, Induced Lactation, and Emergencies

16

RELACTATION AND INDUCED LACTATION

Relactation is the process of increasing milk production in someone who has previously been pregnant.

The decision to relactate is often made when there is some milk production, but it may also be made many years after the last nursing. The difference between relactation and increasing low milk production is one of degree. Most commonly, relactation occurs after nursing parents spent weeks or months nursing very little or not at all. They may or may not have nursed after birth. Unlike those inducing lactation (see next point), those relactating have experienced the development of milk-making tissue during pregnancy. If parents who are relactating can transition the baby to nursing, feed 10 to 12 times each day, spend lots of time every day touching and holding the baby, and there are no physical obstacles to making milk, over several weeks the odds of measurable milk production are good.

> **KEY CONCEPT**
>
> *Growth of milk-making tissue during pregnancy increases the odds that relactation will result in significant milk production.*

• • •

Induced lactation is the process of stimulating milk production in someone who has never been pregnant.

Although induced lactation was once referred to as "adoptive nursing," with the availability of modern reproductive technologies, this term does not always apply. A parent may be adopting a baby or surrogacy may be involved (Farhadi & Philip, 2017). The nursing parent may have been born male and transitioned to female (Reisman & Goldstein, 2018; Sperling & Robinson, 2018). The birthing parent may have a same-sex partner who also wants to nurse, known as co-nursing (Wilson, Perrin, Fogleman, & Chetwynd, 2015). In some families, men decide to nurse (Kunz & Hosken, 2009).

Parents inducing lactation begin without the mammary development that occurs during pregnancy. As two U.S. authors (Marasco & West, 2020, p. 266) wrote:

"Inducing lactation really is more like building a milk factory by hand from bricks and mortar instead of having the construction company--pregnancy--do the job with all their specialized parts and equipment. It's a slower process..."

> **KEY CONCEPT**
>
> *Milk production from induced lactation varies widely by cultural norms..*

Gathering Information

Ask why the parents want to nurse or produce milk, and ask them to describe their goals and expectations.

Reasons for nursing or producing milk. Parents decide to relactate or induce lactation for a variety of reasons. They may want to experience or reclaim the emotional closeness of the nursing relationship. See the later section "Unique to Induced Lactation" for emotional benefits of inducing lactation for an adopted child. The baby may have an intolerance or allergy to human-milk substitutes. The baby may have a medical condition for which human milk is recommended. Parents may be nursing an older baby or toddler and decide to relactate for a newly adopted child, a child born via surrogacy, or a baby birthed by their partner. Some relactate or induce lactation to help provide human milk as a treatment for a sick friend or relative. In parts of the world where HIV is prevalent, relactation may occur when the baby is discovered to be HIV positive, which can only be determined well after birth (Nyati et al.,

2014). In some families, the partner may decide to induce lactation to share in the experience of nursing (see later section "Co-nursing with Partners"). In some parts of the developing world, nursing is key to infant survival, so when breastfeeding is at risk, mothers and babies are hospitalized to provide the information and support to ensure relactation is successful (De, Pandit, Mishra, Pappu, & Chaudhuri, 2002). Discussing the reasons for wanting to produce milk can help clarify feelings and goals.

If nursing parents are relactating for a baby they recently birthed, ask what happened with nursing. In this case, the dynamics that caused milk production to decrease may still exist and need to be addressed. If there were feeding problems, ask about them. The cause may be simple misinformation, such as being told to nurse on a schedule, which led to slow weight gain and supplements. If so, provide information about milk-production dynamics (see Chapter 10, "Making Milk"). If nipple pain and trauma were an issue, discuss possible causes and how to help the baby get a deep latch. Other causes may need to be explored, such as tongue-tie. A U.S. phenomenological study that explored the emotions of 10 women who relactated (Lommen, Brown, & Hollist, 2015) found that half of the women had colicky babies, which contributed to their early feeding problems. Their experimentation with formula (which had no effect on their babies' fussiness) caused their milk production to slow, which led to the need to relactate. If they began formula-feeding after birth, ask why and if these reasons are still important. An Egyptian study of 200 women who attempted relactation (Abul-Fadl, Kharboush, Fikry, & Adel, 2012) reported that the main reasons the study mothers stopped nursing were: low milk supply (67%), baby stopped/nursing strike (27%), and nipple pain (50%).

Nursing goals. When discussing goals, ask what aspect of nursing is most important to the parent. A U.S. study in which 8 of its 10 women reached their milk-production goals (Lommen et al., 2015) found that some gauged success more by the closer bond they formed with their baby rather than the volume of milk produced. In another U.S. survey of 366 women who relactated (Auerbach & Avery, 1980), most were not as concerned about the volume of milk they produced as about their ability to nurture their baby through nursing. Some survey mothers decided to relactate for health reasons (baby's formula intolerance or health problems), but most relactated because they hoped nursing would bring them emotionally closer to their babies. In hindsight, 75% of the women surveyed considered relactation a positive experience and their milk production was unrelated to their feelings of success.

Relactation expectations. Let the family know that depending on how low milk production is when the relactation process starts, it may take a month or more to produce a significant volume of milk. In a study done in India with 1,000 healthy mothers relactating for healthy babies less than 6 weeks old (S. Banapurmath, Banapurmath, & Kesaree, 2003), those who had a "lactation gap" (time since last nursing) of less than 15 days were able to stimulate full milk production within 3 to 5 days. Those whose lactation gap was more than 15 days took longer than the length of the 10-day study to reach full lactation. In another U.S. study, more than half of its 366 mothers who relactated established full production within 1 month (Auerbach & Avery, 1980). It took more than 1 month for full relactation in another 25%. The remaining mothers breastfed with supplements until their babies weaned. If nursing parents are concerned that they might not reach full

> **KEY CONCEPT**
>
> *It may take a month or more for a nursing parent to produce a significant volume of milk.*

relactation, assure them that even partial relactation is a huge boon to families, and if this is the end result, they will know they did everything possible.

Induced lactation expectations. Different families approach induced lactation with different goals. To clarify goals, a good starting point is to ask how important milk production is to that family. Some consider substantial milk production their top priority. Others consider the closeness of nursing and the volume of milk produced as equally important. Still others consider induced lactation primarily a way to increase their emotional closeness to their baby and care little about how much milk they produce. When closeness is the top priority, suggest focusing on the emotional aspects of nursing and think of any milk produced as an added bonus. In this case, success is best gauged by the baby's willingness to nurse and the comfort and security baby receives while sucking. If full milk production is one of the top priorities, offer to discuss possible options.

Also let the family know that all nursing parents inducing lactation who nurse long term eventually reach a stage where their baby's need for milk and their milk production match. Some nursing parents bring in enough milk before the baby arrives that they never need to use formula or donor milk. Some families discontinue supplements during the early months. Some can discontinue supplements after 6 months, when solid foods take their place in the baby's diet. For some, it may be closer to 12 months, when their child is eating more solids. But all nursing parents and babies eventually reach the point when extra milk is unnecessary.

• • •

Ask the baby's age and nursing history, as well as any anatomy or health issues in the baby and the nursing parent.

The baby's age, nursing history, and current response to nursing. The baby's age and willingness to nurse may affect the process. In the survey of 366 U.S. mothers who relactated described in the previous point, the mothers who started relactating within 2 months of birth reported greater milk production than those who relactated more than 2 months after birth. With induced lactation, ask if either nursing parent or child have nursed before. It was once thought the younger the baby, the more smoothly induced lactation was likely to go, but adopted toddlers sometimes take to nursing easily and enthusiastically (K. D. Gribble, 2005a). In Australia, adoptions are not allowed until at the earliest 6 to 12 months after birth, and many parents have successfully transitioned their children to nursing at this age, and even much older.

Health or anatomy issues in nursing parent or baby. Do the parent and baby have any known medical conditions? Are they on any medications? (Be sure to ask about hormonal contraception.) Is there anything unusual about the parent's mammary glands or nipples (mammary size, flat or inverted nipples)? Nursing may go more smoothly with a healthy parent and baby with average anatomy. If unusual anatomy such as inverted nipples, tongue-tie, etc. is a factor, it may or may not affect nursing. See the sections about anatomy issues in the baby on p. 262 in Chapter 8, "Baby's Anatomy and Health" and in the nursing parent, see Chapter 17, "Nipple Issues" or Chapter 18, "Breast or Chest Issues."

• • •

Ask about the nursing parent's availability to the baby, any existing support network, and if relevant, infertility issues.

Daily responsibilities. If there are other children, ask how many and their ages. If nursing parents are employed, how many hours per week are they away from the baby? If they are employed and inducing lactation, are they planning to take parental leave when their child arrives? If so, for how long? What other daily obligations do they have? Is the family under any unusual stress? If there are many commitments, can they take some time off and get help with older children while they focus on increasing milk? Provide full information on all options, as circumstances are not a reliable way to predict which parents will follow through and which will not (K. Gribble, personal communication, August 21, 2018).

Available support. Ask if there is an available partner, and if so how the partner and extended family feel about the plans. A 2010 Korean study of 84 women who relactated with the help of a relactation clinic (Cho, Cho, Lee, & Lee, 2010) found that family support was one factor that the 75% of women who succeeded at fully relactating said was important to their success. Is there household help, or is it possible to arrange for it? Is the nursing parent in contact with other nursing parents, either in person or online? If not, suggest possible resources (see the list of resources at the end of this chapter). Emphasize the value of support and ask if family or friends are available to give day-to-day help and encouragement.

KEY CONCEPT

Family support is an important factor for some in reaching their relactation goals.

Infertility issues. If the family is growing by adoption or surrogacy due to infertility, ask if the issue was with the nursing parent, the partner, or both. Some physical conditions that prevent conception or make it impossible to sustain a pregnancy may affect milk production. For example, Sheehan's syndrome, caused by extreme blood loss (after birth or at any time) that is severe enough to render the pituitary non-functional prevents both pregnancy and lactation (Du et al., 2015). Some types of hormonal imbalances may affect fertility, the development of mammary tissue, and milk production (see p. 411 in Chapter 10, "Making Milk."

Strategies for Increasing Milk Production

One key to both relactation and induced lactation is successfully transitioning the baby to nursing.

Because the process involved in relactating and inducing lactation are essentially the same, they share the same basic strategies. One critical aspect of both is successfully transitioning the baby to nursing. Although some studies found that younger babies take to nursing more readily than older babies, children older than 12 months have also willingly nursed (Phillips, 1993). Research conducted internationally documented inborn feeding behaviors (see Chapter 1) in adopted children between 8 months and school age (K. D. Gribble, 2005d). Recognizing and triggering babies' feeding behaviors can make the transition to nursing easier. But every baby is different, and there is no way to know until nursing is tried how the baby will accept it. For specific strategies, see the later section "Helping Baby Latch and Feed" on p. 680.

Creating a Plan and Cultural Influences

Offer to help the family create a plan tailored to their specific priorities and situation.

The only necessary strategy for both relactation and induced lactation is frequent mammary stimulation by nursing and/or milk expression. In some individuals, galactogogues (milk-boosting substances) can increase the effectiveness of nursing and/or milk expression, but galactogogues are optional. Those considering taking galactogogues should discuss this with their healthcare provider in light of their health history. But preferences also play a role. Some parents may not have the time or money to express their milk with an effective pump, while others prefer milk expression over nursing. If there is a discomfort with nursing, explore this, as any reluctance may undermine baby's eventual transition to nursing.

Offer to help the family formulate a plan that incorporates the strategies with which they are most comfortable. If the plan includes strategies they feel uncomfortable with, they are unlikely to follow through.

Induced lactation. If the goal is to nurse primarily for greater intimacy, the plan may involve waiting until the baby arrives and simply nursing with lots of body contact to induce lactation. But if milk production is a higher priority and the family knows ahead of time when the baby will arrive, one option is the induced lactation protocols described on p. 679. However, as Alyssa Schnell (personal communication, 2018), U.S. lactation consultant and author of *Breastfeeding Without Birthing*, points out:

> "I think it is a common misconception that parents need a few months of lead time to induce lactation or relactate for a baby they didn't birth. Little or no lead time is fine! Certainly, there are fewer options, but it is still very possible."

If the family is adopting, the type of adoption may make a difference. How far in advance will they know for certain of the baby's arrival? Is it a traditional U.S. adoption? In this case, there is usually a required 48- to 72-hour wait time after birth before the adopting family can take custody of the baby. Birth parents may also change their minds right before the baby is scheduled to arrive or after baby's born. For obvious reasons, any uncertainty may affect the desire to produce milk in advance. In Australia, adoption is not allowed until the baby is 6 to 12 months or older, so the focus will be less on milk production than a family adopting a newborn. Is a surrogate carrying the baby? If so, there may be much more time and greater certainty about when the baby will be in their arms.

Discuss the following strategies in light of their priorities and situation and help them create a plan with which they feel comfortable.

• • •

Cultural beliefs about nursing and parenting practices may affect milk production.

In developing countries, there is a long history of successful relactation and induced lactation. Researchers documented full induced lactation in Africa, Indonesia, South America, India, Polynesia, and among Native Americans (Wieschhoff, 1940). In South Africa, researchers reported grandmothers bringing in full or partial lactation for their grandchildren after their mothers left for an extended absence or returned to work (Slome, 1956). A Nigerian article documented that by simply breastfeeding 8 to 10 times per day, six women were able to achieve full lactation within 3 to 4 weeks for babies whose mothers had died (Abejide et al., 1997). In these societies, it is expected that parents can produce enough milk for their babies and because they all know that baby's survival depends on nursing, those around them support them in their efforts.

But in many developed countries, even parents who birth their babies doubt their ability to make enough milk, and parents relactating and inducing lactation are less likely to reach full milk production. In one survey of 65 Western adoptive mothers who induced lactation, they calculated their babies received 25% to 75% of their daily milk intake by nursing (Hormann, 1977). The mothers calculated these percentages by subtracting the amount of formula the baby took per day from the amount needed by an exclusively formula-fed baby. But these estimates were likely low because formula-fed babies, on average, consume 15% more milk at 3 months and 23% more at 6 months than exclusively nursed babies (Heinig, Nommsen, Peerson, Lonnerdal, & Dewey, 1993). Only two of these 65 survey mothers induced full lactation, and two mothers with pituitary disorders produced no milk.

After comparing the differences in outcomes among adoptive parents inducing lactation in developed and developing countries, Australian researcher Karleen Gribble (K. D. Gribble, 2004, p. 5) wrote:

> "Adoptive mothers in developing countries may have greater milk production than mothers in the West because they are more knowledgeable about breastfeeding, practice frequent breastfeeding, remain in close physical contact with their children and live in cultures that are supportive of breastfeeding. They also have reproductive and breastfeeding histories that may make breastfeeding easier, though they are less likely to have pharmaceutical galactagogues available. Adoptive mothers in the West should be encouraged to maximize their milk supply by emulating the mothering styles of women in developing countries and developing a strong support network for breastfeeding. It may be that most adoptive mothers are physically capable of producing sufficient breastmilk for the child but that in the West, sociocultural factors act as preventatives."

Knowledge about nursing. In developing countries, people learn about nursing during their childhood by watching babies nursing around them. But in Western cultures, most either nurse behind closed doors or cover themselves, leaving new parents ignorant and uncertain about how nursing works.

Nursing and parenting practices. Among birthing parents around the world, differences in nursing and parenting practices affect both milk production and return to fertility (see Chapter 12, "Sex, Fertility & Contraception"). As U.S. researcher Kathleen Kennedy noted, a Western parent may think of a "nursing" as a lengthy, ritualized activity involving changing the baby's diaper/nappy, making a drink, muting the phone, settling into a certain chair, and then feeding baby for an extended time. However, nursing parents in a developing country may keep the baby on their body, feeding at the slightest cue for just a few minutes 15 to 20 times each day (Lozoff & Brittenham, 1979). In developing countries, this greater body contact may enhance the hormonal response to milk production. Western parents, on the other hand, are encouraged to feed their babies at regular time intervals, sleep separately, and avoid holding their babies "too much" for fear of "spoiling." As a result, Western babies spend much of their days in infant seats, strollers/prams, and cribs. When relactating or inducing lactation in a developed country, attending nursing peer support groups (such as La Leche League and the Australian Breastfeeding Association), where more responsive feeding is practiced, can provide exposure to parenting practices that enhance milk production.

KEY CONCEPT

In cultures where nursing is the norm, families who relactate or induce lactation keep their babies close, feed more often, and have more support, so they produce more milk.

Attitudes about nursing. In developing countries, birthing and adoptive parents are strongly encouraged and supported in their efforts to nurse because nursing is a matter of life or death. One study of 1,000 relactating mothers in India (S. Banapurmath et al., 2003) estimated that during the first 2 months of life, compared to exclusively breastfed babies, babies not nursed at all were more than 23 times more likely to die. For this reason, when feeding problems arise in India, mothers relactating may be hospitalized to increase their odds of success (De et al., 2002). In Indian culture, mammary glands are considered primarily for feeding and comforting babies, and their exposure in public for feeding is widely accepted (Dettwyler, 1995). Nursing parents also have confidence in their ability to nurse because they are surrounded by nursing parents producing ample milk. In Western countries, the mammary gland has been sexualized and even the parents giving birth doubt their milk-making abilities. Western parents relactating or inducing lactation may be met with amazement, doubt, even criticism.

KEY CONCEPT

The supplemental feeding method used during relactation or induced lactation can promote or undermine the process.

Supplemental feeding methods vary around the world. In developing countries, most parents relactating or inducing lactation supplement their babies with easy-to-clean, temporary methods, such as spoons and cups. Feeding bottles—a long-term feeding method—are rarely used due to contamination risks. In developed countries, however, feeding bottles are common, and due to their fast flow, the baby is more likely to take more supplement than needed. In one study of relactation in 15 mothers in India (C. R. Banapurmath, Banapurmath, & Kesaree, 1993), full relactation was achieved only when feeding bottles were stopped. In a Nigerian study in which six mothers achieved full induced lactation (Abejide et al., 1997), babies were supplemented only by cup or spoon. Also, their healthcare providers and families strongly urged them to induce lactation to ensure their baby's survival and provided practical help to accomplish this. A nursing supplementer (see p. 897 for details) is another supplemental feeding method that is used primarily in developed countries, which—when used optimally—has the advantage of providing extra milk flow during nursing to reinforce nursing and support greater milk production.

• • •

Suggest nursing parents learn the basics of making milk and the physical changes expected as milk production begins.

To understand the reasons behind the "how-tos" of relactation and induced lactation, it is helpful to understand the basic dynamics of milk production (see Chapter 10, "Making Milk"). It also helps to be able to gauge when the baby is getting enough milk and when she needs more supplement. Knowing how to help the baby latch deeply will help avoid nipple pain and increase baby's feeding effectiveness. The more nursing parents know, the easier it is to adapt recommendations to their baby and their own unique situation.

It can also be reassuring to know what physical and emotional changes may occur as milk production increases:

- **Menstrual changes.** With increased mammary stimulation, menstruation may become irregular or stop.
- **Changes in mammary tissue.** The areolae may darken and the mammary tissue may become tender, feel fuller, hotter, or heavier, and increase in size.
- **Mood changes.** With lactation-related hormonal changes, some find that with more oxytocin, prolactin, and other nursing hormones in their

system, their mood improves. Others begin to feel warm, anxious, or nervous or become depressed, fatigued, tearful, or angry. Mood changes may lead to feeling overwhelmed or like giving up. Mood changes are usually a sign of pending milk increase. If a parent is feeling down, suggest tapping into their support network.

• • •

Encourage those relactating or inducing lactation to accept all offers of help and to take good care of themselves.

Getting more rest, eating a more nutritious diet, and drinking more fluids will most likely not boost milk production. But they can be important to a nursing parent's morale and ability to cope. Encourage them to accept all offers of help. Offer to help formulate a daily plan that will maximize the time spent boosting milk production, while allowing the time needed to care for other children and to meet other responsibilities.

Mammary Stimulation and Body Contact

The most effective strategy for relactation and induced lactation is frequent, effective, around-the-clock nursing.

Nurse at least 10 to 12 times per day. Before there is milk to remove, nipple stimulation causes the release of the hormone prolactin, which contributes to milk production and the growth of milk-making tissue. Frequent nursing stimulates milk production in a number of ways. In those producing some milk, it takes advantage of the "drained glands make milk faster" dynamic (explained in Chapter 10, "Making Milk"), which causes an increase in the rate of milk production between feeds by keeping pressure within the mammary glands low and by preventing a build-up of the substance referred to as ***feedback inhibitor of lactation*** which contributes to the slowing of milk production (Kent, Prime, & Garbin, 2012). Over time, frequent milk removal also increases milk production by speeding the metabolic activity of key enzymes used in milk-making and stimulating the growth and development of more milk-making tissue (Czank, Henderson, Kent, Tat Lai, & Hartmann, 2007). For some families,

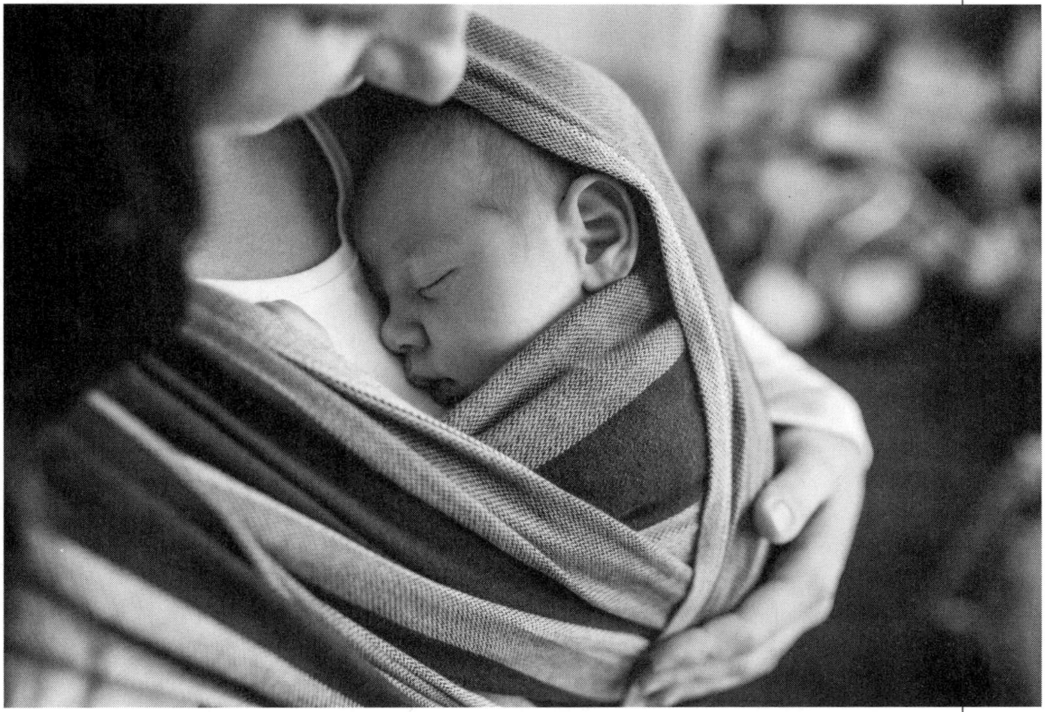

using a nursing supplementer (see p. 879) may be a very important tool when using nursing to relactate or induce lactation. Not every baby will stay interested in nursing without milk flow, and even those who will nurse without flow will nurse longer and more vigorously when there is flow, more effectively stimulating milk production.

KEY CONCEPT

Frequent milk removal increases milk production for relactating parents.

Be sure the baby latches deeply. Frequent nursing can increase the rate of milk production only if the baby actively nurses and removes the milk effectively. Suggest using strategies described in Chapter 1 to find an effective and comfortable feeding position and to be sure the baby latches deeply. A shallow latch can cause nipple pain, and it can reduce the baby's milk intake and drain milk-making glands unevenly, which can slow milk production (Mizuno et al., 2008).

Offer each side more than once at each feed. Suggest that each time the baby comes off to offer the other side. If the baby does not stay active (just mouthing the nipple rather than actively sucking and swallowing) or if she falls asleep quickly, suggest using compression (see next paragraph) to keep baby active longer on that side. To increase the stimulation, if possible, encourage the baby to take each side at least twice.

Use compression or massage to increase time spent actively sucking. If the baby stops sucking actively, compression or massage during feeds can increase milk flow, which helps to keep her feeding actively longer. For a description of breast compression, see p. 889.

Keep baby close at night and guide the sleeping baby to latch. To help increase the number of daily feeds, the baby can be gently guided to latch when drowsy or in a light sleep (known as "dream feeding"). U.K. research found that laying a sleeping baby tummy down on the parent's semi-reclined body triggers inborn feeding behaviors, which can lead to effective feeding during light sleep, even in late preterm babies (S. Colson, DeRooy, & Hawdon, 2003).

Avoid soothers and limit all sucking to the nursing parent to increase the time spent stimulating milk production. Swaddling and soothers, such as pacifiers/dummies and swings, can reduce time spent nursing and lead to poorer nursing outcomes (Buccini, Perez-Escamilla, Paulino, Araujo, & Venancio, 2017). Giving supplements with a nursing supplementer can increase stimulation of milk-making tissue by keeping the baby actively nursing longer.

• • •

Suggest nursing parents keep the baby on their body as much as possible to trigger feeding behaviors and to enhance milk- production.

U.S. and Swedish research found associations between touch, enhanced hormonal responses in the nursing parent, as well as increased milk production. After birth, newborns' touch increased the birthing parents' blood oxytocin levels (Matthiesen, Ransjo-Arvidson, Nissen, & Uvnas-Moberg, 2001). In those exclusively pumping for preterm babies, daily skin-to-skin contact with their baby was associated with greater milk volumes expressed (Hurst, Valentine, Renfro, Burns, & Ferlic, 1997). Skin-to-skin contact before nursing was associated with lower levels of stress hormones in the nursing parent and a greater hormonal response to nursing (Handlin et al., 2009).

It may be easier for nursing parents to keep their baby on their body by using a sling or baby carrier during the day (preferably one that makes nursing possible) and to spend as much time as practical with the nipple accessible to the baby in semi-reclined feeding positions, such as leaning back comfortably on the sofa (see Chapter 1). At night, encourage the parents to keep the baby close and to nurse often.

• • •

Milk expression can also be used to speed the rate of milk production.

If the baby is nursing effectively, suggest making nursing a higher priority than milk expression. But if the nursing parent is away from the baby regularly or the baby is not yet nursing effectively, milk expression can be a useful tool. The first choice for anyone relactating is a rental-grade pump with a double-pump kit, which was found to be more effective at establishing milk production than hand expression alone (Lussier et al., 2015; Slusher et al., 2012). (Although many parents inducing lactation report that the first milk produced is easier to express by hand.) When relactating or inducing lactation, suggest those pumping to double-pump at least once in the middle of the night, when prolactin levels are naturally higher (Neville, 1999).

Use massage and compression during pumping or use hand expression after pumping. A U.S. study found that 86% of its 66 mothers of preterm babies expressed an average of 93% more milk when they used a specific technique called ***hands-on pumping*** that included massage before pumping, massage and compression during pumping, and hand expression or single pumping to drain the glands more fully (Morton et al., 2009). For details on this evidence-based technique, see p. 492.

Where breast pumps are not available or are outside the family's means, hand expression can be used (S. Banapurmath et al., 2003). One case study from Brazil described a mother with low milk production who relactated at 8 weeks by getting a deeper latch and nursing more frequently, hand-expressing her milk after each nursing, and feeding it to her baby (de Melo & Murta, 2009). Her milk volume quickly increased, which led to better weight gain and full milk production.

KEY CONCEPT

If the baby is nursing effectively, suggest giving a higher priority to frequent nursing rather than milk expression.

If the nursing parent chooses to pump, discuss available pump models and pump fit. Double-pumping is a huge time saver (Becker, Smith, & Cooney, 2016). Some pumps offer hands-free options. Also suggest the following strategies.

Express long enough to remove the milk well. The hands-on pumping technique mentioned above takes on average 25 minutes to complete. The more fully drained of milk the mammary glands are during expressions, the faster the rate of milk production increases.

Express milk after or between feeds. After baby arrives, in most cases, parents will stop pumping and focus on nursing. If it is not too overwhelming to express milk in addition to everything else, suggest expressing some milk by hand as many times per day as practical after or between feeds (perhaps when they use the toilet). Even if little or no milk is expressed, its main purpose is to stimulate faster milk production.

From time to time pump intensively. The purpose of pumping intensively in the short term is to give milk production a quick boost. One pumping strategy credited to U.S. lactation consultant Catherine Watson Genna involves putting the pump in an area its user passes often and can sit or stand comfortably.

During a several-day period, every time they pass the pump, use it for 5 to 10 minutes. Another pumping strategy involves double-pumping 10 minutes on and 10 minutes off for an hour, perhaps while watching a show. For a summary of different options for intensive pumping, see p. 447.

• • •

Suggest keeping the longest stretch between milk removals shorter than 8 hours.

When mammary glands become full, they make milk slower, so long stretches between feeds and/or milk expressions (usually at night) can slow milk production. Ask the length of the current longest stretch. To avoid slowing milk production for part of the day, suggest avoiding going longer than 8 hours without either feeding or expressing milk. If the baby sleeps longer than 8 hours at night, ask whether the nursing parent prefers to do a "dream feed" (nursing without baby waking fully) or express milk. For those with a small storage capacity (see p. 447-448), even an 8-hour stretch may be long enough to cause milk production to slow.

• • •

Suggest keeping a record of the volume of milk expressed and spending a few extra minutes to express just a little bit more milk each time.

Many families are unclear about how to increase milk production. It may help to emphasize that draining the milk-making glands more fully and more often is what will send the signal to make milk faster. Let the family know that milk increases slowly and gradually, so keeping a written record (whether digital or on paper) and totaling the volume expressed each day can be incredibly affirming. Without this daily total, they may not realize they are making progress. Also, reviewing these numbers daily will help them put their focus in the right place: on the number of daily milk removals, one key aspect of bringing in more milk. Encourage them, too, to express a little longer, even if they get only a few milliliters more. Every little bit helps in reaching the goal.

Galactogogues

Prescribed and/or herbal galactogogues may help boost milk production.

For details on medications and plant-based galactogues and their recommended doses, see p. 449. When parents express an interest in using them, suggest discussing this with their healthcare provider in light of their health history. Their preferences also play a role. For example, some prefer not to take prescription medicines but are enthusiastic about taking herbs. Others are uncomfortable taking herbs but want to take medications. Still others want to try neither or both.

• • •

In many studies done in developing countries, galactogogues were not necessary for full milk production.

Although galactogogues may be helpful in some cases, relactation and induced lactation can be accomplished without them, especially in certain parts of the world.

Relactation. One study conducted in India randomly assigned relactating women to one of two groups (Seema, Patwari, & Satyanarayana, 1997). Group I breastfed frequently and received ongoing information and support from a health worker. Group II received the same along with metoclopramide, a prescribed galactogogue. Time to full relactation, pattern of weight gain, rate of reduction of supplement, and total weight gain were comparable between the two groups, with 92% of the mothers achieving full relactation and 6% partial relactatation. The researchers concluded that most can fully relactate without using galactogogues.

In a large study done in India in which no galactogogues were used (S. Banapurmath et al., 2003), 83% of its 1,000 mothers with babies younger than 6 weeks reached full milk production within 10 days. These mothers were instructed to breastfeed at least every 2 hours, offer the breast whenever the baby showed interest, use hand expression to stimulate milk production, provide lots of skin-to-skin contact, and sleep with their babies at night. In another study on relactation from India (De et al., 2002), when breastfeeding 10 to 12 times per day for about 10 minutes per breast, 61% of the 139 relactating mothers achieved full milk production (including one mother relactating for twins) and 23% achieved partial milk production. These mothers were encouraged to supplement as needed by cup and spoon, sleep with the babies, and provide lots of skin-to-skin contact.

Induced lactation. Galactogogues may be helpful to some, but like relactation, induced lactation can be accomplished without them. When used, they can be given either before or after the baby arrives (Bryant, 2006). In one study of 27 mothers inducing lactation in Papua, New Guinea (Nemba, 1994), 11 mothers who had never breastfed received a single injection of 100 mg of medroxyprogesterone (Depo-Provera) a week before beginning their efforts to induce lactation, then took 10 mg of metoclopramide (Reglan) or 25 mg of chlorpromazine (Thorazine) four times daily until they had enough milk to sustain their babies. The 16 mothers who had previously breastfed did not receive the injection but took the daily oral medication until adequate lactation was established. In this study, 24 out of the 27 mothers induced full lactation.

KEY CONCEPT

Galactogogues can help with relactation and induced lactation. But they are not necessary.

BOX 16.1 One Pumping Plan to Induce Lactation

1. About 2-4 weeks (or more) before the baby arrives, start manual massage of the nipples and glands for 10 minutes 8-10 times per day for 2 weeks.
2. After 2 weeks, begin double pumping with a rental-grade pump for 10-15 minutes 8-10 times per day. If pumping without milk flow causes discomfort, try lubricating the nipple tunnel with a bit of olive or coconut oil.
3. When baby arrives, use a nursing supplementer (see p. 897) to provide milk while baby nurses. Pump after feeds if desired or as time permits. Monitor baby's weight gain to ensure adequate milk intake.
4. As the mammary glands begin to feel heavy, and tender, see if baby will nurse without supplementation for the first few minutes of the feed. Continue to track weight gain.
5. As long as baby's hunger cues aren't frantic and weight gain is sufficient, gradually decrease either the amount of milk in the supplementer or the length of time the milk is allowed to flow from the supplementer during the feed. A time may come when it's no longer possible to decrease the amount of supplement without leaving baby hungry.

Adapted from (Marasco & West, 2020, p. 267)

Unique to Induced Lactation

Nursing can help an adopted or foster child form a healthy attachment and increase the nursing parent's sensitivity to the child.

The importance of human milk to the normal health and development of any baby (and nursing parent) is well known (AAP, 2012; Louis-Jacques & Stuebe, 2018). But nursing is about much more than milk. The profound effects of nursing on the parent-child relationship are especially valuable to adoptive families. In one Australian review article, researcher Karleen Gribble described the role nursing played in helping adopted children, especially those with a history of abuse or neglect, form a close and healthy relationship with their new family (K. D. Gribble, 2006). The regular, intimate touch and the calming, relaxing, analgesic effect of nursing can be key to an easier transition from the birth family or an institution to the new family. For adoptive parents, the relaxing hormones released during nursing provide stress relief and enhance their sensitivity to their child (Uvnas-Moberg, 2014). In another article, Gribble reports that when children spend time in institutions before adoption, adoptive parents believed that the primal experience of nursing helped their children express grief over the loss of their birth family and comforted them as they adjusted to their new family (K. D. Gribble, 2005d).

KEY CONCEPT

Nursing can help adopted children form a close and healthy bond with their new parents.

Nursing foster children can also promote emotional healing. One case report about a medically fragile foster child described the improvements in physical and emotional health that occurred with nursing (K. D. Gribble, 2005b). Its author suggested that families consider this option when the child is likely to be with the foster family long term, especially for children who were previously nursed or whose birth parent expressed a desire for their child to be nursed. To allay any concerns about transmission of illness, such as HIV and HTLV-1 (see p. 824 and p. 826), she suggested having foster families take blood tests (such as are used by milk banks for milk donors). She noted that the biggest barriers to providing nursing and human milk to foster children is social, as many social services personnel consider nursing "an extra" or "a luxury," rather than a basic human need and right.

• • •

For families inducing lactation who know in advance when their baby will arrive, one option is to stimulate milk production before the baby joins their family.

If a family knows in advance when the baby is expected, they can consider spending some time before the baby comes stimulating milk production. Alyssa Schnell, a U.S. lactation consultant who wrote *Breastfeeding Without Birthing* and specializes in helping families induce lactation, describes in her book and on her website (**sweetpeabreastfeeding.com**) the three basic steps to make milk without pregnancy:

1. Prepare the mammary glands to make milk
2. Stimulate milk production
3. Nurse and make milk

Typically, the first two steps occur before the baby arrives. These first and second steps are optional if there is no time before baby's arrival or the parents prefer to wait until baby arrives to begin bringing in milk. In her book, Schnell describes five generic protocols (or detailed step-by-step plans) that involve variations of these three steps, the Traditional, Avery, Pumping, Herbal, and Newman-Goldfarb (Schnell, 2013). For best results, a lactation supporter can help a family customize a personal protocol for inducing lactation or relactation based on their specific needs and preferences, taking into account their health and fertility history. For example, some families prefer to use only frequent pumping or hand expression to stimulate milk production before the baby's arrival. Others may want to use milk-enhancing herbs and drugs to prepare mammary tissue and to stimulate milk production.

The use of drugs and herbs to promote induced lactation has a long history. A 1940 article that summarized reports of induced lactation and relactation from around the world (Wieschhoff, 1940) described the use of herbs by the indigenous people of British Columbia, Canada to stimulate lactation without the help of pregnancy. A 2007 Israeli review article (Moran & Gilad, 2007) noted that in the 20th century, estrogen, chlorpromazine, and/or oxytocin were given in some countries to those inducing lactation. One well-known protocol for families who have the time to stimulate lactation before the baby arrives was developed by Canadian pediatrician Jack Newman and one of the first parents to use them, Canadian lactation consultant Lenore Goldfarb. The website **asklenore.info** describes these protocols in detail.

Newman-Goldfarb induced lactation protocols. At this writing, three protocols are described:

- **Regular Protocol,** for those with at least 6 months before their baby's arrival
- **Accelerated Protocol,** for those with less than 6 months
- **Menopause Protocol,** for those who have had surgical removal of their reproductive organs or naturally occurring menopause.

To enhance the development of mammary tissue, all three protocols involve taking one active oral contraceptive pill (containing 1 to 2 mg of progesterone and no more than 0.035 mg of estrogen) without interruption each day. To speed milk production, they also include daily domperidone, a prescribed galactogogue (see p. 450-451). Before the baby arrives, the oral contraceptive is stopped (the timing varies among the protocols), which causes a drop in the user's progesterone level, while the domperidone that continues to be taken stimulates an increase in blood prolactin levels, causing milk to increase. This process mimics (at much lower levels) the hormonal changes that naturally occur after birth. After the oral contraceptive is stopped, to further stimulate milk production, herbs are started and the parent inducing lactation begins pumping every 3 hours with an automatic double pump. Possible side effects of these protocols include prolonged breakthrough menstrual bleeding, increased blood pressure, and weight gain.

At this writing, there is no published research on the effectiveness of the Newman-Goldfarb protocols. In Goldfarb's doctoral thesis (Goldfarb, 2010), she analyzed the results of a mixed-methods quantitative and qualitative survey she conducted with 228 women who induced lactation or relactated. However, these survey women did not necessarily use the Newman-Goldfarb protocols. They used a variety of approaches. As described in the previous section, many earlier studies of those inducing lactation in the developing world found that the vast majority of mothers produced enough milk for their babies, some by simply nursing intensively for several weeks. In contrast, Goldfarb's survey found that at peak milk production, only 23% of the 228 mothers produced all the milk their babies needed and about 7% produced "just about all." One noteworthy statistic was the length of time Goldfarb's survey women breastfed. After spending months preparing, the vast majority (about 150) reported a breastfeeding duration of 0 to 30 days. Fewer than 20 breastfed for 31 to 60 days. The number who breastfed for 61 to 120 days was in single digits. Although there is a logic to these protocols, in light of the current lack of evidence, it appears questionable that they produce better or even similar results than other strategies to induce lactation.

Suggest that anyone considering using a protocol that involves drugs or herbs consult with their healthcare provider to review these options in light of their health history. Also, if hormonal contraceptives are contraindicated due to thrombosis (a major health risk if long airplane flights are involved with an adoption), cardiac problems, or severe hypertension, these protocols should not be used.

Be sure to clarify, too, that these protocols are not meant to be used after the baby arrives. As Australian author and researcher Karleen Gribble (personal communication, 2018) wrote:

> "I have seen women who have their child placed with them go on the Newman-Goldfarb protocols because they think this is how they will make the most milk, and so for a period of weeks or months they aren't breastfeeding their baby. The reliance on the medications also distracts from the basics—milk removal for increasing milk production."

That said, these protocols may help some families reach their goals by providing a set schedule of mammary stimulation, which is the most important aspect of any plan.

• • •

The milk produced from induced lactation is comparable to mature milk.

A 2015 U.S. pilot study (Perrin, Wilson, Chetwynd, & Fogleman, 2015) examined weekly milk samples provided by two women who induced lactation without pregnancy and compared these samples to the milk of three control mothers who lactated after pregnancy. The researchers analyzed the milk samples for total protein, secretory immunoglobulin A (sIgA), lysozyme, and lactoferrin. They found the milk of the women who induced lactation was comparable to the milk of the control mothers but slightly higher in protein, secretory IgA, and lysozyme.

Transitioning Baby to Nursing

Helping Baby Latch and Feed

Suggest the adoptive nursing parent focus first on their developing relationship.

Before adoptive parents attempt nursing, suggest they first focus on their developing relationship with the child. Because nursing is an intimate act, children are more likely to latch and feed when they trust and feel close to their new parent. When adoptive parents welcome the child to the family, at first, they are strangers to the child. Before offering to nurse, suggest they first find ways to become emotionally closer, such as holding, carrying, co-sleeping, co-bathing, and being responsive to the child's needs.

For the first few weeks, it may help to make their relationship exclusive, which may mean others do not hold the child (Macrae & Gribble, 2006). The child's personality and past experiences with feeding will also affect her response to nursing. For example, if the child is used to being fed quickly with a fast-flow bottle, it may help to transition gradually by first shifting to a medium-flow teat and then a slow-flow teat. Gradual steps—such as bottle-feeding in a nursing position (see photos on p. 683)—can allow her to experience feeding as something that is less overwhelming and more pleasurable before offering to nurse. Patience and persistence are key.

KEY CONCEPT

Because nursing is hardwired, most babies will eventually latch and feed.

• • •

If the baby balks at nursing, it may help to first trigger the baby's inborn feeding behaviors and be patient.

Some babies latch and feed easily and enthusiastically. Other babies nurse only with patience and encouragement. In one U.S. survey of 366 women who relactated, 39% reported their baby nursed well at the first try, 32% were ambivalent about nursing, and 28% refused to nurse (Auerbach & Avery, 1980). Within 1 week, 54% had latched and fed well, and by 10 days, the rate rose to 74%. On average, babies younger than 3 months and those who had previously nursed latched and fed more easily.

Babies fed for long periods with feeding bottles may at first be more reluctant to nurse than babies fed in other ways (Abejide et al., 1997). But because babies are hardwired to nurse, most will eventually get there. Inborn feeding behaviors have been reported from all over the world in adopted children aged 8 months to school age (K. D. Gribble, 2005d). One Australian article described six children between 12 and 48 months old who stimulated partial relactation in their mothers from sucking alone after being weaned for at least 6 months (Phillips, 1993). Suggest nursing parents start by spending some time each day with baby resting tummy down on their semi-reclined body, as this triggers inborn feeding behaviors (S. D. Colson, Meek, & Hawdon, 2008). (For more details, see Chapter 1.)

• • •

If the baby continues to balk at nursing, suggest trying some basic strategies.

If a baby never nursed or has not nursed for some time, it may take patience before she latches and feeds. At first, suggest the following strategies.

- **Keep the parent's body a pleasant place to be,** not a battleground. If nursing feels stressful, feed another way and instead give baby lots of cuddle time on the parent's chest, especially while asleep (Smillie, 2017).
- **Spend time touching and skin-to-skin.** When not feeding, hold the baby and—if baby likes it—give skin-to-skin contact, perhaps by taking warm baths together.
- **Offer to nurse while baby is in a light sleep or drowsy.** Some babies nurse more easily when in a relaxed, sleepy state (S. Colson et al., 2003).
- **Use feeding positions baby likes best and experiment**, starting first with a semi-reclined position with baby tummy down and supported on the parent's body (see photos of these starter positions on p. 23-29).
- **Try nursing in a private place without distractions.** This could be a quiet, darkened room or an area with dim lighting.

- **Trigger a milk ejection before baby latches** to give an instant reward or try expressing milk first onto baby's lips.
- **Try shaping and/or supporting the mammary tissue.** Using the sandwich technique, nipple tilting, and other techniques may help the baby latch deeper and better trigger active sucking. For details, see p. 884.
- **Try nursing in motion,** while walking or rocking.
- **Spend lots of time nursing** whenever the baby nurses well.
- **Supplement as needed** to make sure the baby gets the milk she needs to feel strong, calm, and open to nursing.
- **If baby is older than 3 to 4 months, spend time with other nursing families,** such as at La Leche League or Australian Breastfeeding Association meetings, where the child can see other babies and children nursing.

• • •

Suggest nursing for comfort as well as for food.

In parts of the world, parents are warned not to let the baby use them "as a pacifier," but nursing for comfort both enhances the parent-child relationship and stimulates milk production. Suggest taking advantage of any and all chances to nurse for comfort.

- Offer to nurse whenever the baby wants to suck, rather than a pacifier/dummy.
- Offer to nurse when the baby is not too hungry or too full.
- When baby is nursing, give lots of cuddling and skin-to-skin contact.
- Approach nursing as a time the child gets special attention and closeness.

• • •

In some situations, tools and other strategies may help make the transition to nursing go more smoothly.

Drip expressed milk during latch. If the baby starts nursing but won't stay latched, ask a helper to use a spoon or eyedropper to drip expressed milk as baby latches or in the corner of her mouth as she begins sucking. Swallowing triggers sucking, which can get baby started nursing. Give more milk if baby comes off. In some studies (S. Banapurmath et al., 2003; Kesaree, 1993), this is called the "drop-and-drip" method and was used effectively to help relactating babies accept nursing.

Feed a little milk first. Some babies are more willing to try nursing if they are not very hungry. Suggest giving one-third to half of a feed the usual way and then attempt nursing.

Try a feeding-tube device. If slow milk flow is frustrating for the baby during nursing, a feeding-tube device—also known as a nursing supplementer (see p. 897)—will increase flow and may help the baby stay active longer. Because latching can be more challenging when using these devices, if slow flow is not an issue, it may not be a good choice. The best way to avoid over-supplementning with a feeding-tube device in this situation is to make sure the flow is not too fast. The flow is just right if baby spends at least 10 to 15 minutes per side at each feed before finishing. A too-fast flow will shorten feeding times by too much, which reduces stimulation, which can delay milk increase and make weaning from the device more difficult. For details, see p. 899.

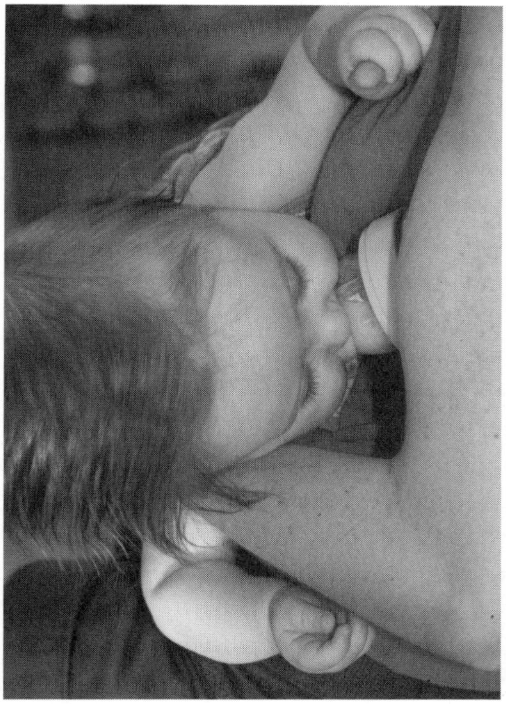

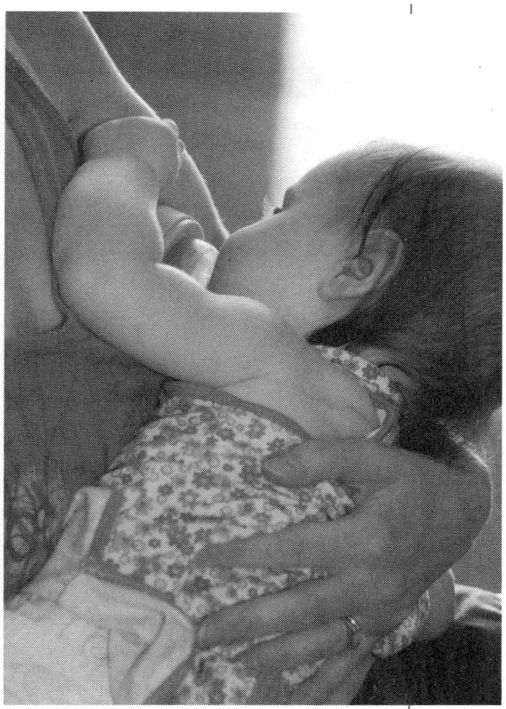

Bottle feeding in a nursing position may help to gradually transition baby to nursing.

Use the feeding bottle as a transitional tool. If the bottle-fed baby will not yet nurse or the family chooses to supplement with a bottle, suggest using the paced bottle-feeding technique described on p. 902-903. These strategies may also help encourage the transition to nursing or the continued acceptance of nursing by the baby:

- When bottle-feeding, suggest nursing parents hold the baby in a nursing position during feeds or hold the bottle against their nipple, so the baby gets used to feeding there.
- Wrap the bottle in a cloth and feed it against the exposed nipple, so the baby cannot touch the hard plastic of the bottle while feeding but can feel the parent's skin.
- Try "bait and switch," where the nursing parent begins by bottle-feeding in a nursing position, and while the baby is actively sucking and swallowing, pulls out the bottle teat and inserts the parent's nipple. (This can also be used with a pacifier/dummy.)

U.S. lactation consultant Dee Kassing describes another approach to bottle-feeding that may ease the transition to nursing by using the bottle to mimic nursing (Kassing, 2002):

- Use a slow-flow nipple.
- Rather than inserting the bottle nipple/teat into the baby's mouth, brush it lightly against the baby's lips and wait for her to open wide before allowing her to draw it into her mouth.
- Use a standard-width bottle nipple/teat and encourage a wide gape as the baby feeds.

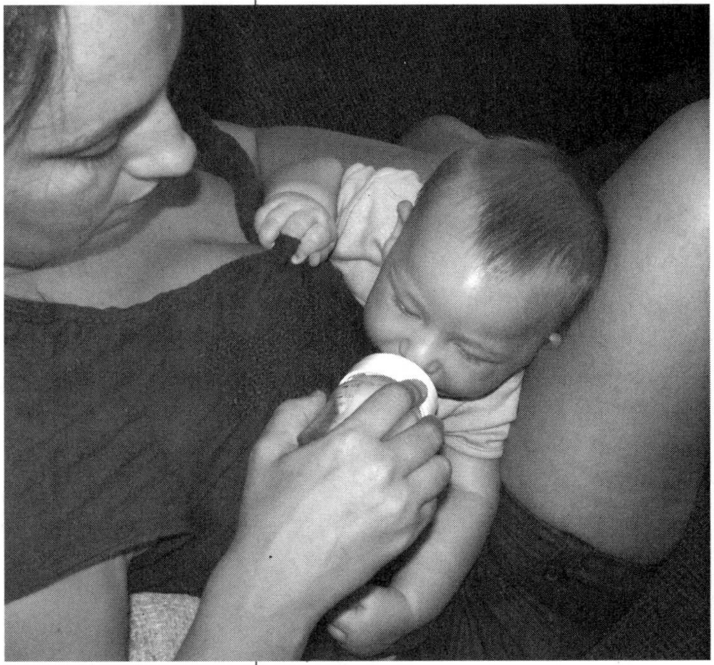

Try a thin, silicone nipple shield. In some situations, nipple shields can help transition a baby to nursing, especially if she was regularly fed by bottle, received a pacifier, or the nursing parent has inverted nipples. For details on use, fit, and application of a nipple shield, see p. 912-917.

Gauging Adequate Milk Intake

Discuss feeding methods for supplementing and their potential impact on milk production.

In the developing world, where relactation and induced lactation are practiced successfully, temporary feeding methods, such as a cup or a spoon, are often used to give supplements when needed. Some studies noted that babies supplemented by bottle have a more difficult time making the transition to full nursing. A 2018 study of 64 mothers in Sudan (Mehta, Rathi, Kushwaha, & Singh, 2018) found that supplementing by bottle reduced the odds of full relactation by nearly 63%. Researchers who studied 15 relactating mothers in India (C. R. Banapurmath et al., 1993, p. 1330) wrote: "It was interesting to note that babies refused to suck at the breast once they were used to bottle feeding....In all these mothers, relactation was successful when bottle feeding was stopped." It may be that the bottle's fast flow can cause babies to take more milk than they need, meaning less active sucking during nursing. Because feeding bottles are a long-term feeding method (and in some parts of the world more socially acceptable than nursing), parents may be less motivated to discontinue them (K. D. Gribble, 2005b).

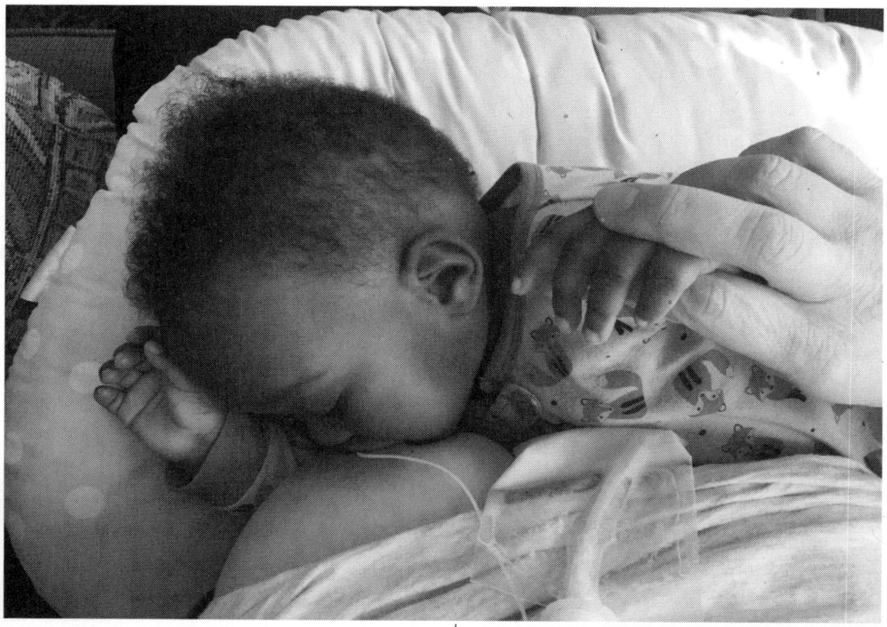

This mother exclusively nursed her biological first child. Her second child joined their family through adoption, feeding exclusively at the breast for her whole first year with a nursing supplementer containing donor human milk provided by milk-sharing families.

An alternative to cups, spoons, and feeding bottles is the nursing supplementer, also known as a feeding-tube device, which can provide the needed supplement while baby nurses. This feeding method may keep the baby actively nursing longer and therefore stimulate more milk production. Another advantage is that it may avoid the need to feed the baby again after nursing. But these devices can also be difficult for parents to use and difficult for some parents and babies to wean from. Alyssa Schnell, U.S. IBCLC and author *Breastfeeding Without Birthing* (personal communication, 2018) found in her practice:

> "Using a nursing supplementer can feel frustrating and overwhelming for parents. When I develop a personal protocol for my clients, I will suggest that they purchase a nursing supplementer before baby arrives and practice filling it with water, assembling, and taking it apart. They can even wear the supplementer with the feeding tube at their breast/chest and have their partner suck the water. Great for practice, nipple stimulation and partner involvement! We surveyed adoptive parents regarding using nursing supplementers to determine what helped them be successful with them. Top response: partner support! Get those partners to fill the supplementers and clean them too."

Not all parents are comfortable using a nursing supplementer (Borucki, 2005), so discuss the range of feeding options and support parents in their choice. Their decision may depend in part on whether they are close to full milk production, making some milk, or making little or no milk. For the pros and cons of each supplemental feeding method, see p. 896.

• • •

As the young baby takes more milk during nursing, suggest checking baby's weight regularly to be sure she gets enough—but not too much—supplement.

As parents notice the young baby is swallowing more milk and nursing longer, they can start the process of gradually decreasing the volume of supplement given (see Box 16.1). Before doing so, however, suggest having the baby weighed by her healthcare provider and schedule weight checks at least weekly on the same scale. If the baby is younger than 3 months and her weight gain slips below about 30 g (about 1 oz.) per day or about 200 g. (7 oz.) per week, this is a sign the baby needs more supplement. (For weight gains appropriate for older children, see Table 6.1 on p. 191.

The goal is to strike the delicate balance of feeding the smallest volume of supplement needed while actively nursing as much as possible to stimulate faster milk production. Babies need to stay well nourished. If the supplement is reduced too quickly and the baby becomes weak from low milk intake, this can compromise her ability to nurse. On the other hand, if baby receives too much supplement, she will be too full to nurse often or long enough to stimulate faster milk production. Regular weight checks will help the parents keep the baby's milk intake in the right range.

KEY CONCEPT

Between birth and 3 months, if babies slip below a weight gain of 30 g (1 oz.) per day or 198 g (7 oz.) per week, more supplement is needed.

• • •

If needed, test-weighing and milk expression can help nursing parents gauge their milk production.

The baby's weight gain is the best indicator of how close the nursing parent's milk production is to meeting the baby's needs. The two strategies that follow provide information about the baby's milk intake and the nursing parent's milk production.

Test-weighing. A reliable way to gauge baby's milk intake while nursing is to use a very accurate (to 2 g) electronic baby scale for pre- and post-feed weights (Rankin et al., 2016). These scales are available in many hospitals and lactation clinics. In some areas, they can be rented for home use from breast-pump rental companies. See Table 6.3 on p. 224 for average milk intake per feed by age. Of course, the volume of milk the baby consumes at one feed will vary by her hunger (just like in adults) and by time of day. Although knowing averages can be helpful, daily milk intake among healthy, thriving nursing babies can vary by as much as three-fold (Kent et al., 2006). Also, one test-weight is not enough information to gauge a baby's 24-hour milk intake. In most cases, though, checking baby's weight gain every few days or weekly is enough information for good decision-making.

Milk expression. Expressing milk can provide clues to milk production, but it is less reliable than test-weighing because not all lactating parents—even those with excellent milk production—can express milk effectively, especially in the beginning. One Australian study of 28 breastfeeding mothers with established and ample milk production found 11% were unable to express much milk using any of the seven pump cycling patterns tested (Kent, Ramsay, Doherty, Larsson, & Hartmann, 2003). Milk expression is a learned skill that often takes time and practice to master. Even when the most effective pump (usually a rental pump) is used, factors unrelated to milk production—such as pump fit and responsiveness—can affect milk yield. For details, see p. 907-908.

• • •

Other signs of milk intake, such as audible swallowing and diaper output, are not completely reliable but can provide clues on a daily basis.

Audible swallowing. When the nursing baby swallows, some describe the sound as "kah…kah…kah." After milk ejection, most babies swallow after every suck or two, with occasional pauses. As nursing continues, milk flow slows, and as a baby's hunger is satisfied, she swallows less often. If the parents can't hear the baby swallow at all, she may just be a quiet feeder. But if the baby's audible swallowing stops early in the feed or she falls asleep quickly, suggest keeping baby actively nursing longer by first helping her latch deeper and then use compression (see p. 889 for compression techniques that stimulate a faster milk flow).

Diaper output. Although studies indicate that diaper output is not a completely reliable gauge of milk intake during the first 14 days of life (DiTomasso & Paiva, 2018; Nommsen-Rivers, Heinig, Cohen, & Dewey, 2008; Shrago, Reifsnider, & Insel, 2006), during the first 6 weeks, the number of stools per day can provide a general idea of whether a baby is getting enough milk. The mean number of stools per day among exclusively nursing newborns was four, but some passed as many as eight per day. Because formula can be constipating, formula supplements can affect the number and consistency of a baby's stools, making diaper output an even less reliable indicator. (Many families find it very encouraging, though, when their baby's stools become more like a nursing baby and less like a formula-fed baby.) When ultra-absorbent disposable diapers/nappies are used, wet diapers can be difficult to count. That said, a baby's urine should always be light colored and not strong-smelling. One Indian study's authors (S. Banapurmath et al., 2003) suggested its 1,000 relactating mothers expect their babies to have at least six urinations during the day and two at night, with the urine staying clear and colorless.

KEY CONCEPT

Between weight checks during the first 6 weeks, number of stools per day can provide a general idea of whether babies are getting enough milk.

Keep track of stools and feeds. Although it is only a rough sign of milk intake, between regular weight checks, suggest that as the supplement is decreased, parents make note every day of:

- The number of the baby's stools at least the size of a U.S. quarter (2.5 cm) or larger
- At how many feeds baby nurses and her response to it (active sucking? accepts nursing well?)
- Volume of supplement given, when given, and total given over 24 hours

It can be reassuring to see the baby's stooling stay steady as the supplements are decreased. Although four stools per day the size of a U.S. quarter (2.5 cm) or larger are average at first, not all thriving babies follow this pattern. A 2014 French study that examined the bowel habits of 283 exclusively breastfed babies (Courdent, Beghin, Akre, & Turck, 2014) found that 37% of the babies in one group went more than 24 hours between stools during their first month. Some healthy, thriving, exclusively nursing babies may go as a long as a week between stools, which is not a cause for concern as long as the baby is gaining weight well. If the baby stooling infrequently is younger than one month, a weight check is recommended. If the weight gain is in the normal range, no change is needed.

• • •

Whenever low milk intake is a possibility in a younger baby, the parents should know the signs of dehydration.

Knowing the signs of dehydration can be reassuring when the baby is thriving and can act as a warning if she's not. The following are signs the baby needs more supplement:

- Two or fewer wet diapers in 24 hours
- When skin is pinched, it stays pinched looking
- Extreme sleepiness or lethargy
- Dry mouth and eyes

• • •

Signs the baby's milk intake while nursing is increasing include less supplement taken, changes in stool consistency, and others.

Less supplement taken. As the baby takes more milk while nursing, she may become more interested in nursing and less interested in finishing the supplement. When the nursing parent notices this, suggest reducing the volume of supplement. If a nursing supplementer is used, try starting the feed without it and ending the feed with it.

Other signs of increasing human-milk intake. When the baby is supplemented with formula, another sign of increasing human-milk intake is looser and milder-smelling stools. If the baby was ill, her health and temperament may improve. A diaper rash or other skin condition may improve. The baby may become more alert and active, or if she was tense before, she may seem more relaxed.

Follow baby's lead. When the baby continues to gain at least 7 oz. (200 g) per week while the amount of supplement decreases, it means human-milk intake is filling the gap. It may be time to decrease the supplement if the baby does any of the following:

- Wants to spend more time nursing
- Lets milk dribble out while sucking
- Seems full faster
- Takes less supplement

If there is supplement left after several feeds in a row, cut back a little on the volume in the container. Unless it is obvious the supplement needs to be decreased faster, cutting back by a half-ounce (15 mL) per feed works well for many families, allowing a day or two in between reductions.

Less supplement in the morning, more in the afternoon. An alternative to cutting back the same volume at every feed is to handle feeds differently at different times of day. Most nursing parents have the most milk available in the morning and less as the day goes on. Reducing supplements may work best by offering less at the first morning feed and more in the evening. As milk production continues to increase, the first morning feed is usually the best time to eliminate the supplement completely. If the baby seems comfortable after receiving less supplement than usual, continue to gradually reduce the volume offered without leaving the baby hungry. Avoid giving her more supplement than she wants.

Same-sex partners co-nurse their daughters, who were born 7 months apart.

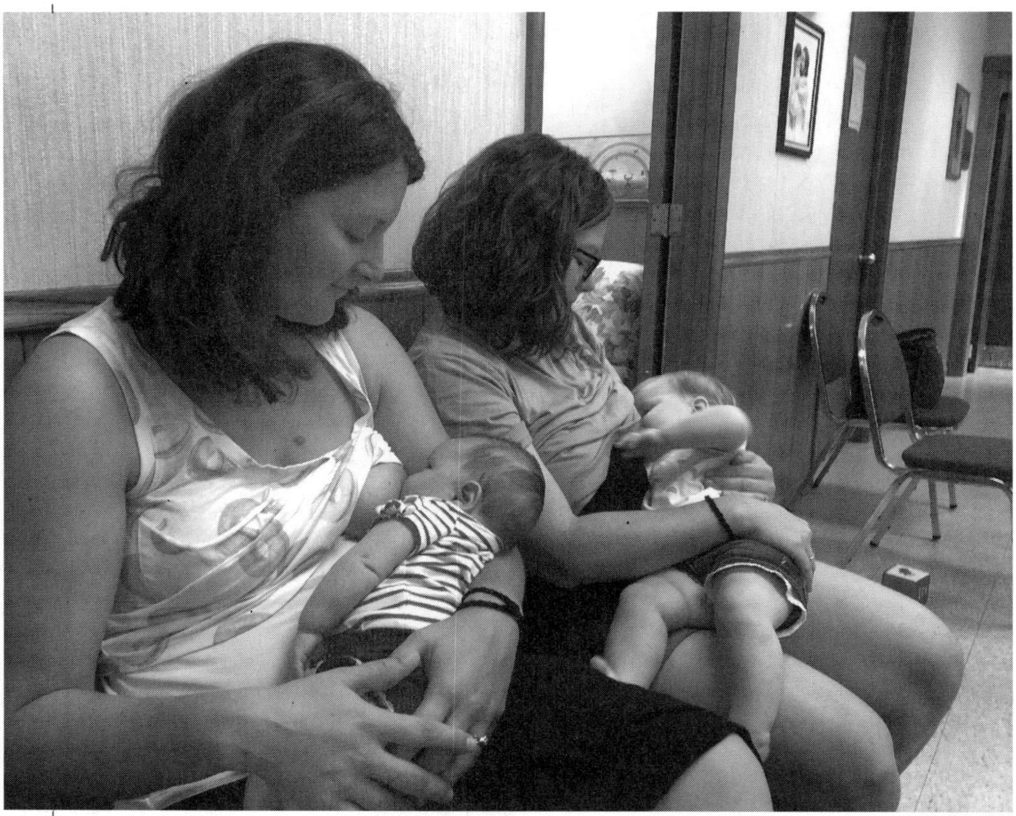

• • •

Milk production may dip slightly as menstruation starts.

Even if the hormonal changes involved in menstruation cause a slight decrease in milk production, with a few days of increased nursing, milk production usually quickly rebounds.

Co-nursing with Partners

In some families, both parents nurse the baby, which is known as co-nursing.

Both partners nurse (known as co-nursing) in a variety of different types of families, some of which are described in online posts and in the medical literature.

Cisgender female couples. In this type of family, both women were assigned as female at birth and both identify as female (cisgender). In some of these families, only the birthing parent breastfeeds or only the non-gestational parent breastfeeds by relactating or inducing lactation. In other families, both women co-nurse, which can happen in different ways.

- Both women give birth within a short time of each other and breastfeed both babies.
- One woman gives birth and the other relactates or induces lactation (Koning, 2011).
- Neither woman gives birth, and the couple adopts a baby or the baby is born via surrogacy, with both women relactating or inducing lactation.

In one case report, a lesbian couple adopted a baby and both induced lactation while co-nursing during the early weeks with the baby's birth mother (Wilson et al., 2015).

Transgender women and their partners. In this type of family, transgender women—those assigned as male at birth who identify as female and transitioned to female—induce lactation. In one case, a transgender woman, who received hormone therapy for 6 years before her adopted baby was born, produced enough milk to fully sustain the baby for the first 6 weeks (Reisman & Goldstein, 2018). Research confirms that estrogen therapy grows mammary tissue (Sonnenblick, Shah, Goldstein, & Reisman, 2018). In another case, a transgender woman induced lactation and shared breastfeeding with her female partner, who was also the baby's birth mother (Sperling & Robinson, 2018). An online article shared the experiences of three transgender women who breastfed their babies (Burns, 2018). This article mentioned several aspects of co-nursing these women appreciated:

- Sharing nursing makes life with a newborn easier and less intense.
- Sharing night feeds means both parents get more sleep.
- The birth parent can go out more easily without worry about the baby being unhappy.
- Nursing affirmed the transgender women's status as a woman, in terms of their ability to nurture the baby at their breast and stimulating more mature breast development.
- Co-nursing prevents feelings of jealousy that are common in non-nursing partners (Pelka, 2009).

Transgender men and their partners. Transgender men are those assigned as female at birth but identify as male and transitioned to male. Transgender men may become pregnant, give birth, and nurse their babies, which some refer to as "chestfeeding" (MacDonald et al., 2016). Their partners may be anywhere on the gender spectrum and may choose to nurse, too. Some transgender men have surgery to reduce their mammary tissue, which may affect milk production (see p. 797).

Birthing mothers and fathers. Male lactation is known in other species, and there are some anecdotal accounts of cisgender men producing milk (Swaminathan, 2007). If a father wants to experience nursing, consider "dry nursing" (described in the next point). In general, any parent who has not experienced a female puberty or estrogen therapy is likely to have much less mammary tissue than those who have, which decreases the chances of producing much milk.

• • •

How to best manage the logistics of co-nursing is something each family works out for itself based on its own goals and priorities.

One aspect of co-nursing that needs to be sorted out is how to balance milk production between the co-nursing partners.

Goals and priorities differ. In some families, one partner may want to co-nurse simply to experience the emotional closeness of a nursing relationship and not necessarily to produce much—if any—milk. In this case, nursing without relactating or inducing lactation, also known as "dry nursing," may satisfy this goal. As Alyssa Schnell, U.S. lactation consultant and author of *Breastfeeding Without Birthing,* wrote about dry nursing on her website **sweetpeabreastfeeding.com**:

> "It is not necessary to bring in milk (induce lactation or relactate) in order to nurse a baby. Some parents may bottle-feed or their partner will breastfeed for nutrition, and they will nurse for comfort and connection

and to meet baby's need for non-nutritive sucking (instead of using a pacifier). Other parents may feed baby at their breast/chest using an at-breast/chest supplementer."

Other families have different goals. In the same-sex female couple described in the previous point who induced lactation for an adopted baby (Wilson et al., 2015), milk production was a higher priority for one partner than the other. However, they ultimately decided that sharing feeds and parenting equally was a higher priority for them than milk production.

Making the birthing parent's milk production a priority. If the family includes one birthing parent, due to the hormonal effects of pregnancy, the birthing parent is likely to have a natural milk-production advantage. In an online article (Koning, 2011), Liesbeth Koning described being the first to nurse baby Grace when her partner Melissa gave birth. Koning started an induced lactation protocol several months before Grace's birth and was producing some milk. She decided, though, to spend the first weeks after the birth pumping, so that Melissa could establish full milk production by nursing Grace. Koning breastfed baby Grace during the workday after Melissa's parental leave ended, and the two mothers produced so much milk, they became milk donors for the local milk bank.

Making the stay-at-home partner's milk production a priority. In some families, deciding how often each partner nurses may be determined in part by the couple's employment plans. If one partner plans to care for the baby while the other works, that couple may put a higher priority on the stay-at-home partner's milk production.

NURSING IN EMERGENCIES

During emergencies, nursing is key to infant health and survival.

Even in developed countries during times of peace and plenty, babies fed non-human milks are at greater risk of illness and death (Bartick et al., 2017). However, during war, famine, drought, flood, earthquake, hurricane, or other natural disasters, the risks of formula-feeding increase exponentially as conditions deteriorate and challenges such as the following occur:

- Poor hygiene
- Limited or contaminated water supplies
- Less available food of all types, including infant formula
- Limited access to refrigeration and heat to sterilize containers
- Increased exposure to illness from crowds
- Decreased availability of medical treatment

A baby fed non-human milks during an emergency is more likely to become ill from exposure to organisms in contaminated water and food and is at risk for underfeeding when formula becomes scarce. The non-nursing baby is also more likely to become ill because she is not receiving the antibodies and other immunities in mother's milk. Formula and other foods also actively facilitate

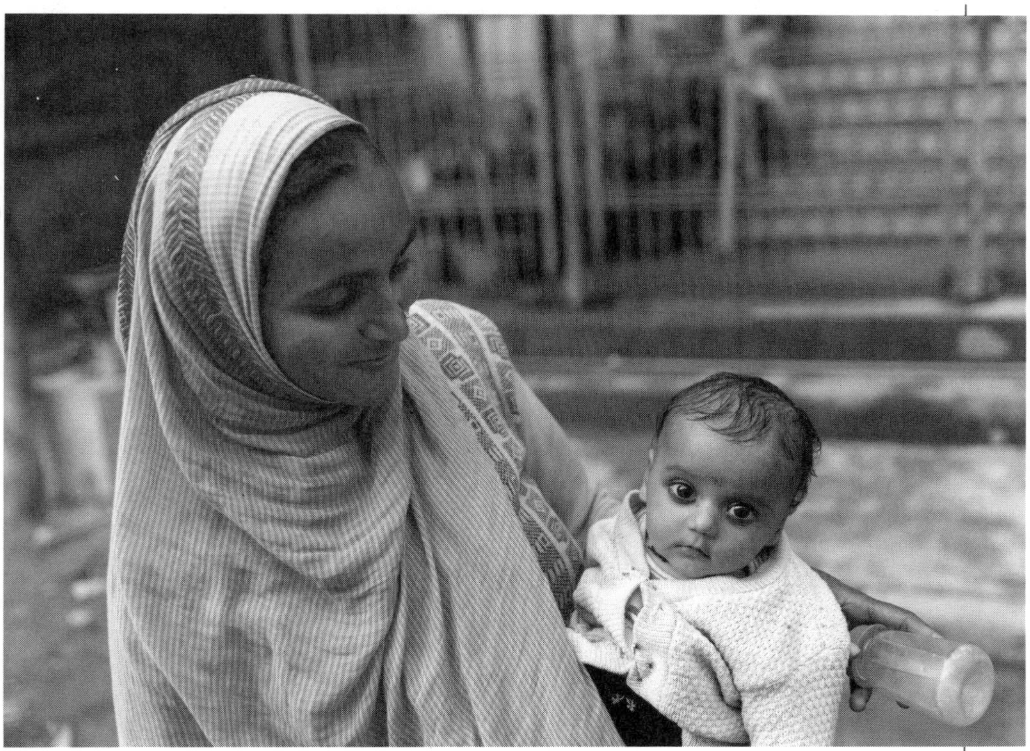

The European refugee crisis that began in 2015 included many nursing families.

infection in infants (K. D. Gribble, 2011). During flooding in Botswana in 2005 and 2006, of its 2 million people, more than 20,000 cases of diarrhea in children under 5 years led to more than 500 deaths (K. Gribble, 2014). Fully formula-fed babies were more than 30 times more likely to be hospitalized than babies who were exclusively nursed, and in one hospital cohort, 32 of 33 babies who died were exclusively formula fed. The remaining baby who died was mixed-fed both formula and human milk.

Nursing becomes vital during emergencies because it provides babies with unlimited safe food and fluids during their first 6 months, a safe partial food and fluids source after 6 months, and protection from illness. Along with all this, nursing also enhances the close, loving parent-child bond and relieves stress in the nursing parent, which can be vital to preventing neglectful care and abandonment during emergencies. Nursing also delays the return to fertility and enables families to nourish the baby with the more limited resources they have available.

KEY CONCEPT

Nursing during emergencies can mean the difference between life and death.

While appropriate nursing practices are important to all families, during an emergency, they may make the difference between life and death. Suggest any nursing parent in an emergency:

- Start nursing within an hour or so of birth.
- Maintain as much parent-baby skin-to-skin contact as possible after birth for increased infant stability.
- Nurse often and well day and night.
- Nurse exclusively for the first 6 months.
- Offer appropriate solid foods to the baby at around 6 months of age.
- Continue nursing for at least the first 2 years (WHO, 2018).

• • •

Even when malnourished and stressed, nursing parents can produce good quality milk for their babies.

Babies sometimes die unnecessarily due to common misconceptions about nursing in emergencies. For example, in Iraq during the Gulf War, the misconception that women could not produce adequate milk when malnourished and under great stress led some officials, journalists, and relief workers to discourage nursing (Burleigh, 1991). Although psychological stress can delay milk ejection, nursing is most definitely possible and milk will continue to be produced if nursing parents keep nursing. One U.S. study found that perceived stress, sleep difficulty, and fatigue were not related to milk volume (Hill, Aldag, Chatterton, & Zinaman, 2005). In 1978 after a devastating earthquake in Guatemala, continued nursing by local mothers played a key role in infant survival (Solomons & Butte, 1978).

KEY CONCEPT

It takes weeks of famine conditions before the quality and quantity of mother's milk begins to suffer.

As described in Chapter 13, "Nutrition, Exercise, and Lifestyle Issues," nursing parents can produce ample milk even on very inadequate diets. A meta-analysis examining research from around the globe found that only when famine or near famine conditions continue for weeks does a mother's milk production or milk quality suffer (Prentice, Goldberg, & Prentice, 1994). A Dutch study found that even in famine conditions, milk production may be only slightly affected among previously well-nourished mothers with good body stores (Smith, 1947). If famine occurs, providing nursing parents with food is less costly and results in better health outcomes than providing formula for babies.

Fluid intake appears to be unrelated to milk production. One U.S. study found that increasing nursing mothers' fluid intake by 25% did not affect their milk production (Dusdieker, Booth, Stumbo, & Eichenberger, 1985). For more details on fluid intake and milk production, see p. 557.

In her article "Infant Feeding in Emergencies," U.K. author Marion Kelly (Kelly, 1993, p. 111) wrote:

> "Since the ability to breastfeed is remarkably resistant to the effects of maternal undernutrition and psychological stress, the notion that many mothers who were breastfeeding pre-crisis will need to use breast-milk substitutes once disaster has struck should be rejected by those with responsibility for relief programmes."

• • •

Trained relief workers and experienced nursing parents can provide nursing support.

In all cultures, nursing support during emergencies is important. The belief that stress or lack of food in emergencies negatively affects milk quality or volume seems to be universal. Even in countries like Canada, where nursing is the norm, nursing parents often worry about not making enough milk, even when their milk production is ample (Galipeau, Dumas, & Lepage, 2017). "Perceived insufficient milk" does not necessarily mean milk production is low. It may be a misinterpretation of normal infant behaviors or unrealistic expectations of how often a newborn should nurse. For this reason, health workers in emergencies need to understand nursing norms, so they can help families learn to gauge adequate milk production and encourage feeding more often if they need to increase milk production.

Part of any relief effort should be the establishment of policies that make nursing information and support a priority. Some found an effective way to support nursing is to find parents who are currently nursing in the affected areas or those who have previously nursed with the knowledge and skills to help others (Rahman et al., 2016). Experienced nursing parents can counsel others on overcoming common challenges, such as nipple pain, worries about low milk production, and mastitis, as well as provide information on increasing milk production for those mostly nursing; and provide information on relactation or induced lactation for those who never nursed or who weaned prior to the emergency.

• • •

Exclusive nursing, wet nursing, induced lactation, and relactation should be encouraged in emergencies, as even partial milk production can save babies' lives.

To prevent infant deaths in an emergency, birthing parents who previously weaned or never nursed can be encouraged to relactate, and adoptive parents can be encouraged to induce lactation. Even partial milk production provides a source of safe, uncontaminated food and protection from illness. See the previous sections in this chapter for the strategies used for relactation and induced lactation.

In an emergency, the main focus should be on basic approaches, such as nursing the baby for food and for comfort and using hand expression to stimulate milk production when the baby is not nursing. Also key is frequent parent-baby skin-to-skin contact day and night.

• • •

During emergencies, infant formula and any other foods that replace nursing should only be given to those caring for babies who cannot fully nurse, along with intensive support to improve survival rates.

When a war or natural disaster occurs, the first impulse among many in developed nations is to offer aid in the form of infant formula (DeYoung, Suji, & Southall, 2018; K. D. Gribble, 2005c). But this can cause more problems than it solves. Because exclusive nursing is not common anywhere in the world, making formula available puts nursing babies at risk (K. Gribble, 2014). Providing formula to the affected areas can increase formula-related deaths, undermine families' confidence in nursing, and create an unnecessary dependence on commercial products. Nursing parents may decide to start giving their babies formula. Researcher Karleen Gribble describes the reasons nursing parents request formula in emergencies (K. Gribble, 2014):

- **The misconception that they are unable to fully nurse** due to stress, food shortages, or their misinterpretation of their baby's behavior.
- **Cultural beliefs,** for example that experiencing trauma (such as the 2010 Haitian earthquake) will make their milk "bad" (Dornemann & Kelly, 2013).
- **An aspiration to bottle-feed.** In developing countries, formula-feeding is associated with higher socioeconomic status, which makes it appealing to some families.
- **Formula costs a lot of money.** Some nursing parents may not plan to feed donated formula to their baby but may be tempted to request formula in order to sell it. In the Philippines, for example, for those in the lowest income group, a full month's supply of formula may be worth three-quarters of their monthly household income.

In 1991, during relief efforts in Iraq, although Kurdish parents were told by British health personnel about the health risks of infant formula, many "expressed skepticism on the grounds that the practice had originated in the West" (Kelly,

1993, p. 116). A 2017 narrative review (Carroll, Lama, Martinez-Brockman, & Perez-Escamilla, 2017) noted that in conflict situations, many families tend to stop nursing, which makes nutritional challenges worse. Relief workers need to know that when nursing babies are fed formula it will decrease the nursing parent's milk production and increase the babies' risk for formula-related illness and death. Use of infant formula actively and passively harms babies' immune systems, making them vulnerable to infection and death from diarrhea and pneumonia.

When an emergency occurs in areas where nursing is not yet the norm, health risks to babies increase when formula is no longer easily available and hygiene deteriorates (Hipgrave, Assefa, Winoto, & Sukotjo, 2012). In these areas, relief workers wanting to support nursing may encounter the extra challenge of dealing with traditional practices that undermine nursing. During the war in Bosnia, for example, many formula-fed babies died when formula became scarce and safe preparation became a challenge. However, traditional practices, such as scheduled feeding and early and regular use of formula, undermined milk production (Ademovic, 1998). Lack of access to infant formula can kill within a few days. After Hurricane Katrina in New Orleans, formula-fed infants died because they did not have access to formula or human milk.

KEY CONCEPT

Unless international guidelines are followed, providing infant formula during emergencies can undermine nursing, increasing the risk of infant death.

If formula is provided in a crisis area, this should be done only under existing international guidelines (IYCFECG, 2017), which include:

- Limiting formula distribution to specifically defined situations
- Guaranteeing its availability as long as the baby requires it (until at least 6 months)
- Providing formula only in unbranded, generic packaging so sales are not promoted
- Distributing the formula only to babies younger than 12 months of age who are partially weaned along with making available clean water, fuel and containers for heating and sterilization, instructions and measuring tools, and extra medical support for formula-related illness, such as treatments for diarrhea, and specific plans for nursing promotion to offset the availability of formula
- Adjust practices as needed to better reflect cultural values (DeYoung et al., 2018)

Easily cleaned feeding cups may also need to be provided in areas where hygiene is poor to avoid the use of feeding bottles and nipples/teats, which are not recommended because they are easily contaminated. Extra food allowances may also be offered to nursing parents as an incentive for continued nursing.

Infant formula is not the only cause for concern. In 2016 during the European refugee crisis, researchers (Theurich & Grote, 2017) noted that commercial infant foods were distributed in the refugee camps that recommended on their packaging that they should be given to babies beginning at 4 months, which was counter to best practice and had the potential to increase health problems in a vulnerable population.

Promoting the survival of babies in emergencies must involve promotion of exclusive nursing and measures that help families achieve this, including:

- Giving nursing parents priority access to food and other resources
- Providing "safe spaces" where nursing parents can care for their babies and receive lactation help
- Preventing the uncontrolled distribution of infant formula or other milk products

Yet despite these guidelines, infant formula continues to be distributed inappropriately in emergencies (Shaker-Berbari, Ghattas, Symon, & Anderson, 2018).

RESOURCES

asklenore.info—Location of the Protocols for Induced Lactation created by Lenore Goldfarb and Canadian pediatrician Jack Newman.

bit.ly/BA2-CDCDisasters—U.S. Centers for Disease Control and Prevention's (CDC) 2018 webpage "Disaster Planning: Infant and Child Feeding."

bit.ly/BA2-WHOEmergencies—2017 publication "Infant and Young Child Feeding in Emergencies" distributed by WHO and created jointly by many international organizations. Free and downloadable.

bit.ly/BA2-WHORelactation—World Health Organization's (WHO) free, downloadable booklet, "Relactation: Review of Experience and Recommendations for Practice."

ennonline.net—U.K.'s Emergency Nutrition Network, whose Infant and Young Child Feeding in Emergencies (IFE) Core Group offers downloadable information for the public and relief workers on protecting nursing during emergencies.

Marasco, L. & West, D. (2020). *Making More Milk: The Breastfeeding Guide to Increasing Your Milk Production,* 2nd ed. New York, NY: McGraw Hill.

Schnell, A. *Breastfeeding Without Birthing: A Breastfeeding Guide for Mothers through Adoption, Surrogacy, and Other Special Circumstances.* Amarillo, TX: Praeclarus Press, 2013.

sweetpeabreastfeeding.com—Website of U.S. lactation consultant Alyssa Schnell, author of *Breastfeeding Without Birthing*, which includes free webinars, podcasts, and articles for parents and professionals on relactation and inducing lactation.

REFERENCES

AAP. (2012). Breastfeeding and the use of human milk. *Pediatrics, 129*(3), e827-e841.

Abejide, O. R., Tadese, M. A., Babajide, D. E., et al. (1997). Non-puerperal induced lactation in a Nigerian community: Case reports. *Annals of Tropical Paediatrics, 17*(2), 109-114.

Abul-Fadl, A. M., Kharboush, I., Fikry, M., et al. (2012). Testing communication models for relactation in an Egyptian setting. *Breastfeeding Medicine, 7,* 248-254.

Ademovic, M. (1998). Breastfeeding during wartime means safe, available food for baby. *BFHI News, 8,* 2-3.

Auerbach, K. G., & Avery, J. L. (1980). Relactation: A study of 366 cases. *Pediatrics, 65*(2), 236-242.

Banapurmath, C. R., Banapurmath, S. C., & Kesaree, N. (1993). Initiation of relactation. *Indian Pediatrics, 30*(11), 1329-1332.

Banapurmath, S., Banapurmath, C. R., & Kesaree, N. (2003). Initiation of lactation and establishing relactation in outpatients. *Indian Pediatrics, 40*(4), 343-347.

Bartick, M. C., Schwarz, E. B., Green, B. D., et al. (2017). Suboptimal breastfeeding in the United States: Maternal and pediatric health outcomes and costs. *Maternal and Child Nutrition, 13*(1).

Becker, G. E., Smith, H. A., & Cooney, F. (2016). Methods of milk expression for lactating women. *Cochrane Database of Systematic Reviews, 9,* CD006170. doi:10.1002/14651858.CD006170.pub5.

Borucki, L. C. (2005). Breastfeeding mothers' experiences using a supplemental feeding tube device: Finding an alternative. *Journal of Human Lactation, 21*(4), 429-438.

Bryant, C. A. (2006). Nursing the adopted infant. *Journal of the American Board of Family Medicine, 19*(4), 374-379.

Buccini, G. D. S., Perez-Escamilla, R., Paulino, L. M., et al. (2017). Pacifier use and interruption of exclusive breastfeeding: Systematic review and meta-analysis. *Maternal and Child Nutrition, 13*(3).

Burleigh, P. (1991, June 10). Watching children starve to death: An exclusive look inside Iraq's devastated hospitals. *Time,* 36-37.

Burns, K. (2018). Yes, transwomen can breastfeed—Here's how. Retrieved from **https://www.them.us/story/trans-women-breastfeed**.

Carroll, G. J., Lama, S. D., Martinez-Brockman, J. L., et al. (2017). Evaluation of nutrition interventions in children in conflict zones: A narrative review. *Advances in Nutrition, 8*(5), 770-779.

Cho, S. J., Cho, H. K., Lee, H. S., et al. (2010). Factors related to success in relactation. *Journal of the Korean Society of Neonatology, 17,* 232-238.

Colson, S., DeRooy, L., & Hawdon, J. (2003). Biological Nurturing increases duration of breastfeeding for a vulnerable cohort. *MIDIRS Midwifery Digest, 13*(1), 92-97.

Colson, S. D., Meek, J. H., & Hawdon, J. M. (2008). Optimal positions for the release of primitive neonatal reflexes stimulating breastfeeding. *Early Human Development, 84*(7), 441-449.

Courdent, M., Beghin, L., Akre, J., et al. (2014). Infrequent stools in exclusively breastfed infants. *Breastfeeding Medicine, 9*(9), 442-445.

Czank, C., Henderson, J. J., Kent, J. C., et al. (2007). Hormonal control of the lactation cycle. In T. W. Hale & P. E. Hartmann (Eds.), *Hale & Hartmann's Textbook of Human Lactation* (p. 89-111). Amarillo, TX: Hale Publishing.

de Melo, S. L., & Murta, E. F. (2009). Hypogalactia treated with hand expression and translactation without the use of galactagogues. *Journal of Human Lactation, 25*(4), 444-447.

De, N. C., Pandit, B., Mishra, S. K., et al. (2002). Initiating the process of relactation: An Institute based study. *Indian Pediatrics, 39*(2), 173-178.

Dettwyler, K. A. (1995). Beauty and the breast. In P. Stuart-Macadam & K. A. Dettwyler (Eds.), *Breastfeeding: Biocultural Perspectives* (pp. 39-73). New York, NY: Aldine de Gruyter.

DeYoung, S., Suji, M., & Southall, H. G. (2018). Maternal perceptions of infant feeding and health in the context of the 2015 Nepal earthquake. *Journal of Human Lactation, 34*(2), 242-252.

DiTomasso, D., & Paiva, A. L. (2018). Neonatal weight matters: An examination of weight changes in full-term breastfeeding newborns during the first 2 weeks of life. *Journal of Human Lactation, 34*(1), 86-92.

Dornemann, J., & Kelly, A. H. (2013). 'It is me who eats, to nourish him': A mixed-method study of breastfeeding in post-earthquake Haiti. *Maternal and Child Nutrition, 9*(1), 74-89.

Du, G. L., Liu, Z. H., Chen, M., et al. (2015). Sheehan's syndrome in Xinjiang: Clinical characteristics and laboratory evaluation of 97 patients. *Hormones (Athens), 14*(4), 660-667.

Dusdieker, L. B., Booth, B. M., Stumbo, P. J., et al. (1985). Effect of supplemental fluids on human milk production. *Journal of Pediatrics, 106*(2), 207-211.

Farhadi, R., & Philip, R. K. (2017). Induction of lactation in the biological mother after gestational surrogacy of twins: A novel approach and review of literature. *Breastfeeding Medicine, 12*(6), 373-376.

Galipeau, R., Dumas, L., & Lepage, M. (2017). Perception of not having enough milk and actual milk production of first-time breastfeeding mothers: Is there a difference? *Breastfeeding Medicine, 12,* 210-217.

Goldfarb, L. E. (2010). An assessment of the experiences of women who induced lactation. *(Doctor of Philosophy in Interdisciplinary Studies with a Concentration in Arts & Sciences and a specialization in Human Lactation and Reproductive Counseling)*, Union Institute & University, Cincinnati, OH.

Gribble, K. (2014). Formula feeding in emergencies. In V. R. Preedy & R. R. Watson (Eds.), *Handbook of Dietary and Nutritional Aspects of Bottle Feeding* (pp. 143-161). The Netherlands: Wageningen Academic Publishers.

Gribble, K. D. (2004). The influence of context on the success of adoptive breastfeeding: Developing countries and the west. *Breastfeeding Review, 12*(1), 5-13.

Gribble, K. D. (2005a). Adoptive breastfeeding. *Breastfeeding Review, 13*(3), 6.

Gribble, K. D. (2005b). Breastfeeding of a medically fragile foster child. *Journal of Human Lactation, 21*(1), 42-46.

Gribble, K. D. (2005c). Infant feeding in the post-Indian Ocean tsunami context: Reports, theory and action. *Birth Issues, 14*(4), 121-127.

Gribble, K. D. (2005d). Post-institutionalized adopted children who seek breastfeeding from their new mothers. *Journal of Prenatal & Perinatal Psychology & Health, 19*(3), 217-235.

Gribble, K. D. (2006). Mental health, attachment and breastfeeding: Implications for adopted children and their mothers. *International Breastfeeding Journal, 1*(1), 5.

Gribble, K. D. (2011). Mechanisms behind breastmilk's protection against, and artificial baby milk's facilitation of, diarrhoeal illness. *Breastfeeding Review, 19*(2), 19-26.

Handlin, L., Jonas, W., Petersson, M., et al. (2009). Effects of sucking and skin-to-skin contact on maternal ACTH and cortisol levels during the second day postpartum-Influence of epidural analgesia and oxytocin in the perinatal period. *Breastfeeding Medicine, 4*(4), 207-220.

Heinig, M. J., Nommsen, L. A., Peerson, J. M., et al. (1993). Energy and protein intakes of breast-fed and formula-fed infants during the first year of life and their association with growth velocity: The DARLING Study. *American Journal of Clinical Nutrition, 58*(2), 152-161.

Hill, P. D., Aldag, J. C., Chatterton, R. T., et al. (2005). Psychological distress and milk volume in lactating mothers. *Western Journal of Nursing Research, 27*(6), 676-693; discussion 694-700.

Hipgrave, D. B., Assefa, F., Winoto, A., et al. (2012). Donated breast milk substitutes and incidence of diarrhoea among infants and young children after the May 2006 earthquake in Yogyakarta and Central Java. *Public Health Nutrition, 15*(2), 307-315.

Hormann, E. (1977). Breastfeeding the adopted baby. *Birth and the Family Journal, 4,* 165.

Hurst, N. M., Valentine, C. J., Renfro, L., et al. (1997). Skin-to-skin holding in the neonatal intensive care unit influences maternal milk volume. *Journal of Perinatology, 17*(3), 213-217.

IYCFECG. (2017). Infant and young child feeding in emergiecies: Operational guidance for emergency relief staff and programme managers, version 3. Retrieved from **https://www.ennonline.net/operationalguidance-v3-2017**.

Kassing, D. (2002). Bottle-feeding as a tool to reinforce breastfeeding. *Journal of Human Lactation, 18*(1), 56-60.

Kelly, M. (1993). Infant feeding in emergencies. *Disasters, 17*(2), 110-121.

Kent, J. C., Mitoulas, L. R., Cregan, M. D., et al. (2006). Volume and frequency of breastfeedings and fat content of breast milk throughout the day. *Pediatrics, 117*(3), e387-395.

Kent, J. C., Prime, D. K., & Garbin, C. P. (2012). Principles for maintaining or increasing breast milk production. *Journal of Obstetric, Gynecologic & Neonatal Nursing, 41*(1), 114-121.

Kent, J. C., Ramsay, D. T., Doherty, D., et al. (2003). Response of breasts to different stimulation patterns of an electric breast pump. *Journal of Human Lactation, 19*(2), 179-186; quiz 187-178, 218.

Kesaree, N. (1993). Drop and drip method. *Indian Pediatrics, 30*(2), 277-278.

Koning, L. (2011). How two lesbian mamas share breastfeeding duties. Retrieved from **https://offbeathome.com/co-breastfeeding/**.

Kunz, T. H., & Hosken, D. J. (2009). Male lactation: Why, why not and is it care? *Trends in Ecology & Evolution, 24*(2), 80-85.

Lommen, A., Brown, B., & Hollist, D. (2015). Experiential perceptions of relactation: A phenomenological study. *Journal of Human Lactation, 31*(3), 498-503.

Louis-Jacques, A., & Stuebe, A. M. (2018). Long-term maternal benefits of breastfeeding. *Contemporary OB-GYN, 64*(7).

Lozoff, B., & Brittenham, G. (1979). Infant care: Cache or carry. *Journal of Pediatrics, 95*(3), 478-483.

Lussier, M. M., Brownell, E. A., Proulx, T. A., et al. (2015). Daily breastmilk volume in mothers of very low birth weight neonates: A repeated-measures randomized trial of hand expression versus electric breast pump expression. *Breastfeeding Medicine, 10*(6), 312-317.

MacDonald, T., Noel-Weiss, J., West, D., et al. (2016). Transmasculine individuals' experiences with lactation, chestfeeding, and gender identity: A qualitative study. *BMC Pregnancy and Childbirth, 16,* 106.

Macrae, S., & Gribble, K. D. (2006). Why grandma can't pick up the baby. In S. Macrae & J. MacLeod (Eds.), *Adoption Parenting: Building a Toolbox, Creating Connections.* Warren, NJ: EMK Press.

Marasco, L. & West, D. (2020). *Making More Milk: The Breastfeeding Guide to Increasing Your Milk Production,* 2nd ed. New York, NY: McGraw Hill.

Matthiesen, A. S., Ransjo-Arvidson, A. B., Nissen, E., et al. (2001). Postpartum maternal oxytocin release by newborns: Effects of infant hand massage and sucking. *Birth, 28*(1), 13-19.

Mehta, A., Rathi, A. K., Kushwaha, K. P., et al. (2018). Relactation in lactation failure and low milk supply. *Sudan Journal of Paediatrics, 18*(1), 39-47.

Mizuno, K., Nishida, Y., Mizuno, N., et al. (2008). The important role of deep attachment in the uniform drainage of breast milk from mammary lobe. *Acta Paediatrica, 97*(9), 1200-1204.

Moran, L., & Gilad, J. (2007). From folklore to scientific evidence: Breast-feeding and wet-nursing in Islam and the case of non-puerperal lactation. *International Journal of Biomedical Science, 3*(4), 251-257.

Morton, J., Hall, J. Y., Wong, R. J., et al. (2009). Combining hand techniques with electric pumping increases milk production in mothers of preterm infants. *Journal of Perinatology, 29*(11), 757-764.

Nemba, K. (1994). Induced lactation: A study of 37 non-puerperal mothers. *Journal of Tropical Pediatrics, 40*(4), 240-242.

Neville, M. C. (1999). Physiology of lactation. *Clinics in Perinatology, 26*(2), 251-279, v.

Nommsen-Rivers, L. A., Heinig, M. J., Cohen, R. J., et al. (2008). Newborn wet and soiled diaper counts and timing of onset of lactation as indicators of breastfeeding inadequacy. *Journal of Human Lactation, 24*(1), 27-33.

Nyati, M., Kim, H. Y., Goga, A., et al. (2014). Support for relactation among mothers of HIV-infected children: A pilot study in Soweto. *Breastfeeding Medicine, 9*(9), 450-457.

Pelka, S. (2009). Sharing motherhood: Maternal jealousy among lesbian co-mothers. *Journal of Homosexuality, 56*(2), 195-217.

Perrin, M. T., Wilson, E., Chetwynd, E., et al. (2015). A pilot study on the protein composition of induced nonpuerperal human milk. *Journal of Human Lactation, 31*(1), 166-171.

Phillips, V. (1993). Relactation in mothers of children over 12 months. *Journal of Tropical Pediatrics, 39*(1), 45-48.

Prentice, A. M., Goldberg, G. R., & Prentice, A. (1994). Body mass index and lactation performance. *European Journal of Clinical Nutrition, 48 Suppl 3,* S78-86; discussion S86-79.

Rahman, A., Hamdani, S. U., Awan, N. R., et al. (2016). Effect of a multicomponent behavioral intervention in adults impaired by psychological distress in a conflict-affected area of Pakistan: A randomized clinical trial. *Journal of the American Medical Association, 316*(24), 2609-2617.

Rankin, M. W., Jimenez, E. Y., Caraco, M., et al. (2016). Validation of test weighing protocol to estimate enteral feeding volumes in preterm infants. *Journal of Pediatrics, 178,* 108-112.

Reisman, T., & Goldstein, Z. (2018). Case report: Induced lactation in a transgender woman. *Transgender Health, 3*(1), 24-26.

Schnell, A. (2013). *Breastfeeding Without Birthing: A Breastfeeding Guide for Mothers through Adoption, Surrogacy, and Other Special Circumstances.* Amarillo, TX: Praeclarus Press.

Seema, Patwari, A. K., & Satyanarayana, L. (1997). Relactation: An effective intervention to promote exclusive breastfeeding. *Journal of Tropical Pediatrics, 43*(4), 213-216.

Shaker-Berbari, L., Ghattas, H., Symon, A. G., et al. (2018). Infant and young child feeding in emergencies: Organisational policies and activities during the refugee crisis in Lebanon. *Maternal and Child Nutrition, 14*(3), e12576.

Shrago, L. C., Reifsnider, E., & Insel, K. (2006). The Neonatal Bowel Output Study: Indicators of adequate breast milk intake in neonates. *Pediatric Nursing, 32*(3), 195-201.

Slome, C. (1956). Nonpuerperal lactation in grandmothers. *Journal of Pediatrics, 49*(5), 550-552.

Slusher, T. M., Slusher, I. L., Keating, E. M., et al. (2012). Comparison of maternal milk (breastmilk) expression methods in an African nursery. *Breastfeeding Medicine, 7*(2), 107-111.

Smillie, C. M. (2017). How infants learn to feed: A neurobehavioral model. In C. W. Genna (Ed.), *Supporting Sucking Skills in Breastfeeding Infants* (3rd ed., pp. 89-111). Burlington, MA: Jones & Bartlett Learning.

Smith, C. (1947). Effects of maternal undernutrition upon newborn infants in Holland (1944-1945). *Journal of Pediatrics, 30,* 229-243.

Solomons, N. W., & Butte, N. (1978). A view of the medical and nutritional consequences of the earthquake in Guatemala. *Public Health Reports, 93*(2), 161-169.

Sonnenblick, E. B., Shah, A. D., Goldstein, Z., et al. (2018). Breast imaging of transgender individuals: A review. *Current Radiology Reports, 6*(1), 1.

Sperling, D., & Robinson, L. (2018). Induced lactation in a transgendered female partner. *Journal of Obstetric, Gynecologic & Neonatal Nursing, 47*(Supplement 3S), S61.

Swaminathan, N. (2007). Strange but true: Men can lactate. *Scientific American* (September 6).

Theurich, M. A., & Grote, V. (2017). Are commercial complementary food distributions to refugees and migrants in Europe conforming to International Policies and Guidelines on Infant and Young Child Feeding in Emergencies? *Journal of Human Lactation, 33*(3), 573-577.

Uvnas-Moberg, K. (2014). *Oxytocin: The Biological Guide to Motherhood.* Amarillo, TX: Praeclarus Press.

WHO. (2018). Infant and young child feeding. Retrieved from **http://www.who.int/mediacentre/factsheets/fs342/en/index.html**.

Wieschhoff, H. (1940). Artificial stimulation of lactation in primitive cultures. *Bulletin of the History of Medicine, VIII*(10), 1403-1415.

Wilson, E., Perrin, M. T., Fogleman, A., et al. (2015). The intricacies of induced lactation for same-sex mothers of an adopted child. *Journal of Human Lactation, 31*(1), 64-67.

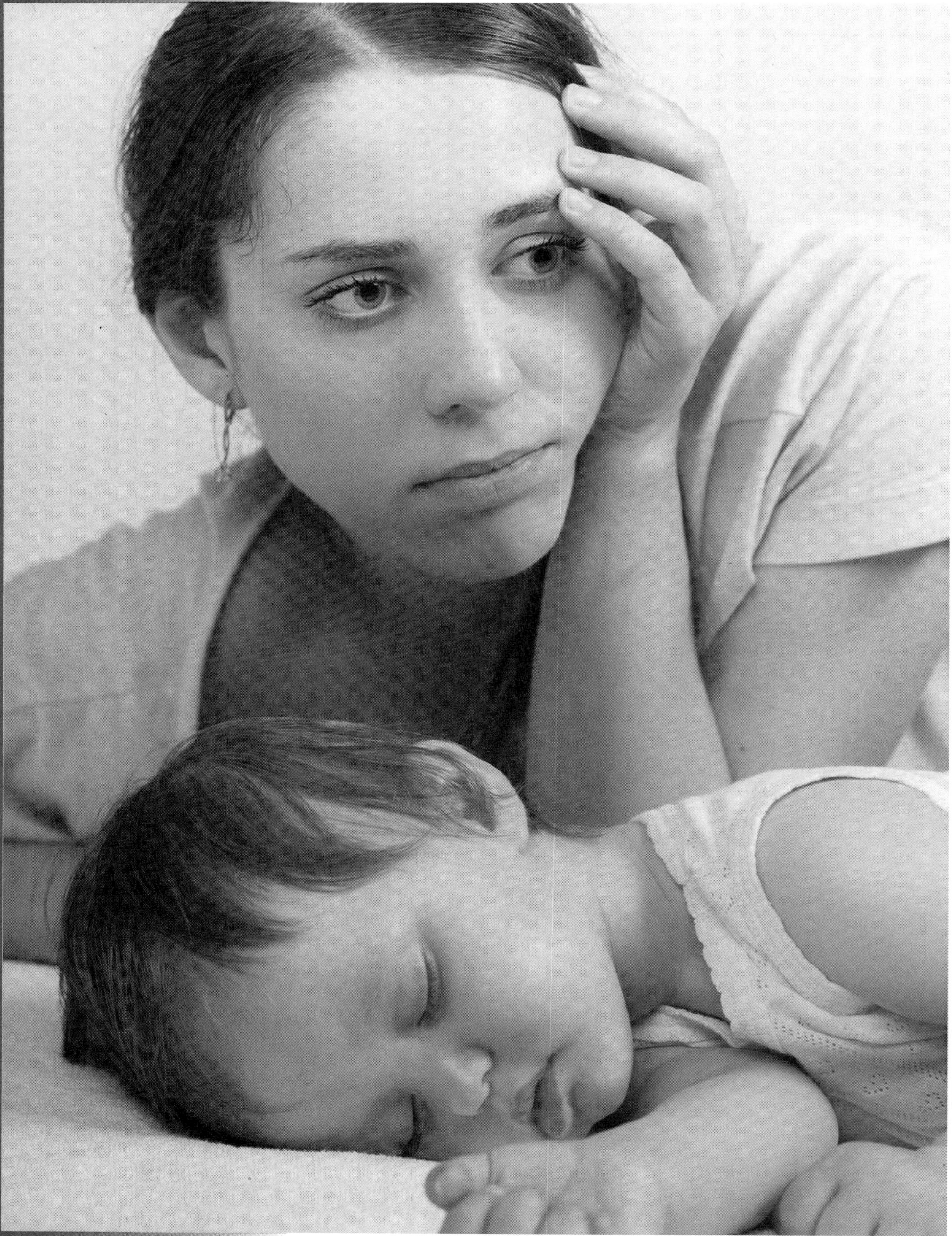

Nipple Issues

17

NIPPLE PAIN

In most cases, nipple pain is a solvable problem.

Mild nipple pain is common during the first 2 weeks of nursing (M. L. Buck, Amir, Cullinane, Donath, & Team, 2014; Niazi et al., 2018), especially when the pain resolves with milk ejection (see next section). But nipple pain that lasts throughout a feed or moderate-to-severe pain and skin trauma are signs that damage is being done. Or they may indicate the presence of a condition requiring treatment, such as mastitis or a bacterial or yeast infection. Unfortunately, many nursing parents with moderate-to-severe nipple pain do not seek help because they mistakenly believe that nipple pain is a normal part of nursing.

• • •

Nipple pain—especially when it is intense and ongoing—can interfere with activity, sleep, and mood and may contribute to depression.

When nursing is painful, parents may dread feeds. This dread and the anxiety that accompanies it can lead to depression. Nipple pain is one of the most common reasons given for premature weaning (Gianni et al., 2019; Odom, Li, Scanlon, Perrine, & Grummer-Strawn, 2013).

A 2011 U.S. retrospective study (Watkins, Meltzer-Brody, Zolnoun, & Stuebe, 2011) noted the link between nipple pain and depression. The dynamics of this association were described in more detail in a prospective Australian study of 65 breastfeeding mothers who were asked to complete a written mood evaluation (L.H. Amir, Dennerstein, Garland, Fisher, & Farish, 1997). More than twice as many mothers with nipple pain rated as depressed compared with those without nipple pain (38% vs. 14%). After the nipple pain resolved, about the same percentage of women in both groups rated as depressed. In other words, when a parent in pain is depressed, in some cases resolving the pain may also resolve the depression.

KEY CONCEPT

Severe nipple pain and/or pain that lasts throughout a nursing session is a sign that some adjustment is needed.

A 2012 Australian study (H. L. McClellan, Hepworth, Garbin, et al., 2012) compared two groups of breastfeeding mothers, one with nipple pain and trauma and another without. The researchers found that the more intense the mothers' pain levels and the longer their pain lasted, the more it interfered with their lives. Not surprisingly, the effect of the continuing pain was to decrease activity levels, increase the incidence of sleep problems, and negatively affect mood.

• • •

The intensity of nipple pain is determined in part by degree of trauma, but many other factors affect pain levels, too.

It seems obvious that more nipple trauma leads to higher pain levels, but the picture is much more complex. A 2019 systematic review of 25 studies, 23 of which were randomized controlled trials (Coca et al., 2019), found that the study mothers with nipple trauma consistently reported higher levels of pain intensity than those without trauma. However, there are many other factors that also affect the level of perceived pain in nursing parents. In 2015, an Australian physician and a pain specialist (L. H. Amir, Jones, & Buck, 2015) collaborated to create the Breastfeeding Pain Reasoning Model (Figure 17.1). This tool summarizes many of the factors other than skin damage that can affect perception of pain. These factors help explain why one nursing parent appears to have severe trauma but considers the pain manageable while another has no nipple damage but finds the nursing pain overwhelming. Fatigue, the use of inflammatory medication, a history of trauma, poor social support, and many of the other factors listed in Figure 17.1 can increase the perceived pain of nursing.

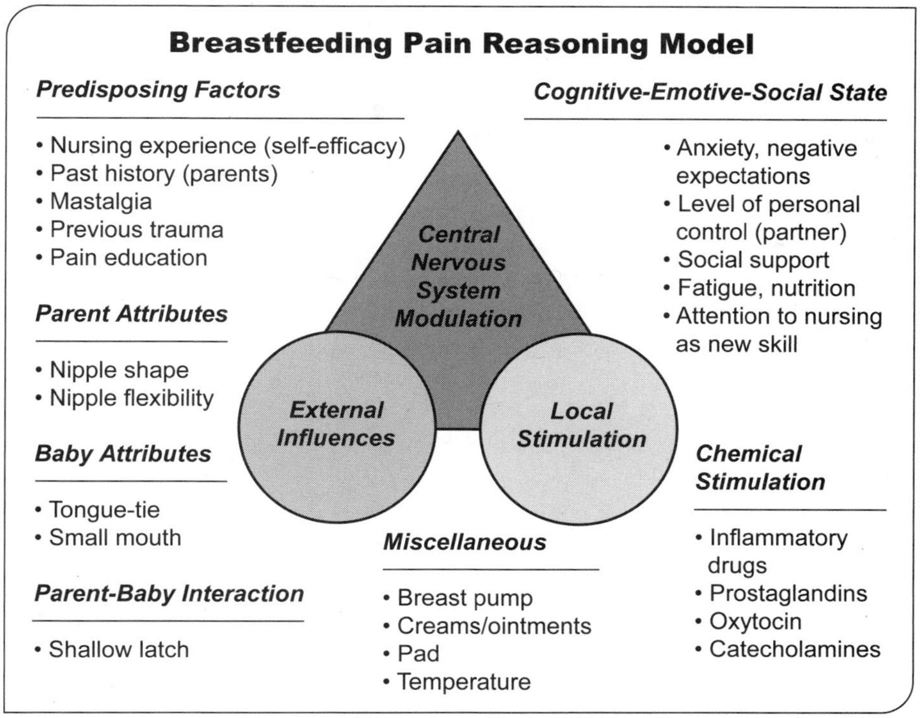

Figure 17.1 The Breastfeeding Pain Reasoning Model.
Adapted from (L. H. Amir et al., 2015).

What's Normal after Birth?

Some mild nipple pain in the first 2 weeks is normal if it resolves with milk ejection and there is no skin damage.

According to some studies (M. L. Buck et al., 2014; Niazi et al., 2018), about 80% of nursing parents experience some nipple pain during the early weeks of nursing. Called "transient soreness" by some (Smith, 2021), according to a Cochrane systematic review (Dennis, Jackson, & Watson, 2014), nipple pain usually peaks around the third day after birth and is mostly resolved by about 10 days. However, the incidence of nipple pain varies in different parts of the world and in different studies. For example, one large Thai study prospectively followed 1,649 women after singleton pregnancies (Puapornpong, Paritakul, Suksamarnwong, Srisuwan, & Ketsuwan, 2017) and found that by Day 7, just under 10% experienced nipple pain at more than half their nursing sessions. The risk factors for nipple pain were first-time birth and receiving no information about breastfeeding. In 72% of these cases, shallow latch was the cause, in 23% tongue-tie was a factor, and in 4% oversupply contributed to nipple pain (see later section).

> **KEY CONCEPT**
>
> *According to the "30-second rule," it is safe to ignore early nipple pain only if the latch seems deep and the pain resolves within 30 seconds.*

One possible reason early nipple pain is so common is the increased sensitivity of the nipples and mammary glands post-delivery. Some theorize that this heightened sensitivity to touch from hormonal changes may be important to the establishment of early milk production (Prime, Geddes, & Hartmann, 2007).

To reassure parents experiencing this initial pain, U.S. lactation consultants Barbara Wilson-Clay and Kay Hoover share what they call the "30 second rule" (Wilson-Clay & Hoover, 2017, p. 55). They tell parents it is safe to ignore nipple pain if the latch seems deep and the pain resolves within 30 seconds. But if skin trauma develops or the pain lasts longer than 30 seconds, it's time to seek help.

• • •

Suggest seeking help as soon as possible if nipple pain is intense or skin trauma develops.

If a parent experiences any of the following, suggest seeking help as soon as possible:

- Intense, toe-curling pain
- Pain lasting throughout the feed
- Pain or a burning sensation between feeds
- Damaged skin (cracks, bleeding, lesions) on the nipple
- Continuing pain with no improvement after a day or two of consistently trying to address the cause

Allowing pain to continue unaddressed increases the risk that complications—such as infection—may develop (Kent et al., 2015), which can lead to persistent pain that may intensify over time. Continuing pain may also be a sign the baby is not transferring milk well during nursing.

Nipple Pain During the First Week

Ask what day the pain started, when during the feed it occurs, its intensity, and if there is trauma, where it is and what it looks like.

When the pain started may provide clues to possible causes (see Box 17.1).

- **After a couple days of comfortable nursing.** Explore the possibility that mammary fullness from milk increase after birth may be contributing to a shallow latch. Suggest nursing more often and using reverse pressure softening (RPS, see p. 885) or expressing a little milk to soften the nipple and areola before latching.
- **At the beginning of the feed.** If the baby is younger than 2 weeks old and the discomfort resolves after the milk starts to flow, this may be "transient soreness" or a sign of a shallow latch. If it lasts longer than about 30 seconds, suggest trying some of the positioning strategies in the next section.
- **During the entire nursing session.** This parent needs help now. Possible causes include shallow latch, variations in infant oral anatomy (tongue-tie, unusual palate, small or recessed lower jaw, etc.), strong sucking, or variations in nipple anatomy.
- **After feeds or in between.** If nursing is comfortable and the pain starts after feeds, ask the parent to look at the nipple when the pain begins for any color changes. If there are color changes, consider vasospasm (white) or Raynaud's phenomenon (white, blue, and/or red).

The intensity and timing of the pain will provide more clues. Again, transient nipple soreness typically peaks around the third day.

There can also be visual clues to the cause of nipple pain and trauma:

- **Misshapen nipple after feeds.** The nipple may look like the tip of a new tube of lipstick, flattened and pointed. If this happens consistently, this is a sign of a shallow latch that can lead to the damage described in the next point.
- **Cracks, bleeding, or a compression stripe** (a white line across the nipple face)—usually a sign of a shallow latch (see the next section).

BOX 17.1 Factors Contributing to Nipple Pain or Trauma during the First Week

Interactive Factors
• Shallow latch—Nipple may look pinched or misshapen after feeds or the areola may be bruised • Suction—Baby pulled off without first breaking the suction • Fit—Due to a small mouth and/or large nipple, baby can fit only the nipple in his mouth
Baby Factors
• Variations in oral anatomy—Tongue-tie, lip-tie, unusual palate shape, short or recessed jaw • Strong or unusual sucking, clamping, biting, or clenching
Parent Factors
• Engorgement—Shallow latch due to taut mammary tissue • Vasospasm or Raynaud's phenomenon—Nipple changes color after feed • Nipple anatomical variations—Nipple inverted, dimpled, etc. • Use or misuse of pumps or products—(see next section) for pumps: check fit, level of suction, use of bottles or pacifiers/dummies; poorly fitting bras; wet breast pads, irritating creams/ointments

More than one factor may contribute to nipple pain, so consider multiple factors.

Other possible causes include variations in infant oral anatomy, variations in nipple anatomy, or fast milk flow (baby squeezes the nipple in his mouth to slow the flow).

- **Starburst-shaped lesions in the center of the nipple** were reported (Wilson-Clay & Hoover, 2017, p. 56) in an engorged mother, when milk flow was slowed by mammary swelling.

• • •

Ask for a description of the pain.

The words used to describe nipple pain are not always reliable clues to its cause. But how nursing parents describe their pain may reflect their emotions, which gives lactation supporters the chance to respond with empathy and understanding. One mixed-methods Canadian study that used a descriptive qualitative approach (Jackson, O'Keefe-McCarthy, & Mantler, 2019) interviewed breastfeeding mothers about their experiences of nipple pain and concluded that many found their pain severe and distressing. Pain associated with nursing did not fall into specific pain types, and the researchers referred to it as "multidimensional." They concluded that current pain measurement tools may be inadequate to provide a clear sense of this experience, which may make it difficult for healthcare providers to respond appropriately.

• • •

When nipple pain—with or without skin trauma—persists beyond the first 7 to 10 days, there is often more than one contributing cause.

It is tempting to assume when one cause of nipple pain is identified and addressed that the problem is solved. But as one 2015 Australian study (Kent et al., 2015) found, there is often more than one contributing factor. This study examined the records of the 708 lactation consults that occurred during two 6-month periods in an infant feeding center in Western Australia. Of these lactation consults, 36% involved nipple pain. The researchers recorded the attributed causes, results of cultures, treatment, and resolution. The top four factors contributing to persistent nipple pain—from most to least common—were:

1. Shallow latch (attachment and positioning issues) (90%)
2. Tongue-tie (67%, 25% of the initial consults)
3. High or arched palate (44%)
4. Infection (26%)

In 89% of the cases, there was more than one contributing cause of persistent nipple pain. In some cases (such as infection and vasospasm), these causes arose as complications of nipple trauma. The researchers concluded that because persistent nipple pain can occur as a result of "cascading events," early and effective lactation help is vital.

Interactive Factors

Depth of Baby's Latch

During the early weeks, shallow latch is the most common cause of nipple pain and trauma.

As described in the previous point, the most common cause of nipple pain and trauma is a shallow latch. When a baby latches shallowly, the nipple is pressed against his hard palate, which if done consistently, can cause pain and damage. With a shallow latch, the baby may also receive less milk with every suck.

How is a deep latch defined? Ultrasound research (Douglas & Geddes, 2018; Elad et al., 2014; L. A. Jacobs, Dickinson, Hart, Doherty, & Faulkner, 2007) revealed that when nursing is going normally, on average, the nipple extends to within about 5 mm of the junction of baby's hard and soft palates. (Parents can explore their own mouths using their finger or tongue to find the location of this area where the roof of their mouth turns from hard to soft.) If the nipple reaches this depth, the nipple experiences little friction or pressure, and nursing is comfortable. This author nicknamed this area in the baby's mouth the comfort zone (Mohrbacher & Kendall-Tackett, 2010). Early nipple pain and trauma can usually be quickly resolved once the nipple consistently reaches the comfort zone at every feed. When this happens, traumatized nipples can heal, even with continued nursing.

KEY CONCEPT

When the nipple reaches the comfort zone consistently, traumatized nipples can heal, even with continued nursing.

How often do latch adjustments help? A French lactation consultant in private practice examined the records of the 61 consults she did over a 13-month period (Darmangeat, 2011) and found that about two thirds of the consults involved nipple pain. Getting a deeper latch resolved the pain in 65%. She noted that the main issues were the baby not opening wide while latching and the baby was held too far away from the nipple.

• • •

Ask what feeding positions they are using and whether the parent supports the mammary tissue during nursing sessions.

In addition to the baby not opening wide at latch and being held too far away, other dynamics that can contribute to shallow latch include the following.

Upright feeding position, especially during the early weeks. In these positions, gaps form easily between the nursing couple, which can disorient baby and lead to feeding struggles. See next point for more.

Unstable or "head below bottom" position. If a baby is held in a precarious position or his head is lower than his bottom, the baby may shift to try to stabilize himself, which can pull the nipple out of the comfort zone. If a baby feels unstable, he may also pull at the nipple or clamp down.

Supporting the mammary gland at an unnatural level. If the gland is not at its usual resting place, supporting the tissue can become tiring. Releasing the gland after latch may cause its weight to pull the nipple out of the comfort zone, turning a deep latch into a shallow one. If this happens, suggest either supporting the gland throughout the feed or—even easier—use a feeding position that allows the baby to latch while the gland is at its natural level.

• • •

At first, using starter positions and allowing the baby to do the latching may make nursing easier and more comfortable.

While a nursing couple is in the learning phase, suggest the parent lean back into a semi-reclined feeding position (see pp. 23-29 in Chapter 1). These ***starter positions*** simplify latching and usually lead to more comfortable nursing. When the baby rests tummy down on the parent's body, this full frontal body contact activates his inborn feeding behaviors (S. Colson, 2019). Baby's head bobs on the parent's body, which triggers a wide-open mouth with a relaxed jaw and baby's tongue forward (Figure 17.2. In this position, most babies can latch comfortably with little help. Free, short videos of nursing couples using these positions are available to share with families at **YouTube.com/NancyMohrbacher**.

In a study of 40 English and French mothers during the first month post-delivery, when mothers used these starter positions (S. D. Colson, Meek, & Hawdon, 2008, p. 448):

> "...there was no need to line up nose to nipple and wait for mouth gape or to assess tongue position as suggested by those teaching [positioning and attachment] skills. Gravity pulled the baby's chin and tongue forward. Together the anti-gravity reflexes often triggered the degree of mouth opening needed to achieve pain-free, neonatal self-attachment even when the baby appeared to be in light sleep."

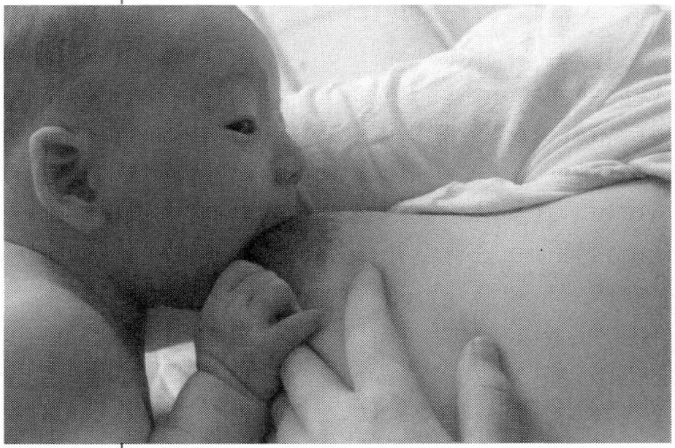

Figure 17.2 Baby self-attaches with a wide-open mouth, a relaxed jaw, and tongue forward. ©2020 Melanie Ham, used with permission

In upright feeding positions, gravity pulls baby's body down and away, so a deep latch is more difficult to achieve and maintain. Keeping baby latched deeply at nipple height throughout the feed requires effort by the parent, which can be tiring over time.

• • •

If nipple pain occurs when using the starter positions, the baby may need more help, or there may be other contributing factors.

Despite good feeding dynamics, nipple pain and trauma can occur when there are fit issues or if nursing couples have the anatomical variations described in later sections, such as tongue-tie, unusual palate shape, and variations in nipple shape and size. After achieving a deep latch, if the parent does not have a noticeable improvement in comfort, it's time to consider other contributing factors.

How Baby Comes Off

Taking the baby off the nipple without first breaking suction can cause nipple pain.

Whenever possible, encourage parents to let the baby nurse until he comes off on his own. But if it's necessary to take the baby off before he is finished, suggest first breaking the suction. Do this by gently inserting a finger into the corner of the baby's mouth, pulling down on the baby's chin, or pressing down gently on the mammary tissue near baby's mouth.

Nipple-Baby Fit

If the nipples are so wide or long that the baby can't take in more than just the nipple, this may cause nipple pain.

When nursing is going well, at latch, the baby usually takes the nipple and some of the areola into his mouth. But if the nipple is so wide or long that the baby can't accommodate more than just the nipple itself (often called a "poor fit," see p. 103 and 113), this can cause pain and trauma, as well as feeding aversion and ineffective milk removal (Wilson-Clay & Hoover, 2017, p. 55).

If the combination of a large nipple and a small mouth leads to pain and trauma, first try to make nursing work (optimizing how baby latches, use of a nipple shield, or any other strategy that works). If there's no improvement, reassure the parent that babies grow very quickly and that it's possible to establish full milk production by expressing milk until the baby's mouth grows enough to comfortably nurse, which will usually be within a few weeks. See p. 497-507 for strategies on how to establish full milk production with a pump.

Baby Factors

Variations in Oral Anatomy

Even if a baby has an identified tongue-tie and/or lip-tie, because not all affected babies have nursing problems, it's important to start with the basics.

The string-like membrane that attaches the tongue to the floor of the mouth is called the ***lingual frenulum***. The membrane that attaches the upper lip to the upper gum line is called the ***labial frenulum***. If either or both of these membranes are tight, fibrous, or thick enough to restrict normal tongue or lip movements, this is called tongue-tie (ankyloglossia) or lip-tie. They may or may not affect comfort during nursing.

Start with the basics. A 2015 review of the literature (Power & Murphy, 2015) concluded that at most about 50% of tongue-tied babies have nursing problems. In other words, even if a baby is identified as tongue-tied, if the nursing parent has nipple pain or trauma, start with the usual strategies, such as trying to get a deeper latch, before assuming the tongue-tie is the cause of the pain. It's very possible that the painful nursing can be resolved without treating the tongue-tie.

Symptomatic tongue-tie and nipple pain. Symptomatic tongue-tie is the term used when the baby's restricted tongue movements are causing feeding problems. Nipple pain and/or trauma are common among parentss of babies with symptomatic tongue-tie. One U.K. study of 215 tongue-tied babies with nursing problems (Griffiths, 2004) found:

- 88% of the babies had difficulty latching
- 77% of the mothers had nipple pain or trauma
- 72% of the babies fed continuously while awake due to inadequate milk intake
- 52% of the nursing couples experienced all three of these symptoms

KEY CONCEPT

Because many tongue-tied babies nurse without problems, if the mother of a tongue-tied baby has nipple pain, it's always best to start with basic strategies.

For suggestions on how to resolve nipple pain and trauma in nursing babies with symptomatic tongue-tie, see p. 271-276.

Lip-tie and nipple pain. At this writing, very little is known about the impact of lip-tie on nursing. For details, see p. 277-279.

• • •

An unusual palate shape—high, bubble, grooved—or a small or recessed jaw may contribute to painful nursing, but positioning strategies may help.

Other aspects of the baby's oral anatomy may affect nursing comfort.

Unusual palate shapes do not always cause painful nursing. Types of palates reported to contribute to nipple pain include: bubble palate, grooved or channel palate, and high palate (Snyder, 1997). Babies who are intubated for long periods may develop grooves in their palates or high, narrow arches (Wilson-Clay & Hoover, 2017; Wolf & Glass, 1992).

The baby with a grooved palate has a thin channel along its length, which may affect the baby's ability to maintain suction during feeds. Like a bubble palate, the groove may affect how deeply the baby draws the nipple into his mouth.

A small or recessed jaw (micronathia or retrognathia) may contribute to nipple pain because it affects tongue placement. Tips to try include:

- A very asymmetrical latch (see p. 878) with head tilted back and baby's body pulled in close to the nursing parent's opposite nipple
- Side-lying positions or semi-reclined starter positions (see pp. 23-29) may help increase the baby's head extension for easier breathing

For more strategies, see p. 291-292.

• • •

The baby's oral anatomy is just one part of the story. Feeding position and how parent and baby fit together also affect nursing comfort.

With tongue-tie, lip-tie, an unusual palate shape, and a small or recessed jaw, the infant's anatomy is only part of the story. Comfort during nursing is also affected by the parent's anatomy and how they fit together. If the nipple and mammary gland are taut or inflexible, for example, the fit between parent and baby with a variation in oral anatomy may be less than ideal. But if the mammary gland and nipple are more pliable, nursing may be comfortable. Engorgement or tissue swelling (edema) after birth may contribute to painful nursing, but feeds may become more comfortable quickly as the tissue swelling subsides. Nursing position can also be a factor. Positions in which the nursing couple struggles against gravity (upright positions) may make a challenging fit even more difficult.

Torticollis

If baby keeps his head turned to one side, consider torticollis as a possible contributor to nipple pain.

U.S. research (Boere-Boonekamp & van der Linden-Kuiper, 2001) estimated that 10% of babies younger than 8 weeks old prefer to hold their heads to one side. In some cases, this may be a sign of torticollis, from the Latin words meaning "twisted neck," which is caused by a confined position in the womb. When a baby's neck muscles are pulled to one side, this pulls the baby's lower jaw and affects jaw development in utero, which may give the baby's jaw an asymmetrical look. In some cases, the baby also may be in pain (Mojab, 2007).

A review of the literature (Wall & Glass, 2006) described 11 babies with asymmetrical lower jaws (mandibles) whose lower gumlines were tilted to one side rather than parallel. Ten of the 11 mothers had birth complications. All had nursing problems, including nipple pain, latching struggles, and ineffective feeding. Nine of the 11 babies needed supplements. The authors suggested that nursing problems may be the first symptom of undiagnosed torticollis.

For babies with this condition, encourage parents to experiment with different feeding positions until they find the positions most comfortable for them both. If one position is clearly best, encourage them to use that one for now. U.S. lactation consultant Catherine Watson Genna described how to best support nursing for the baby with torticollis (Genna, 2015, p. 217):

> "The mechanistic approach to positioning and latch (place tab A into slot B) can exacerbate breastfeeding difficulties. Infants are more likely to achieve comfortable stable positions if placed prone on their reclining mother. Postpartum women respond to support for their intuition and language that paints a picture rather than 'left-brained' lists of instruction."

Very different positions may work best on each side. But sometimes the baby may need to keep his body in the same position on both sides (LeVan, 2011). This can often be done by simply sliding baby's body to the other side. An occupational or physical therapist can recommend therapeutic exercises to help improve the baby's range of motion.

Strong or Unusual Suck

Some babies generate unusually high suction levels during nursing, which may contribute to painful feeds.

Most parents can resolve painful nursing by getting a deeper latch, reducing their engorgement, or with practice over time. But there are some who continue to suffer painful feeds for weeks and even months, despite all efforts.

One Australian study of 60 nursing couples (H. McClellan et al., 2008) compared suction levels in the mouths of 30 nursing babies whose mothers were comfortable with 30 whose mothers had continuing pain after other causes—candida, bacterial infection, vasospasm, dermatitis, infant tongue-tie, and torticollis—were ruled out.

The babies in both groups spent about the same amount of time at the breast and about the same amount of time actively sucking. In the pain group, half of the mothers felt pain throughout the feed, while the other half felt pain either at the beginning of the feed or after a few minutes.

The researchers found that the babies in the pain group generated significantly higher mean suction levels, both while actively sucking (152 mmHg vs. 97 mmHg) and when the suction was lowest (91 mmHg vs. 55 mmHg), as compared with the babies in the comfortable group. The babies whose mothers were in pain also took less milk during breastfeeding despite the higher suction levels, which the researchers thought might be because the pain interfered with milk ejection. The researchers suggested high suction levels may be one reason some parents find nursing painful even after seeking help.

Another study by the same team (H. L. McClellan, Hepworth, Kent, et al., 2012) examined 24-hour milk intake in a group of 21 mothers with persistent nipple pain and 21 mothers without pain. They found the babies in the pain group who fed longer took less milk at feeds. However, those in pain were able to produce adequate milk for their babies.

Using ultrasound to monitor movements and suction levels inside these babies' mouths (H. L. McClellan, Kent, Hepworth, Hartmann, & Geddes, 2015), a research team attempted to better understand the dynamics causing the pain and slower milk flow. In this study, 25 mothers in pain were compared with 25 mothers not in pain. The researchers found that the babies in the pain group generated about double the level of suction during nursing and used different tongue movements, which resulted in less nipple expansion and slower milk flow. Another difference was that the babies in the pain group were introduced to bottle-feeding earlier than the babies in the control group. The researchers didn't know if the babies were introduced to the bottle earlier because the mothers were in pain or if the earlier introduction of the bottle might have altered the babies' sucking. More research is needed.

• • •

Painful feeds can occur during nursing when babies bunch or hump their tongue, clamp or clench their jaws, or do other kinds of unusual sucking.

From birth, some babies clench or clamp down whenever the inside of their mouth is touched. This response (also known as "gum biting") is common in preterm babies, especially those born between 32- and 36-weeks gestation. But it may occur in a term baby, too, perhaps due to temporary immaturity.

The best first strategy in this situation is to use the starter positions (see p. 23-29), allowing the baby to latch, rather than helping him on (Figure 17.2). Allowing the baby to control latching may eliminate clenching. When the baby self-attaches, he naturally extends his tongue first with a relaxed jaw. This eliminates the contact of the mammary tissue with the baby's lower gum ridge, which sometimes triggers this behavior.

If a baby bunches, humps, or sucks his tongue, suggest having him evaluated for tongue-tie. Also consider the tongue exercises described on p. 890-891.

KEY CONCEPT

Some characteristics of the nursing parent's mammary tissue or nipple may also lead to soreness.

Parent Factors

Taut Mammary Tissue

Taut mammary tissue can make it difficult for the baby to draw the nipple back to the comfort zone, leading to nipple pain and trauma.

When mammary tissue is taut (either naturally or due to temporary factors like engorgement or tissue swelling from excess IV fluids during labor), the baby may be limited to drawing only the nipple into his mouth. This leads to a shallow latch, pain during feeds, and lower milk intake, which can aggravate engorgement. Strategies to try include:

- Reverse pressure softening (RPS)—a simple technique described on p. 885 that gently pushes the swelling further back into the mammary gland, softening the nipple and areola for easier latching.
- Expressing a little milk to soften nipple and areola.
- Mammary shaping—see p. 884-885 for descriptions.

When the baby is able to latch deeply and comfortably, suggest nursing more often to more quickly relieve the engorgement. See p. 751-753 for more strategies.

Variations in Nipple Anatomy

Ask if one or both nipples are flat or inverted or if there is anything unusual about the nipples.

Protruding (everted) nipples are not necessary for comfortable and effective nursing, as many nursing parents can attest. Some studies (Dewey, Nommsen-Rivers, Heinig, & Cohen, 2003; Moore & Anderson, 2007) found nursing problems were more common among those with flat or inverted nipples and concluded that these parents may benefit from extra lactation support and help during the early days. For details, see the later section "Flat and Inverted Nipples" on p. 736.

If the nipple changes color after feeds and the parent experiences burning or shooting pain, consider vasospasm or Raynaud's phenomenon.

Vasospasm and Raynaud's Phenomenon

Both vasospasm and Raynaud's phenomenon involve color changes of the nipple after nursing due to restricted blood flow, but they are different conditions with different causes.

Vasospasm is caused by compression of the nipple, which constricts the blood vessels and causes the nipple to blanch, or turn white. One prospective Australian cohort study of 360 mothers (M. L. Buck et al., 2014) found that 23% of its study mothers experienced vasospasm during the early weeks post-birth. Vasospasm is most commonly caused by either a shallow latch or the baby compressing the nipple to slow a fast milk flow. When the nipple is compressed, it may look misshapen after feeds—pointed or creased, like the tip of a new tube of lipstick (Wilson-Clay & Hoover, 2017, p. 44). The blood flowing back to the nipple may cause a burning sensation, intense throbbing, or shooting pain.

Strategies for nursing with vasospasm:

- **Try to get a deeper latch** to avoid nipple compression. If shallow latch is the cause, a good place to begin is to try using starter positions (p. 23-29), and allowing baby to do the latching (Figure 17.2). If using upright feeding positions, try mammary shaping, an asymmetrical latch, and other strategies for achieving a deeper latch.
- **Apply warmth after feeds** via warm compresses, a heating pad, taking a warm shower, immersing the glands in warm water (Walker, 2017), or using a hair dryer on warm. Warmth can prevent or relieve pain by increasing blood flow to the nipple.
- **Gently massage the nipple after feeds** to more quickly return blood flow.
- **Take pain medication,** such as ibuprofen or whatever analgesia the parent's healthcare provider recommends.

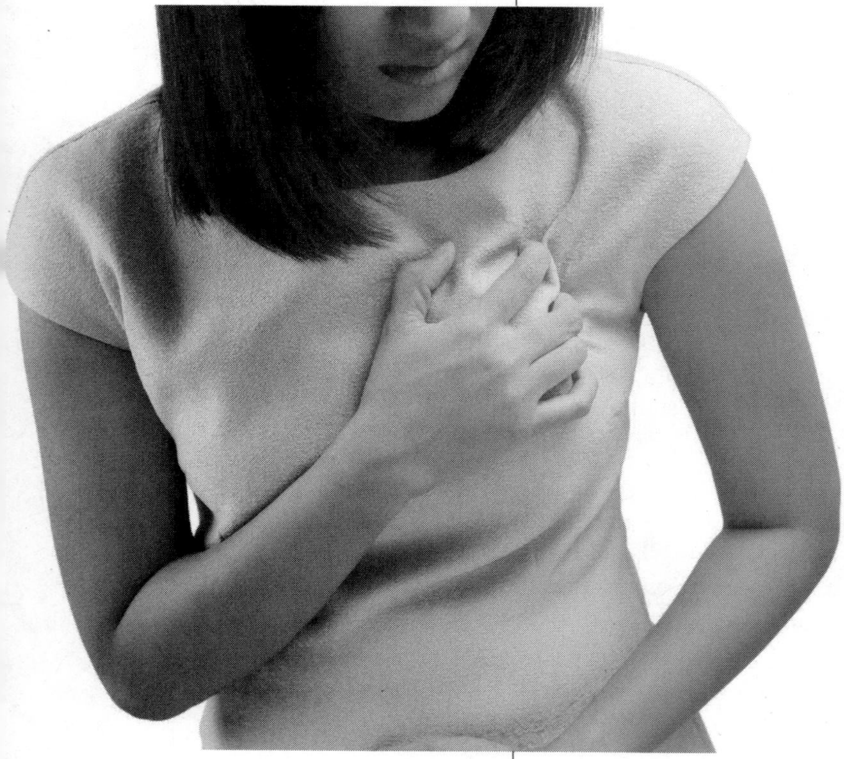

In one prospective Canadian study of 84 mothers with persistent nipple pain (V. Livingstone & Stringer, 1999) 5 of the 84 study mothers suffered from vasospasms. The interventions that resolved the vasospasms were getting a deeper latch and avoiding nipple exposure to cold.

Raynaud's phenomenon is a circulatory disorder that affects many individuals of childbearing age (Stringer & Femia, 2018). Its symptoms include color changes in the extremities (fingers, toes, nipples), which may turn red, white, and/or blue from restricted blood flow. Raynaud's phenomenon has a variety of triggers: exposure to cold, nicotine, caffeine, emotional stress, and certain medications (beta blockers, oral contraceptives, pseudoephedrine) (Avila-Vega, Urrea-Mendoza, & Lee, 2019). Those with Raynaud's phenomenon likely experienced its symptoms before giving birth and nursing (Anderson, Held, & Wright, 2004). They also may have a history of migraine headaches or autoimmune disorders (Hughes & Herrick, 2016).

The following strategies may help when nursing with Raynaud's phenomenon:

- **Dress warmly.** Some find wool breast pads helpful, or nursing with a blanket, sweater, or jacket around the shoulders.
- **After feeds, apply dry warmth to the nipples** with a heating pad, a hair dryer set on warm, or microwaveable warm pads. Avoid moist heat, as evaporation can cool the nipples and trigger symptoms. Warmth can prevent or relieve pain by increasing blood flow to the nipples.
- **After feeds, gently massage the nipples** to more quickly return blood flow.
- **Discuss over-the-counter analgesia and prescribed medications with a healthcare provider.** Some find over-the-counter pain relievers helpful. Nifedipine, a prescribed calcium channel blocker that increases blood flow, is an effective treatment (T.W. Hale & Berens, 2010). A recommended dose of 30 to 60 mg/day of sustained-release formulation is considered compatible with nursing (T.W. Hale, 2019, pp. 553-554). A 2-week course is usually long enough to relieve the pain for most without recurrence, but some may need to take it longer (Garrison, 2002).
- **Other Raynaud's treatments.** Nitroglycerin ointment or spray (2%) is another possible treatment, although it may only be effective in 50% of the cases (Garrison, 2002). It is applied sparingly after feeds for 24 hours and after that only when blanching occurs. The effectiveness of taking vitamin B_6 supplements is unknown.

Nipple Pain at Any Time

Ask the baby's age, when the pain started, if there's a history of nipple trauma, and if there are any skin changes.

The baby's age can provide clues to the cause of the pain. If the baby is older than about 4 months old, for example, teething may be a factor.

When the pain started. If nipple pain starts after weeks or months of comfortable nursing, something changed and the key is to find out what (see Box 17.2). In an article for doctors (L. Amir, 2004), Australian physician and lactation consultant Lisa Amir asked the question: "What are the likely causes of the sudden onset of nipple pain in a breastfeeding woman?" and answered: candida infection, eczema/dermatitis, vasospasm, pregnancy, trauma (such as a bite), and herpes infection.

KEY CONCEPT

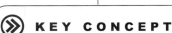

Timing of nipple pain can help determine its cause.

Prior nipple trauma. Broken skin on the nipple increases the risk of developing mastitis, as well as fungal and bacterial infections (Berens, Eglash, Malloy, & Steube, 2016; L. Fernandez, Mediano, Garcia, Rodriguez, & Marin, 2016).

Visible skin changes. The type of skin changes provides clues to possible causes. For example, an areola that looks inflamed, shiny, or appears to have white plaque may indicate candida or thrush (Francis-Morrill, Heinig, Pappagianis, & Dewey, 2004). Yellow pus in a traumatized nipple indicates a bacterial infection, a sore or lesion could be a herpes infection (Berens et al., 2016) or an infected Montgomery gland (Wilson-Clay & Hoover, 2017, p. 65), yellow crusting or tiny pin-sized vesicles could be signs of impetigo (Khan & Ramirez, 2017; Thorley, 2000).

• • •

Ask for a description of the pain and what the parent thinks is the cause.

Type of pain. If the pain is extreme and there is no broken skin or visible skin color change, consider candida or mastitis. See also Figure 17.1 for other factors that intensify the perception of pain.

Parent's idea of the cause. Was there an incident that caused skin damage, such as biting or pulling off the nipple without breaking the suction?

• • •

Ask if the timing of the pain coincided with the use of a breast pump or other product.

Breast pumps and other products can contribute to nipple pain. For example, if a pump user turns up its suction too high (thinking that will pump more milk) or uses a pump with a too-large or too-small nipple tunnel (see p. 907-908), it may contribute to nipple pain and trauma. Any product applied to the nipple—such as creams or ointments—can cause a reaction, such as dermatitis or eczema (Heller, Fullerton-Stone, & Murase, 2012). When wet nursing pads are left against the skin for too long, this can cause a skin breakdown called "maceration."

Interactive Factors

Candida/Thrush

Candidiasis is a fungal infection that can cause mild or severe nipple pain.

The pain associated with this fungal infection may be described as itching, burning, or stabbing (L. H. Amir et al., 2013). For details, see the later section, "Candida/Thrush." This is considered an "interactive factor" because it can be passed between nursing parent and baby.

Baby Factors

Teething and Biting

When a baby's teeth are about to erupt, his gums feel sore, and applying pressure feels soothing but may temporarily cause nipple pain.

When a baby is teething, his gums may feel swollen and sore. As a result, he may nurse differently or chew on the nipple, as applying pressure to his gums can ease his discomfort. If the nursing parent is experiencing pain or discomfort, discuss the parent's feelings and share this information.

Teething is temporary. Nipple pain from teething will pass as the baby's teeth erupt.

Before nursing, use cold to numb baby's gums. Until baby's teething pain subsides, suggest giving the baby something cold to chew on before nursing, such as a cold, wet washcloth or a cold teething toy. For the baby eating solid foods, a frozen bagel or frozen peas or berries may help soothe baby's gums and make nursing more comfortable.

Try other options before using numbing preparations on baby's gums. One risk of using over-the-counter numbing products on baby's gums is that they may also numb the baby's tongue and the nipple, complicating nursing.

BOX 17.2 Possible Causes of Nipple Pain Starting After 1 Month

Interactive Factors

- Shallow latch—Older babies/toddlers may nurse acrobatically
- Candida/thrush—Diagnosis/treatment needed

Baby Factors

- Teething and biting
- Pulling off the nipple without first breaking the suction
- Unusual feeding positions—Most often, an older baby or toddler

Parent Factors

- Overabundant milk production—Baby may clamp or clench to slow flow
- Blebs, blisters
- Skin problems—Dermatitis, impetigo, eczema, psoriasis, poison ivy/oak
- Sores—Herpes, infected Montgomery glands
- Pregnancy—Hormonal changes may cause nipple discomfort
- Referred pain—From mastitis, fibromyalgia, pulled muscle, pinched nerve, etc.
- Use or misuse of pumps or products—Pumps: fit and suction level, use of bottles or pacifiers/dummies; wet nursing pads, creams/ointments

Complications of Nipple Trauma

- Mastitis
- Bacterial or fungal infection
- Bacterial dysbiosis or lactiferous ductal infection

Before using these products, suggest consulting the baby's healthcare provider about using pain medication or other strategies.

• • •

It is not necessary to stop nursing after baby's teeth erupt because while a baby is actively nursing, he can't bite.

Many parents are warned to stop nursing when their baby gets his first tooth, but many babies never bite, and those who try once usually never bite again.

During nursing, the nipple is positioned deeply in baby's mouth, with the baby's lips and gums on the areola and the baby's tongue covering his lower gum, so even if a baby has teeth, he cannot bite while actively nursing.

• • •

If a baby bites, suggest trying to stay calm and break the suction with a finger.

Most nursing parents' first reaction to biting is to startle and pull the baby off. After this reaction, most babies never bite again. But if it happens again, suggest trying to stay calm. Pulling the baby off the nipple with his teeth clamped down can cause more damage than the bite itself. If the parent yells, many babies will be startled. This can backfire in sensitive babies, who may respond by becoming distressed at feeds or not latching at all. (For strategies, see the section "Nursing Strike" on p. 128-129.) Because bringing a baby "on strike" back to nursing can be a stressful process, suggest trying to stay calm if the baby bites again.

Rather than pulling the baby off the nipple when he bites, suggest slipping a finger between the baby's gums or teeth, which will also release the nipple.

• • •

If the nursing parent is worried or stressed about biting, discuss ways to prevent it.

If the baby is biting persistently, suggest the following strategies:

- **Give the baby complete attention during nursing.** Eye contact, stroking, and talking decrease the odds the baby will bite to get attention.
- **Learn to recognize the end of a feed.** Most biting occurs when the baby loses interest in nursing. Parents who are alert may notice, for example, that tension develops in baby's jaw before he bites down. When this sign occurs, break the suction and take him off before he bites. Some babies chew or bite down near the end of a nursing session as a sign they are done.
- **Don't pressure a disinterested baby to nurse.** If the baby pushes away, suggest offering to nurse again later.
- **Make sure the baby latches deeply.** Getting the nipple deeply into baby's mouth triggers active sucking and lessens the odds of biting.
- **Remove a sleeping baby who is not actively sucking.** To do this, suggest gently inserting a finger between baby's gums to release the nipple. If baby bites, he'll bite the finger instead of the nipple.
- **Keep the milk production abundant.** Some babies bite when they are frustrated by slow milk flow. Unnecessary supplements of formula, water, or juice can decrease milk production.
- **Note behaviors that lead to biting.** Some babies bite when teased, pressured to nurse, or when someone is yelling nearby. Suggest the parent notice what happened before the bite. Knowing the trigger can prevent future biting.
- **Keep nursing relaxed and positive.** Some babies bite when the nursing parent is tense. If the parent is frazzled, suggest trying deep breathing, relaxing music, or nursing lying down or in a darkened room.
- **Give praise when baby doesn't bite.** Suggest saying, "Thank you" and "good baby" when he is gentle during nursing. Smiles, hugs, and kisses can help gently teach baby to nurse comfortably.

• • •

If biting becomes persistent, other strategies may help.

In addition to breaking the suction, the following strategies may discourage biting:

- **Stop the feed.** Remove the temptation for baby to make the parent jump or startle again.
- **Offer a teether,** such as a teething ring, a toy, or anything acceptable to bite.
- **Set baby quickly on the floor to give the message that biting brings negative consequences.** After allowing a few seconds of distress, comfort the baby.
- **Keep a finger near the baby's mouth ready to break the suction, if needed.** Some distractible babies try to turn and look with the nipple still in their mouth. If the parent responds consistently by breaking the suction, baby will learn quickly that turning away means losing the nipple.

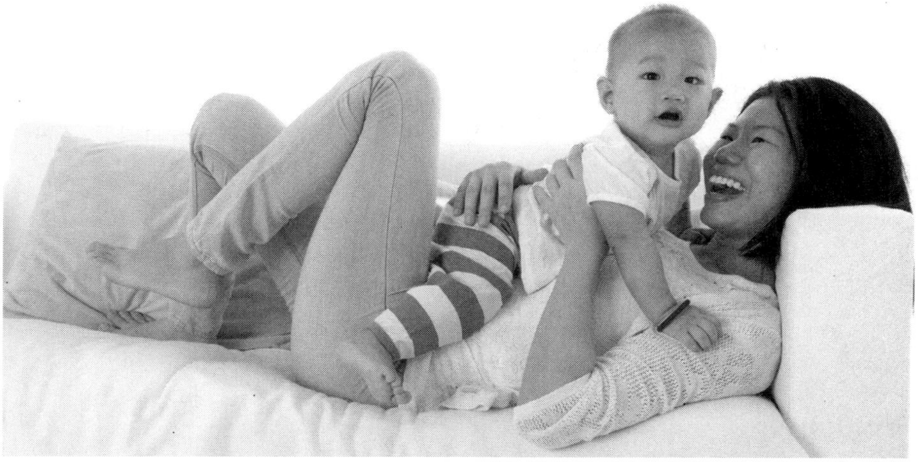

A baby needs to learn what to do with new teeth while nursing. Babies don't understand that biting causes pain. They don't bite to be mean. Nursing babies learn to associate their nursing parent with feelings of security and comfort, as well as relief from hunger. These positive associations should help baby learn quickly not to bite.

Distractibility and Acrobatic Nursing Positions

If a distractible baby's pulling off the nipple causes nipple pain, suggest having a finger ready to break the suction when needed.

As babies grow and become more aware of their surroundings, they may turn their heads while nursing to look at distractions without first breaking the suction. If so, encourage the parent to be ready to break the suction. Over time, consistent removal from nursing discourages this behavior.

• • •

If an older baby's acrobatic nursing causes nipple pain, encourage the parent to set limits.

Babies old enough to crawl and walk may want to latch in unusual positions that pull on the nipple, causing discomfort. Reassure the parent that nursing needs to feel good for them both and that it is fine to let the baby know that they will nurse only in positions that are comfortable.

Parent Factors

Overabundant Milk Production or Fast Milk Flow

Nipple pain can occur when the baby changes his suck to make a fast milk flow more manageable.

When a parent has overabundant milk production or a very fast milk flow, the baby may use his mouth or tongue to compress or crimp the nipple to avoid being overwhelmed by milk. In some cases, these sucking changes cause nipple pain and trauma. In a large 2017 Thai study (Puapornpong et al., 2017), among the mothers experiencing nipple pain at 7 days, the researchers attributed 4% of these cases to oversupply.

If fast milk flow may be a contributing cause, suggest trying starter feeding positions (see p. 23-29), as nursing "uphill" (with baby's head higher than the nipple) gives him better control over milk flow and reduces the need to compress the nipple. Some babies prefer side-lying positions, which allow them to easily let milk run out of the side of their mouth during fast flow. When using side-lying positions in this situation, some parents find that putting a folded towel under baby's head during nursing minimizes their laundry load.

Mastitis

Mastitis is sometimes perceived as nipple pain.

Depending on the location of the plugged duct, infection, or abscess, nipple pain may be a type of ***referred pain*** (see later section). This means the source of the pain is elsewhere, but it is perceived in the nipple. In this case, the nipple pain will resolve when the mastitis resolves.

Blisters, Sores, Blebs, and Other Skin Problems

Blisters, sores, blebs, and any other skin problem can cause nipple pain.

For details, see these later sections in this chapter.

Pregnancy

Due to hormonal changes, nipple pain during pregnancy is common.

Nipple tenderness may be one of the first symptoms of pregnancy. Some feel nipple tenderness before missing their first menstrual period, while others experience it later. For strategies to make this type of nipple pain more manageable, see p. 621 in Chapter 14, "Pregnancy and Tandem Nursing."

Breast Pumps, Bottles, Pacifiers, and Other Products

Using a breast pump should not hurt, but if it doesn't fit well or the suction is set too high, pain and trauma can result.

Many parents think "more is better" when it comes to pump suction. They mistakenly think that milk expression with a pump is like sucking a drink through a straw—the stronger the suction, the greater their milk yield. But that's not the way it works. Australian research (Kent et al., 2008; Ramsay et al., 2006) found that setting the pump suction too high resulted in less expressed milk, because users became tense, inhibiting their milk ejection. The most effective suction setting is the highest that is comfortable, which for some users, may even be the pump's lowest setting. If a parent feels pain during or after pumping, first suggest trying a lower suction setting.

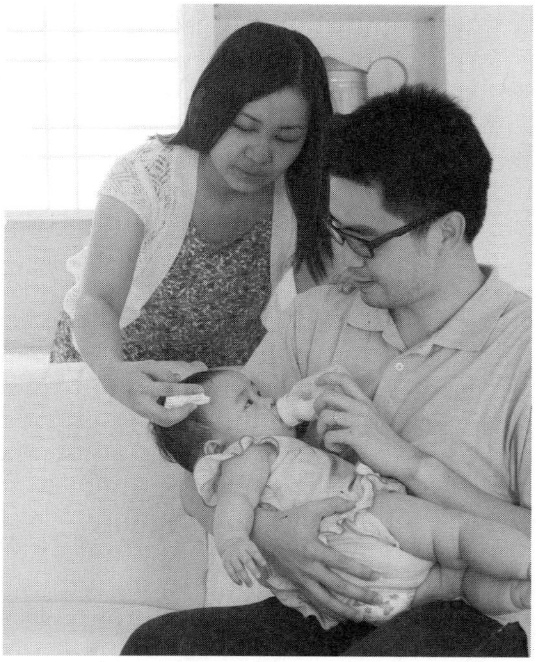

Pump fit is determined by how well a user's nipple fits into the pump's nipple tunnel. Good fit is necessary for comfortable and effective milk flow. If the nipple tunnel is too small, the nipple may rub along its sides or get wedged. If the nipple tunnel is too large, too much areola may rub along its sides, causing pain and trauma. Many pump companies offer a variety of nipple-tunnel sizes, which can be purchased separately. For more details, see p. 907-908.

• • •

The use of artificial teats and pacifiers may change baby's suck, causing nipple pain.

Does using feeding bottles and pacifiers/dummies change babies' suck and contribute to nipple pain? An Australian study cited earlier (H. L. McClellan et al., 2015) found that babies generating higher suction levels during nursing (whose mothers suffered persistent nipple pain) received feeding bottles earlier than the babies whose nursing mothers were not in pain. One Italian study of 219 mothers (Centuori et al., 1999) found that the use of a pacifier or feeding bottle in the hospital after birth was associated with nipple pain at discharge. Two Swedish studies (Righard, 1998; Righard & Alade, 1997) found an association between bottle and pacifier use and the development of an "incorrect" sucking pattern during nursing that the researchers called "superficial nipple sucking," which could lead to nipple pain. A U.S. study of 328 mothers and newborns (Dewey et al., 2003) also found an association between bottle and pacifier use in the first 48 hours and what they called "suboptimal breastfeeding behaviors" on Days 3 and 7.

If this may be contributing to nipple pain, suggest discontinuing the use of pacifiers. If the baby received bottles, suggest that a period of either exclusive nursing or the use of another feeding method may help the baby learn to suck without causing pain. Discuss the pros and cons of other feeding methods, which are described on p. 896.

• • •

Other products may also contribute to nipple pain and trauma.

Other possible products that might contribute to nipple pain include:

- Bras that are so tight they compress the nipple or bras with a rough seam that rubs and irritates the nipple
- Topical creams or ointments (prescribed or over-the-counter), which can cause skin reactions (Cooper & Shaw, 1999; Huggins & Billon, 1993)
- Breast pads, when left wet for too long against the nipple, can cause skin breakdown known as maceration (why our skin turns white and wrinkly after we've stayed in a bath too long)
- Any product that requires washing the nipple after use, which can cause further irritation

If any of these could be a contributing cause of the nipple pain, suggest making a change, such as wearing a different bra, trying a different product, discontinuing the nipple cream or ointment, or asking the healthcare provider for a substitute.

Referred Pain or a History of Pain Disorder

An injury or condition elsewhere in the body may be perceived as nipple pain, or the parent may have a history of pain disorder in which normal touch is perceived as pain.

When an injury or condition occurs along the same nerve pathway as the nipple, it may be perceived as nipple pain. Called referred pain, this could be due to mastitis or an injury elsewhere in the body. If other causes are ruled out, ask if parents pulled a back, shoulder, or neck muscle, or if they have pain elsewhere in their body.

In the Academy of Breastfeeding Medicine Clinical Protocol #26 on persistent pain with nursing (Berens et al., 2016), its authors note that those with pain disorders, such as allodynia, may perceive light touch as painful. When a nursing parent is in pain and the cause in unclear, ask about a history of allodynia or other pain disorders, such as fibromyalgia, irritable bowel syndrome, migraines, or others.

Strategies for Nipple Pain and Trauma

When considering strategies, using a standardized rating scale to describe nipple trauma has several benefits.

The following four-stage system for rating nipple trauma was developed by this author in consultation with a wound specialist as a starting point for developing and validating a standardized rating system. Benefits of a standardized rating system for nipple trauma include:

- Streamlining communication among the healthcare team
- Allowing researchers to more easily compare study results
- Dispelling the common misconception that nipple trauma is a normal part of nursing
- Making it possible to differentiate possible treatment options by severity of trauma

This rating scale was incorporated into lactation texts and used by some researchers (Lauwers & Swisher, 2015; Wilson-Clay & Hoover, 2017).

- **Stage I—Superficial Intact.** Includes pain or irritation without skin breakdown. May include redness (erythema), bruising, red spots (petechiae), swelling (edema).
- **Stage II—Superficial with Tissue Breakdown.** May include pain with possible abrasion, shallow crack or fissure, compression stripe, hematoma, and shallow ulceration.
- **Stage III—Partial Thickness Erosion.** Includes skin breakdown involving the destruction of the epidermis to the lower layers of the dermis. May include deep fissure, blister, deep ulceration with more advanced erosion.
- **Stage IV—Full Thickness Erosion.** Includes deeper damage through the dermis. May include full erosion of some parts of the dermis.

Comfort Measures

Comfort measures may reduce pain during and after nursing.

With nipple pain, the best first step is to find the causes and—if possible—correct them. After that, depending on the causes, comfort measures and treatments may help.

Commonly recommended comfort measures for nipple pain include:

- Take an analgesia that is compatible with the parent's health history (consult with the healthcare provider) and is compatible with nursing.
- Stimulate a milk ejection first by expressing milk or pumping before baby latches.
- Nurse first on the least sore side until the milk ejection occurs, then move the baby gently to the more painful side.
- Wear breast shells between feeds to reduce clothing friction or pressure.

If breast shells (see p. 908-910) are used, suggest choosing the shell backings with the large nipple openings (not the smaller openings designed for use with inverted nipples). For safe use, if the shells are worn inside a bra cup, make sure it is large enough to accommodate the shells without putting too much pressure on the mammary gland. Consistent pressure on the gland can increase risk of mastitis. (A parent with nipple trauma is already at increased risk for mastitis.) Red circles on the skin when the breast shells are removed indicate a larger size bra cup is needed.

• • •

When the causes of painful nursing cannot be corrected quickly, it may help to vary positions at each feed.

Although varying positions at each feed is not recommended when nursing is going well (see p. 22), if the causes of the nipple pain cannot immediately be corrected, such as symptomatic tongue-tie or an unusually shaped palate, varying nursing positions may make direct nursing more tolerable by spreading the pain and damage more evenly. If the starter positions are used (see pp. 23-29), the parent can adjust the baby's lie, so he approaches the nipple from different angles at each feed—vertically, horizontally, and diagonally. If they use upright positions, the baby can be positioned at various angles in front and along the parent's side. For another option, see the photo and description of the all-fours dangle hold on p. 35.

• • •

If the pain is severe enough that the parent wants to take a break from direct nursing, suggest expressing milk while the nipples heal.

If the nipple pain is too intense to continue nursing or the pain is interfering with the parent-child relationship, one option is to express milk and feed it to the baby for a short while with one of the alternative feeding methods described on p. 896. For expression strategies to maintain milk production, see p. 504.

Treatments for Nipple Trauma

Due to the poor quality of much of the research on treatments for nipple trauma, it is not clear if one treatment option is more effective than another.

Treatments for nipple trauma are not always necessary. In some cases, getting a deeper latch may be all that's needed to make nursing comfortable. With a deeper latch, it is often possible to continue nursing while the nipples heal. If the pain is more severe, sharing comfort measures may be helpful.

Conclusions of a Cochrane Review. A major challenge in evaluating treatment options for nipple trauma is the low quality of evidence. Of the thousands of studies comparing treatments for nipple pain and trauma, a 2014 Cochrane Review found only four worthy of closer examination. And of those four (which included a total of 656 women), none of the five treatments evaluated—glycerin gel pads, lanolin with breast shells, lanolin alone, expressed milk, and all-purpose nipple ointment (APNO)—proved to be more effective than doing nothing. The authors wrote (Dennis et al., 2014, p. 2):

> "Currently, there is not enough evidence to recommend any specific type of treatment for painful nipples among breastfeeding women. These results suggest that applying nothing or expressed breast milk may be equally or more beneficial in the short-term experience of nipple pain than the application of an ointment such as lanolin. One important finding in this review was that regardless of the treatment used, for most women, nipple pain reduced to mild levels approximately 7 to 10 days after giving birth."

Research on all-purpose nipple ointment (APNO). Developed by Canadian pediatrician Jack Newman, this ointment requires a prescription, and the pharmacist mixes a precise proportion of antibiotic, antifungal, and anti-inflammatory medications. Those who recommend APNO suggest applying it sparingly to the affected nipples after feeds, and when the pain is gone, the parent weans from it gradually over a week. However, research found no benefit to using APNO. A Canadian double-blind randomized clinical trial (Dennis, Schottle, Hodnett, & McQueen, 2012) included 151 mothers with damage to one or both nipples. All mothers received help in getting a deeper latch. They were then assigned to one of the two treatment groups: 1) APNO or 2) lanolin. The researchers followed the mothers for 12 weeks. At 1 week there was no difference in pain scores between the two groups, and at 12 weeks there were no significant differences in breastfeeding exclusivity and duration. They concluded that APNO was no better than lanolin in treating nipple trauma.

Research on lanolin. Some studies that compared using lanolin to expressed milk for nipple pain and trauma (Abou-Dakn, Fluhr, Gensch, & Wockel, 2011; Mariani Neto et al., 2018) found lanolin more effective than expressed milk, but the research is mixed. In 2017, the same research team that studied APNO published another randomized controlled trial (Jackson & Dennis, 2017) in which all 186 mothers received breastfeeding education and help. They then assigned the mothers to one of two groups: 1) lanolin along with usual care or 2) usual care alone, which could include warm compresses, analgesia, air-drying the nipples, use of breast shells. The researchers found no significant differences in pain levels or breastfeeding outcomes between the two groups. However, significantly more mothers in the lanolin group were satisfied with their treatment, as compared with the usual-care group.

• • •

The use of topical treatments—creams, ointments, oils, gel pads, and tea bags—to treat painful nipple is nearly universal in some areas but has drawbacks.

The use of topical creams and ointments for nipple pain and trauma is nearly universal in some areas. One Australian prospective cohort study of 360 women planning to breastfeed their expected first baby (Miranda L. Buck, Amir, & Donath, 2015) found that during the first week after birth, 91% used a topical treatment on their nipples. Purified lanolin was used by 74% and hydrogel pads were used by 12%. By 8 weeks, 37% continued to use topical nipple treatments.

Depending on the ingredients in the topical treatment, some drawbacks to using these products may include:

- An unfamiliar taste on the nipple, which may cause fussiness or distress in the baby during latch
- If the product is unsafe for baby to ingest, removing it from the nipple before nursing may cause more damage
- Clogging nipple pores or reducing oxygen to the wound may occur, slowing healing
- Dry skin may result if alcohol is one of the ingredients
- If anesthetic agents are included, such as those found in teething gels, they may numb baby's mouth or delay milk ejection

Virgin olive oil and virgin coconut oil. In animal studies (Donato-Trancoso, Monte-Alto-Costa, & Romana-Souza, 2016; Nevin & Rajamohan, 2010), both olive oil and coconut oil (which are antioxidants) reduced inflammation, which promotes wound healing. Some lactation supporters recommend the use of these plant oils for preventing nipple cracks and pain or for treating nipple pain and trauma (Cordero, Villar, Barrilao, Cortes, & Lopez, 2015; Karacam & Saglik, 2018). In a Turkish study that compared the use of olive oil with lanolin to prevent nipple pain (Gungor et al., 2013), the researchers found that 53% of the study mothers preferred the olive oil and only 16% preferred the lanolin. Olive and coconut oils seem like a logical choice because they are inexpensive, and many families already have them on hand in their kitchens. But even natural plant oils can cause skin reactions. A U.K. study that involved the twice-daily application of 6 drops of olive oil to the forearms of adult volunteers (Danby et al., 2013) found that after 4 weeks of use, it led to redness and skin breakdown. They concluded that regular use of olive oil may contribute to contact dermatitis in those with and without a family history of allergy.

Vitamin E is not recommended. Applying vitamin E to a painful nipple by puncturing vitamin E capsules and squeezing the contents onto the nipple—once a commonly recommended treatment—is no longer recommended because it may cause:

- ***Skin reactions in users.*** Although vitamin E rarely causes allergic reactions when taken orally, it can when applied topically (Aeling, Panagotacos, & Andreozzi, 1973; Fisher, 1986, p. 151).
- ***Elevated vitamin E levels in baby*** were found after vitamin E was applied to damaged nipples (Marx, Izquierdo, Driscoll, Murray, & Epstein, 1985).

Warm water compresses. Although warm-water compresses are easily available to everyone, they do not appear to be an effective treatment for nipple pain. In one Canadian study of 65 first-time mothers with nipple pain (Lavergne, 1997), warm water and tea-bag compresses were compared with no treatment. No differences were found in the effectiveness of the two types of compresses, and nearly 45% of the mothers dropped out of the study.

• • •

Since the publication of the 2014 Cochrane Review on treatment options for nipple pain (Dennis et al., 2014), research on new and different options were published.

Research is emerging on other possible treatments for nipple pain and damage, such as the use of silver cups and phototherapy with low-level lasers and LED light.

Silver cups. Silver is a natural antibacterial and non-toxic material that is not absorbed by the skin. Wound dressings impregnated with silver are used as topical treatments for infected wounds elsewhere on the body (Beam, 2009). Now washable and reusable silver nipple cups are being marketed as a treatment for nipple pain and trauma. They are significantly more expensive than other options. But are they effective? As yet we don't have enough information to say. In 2015, an Italian pilot study examined the use of silver nipple cups in breastfeeding women with nipple pain and fissures (Marrazzu et al., 2015). The researchers randomly assigned 40 women into one of its two groups: 1) the control group, which used expressed milk as a treatment, and 2) the experimental group, which wore the silver cups between feeds. At 2 days, there was no difference in pain scores. On Days 7 and 15, the pain scores were significantly lower in the silver-cup group, and the silver-cup group appeared to heal faster. More research is needed.

Light treatments (phototherapy). Different types of light treatment are used successfully to speed wound healing and reduce pain in other parts of the body, including episiotomy (Kymplova, Navratil, & Knizek, 2003). The two phototherapy treatments below involve access to costly equipment, which is not available everywhere. Animal studies (de Sousa et al., 2010) found low-level laser therapy speeds healing. In the following studies, two light treatments were used in nursing parents with nipple trauma.

- ***Low-level laser phototherapy*** was found in two case reports (M.L. Buck, Eckereder, & Amir, 2016) to hasten healing of badly traumatized nipples and significantly reduce pain. A triple-blind, randomized controlled trial of 59 women (Coca et al., 2016) found that two low-level laser therapy sessions significantly reduced pain scores by a full 2 points on a 10-point scale. A third session had little effect. A 2019 randomized controlled trial (Camargo et al., 2019) found that one phototherapy session was not enough to reduce nipple pain. Animal research (Kovalyov, 2001) found lower prolactin levels to be a possible side effect of this light therapy. For this reason, Iranian researchers monitored the prolactin levels of women receiving low-level laser therapy for their cesarean wounds (Mokmeli, Khazemikho, Niromanesh, & Vatankhah, 2009) and found no differences in prolactin levels between the laser therapy group and the controls.
- ***LED phototherapy.*** A 2012 Brazilian pilot study compared the effects of daily LED phototherapy over the course of a week with a sham light therapy (Chaves, Araujo, Santos, Pinotti, & Oliveira, 2012). All 16 of its study mothers received help in getting a deeper latch. The researchers found that in those who received the real LED phototherapy the nipple trauma healed faster than in those who received the sham treatment. At this writing, a larger randomized controlled trial on the effectiveness of LED phototherapy is underway (Campos et al., 2018). More research is needed.

• • •

In unusual cases, a nipple shield may help reduce pain during nursing.

Although a nipple shield may provide some pain relief, its use is not the best first choice. If pain and trauma are caused by shallow latch, using a nipple shield without first trying to get a deeper latch may not help. If the baby latches to the tip of the shield, rather than its soft brim, this compresses the nipple through the shield tip, which would cause continued pain.

If the causes of the nipple pain and trauma cannot be corrected quickly, a nipple shield may decrease the pain enough to make direct nursing tolerable until the baby either outgrows the problem or until it is corrected later. One example is a baby with symptomatic tongue-tie who is scheduled for a frenotomy at a later date.

• • •

Blood swallowed from traumatized nipples is not harmful to the baby.

Assure the family that any blood their baby swallows from damaged nipples will not be harmful. Emphasize that finding and correcting the causes of the nipple damage will allow it to heal, which will stop the bleeding.

Preventing Infection

Broken skin on the nipple increases a nursing parent's risk of nipple infection, mastitis, and other complications.

Our skin acts as a protective layer so that organisms cannot enter the body. Cracks or bleeding nipples create a point of entry for bacteria, fungi, and viruses on the nipple and within the mammary gland. Research found an association between broken nipple skin and an increased incidence of mastitis (L. H. Amir & Academy of Breastfeeding Medicine Protocol, 2014; L. Fernandez et al., 2016).

• • •

Daily washing. Whenever there is skin damage anywhere on the body, a standard recommendation is to wash the wound once a day with soap and water to prevent infection. In years past, nursing parents were cautioned to avoid soap on their nipples, because it could be drying. But when there is nipple trauma, daily washing with warm soapy water and a warm water rinse in a bath or shower only makes sense.

To prevent infection, some suggest washing damaged nipples daily with mild soap, and after nursing, rinse the nipples and apply an antibiotic ointment.

Biofilm. When bacteria enter a wound, these organisms create a sticky goo called a ***biofilm***, which protects the bacteria and reduces the effectiveness of topical treatments (Harriott & Noverr, 2009). A baby's saliva stimulates biofilm production. But gentle washing (known as "wound debridement") dislodges this biofilm to help prevent infection and promote healing (Ryan, 2007).

Rinse with water after nursing. Based on the conclusions of a Cochrane Review (R. Fernandez & Griffiths, 2012), lactation textbooks recommend parents with nipple trauma use tap or saline water to rinse their nipples after every feed (Smith, 2021, p. 257; Wilson-Clay & Hoover, 2017, p. 59). The purpose of this practice is to prevent the organisms in the baby's mouth from colonizing the wound.

Apply an antibiotic ointment. After rinsing, another way to prevent infection is to apply a thin layer of mupirocin (Bactroban®) ointment to help prevent infection. The ointment does not have to be removed and is compatible with continued nursing (T.W. Hale, 2019, p. 531-532). Mupirocin ointment was used with positive results in a 2014 U.S. prospective study that followed a group of 83 nursing mothers with nipple pain at a lactation practice (A. M. Witt, Burgess, Hawn, & Zyzanski, 2014). For more details about this study, see p. 725.

At this writing, an emerging treatment to prevent mastitis is the use of specific probiotics (Walker, 2019). For details, see p. 763-764.

KEY CONCEPT

Cracked or bleeding nipples increase risk of infection.

BACTERIAL, FUNGAL AND VIRAL NIPPLE INFECTIONS

Although good hygiene and antibiotic ointments may prevent infections from developing while nipple trauma is healing, once an infection is present, other treatments may be needed to resolve it.

When nipple trauma does not heal quickly or nipple pain continues or even intensifies despite correcting the cause, an infection may be present.

Infection is one possible complication of nipple trauma. If healing slows or stops and/or the pain increases rather than decreases, these are signs of a bacterial infection, a fungal infection, or both. Over the years, many researchers compared the prevalence of bacterial and fungal infections in nursing parents suffering from persistent nipple and/or breast pain, and it appeared that bacterial infections were much more common than fungal infections (L. H. Amir, Garland, Dennerstein, & Farish, 1996; Graves, Wright, Harman, & Bailey, 2003; Thomassen, Johansson, Wassberg, & Petrini, 1998).

Bacteria can be cultured in those with and without symptoms. However, more recent research called these conclusions into question. A 2013 Australian longitudinal, prospective cohort study followed 360 first-time mothers four times in person after delivery and again at 8 weeks by phone (L. H. Amir et al., 2013). At 4 weeks, when they cultured the mothers' milk and nipples for bacteria and fungi, they found at least 50%—both those with and without nipple pain—cultured positive for the bacterium *Staphylococcus aureus*. Many also cultured positive for the fungus *Candida albicans*, most commonly responsible for thrush. The authors of the Academy of Breastfeeding Medicine Clinical Protocol #26 on persistent pain during nursing wrote (Berens et al., 2016, p. 48):

> "Although a number of studies have attempted to identify what, if any, microbe may cause persistent nipple/breast pain during lactation, the roles of bacteria and yeast remain unclear. Both *Staphylococcus aureus sp* and Candida can be found on nipples and in breast milk of women with no symptoms. Additional theories suggest a role for virulence traits that make detection and elimination of potentially causative microbes extremely difficult."

In other words, there's a lot about these dynamics that have today's most knowledgeable experts stumped. Hopefully, future research will clarify the mechanisms at work so more effective treatments can be found. In the meantime, the following sections provide suggestions based on what we currently know.

Bacterial Infections

Bacterial and fungal infections of the nipple have some symptoms in common, but other symptoms set them apart.

As described in the previous point, the telltale signs of a nipple infection are:

- Healing slowed or even stopped
- Pain continues or intensifies

These two symptoms can occur with both a bacterial and fungal infection. Symptoms that distinguish a bacterial infection of the nipple from a fungal infection include:

- Obvious yellow pus in the traumatized area
- Yellow scabs or crusty areas on the nipple

Yellow areas on the nipple from pus, scabbing, or crustiness are signs of a bacterial infection (Khan & Ramirez, 2017; Wilson-Clay & Hoover, 2017). However, even if no yellow is visible on the nipple, a bacterial infection is still possible. See the next section for a description of the symptoms of a fungal infection of the nipple that distinguish it from a bacterial infection, keeping in mind that both may be present.

• • •

One effective treatment for a bacterial infection of the nipple is oral antibiotics.

Use of a topical antibiotic ointment on traumatized areas may help prevent a bacterial infection from developing (Wilson-Clay & Hoover, 2017; A. Witt, Mason, Burgess, Flocke, & Zyzanski, 2014), but once a bacterial infection develops, research found topical treatments less effective than other options.

Early research on treatment options for bacterial infections. In one Canadian study of 227 mothers with babies younger than 1 month, 64% of those with moderate to severe pain along with nipple cracks, fissures, ulcers, and/

or visible pus were diagnosed with *Staphylococcus aureus* bacterial infections (V. Livingstone & Stringer, 1999; V. H. Livingstone, Willis, & Berkowitz, 1996).

To determine the most effective treatment for these infections, these Canadian researchers divided 84 mothers whose nipples cultured positive for *Staphylococcus aureus* into four groups, each with a different treatment plan. They then checked their progress 5 to 7 days later (V. Livingstone & Stringer, 1999). All of the treatment groups received help in getting a deeper latch. The percentage that improved varied by group:

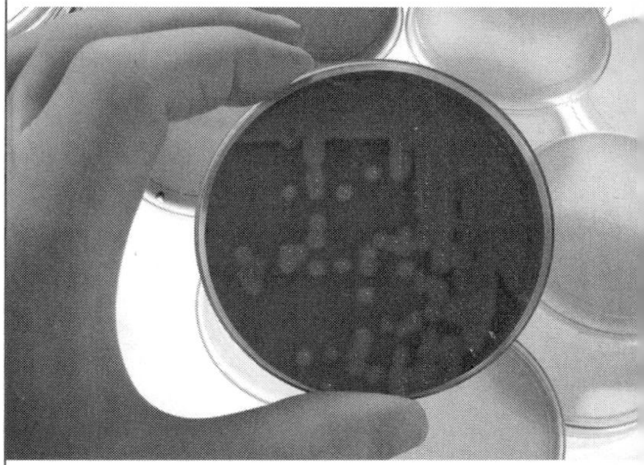

- 9% in the instruction-only group
- 16% in the group that applied the mupirocin antibiotic ointment after every feed
- 36% in the group that applied topical fusidic acid after every feed
- 79% in the group that received a 10-day course of oral antibiotics (dicloxacillin, cephalosporins, or erythromycin)

The researchers found that within 7 days, 25% of those not taking oral antibiotics developed mastitis (another possible complication of nipple trauma), compared with 5% of those taking oral antibiotics, so they stopped the study early due to ethical concerns. The researchers concluded that oral antibiotics are an effective treatment in those with extremely sore, cracked nipples.

Later research on treatment options for bacterial infections. A 2014 U.S. prospective study followed a group of 89 nursing mothers seen at a lactation practice for chronic nipple pain (A. M. Witt et al., 2014). A small number (7) of these mothers either planned to wean or were showing obvious signs of a bacterial infection, so they were started immediately on oral antibiotics. The large majority (82) were started on a conservative treatment plan, which involved:

- Help in getting a deeper latch
- Prescription mupirocin ointment applied after every feed or if inflammation or dermatitis is present, prescribe Triamcinolone 0.1%

Among the 82 mothers who started with this conservative treatment, 38 did well, meaning their nipple pain resolved within 5 days of beginning treatment. The pain did not resolve for the remaining 44. Three of these mothers were diagnosed with a fungal infection and treated with fluconazole. The remaining 41 mothers who "failed" the conservative treatment had some characteristic in common.

- They were in greater pain at first
- The latch help reduced their pain less

But fortunately, after they were prescribed oral antibiotics (the most common was dicloxacillin and for penicillin-allergic women either trimethoprim-sulfamethoxazole or clindamycin) pain levels dropped quickly. At follow-up between 6 and 12 weeks later, the group that did well with the conservative treatment developed no more complications. The pain levels were low in both groups, and their nursing rates were equal. The median length of antibiotic use in this study was 14 days. The researchers concluded that when pain continues despite getting a deeper latch and treating it with topical mupirocin, oral antibiotics are a logical next step.

• • •

Impetigo, another type of bacterial infection, can be treated without interrupting nursing.

A 2017 U.S. summary of common lactation problems and their treatments (Khan & Ramirez, 2017) noted that impetigo is often caused by *Staphylococcus aureus* (staph) and group A beta-hemolytic streptococcus. Impetigo can cause nipple pain and appear as honey-crusted cracks and reddened nipples. The colonizing staph crusting may also block a nipple pore, causing mastitis. These authors recommend cleaning the nipple with a washcloth containing soap and water to remove the crusting, rinse, then apply prescribed mupirocin antibiotic ointment. In some cases, a topical ointment may be enough to clear the impetigo. In other cases, oral antibiotics may be necessary (dicloxacillin, cephalexin, or erythromycin 500 mg every 6 hours for 10 days).

Impetigo can happen later in lactation, too. In one Australian case report (Thorley, 2000), a mother reported unbroken, watery, pinhead-sized blisters in a line on her areola and nipple and waves of pain in her breast. When asked if her 15-month-old nursing toddler had any blisters like this, she said she had seen some on his face but thought they were chickenpox. The sores eventually scabbed over. The mother was diagnosed with impetigo and treated by her healthcare provider without interrupting nursing.

Candida/Thrush

A yeast infection, also known as thrush or candidiasis, is an overgrowth of a fungus that normally lives in our bodies.

Candida albicans, a one-celled organism, is a fungus involved with most cases of thrush and vaginal yeast infections. It thrives in moist, dark environments, such as on the nipples, in the vagina, in the mouth, and in the baby's diaper area. This fungus normally lives in our bodies in balance with other organisms, but illness, pregnancy, antibiotic use, and other factors that throw the body out of balance can cause an unhealthy overgrowth. One U.S. study (Morrill, Heinig, Pappagianis, & Dewey, 2005) found the use of bottles during the early weeks of nursing to be associated with an increased incidence of candidiasis.

• • •

A lot is still unknown about the prevalence of candida infections among nursing parents.

How often do fungal infections occur in nursing parents? Because *Candida albicans* is naturally present in our bodies, confirming its overgrowth can be challenging. Candida also can be cultured from the mouths of 80% to 90% of babies (Strong & Mele, 2013). Concern about possible overtreatment of nipple and breast pain with antifungal drugs led researchers to learn more about the prevalence of yeast infections of the nipple and reliable ways to confirm it.

One U.S. study (Morrill et al., 2005) attempted to determine the prevalence of thrush by comparing a control group of 40 non-pregnant, non-lactating women with a group of 100 low-income new mothers being seen at a Nevada lactation clinic. None of the women in the control group tested positive for candida. In the nursing group, however, 2 weeks after birth, after culturing the babies' mouths and the mothers' nipples/areolae, breast folds, and milk, the researchers found that 23% of the nursing group tested positive for candida, and 8% of these mothers already had thrush symptoms, such as burning nipples, painful breasts, stabbing pain in the breast, and shiny or flaky skin on the nipples/areolae. By 9 weeks, 87% of these mothers had symptoms of a candida infection and 18% of their babies had obvious white patches in their mouths. Of the mothers and babies who cultured positive, 43% were still breastfeeding at 9 weeks, compared with 69% who did not culture positive. Of those who cultured positive at 2 weeks, 65% weaned by 9 weeks, all reportedly due to pain. Of those who cultured negative at 2 weeks, 31% weaned by 9 weeks, 38% due to pain and the other 62% for other reasons. The researchers acknowledged that this prevalence of candida may not apply to other populations.

Few of the study mothers with symptoms received treatment from their healthcare providers. Of those who were treated for candida, 40% who received treatment weaned before 9 weeks due to continuing pain. This may be in part because the candida infection was treated with nystatin, which in many cases is ineffective. One U.S. study (Goins, Ascher, Waecker, Arnold, & Moorefield, 2002) found nystatin effective in babies in only 32% of cases, while oral fluconazole suspension was effective in 100%.

In an attempt to sort out the role bacteria and yeast play in early nipple and breast pain, a 2013 Australian prospective, longitudinal cohort study (L. H. Amir et al., 2013) followed 360 first-time mothers from 36 weeks of pregnancy through 8 weeks after delivery. They cultured the mothers' nipples and milk and babies' mouths and found that at 4 weeks post-delivery, at least 50% cultured positive for the bacterium *Staphylococcus aureus* (staph), unrelated to symptoms. In other words, at 4 weeks, most mothers cultured positive for staph whether or not they had nipple pain or any other symptoms of infection. To confirm the role of candida in nipple pain, they used both microbial cultures and a molecular technique (real-time polymerase chain reaction, or PCR, samples) designed to be more sensitive than cultures. They found the molecular technique more effective at identifying candida than cultures, but this method is not generally available to practitioners. More of the women with the burning pain often associated with thrush tested positive for candida (86% versus 57% of those without burning pain).

• • •

The existence of burning or shooting pain alone is not enough to confirm that a yeast infection is the cause of pain. A combination of symptoms is more reliable.

Many nursing parents are mistakenly treated for thrush only to discover the cause of their pain was Raynaud's phenomenon (Anderson et al., 2004; Strong & Mele, 2013) or a bacterial infection (Thomassen et al., 1998). One U.S. survey of physicians (Brent, 2001) found that 93% diagnose thrush based on symptoms only and do not use diagnostic tests. As noted in the previous point, this is likely because culture results are often unreliable.

The 2013 Australian study cited in the previous point (L. H. Amir et al., 2013) concluded that the best approach is to identify thrush by its symptoms. In an effort to clarify which symptoms are reliable signs of thrush, U.S. researchers studied 100 mothers (Francis-Morrill et al., 2004) and found that thrush is more likely to be a cause of painful nursing if the following symptoms occur together:

- Shiny nipple/areola skin with stabbing pain
- Flaky nipple/areola skin and mammary pain

If these symptoms appear alone, they are much less likely to indicate candida. Other symptoms of candida infections include white plaques on the nipples and areolae or red or inflamed-looking nipples and areolae.

In the baby, possible symptoms include:

- White patches on the baby's gums, cheeks, palate, tonsils, and/or tongue (if wiped off, they may look red or bleed)
- Diaper rash (may be simply red or red with raised dots)

Most nursing babies have a white, milky coating on their tongue. This is not a sign of thrush unless white patches spread to the baby's cheeks and gums (Wilson-Clay & Hoover, 2017, p. 176). Some babies have a yeast rash on their bottom but not in their mouth.

Before a parent is treated for candida —especially if the baby has no symptoms— rule out other possible causes of nipple pain, such as shallow latch, bacterial infection, mastitis, vasospasm, Raynaud's phenomenon, and skin problems, such as eczema, psoriasis, and dermatitis (see later section).

• • •

With shooting or burning mammary pain, consider possibilities other than yeast first.

Once it was believed that the most likely cause of shooting or burning pain in the mammary gland was a secondary yeast infection in or around the milk ducts. But researchers questioned the existence of this condition (T. W. Hale, Bateman, Finkelman, & Berens, 2009; Jimenez et al., 2017), and other causes for these symptoms were identified (Anderson et al., 2004; Berens et al., 2016; Eglash, Plane, & Mundt, 2006). For details, see p. 776-778.

• • •

Nursing parents with nipple damage may develop both bacterial and fungal infections and need treatment for both.

Persistent nipple and mammary pain often has multiple causes (Kent et al., 2015). Follow-up is important because even if one cause is found and addressed, more treatment may be needed.

• • •

Treatment options for thrush vary by local practice and availability.

If thrush is diagnosed by a healthcare provider, discuss treating both parent and baby, even if one has no symptoms, to prevent a recurrence (Chetwynd, Ives, Payne, & Edens-Bartholomew, 2002). If after treatment, thrush persists, treating the nursing couple at the same time may be more effective (Wambach, 2021, p. 293). Over-the-counter and prescribed treatments are available for yeast infections (Berens et al., 2016).

Thrush Treatment Options for the Baby:

Over-the-counter treatments

- **Gentian violet.** This dye was once recommended as an over-the-counter treatment for thrush. in both parents and babies. However, because it can cause cancer, the World Health Organization and Health Canada now advise against its use. For details, see **bit.ly/BA2-Gentian**.

Treatments requiring a prescription

- **Nystatin suspension.** Apply 1 dropperful in each cheek 4 to 8 times daily for at least 2 weeks. It is most effective if used after every feed. One U.S. study (Goins et al., 2002) found nystatin effective in only 32% of its cases, while oral fluconazole suspension was effective in 100%.

- **Miconazole gel.** Apply the 25 mg gel (not available in the U.S.) 4 times daily. One German study (Hoppe, 1997) found it faster and more effective than nystatin.
- **Clotrimazole gel.** Pharmacists make this oral gel by crushing a 10 mg clotrimazole lozenge and mixing it with 5 mL of glycerin or 3 mL of methylcellulose. Apply to baby's mouth every 3 hours for five applications (L. Amir & Hoover, 2002).
- **Fluconazole.** Give 6 mg/kg oral suspension via dropper as a first dose followed by 3 mg/kg/day once daily for 2 weeks (L. Amir & Hoover, 2002).

Thrush Treatment Options for the Nursing Parent:

Over-the-counter treatments

- **Gentian violet.** This dye was once recommended as an over-the-counter treatment for thrush. in both parents and babies. However, because it can cause cancer, the World Health Organization and Health Canada now advise against its use. For details, see **bit.ly/BA2-Gentian**.
- **Miconazole.** Cream or lotion (2%). Apply to nipples/areolae 2 to 4 times daily for 7 days (L. Amir & Hoover, 2002).
- **Ketoconazole.** Cream (2%). Apply to nipples/areolae 2 to 4 times daily at least 2 days after symptoms disappear (L. Amir & Hoover, 2002).

Treatments requiring a prescription

- **Clotrimazole.** Over-the-counter (OTC) and prescription versions are available. For OTC versions: Apply to nipples/areolae after feeds 2 to 4 times daily for at least 2 days after symptoms disappear. Prescribed version: Pharmacists make a gel by crushing a 10 mg clotrimazole lozenge and mixing it with 5 mL of glycerin or 3 mL of methylcellulose. Apply to nipples/areolae every 3 hours for five applications (L. Amir & Hoover, 2002).
- **Nystatin cream or ointment.** Apply 4 times per day for 14 days. Note: Nystatin is much less effective than other treatment options (see "baby" above).
- **Nystatin with triamcinolone (corticosteroid).** Use cream or ointment. Apply to nipples/areolae 4 times daily until at least 2 days after symptoms disappear.
- **Oral fluconazole.** Used when topical treatments are ineffective. Take either a 200 mg or 400 mg loading dose, then 100 mg 2 times daily for at least 2 weeks. Continue for 1 week after pain is gone (Berens et al., 2016; Forster et al., 2011; Khan & Ramirez, 2017; Wambach, 2021, p. 294). The single-dose treatment for vaginal yeast infections is not usually effective (Moorhead, Amir, O'Brien, & Wong, 2011).

For those who prefer a more "natural" treatment, a U.S. physician (Khan & Ramirez, 2017) suggests the nursing parent mix 1 teaspoon (5 mL) of vinegar with 1 cup (236 mL) of water and apply after each nursing session to nipple and allow to air dry.

• • •

Nursing can continue during thrush treatment. In some cases, the parent may first feel worse before feeling better.

In mild cases of thrush, once treatment starts, there may be some relief in 1 to 2 days. In more severe cases, it may take 3 to 5 days or longer. While taking oral fluconazole, it may take a week or longer for the pain to disappear, because rather than killing the yeast, fluconazole prevents it from reproducing. Encourage the parent to use the medication for the full course, since thrush may recur if it is stopped when the symptoms disappear.

During treatment, the symptoms may seem worse for a day or two before they improve. Suggest rinsing the nipples with clear water and air drying them after each nursing, as thrush thrives on milk and moisture. Before the pain has gone, suggest using the comfort measures described earlier in this chapter.

• • •

After treatment, if there is a recurrence of thrush, suggest taking precautions to prevent future recurrence.

Thrush can be harbored in many places, and it can spread to other members of the family. If it recurs, suggest parents:

- Ask for treatment for their partner and, if nursing more than one, the other sibling.
- Wash their hands often, especially after changing diapers and using the toilet.
- Wash baby's hands often if he sucks thumb or fingers.
- If pacifiers, bottle nipples/teats, or teethers are used, boil them once a day for 20 minutes to kill the yeast. After 1 week of treatment, discard them and buy new ones.
- If breast pumps are used, boil daily for 20 minutes all parts that touch the milk.
- If nursing pads are used, use disposable pads and discard after each feed.
- Wash toys that baby puts in his mouth in hot, soapy water and rinse well.
- Use paper towels for hand drying. Discard after use.

Parents sometimes feel anxious about using expressed milk frozen during a thrush outbreak. A Brazilian study (Rosa, Novak, de Almeida, Medonca-Hagler, & Hagler, 1990) found low levels of live yeast in human milk that was previously frozen and thawed. The researchers concluded that freezing does not kill yeast. But they acknowledged the possibility that the milk became contaminated with live yeast during its handling, There is currently no evidence to indicate that milk expressed and stored during a bout of nipple thrush or thrush in baby's mouth can cause a recurrence. In the Academy of Breastfeeding Medicine's Clinical Protocol #8 on storage and handling of human milk, its authors wrote (Eglash, Simon, & Academy of Breastfeeding, 2017, p. 393):

> "If a mother has breast or nipple pain from a bacterial or yeast infection, there is no evidence that her stored expressed milk needs to be discarded."

If parents are still concerned about using the milk, an alternative to discarding it is to use it while parent and baby are being treated for thrush. If that's not possible, another alternative is to warm the expressed milk to temperatures that kill yeast. Milk banks heat milk to 63 degrees C (144.5 degrees F) for 30 minutes, which will kill bacteria and yeast. According to one reference (L. Amir & Hoover, 2002), candida dies within minutes at a temperature of 122 degrees F (60 degrees C). Of course, if the milk is heated, cool it to between room temperature and body temperature before feeding.

Viral Herpes Infections

Herpes sores, which are spread by contact, can occur on or near the nipple and can be fatal to the newborn.

Herpes simplex 1 (cold sores or fever blisters) and 2 (genital herpes) are two different herpes viruses spread by contact with the sores. They are small, painful, fluid-filled, red-rimmed blisters that dry after a few days and form a scab. Genital herpes sores can be spread to other body parts, including the nipple, by touch.

These herpes viruses are often fatal when contracted by newborn babies up to 3 weeks of age (Field, 2016; Sullivan-Bolyai, Fife, Jacobs, Miller, & Corey, 1983). One 2019 case report (D'Andrea & Spatz, 2019) described a nursing newborn who survived a life-threatening herpes infection contracted during his second week from contact with his mother's breast lesions. Because it was not possible for the baby to breastfeed without touching the mother's breast lesions, breastfeeding was interrupted for 11 days while mother and baby were hospitalized and treated with the IV antiviral drug acyclovir. The mother pumped often during those 11 days, and they resumed breastfeeding after discharge, eventually meeting her goal of breastfeeding for 2 years.

If pregnant parents or their partners have recurrent herpes, they should talk to a healthcare provider knowledgeable about herpes and nursing to decide what precautions to take. If a sore on the nipple or mammary gland could be herpes, it should be cultured. Culture results should be available within a few days at most.

If a nursing parent is waiting for the results of a culture or herpes on the nipple or gland is confirmed, nursing can continue if the sores can be covered, so the baby does not touch them. A 2019 Indian case report described the experience of a breastfeeding mother who developed active herpes in her eyes (Agarwal, Maharana, Titiyal, & Sharma, 2019). During and after her drug treatment, her healthcare providers encouraged her to keep nursing, and at 2 months, her breastfeeding baby was healthy. But if the sores are on the nipple, areola, or anywhere else the baby might touch while nursing, it's better to express milk from that side until the sores heal. In the meantime, it's fine to nurse on the unaffected side. If the nursing parent's hand or breast-pump parts touch the sores while expressing milk, they may contaminate the expressed milk with the virus, and it should be discarded. If the hands or breast-pump parts do not come in contact with the sores, the newborn may be fed the milk.

• • •

Serious complications from contracting herpes are much less likely in babies older than 1 month.

Although herpes can be dangerous to a baby younger than 1 month, there are case reports of older babies touching their nursing parent's herpes sores while nursing without developing complications. There is also a documented case of a nursing 15-month-old with a cold sore in his mouth who passed herpes to his mother's breast (Sealander & Kerr, 1989). Although an older baby is not likely to develop life-threatening complications from herpes, suggest taking steps to avoid spreading it to the child, as the sores can be very painful for a week or more and may make eating and drinking difficult.

• • •

When a nursing parent contracts other herpes infections, such as shingles and chickenpox, contagious sores may erupt on the nipple and mammary gland.

For details on how to prevent transmission of shingles (herpes zoster) and chickenpox (varicella zoster) to a nursing baby, see p. 821 and 823.

OTHER SKIN PROBLEMS

Skin problems that occur anywhere else on the body can also occur on the nipple and mammary gland and may be unrelated to nursing.

Skin conditions and rashes that appear on the nipple or mammary gland may be completely unrelated to nursing. One example is hives, which is caused by an allergic reaction to a substance touched or consumed. Asking the questions that follow may help provide clues to whether a skin problem is related or unrelated to lactation.

• • •

Ask the parent to describe the skin problem and gather other information to help determine next steps.

Some questions to ask nursing parents with skin problems include:

Have they recently used any cream, ointment, pads, or other product on or near their nipples? Eczema and other types of dermatitis (inflammation of the skin) can develop on or around the nipples when topical cortisone, antifungals, and mupirocin are used, triggering a secondary rash (T.W. Hale, 2019). In some articles (Cooper & Shaw, 1999; Huggins & Billon, 1993) nipple inflammation occurred as a reaction to ingredients in nystatin cream, a prescribed candida treatment.

Have they used a new laundry product or toiletry product, like cologne, deodorant, hair spray, or powder near their mammary glands? In some parents, products applied to the skin may cause irritation.

Have they used any tools or devices on their nipples, like a breast pump, breast shells, nipple shields, or nipple everters? Too-high suction levels can sometimes cause skin damage, and exposure to the plastics of breast shells or pump parts may cause a reaction in some sensitive parents (Wilson-Clay & Hoover, 2017, p. 61).

Do they have a health problem and/or are they taking any medication? Skin problems can indicate an allergic reaction or a sensitivity to some medications. Certain health problems increase the risk of skin reactions. For example, one mother with celiac disease, which increases the risk of dermatitis, developed painful eczema on her nipples while breastfeeding (L. Amir, 1993). With her second child, medical treatment resolved the eczema. When eczema is the cause, parents may notice vesicles that erupt and become crusted (Wiener, 2006).

Is the baby eating solid foods, teething, or taking medication? Parents can react to medication and/or teething gels in a baby's mouth. If parents are sensitive to certain foods, eczema can develop on the nipples when the baby nurses with particles of these foods still in his mouth. Rinsing the baby's mouth with water before nursing or eliminating the irritating food from the baby's diet for a while may help.

Do both parent and child have a similar skin problem anywhere else on their bodies, or do they have a history of allergic skin reactions? Skin problems unrelated to nursing can spread to the nipple area. In that case, parents may be familiar with the problem and the treatments that work for them. One example is psoriasis, which is often triggered 4 to 6 weeks after birth or by a skin injury (Berens et al., 2016). If a parent has an ongoing skin condition, they may just want to know the effect, if any, of their usual treatments on nursing. Parents with poison ivy on their nipple probably have the rash in other areas, too. With poison ivy, as long as the glands and nipples have been washed and the oil from the plant removed, it is safe for the baby to nurse (Wilson-Clay & Hoover, 2017, p. 62). See also the example on p. 726 in the previous section of the mother and child with impetigo (Thorley, 2000). A history of allergic rashes or other skin reactions raises the strong possibility that the problem is dermatological rather than lactation-related (Porter & Schach, 2004).

For unexplained skin problems, suggest basic strategies (Wambach, 2021, p. 289) such as: discontinue products that might irritate, take showers often, wear all-cotton bras, expose the nipple to sunlight and air for 15 minutes, and after nursing, rinse the affected nipple and areola with warm water, pat dry, and dry with a hair dryer set on low.

KEY CONCEPT

In some cases, topical treatments for nipple pain—such as lanolin and nystatin cream—can cause skin reactions.

• • •

Eczema-like skin irritations fall into several main categories, which have different triggers.

In Clinical Protocol #26 from the Academy of Breastfeeding Medicine (Berens et al., 2016), its authors explain that eczema-like skin conditions fall into several basic categories:

- **Atopic dermatitis**—Eczema usually occurs in those with allergic tendencies and is triggered by skin irritants and environmental factors, like a change in weather.
- **Irritant contact dermatitis**—Triggered by friction and direct contact with traces of solid foods or medication in baby's mouth, wet nursing pads, laundry detergent, fabric softener, dryer sheets, fragrances, topical treatments for nipple pain.
- **Allergic contact dermatitis**—Common triggers are lanolin, topical antibiotics, chamomile, vitamins A and E, and fragrance.

• • •

Continued pain and slow healing are signs it's time to consult a healthcare provider.

A dermatologist who is knowledgeable about lactation-related issues can be a tremendous ally to lactation supporters and the families they help (Heller et al., 2012). In a U.S. report of 20 mothers who saw a lactation consultant for unusual skin problems on or near the nipple and who were later referred to a dermatologist (Huggins & Billon, 1993), the authors concluded that with appropriate treatment parents with these unusual skin conditions were able to resume nursing without pain within a few days. They suggest those with skin problems consider seeing a dermatologist, if possible, or another healthcare provider when:

- They continue to feel significant pain during nursing, even when baby is latching deeply.
- Nipple trauma heals unusually slowly or has stopped completely.
- Blisters, rash, scaling, crusting, or oozing sores appear on the nipples, are healing slowly, or healing has stopped.
- Nipples show no sign of improvement, even after treatment.

If parents with eczema on their nipples do not improve with treatment, they should be seen soon by their healthcare provider to rule out Paget's disease.

• • •

Paget's disease accounts for 1% to 3% of breast cancers and is sometimes mistaken for nipple eczema (Chen, Sun, & Anderson, 2006). It usually appears on one nipple, comes on gradually, has an irregular but distinct edge, and the nipple is almost always affected, sometimes seeming to disappear. When eczema does not clear within 3 weeks of treatment, parents should see their healthcare provider right away to rule out this possibility (Barankin & Gross, 2004). Because its symptoms seem minor, many postpone seeing their healthcare provider. One study found the average wait before seeking treatment for Paget's disease was 30 weeks (Duff, 1998). Waiting this long decreases the odds of survival. Early detection is vital.

NIPPLE BLISTERS AND BLEBS

Blisters

A clear blister is usually caused by friction and/or high vacuum.

A blister may form on the tip of the nipple if the baby is latched shallowly and putting undue pressure on the end of the nipple. Discuss the basics of getting a deeper latch (see the first chapter). Starter positions may help a young baby latch deeper, especially if baby is allowed to self-attach (Figure 17.2). This adjustment may be all that's needed to reduce the pain and prevent the blister from recurring.

• • •

To open a blister, suggest first applying warm, wet compresses before nursing.

The moisture of a warm, wet compress before nursing will soften the nipple skin, and the heat will thin the skin, which may cause the blister to open. If not, see the later point on opening a bleb for more suggestions.

Blebs or Milk Blisters

A milk blister, or bleb, may or may not be painful and appears to be associated with plugged milk ducts.

One type of white spot on the nipple is called a ***bleb*** or ***milk blister.*** Its cause is still not fully understood. Some think a bleb could be a plug— perhaps caused by a granule of thickened milk—blocking the milk from flowing at the nipple. Some think blebs may be caused by a thin layer of skin blocking the opening of a milk duct from the outside. One medical textbook suggests they may be small pressure cysts that form at the end of the milk duct (Lawrence & Lawrence, 2016, p. 270).

Many observed that these white spots sometimes coincide with bouts of mastitis, but the cause and effect is unclear (Noble, 1991; Wambach, 2021, p. 295). Does the bleb cause the mastitis by blocking the flow of milk from the duct? Or does the bleb form as a result of the mastitis, which caused the milk to thicken in a duct? At this writing, no one knows for sure.

If the bleb is not painful, no treatment is needed. It may resolve on its own over time.

• • •

A white spot on the nipple may be due to other causes.

White nipple spots that are not blebs may or may not be painful. These could be caused by a build-up of dead skin, like cradle cap, which can be removed by rubbing it with a lubricating oil like lecithin (Lawrence & Lawrence, 2016, p. 270). In *The Breastfeeding Atlas*, U.S. lactation consultants Barbara Wilson-Clay and Kay Hoover (Wilson-Clay & Hoover, 2017, p. 63) note that some report a white spot after the baby bit the nipple, which is caused by an accumulation of saliva and milk moisture under skin edges. They recommend cleaning the area with soap and water like any bite wound and applying topical antibiotic ointment to prevent infection (for details, see "Preventing Infection" on p. 722).

Possible cause of a white spot on the nipple is candida or thrush. With thrush, a small blister-like sore may develop on the nipple. Before assuming a white spot is a bleb, first rule out these other possibilities.

• • •

If a bleb is painful, there are several ways parents can try to resolve it on their own.

For home bleb treatment, first, suggest applying wet heat to it, either with warm compresses or by soaking the nipple in warm water (side-lying in a bathtub or leaning forward into a sink or basin of warm water). Then suggest rubbing the nipple with a damp cloth to remove any excess skin (Wambach, 2021, p. 295). Some also suggest lubricating the nipple with olive oil (Wilson-Clay & Hoover, 2017, p. 63). After this, suggest trying to express milk from that duct by compressing the areola behind the plug. In some cases, it may be possible to express a thickened string of milk, which may help open the duct and keep it open.

• • •

If the bleb is painful and persists despite these treatments, suggest seeing a healthcare provider to treat it.

One way to treat a bleb is to have a healthcare provider open it with a sterile needle. In some cases, when the duct is opened, milk from behind the plug will flow and bring relief. After the bleb is opened, to prevent infection, suggest washing it daily with a mild soap and water and rinsing well with water. Another way to help prevent infection is to apply a thin layer of a topical antibiotic ointment, such as mupirocin, to the affected nipple after feeds.

In other cases, a bleb may be dry. U.S. physician Maryann O'Hara analyzed the tissue from the dry blebs she excised from five women (O'Hara, 2012). She found no bacteria or fungi and concluded the dry blebs were an inflammatory tissue reaction to nipple trauma. She treated them with a very thin layer of mid-potency steroid ointment applied after nursing and covered with plastic wrap until the next feed. Within a few days, the blebs were healed.

Another treatment for a persistent bleb was described in a 2019 case report (Mitchell, Eglash, & Bamberger, 2019). At 6 months post-delivery, this breastfeeding mother had worsening breast pain, recurring plugged ducts, and persistent blebs in her left breast. Her milk cultured positive for a multiple drug-resistant strain of *Staphylococcus aureus* (MRSA). Over the next 8 weeks, several treatments of IV antibiotics completely resolved the bleb, plugged ducts, and pain.

• • •

To prevent recurring blebs, some dietary changes and lecithin supplements may help.

If blebs and/or plugged ducts continue to recur, some suggest reducing saturated fats in the diet and taking a lecithin supplement (Eglash, 1998). Suggested dosages of lecithin range from 1 tablespoon per day to 1 tablespoon 3 to 4 times a day or one to two 1,200 mg capsules 3 or 4 times per day.

NIPPLE TYPES AND PROCEDURES

Flat and Inverted Nipples

Flat nipples do not protrude or become erect when stimulated or cold. Many babies latch and nurse well from flat nipples.

Protruding (everted) nipples are not necessary for effective nursing, as many nursing parents with flat (Figure 17.3) and inverted (Figure 17.4) nipples can testify. Most babies are happy to suck on anything they can get into their mouths, including adult arms, shoulders, and necks, none of which have protruding nipples. See the following points for strategies if nursing problems occur.

• • •

Inverted nipples retract rather than protrude when the areola is compressed.

A nipple may appear everted at rest but retract when stimulated. The ***pinch test*** will reveal this by gently compressing near the edge of the areola, about an inch (2.5 cm) behind the base of the nipple. If the nipple protrudes, it is not inverted (even if it appears inverted at rest). If the nipple retracts or becomes concave (Figure 17.4), it is an inverted nipple.

• • •

There are different types of inverted nipples and explanations for their cause.

Some attribute nipple inversion to very short milk ducts that draw the nipple in (Chandler & Hill, 1990). Others assert that nipples invert because they contain less dense connective tissue beneath the nipple (Terrill & Stapleton, 1991).

Inverted nipple classification system. Plastic surgeons—who are asked to surgically correct some inverted nipples—created an inverted nipple classification system based on the amount of connective tissue they contain (called ***degree of fibrosis***) and how easily they can be made to protrude (Han & Hong, 1999). What plastic surgeons call a Grade I inverted nipple can be easily everted manually and may stay everted after nursing. A nursing baby who sucks normally will draw them out with no difficulty. Grade II inverted nipples are considered moderately inverted. While a healthy term baby may draw them out, they will retract again after feeds. At first, some preterm or sick babies may find Grade II inverted nipples challenging. Severely inverted nipples, or Grade III, can barely be pulled out. While rare, these Grade III inverted nipples

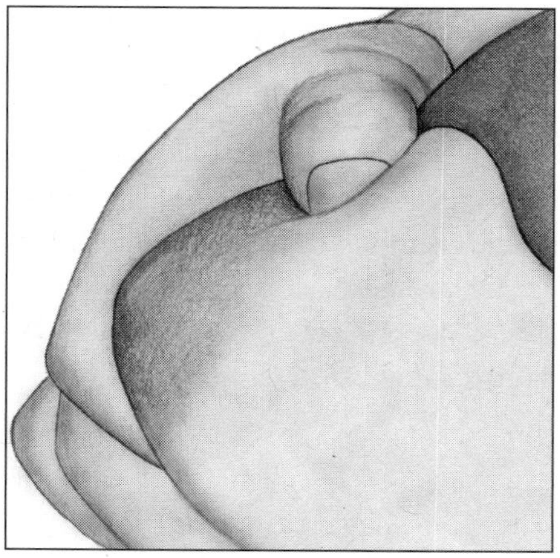

Figure 17.3 Flat nipple

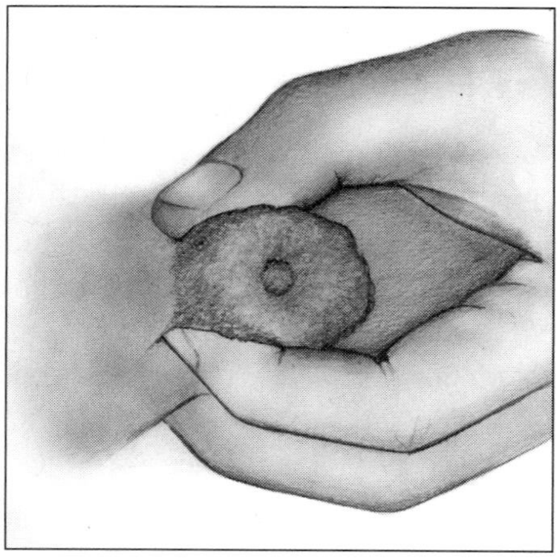

Figure 17.4 Inverted nipple

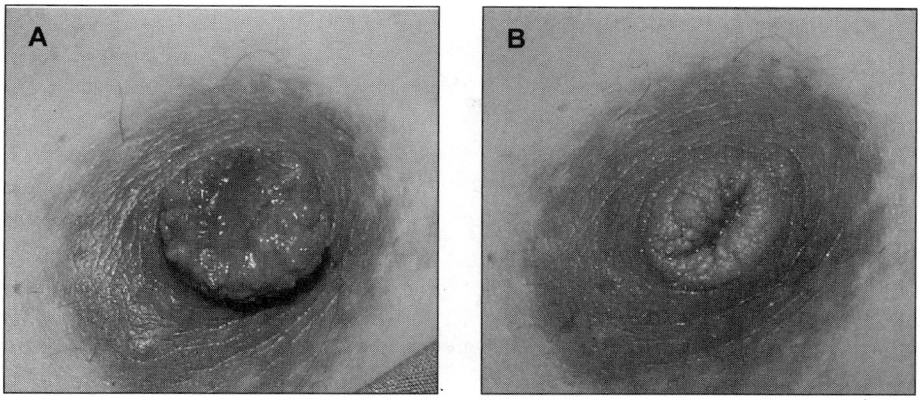

Figure 17.5 This dimpled nipple is open (left) after pumping then closed (right). Barbara Wilson-Clay, Kay Hoover, from *The Breastfeeding Atlas,* 6th ed, 2017. Used with permission.

may make drawing the nipple out during nursing difficult or in extreme cases impossible.

Dimpled nipples. A dimpled or folded nipple (Figure 17.5) is a type of inverted nipple in which only a part of the nipple is inverted. It will not protrude or harden when stimulated, but it can be manually opened or drawn out during nursing or pumping. It does not, however, stay open afterwards.

Inverted nipples and nipple pain. Some types of dimpled and inverted nipples can cause nipple pain, especially during the early weeks. U.S. lactation consultants Barbara Wilson-Clay and Kay Hoover describe the experience of one mother with dimpled nipples whose nipple tissue inside the fold was adhered, and breastfeeding and pumping left this inner tissue moist, causing skin breakdown from too much moisture (maceration) and bleeding (Wilson-Clay & Hoover, 2017, p. 48). In this case, the mother was able to resolve her problem by holding the nipple open after nursing or pumping until it dried and by keeping this area very clean. A hair dryer set on warm can also be used to speed the drying process.

KEY CONCEPT

Treating flat or inverted nipples during pregnancy may cause more problems than it solves.

• • •

One nipple may be flat or inverted while the other nipple protrudes.

It is not unusual for nipples to vary in the same nursing parent. One nipple may protrude while the other is flat or inverted. Both nipples may be flat, but one may protrude more than the other. Both nipples may be inverted but one may be more inverted than the other. The baby may show a preference for the nipple that is less inverted or more protruding.

• • •

During pregnancy, treatments to draw out flat and inverted nipples may cause more nursing problems than they solve.

Treatments during pregnancy to treat flat and inverted nipples—such as daily practice of the Hoffman technique (in which the fingers are used to draw out inverted nipples) or wearing breast shells—were once recommended. However, two U.K. studies (Alexander, Grant, & Campbell, 1992; MAIN, 1994) found that the groups in which flat or inverted nipples were identified during pregnancy and treated had more nursing problems after birth than the control groups. The researchers expressed concern that identifying "problem" nipples during pregnancy may "act as a disincentive" to successful nursing because it calls into question the parent's ability to nurse. They concluded that during pregnancy recommending "breast shells may reduce the chances of successful breastfeeding" (Alexander et al., 1992, p. 1030).

• • •

Nipple shape may change at different times and in different situations.

Nipple shape is not static, and it may change. For example, during the early days after birth, engorgement or excess IV fluids received during labor may cause tissue swelling that flattens previously protruding nipples. If this presents nursing challenges, to make latching easier, try hand-expressing some milk (p. 484) or try reverse pressure softening (p. 885), which moves tissue swelling away from the nipple and areola.

Previously inverted nipples that were drawn out by nursing may stay everted for the next baby, or they may invert again after weaning. Gaining weight can add fatty tissue to the mammary glands, which can flatten a previously protruding nipple.

• • •

Even if flat and inverted nipples increase the risk of latching struggles, it is not helpful to tell nursing parents their nipples are the problem.

Some U.S. studies (Dewey et al., 2003; Moore & Anderson, 2007) found an association between flat and inverted nipples and early nursing struggles. These studies were published before research on the starter positions appeared (see p. 23-29), so it is likely the study mothers used upright nursing position, which may make early nursing more challenging.

In some countries, such as India, cultural beliefs about the importance of protruding nipples to nursing success influences practices. One Indian study (Chanprapaph, Luttarapakul, Siribariruck, & Boonyawanichkul, 2013) examined the effects of a commercial product designed to elongate "short nipples" (defined as less than 7 mm long) during pregnancy. Another Indian study described the belief that if faced with an inverted nipple after birth, the newborn will be unable to nurse until the nipple is drawn out. According to the nursing staff quoted in this study, this belief contributes to delays in the first feed (Majra & Silan, 2016, p. 18):

> "Just imagine everything (delivery) went well and mother is ready for feeding and all of sudden she comes to know (that) you have breast abnormality that need to correct. Without that, don't expect to breastfeed."

During the early days and weeks, nursing struggles are common in all families (Feenstra, Jorgine Kirkeby, Thygesen, Danbjorg, & Kronborg, 2018; Wagner, Chantry, Dewey, & Nommsen-Rivers, 2013). If nursing parents are told their nipple anatomy is to blame, this can be incredibly demoralizing. After all, there is little they can do about their nipple shape. They may feel as though their nipples are "defective" and that nursing is an impossibility. Keep in mind, there's no way to know for sure if their nipple shape is the cause of the nursing struggle. If parents express concern about their nipple shape, a more supportive (and accurate) response is: "Your nipples are great for nursing. Often nursing takes time and practice to master. Give it some time"

• • •

In parents with flat and inverted nipples, several basic strategies can help minimize early nursing problems.

What should a parent with flat or inverted nipples do to minimize nursing struggles after birth?

Follow best practices. Review p. 45-65 in Chapter 2 for the basic recommendations for getting nursing off to the best start. They include:

- Immediate and uninterrupted skin-to-skin contact
- Allowing the baby to do the breast crawl for the first feed

- Encouraging early and frequent nursing
- Providing a private, comfortable, and supportive environment
- Keeping nursing couples together and in body contact as much as possible day and night

An Indian study (Girish et al., 2013) found that babies allowed to do the breast crawl for their first feed after birth had significantly fewer nursing problems during the hospital stay. At the following link, scroll to 6:30 to watch the first feed of a newborn who latched easily to a mother with flat, dimpled nipples: **bit.ly/BA2-BF1stHours.**

Suggest trying the starter positions during the early learning period. The feeding positions described on p. 23-29 take maximum advantage of babies' inborn feeding behaviors to make early nursing easier.

If possible, avoid artificial nipples during the first weeks. In *The Breastfeeding Atlas* (Wilson-Clay & Hoover, 2017, p. 47), authors Wilson-Clay and Hoover suggest that after the "supernormal stimulus" of bottles and pacifiers/dummies, babies whose parents have flat or inverted nipples may be more prone to nursing problems than the average baby. If possible, suggest avoiding exposure to artificial nipples during the early weeks, while baby is learning to nurse.

• • •

If the baby takes only one side, suggest feeding often from that side and continue to try the other side.

Most nursing parents have one nipple that is easier for the baby to take. If the baby takes one side well, suggest feeding often from that side and expressing milk from the unused side, while trying the following strategies when offering the unused side.

Express some milk on the nipple or in baby's mouth to entice him. If there's a helper, suggest they drip some milk near the nipple with a spoon or eyedropper, while the parent leans back and helps baby attach to that side.

Draw out the nipple on the unused side by

- ***Pulling back slightly on the tissue to help the nipple protrude*** (Figure 17.6). Rarely, it may be necessary to pull back throughout the feed at first.
- ***Nipple rolling.*** If the nipples can be grasped, suggest rolling the nipple between thumb and index finger for a minute or two and then quickly touch it with a moist, cold cloth or ice wrapped in a cloth. (Avoid prolonged ice on the nipple, as it can numb it and inhibit milk ejection.)
- ***Mammary shaping or support.*** Breast sandwich, nipple tilting, and other techniques may help the baby latch deeper to trigger active sucking. For details, see p. 884-885.
- ***Breast shells.*** These plastic devices—worn in the bra before feeds—include a dome and a snap-on backing with a small opening designed to apply pressure to the areola and draw out the nipple. If used, suggest restricting wear time to no longer than 30 minutes before a feed, as consistent pressure on the tissue increases the risk of mastitis. Also suggest using shells only if the bra cup is large enough to comfortably accommodate them. If the shells leave obvious red rings on the gland, the bra cup may be too small for safe use.

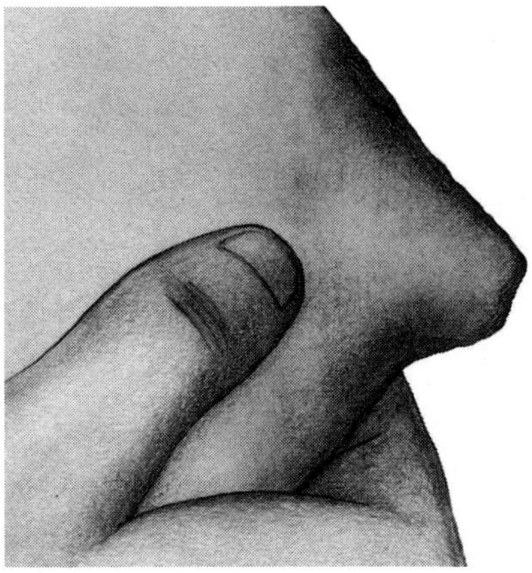

Figure 17.6 While the baby latches, try pulling back slightly on the mammary tissue to make the nipple more protruding. ©2020 Nancy Mohrbacher Solutions, Inc.

- ***Breast pump.*** Using a breast pump before nursing can soften the areola and help draw out the nipple. The suction generated by the pump pulls out the nipple uniformly from the center, which may make it easier for baby to latch.
- ***Modified syringe.*** An alternative to a commercial nipple everter is a modified disposable syringe, which is available worldwide. In one Indian study (Kesaree, Banapurmath, Banapurmath, & Shamanur, 1993), the researchers describe how to transform a 10 or 20 mL syringe (depending on nipple size) into a small suction device that can be used to draw out an inverted nipple before feeds. (For details, see p. 909-910.) These researchers followed eight mothers with inverted nipples whose babies were unable to latch and who were bottle-feeding for 28 to 103 days. After receiving positioning help and using the modified syringe for 30 to 60 seconds several times a day, seven of eight babies latched. Within 4 to 6 weeks, six of the eight women were exclusively breastfeeding. Another Indian study described the use of rubber bands that were applied to the base of the nipple with a modified syringe (Chakrabarti & Basu, 2011) to improve nursing outcomes among mothers with flat or inverted nipples. These rubber bands were left in place while the babies nursed.
- ***Commercial nipple everters.*** Along with the makeshift devices described above, commercial products are available in some areas that are specifically designed to draw out inverted nipples. A U.S. study (Boucher-Horwitz, 2011) found one product (supple cups) effective at helping women with inverted nipples overcome early nursing challenges.

• • •

Using a nipple shield may help a non-latching baby nurse directly.

If the previous strategies do not work, suggest trying a nipple shield, a flexible silicone nipple worn over the parent's nipple during feeds. A nipple shield provides a protruding nipple and has holes in the tip, so the milk flows through it while baby nurses. For details on fit, applying the shield, latching with the shield, and weaning from the shield, see p. 912-917.

• • •

If none of these strategies work, suggest expressing milk and feeding it using an alternative feeding method.

In some cases, depending on the type and degree of nipple inversion, manual expression may not be effective. In this case, a breast pump may not only express milk more effectively, it may also help draw out the nipple when the usual strategies fail. With some types of severely inverted nipples, when the baby tries to latch, rather than compressing the mammary tissue under the areola, he may compress the buried nipple instead. In this case, the baby may not receive much milk and nursing may be painful for the parent. A breast pump does not compress the areola. It provides uniform suction on the nipple, drawing the nipple out and, in some cases, stretching the fibrous tissue that holds it in.

How long pumping is necessary will depend on the type of inverted nipple and the degree of inversion. For some, one pump session is enough for the nipple to stay out. If so, the parent can start nursing on that side immediately. But more pumping may be needed. Rarely, pumping may be needed exclusively.

In some cases, after the nipple is drawn out by the pump, it may invert again when the baby pauses during nursing. If this happens, suggest a short pump session to draw out the nipple and use a feeding-tube device (e.g., a nursing supplementer, see p. 897-900) to encourage more continuous sucking as a temporary transition to exclusive nursing.

If it's necessary to pump exclusively--either for a time or indefinitely—and feed the baby in other ways, discuss pumping and feeding methods. For details on how to establish full milk production with a pump, see p. 498-507.

• • •

Depending on the type and degree of nipple inversion, some parents experience persistent nipple pain.

A true inverted nipple or dimpled nipple may cause nipple soreness, depending on its type and severity. Normal nursing may even cause trauma in some types of inverted nipples. If the nipple retracts between feeds, the skin may stay moist, contributing to chapping. If so, see the point on p. 737 about drying the nipple after feeds.

Some nursing parents experience nipple pain for about 2 weeks, as their baby's sucking gradually draws out their nipples. Others have persistent sore nipples for a longer time. Sometimes, instead of stretching, the fibrous tissue that inverts the nipple remains tight, creating a point of stress that can cause cracks or blisters. When the nipple can be drawn into the back of the baby's mouth and the baby begins nursing effectively, many are able to nurse without discomfort. Rarely, some nursing parents continue to feel some discomfort even after the baby begins nursing well, because the nipple underwent a radical change. In this case, suggest the comfort measures on p. 718.

Less Common Nipple Types

Some nursing parents have extra nipples and mammary glands.

Between 0.2% and 6% of all people have extra mammary tissue and/or nipples (also called ***accessory*** or ***supernumerary nipples***), although they are more common among women (Loukas, Clarke, & Tubbs, 2007). These extra glands and nipples are remnants from the embryonic development of the mammary ridge (Wambach & Genna, 2021, p. 54). Some extra glands are mammary tissue with no nipples; some are nipples with no mammary tissue. Some have ducts that leak milk through the skin without a nipple (Wilson-Clay & Hoover, 2017, p. 68). For more details, along with comfort measures after birth when needed, see p. 784.

• • •

When two nipples emerge from one areola, this is called a double or bifurcated nipple.

If the nursing parent has two nipples in their areola (known as a ***double*** or ***bifurcated nipple***), this should not affect nursing, as long as they are close enough together that the baby can latch to both nipples at the same time. Positioning adjustments may make this easier (Wilson-Clay & Hoover, 2017, p. 75). When pumping, ideally, the nipple tunnel would be large enough to comfortably accommodate both nipples during pumping.

• • •

In rare cases, a nipple may have no nipple pores, making milk flow impossible.

In the textbook, *Breastfeeding and Human Lactation* (Wambach, 2021, pp. 282-283), the author reported the experiences of two women who were born with one breast missing nipple pores and ducts leading to the nipple. In both cases, during the third month of pregnancy the affected breast became abnormally enlarged. After birth, that breast became severely engorged. Ultrasound revealed the missing ducts and pores.

Pierced Nipples

Mothers with pierced nipples have successfully nursed.

Over the years, nipple piercing has become more common (Sadove & Clayman, 2008). One U.K. study of more than 10,000 people, aged 16 and older (Bone, Ncube, Nichols, & Noah, 2008) found that 10% (1,934) had body piercings other than the earlobe. Of these, 9% (143) had nipple piercings, with twice as many men as women and most in the 16-to-24 age group.

The literature includes several examples of parents successfully nursing with pierced nipples (Wilson-Clay & Hoover, 2017, pp. 75, 181). One case report describes a mother who removed the ring from one of her nipples after birth and breastfed from one breast only (Lee, 1995).

• • •

Possible nursing complications from nipple piercing include altered nipple sensation, milk flow problems, and mastitis.

After a nipple piercing occurs, healing usually takes 6 to 12 months, and there is a 10% to 20% increased risk of mastitis unrelated to lactation (V. R. Jacobs, Golombeck, Jonat, & Kiechle, 2003). In a review of 12 cases of infection and one case of abscess (Bengualid, Singh, Singh, & Berger, 2008), the authors noted that all infections occurred between 3 and 9 months after the piercing. In the U.K. study described in the previous point, 38% had complications after a nipple piercing, with swelling, infection, and bleeding the most common. About 25% saw a healthcare provider as a result of the complications, with 1 in 100 hospitalized.

In a 2009 letter to the editor of the *Journal of the American Medical Association* (Garbin, Deacon, Rowan, Hartmann, & Geddes, 2009), Australian lactation consultant Cathy Garbin and members of her research team described three cases of low milk production in women with a history of nipple piercing. The researchers attributed the low milk production to scar tissue blocking the milk ducts.

Ask nursing parents with pierced nipples:

- Were there any complications from the nipple piercing?
- Do they remove the nipple jewelry before nursing?
- Are their nipples either numb or hypersensitive?
- Is there any obvious scarring on the nipples? If so, where?
- How much weight has the baby gained?
- Have they seen any nipple discharge other than milk?

Numbness of the nipples may affect milk ejection during nursing and pumping. The nursing baby's healthy weight gain rules out these potential problems. Hypersensitivity could make nursing painful. Scarring could affect milk flow. Encourage all parents to remove their nipple jewelry before nursing to prevent choking. If parents are concerned about their nipple piercing closing before the baby weans, suggest using temporary jewelry to keep it open (Martin, 2004).

RESOURCES

bfmed.org/protocols—Free, downloadable fully referenced protocols in multiple languages are ideal for sharing with healthcare providers from the Academy of Breastfeeding Medicine:

- #26 Persistent pain with breastfeeding

Wilson-Clay, B. and Hoover, K. (2017). *The Breastfeeding Atlas,* 6th edition. LactNews Press: Manchaca, TX. A treasure-trove of clinical photos showing common and unusual nipple issues, including anatomical variations, clinical conditions, and strategies.

REFERENCES

Abou-Dakn, M., Fluhr, J. W., Gensch, M., et al. (2011). Positive effect of HPA lanolin versus expressed breastmilk on painful and damaged nipples during lactation. *Skin Pharmacology and Physiology, 24*(1), 27-35.

Aeling, J. L., Panagotacos, P. J., & Andreozzi, R. J. (1973). Letter: Allergic contact dermatitis to vitamin E aerosol deodorant. *Archives of Dermatology, 108*(4), 579-580.

Agarwal, R., Maharana, P. K., Titiyal, J. S., et al. (2019). Bilateral herpes simplex keratitis: Lactation a trigger for recurrence! *BMJ Case Reports, 12*(3).

Alexander, J. M., Grant, A. M., & Campbell, M. J. (1992). Randomised controlled trial of breast shells and Hoffman's exercises for inverted and non-protractile nipples. *British Medical Journal, 304*(6833), 1030-1032.

Amir, L. (1993). Eczema of the nipple and breast: A case report. *Journal of Human Lactation, 9*(3), 173-175.

Amir, L. (2004). Test your knowledge. Nipple pain in breastfeeding. *Australian Family Physician, 33*(1-2), 44-45.

Amir, L., & Hoover, K. (2002). Candidiasis and breastfeeding. Schaumburg, IL: La Leche League International.

Amir, L. H., & Academy of Breastfeeding Medicine Protocol, C. (2014). ABM Clinical Protocol #4: Mastitis, revised March 2014. *Breastfeeding Medicine, 9*(5), 239-243.

Amir, L. H., Dennerstein, L., Garland, S. M., et al. (1996). Psychological aspects of nipple pain in lactating women. *Journal of Psychosomatic Obstetrics and Gynaecology, 17*(1), 53-58.

Amir, L. H., Dennerstein, L., Garland, S. M., et al. (1997). Psychological aspects of nipple pain in lactating women. *Breastfeeding Review, 5*, 29-32.

Amir, L. H., Donath, S. M., Garland, S. M., et al. (2013). Does Candida and/or Staphylococcus play a role in nipple and breast pain in lactation? A cohort study in Melbourne, Australia. *BMJ Open, 3*(3).

Amir, L. H., Garland, S. M., Dennerstein, L., et al. (1996). Candida albicans: Is it associated with nipple pain in lactating women? *Gynecologic and Obstetric Investigation, 41*(1), 30-34.

Amir, L. H., Jones, L. E., & Buck, M. L. (2015). Nipple pain associated with breastfeeding: Incorporating current neurophysiology into clinical reasoning. *Australian Family Physician, 44*(3), 127-132.

Anderson, J. E., Held, N., & Wright, K. (2004). Raynaud's phenomenon of the nipple: A treatable cause of painful breastfeeding. *Pediatrics, 113*(4), e360-364.

Avila-Vega, J., Urrea-Mendoza, E., & Lee, C. (2019). Raynaud's phenomenon of the nipple as a side-effect of labetalol: Case report and literature review. *Case Reports in Women's Health, 23*, e00135.

Barankin, B., & Gross, M. S. (2004). Nipple and areolar eczema in the breastfeeding woman. *Journal of Cutaneous Medicine and Surgery, 8*(2), 126-130.

Beam, J. W. (2009). Topical silver for infected wounds. *Journal of Athletic Training, 44*(5), 531-533.

Bengualid, V., Singh, V., Singh, H., et al. (2008). Mycobacterium fortuitum and anaerobic breast abscess following nipple piercing: Case presentation and review of the literature. *Journal of Adolescent Health, 42*(5), 530-532.

Berens, P., Eglash, A., Malloy, M., et al. (2016). ABM Clinical Protocol #26: Persistent pain with breastfeeding. *Breastfeeding Medicine, 11*(2), 46-53.

Boere-Boonekamp, M. M., & van der Linden-Kuiper, L. L. (2001). Positional preference: Prevalence in infants and follow-up after two years. *Pediatrics, 107*(2), 339-343.

Bone, A., Ncube, F., Nichols, T., et al. (2008). Body piercing in England: A survey of piercing at sites other than earlobe. *British Medical Journal, 336*(7658), 1426-1428.

Boucher-Horwitz, J. (2011). The use of supple cups for flat, retracting, and inverted nipples. *Clinical Lactation, 2*(3), 30-33.

Brent, N. B. (2001). Thrush in the breastfeeding dyad: Results of a survey on diagnosis and treatment. *Clinical Pediatrics (Philadelphia), 40*(9), 503-506.

Buck, M. L., Amir, L. H., Cullinane, M., et al. (2014). Nipple pain, damage, and vasospasm in the first 8 weeks postpartum. *Breastfeeding Medicine, 9*(2), 56-62.

Buck, M. L., Amir, L. H., & Donath, S. M. (2015). Topical treatments used by breastfeeding women to treat sore and damaged nipples. *Clinical Lactation, 6*(1), 16-23.

Buck, M. L., Eckereder, G., & Amir, L. H. (2016). Low level laster therapy for breastfeeding problems. *Breastfeeding Review, 24*(2), 27-31.

Camargo, B. T. S., Coca, K. P., Amir, L. H., et al. (2019). The effect of a single irradiation of low-level laser on nipple pain in breastfeeding women: A randomized controlled trial. *Lasers in Medical Science.* doi:-5.

Campos, T. M., Dos Santos Traverzim, M. A., Sobral, A. P. T., et al. (2018). Effect of LED therapy for the treatment nipple fissures: Study protocol for a randomized controlled trial. *Medicine (Baltimore), 97*(41), e12322.

Centuori, S., Burmaz, T., Ronfani, L., et al. (1999). Nipple care, sore nipples, and breastfeeding: A randomized trial. *Journal of Human Lactation, 15*(2), 125-130.

Chakrabarti, K., & Basu, S. (2011). Management of flat or inverted nipples with simple rubber bands. *Breastfeeding Medicine, 6*(4), 215-219.

Chandler, P. J., Jr., & Hill, S. D. (1990). A direct surgical approach to correct the inverted nipple. *Plastic and Reconstructive Surgery, 86*(2), 352-354.

Chanprapaph, P., Luttarapakul, J., Siribariruck, S., et al. (2013). Outcome of non-protractile nipple correction with breast cups in pregnant women: A randomized controlled trial. *Breastfeeding Medicine, 8*(4), 408-412.

Chaves, M. E., Araujo, A. R., Santos, S. F., et al. (2012). LED phototherapy improves healing of nipple trauma: A pilot study. *Photomed Laser Surg, 30*(3), 172-178.

Chen, C. Y., Sun, L. M., & Anderson, B. O. (2006). Paget disease of the breast: Changing patterns of incidence, clinical presentation, and treatment in the U.S. *Cancer, 107*(7), 1448-1458.

Chetwynd, E. M., Ives, T. J., Payne, P. M., et al. (2002). Fluconazole for postpartum candidal mastitis and infant thrush. *Journal of Human Lactation, 18*(2), 168-171.

Coca, K. P., Amir, L. H., Alves, M., et al. (2019). Measurement tools and intensity of nipple pain among women with or without damaged nipples: A quantitative systematic review. *Journal of Advanced Nursing, 75*(6), 1162-1172.

Coca, K. P., Marcacine, K. O., Gamba, M. A., et al. (2016). Efficacy of low-level laser therapy in relieving nipple pain in breastfeeding women: A triple-blind, randomized, controlled trial. *Pain Management in Nursing, 17*(4), 281-289.

Colson, S. (2019). *Biological Nurturing: Instinctual Breastfeeding* (2nd ed.). Amarillo, TX: Praeclarus Press.

Colson, S. D., Meek, J. H., & Hawdon, J. M. (2008). Optimal positions for the release of primitive neonatal reflexes stimulating breastfeeding. *Early Human Development, 84*(7), 441-449.

Cooper, S. M., & Shaw, S. (1999). Contact allergy to nystatin: An unusual allergen. *Contact Dermatitis, 41*(2), 120.

Cordero, M. J., Villar, N. M., Barrilao, R. G., et al. (2015). Application of extra virgin olive oil to prevent nipple cracking in lactating women. *Worldviews on Evidence-Based Nursing, 12*(6), 364-369.

D'Andrea, M. A., & Spatz, D. L. (2019). Maintaining breastfeeding during severe infant and maternal HSV-1 infection: A case report. *Journal of Human Lactation, 35*(4), 737-741.

Danby, S. G., AlEnezi, T., Sultan, A., et al. (2013). Effect of olive and sunflower seed oil on the adult skin barrier: Implications for neonatal skin care. *Pediatric Dermatology, 30*(1), 42-50.

Darmangeat, V. (2011). The frequency and resolution of nipple pain when latch is improved in a private practice. *Clinical Lactation, 2*(3), 22-24.

de Sousa, A. P., Santos, J. N., Dos Reis, J. A., Jr., et al. (2010). Effect of LED phototherapy of three distinct wavelengths on fibroblasts on wound healing: A histological study in a rodent model. *Photomedicine and Laser Surgery, 28*(4), 547-552.

Dennis, C. L., Jackson, K., & Watson, J. (2014). Interventions for treating painful nipples among breastfeeding women. *Cochrane Database of Systematic Reviews, 12*, Cd007366. doi:10.1002/14651858.CD007366.pub2

Dennis, C. L., Schottle, N., Hodnett, E., et al. (2012). An all-purpose nipple ointment versus lanolin in treating painful damaged nipples in breastfeeding women: A randomized controlled trial. *Breastfeeding Medicine, 7*(6), 473-479.

Dewey, K. G., Nommsen-Rivers, L. A., Heinig, M. J., et al. (2003). Risk factors for suboptimal infant breastfeeding behavior, delayed onset of lactation, and excess neonatal weight loss. *Pediatrics, 112*(3 Pt 1), 607-619.

Donato-Trancoso, A., Monte-Alto-Costa, A., & Romana-Souza, B. (2016). Olive oil-induced reduction of oxidative damage and inflammation promotes wound healing of pressure ulcers in mice. *Journal of Dermatological Science, 83*(1), 60-69.

Douglas, P., & Geddes, D. (2018). Practice-based interpretation of ultrasound studies leads the way to more effective clinical support and less pharmaceutical and surgical intervention for breastfeeding infants. *Midwifery, 58*, 145-155.

Duff, M. (1998). Paget's disease of the nipple: A 14 year experience. *Irish Medical Journal, 91*(4), 1-5.

Eglash, A. (1998). Delayed milk ejection reflex and plugged ducts: Lecithin therapy. *ABM News and Views, 3*(1), 4.

Eglash, A., Plane, M. B., & Mundt, M. (2006). History, physical and laboratory findings, and clinical outcomes of lactating women treated with antibiotics for chronic breast and/or nipple pain. *Journal of Human Lactation, 22*(4), 429-433.

Eglash, A., Simon, L., & Academy of Breastfeeding, M. (2017). ABM Clinical Protocol #8: Human milk storage information for home use for full-term infants, revised 2017. *Breastfeeding Medicine, 12*(7), 390-395.

Elad, D., Kozlovsky, P., Blum, O., et al. (2014). Biomechanics of milk extraction during breast-feeding. *Proceedings of the National Academy of Sciences of the USA, 111*(14), 5230-5235.

Feenstra, M. M., Jorgine Kirkeby, M., Thygesen, M., et al. (2018). Early breastfeeding problems: A mixed method study of mothers' experiences. *Sexual & Reproductive Healthcare, 16,* 167-174.

Fernandez, L., Mediano, P., Garcia, R., et al. (2016). Risk factors predicting infectious lactational mastitis: Decision tree approach versus logistic regression analysis. *Maternal and Child Health Journal, 20*(9), 1895-1903.

Fernandez, R., & Griffiths, R. (2012). Water for wound cleansing. *Cochrane Database of Systematic Reviews(2),* CD003861. doi:10.1002/14651858.CD003861.pub3

Field, S. S. (2016). Fatal neonatal herpes simplex infection likely from unrecognized breast lesions. *Journal of Human Lactation, 32*(1), 86-88.

Fisher, A. (1986). *Contact Dermatitis.* Philadelphia, PA: Lea & Febiger.

Forster, D. A., McEgan, K., Ford, R., et al. (2011). Diabetes and antenatal milk expressing: A pilot project to inform the development of a randomised controlled trial. *Midwifery, 27*(2), 209-214.

Francis-Morrill, J., Heinig, M. J., Pappagianis, D., et al. (2004). Diagnostic value of signs and symptoms of mammary candidosis among lactating women. *Journal of Human Lactation, 20*(3), 288-295; quiz 296-289.

Garbin, C. P., Deacon, J. P., Rowan, M. K., et al. (2009). Association of nipple piercing with abnormal milk production and breastfeeding. *Journal of the American Medical Assocation, 301*(24), 2550-2551.

Garrison, C. P. (2002). Nipple vasospasms, Raynaud's syndrome, and nifedipine. *Journal of Human Lactation, 18*(4), 382-385.

Genna, C. W. (2015). Breastfeeding infants with congenital torticollis. *Journal of Human Lactation, 31*(2), 216-220.

Gianni, M. L., Bettinelli, M. E., Manfra, P., et al. (2019). Breastfeeding difficulties and risk for early breastfeeding cessation. *Nutrients, 11*(10).

Girish, M., Mujawar, N., Gotmare, P., et al. (2013). Impact and feasibility of breast crawl in a tertiary care hospital. *Journal of Perinatology, 33*(4), 288-291.

Goins, R. A., Ascher, D., Waecker, N., et al. (2002). Comparison of fluconazole and nystatin oral suspensions for treatment of oral candidiasis in infants. *Pediatric Infectious Disease Journal, 21*(12), 1165-1167.

Graves, S., Wright, W., Harman, R., et al. (2003). Painful nipples in nursing mothers: Fungal or staphylococcal? A preliminary study. *Australian Family Physician, 32*(7), 570-571.

Griffiths, D. M. (2004). Do tongue ties affect breastfeeding? *Journal of Human Lactation, 20*(4), 409-414.

Gungor, A. N., Oguz, S., Vurur, G., et al. (2013). Comparison of olive oil and lanolin in the prevention of sore nipples in nursing mothers. *Breastfeeding Medicine, 8*(3), 334-335.

Hale, T. W. (2019). *Hale's Medications & Mothers' Milk: A Manual of Lactational Pharmacology* (18th ed.). New York, NY: Springer Publishing Company.

Hale, T. W., Bateman, T. L., Finkelman, M. A., et al. (2009). The absence of Candida albicans in milk samples of women with clinical symptoms of ductal candidiasis. *Breastfeeding Medicine, 4*(2), 57-61.

Hale, T. W., & Berens, P. D. (2010). *Clinical Therapy in Breastfeeding Patients.* Amarillo, TX: Hale Publishing.

Han, S., & Hong, Y. G. (1999). The inverted nipple: Its grading and surgical correction. *Plastic and Reconstructive Surgery, 104*(2), 389-395; discussion 396-387.

Harriott, M. M., & Noverr, M. C. (2009). Candida albicans and Staphylococcus aureus form polymicrobial biofilms: Effects on antimicrobial resistance. *Antimicrobial Agents and Chemotherapy, 53*(9), 3914-3922.

Heller, M. M., Fullerton-Stone, H., & Murase, J. E. (2012). Caring for new mothers: Diagnosis, management and treatment of nipple dermatitis in breastfeeding mothers. *International Journal of Dermatology, 51*(10), 1149-1161.

Hoppe, J. E. (1997). Treatment of oropharyngeal candidiasis and candidal diaper dermatitis in neonates and infants: Review and reappraisal. *Pediatric Infectious Disease Journal, 16*(9), 885-894.

Huggins, K. E., & Billon, S. F. (1993). Twenty cases of persistent sore nipples: Collaboration between lactation consultant and dermatologist. *Journal of Human Lactation, 9*(3), 155-160.

Hughes, M., & Herrick, A. L. (2016). Raynaud's phenomenon. *Best Practice and Research: Clinical Rheumatology, 30*(1), 112-132.

Jackson, K. T., & Dennis, C. L. (2017). Lanolin for the treatment of nipple pain in breastfeeding women: A randomized controlled trial. *Maternal & Child Nutrition, 13*(3).

Jackson, K. T., O'Keefe-McCarthy, S., & Mantler, T. (2019). Moving toward a better understanding of the experience and measurement of breastfeeding-related pain. *Journal of Psychosomatic Obstetrics & Gynaecology, 40*(4), 318-325.

Jacobs, L. A., Dickinson, J. E., Hart, P. D., et al. (2007). Normal nipple position in term infants measured on breastfeeding ultrasound. *Journal of Human Lactation, 23*(1), 52-59.

Jacobs, V. R., Golombeck, K., Jonat, W., et al. (2003). Mastitis nonpuerperalis after nipple piercing: Time to act. *International Journal of Fertility and Women's Medicine, 48*(5), 226-231.

Jimenez, E., Arroyo, R., Cardenas, N., et al. (2017). Mammary candidiasis: A medical condition without scientific evidence? *PLoS One, 12*(7), e0181071.

Karacam, Z., & Saglik, M. (2018). Breastfeeding problems and interventions performed on problems: Systematic review based on studies made in Turkey. *Turk Pediatri Arsivi, 53*(3), 134-148.

Kent, J. C., Ashton, E., Hardwick, C. M., et al. (2015). Nipple pain in breastfeeding mothers: Incidence, causes and treatments. *International Journal of Environmental Research and Public Health, 12*(10), 12247-12263.

Kent, J. C., Mitoulas, L. R., Cregan, M. D., et al. (2008). Importance of vacuum for breastmilk expression. *Breastfeeding Medicine, 3*(1), 11-19.

Kesaree, N., Banapurmath, C. R., Banapurmath, S., et al. (1993). Treatment of inverted nipples using a disposable syringe. *Journal of Human Lactation, 9*(1), 27-29.

Khan, T. V., & Ramirez, M. (2017). Management of common breastfeeding problems: Nipple pain and infections--A clinical review. *Clinical Lactation, 8*(4), 181-188.

Kovalyov, M. I. (2001). Dynamics of prolactin, gonadotropin, and of sex steroids in the blood serus of parturients during laster therapy. *Proceedings of SPIE, 4422,* 49-52.

Kymplova, J., Navratil, L., & Knizek, J. (2003). Contribution of phototherapy to the treatment of episiotomies. *Journal of Clinical Laser Medicine & Surgery, 21*(1), 35-39.

Lauwers, J., & Swisher, A. (2015). Breastfeeding in the early weeks. In *Counseling the Nursing Mother* (6th ed., pp. 403). Burlington, MA: Jones & Bartlett Learning.

Lavergne, N. A. (1997). Does application of tea bags to sore nipples while breastfeeding provide effective relief? *Journal of Obstetric, Gynecologic, and Neonatal Nursing, 26*(1), 53-58.

Lawrence, R. A., & Lawrence, R. M. (2016). *Breastfeeding: A Guide for the Medical Profession* (8th ed.). Philadelphia, PA: Elsevier.

Lee, N. (1995). More on pierced nipples. *Journal of Human Lactation, 11*(2), 89.

LeVan, J. (2011). Helping your baby with torticollis. *Journal of Human Lactation, 27*(4), 399-400.

Livingstone, V., & Stringer, L. J. (1999). The treatment of Staphyloccocus aureus infected sore nipples: A randomized comparative study. *Journal of Human Lactation, 15*(3), 241-246.

Livingstone, V. H., Willis, C. E., & Berkowitz, J. (1996). Staphylococcus aureus and sore nipples. *Canadian Family Physician, 42,* 654-659.

Loukas, M., Clarke, P., & Tubbs, R. S. (2007). Accessory breasts: A historical and current perspective. *American Surgeon, 73*(5), 525-528.

MAIN. (1994). Preparing for breast feeding: Treatment of inverted and non-protractile nipples in pregnancy. The MAIN Trial Collaborative Group. *Midwifery, 10*(4), 200-214.

Majra, J. P., & Silan, V. K. (2016). Barriers to early initiation and continuation of breastfeeding in a tertiary care institute of Haryana: A qualitative study in nursing care providers. *Journal of Clinical and Diagnostic Research, 10*(9), LC16-LC20.

Mariani Neto, C., de Albuquerque, R. S., de Souza, S. C., et al. (2018). Comparative study of the use of HPA lanolin and breast milk for treating pain associated with nipple trauma. *Revista Brasileira de Ginecolgia Obstetricia, 40*(11), 664-672.

Marrazzu, A., Sanna, M. G., Dessole, F., et al. (2015). Evaluation of the effectiveness of a silver-impregnated medical cap for topical treatment of nipple fissure of breastfeeding mothers. *Breastfeeding Medicine, 10*(5), 232-238.

Martin, J. (2004). Is nipple piercing compatible with breastfeeding? *Journal of Human Lactation, 20*(3), 319-321.

Marx, C. M., Izquierdo, A., Driscoll, J. W., et al. (1985). Vitamin E concentrations in serum of newborn infants after topical use of vitamin E by nursing mothers. *American Journal of Obstetrics and Gynecology, 152*(6 Pt 1), 668-670.

McClellan, H., Geddes, D., Kent, J., et al. (2008). Infants of mothers with persistent nipple pain exert strong sucking vacuums. *Acta Paediatrica, 97*(9), 1205-1209.

McClellan, H. L., Hepworth, A. R., Garbin, C. P., et al. (2012). Nipple pain during breastfeeding with or without visible trauma. *Journal of Human Lactation, 28*(4), 511-521.

McClellan, H. L., Hepworth, A. R., Kent, J. C., et al. (2012). Breastfeeding frequency, milk volume, and duration in mother-infant dyads with persistent nipple pain. *Breastfeeding Medicine, 7,* 275-281.

McClellan, H. L., Kent, J. C., Hepworth, A. R., et al. (2015). Persistent nipple pain in breastfeeding mothers associated with abnormal infant tongue movement. *International Journal of Environmental Research and Public Health, 12*(9), 10833-10845.

Mitchell, K. B., Eglash, A., & Bamberger, E. T. (2019). Mammary dysbiosis and nipple blebs treated with intravenous daptomycin and dalbavancin. *Journal of Human Lactation.* doi:10.1177/0890334419862214.

Mohrbacher, N., & Kendall-Tackett, K. (2010). *Breastfeeding Made Simple: Seven Natural Laws for Nursing Mothers* (2nd ed.). Oakland, CA: New Harbinger Publications.

Mojab, C. G. (2007). Congenital torticollis in the nursling. *Journal of Human Lactation, 23*(1), 12.

Mokmeli, S., Khazemikho, N., Niromanesh, S., et al. (2009). The application of low-level laser therapy after cesarean section does not compromise blood prolactin levels and lactation status. *Photomedicine and Laser Surgery, 27*(3), 509-512.

Moore, E. R., & Anderson, G. C. (2007). Randomized controlled trial of very early mother-infant skin-to-skin contact and breastfeeding status. *Journal of Midwifery & Women's Health, 52*(2), 116-125.

Moorhead, A. M., Amir, L. H., O'Brien, P. W., et al. (2011). A prospective study of fluconazole treatment for breast and nipple thrush. *Breastfeeding Review, 19*(3), 25-29.

Morrill, J. F., Heinig, M. J., Pappagianis, D., et al. (2005). Risk factors for mammary candidosis among lactating women. *Journal of Obstetric, Gynecologic & Neonatal Nursing, 34*(1), 37-45.

Nevin, K. G., & Rajamohan, T. (2010). Effect of topical application of virgin coconut oil on skin components and antioxidant status during dermal wound healing in young rats. *Skin Pharmacology and Physiology, 23*(6), 290-297.

Niazi, A., Rahimi, V. B., Soheili-Far, S., et al. (2018). A systematic review on prevention and treatment of nipple pain and fissure: Are they curable? *Journal of Pharmacopuncture, 21*(3), 139-150.

Noble, R. (1991). Milk under the skin (milk blister)--A simple problem causing other breast conditions. *Breastfeeding Review, 2*(3), 118-119.

O'Hara, M. A. (2012). Bleb histology reveals inflammatory infiltrate that regresses with topical steroid: A case series [abstract]. *Breastfeeding Medicine, 7*(Supplement 1), S2-S17.

Odom, E. C., Li, R., Scanlon, K. S., et al. (2013). Reasons for earlier than desired cessation of breastfeeding. *Pediatrics, 131*(3), e726-732.

Porter, J., & Schach, B. (2004). Treating sore, possibly infected nipples. *Journal of Human Lactation, 20*(2), 221-222.

Power, R. F., & Murphy, J. F. (2015). Tongue-tie and frenotomy in infants with breastfeeding difficulties: Achieving a balance. *Archives of Disease in Childhood, 100*(5), 489-494.

Prime, D. K., Geddes, D. T., & Hartmann, P. E. (2007). Oxytocin: Milk ejection and maternal-infant well-being. In T. W. a. H. Hale, P.E. (Ed.), *Hale & Hartmann's Textbook of Human Lactation.* Amarillo, TX: Hale Publishing.

Puapornpong, P., Paritakul, P., Suksamarnwong, M., et al. (2017). Nipple pain incidence, the predisposing factors, the recovery period after care management, and the exclusive breastfeeding outcome. *Breastfeeding Medicine, 12,* 169-173.

Ramsay, D. T., Mitoulas, L. R., Kent, J. C., et al. (2006). Milk flow rates can be used to identify and investigate milk ejection in women expressing breast milk using an electric breast pump. *Breastfeeding Medicine, 1*(1), 14-23.

Righard, L. (1998). Are breastfeeding problems related to incorrect breastfeeding technique and the use of pacifiers and bottles? *Birth, 25*(1), 40-44.

Righard, L., & Alade, M. O. (1997). Breastfeeding and the use of pacifiers. *Birth, 24*(2), 116-120.

Rosa, C. A., Novak, F. R., de Almeida, J. A., et al. (1990). Yeasts from human milk collected in Rio de Janeiro, Brazil. *Revista de Microbiologia, 21*(4), 361-363.

Ryan, T. J. (2007). Infection following soft tissue injury: Its role in wound healing. *Current Opinions in Infectious Diseases, 20*(2), 124-128.

Sadove, R., & Clayman, M. A. (2008). Surgical procedure for reversal of nipple piercing. *Aesthetic Plastic Surgery, 32*(3), 563-565.

Sealander, J. Y., & Kerr, C. P. (1989). Herpes simplex of the nipple: Infant-to-mother transmission. *American Family Physician, 39*(3), 111-113.

Smith, L. (2021). Postpartum care. In K. Wambach & B. Spencer (Eds.), *Breastfeeding and Human Lactation* (6th ed., pp. 247-280). Burlington, MA: Jones and Bartlett Learning.

Snyder, J. (1997). *Variations in Infant Palatal Structure and Breastfeeding.* Encino, CA: Lactation Institute.

Stringer, T., & Femia, A. N. (2018). Raynaud's phenomenon: Current concepts. *Clinical Dermatology, 36*(4), 498-507.

Strong, G. D., & Mele, N. (2013). Raynaud's phenomenon, candidiasis, and nipple pain: Strategies for differential diagnosis and care. *Clinical Lactation, 4*(1), 21-17.

Sullivan-Bolyai, J. Z., Fife, K. H., Jacobs, R. F., et al. (1983). Disseminated neonatal herpes simplex virus type 1 from a maternal breast lesion. *Pediatrics, 71*(3), 455-457.

Terrill, P. J., & Stapleton, M. J. (1991). The inverted nipple: To cut the ducts or not? *British Journal of Plastic Surgery, 44*(5), 372-377.

Thomassen, P., Johansson, V. A., Wassberg, C., et al. (1998). Breast-feeding, pain and infection. *Gynecologic and Obstetric Investigation, 46*(2), 73-74.

Thorley, V. (2000). Impetigo on the areola and nipple. *Breastfeeding Review, 8*(2), 25-26.

Wagner, E. A., Chantry, C. J., Dewey, K. G., et al. (2013). Breastfeeding concerns at 3 and 7 days postpartum and feeding status at 2 months. *Pediatrics, 132*(4), e865-875.

Walker, M. (2017). *Breastfeeding Management for the Clinician: Using the Evidence* (4th ed.). Burlington, MA: Jones & Bartlett Learning.

Walker, M. (2019). Novel innovations and recent findings in lactation support. *Clinical Lactation, 10*(4), 175-182.

Wall, V., & Glass, R. (2006). Mandibular asymmetry and breastfeeding problems: Experience from 11 cases. *Journal of Human Lactation, 22*(3), 328-334.

Wambach, K. (2021). Breast-related problems. In K. Wambach & B. Spencer (Eds.), *Breastfeeding and Human Lactation* (6th ed., pp. 281-312). Burlington, MA: Jones & Bartlett Learning.

Wambach, K., & Genna, C. W. (2021). Anatomy and physiology of lactation. In K. Wambach & B. Spencer (Eds.), *Breastfeeding and Human Lactation* (6th ed., pp. 49-83). Burlington, MA: Jones & Bartlett Learning.

Watkins, S., Meltzer-Brody, S., Zolnoun, D., et al. (2011). Early breastfeeding experiences and postpartum depression. *Obstetrics & Gynecology, 118*(2 Pt 1), 214-221.

Wiener, S. (2006). Diagnosis and management of Candida of the nipple and breast. *Journal of Midwifery & Women's Health, 51*(2), 125-128.

Wilson-Clay, B., & Hoover, K. (2017). *The Breastfeeding Atlas* (6th ed.). Manchaca, TX: LactNews Press.

Witt, A., Mason, M. J., Burgess, K., et al. (2014). A case control study of bacterial species and colony count in milk of breastfeeding women with chronic pain. *Breastfeeding Medicine, 9*(1), 29-34.

Witt, A. M., Burgess, K., Hawn, T. R., et al. (2014). Role of oral antibiotics in treatment of breastfeeding women with chronic breast pain who fail conservative therapy. *Breastfeeding Medicine, 9*(2), 63-72.

Wolf, L., & Glass, R. (1992). *Feeding and Swallowing Disorders in Infancy.* Tucson, AZ: Therapy Skill Builders.

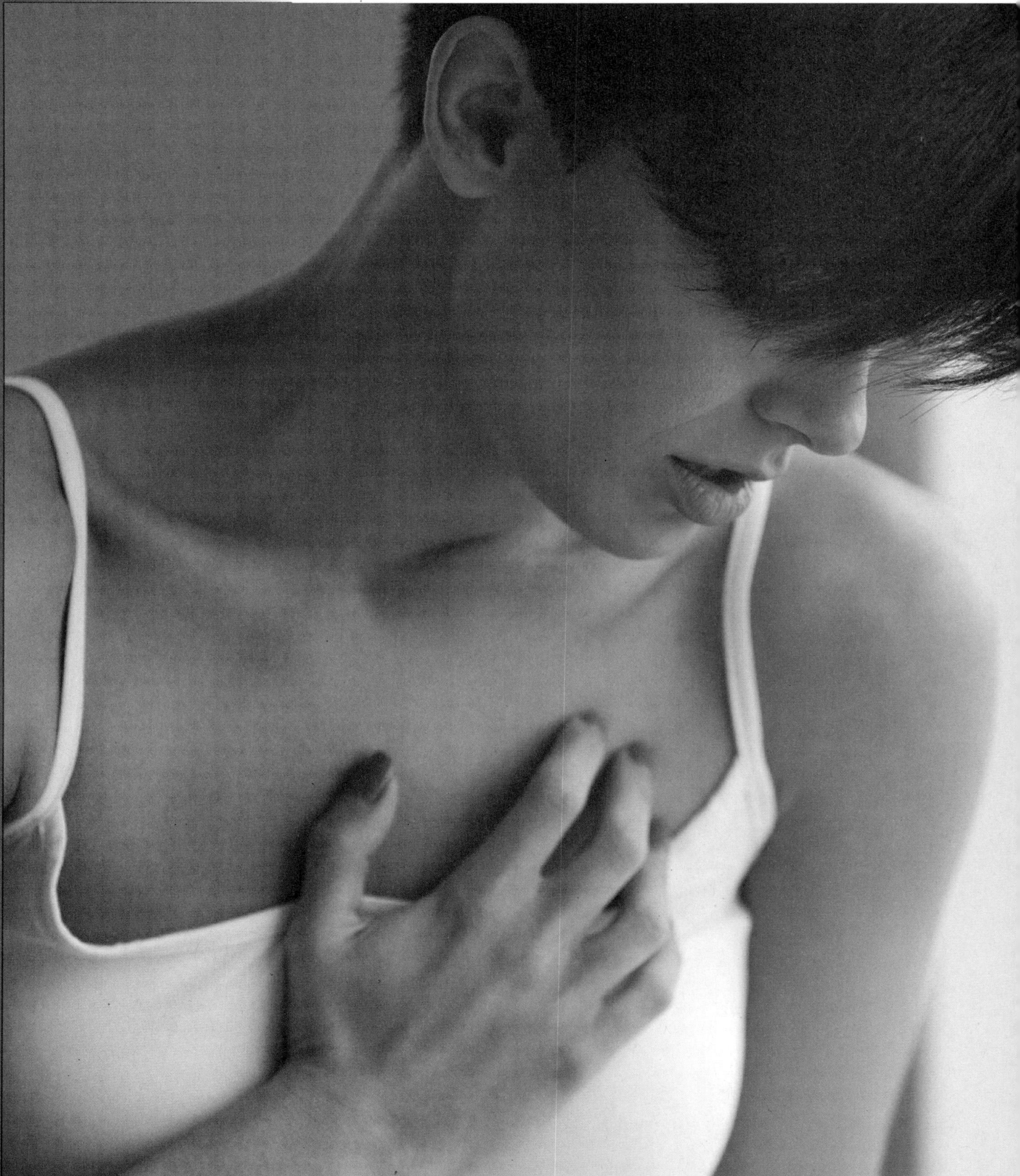

Breast or Chest Issues

18

ENGORGEMENT

As milk production increases after birth, most nursing parents feel some mammary fullness or engorgement, which usually subsides within a few days.

Between the 2nd and 6th day after birth, the mammary glands usually begin to feel tender, larger, and heavier. These sensations are caused by an increasing production of milk, as well as an increased flow to the glands of blood and lymph, which play a role in milk production. If the baby latches deeply and removes colostrum early, often, and effectively, these extra fluids will drain easily from the glands. Within the next few weeks as milk production is established and the hormones of childbirth decrease to lower levels, the mammary glands begin to feel softer most of the time, even with abundant milk production.

Causes of engorgement. After birth, some mammary fullness or engorgement is considered "physiologic," or normal. At this writing, as milk production increases, no standardized method exists that can distinguish normal mammary fullness from engorgement (P. Berens & Brodribb, 2016). The difference is a matter of degree. If milk is removed early, often, and effectively by the baby or by milk expression, normal fullness is less likely to become painful engorgement (Alekseev, Vladimir, & Nadezhda, 2015; Moon & Humenick, 1989). But if nursing is delayed or the baby nurses infrequently or ineffectively and the glands stay full of milk for too long (sometimes called ***milk stasis***), blood circulation slows.

KEY CONCEPT

Infrequent or ineffective nursing can lead to engorgement.

Symptoms of engorgement. As pressure builds in the gland, the spaces between the milk-producing cells open and proteins from the blood and milk seep into the mammary tissues, causing swelling (C. Fetherston, 2001). This swelling can cause discomfort, warmth, and throbbing, which may extend into the armpit area, where some milk-producing glands (called the ***tail of Spence***) are located. The skin on the glands may appear taut and shiny. When pressure builds inside the gland, as discussed in Chapter 10, "Making Milk," this causes milk production to slow. If pressure keeps building, eventually continued pressure will cause the milk-making cells (mammary epithelial cells, also known as lactocytes) to shut down operations entirely and over time self-destruct (a process called ***apoptosis***). Engorgement may also cause a fever of up to 101ºF/38.3ºC which is sometimes confused with a post-delivery infection, resulting in unnecessary separation of the nursing couple.

Types of engorgement. Engorgement may occur only in the areola (***areolar engorgement***), only in other areas (***peripheral engorgement***), or in both. It may also occur in one or both glands.

• • •

Excess IV fluids given during labor can aggravate and prolong engorgement.

Within the first 48 hours of giving birth, if swelling (known as ***edema***) occurs in the mammary tissue (and ankles)—even before the milk increases—excess IV fluids given during labor may be the cause.

Sometimes laboring parents receive excess IV fluids (Noel-Weiss, Woodend, & Groll, 2011). This may happen when more is given than ordered by their healthcare provider (G. Gonik & Cotton, 1984). Also, one type of commonly used IV fluid (crystalloid) both adds to the body's fluid load and reduces the ability to process excess fluid, extending the amount of time it takes for swelling to resolve. If a parent with this type of tissue swelling also becomes engorged, this dynamic can delay the resolution of engorgement for up to 10 to 14 days (Cotterman, 2004; G. Gonik, Cotton, D.B., 1984; Park, Hauch, Curlin, Datta, & Bader, 1996).

A 2015 Canadian prospective, longitudinal cohort study of first-time mothers of a healthy term baby (Kujawa-Myles, Noel-Weiss, Dunn, Peterson, & Cotterman, 2015) found that the mothers who received IV fluids during labor had more breast swelling than those who didn't receive IV fluids during labor.

• • •

Frequent nursing removes colostrum and later milk, which allows the extra blood and lymph to drain more easily from the mammary glands. Effective milk removal makes fullness less likely to become painful engorgement (Alekseev et al., 2015; Moon & Humenick, 1989).

To help prevent or minimize engorgement, keep the nursing couple together after birth and encourage early, frequent, and long nursing sessions and express colostrum after nursing.

Early nursing patterns. With unrestricted access to nursing, a newborn may feed often for short periods, such as a few minutes every hour, or for long stretches, even hours at a time, until the milk becomes more abundant, or "comes in" (Benson, 2001). When a baby's inborn feeding reflexes are triggered, she can even feed effectively while in a light sleep (Colson, 2019; Colson, DeRooy, & Hawdon, 2003). If the baby sleeps for long stretches, encourage parents to keep the baby on their body or nearby and guide her to the nipple whenever she shows feeding behaviors. This helps relieve fullness while providing the milk the baby needs.

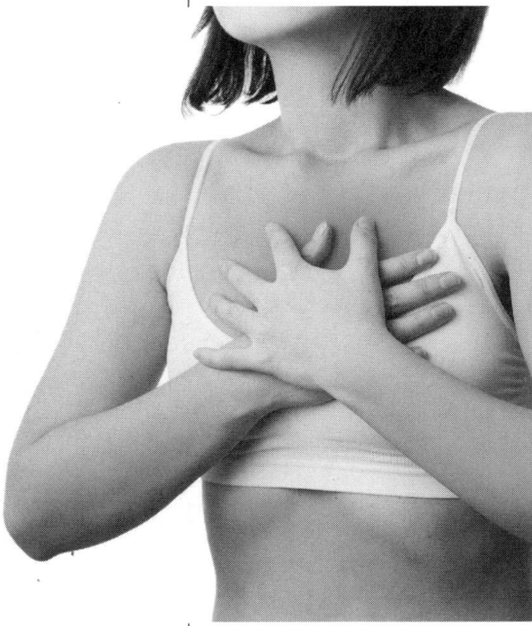

Finish the first side first and alternate the starting side. One Australian study of 152 mothers and babies (Evans, Evans, & Simmer, 1995) found that when babies breastfed from one breast for as long as they wanted before taking the second side, their mothers experienced significantly less engorgement than those who were told to be sure their babies took both sides per feed. A 2016 U.S. study (Witt, Bolman, Kredit, & Vanic, 2016) found that alternating which side the baby nursed from first also reduced the incidence of engorgement.

Another U.S. study of 54 women (Moon & Humenick, 1989) found that more mothers became engorged when they followed hospital instructions to restrict their baby's early feeding time. In other words, the more minutes spent at each breast during early nursing, the less engorgement they experienced later. Limiting early feeding times was common advice during the 1980s when it was erroneously thought to reduce early nipple pain.

Express colostrum after nursing at least twice a day. A 2015 Russian study of 146 women—70 with severe engorgement and 76 controls (Alekseev et al., 2015)— found that when its study mothers expressed colostrum for 20 to 25 minutes at least once or twice per day during the first 2 to 3 days after birth, this effectively prevented severe engorgement from developing. Although the study mothers used a breast pump to express their colostrum, another option is to use hand expression. U.S. pediatrician Jane Morton (J. Morton, 2019) created the website **firstdroplets.com** to encourage new parents to learn hand expression during the last month of pregnancy (see p. 474 for research on its safety) and use this technique after birth to feed their newborn the expressed colostrum by spoon after nursing to prevent excess weight loss. This website features demonstration videos on hand expression.

• • •

Engorgement may manifest differently in different parents and in the same parent with the first and subsequent babies.

One U.S. study (Hill & Humenick, 1994) found that mothers who nursed previous babies became engorged sooner and more severely than first-time nursing mothers. A study done in Russia by Swedish, Canadian, and Russian researchers (Bystrova et al., 2007) also found that engorgement was significantly more pronounced and occurred earlier among those who gave birth previously. A 2015 Russian study (Alekseev et al., 2015) noted that 90% of its 70 severely engorged mothers also previously experienced severe breast engorgement just before menstruation began.

With hospital discharge occurring in most places during the first few days after delivery, when engorgement occurs, it usually happens at home, complicating early nursing (Johansson, Fenwick, & Thies-Lagergren, 2019). A 2016 prospective study of 73 engorged mothers who were seen at a U.S. lactation practice (Witt, Bolman, Kredit, et al., 2016) found that on average, engorgement peaked at around 5 days and with effective treatment (see later point) lasted an average of 4 days.

• • •

If a parent reports feeling engorged, ask for more information.

Questions to ask an engorged parent include:

- **Baby's age.** Engorgement usually starts 3 to 6 days after birth. If the baby is older than about 2 weeks, mammary fullness may occur from missed or delayed feeds or from other causes such as mastitis (P. Berens & Brodribb, 2016).
- **How often and long they nurse.** If the baby is not nursing often or falls asleep quickly during feeds, this may intensify engorgement.
- **How the mammary glands feel.** Is the skin on the mammary glands soft and elastic or stretched tight? Does the areola feel soft and elastic like an earlobe or hard like the tip of a nose? If the areola is soft and elastic, the techniques described in a later point to soften the areola before nursing may not be helpful. If the areola is hard, these techniques may help the baby get a deeper latch.

• • •

When it occurs, engorgement should be treated as soon as possible to reduce discomfort and prevent complications.

By treating engorgement promptly, its most extreme symptoms can usually be prevented or resolved within 12 to 48 hours. However, if engorgement is not treated promptly, it can take up to 7 to 14 days or longer for symptoms to resolve (Humenick, Hill, & Anderson, 1994).

Because taut mammary tissue makes getting a deep latch more difficult, possible complications of engorgement include:

- Feeding problems and weight gain issues in baby
- Nipple pain and trauma
- Mastitis

In extreme cases, unrelieved pressure can damage the milk-making tissue, which may compromise long-term milk production (Wilson-Clay & Hoover, 2017, p. 86).

If a parent has a history of breast or chest surgery or injury, sections of the mammary gland may not drain at all. If so, mention that milk ducts that are no longer connected to the nipple are unlikely to increase the risk of mastitis, because they are not exposed to outside organisms. Like parents who do not nurse after birth, those areas will quickly stop producing milk and revert to their prepregnancy state. For details, see the later section of this chapter "Breast or Chest Surgery or Injury."

• • •

Basic strategies to treat engorgement reduce swelling and pain and help drain the milk more often and/or more fully.

Any strategies that more fully drain the milk and reduce swelling will help resolve engorgement more quickly. Encourage families to use any of the following basic strategies that are soothing and work well for them (Westerfield, Koenig, & Oh, 2018).

Nurse often and long with a deep latch. Suggest nursing as often as the baby is willing, at least every couple of hours or more often if baby shows interest. Allow the baby to "finish the first side first," which means letting baby stay on one side until she comes off on her own, rather than trying to drain both sides equally (Evans et al., 1995). Also suggest alternating which side baby takes first at each feed (Witt, Bolman, Kredit, et al., 2016).

After nursing, if still feeling full, express milk. Some parents are told they should not express milk, because it will increase their milk production and worsen their engorgement. However, the opposite is true. Draining milk more fully helps reduce fluid congestion in the glands and resolves the engorgement more quickly. If the baby doesn't soften both sides after nursing, suggest hand-expressing milk or pumping "to comfort" with an effective breast pump just long enough to make both sides feel softer. If a pump is not available, another option is the warm bottle method of milk expression described on p. 486, which simply requires a wide-mouthed glass bottle. If a pump is used, suggest first using massage (Witt, Bolman, Kredit, et al., 2016) (see below) or reverse pressure softening (Cotterman, 2004), which is described on p. 885. Rather than using a pump just until comfortable, another milk expression strategy involves draining the glands as fully as possible with the pump just once or twice but no more. If only done once or twice, this may help reduce fluid congestion in the glands without stimulating an oversupply.

KEY CONCEPT

Expressing milk can resolve engorgement more quickly.

Relax and use warmth to stimulate milk flow for better milk drainage.

- ***Apply heat briefly*** before nursing or milk expression by taking a warm shower or applying warm, moist heat for a minute or two. Prolonged heat is not recommended, because it may increase swelling, making the engorgement worse. The purpose of this brief application of heat is to stimulate milk flow.
- ***Use massage.*** Share with families the video at **bit.ly/BA2-BolmanMassage**, which includes a section starting at the 2:50 timestamp on massage with olive oil during engorgement. This video also demonstrates ways to knead the gland with one or both hands and how to use fingertip tapping to prepare the gland for better milk flow during hand expression or pumping. Two 2016 U.S. studies (Witt, Bolman, & Kredit, 2016; Witt, Bolman, Kredit, et al., 2016) found therapeutic breast massage during lactation (TBML) effectively decreased pain and resolved engorgement more quickly. The study mothers found this an effective technique. Massaging when the baby's sucking slows down during nursing may help

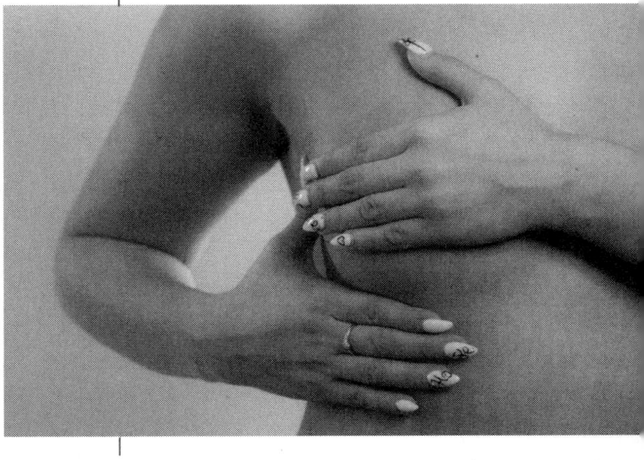

BOX 18.1 Massage Techniques Recommended for Engorgement

1. Find a comfortable position, preferably reclining or leaning back.
2. To soften the areola, alternate gentle fingertip massage within the areola with reverse pressure softening (p. 885).
3. Include gentle stroking massage from the areola toward the armpit, using olive oil to reduce friction if desired.
4. When the areola is soft enough, encourage baby to latch, continuing with the gentle stroking massage while nursing, as well as soft vibrating or circular motions.
5. Follow nursing with massage and hand expression to drain the milk more fully.

Adapted from (Bolman, Saju, Oganesyan, Kondrashova, & Witt, 2013, p. Appendix A). See video at **bit.ly/BA2-BolmanMassage**.

relieve engorgement, too, by increasing milk intake and milk drainage (Bowles, 2011). Some combine warmth and massage by massaging in the shower or while leaning over a basin of warm water. See also the Chinese manual therapy techniques described on p. 881-884.

Apply cold compresses between feeds to reduce swelling and relieve pain. When using cold compresses, suggest protecting the skin by wrapping ice packs, chilled gel packs, or a bag of frozen vegetables in a cloth. Apply them to the glands for about 20 minutes or so (P. Berens & Brodribb, 2016). In addition to feeling soothing, applying cold constricts the mammary tissue and allows blood and lymph to drain more easily. In some Far Eastern cultures, such as China, South Korea, and Thailand (Chiu et al., 2010; Ketsuwan, Baiya, Paritakul, Laosooksathit, & Puapornpong, 2018; Lim, Song, Hur, Lee, & Lee, 2015; Wong et al., 2017), cold may be considered culturally inappropriate during the early weeks after birth.

• • •

Only low-quality studies were conducted on other treatments for engorgement, but some treatments may have promise, and nursing parents may find them soothing.

The authors of a 2016 Cochrane Review (Mangesi & Zakarija-Grkovic, 2016) concluded that all 13 of the studies on engorgement treatments they reviewed were of low quality. Although more research is needed on the following treatments, they noted that some seemed promising.

Acupuncture was compared in a Swedish randomized controlled trial of 205 women (Kvist, Hall-Lord, Rydhstroem, & Larsson, 2007) with usual care. Significantly fewer women in the acupuncture group became engorged on Days 4 and 5, but there was no difference on Day 6. Fewer women in the acupuncture group experienced fever compared with the usual-care group.

Cabbage leaves have long been recommended as a home remedy for engorgement. They are inexpensive, soothing, and unlikely to have harmful side effects. When chilled cabbage leaves were compared with cold packs (K. L. Roberts, 1995), the results were the same, but most of the study mothers preferred the cabbage leaves. A 2017 randomized controlled trial done in Singapore (Wong et al., 2017) had different results. Among its 227 mothers, breast hardness was less at all time points in the cabbage-leaves group but only at two time points in the cold-packs group. Both cold packs and cabbage leaves produced better results than the no-care control group, but mothers preferred the cabbage leaves treatment to the cold packs. An Australian double-blind study (K. L. Roberts, Reiter, & Schuster, 1998) compared the use of a cream containing cabbage leaf extract with a placebo cream in 21 engorged women and found no differences in outcome. A 2015 South Korean controlled clinical trial of 66 women after a cesarean birth (Lim et al., 2015) found that adding cabbage leaves to early breast care (which involved heat, breast massage, and acupuncture) produced no additional engorgement relief, but both the early-care-alone and the early-care-plus-cabbage- leaves groups experienced less engorgement than the no-care group.

To use cabbage leaves as a treatment for engorgement, rinse either refrigerated or room temperature cabbage leaves, strip the large vein, and cut a hole for the nipple (K. L. Roberts, Reiter, & Schuster, 1995). Apply the cabbage leaves directly to the glands, if possible, wearing them inside a bra. When they wilt, usually within 2 to 4 hours, suggest removing them and reapplying fresh leaves. In some studies (K. L. Roberts, 1995), any relief reported from the use of cabbage leaves occurred within 8 hours of application.

Gua-Sha therapy, a scraping technique, was compared in a Taiwanese randomized controlled trial with traditional care (massage and heat) (Chiu et al., 2010). The differences between the two groups were not statistically significant, but the engorgement symptoms in the Gua-Sha group showed more improvement.

Herbal compresses, such as hollyhock leaf, and herbal mixtures are used in some cultures to treat engorgement. A 2017 Iranian randomized controlled clinical trial of 40 engorged women (Khosravan, Mohammadzadeh-Moghadam, Mohammadzadeh, Fadafen, & Gholami, 2017) found that when hollyhock-leaf compresses were used along with usual care (warm compresses before nursing and cold compresses after), the hollyhock group had a significantly better outcome. A 2018 Thai randomized controlled trial compared the effects of herbal compresses that used a variety of traditional herbs and compared the results to hot compresses (Ketsuwan et al., 2018). The herbal compresses were more effective at reducing pain in engorged mothers.

Engorgement treatments found ineffective. Several studies found the following treatments no more effective than usual care:

- ***Kinesio-elastic therapeutic taping*** (K-ETT) was studied in the U.S. using a quasi-experimental and comparative design with 34 mothers who had one breast taped and the other untaped (Brown & Langdon, 2014). No difference was found in the incidence of engorgement among the 65% who became engorged.
- ***Progesterone gel*** was studied in Russia (Alekseev, 2017) and found to have no effect on mammary density.
- ***Ultrasound*** was studied using a randomized double-blind controlled trial in Australia in which 197 engorged breasts were treated, the experimental group with a thermal continuous ultrasound machine and the control group with a sham machine that generated only heat (McLachlan, Milne, Lumley, & Walker, 1993). The engorgement resolved equally quickly in both groups.

Older treatments. Both the 2016 Cochrane Review (Mangesi & Zakarija-Grkovic, 2016) and Clinical Protocol #20 on engorgement from the Academy of Breastfeeding Medicine (P. Berens & Brodribb, 2016) mentioned a medical treatment for engorgement—enzyme therapy with a protease complex—that some studies found effective, but the research supporting it is now more than 50 years old.

If taut, engorged glands make it difficult for the baby to get a deep latch, suggest softening the areola before baby latches.

• • •

If the nipple and areola become so flat and taut that the baby can latch only to the nipple, nursing may become both painful and ineffective, aggravating the engorgement. If this happens, the following strategies may help:

- **Try reverse pressure softening**, which involves applying gentle consistent pressure with the fingers to move the swelling back into the body of the mammary gland, softening the areola. For details, see p. 885.
- **Massage and express just enough milk to soften the areola.** Share the video at **bit.ly/BA2-BolmanMassage** which demonstrates techniques based on traditional Russian massage and hand-expression (Bolman et al., 2013). Another milk-expression option is the warm bottle method (see p. 486), or an effective breast pump, using massage or reverse pressure softening first. Make sure the family knows that expressing milk will help resolve engorgement more quickly.
- **Wear breast shells.** Worn for about a half hour before feeding, they can soften the areola and draw out the nipple. For this purpose, use the breast shells with the smaller hole designed to draw out inverted nipples, rather than the shell backings used for sore nipples.
- **Try a nipple shield.** Short-term use may help the baby latch and drain milk well. As the engorgement resolves, suggest weaning from the shield. (For details on fit, application, and weaning from the shield, see p. 912-917.)

• • •

If baby still cannot latch, despite trying all of the above strategies, suggest expressing milk and feeding it to the baby.

If milk expression must temporarily substitute for nursing, see p. 487 for details on choosing an effective breast pump and p. 498 for pumping strategies.

• • •

If engorgement continues on one side despite consistent treatment, suggest seeing a healthcare provider to rule out other causes.

In rare cases, continued engorgement may be a warning sign of another type of breast problem, such as mastitis, a cyst, or even breast cancer (P. Berens & Brodribb, 2016). If there is no other obvious cause, suggest seeing a healthcare provider as soon as possible.

MASTITIS

Mastitis means inflammation of the mammary gland, which includes a range of conditions from the mild to the severe.

"Itis" means inflammation, so "mastitis" refers to inflammation of the mammary gland, which may or may not include a bacterial infection. As we learn more about mastitis, the terms used to describe its different forms are changing. For many years, the general term mastitis was used by many to mean one type of breast inflammation that also involved broader, more general symptoms, such as fever, body aches and lethargy (Amir, Trupin, & Kvist, 2014). In recent years, some Spanish researchers suggested the term ***acute mastitis*** to refer to the mastitis that involves these broader symptoms and suggested the term ***subacute mastitis*** for the milder, more localized version that some refer to as ***plugged*** or ***blocked ducts***. The dictionary definition of "subacute" is "falling between acute and chronic in character, especially when closer to acute" (Baeza, 2016). Subacute mastitis as described by these Spanish researchers include "breast inflammation, painful breastfeeding" in one article (Arroyo et al., 2010, p. 1552) and "needle-like and burning pain, engorgement" in another (Jimenez et al., 2015, p. 407). But what sets subacute mastitis apart from acute mastitis is the absence of fever, body aches, or other general symptoms. Its symptoms are all confined to the mammary gland.

The Academy of Breastfeeding Medicine and the World Health Organization acknowledge that blocked or plugged ducts are part of the mastitis continuum (Amir & Academy of Breastfeeding Medicine Protocol, 2014; WHO, 2000). Often, when working with families, it may be difficult to be absolutely sure that a particular case is subacute or acute mastitis. But as the following sections describe, the recommendations for both are similar.

KEY CONCEPT

Approximately 15-20% of nursing parents experience mastitis.

It may help to imagine each case of mastitis as being on a spectrum. At the least severe end of this spectrum is ***subclinical mastitis***, which the next section describes as a type of mastitis that has no obvious symptoms. It involves changes in milk composition that can only be detected by laboratory tests. Subclinical mastitis is a concern, because in HIV-positive nursing parents, it increases the risk of HIV transmission to the baby (S. Filteau, 2003; S. M. Filteau et al., 1999; Li, Solomons, Scott, & Koski, 2018). It also may be significant as a precursor to other types of mastitis. Next along the mastitis spectrum is subacute mastitis, or a blocked or plugged duct. The least severe type of plugged duct can be cleared with one good nursing or pump session. Others may last longer and take more home treatment to resolve. Further along this spectrum is acute mastitis, which some call ***breast infections***, which usually involve a hardened area in the gland with red streaks and a fever, which may or may not involve a bacterial infection. At the most severe end of the mastitis spectrum is an abscess, a pus-filled cyst that requires drainage, either in a healthcare provider's office or in the hospital. The following sections cover them all in detail.

Subclinical Mastitis

Subclinical mastitis in humans involves no obvious symptoms but is important in HIV-positive parents and may increase the risk of other types of mastitis.

The word "subclinical" means having no obvious symptoms. In the dairy industry, subclinical mastitis is well known and linked to decreased milk production in cows, but it appears this is not the case in humans (Aryeetey, Marquis, Brakohiapa, Timms, & Lartey, 2009).

Subclinical mastitis involves a change in the composition of human milk, specifically in the ratio of sodium to potassium in the absence of weaning, with sodium levels going up and potassium levels going down (Aryeetey, Marquis, Timms, Lartey, & Brakohiapa, 2008; S. M. Filteau et al., 1999; Kasonka et al., 2006). Levels of pro-inflammatory cytokines and trace elements like selenium and phosphorus are also affected (Li et al., 2018), as well as milk-enzyme levels (Rasmussen et al., 2008).

Subclinical mastitis is of interest and concern, because when the milk of HIV-positive lactating parents undergoes these changes, the viral load of HIV in the milk increases, putting the nursing baby at greater risk of becoming infected with

HIV. U.K. research on Bangladeshi women (Flores & Filteau, 2002) found that basic breastfeeding counseling—promoting early and exclusive nursing, feeding on cue, and good nursing technique—reduces the percentage of mothers whose milk composition changed in these ways. In other words, the more optimal the nursing dynamics, the less likely the mothers were to develop subclinical mastitis. Other research on breastfeeding mothers of 3- to 6-month-olds (Aryeetey et al., 2009) found no significant decrease in milk production among mothers whose milk showed signs of subclinical mastitis.

At least one Australian researcher (C. Fetherston, 2001) questioned the current interpretations of these changes in milk composition, because as she pointed out, these same changes occur for reasons other than mastitis and weaning. Higher sodium and lower potassium levels are also normal during pregnancy and when milk production increases rapidly after birth (J. A. Morton, 1994). Even when mammary glands are healthy, there are other situations in which this change in sodium/potassium ratios occur, including preterm birth, nipple trauma, overabundant milk production, low milk production, and a systemic infection in the nursing parent (C. M. Fetherston, Lai, & Hartmann, 2006). More research is needed.

Blocked Ducts and Infections

Mastitis is a common problem, especially during the early weeks of nursing.

As mentioned in the first point in this section, definitions of mastitis are shifting. Subacute mastitis is a new term intended to differentiate blocked ducts from more severe forms of mastitis. The prevalence of symptomatic mastitis—both subacute (without a fever or body aches) and acute—varies from study to study and depends in part on whether the study was limited to a specific time period or whether it included mastitis at any stage of lactation (Kvist, 2013). Its prevalence also depends on whether the study included only those whose mastitis was diagnosed by a healthcare provider or whether it included all nursing parents with symptoms of mastitis, even if the parents treated it on their own at home without consulting their healthcare provider. According to some research (Riordan & Nichols, 1990; Scott, Robertson, Fitzpatrick, Knight, & Mulholland, 2008), only about half of parents with mastitis symptoms contact their healthcare providers.

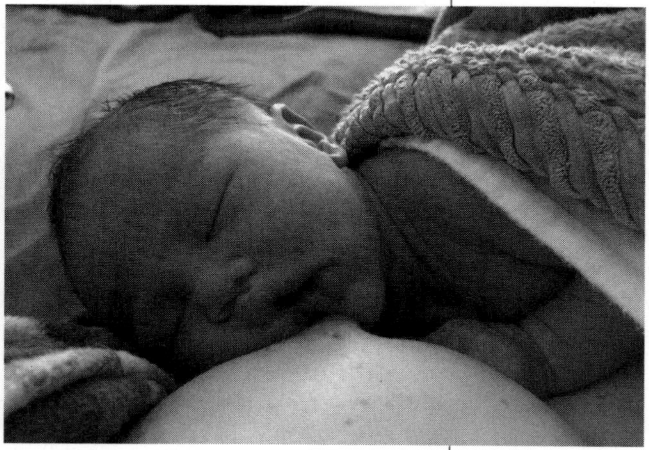

Table 18.1 lists many prospective studies with large groups of nursing parents and sheds light on the factors that increase risk for mastitis. In a U.S. prospective study (Foxman, D'Arcy, Gillespie, Bobo, & Schwartz, 2002), the incidence of mastitis (9.5%) was about half that of other Western studies, but this study reported only "healthcare provider-diagnosed mastitis," which did not include those who treated mastitis on their own.

Mastitis is not unknown in developing countries. However, as Table 18.1 illustrates, in areas where nursing is the cultural norm, rates of mastitis are much lower than in many Western countries. This may be in part because families and healthcare providers are more familiar with nursing norms.

A 2017 U.K. study that analyzed 110 milk samples from 44 healthy breastfeeding mothers (Tuaillon et al., 2017) found that the milk from nearly one quarter (23%) of these mothers had the inflammatory markers that indicated subclinical mastitis (see previous point), putting them at risk for developing mastitis

TABLE 18.1 Incidence of Mastitis and Risk Factors

Study	Country	Number	Time Period	% with Mastisis	Risk Factors/Comments
Western Countries					
Cullinane, 2015	Australia	346	0-8 wk	20	Oversupply, nipple-shield use, expressing several times/day, Staph aureus on nipple or in milk
Scott, 2008	Scotland	420	6 mo	18	53% of episodes in 1st 4 weeks, 10% told to wean
Amir, 2007	Australia	1,193	6 mo	17	Longer duration of nipple pain and cracks
Foxman, 2002	U.S.	946	12 wk	9.5 (included only cases reported to providers)	History of mastitis with previous child, nipple pain or cracks in the same week as the mastitis
Kinlay, 2001	Australia	1,075	6 mo	20	Cracked nipples
Fetherston, 1998	Australia	306	3 mo	27 (6.5 recurred)	Stress, blocked ducts, tight bra, nipple pain or nipple looking misshapen after feed, history of mastitis, milk thicker than normal, latching struggles
Non-Western Countries					
Dutta, 2018	India	3,117	1 yr	5	1st child, low socioeconomic status, anemia, engorgement, cracked nipple, inverted nipple, shallow latch, infrequent nursing
Khanal, 2015	Nepal	338	1 mo	8	Cesarean birth, prelacteal feeds
Tang, 2014	China	670	6 mo	6	Nipple pain and cracks, stress

Adapted from (Amir, Forster, Lumley, & McLachlan, 2007; Cullinane et al., 2015; Dutta & Gowder, 2018; C. Fetherston, 1998; Foxman et al., 2002; Khanal, Scott, Lee, & Binns, 2015; Kinlay, O'Connell, & Kinlay, 2001; Scott et al., 2008; Tang, Lee, Qiu, & Binns, 2014)

symptoms. One 2014 European review article (Bergmann, Rodriguez, Salminen, & Szajewska, 2014) suggested that the use of antibiotics during the perinatal period may increase risk of mastitis in part by disrupting levels of healthy bacteria in the mammary gland.

• • •

When nursing parents develop mastitis, they may feel discouraged about nursing and worried about both themselves and their baby.

A U.S. researcher (Kendall-Tackett, 2007) described the association found between physical inflammation and depression. Because mastitis increases mammary inflammation, it may also negatively affect a parent's mood and increase the risk of depression.

If parents with mastitis are worried about continuing to nurse, reassure them that nursing is a vital part of mastitis treatment (see later section) and that some immunological components in the milk are elevated during mastitis to protect the baby's health (Buescher & Hair, 2001). Keeping the milk flowing will prevent mastitis from worsening and will speed recovery. Discuss possible causes of mastitis to help parents determine why it happened and how to prevent it from recurring.

If parents are in pain, encourage them to talk to their healthcare provider about pain medication compatible with nursing, such as ibuprofen (T.W. Hale, 2019, pp. 374-375), an anti-inflammatory that may also help reduce tissue swelling more quickly. For details, see later section "Mastitis Treatments." If the parent wants to wean, see this same section for specific strategies on preventing abscess during gradual weaning.

Symptoms of Mastitis

Tenderness, lumps, or redness in the gland are symptoms of a blocked duct.

Redness and tenderness occur when a milk duct or lobe is not draining well and becomes inflamed. A 2018 review article (Angelopoulou et al., 2018) described the narrowing of the milk ducts that can occur, contributing to this condition. Just like the gut (Madan et al., 2016), both the mammary gland and human milk have their own ***microbiome*** (Fernandez et al., 2013), a term referring to the interactions of the organisms (bacteria, fungi, and viruses) with the host body.

How bacteria may cause a plugged duct. When there is an overgrowth of the bacteria that is normally present in the body, these bacteria (such as *Staphylococcus aureas*) may produce a thicker ***biofilm***, a sticky substance the bacteria produce to protect themselves. This thicker-than-normal biofilm may cause the milk ducts to narrow, forming a plug. When pressure builds behind the plug, it causes the junctions between the milk-producing cells to open and milk components to leak into surrounding tissue, causing inflammation.

When the microbiome of the mammary gland is altered to the point that the population of unhealthy (pathogenic) organisms in the gland increases at the expense of the normal microbiome, some call this condition ***mammary dysbiosis*** (Mitchell, Eglash, & Bamberger, 2019; Walker, 2018). This simply means a disruption of the gland's normal microbiome that increases risk of inflammation, pain, and mastitis. Possible causes of mammary dysbiosis include nipple trauma (which provides an entry point for organisms into the gland) and the use of antibiotics (which changes the balance of healthy and unhealthy bacteria in the body). Even the parent's blood type and the types of some specific components in the milk (oligosaccharides, for example) were linked to increased risk of mastitis (Angelopoulou et al., 2018; Walker, 2018).

• • •

In some cases, expressed milk from a blocked duct may look thick or stringy, or this may be a sign of an impending blocked duct.

When some milk components leak from the ducts into the gland's surrounding tissues (see previous point), this may leave behind thickened or stringy milk that may be visible in expressed milk (Figure 18.1). Some parents express what looks like a crystal, a grain of sand, or a long, thin strand of spaghetti, which may be accompanied by mucus. None of these are harmful to the baby. One Australian researcher (C. Fetherston, 1998) suggested that thickened expressed milk may be a predictor of future mastitis.

Regarding milk expressed during a bout of mastitis, in Clinical Protocol #4 from the Academy of Breastfeeding Medicine on human milk storage, its authors (Eglash, Simon, & Academy of Breastfeeding, 2017, p. 393) wrote:

> "If a mother has breast or nipple pain from a bacterial or yeast infection, there is no evidence that her stored expressed milk needs to be discarded."

However, it also recommends that if expressed milk smells foul or contains visible pus, it should be discarded rather than fed to the baby.

• • •

Those with mastitis may run a fever, even without a bacterial infection, and cultures cannot reliably tell the difference.

Because the bacteria involved in most cases of mastitis is normally present in the body (Angelopoulou et al., 2018), it is not always possible to know if mammary inflammation is caused by an infection or simply an inflamed blocked duct. The components of the milk, such as cytokines, that leak into surrounding tissues cause inflammation, which can cause a fever, even without bacterial infection (C. Fetherston, 2001; Kvist, Hall-Lord, & Larsson, 2007; Michie, Lockie, & Lynn, 2005). For this reason, blocked ducts can also cause flu-like symptoms, such as feeling achy and run-down, and make the mammary glands feel warmer to the touch.

The test routinely used to culture milk does not reliably distinguish a bacterial infection from an inflamed blocked duct, because skin and milk are not sterile, and bacteria will always be present in both (Angelopoulou et al., 2018; Kvist, Larsson, Hall-Lord, Steen, & Schalen, 2008; Matheson, Aursnes, Horgen, Aabo, & Melby, 1988). In dairy cows, cultures are used successfully, in part because all the lobes drain into one udder. But in humans, mammary lobes are anatomically separate, so during milk expression, milk from the healthy lobes mixes with milk from the infected lobe, diluting bacterial counts (Kvist, 2016). Thankfully, the basic treatments for a blocked duct (subacute mastitis) and an infection (acute mastitis) are nearly the same, so except in extreme cases, it is not necessary to tell the difference.

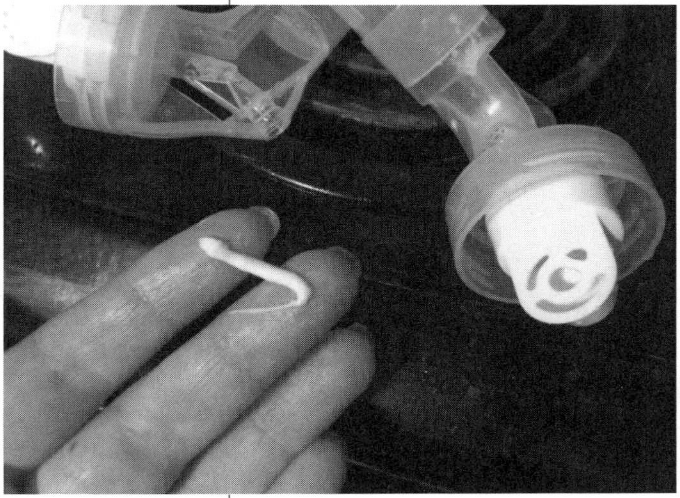

Figure 18.1 Thickened or stringy-looking expressed milk may be a sign of an existing or impending blocked duct.

A Swedish study of 210 episodes of mastitis found that having a fever made no difference in how long the mastitis lasted (Kvist, Hall-Lord, & Larsson, 2007). Mastitis symptoms resolved in about the same length of time whether there was a fever or not. Those with nipple damage, however, took longer to feel better than those without broken skin on the nipple.

• • •

Some symptoms are specific to a bacterial infection.

If the symptoms become severe, no matter what the cause, suggest contacting a healthcare provider. Symptoms that indicate a bacterial infection and may require medical treatment include (Amir & Academy of Breastfeeding Medicine Protocol, 2014):

- Visible pus in a nipple crack or fissure
- Pus or blood in the milk
- Red streaks on the mammary gland
- Any other sudden symptoms with no obvious cause, such as nausea and vomiting

With these symptoms of a bacterial infection, encourage nursing parents to contact their healthcare provider to evaluate whether medication is needed. Whether or not a parent needs antibiotics, nursing can and should continue. Sudden weaning puts nursing parents at risk of the mastitis worsening into an abscess, a much more serious condition.

• • •

Severe mastitis in both sides that occurs during the first 2 weeks after birth may be a hospital-acquired infection.

Usually mastitis occurs in only one side. Hospital-acquired (or ***nosocomial***) infections are often more severe than other types, because they tend to be drug-resistant strains. In this case, mastitis may result from exposure to virulent bacteria after a hospital birth or after a hospital stay for other reasons. This was once a major problem for all parents when hospital stays after birth were longer.

However, now infections that once existed only in the hospital, such as MRSA (methicillin-resistant *Staphylococcus aureus*), have spread to some communities as well, particularly in the U.S. and Taiwan (P. Berens, Swaim, & Peterson, 2010; Chen, Anderson, Lo, Lin, & Chen, 2010). **If a nursing parent develops a MRSA infection, the baby has already been exposed to it before the parent's symptoms became obvious, so there is no reason to stop nursing unless the baby is compromised (ill or born preterm)**. If the baby's health is fragile due to illness or prematurity, expressed milk could be pasteurized before feeding it to her (Gastelum, Dassey, Mascola, & Yasuda, 2005). If heat-treating the milk is not an option, the expressed milk may need to be discarded until it is clear of infection. Recommend handwashing and other routine hygiene practices to help stop the spread of infection (Amir & Academy of Breastfeeding Medicine Protocol, 2014).

• • •

If the baby balks at nursing from the affected side, suggest expressing the milk from that side and continue nursing on the other side.

During mastitis, changes in the taste of mother's milk cause some babies to show a strong preference for the unaffected side, sometimes rejecting the affected side altogether. In a 2014 study (Yoshida et al., 2014), Japanese scientists analyzed the change in taste and concluded that during a bout of mastitis, the milk tastes saltier. If the baby balks at taking the affected side, see p. 125 for strategies. Suggest continuing to nurse on the unaffected side, expressing milk often from the affected side to help clear the mastitis and prevent that side from becoming painfully full. Within a week after the symptoms have cleared, the milk should lose its salty taste (C. M. Fetherston et al., 2006) and the baby should go back to nursing on that side as usual.

• • •

Milk production may be slowed in the affected side for about a week, but it can be brought back to its previous level quickly.

Because the inflammation of mastitis slows milk flow, this signals the nursing parent's body to decrease milk production in the affected side (K. A. Wambach, 2003). The pressure in the gland may also contribute to reduced milk production (Say et al., 2016). An Australian study (C. M. Fetherston et al., 2006) found that within 7 days after the mastitis symptoms were gone, the milk composition was back to normal. To bring milk production back to its previous level, suggest nursing and/or expressing milk often on the affected side.

Mastitis Treatments

Mastitis treatment basics include analgesia, heat and/or cold, frequent milk removal, and rest.

If the symptoms appeared within 24 hours and are not severe, suggest starting with the following basic mastitis home treatments (Amir & Academy of Breastfeeding Medicine Protocol, 2014).

Remove the milk often and well, loosening any tight clothing, including a bra, for better milk flow (Osterman & Rahm, 2000). Suggest going without a bra for a few days, if that would be comfortable.

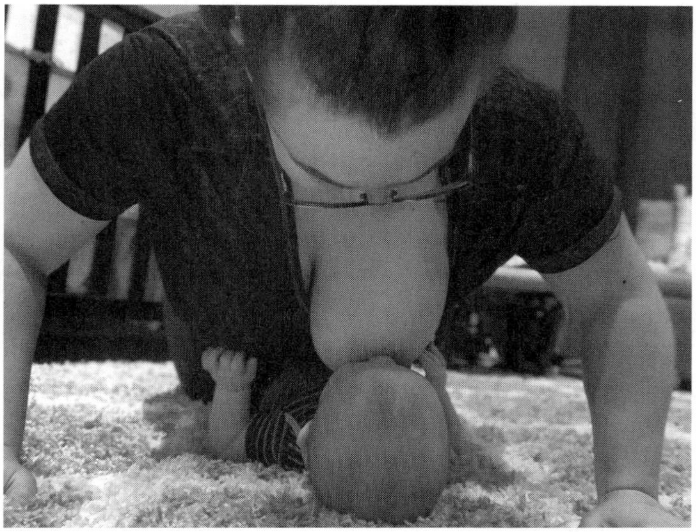

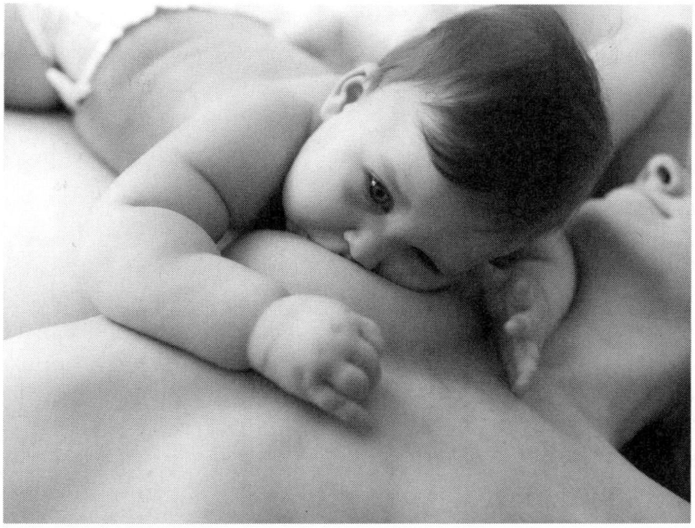

Figure 18.2 Unusual feeding positions like these may make it easier to nurse with baby's nose or chin pointing toward the affected area, which may clear the mastitis more quickly.

- ***Before nursing, apply heat*** for a few minutes (in the shower or with a warm compress) for better milk flow. Suggest removing any dried milk from the nipple with water before nursing or expressing. If the baby is not nursing directly, encourage parents to express milk after applying heat.
- ***Massage gently*** before nursing while the gland is warm and during nursing, concentrating on any lumps or sore areas by using fingertips or the palm, moving from the armpit toward the nipple. U.S. research (Witt, Bolman, Kredit, et al., 2016) found that parents consider massage an effective tool to help resolve mastitis. A video demo of massage techniques is available at **bit.ly/BA2-BolmanMassage**. See also the Chinese manual therapy techniques on p. 881-884.
- ***Remove milk well from the affected side at least every couple of hours, day and night*** to reduce fullness and keep the milk flowing. Nurse on the affected side first for as long as that side feels tender or warm, making sure the baby is latching deeply to more evenly drain the lobes (Mizuno et al., 2008).
- ***Vary feeding positions*** to help unplug the affected area. Whatever position is used, make sure baby latches deeply and at least once during each feed, suggest positioning the baby so her nose or chin points toward the plug (Amir & Academy of Breastfeeding Medicine Protocol, 2014). Some may benefit from occasionally using the all-fours dangle position or over the shoulder (Figure 18.2) (Marmet & Shell, 2017). Suggest using only positions that work well and are comfortable. If parents are not nursing directly, suggest using the tips for increasing milk flow during milk expression that begin on p. 491.

Take analgesia. Encourage any parents in pain to talk to their healthcare provider about appropriate analgesia that is compatible with nursing. Ibuprofen, for example, is also an anti-inflammatory, which can help decrease symptoms, as well as reduce pain, and is considered compatible with nursing (T.W. Hale, 2019, pp. 374-375).

Between feeds, apply heat and/or cold. Because heat can increase swelling, suggest limiting its use to short periods. Wet or dry heat can be applied to the affected area for 10 minutes or so before feeds, at least 3 times each day. Warm showers, warm compresses, a heating pad, or a water bottle can be used. Some find it soothing to soak the gland by leaning over a basin of warm water or lying on their side in a warm bathtub. Between feeds, apply cold to reduce swelling, making sure to wrap any cold packs or packages of frozen vegetables in a cloth to protect the skin. Encourage families to choose heat and/or cold based on what feels most effective and soothing. In some Far Eastern cultures, using cold as a treatment after birth is considered inappropriate (Chiu et al., 2010; Ketsuwan et al., 2018; Lim et al., 2015; Wong et al., 2017).

Rest. Mastitis may be one sign of fatigue or stress. When resistance to illness decreases, other risk factors are more likely to lead to mastitis. If possible, suggest taking the baby to bed and staying there until the mastitis diminishes. If that's not possible, suggest postponing extra activities and plan to spend an hour or two each day with feet up relaxing with the baby. Convey that rest is the key to recovery.

• • •

The use of antibiotics to treat mastitis varies widely by country, and their effectiveness as a treatment is uncertain.

The home treatments described in the previous point are the best first approach for any parent with less-than-severe symptoms of mastitis, especially within the first day the symptoms appear (Amir & Academy of Breastfeeding Medicine Protocol, 2014). Antibiotics will not address the underlying cause of the mastitis but may be appropriate in severe cases and when an infection is obvious. The research on antibiotic use to treat mastitis is mixed. The authors of the Academy of Breastfeeding Medicine's mastitis protocol (Amir & Academy of Breastfeeding Medicine Protocol, 2014, p. 240) recommends: "If symptoms are not improving within 12-24 hours or if the woman is acutely ill, antibiotics should be started."

However, Swedish research (Kvist et al., 2008) calls this recommendation into question. Researchers cultured the milk of 192 women with mastitis and 466 milk donors without mastitis in an attempt to learn more about the role various organisms play in this condition. They found *Staphylococcus aureus* and Group B streptococci in the milk of mothers both with and without mastitis, and they found no correlation between the severity of the symptoms and the levels of bacteria in their milk. They also found that bacterial counts did not differ between those treated with antibiotics and those using only home treatments. They concluded that milk cultures may not be an accurate gauge for determining whether or not a parent with mastitis has a bacterial infection and questioned the use, and especially the frequent use, of antibiotics to treat mastitis.

In some studies, U.S. (Foxman et al., 2002; K. A. Wambach, 2003) and Australian (C. Fetherston, 1997; Kinlay, O'Connell, & Kinlay, 1998) healthcare providers used antibiotic treatment for mastitis in 77% to 97% of their cases. In contrast, a Finnish study that followed 664 women with mastitis (Jonsson & Pulkkinen, 1994) reported 38% were treated with antibiotics. In comparison, 15% of the mothers in a Swedish study (Kvist, Hall-Lord, & Larsson, 2007) were prescribed antibiotics, 3% due to the severity of their symptoms and 11% due to the results of their milk cultures. After the study, only 2% of the study mothers who didn't receive antibiotics during the study appeared to need them later.

A 2013 Cochrane Review (Jahanfar, Ng, & Teng, 2013) found only two studies met their quality criteria and neither found antibiotics more effective than treatments such as frequent milk removal. It concluded that there is very little evidence on the effectiveness of antibiotics for treating mastitis and more research is needed.

• • •

In some cases, treatment with antibiotics may be appropriate.

When parents have a sore gland, fever, and flu-like symptoms, suggest they begin home treatment right away. Suggest they contact their healthcare provider if:

- After 24 hours of home treatment, their symptoms are the same or worse.
- They were running a fever for some time.
- They have obvious signs of a bacterial infection, such as visible pus.
- Their temperature suddenly spikes higher.

If parents have any of these signs, their healthcare provider may prescribe an antibiotic compatible with nursing (Table 18.2). The drugs usually given for a 10 to 14 day course (K. Wambach, 2021, p. 286) are a penicillinase-resistant penicillin (such as flucloxacillin, dicloxacillin) or a cephalosporin, such as cephalexin, taken 500 mg 4 times per day (K. Wambach, 2021, p. 285). Parents taking a shorter course of antibiotics may be at greater risk of recurrence. Encourage parents to take the full course of antibiotics even after they feel better. Antibiotics may help resolve symptoms, even without an infection, because they also have an anti-inflammatory effect.

• • •

Treatments that may complement or substitute for antibiotics include taking specific probiotics, swabbing the nipple and areola with a nisin solution, and topical curcumin.

As mentioned in the previous points, antibiotics are not always an effective mastitis treatment. Also, frequent use of antibiotics has produced many resistant strains of bacteria, which is one reason to use them sparingly. Antibiotics also reduce the diversity of the microbiome (Angelopoulou et al., 2018). Promising research was published on the following mastitis treatment alternatives (Table 18.2).

The use of specific probiotics to prevent or treat mastitis. As mentioned in a previous point, the microbiome of the mammary gland consists of organisms such as beneficial bacteria that contribute to its health and the health of the nursing baby (Collado, Delgado, Maldonado, & Rodriguez, 2009; Hunt et al., 2011). By analyzing milk samples from healthy parents and those suffering from mastitis, Spanish research (Jimenez et al., 2015) found that during bouts of mastitis, the type of bacteria in the milk changes markedly. For more than a decade, researchers (Arroyo et al., 2010; Bergmann et al., 2014; Hurtado et al., 2017; Jimenez et al., 2008) tested the theory that giving lactating parents the specific probiotics (live beneficial organisms) found in healthy mammary glands may help prevent and treat mastitis.

Taking just any random probiotics found online or on store shelves will not effectively treat mastitis. The probiotics used as treatments are specific strains, which are referred to by the name of their genetic variant or subtype (usually capitalized and in italics), the code for the lab where the product was made (a combination of numbers and capital letters), and the serial number of the strain

TABLE 18.2 Mastitis Treatment Options

Options	Specifics	When Used
Antibiotics	• Penicillinase-resistant penicillins: dicloxacillin, flucloxacillin • Penicillin alternatives for allergic parents: cephalexin, clindamycin • MRSA-effective treatment: vancomycin	Prescribe when home treatment does not improve symptoms ≤24 hr or parent is severely ill
Probiotics	• *L. salivarius PS2*—As a preventive: 9 log10CFU daily from 30 wk of pregnancy • *L. fermentum CECT5716*—As a preventive: 3 log10CFU daily from birth to 16 wk; or as a treatment: 9 log10CFU daily for 21 days • *L. salivarius CECT5713*-- As a treatment: 9 log10CFU daily for 21 days	To prevent mastitis, as a home treatment, as an alternative or complement to antibiotics
Bacteriocins	• *L. lactis ES1515* (nisin source)—Apply 0.1 mL to nipple and areola after each nursing for 14 days	As an alternative or complement to antibiotics
Curcumin Cream	• Curcumin cream 200 mg--Apply to the gland every 8 hr for 3 days	To relieve inflammation and breast pain from mastitis

Adapted from (Walker, 2018)

(see Table 18.2). More studies are definitely needed (Amir, Griffin, Cullinane, & Garland, 2016). In the meantime, these products may be used along with antibiotics (as a complementary treatment) to help offset their effects on the parent's microbiome. Examples of specific products that contain the studied probiotics and the city where they are manufactured (Walker, 2019) include:

- Lactanza herediturn (Angelini, Barcelona, Spain)
- Qiara (Puremedic, Kew, Victoria, Australia)
- Target b2 (Klaire Labs, Reno, NV USA)

Swabbing the nipple and areola with a nisin solution after nursing. A Spanish pilot study (Fernandez, Delgado, Herrero, Maldonado, & Rodriguez, 2008) examined an alternative mastitis treatment: the topical application of nisin, a food-grade antimicrobial produced by the lactic acid bacterium *Lactococcus lactis*. Nisin is a bacteriocin, a substance produced by bacteria that kills other bacteria. This substance is commonly found in the milk of healthy lactating parents (Fernandez et al., 2014; Martin et al., 2007). In the 2008 Fernandez study, eight mothers with mastitis in both breasts were divided into two groups. One group of four mothers applied a small amount of nisin solution (~0.1 mL) to the nipple and areola after every nursing session for 2 weeks. The control group of four applied a solution without nisin. After 2 weeks, the symptoms completely resolved in the nisin group, whereas symptoms continued in the control group.

Staphylococcus aureus—even methicillin-resistant strains (MRSA)—responded to the nisin, and the level of *Staphylococcus aureus* in the milk of the nisin group declined throughout the 2 weeks of the study. In the non-nisin group, though, the level of Staph aureus in the milk increased slightly.

Topical curcumin. One topical treatment found to ease the symptoms of mastitis is topical curcumin (turmeric), which has anti-inflammatory properties. A 2014 Iranian double-blind randomized placebo-controlled clinical trial (Afshariani,

Farhadi, Ghaffarpasand, & Roozbeh, 2014) divided its 64 breastfeeding mothers with acute mastitis into two groups. One group applied curcumin cream 200 mg (Neurobiologix, TX, USA) to the affected breasts every 8 hours for 3 days. The other group applied a placebo cream. After the 3 days, 72% of those using the curcumin cream had no symptoms, as compared with 39% of those using the placebo cream.

• • •

If parents do not respond to antibiotics or the other alternative or complementary treatments within 2 days, the World Health Organization and the Academy of Breastfeeding Medicine (Amir & Academy of Breastfeeding Medicine Protocol, 2014; WHO, 2000) recommend culturing the milk so another drug can be chosen that targets the specific organism involved. If resistant bacteria, such as MRSA, are prevalent in that geographical area, a culture is needed to identify this. It is also possible the problem is not mastitis but one of the following conditions.

If there is no improvement within 2 days of antibiotic or alternative treatments, consider the need for a different antibiotic and rule out other mammary disease.

Cellulitis is sometimes mistaken for mastitis. It is an inflammation of the skin and underlying tissues, and a different organism is usually involved. The organism usually enters the body through broken skin, such as nipple trauma. It affects the connective tissue of the mammary gland, rather than the milk-making tissue (K. Wambach, 2021, p. 286). The areas affected may look red and swollen and appear raised. Heat and massage can aggravate cellulitis, rather than helping resolve it, and parents will need different antibiotics to treat it. When the usual treatments are not working, suggest a healthcare provider evaluate the parent for cellulitis.

KEY CONCEPT

Cellulitis may look like mastitis, but has a different cause and treatment.

Idiopathic granulomatous mastitis is a rare benign inflammatory breast disorder that most often occurs after pregnancy in those of childbearing age and is sometimes mistaken for bacterial mastitis or breast cancer (Barreto, Sedgwick, Nagi, & Benveniste, 2018). Symptoms include breast swelling, redness, and abscess formation. It is diagnosed by ruling out infectious mastitis and doing a biopsy to rule out cancer (Mitchell, Johnson, Eglash, & Academy of Breastfeeding, 2019). At this writing, much is still unknown about its causes and the most effective treatments (Haitz, Ly, & Smith, 2019; Lei et al., 2017), as well as its recurrence (Uysal, 2018; Wolfrum, Kummel, Theuerkauf, Pelz, & Reinisch, 2018).

Inflammatory breast cancer. If a red and swollen mammary gland does not improve within at least 72 hours of treatment with antibiotics, suggest seeing a healthcare provider to rule out this life-threatening condition. The early stages of inflammatory breast cancer account for 1% to 5% of all breast cancers in the U.S. and can mimic mastitis (NCI, 2020). Its symptoms include redness, swelling and warmth in the gland without an obvious lump. These symptoms occur when cancer cells block the lymph nodes. As the disease progresses, the skin may change color, appearing pink, purple, or bruised. Areas may also form ridges or look pitted, like the skin of an orange (called ***peau d'orange***). The nipple may become flattened, red, and crusty. Inflammatory breast cancer can be diagnosed by exam and diagnostic imaging confirmed with biopsy.

For a more complete list of possible conditions that may be mistaken for mastitis, see the Clinical Protocol #30 on breast masses and complaints from the Academy of Breastfeeding Medicine (Mitchell, Johnson, et al., 2019). which is free, downloadable, and available in multiple languages at **bfmed.org/protocols**.

• • •

If a breast or chest lump doesn't shrink within a few days of treatment, suggest contacting a healthcare provider to rule out other causes.

Most lumps are not caused by cancer, but this possibility and others, such as galactoceles, fibroadenomas, and cysts, need to be ruled out when the lump does not decrease in size after treatment. For details, see the later section "Breast Lumps" and the Clinical Protocol #30 on breast masses from the Academy of Breastfeeding Medicine (Mitchell, Johnson, et al., 2019) at **bfmed.org/protocols**.

Causes of Mastitis

The most common risk factors for mastitis are periods of mammary fullness, nipple trauma, and sustained pressure on the mammary gland.

The following are the most common causes of mastitis.

Periods of mammary fullness can sometimes occur even when nursing is going well, but discuss other possible causes, such as.

- ***Ineffective nursing**, **leaving the gland full after feeds***—This may be from a shallow latch, engorgement, or anatomical issues, such as inverted nipples, tongue-tie, or an unusually shaped palate. In one Australian study (C. Fetherston, 1998), all five mothers of babies with symptomatic tongue-tie (see p. 263) developed mastitis.
- ***Overabundant milk production***—Even when a baby nurses effectively, if parents produce much more milk than the baby takes, the glands may feel full much of the time. If the baby's weight gain is well above average, this may be a possibility. For details, see p. 459.
- ***Restricted nursing***—This may occur when parents schedule feeds or limit feeding length. Ask parents to describe how a typical nursing session unfolds.
- ***Missed feeds, supplements, or irregular feeding patterns***—Is the baby fed by bottle or does she take a pacifier/dummy? Supplements and pacifiers can delay nursing. Some babies are just naturally irregular feeders. Suggest parents nurse or express milk before mammary fullness develops.
- ***Baby sleeps for long stretches day or night***—This may be due to normal growth and development. Ask whether the baby's nursing pattern changed before the mastitis occurred. Babies can nurse effectively even in light sleep (Colson, 2003, 2019), such as during "dream feeds."
- ***Ineffective milk expression***—This may happen during an extended time away from baby when a new method or an ineffective breast pump is used.
- ***Outside distractions that prevent or delay nursing***—Ask if the parents were unusually busy. A prime time for mastitis is around the holidays, when families are busy, distracted, and fatigued.
- ***Too-rapid weaning***—This may leave the mammary glands full of milk for too long.
- ***Uneven milk removal***—This is usually caused by a shallow latch, during which the baby may drain some areas of the gland more than others.

One Japanese study of 37 mothers and babies (Mizuno et al., 2008) found that when babies latch shallowly, the gland may not drain evenly, leaving some areas more drained and other areas less drained. Researchers determined the degree of drainage of different lobes by drawing milk from their corresponding nipple pores and measuring their milk fat content. High fat content indicated that the lobe was well drained during nursing. Low fat content indicated not as much milk was taken from that lobe. The researchers found that the study babies who achieved a deep latch drained the gland more evenly than those who latched shallowly.

Nipple trauma. Broken skin on the nipple provides a point of entry for bacteria. Ultrasound research (Ramsay, Kent, Owens, & Hartmann, 2004) found that after milk ejection, milk flows back into the ducts, making it possible for bacteria to be carried back with the milk. Most studies that examined risk factors for mastitis found an association between broken skin on the nipple and increased risk of mastitis.

Consistent pressure on the gland. Firm, sustained pressure on the gland can restrict milk flow, which can cause milk components to leak into the surrounding tissue and trigger inflammation. Examples include:

- ***An ill-fitting bra*** that binds part of the breast or one that provides little support, allowing the weight of heavy breasts to constrict milk ducts (C. Fetherston, 1998).
- ***Breast shells*** worn for hours in a bra with too-small cups, leaving indentations on the breast when removed (C. Fetherston, 1998).
- ***Stomach-sleeping*** (Figure 18.3), which can cause long-term breast tissue compression.
- ***Straps from a tote or baby carrier*** that apply sustained pressure to the gland.

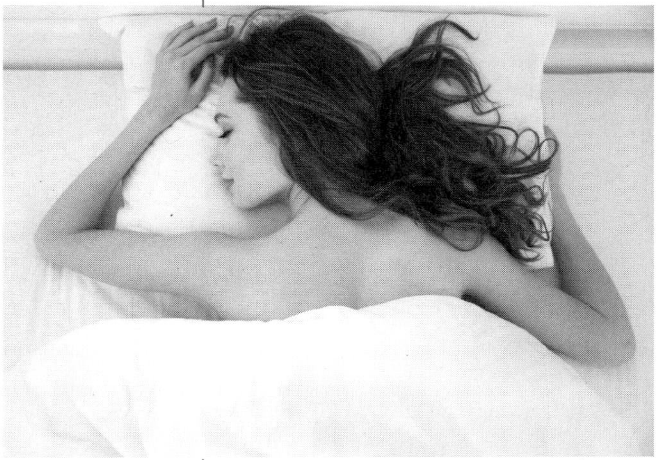

Figure 18.3 Stomach sleeping puts consistent, sustained pressure on the mammary glands, which is one possible cause of mastitis.

Fatigue often precedes mastitis (C. Fetherston, 1998; Riordan & Nichols, 1990). For other, more unusual factors that can increase the risk of mastitis, see the next section.

• • •

If parents with mastitis decide to wean, help them do it gradually and safely.

If parents with mastitis wean too quickly, this may cause their mastitis to worsen or to develop into an abscess (see later section). To avoid a more serious health problem, suggest parents wait to wean until mastitis clears, and then wean very slowly to avoid a recurrence.

U.S. lactation consultants Barbara Wilson-Clay and Kay Hoover describe a slow-weaning plan after the surgical drainage of a breast abscess in *The Breastfeeding Atlas* (Wilson-Clay & Hoover, 2017, p. 96). The mother exclusively expressed her milk with a breast pump and alternated between

- Dropping a daily pump session and
- Gradually decreasing the length of each pumping by a couple of minutes

Each time she implemented one of the above strategies, she kept her pumping routine the same for several days to give her milk production a chance to decrease before implementing the alternate strategy. With this method, the mother ceased milk production safely and comfortably over a period of several weeks. Any time during the weaning the mother felt any fullness, she pumped just enough milk to soften her breasts. That way she was able to stop milk production without causing more health problems.

Recurring Mastitis

Recurring mastitis can be demoralizing, even to a motivated parent.

Chronic mastitis can cause even the most dedicated parents to question their commitment to nursing. It's important to listen carefully and acknowledge parents' feelings, no matter how negative. Offer to help determine the cause of the recurrences, and assure them that in most cases the cause can be found and eliminated or treatment can be started that can break the cycle. If they decide to wean, emphasize the importance of weaning slowly and carefully (see previous point).

• • •

To determine the cause, first ask about the treatments previously tried.

Failure to fully recover from a previous mastitis is a common cause of recurring mastitis. It is especially likely if the last episode of mastitis was within the previous few weeks, although previous mastitis anytime puts parents at greater risk of recurrence. Encourage parents to be vigilant with home treatment until the mastitis is completely gone.

If mastitis recurs even after treatment with antibiotics, it is still possible that the original mastitis did not completely resolve. Repeated mastitis can happen—especially if the same risk factors are still present—but it is usually a recurrence of the original mastitis, rather than a new case. Other possibilities include:

- **A too-short course of antibiotics** of less than 10 to 14 days (K. Wambach, 2021, p. 286), either due to the healthcare provider's order or because the antibiotics were stopped too soon.
- **Use of an inappropriate antibiotic** that did not treat the responsible organism
- **Reinfection after finishing the medication** by an organism carried in the baby's throat or nose (Wust, Rutsch, & Stocker, 1995).

If mastitis recurs after parents took an antibiotic for at least 10 days, the Academy of Breastfeeding Medicine (Amir & Academy of Breastfeeding Medicine Protocol, 2014) suggests asking a healthcare provider to culture the milk to determine if another antibiotic might be more effective. Because *Staphylococcus aureus* is the most common organism associated with mastitis, it is typically treated with the antibiotics effective against it. But sometimes other bacteria are involved, such as *Streptococcus pneumoniae* (Wust et al., 1995), *Escherichia coli,* Group B Streptococcus, or even tuberculosis (Farrokh, Alamdaran, Feyzi Laeen, Fallah Rastegar, & Abbasi, 2019; Gupta, Gupta, & Duggal, 1982), and another drug would be more effective. If drug-resistant strains such as MRSA (methicillin-resistant staph aureus) are common in the area, this should also be considered (P. D. Berens, 2015). For recommendations of specific drugs and doses that parents can share with healthcare providers, see the Clinical Protocol #4 from the Academy of Breastfeeding Medicine (Amir & Academy of Breastfeeding Medicine Protocol, 2014), which is available for free download in multiple languages at **bfmed.org/protocols**.

• • •

Talk to parents about their usual nursing patterns to see if any of the common causes of mastitis may be contributing to its recurrences.

Most often, recurring mastitis is triggered by one of its common causes:

- Intermittent periods of mammary fullness
- Entry of bacteria in the gland via nipple trauma
- Sustained pressure on the gland

See the previous section for more specific areas to explore, such as overabundant milk production, a change in feeding or sleeping patterns, starting a new job, a recent nipple bite, trauma from an ill-fitting breast pump, constrictive clothing, stomach-sleeping, a new baby carrier, etc. One of these may be the underlying cause responsible for recurring mastitis.

• • •

Other, more unusual risk factors, along with fatigue and stress, may also contribute to recurring mastitis.

Fatigue or feeling "run down" often precedes mastitis (Riordan & Nichols, 1990), especially in parents with more than one child (C. Fetherston, 2001). Anything that decreases parents' resistance to illness or infection may make them more prone to mastitis, especially if other risk factors are present. In one survey of 91 breastfeeding mothers (Riordan & Nichols, 1990), those who had mastitis (about one-third) ranked fatigue first and stress second as major contributing factors. Several described family travel, hectic holidays, christenings, parties, and household moves as triggers. In a German review of 16 studies (Wockel, Abou-Dakn, Beggel, & Arck, 2008), its authors suggested that stress contributes to mastitis by releasing cytokines, which trigger inflammation in the body.

Other, more unusual factors that can contribute to recurring mastitis include:

- **Nipple bleb**, or milk blister, blocking milk flow from one or more nipple pores (for details, see p. 734)
- **Exclusive pumping**, which often leads to longer periods of mammary fullness than are common with direct nursing
- **Health issues** that increase parents' susceptibility to infection, such as diabetes, IgA deficiency (C. M. Fetherston, Lai, & Hartmann, 2008), or anemia (C. Fetherston, 1998)
- **Nipple shield use.** Was it used because the baby nursed ineffectively, or could poor hygiene of the shield be a factor (C. Fetherston, 1998)?
- **Breast or chest injury** from intense exercise or trauma, which may cause mammary swelling and block milk flow (C. Fetherston, 1998)
- **Nipple piercing**, which allows bacteria to enter the gland (Garbin, Deacon, Rowan, Hartmann, & Geddes, 2009; Jacobs, Golombeck, Jonat, & Kiechle, 2003; Trupiano et al., 2001)
- **Internal breast or chest abnormalities**, such as scar tissue from previous surgery, abscess, cyst, or cancer that causes internal pressure on ducts and blocks milk flow (Dahlbeck, Donnelly, & Theriault, 1995; Meguid, Oler, Numann, & Khan, 1995; Wang et al., 2012)

If the mastitis always recurs in the same area, there may be an internal cause. Any breast or chest surgery—biopsy, breast reduction or top surgery, implants, tumor, or cyst removal—increases the risk of mastitis due to internal scarring, which can put pressure on the milk ducts. Unusual anatomy in a duct is another possible cause. Due to pressure on milk ducts, an existing lump from any cause may put a parent at increased risk for mastitis. Since these causes cannot be easily corrected, a parent may choose to nurse only on the unaffected side, gradually allowing milk production to stop on the affected side.

Recurring mastitis in the same location is also a warning sign of possible breast cancer. If the mastitis always occurs in the same gland and at the same spot, suggest seeing a healthcare provider for diagnostic imaging to rule out this cause.

• • •

Three possible treatments for chronic recurring plugged ducts or more severe forms of mastitis are lecithin supplements, ultrasound therapy, and low-dose, long-term antibiotics.

If the previous strategies don't provide long-term resolution of recurring mastitis and it continues to recur, consider the following treatments.

Lecithin supplements have been recommended as a home remedy for recurring plugged ducts for many years, although how this works is unclear. The popular lactation website **KellyMom.com** (Bonyata, 2018) recommends taking 3,600 to 4,800 mg of lecithin per day, or one 1,200 mg capsule three to four times daily. After 1 to 2 weeks at this dose with no plugged ducts, reduce it by one capsule per day. If the plugged ducts do not return during the next 2 weeks, reduce it again by one capsule per day. If the plugged ducts return, the nursing parent can continue taking one to two capsules per day indefinitely. Lecithin is a common food additive and occurs naturally in many foods. Therefore, it is compatible with nursing.

Ultrasound therapy. Therapeutic ultrasound involves sending noninvasive vibrating particles into the body and is used in some parts of the world to treat tissues damaged by disease or injury.(Rothenberg, Jayaram, Naqvi, Gober, & Malanga, 2017). In Australia, ultrasound is commonly used by physiotherapists to treat recurring mastitis, although a 2019 survey of practitioners (Diepeveen et al., 2019) found that the dosages used varied greatly among providers. A small Canadian pilot study (Lavigne & Gleberzon, 2012) found that ultrasound therapy (an average of three sessions) benefited more than half of the 25 nursing parents treated for recurring plugged ducts. A 2016 interview (Robertson, 2016) described the practice of a U.S. occupational therapist (who struggled with plugged ducts while nursing her own baby), who trained as an ultrasound provider and offers this service to nursing parents in her local area.

Long-term, low-dose antibiotics. According to U.S. physicians Ruth and Robert Lawrence (Lawrence & Lawrence, 2016, p. 571), if chronic bacterial infection is a possible underlying cause of recurring mastitis, these doctors suggest breaking the cycles with a preventive, low-dose, long-term antibiotic treatment. Here's how it works. Begin with a 10- to 14-day course of antibiotics to treat the current bout of mastitis, which is followed by low doses of antibiotics (i.e., 500 mg. erythromycin) taken daily for 2 to 3 months to prevent recurrence.

Abscess

Abscesses in the mammary gland are uncommon and usually occur when mastitis is not treated promptly and appropriately or doesn't respond to treatment.

An abscess is a walled-off area of pus in the body with no opening for drainage. To resolve an abscess, it must be either aspirated or surgically drained. It is a serious and often painful condition that needs immediate medical attention.

Abscesses in the mammary gland are categorized by location. ***Subareolar abscesses*** are just under the areola. ***Intrammamary unilocular abscesses*** are deeper within the mammary tissue and contain just one pocket of pus. Abscesses may have one pocket or multiple pockets, called ***multiocular abscesses***. Thankfully, mammary abscesses are relatively uncommon. When both self-reported and healthcare provider-treated mastitis are considered, they occur in about 3% of nursing parents with a history of mastitis (Amir, Forster, McLachlan, & Lumley, 2004). One Swedish study (Kvist & Rydhstroem, 2005) found that among the more than 1.4 million women who gave birth in Sweden between 1987 and 2000 (not just those who had mastitis), the rate of abscess was 0.1%. When an abscess occurs in nursing parents, it is usually the result of untreated mastitis, a delay in treatment, or incorrect treatment.

• • •

In some areas, most abscesses culture positive for MRSA, an organism resistant to common antibiotics.

As resistant strains of bacteria spread into communities, incorrect treatment of mastitis may become more of an issue. One U.S. study (Stafford et al., 2008) reported that cases of community-acquired methicillin-resistant *Staphylococcus aureus* (MRSA) increased nine-fold in the Dallas, Texas area between 2003 and 2008 and that 63% of the breastfeeding study mothers diagnosed with breast abscesses cultured positive for MRSA. Two other U.S. studies conducted in Houston, Texas, (P. Berens et al., 2010; Peterson, 2007) found similar percentages of MRSA (63% to 64%) among its study mothers with breast abscesses. Although MRSA is most common in the U.S. and Taiwan, it may also occur elsewhere. Case reports identified MRSA in other areas where it is uncommon, such as Japan (Hagiya, Shiota, Sugiyama, & Otsuka, 2014), Italy (Rimoldi et al., 2019), Germany (Lukassek, Ignatov, Faerber, Costa, & Eggemann, 2019), and Australia (Montalto & Lui, 2009). When an abscess develops, keep this possibility in mind.

Where community-acquired MRSA is prevalent, practicing good hygiene is vital. Suggest parents wash their hands often. Healthcare providers need to be vigilant about using gloves and routinely disinfecting the everyday objects they touch, such as clipboards, pens, and keyboards, as well as the surfaces parents and babies touch, such as baby scales and breast pumps (Wilson-Clay, 2008).

• • •

An ultrasound is preferred over a mammogram to identify an abscess and may be used during treatment.

In many cases, the parent's healthcare provider may be unable to confirm an abscess by examination alone. Often, when an abscess develops, there is no fever or other more generalized symptoms. A mammogram cannot distinguish an abscess from other masses, such as a tumor, and the tissue squeezing involved in this procedure can be very painful for parents with an inflamed mammary gland. Ultrasound, on the other hand, is not only more comfortable to the parent, but it can also distinguish an abscess from solid masses, especially when performed by a technician familiar with the lactating mammary gland (Haliloglu, Ustuner, & Ozkavukcu, 2019). Confirming the existence, size, and location of the abscess allows the healthcare provider to determine whether or not surgical drainage is necessary or whether a less-invasive treatment is an option.

• • •

For most abscesses, treatments are available that are less invasive than surgical incision and drainage and make continued nursing more likely.

Until recent years, abscesses were usually treated by surgical incision and drainage, which required hospitalization. But research (Christensen et al., 2005) found that a combination of ultrasonic imaging to locate the abscess and aspiration and flushing with a needle, catheter, or suction device can eliminate the need for surgery. These procedures are much less invasive and can typically be done as an outpatient, which minimizes separation of nursing couples. Culturing the aspirated fluid for organisms and treating the nursing parent with appropriate antibiotics for at least 10 days is also a vital part of this treatment.

Abscess drainage with fine-needle aspiration, catheters, and suction devices. Swedish research (Ulitzsch, Nyman, & Carlson, 2004) found that fine-needle aspiration worked well with abscesses 3 cm and smaller in 97% of its study mothers. This study followed 43 breastfeeding women diagnosed with 56 abscesses. In those 3 cm or smaller, the researchers used fine-needle aspiration guided by ultrasound to aspirate and flush them with saline solution. For abscesses larger than 3 cm, they inserted catheters to drain and flush them. Some mothers (48%) needed the aspiration and flushing done only once for their abscesses to resolve; others needed multiple aspirations and flushing (2 to 5) before their abscesses resolved. Catheters were left in the breast an average of 6 days (range: 1 to 25 days) before removal. Only one (2%) of the 43 mothers subsequently needed surgical incision and drainage. A similar but larger Danish study had similar results, and its authors concluded that because these procedures do not require hospitalization or affect nursing, they "should replace surgery as the first line of treatment in uncomplicated…breast abscess" (Christensen et al., 2005, p. 188).

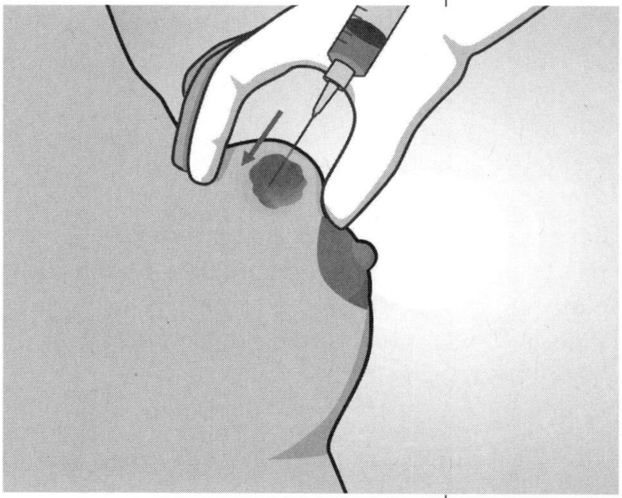

A 2019 French retrospective study examined the medical records of 92 consecutive women who were treated for 105 abscesses in a single institution (Colin, Delov, Peyron-Faure, Rabilloud, & Charlot, 2019). Among the abscesses drained, 78% were larger than 3 cm and 38% were larger than 5 cm. (The largest abscess was 15 cm.) By using ultrasound to guide them, the providers successfully drained these abscesses without surgical incisions by using fine-needle aspiration, catheters, or suction-assisted biopsy devices. The researchers noted that draining the abscesses without surgery allowed nursing to continue.

Mini-incision and suction drain. Even if surgical incision and drainage is recommended, there are still options that make continued nursing more likely. A 2016 Chinese retrospective study compared the results in two groups of women who were hospitalized with breast abscesses for surgical incision and drainage (Wei, Zhang, & Fu, 2016). One group of 32 had traditional incision and drainage performed, while 30 women had their abscesses drained using a mini-incision on the edge of the areola and a drain employing suction to remove the abscess contents. The mini-incision group had an average hospital stay 3 days shorter than the other group. None of the 32 women who received the traditional incision and drainage breastfed afterward, while 28 of the 30 women in the mini-incision group continued to nurse their babies after leaving the hospital.

A 2015 Cochrane systematic review (Irusen, Rohwer, Steyn, & Young, 2015) rated the quality of evidence on abscess treatments as poor and could not come to any conclusions about which method and which antibiotics should be used.

• • •

When nursing continues during abscess treatment, the parent may need to make some adjustments.

Aspiration of the contents of the abscess should not affect nursing. If a catheter or surgical incision and drainage is used near the areola, the parent can continue nursing on the unaffected side. If the catheter or surgical incision is far enough from the areola so that the baby's mouth does not touch it when she nurses, nursing may continue on the affected side. An abscess that is surgically drained is not usually closed. Rather, it remains open and is allowed to drain and heal from the inside out. As with any parent with mastitis, rest is a vital part of the treatment.

If nursing does not continue on the affected side, encourage the parent to express milk from that side while the incision is healing to prevent engorgement. (To help create a milk-expression plan, see p. 504.)

Nursing can continue on the affected side after surgical drainage (Amir & Academy of Breastfeeding Medicine Protocol, 2014) and will not prevent healing, even though milk may seep out of the incision. The incision may heal more slowly, but continuing to nurse prevents the affected gland from becoming painfully full, which prevents the mastitis from recurring and decreases the odds that the baby will prefer the unaffected side after healing.

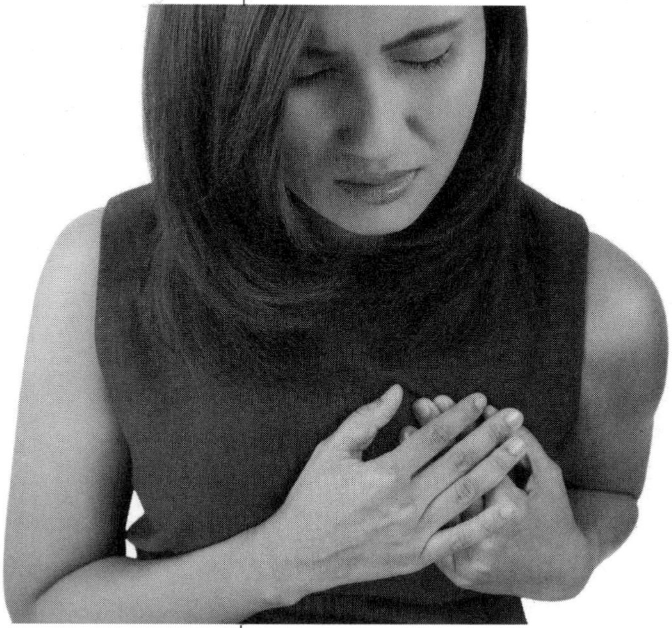

DEEP BREAST PAIN

Nursing parents with continuing breast and/or nipple pain may feel worried and upset.

Dealing with pain is difficult in any case, but in addition to the discomfort suffered and the negative impact ongoing pain can have on many aspects of daily life (McClellan et al., 2012), there is also the worry that the pain may be a sign of a serious physical problem, such as breast cancer. Continuing pain gives many parents second thoughts about nursing. Listen and acknowledge these feelings. Offer to help parents determine the cause of the pain. Assure them that in most cases the cause of deep breast pain can be found and the pain relieved. Also encourage parents to contact their healthcare provider for appropriate pain medication.

Perception of pain can vary tremendously from person to person, too, depending on a wide variety of factors. See Figure 17.1 on p. 701 for an overview of the variables that may cause pain to be perceived as more or less intense.

• • •

Ask the age of the baby, where and when the pain is felt, and if they have a history of nursing problems, especially nipple trauma, which can lead to painful complications.

Some causes of deep breast pain can occur at any stage of lactation, but some are more likely during the first weeks, while nursing is getting established. For example, nipple pain and trauma, mastitis, vasospasm, and strong milk ejection are more common during early nursing. Referred pain from an injury can happen at any time.

History of nipple trauma. Broken skin on the nipple allows organisms to enter the mammary gland, making it a major risk factor for mastitis (Amir & Academy of Breastfeeding Medicine Protocol, 2014), as well as bacterial and fungal nipple infections (see the previous chapter). Nipple damage—especially if it continues for weeks or months— also can negatively affect the microbiome of the mammary gland. Just like the gut, both the mammary gland and human milk have their own microbiome, a population of organisms (bacteria, fungi, and viruses) that interact with the host's body either positively or negatively. If the normal microbiome of the mammary gland increases in unhealthy (pathogenic) organisms, this can lead to condition known as mammary dysbiosis (P. Berens,

Eglash, Malloy, & Steube, 2016; Walker, 2018). This change may lead to a ***lactiferous ductal infection***, when nursing parents suffer from persistent sore, tender, throbbing breasts and nipples that may last for months (P. Berens et al., 2016). For treatment options, see next page.

Other questions to ask. Parents with deep breast pain may feel it in one or both sides. It may be localized in one area or radiate throughout the gland. If parents have (or had) nipple trauma or mastitis, this may be a clue to its cause. The following are the most common causes of deep breast pain, along with how the symptoms of each may be perceived.

If the pain is in one side during or between feeds, consider these common causes:

- ***Nipple pain and/or trauma***—The damage may be limited to nipple, but the pain is usually radiating into the mammary tissue (Amir et al., 2013). It resolves when nursing no longer hurts and the nipples are healed. Ask if the nipples look misshapen after feeds. For more, see the previous chapter, "Nipple Issues."
- ***Mastitis***—The pain is usually localized, but it could be radiating. In severe cases, it could occur in both sides. Most cases occur during the early weeks of nursing (Amir et al., 2007) but it can also happen later. Ask if there is a hard area in the gland or if putting pressure on it is painful. If the pain continues after treatment for mastitis, suggest seeing a healthcare provider to rule out abscess and other mammary issues (Amir, 2003). See earlier section, "Mastitis."
- ***Nipple infection***—The pain may be localized or radiating. Bacterial or fungal infection may develop after nipple damage and may include visible pus or yellow scabbing or crusting. To distinguish bacterial from fungal infection, see pp. 724 and 727.

If the pain is in both sides during feeds, consider:

- ***Engorgement***—The pain is usually radiating and will resolve with engorgement. It usually occurs during the first 2 weeks of nursing, and the tissue feels taut. It can occur later if feeds are missed or baby sleeps for unusually long stretches. See previous section, "Engorgement."
- ***Strong milk ejection***—The pain is usually radiating. A German study of 335 non-lactating women (Peters, Diemer, Mecks, & Behnken, 2003) found a strong association between milk duct dilation and breast pain unrelated to menstrual cycles. The wider the milk ducts while dilating, the greater the pain. Ultrasound research on breastfeeding women (Ramsay et al., 2004) found a large variation in duct size and a significant increase in ductal diameter during milk ejection, which may contribute to breast pain during feeds in some parents. Ask if the pain starts shortly after feeds begin, when baby's audible gulping is heard. Overabundant milk production may increase the pain. This pain usually decreases over time, disappearing within a month or so after birth (K. Wambach, 2021, p. 295).
- ***Pain disorder***—Those with the condition ***allodynia*** feel pain even with the type of light touch that does not usually cause pain. The authors of the Academy of Breastfeeding Medicine Clinical Protocol

#26 on persistent pain during nursing (P. Berens et al., 2016) noted that this unusual response to touch may occur in parents with other pain disorders, such as irritable bowel syndrome, fibromyalgia, migraines, interstitial cystitis, temporomandibular joint (TMJ) disorder, and painful intercourse. The authors also note that pain disorders are associated with depression, anxiety, and other psychological issues and those with these disorders may benefit from the type of psychological treatment given to those with chronic pain.

If the pain is in both sides between feeds, consider:

- ***Vasospasm or Raynaud's phenomenon***—The pain is usually radiating. The nipple may turn white (blanch) after the baby releases it. One large prospective Australian study (Buck, Amir, Cullinane, Donath, & Team, 2014) found that 23% of its 360 first-time mothers experienced vasospasm during the first 8 weeks after birth. If Raynaud's phenomenon is involved, the nipple may also turn red and/or blue, and the parent may have a history of pain and blanching when fingers or toes are exposed to cold. Symptoms usually begin during the early weeks of nursing. For details and treatment options, see p. 710.
- ***Oversupply***—Sharp pain or dull, aching pain may occur as the glands become full of milk (P. Berens et al., 2016).
- ***Referred pain from nipple pain and/or trauma***—The pain may be localized or radiating and will resolve when nipple pain and/or trauma resolves (Amir et al., 2013). It usually occurs during the early weeks of nursing but may occur later if nipple damage happens when baby is teething.

• • •

If the pain is in one side during or between feedings, consider:

If the common causes don't seem to fit, explore less-common causes of deep breast pain.

- ***Bacterial dysbiosis*** or ***lactiferous ductal infection.*** As mentioned on the previous page, a parent with a history of nipple trauma may develop sore, tender glands and/or nipples that can last for months. This could also occur on both sides. Due to an overgrowth of bacteria, yeast, or both, this condition is caused by an alteration in the mammary microbiome and can be challenging to resolve. In the Academy of Breastfeeding Medicine Clinical Protocol #26 on persistent pain during nursing (P. Berens et al., 2016), its authors refer to this as bacterial dysbiosis or a lactiferous ductal infection. Its authors suggest treating it with oral antibiotics (cephalosporin, amoxicillin/clavulanate, dicloxacillin, or erythromycin) for 2 to 6 weeks. To download a copy of this protocol to share with healthcare providers, go to **bfmed.org/protocols**. Treating this condition with a specific probiotic (L. fermentum CECT 5716) was tested in a 2015 Spanish randomized double-blinded controlled study (Maldonado-Lobon et al., 2015). This study found that the groups receiving the probiotic (no matter what the dose) had a significant decrease in the bacterial load of their expressed milk and significantly decreased mammary pain.
- ***Internal scarring from previous breast or chest surgery or injury***—The pain is usually localized. Ask if there is a history of any breast or chest surgery or injury. If so, see last section in this chapter.

- ***Ruptured breast implant***—The pain is usually localized. Breast shape may change or there may be skin changes. If this is the problem, removal surgery may be needed.
- ***Galactocele***—The pain is usually localized. An obvious lump can usually be felt within the gland and easily moved. For details, see p. 781.
- ***Duct ectasia***—The pain is usually localized and may also include burning, itching, and swelling of the nipple. For details, see p. 783.
- ***Referred pain from muscle strain or injury***—The pain may be localized or radiating and resolves when the injury heals. An injury elsewhere in the body may be felt as breast pain if it occurs along the same nerve pathways. During the early weeks, this could be due to a birth injury, such as a pulled back or neck muscle. Later, it may be due to any injury, joint pain, or muscle strain, such as leaning over to nurse in uncomfortable positions. It may be felt in both sides. Ask if the parent has a pulled muscle, muscle strain, or any other injury. If so, suggest using starter positions (see p. 23-29) so it's possible to relax all muscles during nursing rather than supporting baby's weight in arms.
- ***Breast cancer***—The pain may be localized or radiating. If breast pain does not resolve after a couple of weeks, suggest seeing a healthcare provider to rule this out. Between 8% and 15% of those later diagnosed with breast cancer report breast pain as one of their symptoms (Ohene-Yeboah & Amaning, 2008).

If the pain is in both sides during feeds, consider:

- ***Premenstrual pain***—The pain is usually radiating and peaks before a menstrual period when mammary glands swell with extra blood and lymph fluids (Ader, South-Paul, Adera, & Deuster, 2001). It can be felt during or between feeds and includes feelings of heaviness, fullness, and tenderness. Symptoms usually resolve soon after menstruation starts. If fibrocystic breast changes are a contributing factor, eliminating caffeine may help.

If the pain is in both sides between feeds, consider:

- ***Very large mammary glands*** are heavy and can pull on the connective tissues above the glands. Ask parents if they feel tenderness where the glands join the chest wall and near the third rib when they apply gentle pressure above the gland. If appropriate, a different style or better fitting bra may help relieve the pain. Also, Canadian researchers (Kernerman & Park, 2014) found that using pectoral muscle massage and other stretching techniques before feeds improved comfort.

• • •

Shooting, burning pain between feeds is unlikely to be from a ductal yeast infection and more likely to have other causes.

Once it was thought that the most likely cause of shooting or burning breast pain between feeds was a secondary yeast infection in or around the milk ducts (often referred to as ***mammary*** or ***ductal candidiasis***), but research found this questionable.

U.S. research. A U.S. study (Anderson, Held, & Wright, 2004) reported that 8 of 12 women with deep breast pain were treated with repeated courses of an effective antifungal drug with no improvement before their health history

TABLE 18.3 Possible Causes of Deep Breast Pain Based on Location and Timing

Breast Pain Occurs	During a Feed	Between Feeds
In One Side	• Nipple trauma • Mastitis/abscess • Nipple infection (bacterial, fungal, viral) • Referred pain from elsewhere • Internal scarring from breast/chest surgery/injury • Ruptured breast implant • Galactocele • Ductal ectasia • Other mammary disease/disorder • Breast cancer	• Referred pain from nipple trauma • Mastitis/abscess • Bacterial dysbiosis, lactiferous ductal infection • Referred pain from elsewhere • Internal scarring from breast/chest surgery/injury • Ruptured breast implant • Galactocele • Ductal ectasia • Other mammary disease/disorder
In Both Sides	• Engorgement (if baby ≤2 wk) • Strong milk ejection • Premenstrual pain • Muscle strain from large breasts • Pain disorder	• Referred pain from nipple trauma • Vasospasm/Raynaud's phenomenon • Oversupply • Bacterial dysbiosis, lactiferous ductal infection • Muscle strain from large breasts • Pain disorder

Adapted from (P. Berens et al., 2016; Mitchell, Johnson, et al., 2019)

revealed that Raynaud's phenomenon (see p. 710) was the cause of their pain. After treatment with prescription nifedipine for this circulatory disorder, the pain resolved in most.

Another U.S. study compared the cultures of expressed milk from 18 breastfeeding mothers without breast pain or other symptoms with milk cultures of 16 mothers with stabbing or burning breast pain between feeds, as well as nipple pain or trauma (T. W. Hale, Bateman, Finkelman, & Berens, 2009). Accurate assay methods were unable to detect candida in the milk of either group.

Spanish research used a similar approach and found the same results. In a study that analyzed expressed milk samples, nipple swabs, and nipple biopsy samples from 529 women with symptoms consistent with nipple thrush and ductal yeast, such as shooting pains in the breast (Jimenez et al., 2017) were analyzed. The researchers concluded that if yeast played any role in these symptoms, it was minor. Rather, bacteria, such as coagulase-negative staphylococcus and streptococci appeared to be most prominent.

Swedish research, using a case-control study design, followed two groups of 35 women, one group with and one group without symptoms of yeast overgrowth, such as deep breast pain (Kaski & Kvist, 2018). The researchers concluded that although 23% of those in the group with deep breast pain cultured positive for candida in their milk (0% in the control group), neither clinical symptoms nor milk cultures are reliable for diagnosing candida infections. They suggested that when parents experience breast pain, the best strategy is to start with basic nursing dynamics, such as positioning and latch (see Chapter 1).

Australian research. One exception to the previous studies was the prospective longitudinal cohort CASTLE study of 360 first-time mothers who were followed from the end of pregnancy through the first 8 weeks after birth (Amir et al., 2013). Its purpose was to investigate the role that staph bacteria and candida yeast play in the development of nipple and breast pain. The researchers cultured the milk, nipples, and babies' mouth using the ultra-sensitive PCR technology that is not available to most clinicians. They found that the women with the classic symptoms of nipple or breast thrush were more likely to have candida species in their nipple, milk, and baby's mouth (54%) compared with the controls (36%). Nipple damage predicted these symptoms.

When parents experience burning or shooting mammary pain between feeds, before considering yeast as the likely cause, first rule out other causes, such as

- Engorgement
- Referred pain from nipple trauma
- Mastitis
- Oversupply
- Premenstrual pain
- Strong milk ejection
- Vasospasm or Raynaud's phenomenon
- Muscle strain from large breasts
- If there is a history of nipple trauma, mammary or bacterial dysbiosis (p. 775).

BREAST LUMPS

During lactation, the mammary glands typically feel lumpier than at other times.

During lactation, the texture of the mammary glands changes because the milk ducts fill and empty many times each day and more blood and lymph flow to the glands. Suggest parents become familiar with the way their glands feel during lactation by examining them regularly. With practice, they can learn to distinguish normal lumpiness from a lump that might need medical attention by noticing if it decreases in size after nursing. If a lump's size stays constant or increases after nursing, suggest it be checked by a healthcare provider.

• • •

If a lump does not decrease in size after careful home treatment for mastitis, suggest seeing a healthcare provider.

During lactation, most lumps are either milk-filled lobes or inflammation, such as mastitis. Some are benign tumors (fibromas) or milk-retention cysts (galactoceles). Only rarely are they cancerous.

If healthcare providers are not familiar with lactating mammary glands, suggest they consult with a knowledgeable colleague or that the parent seek a second opinion from a healthcare provider experienced with lactation. See Table 18.4 for the most common masses diagnosed during lactation.

• • •

Suggest nursing right before a breast exam or procedure.

Nursing right before an exam or procedure reduces the amount of milk in the mammary glands, making it easier to feel a lump and to perform procedures. If possible, suggest bringing the baby to the appointment along with a helper so baby can nurse while they wait, keeping the volume of milk to a minimum.

TABLE 18.4 Most Common Breast Masses Diagnosed During Lactation

Condition	Description/Test	Treatment
Lactating Adenoma	Painless, rubbery and easily moved mass that may grow quickly. Test: core needle biopsy	None, will resolve after weaning
Galactocele (milk-filled cyst)	Often painless lump(s). Test: fine-needle aspiration.	Either none or, if painful, serial aspiration or drainage with a catheter
Phlegmon (collection of fluid usually after mastitis)	Tender, persistent, irregularly shaped mass may be infected. Test: core needle biopsy to rule out cancer.	Apply cold, treat with antibiotics, monitor as may become an abscess
Abscess (pus-filled cyst)	Tender mass, often with skin redness. Test: fine-needle aspiration.	Drainage with or without antibiotics
Fibroadenoma (benign mass)	Rubbery, smooth mass that moves easily, grows during pregnancy and lactation. Test: If >2-3 cm, core needle biopsy.	Observe and treat symptoms
Breast Cancer (cancerous tumor)	Usually non-tender mass, may include skin dimpling, nipple retraction, bloody nipple discharge. Test: core needle biopsy	Varies by stage and tumor characteristics

Adapted from (Mitchell, Johnson, et al., 2019). For more details, see Clinical Protocol #30 at **bfmed.org/protocols**.

• • •

Nursing is compatible with most diagnostic tests.

Some of the diagnostic tests that might be used to diagnose a breast lump include:

X-rays. Human milk is not affected and it's fine to nurse right after an x-ray.

Imaging scans (PET, MIBI, and EIT scans, and ultrasound). These imaging techniques do not interfere with nursing or affect the milk. Unlike mammograms, ultrasound can effectively distinguish solid lumps from fluid-filled cysts, galactoceles, and abscesses (Haliloglu et al., 2019). In the Academy of Breastfeeding Medicine Clinical Protocol #30 on breast masses and diagnostic breast imaging (Mitchell, Johnson, et al., 2019), its authors recommend the use of ultrasound as the first diagnostic tool with any breast lump or mass.

CAT scan or MRI does not interfere with nursing or affect the milk, but as part of these procedures, parents may be injected with a radiopaque or radiocontrast agent, which allows blood vessels to be seen more clearly. The agents often used with CAT scans are iodinated radiocontrast agents, but unlike other iodine agents, the iodine in these products stays bound to the molecule, which prevents the iodine from going into the milk. Agents used with an MRI typically contain gadolinium. Only miniscule amounts of gadolinium contrast agent reach the milk compartment and virtually none is absorbed orally by the infant (T.W. Hale, 2019, p. 330). According to the 2018 American College of Radiology *Manual for Contrast Media* (ACR, 2018, p. 100):

> "Because of the very small percentage of gadolinium-based contrast medium that is excreted into the breast milk and absorbed by the infant's gut, we believe that the available data suggest that it is safe for the mother and infant to continue breast-feeding after receiving such an agent."

Some package inserts for these products suggest interrupting nursing for 24 hours after use, but this is unnecessary, as these preparations are also used in children for diagnostic purposes.

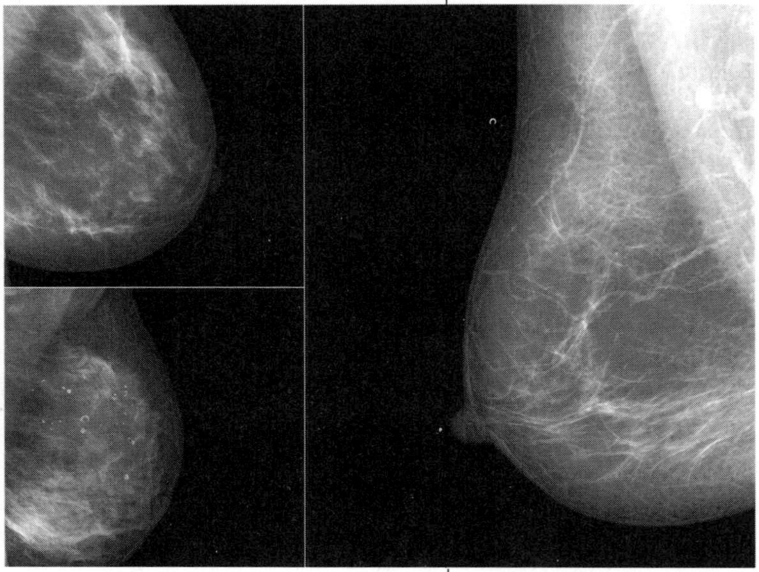

Mammograms use low-level x-rays and can be done on a lactating mammary gland. Like other x-rays, mammograms do not affect the milk, so nursing can continue immediately afterward. But mammograms are usually more difficult to read in younger patients and during lactation, because mammary tissue is denser at those times. The aging process causes mammary tissue to lose density, making mammography a more effective diagnostic tool. A mammogram can help determine the size and location of a known lump, but may not show early lumps or soft-tissue changes in the lactating gland.

The level of milk production affects the quality of a mammogram. Greater milk production causes greater tissue density, making a mammogram harder to read. Conversely, lower milk production makes a mammogram easier to read. But tissue changes take time. It would take about a month after weaning before a difference would be noticeable in the quality of a mammogram.

If nursing parents need a mammogram, encourage them to find a radiologist with experience reading mammograms of lactating parents, bring the baby to the testing site, and nurse before the mammogram.

If an ultrasound shows a suspicious mass, in the Academy of Breastfeeding Medicine Clinical Protocol #30 on breast masses and diagnostic imaging (Mitchell, Johnson, et al., 2019), its authors recommend that a mammogram—specifically the 3D type known as DBT—be done as the next step, because it can show aspects of the mass that an ultrasound cannot.

Fine-needle aspiration cytologic study. This quick, nearly painless procedure can determine the nature of a fluid-filled lump (such as a galactocele or abscess) and can often be done using local anesthesia in an office or clinic without interrupting nursing.

Core needle biopsy is recommended by the Academy of Breastfeeding Medicine (Mitchell, Johnson, et al., 2019) for a solid mass with the guidance of either ultrasound or an MRI.

• • •

A biopsy can usually be done without interrupting nursing.

Suggest nursing parents make sure their healthcare provider knows they are nursing before a breast biopsy. One of the risks sometimes cited for doing a biopsy before weaning is the small risk of a milk fistula forming. A milk fistula occurs when a connection forms between a milk duct and the skin's surface, causing constant milk flow. The authors of the Academy of Breastfeeding Medicine Clinical Protocol #30 on breast masses and diagnostic imaging (Mitchell, Johnson, et al., 2019, p. 6) wrote:

> "We do not recommend discontinuation of breastfeeding before biopsy in an effort to minimize [the risks of milk fistula formation and bleeding

> [due to extra blood flow to the mammary gland]. In fact, the inflammation related to abrupt weaning could increase the risk of fistula formation, and lack of alternative drainage routes could promote fistula formation through the biopsy tract."

• • •

Fibrocystic changes in the mammary gland are common; pregnancy and nursing may reduce the severity of their symptoms.

As parents age, the hormones of menstruation contribute to the development of benign cysts in the mammary glands. Sometimes these changes feel like dense, fibrous areas. At other times, they may feel like a smooth, round lump that can be easily moved around. Some feel pain and tenderness as well, often intensified during menstruation. Because pregnancy and nursing prevent or delay menstruation, many feel relief from their symptoms then. Reducing caffeine may reduce symptoms (Ader et al., 2001).

Any breast lump should be checked by a healthcare provider if it hasn't disappeared within a couple of weeks. Diagnostic imaging and fine-needle aspiration will determine whether or not a lump is a benign cyst.

• • •

Galactoceles, or milk-filled cysts, are uncommon and harmless.

One of the less common causes of breast lumps during lactation (Couto, Glassman, Batista Abreu, & Paes, 2016) is the galactocele, a milk-filled cyst. In the 2016 8th edition of *Breastfeeding: A Guide for the Medical Profession*, U.S. physicians Ruth and Robert Lawrence describe the cause and treatment of galactoceles (Lawrence & Lawrence, 2016, p. 269):

> "Milk-retention cysts are uncommon and, when found, are almost exclusively a problem in lactating women. The contents at first are pure milk. Because of fluid absorption, they later contain thick, creamy, cheesy, or oily material. The swelling is smooth and rounded, and compression of it may cause milky fluid to exude from the nipple. Galactoceles are thought to be caused by blockage of a milk duct. The cyst may be aspirated to avoid surgery, but will fill up again. It can be removed surgically under local anesthesia without stopping breastfeeding. Thus its presence does not require cessation of lactation. Firm diagnosis can be made by ultrasound; a cyst and milk will appear the same, whereas a tumor will be distinguishable."

To avoid surgery, fine-needle aspiration, using a local anesthetic, can usually be done in a healthcare provider's office or clinic, which allows the contents of the cyst to be removed and checked. Once a galactocele is confirmed, if it is not painful or growing, nothing need be done.

KEY CONCEPT

When the milk in a galactocele is aspirated, it will usually refill. If it is not painful, nothing needs to be done.

When a galactocele is painful, however, waiting is not a good strategy. Preliminary Thai research on 16 women with galactoceles (Auvichayapat et al., 2003) found that using a nylon probe to remove the obstruction in the milk duct that caused the galactocele can reduce the incidence of recurrence. In this study, none of the 11 women whose galactoceles were treated with the nylon probe had a recurrence, whereas 2 of the 5 who were treated with fine-needle aspiration had a recurrence.

Galactoceles also sometimes become infected (Ghosh, Morton, Whaley, & Sterioff, 2004). If an infection develops, the Academy of Breastfeeding Medicine (Mitchell, Johnson, et al., 2019) recommends drainage by a healthcare provider.

• • •

Calcifications in the mammary gland occur more often with aging.

During the aging process, calcium leaves the bones and travels to other areas of the body, landing in the arteries, joints, and mammary glands. Calcifications or microcalcifications in the gland are tiny deposits of calcium that can be detected only with a mammogram and occur in about 4% of women (Sickles & Abele, 1981). They appear to be more common in women who breastfed. If a mammogram shows calcifications that are evenly distributed in both sides, this is usually not a cause for concern. However, when they appear in clusters, this is considered a risk factor for cancer, so another mammogram is recommended within a few months (Uematsu, Kasami, & Yuen, 2009).

BLOOD IN THE MILK OR NIPPLE DISCHARGE

Assure the family that blood in the milk usually disappears quickly and will not harm the baby.

When nursing parents see blood in their milk, they may worry they have a serious health problem and that the blood will harm the baby. Suggest they contact their healthcare provider to discuss the blood, but assure them that bleeding from the nipple in late pregnancy and the first few weeks after delivery is usually due to more harmless causes (see next point). Also assure them that it is fine to continue nursing and that the bleeding will not harm the baby.

• • •

Blood in the milk is not uncommon and has several likely causes.

Blood in the milk is probably much more common than we realize. When U.S. researchers examined under a microscope the early milk of 72 women (Kline & Lash, 1964), they detected red blood cells in 17, or 24%, of the asymptomatic breastfeeding women.

Rusty-pipe syndrome, also known as ***vascular engorgement***, is one common cause of blood in the milk during pregnancy and early nursing. It is caused by slight internal bleeding from a combination of increased blood flow to the mammary glands and rapid development of the milk-producing tissues (Barco et al., 2014). Most common in first-time nursing parents, this usually occurs in both sides, although it may occur in one side at first. With this condition, usually there is little or no discomfort and it resolves spontaneously within the first few weeks of lactation (Cizmeci, Kanburoglu, Akelma, & Tatli, 2013; Mitchell, Johnson, et al., 2019; Silva, Carvalho, Maia, Osorio, & Barbosa, 2014). An Australian survey (O'Callaghan, 1981) followed 32 women who reported blood in the milk during pregnancy and early lactation that could not be explained by other causes. Most reported that the blood cleared within 3 to 7 days after birth, with a few reporting a brief reappearance a few weeks later.

Intraductal papilloma is another common cause of blood in the milk. An intraductal papilloma is a benign wart-like growth in a milk duct that causes bleeding as it erodes. It usually occurs in only one side, cannot be felt as a lump, and may or may not be accompanied by discomfort. The bleeding often stops spontaneously within a couple weeks of birth without treatment. However, because these benign growths can become cancerous, diagnostic imaging of the mammary gland is recommended by the Academy of Breastfeeding Medicine (Mitchell, Johnson, et al., 2019) when intraductal papilloma is suspected (de Paula & Campos, 2017).

Fibrocystic changes within the gland, which are common with aging, may cause a bloody nipple discharge. In one case report (Aksoy, Eras, Erdeve, & Dilmen, 2013), the fibrocystic changes were identified by ultrasound, and breastfeeding continued. In this case, the mother's milk continued to appear bloody for several months and then resolved.

Mammary or nipple trauma can cause blood in the milk when broken capillaries in the mammary gland occur from rough handling or too-high breast pump suction levels. If a nursing parent has nipple damage, it may be difficult to know whether blood is coming from the nipple or from inside the gland.

Milk that looks bloody may not be what it seems. If expressed milk has a reddish tinge, it is easy to assume it contains blood. But milk can look reddish for other reasons. U.S. authors (Quinn, Ailsworth, Matthews, Kellams, & Shirley, 2018) described a 9-week-old baby with pink stools whose nursing mother produced pink milk because they were colonized with the bacterium *Serratia marcescens*. After a literature search, these authors found 10 similar cases, all of whom had positive outcomes whether or not antibiotics were prescribed.

• • •

To rule out other, more serious causes, if the blood in the milk doesn't clear within a few weeks of birth, suggest nursing parents see their healthcare provider.

With the previously described causes, blood in the milk usually clears without treatment within a few weeks or so after birth. However, if parents continue to see blood in the milk after that, more serious causes, such as Paget's disease and other types of breast cancer, should be ruled out. Although breast cancer is unlikely, suggest nursing parents see their healthcare provider as soon as possible (Mitchell, Johnson, et al., 2019). Non-invasive tests, such as ultrasound are recommended to help determine the cause of the blood.

• • •

A nipple discharge that is not bloody can be due to a variety of causes.

According to the Academy of Breastfeeding Medicine (Mitchell, Johnson, et al., 2019), a yellow or green nipple discharge that seems to come from multiple ducts on both sides "is generally not concerning" and is considered "physiologic" or within the normal range (Stone & Wheeler, 2015).

Expressed milk comes in a variety of colors—blue, green, brownish, yellow, gold, and clear—which are considered normal for both colostrum and mature milk. For more details, see p. 517-518.

Stringy-looking milk or granules can sometimes be expressed during or right before a bout of mastitis. See Figure 18.1 and p. 758-759 in the previous section for more details.

A multi-colored, sticky discharge may occur in those with ***duct ectasia***, or ***comedomastitis***, which is caused by an inflammation in a milk duct (Lawrence & Lawrence, 2016, pp. 608-609). Nursing parents with this condition may have no discomfort, or they may have burning pain, itching, and nipple swelling. Over time, the affected duct may feel like a hardened tube or a mass under the nipple. Treatment includes warm compresses and antibiotics. If duct ectasia is painful or the discharge appears bloody, surgical removal of the duct is an option.

UNUSUAL BREAST DEVELOPMENT

Extra Nipples and Breast Tissue

Extra nipples, areolae, and/or milk-making tissue sometimes develop, usually along the milk line, which runs from the armpit to the groin.

All mammals have what's called a ***milk line*** (Figure 18.4), the area of the body where nipples form. In some mammals, many nipples form along this line. (Typically, each species has twice the number of nipples as their average litter size.) In humans, although the usual number of nipples is two, some parents have extra ***accessory*** or ***supernumerary nipples***, which usually form along the milk line as remnants from embryonic development of the mammary ridge (K. Wambach & Genna, 2021, p. 54). In some cases, though, these extra glands and nipples develop elsewhere on the body, such as on the buttocks or the back (Lawrence & Lawrence, 2016, p. 39). A 2013 case report and review article (Pieh-Holder, 2013) described the experience of a U.S. woman whose biopsy revealed that a growth on her vulva was active mammary tissue.

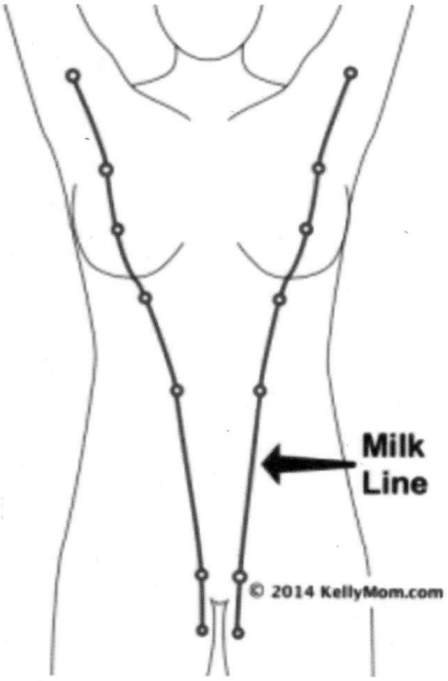

Figure 18.4 The milk line on which most extra nipples and glands develop. ©2014 **KellyMom.com**. Used with permission.

Between 0.2% and 6% of all people have extra mammary tissue and/or nipples, although this is more common in women than in men (Loukas, Clarke, & Tubbs, 2007). Some include milk-making tissue and no nipples; some include nipples but no milk-making tissue. Some have ducts that leak milk through the skin without a nipple (Wilson-Clay & Hoover, 2017, p. 68). Some develop multiple mammary glands. Often, extra nipples look like moles, but some look like full-fledged nipples. In most cases, no milk-producing tissue accompanies extra nipples. But some parents have glandular tissue connected to their extra nipple, which can lead to feelings of fullness and engorgement after birth.

Nursing with extra glands and nipples. The existence of extra glands or nipples should not have much effect on nursing, although they may become engorged and even develop mastitis. Milk-making tissue normally extends into the armpit (known as the tail of Spence), which may become engorged as milk production increases after birth. But when extra glands and/or nipples develop in the armpit or elsewhere, the milk may not drain into the main ductal system.

Staying comfortable after birth. If no glandular tissue is attached to extra nipples, nothing special needs to be done to keep the parent comfortable. If no nipples are attached to extra milk-making tissue, use the same strategies to treat these areas as are recommended to keep newly delivered parents comfortable who do not plan to nurse:

- Avoid wearing clothing that constricts that area.
- Keep stimulation to a minimum.
- Apply cool or cold compresses to reduce swelling.
- Discuss anti-inflammatory medication with the healthcare provider.

When the milk is not removed, the tissue will stop milk production and will quickly involute, or go back to its prepregnancy state.

If extra glands have a nipple attached, milk may leak from the nipple, and it may be possible to express a little milk to relieve feelings of fullness. If they leak during nursing, suggest using pads or cloths to absorb the leaked milk. If mastitis develops in extra milk-making tissue, it may need to be treated (Wilson-Clay & Hoover, 2017, p. 69).

Underdeveloped Mammary Glands

If the mammary glands did not fully develop, nursing parents may be unable to produce enough milk to exclusively nurse their baby.

The normal development of milk-making tissue happens in two ways. Some of this development occurs during puberty, when the glands begin to develop. But it also occurs during pregnancy and after birth. While certain issues—such as placental problems or low prolactin levels—can prevent normal mammary development during pregnancy and affect milk production, what most refer as insufficient glandular tissue is different. As described in the book, *Making More Milk*, U.S. lactation consultants Lisa Marasco and Diana West (Marasco & West, 2020, p. 133) describe it this way:

> "True insufficient glandular tissue (IGT), or mammary hypoplasia, refers to what you started with before pregnancy and typically involves a lack of fullness in part or all of the breast. Small IGT breasts may look as if they never finished puberty and are often less than an A cup, with little palpable tissue. Larger IGT breasts may look 'deflated' or have an unusually long tubular or bowed shaped, with the nipples pointing down or away from the body. This is caused by the missing tissue that would normally provide support."

With some of the normal milk-making tissue missing, they often feel like obvious patches of milk-making tissue in a mostly soft gland (Wilson-Clay & Hoover, 2017, p. 69).

Why does this condition occur? It depends on whether the hypoplasia is congenital (present at birth) or acquired (due to influences after birth). Examples of congenital hypoplasia include some syndromes, like Jeune and Poland (Winocour & Lemaine, 2013) and conditions during fetal development that involve the same area and tissues as the mammary glands, such as mitral-valve prolapse (Rosenberg , Derman , Grabb , & Buda 1983) and scoliosis (Tsai, Hsieh, Liao, & Wu, 2010).

Acquired hypoplasia may affect mammary development before or after puberty. Some possible causes that occur before puberty include chest surgery that cuts through mammary buds (Goyal & Mansel, 2003) and chest traumas (Sadove & van Aalst, 2005). In a baby or child, radiation treatments of the chest may affect mammary development later (Skalkeas, Gogas, & Pavlatos, 1972). During puberty, conditions that may affect mammary development include:

- Hypothyroidism (Pringle, Stanhope, Hindmarsh, & Brook, 1988)
- Ovarian cysts (Sharma, Bajpai, Mittal, Kabra, & Menon, 2006) and other hormonal or ovarian problems (Balcar, Silinkova-Malkova, & Matys, 1972)

In some parts of the world, a greater incidence of altered breast development was found in girls exposed in utero to agricultural chemicals in their environment (Guillette et al., 2006).

Although lactating parents in this situation may not be able to fully nourish their baby without supplementing, the baby can partially nurse along with receiving either donor milk or formula while nursing with a nursing supplementer or using another feeding method (Thorley, 2005). For many of these parents, the biggest challenge is keeping the baby interested in nursing long enough to provide the necessary stimulation to grow more mammary tissue. A nursing supplementer provides continuous flow to keep baby nursing longer.

Depending on how much milk-making tissue is present and their nursing dynamics, parents may also be able to continue to increase milk production over time (Huggins, Petok, & Mireles, 2000) and eventually exclusively nurse later babies (Wilson-Clay & Hoover, 2017, p. 70). One case report (Bodley & Powers, 1999) described a mother who exclusively breastfed a subsequent baby after receiving progesterone treatment during pregnancy to treat a luteal-phase defect.

To read more about how long-term mammary stimulation can grow milk-making tissue, see this author's story of her own experience of nursing with one breast that didn't develop during puberty at **bit.ly/BA2-Magical**.

• • •

The appearance and spacing of the mammary glands and lack of tissue changes during pregnancy are red flags but not completely reliable indicators of future low milk production.

Among individuals, there is great variability in mammary size and shape, as well as how much of the tissue is glandular versus fatty (Geddes, 2007). One U.S. prospective study of 34 mothers (Huggins et al., 2000) found the following visual indicators among those unable to produce enough milk to fully nourish their babies:

- Widely spaced breasts (more than 1.5 inches or about 4 cm apart)
- Large differences in breast size (asymmetry)
- Tubular or cone-shaped (hypoplastic) rather than rounded breasts

Some also had bulbous-looking areolae. Many of the study mothers with low milk production noticed no breast changes during pregnancy or breast fullness after birth. The researchers adapted a rating system from another study (von Heimburg, Exner, Kruft, & Lemperle, 1996) to describe four categories of breast shapes:

1. Round, normal breasts
2. Breasts lacking tissue underneath
3. Breasts lacking tissue underneath and along the sides,
4. Breasts with little tissue anywhere.

It is important, however, never to assume from the shape of the mammary glands or lack of tissue changes during pregnancy that parents will not produce enough milk for their baby. A 2018 Polish study that measured mammary growth during pregnancy in 93 women and analyzed their milk after delivery (Zelazniewicz & Pawlowski, 2019) found no correlation between tissue growth and successful lactation. An Australian study (Cox, Kent, Casey, Owens, & Hartmann, 1999) found that mammary tissue growth continues during nursing throughout the first month after birth. One of its study mothers had no noticeable breast tissue growth before birth but produced plenty of milk for her baby and experienced significant breast tissue growth during the month after delivery.

KEY CONCEPT

Over time, nursing can increase milk production and grow milk-making tissue in parents with mammary hypoplasia.

Whenever possible, parents with these anatomical red flags should be monitored closely, without planting the seeds of doubt (Arbour & Kessler, 2013). Even closer follow-up is crucial if both the nursing parent and the baby have risk factors for inadequate milk intake (Duran & Spatz, 2011). *The Breastfeeding Atlas* features photos of women with these physical characteristics who made ample milk. Its authors (Wilson-Clay & Hoover, 2017, pp. 70-71) wrote:

> "Good counseling skills are critical when a woman presents with abnormal breast markers, because they may not always predict difficulty with breastfeeding. The LC must avoid creating anxiety or a loss of confidence, as this in itself may create breastfeeding problems. Mothers should be urged to try breastfeeding with subsequent children, because often these lactations are more successful for a variety of reasons, including potentially more glandular development with each pregnancy and increased maternal confidence. Because the calibration of the milk supply occurs early in lactogenesis II, women with unusual breasts deserve extra attention and extended follow-up to make sure they reach their full lactation potential with each lactation."

For more insights into the experiences of these families, see the 2014 book by Diana Cassar-Uhl, *Finding Sufficiency: Breastfeeding with Insufficient Glandular Tissue.*

Rapid Mammary Overdevelopment

Some mammary growth is normal, but one type of rapid growth, called gigantomastia, can be disabling.

With pregnancy and early nursing, most parents experience some mammary growth. However, ***gestational gigantomastia*** is an unusual condition that falls far outside the norm. During pregnancy, this condition is triggered when the parent's mammary tissue becomes hypersensitive to pregnancy hormones and grows to double or triple their previous size (8 to 20 bra cup sizes or more), which is often completely incapacitating (Rezai et al., 2015). Although it can occur during a first pregnancy, it usually happens first during a second or third pregnancy and occurs equally in those with small and large mammary glands. Once considered extremely rare, it is becoming more common (Craig, 2008).

The three types of gestational gigantomastia, which have different hormonal triggers, can be distinguished by the timing of the excessive mammary growth. In the first type, which is most common and responds well to antiprolactin hormone therapy, mammary growth occurs in the beginning of pregnancy and continues through all three trimesters. In the second type, the next most common, rapid growth begins in the second trimester, lasts for 3 to 6 weeks, then slows. This second type is usually accompanied by high insulin blood levels. In the third type, the rarest, rapid growth occurs right before or right after birth and, at this writing, a hormone sensitivity has not yet been identified.

• • •

Medical therapies other than surgery are available to treat gestational gigantomastia, which typically recurs with each pregnancy.

In more than 80% of the cases, the mammary glands return to normal size after the baby is born, but gigantomastia recurs with each subsequent pregnancy, even if breast reduction surgery is performed. In cases of extreme incapacitation, mastectomies or breast reduction surgeries are done during pregnancy or afterward (B. Antevski, Jovkovski, Filipovski, & Banev, 2011; B. M. Antevski, Smilevski, Stojovski, Filipovski, & Banev, 2007).

In one case report (Poojari, Pupadhya, Pai, Ramachandra, & Monappa, 2018), the affected mother nursed her baby but developed an abscess.

BREAST OR CHEST SURGERY OR INJURY

Basic Considerations

Discuss goals and options with nursing parents who have a history of breast or chest surgery or injury.

Some parents don't give much thought to their nursing goals, so it may help to first get a sense of what is important to them. Some types of breast surgery or injury (such as breast lifts and liposuction) are unlikely to have much effect on milk production and nursing. But others, such as breast reduction and top surgery, have the potential to significantly reduce milk production. In situations like this, be sure parents understand that nursing does not have to be "all or nothing." From a health standpoint, some nursing is almost always better than none. In terms of health outcomes, babies partially nursed or human-milk fed usually fall between those exclusively nursed and those who have never nursed. Ask how they would feel about partial nursing and let them know that any amount of human milk is a boon to their health and the health of their baby. Some may embrace this idea and others reject it.

Discuss the emotional aspects of nursing, so they are aware that there is more involved than milk. Nursing calms and comforts a baby, and the hormones of nursing enhance the intimacy of the nursing couple. Understanding parents' values, goals, and what aspects of nursing are most important can help them make decisions that feel right for them

Factors That Affect Nursing

Ask for the date and the details of any surgeries or injuries, as well as any complications.

In the book, *Making More Milk* (Marasco & West, 2020), U.S. lactation consultants Lisa Marasco and Diana West describe the "Milk Supply Equation" (below). Breast surgery and injury primarily affect the first two physical dynamics needed for milk production:

Sufficient glandular tissue

\+ **Enough intact nerve pathways and milk ducts**

\+ Adequate normal hormones and receptors

\+ Adequate lactation-critical nutrients

\+ Frequent, effective milk removal, transfer, and mammary stimulation

\+ No lactation inhibitors

= Good milk production

> **KEY CONCEPT**
>
> *Surgeries that remove glandular tissue, such as most breast reductions and top surgeries, are more likely to negatively affect milk production than those that don't.*

Surgery or injury details. If the surgery involved removing some milk-making glands (such as most breast reductions and top surgeries, see later the points about them), there is a good chance it will affect the volume of milk produced. If parents are unsure about how their surgery was done, suggest contacting the surgeon. If they are unclear on injury details, suggest contacting the healthcare provider.

Their sensitivity to touch and temperature. For good milk flow during nursing, intact nerve pathways allow nerve impulses to travel from the mammary gland to the brain and trigger the release of hormones needed for milk ejection. If critical nerve pathways are not functional, achieving normal milk flow can be more challenging. When facing the mammary glands, the primary nerve responsible for sensation of touch and temperature—the fourth intercostal—enters the areola between 1 o'clock and 4 o'clock when facing the left side and 8 o'clock and 11 o'clock when facing the right side (Schlenz, Kuzbari, Gruber, & Holle, 2000). An incision or injury affecting that part of the areola is more likely to cause nerve damage than an incision or injury elsewhere.

Time elapsed since the surgery or injury occurred. Nerves can regenerate (or grow back) over time. This ***reinnervation*** happens at a set rate (about 1 mm per month) and is not influenced by pregnancy or nursing. Therefore, the greater the passage of time since the surgery or injury, the more sensitive the glands and nipples are likely to become and the less likely it is that nerve damage will affect nursing (West & Hirsch, 2008).

Milk ducts affected. In addition to nerve function, the number of intact milk ducts is also important to milk production. Whether cutting milk ducts affects milk production depends in part on how many milk ducts with openings on the nipple existed before the surgery. The average number of milk ducts with nipple-pore openings is 9, but some have as few as 4 and as many as 14 (Ramsay, Kent, Hartmann, & Hartmann, 2005). In parents with 14 milk ducts leading to nipple pores, losing access to a couple of ducts may not have much effect on overall milk production. But in those with 4 ducts leading to openings, losing 2 may have a major impact. Unfortunately, these nipple pores are so small, it's not possible to determine the number in an individual parent. But understanding this dynamic explains why one parent may have no problem after surgery while another struggles. Unlike nerves, the regrowth of milk ducts occurs faster during pregnancy and nursing. If parents have milk-production issues with one child, they will likely produce more milk with each subsequent child.

Complications can occur with any surgery or injury. Ask about changes in nipple sensation and any noticeable scarring, infection, or any subsequent surgeries. Complications and additional surgeries may mean lower milk production (N. Hurst, 2003).

• • •

If there is a history of breast surgery, ask why it was done and if there are any other health issues.

If the surgery was performed to create a more normal appearance because the mammary glands did not develop normally, milk production problems may be due to a lack of glandular tissue rather than the surgery. (For details, see the previous section "Underdeveloped Mammary Glands.") Parents with a history of breast reduction surgery may have other health conditions that affect milk production, such as obesity, diabetes, hypothyroidism, or polycystic ovary syndrome.

• • •

If only one side was affected by surgery or injury, full milk production is more likely.

If surgery or injury occurred on only one side, nursing may not be affected, as most nursing parents are capable of exclusively nursing twins, triplets, and more. Even after the complete removal of one side via mastectomy, some parents have produced enough milk for their babies (even twins!) by nursing often on the remaining side (Michaels & Wanner, 2013).

The exception is the parent who had surgery on one side due to asymmetry, one sign of possible insufficient glandular tissue.

• • •

Ask if sensation in the nipple or gland is either reduced or heightened.

Whenever breast or chest surgery is performed, loss of sensation can happen. When it does, it is an indication of nerve damage. The more extensive the surgery or the larger the breast implant, the greater the risk of loss of sensation (Mofid, Klatsky, Singh, & Nahabedian, 2006). After breast or chest surgery, another possibility is altered sensation. Some experience unusual sensations or heightened sensitivity.

• • •

For parents considering breast or chest surgery, suggest talking to the surgeon about preserving mammary function.

No matter what type of surgery parents are considering—tumor or cyst removal, breast lift, reduction, top surgery, augmentation—encourage them to talk to their surgeon about their desire to nurse and ask about avoiding as much as possible cutting milk ducts and nerves during the surgery. See the impact of specific procedures and recommended techniques in the later sections.

Preparing During Pregnancy

Discuss nursing goals and options.

For details, see the first point in the previous section.

• • •

During pregnancy, encourage parents to learn all they can about normal nursing.

Parents with a history of breast or chest surgery or injury are often overly focused on their special situation and assume that nursing information geared toward the average parent does not apply to them. But they have an even greater need than most to understand nursing norms. Without realistic expectations, when parents have doubts about their ability to produce milk, they may assume that even normal behaviors and feeding patterns are signs that nursing is not working.

Worries about insufficient milk are common worldwide, even among those without a history of breast or chest surgery or injury. In fact, these worries are the most common reason parents give for early weaning and are often unrelated to actual milk production (Galipeau, Dumas, & Lepage, 2017). After breast or chest surgery or injury, parents are even more likely to doubt nursing. For this reason, encourage them to become familiar with nursing norms, how milk production works, and, if possible, participate in peer-support groups.

• • •

Suggest parents use knowledgeable and supportive healthcare providers and breastfeeding-friendly birthing facilities.

During and after birth, families need people around them who can help them accurately evaluate how nursing is going based on reliable indicators. To help get nursing off to the best possible start, encourage them to:

- Give birth at a Baby-Friendly birthing facility.
- Learn how to minimize interventions during labor and birth.
- Find skilled lactation help, meet these support people during pregnancy, and keep their contact information on hand.
- Plan to see the baby's healthcare provider at least weekly for weight checks during the first month.
- Learn when supplements are needed and discuss feeding options.

• • •

Ask if the sensitivity of the nipple or gland decreased after the surgery or injury.

Loss of sensitivity to temperature and touch in the gland indicates nerve damage and may inhibit milk ejection. Knowing this in advance may be helpful, so they can plan ahead. If this is an issue, see p. 480.

Initiating Nursing

To avoid early problems, encourage parents to focus on learning hand expression during the last month of pregnancy, getting a deep latch after birth, and minimizing engorgement.

Nursing early, often, and effectively is important to all nursing parents. But for parents with a history of breast or chest surgery or injury, it is vital to avoid common early nursing problems. As for all nursing parents, suggest learning hand expression during the last month of pregnancy by going to the website of U.S. pediatrician Dr. Jane Morton at **firstdroplets.com**, which provides free videos that demonstrate hand expression. It is a huge advantage to gain this skill before the baby comes. It also gives parents the chance during pregnancy to store some extra milk for supplementation, if needed. After the baby is born, Dr. Morton recommends after nursing sessions for parents to hand-express colostrum, the first milk, and feed it to their baby by spoon as "dessert." This stimulates more milk production and may help prevent excess weight loss in the baby.

Nursing parents with any active mammary tissue in areas where the milk is unable to drain due to severed ducts may experience some engorgement. However, if this happens, reassure them that milk ducts that do not connect to the nipple have a lower risk for infection. Like parents who do not nurse after birth, those areas of the gland will quickly stop producing milk and revert to their pre-pregnancy state. Suggest parents consider any tissue swelling as positive signs that the glands are making milk and use the comfort measures described in the previous "Engorgement" section to ease any discomfort.

• • •

If nerve damage inhibits milk ejection, discuss strategies.

Parents who can feel both touch and temperature on the areola and nipple are likely to experience normal milk ejection during nursing (West & Hirsch, 2008). But parents who have lost all sensation are at risk of impaired or inhibited milk ejection, at least until the nerves grow back.

Parents whose nerve pathways are impaired may need help achieving milk ejection, with strategies such as mental imagery (Cowley, 2014), the use of a synthetic oxytocin nasal spray, or by applying pressure to the gland during nursing (Bolman et al., 2013). Discuss these and see p. 480 for more details.

• • •

In some cases, nipple pain, blanching, and/or feeding problems may be related to nerve damage or scarring.

Sharp nipple pain sometimes occurs when scar tissue is pulled during nursing, especially with the first child nursed after surgery. But if nipple pain becomes an issue, other causes are more likely. Suggest parents in pain first rule out more common and treatable causes, such as shallow latch, bacterial nipple infection, vasospasm, and others described in Chapter 17, "Nipple Issues."

Those who work extensively with nursing parents after breast or chest surgery report that nipple blanching is common, perhaps due to disruption of nerves and/or blood supply (Marasco & West, 2020; West & Hirsch, 2008). No matter what the cause, the treatments for vasospasm may be helpful (see p. 710).

Another commonly reported issue is difficulty latching, because the nipple and areola feel less "full." Use good nursing dynamics to help overcome this challenge.

• • •

If milk production is likely to be low, suggest strategies that can help maximize milk stimulation after birth.

In parents likely to have less-than-full milk production, discuss ways to maximize their milk-making potential that will activate as many prolactin receptors as possible during the critical first few weeks. Not all parents will want to try all the possibilities, but some options include using compression or massage before and during nursing to increase milk removal, increasing feeding frequency, taking herbal or prescribed galactagogues, and expressing milk after and/or between nursing sessions. For details, see p. 442.

The Need for Supplementation

Suggest parents keep close tabs on the baby's weight and diaper output to gauge whether supplements are needed.

The most accurate way to determine whether a baby is getting enough milk is by monitoring her weight. Loss of up to 10% of birth weight within the first 3 to 4 days after birth is considered in the normal range. After that, when nursing is going well, most babies gain on average about 1 ounce (28 g) per day or about 7 ounces (198 g) per week. The need for supplements will depend on the baby's weight. If the baby loses more than 10% of birth weight, supplements are needed right away. However, if the baby's weight gain is slightly below average, there is time to try milk-enhancing strategies first. Diaper output, while not as reliable, can also be used as a rough gauge (DiTomasso & Paiva, 2018; Nommsen-Rivers, Heinig, Cohen, & Dewey, 2008). For details, see p. 202-204.

• • •

Offer to discuss common nursing outcomes after birth.

After breast or chest surgery or injury, possible nursing outcomes include:

- Full milk production with no need for supplements.
- Milk production sufficient for the first few days or weeks, but as the hormones of childbirth settle down and milk production becomes more dependent on the stimulation of milk removal, supplements become necessary (West & Hirsch, 2008).
- Little to no milk production, with supplements needed soon after birth.

Even parents producing little milk may be able to exclusively nurse during the first few days. Some parents with nerve damage find that even with frequent nursing, reduced nerve stimulation results in decreased milk production over time.

If a baby is not receiving adequate milk during nursing, it is vital to rule out other causes—such as shallow latch, tongue-tie, and others—before assuming it is due to surgery or injury. See section beginning on p. 208 for other possibilities.

> **KEY CONCEPT**
>
> *Before assuming a baby's low milk intake is due to low milk production, carefully assess the basics and other possibilities.*

If a baby doesn't need supplements within the first 5 or 6 weeks, chances are good they won't be needed. Babies' milk intake typically increases during the first 5 weeks or so (Hill, Aldag, Chatterton, & Zinaman, 2005; Kent, Gardner, & Geddes, 2016), then plateaus until solid foods are started (Neville et al., 1988). So unless other changes that affect milk production occur, such as decreasing feeding frequency, if a baby is still growing and thriving without supplements by 5 to 6 weeks of age, the baby will probably not need them.

• • •

To stimulate the maximum milk production possible, parents need to strike a delicate balance between giving the baby the smallest volume of supplements needed while actively nursing as much as possible. Babies need to be well nourished to gain weight and thrive, and also to nurse effectively. If a baby does not get enough milk, she can become weak, which can compromise her ability to nurse.

When supplements are needed, encourage parents to give enough—but not too much—and to consider their feeding options.

If supplements are needed, suggest parents consider using a nursing supplementer, also known as a feeding-tube device, which can keep the baby actively nursing longer, thereby stimulating more milk production. It also provides extra milk during nursing, so parents don't have to spend more time feeding the baby again afterward. Not all parents are comfortable using a nursing supplementer (Borucki, 2005), so discuss other feeding options and support them in their choice. Their decision may depend in part on whether they are close to full milk production, making some milk, or making little to no milk. For details on different feeding options, see p. 223.

Breast Lift

In most cases, a breast lift will not affect nursing.

Also known as ***mastopexy***, a breast lift is used to reshape and reposition sagging mammary glands so they appear higher and more rounded (Figure 18.5). This procedure involves removing excess skin, but the nerves and milk-making glands are not usually affected and no mammary tissue is removed. If a breast lift is done along with a breast augmentation, the risks would be the same as the two procedures combined (West & Hirsch, 2008).

Breast Augmentation Surgery

Breast augmentation is one of the most common types of plastic surgery performed.

Also known as ***augmentation mammaplasty***, breast augmentation surgery is performed on millions worldwide. In most of these surgeries, silicone- or saline-filled sacs (Figure 18.6) are inserted into a pocket that is formed either between the chest muscles and the glandular tissue or under the muscle (Figure 18.5). The incision may be in the fold under the breast, near the armpit, around

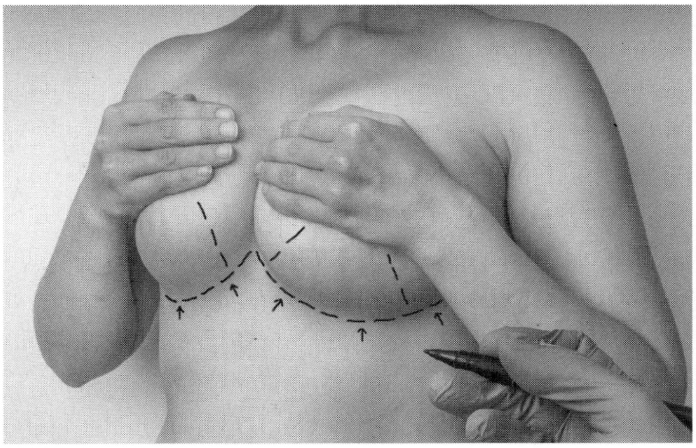

Figure 18.5 A breast lift is used to reshape and reposition sagging mammary glands.

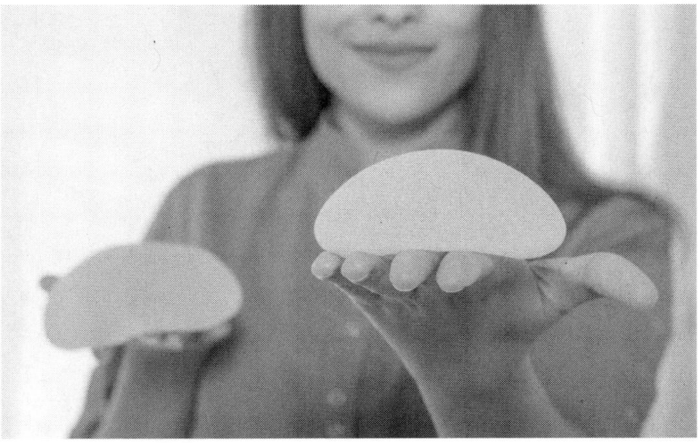

Figure 18.6 Breast implants are sacs filled with either silicone or saline.

the edge of the areola, or rarely, through the navel. Another technique called ***biocompartmental breast lipostructuring*** involves injecting the person's own fat from other parts of the body into the breasts for an increase of up to two cup sizes (Zocchi & Zuliani, 2008). Another injectable option is PAAG (polyacrylamide hydrogel). Injectables are likely to have less impact on lactation than techniques involving incisions.

• • •

Those with a history of breast augmentation surgery are less likely to exclusively nurse their babies than those without a history of breast augmentation surgery.

Large studies and meta-analyses examined the effects of breast augmentation on nursing. One 2015 Australia population-based study compared lactation outcomes among nearly 380,000 mothers (C. L. Roberts, Ampt, Algert, Sywak, & Chen, 2015) and found reduced rates of human-milk feeding among those with a history of breast augmentation.

A 2018 Chinese meta-analysis compiled the data from four cohort studies and one cross-sectional study to compare lactation outcomes among those with and without a history of breast augmentation (Cheng et al., 2018). Its authors concluded that those who had breast augmentation were less likely to successfully establish nursing, especially exclusive nursing. A 2014 Australian systematic review and meta-analysis (Schiff, Algert, Ampt, Sywak, & Roberts, 2014) also found less human-milk feeding among those with a history of breast augmentation.

• • •

Although early studies found a link between incision location and milk production, newer and larger studies do not show this association.

Incision locations. In the 1990s, two small U.S. studies (N. M. Hurst, 1996; Neifert et al., 1990) found an association between low milk production in those with a history of breast surgery and incisions around the areola (***periareolar***). In these older studies, the periareolar groups were at least 5 times more likely to have insufficient milk as those who did not have breast surgery. However, these studies were questionable for several reasons. One did not differentiate between breast augmentation and breast reduction surgery and the other did not control for other factors that might affect milk production.

If the surgical incision is made around the edge of the areola, its specific location does matter. Nipple sensitivity (and therefore milk ejection) depends on an intact fourth intercostal nerve, which usually enters the areola on its outer, lower edge. But many modern surgeons consider maintaining nipple sensitivity an indicator of successful surgery and are aware of the importance of avoiding that specific area to preserve sensitivity (Al Hetmi et al., 2019).

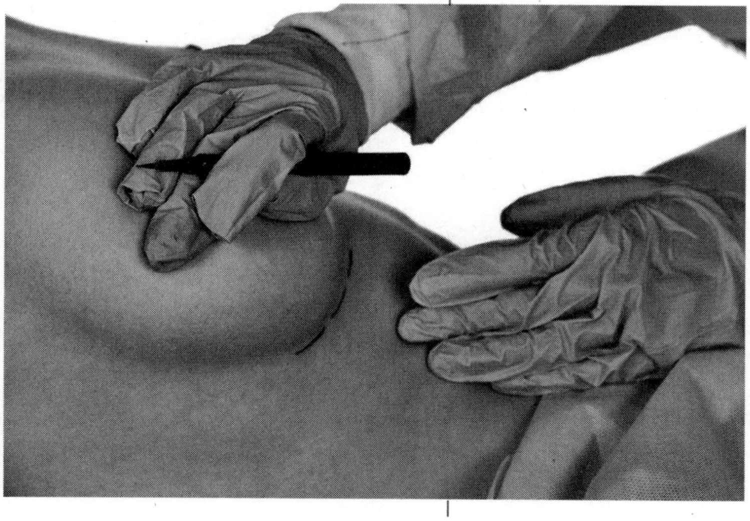

Newer research did not find an association between incision location and lactation outcomes. A 2018 Chinese meta-analysis of four cohort studies and one cross-sectional study (Cheng et al., 2018) found no evidence that periareolar incisions reduce exclusive nursing.

Implant size. A small U.S. study of 20 women with implants (Mofid et al., 2006) found no difference in nipple sensitivity among women who had breast implants inserted around the areola or in the fold under the breast, but this and a Brazilian study (Pitanguy, Vaena, Radwanski, Nunes, & Vargas, 2007) did find an association between larger implants in previously small-breasted women and reduced nipple sensitivity.

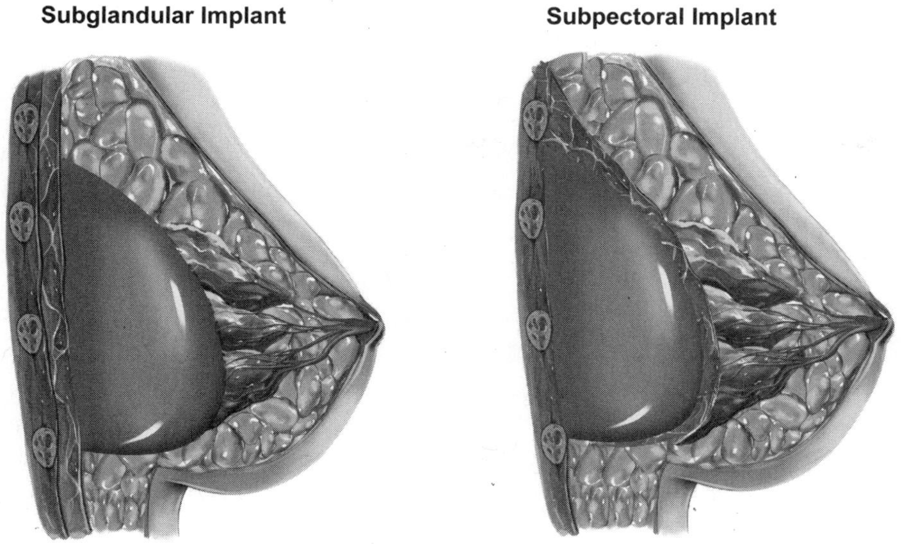

Figure 18.7 Implants inserted under the muscle (right) are less likely to affect lactation than those inserted above the muscle and directly below the milk-making glands.

• • •

The placement of the implants above or below the chest muscles may also affect lactation.

Whether a breast implant is placed above or below the chest muscle may affect nursing. Placing an implant above the chest muscle and directly below the milk-making tissue (***subglandular***) may put more pressure on this glandular tissue, which may possibly reduce milk production or block milk flow. One 2018 French retrospective multicenter study (Bompy et al., 2019) found that those with implants inserted above the chest muscle were significantly less able to nurse successfully compared with those whose implants were inserted below the chest muscle. The alternatives to placing the implant directly under the mammary tissue are to place it either partially covered by the chest muscle (***subpectoral***) (Figure 18.7) or almost completely covered by the chest muscle (***transrectus***). If parents are unsure about how the surgery was done, suggest they contact their surgeon.

• • •

After breast-implant surgery, significant scarring and any subsequent surgery to treat complications may reduce milk production.

Scarring is the body's natural reaction to surgery. Severe scarring, known as capsular contracture, can cause discomfort during nursing or put enough pressure on the milk-producing glands to cause a reduction in milk production (Strom, Baldwin, Sigurdson, & Schusterman, 1997). When scarring is severe, it may require more surgery to remove it, which can cause damage to nerves and milk ducts (Henriksen et al., 2003; Michalopoulos, 2007).

• • •

Concerns about silicone in the milk of those with silicone implants proved to be unfounded.

Silicone is a "ubiquitous substance found in all food, liquids, etc." (T.W. Hale, 2019, p. 688), including lipsticks, other cosmetics, and over-the-counter colic remedies such as Mylicon® drops that are given directly to tiny babies. In addition, absorption of silicone by the babies' digestive tract is considered unlikely.

If parents with silicone breast implants are concerned about silicone in their milk, let them know that research (Semple, Lugowski, Baines, Smith, & McHugh, 1998) found that formula and cow's milk contain levels of silicon (silicone is elemental silicon bonded to oxygen) more than 10 times higher than the milk of mothers with silicone implants.

In the 1990s, some concerns were raised about potential health risks to breastfed children of mothers with silicone breast implants (Levine & Ilowite, 1994; Teuber & Gershwin, 1994). But large studies (Kjoller et al., 1998) later proved these concerns unfounded. In 2001, the American Academy of Pediatrics' Committee on Drugs (AAP, 2001) wrote that when milk from mothers with silicone implants was compared with milk from mothers without implants, there were no differences found in the levels of silicon. The chair of this committee (Berlin, 1994) wrote: "It is unlikely that elemental silicon causes difficulty, because silicon is present in higher concentrations in cow's milk and formula than in the milk of humans with implants."

Breast Reduction Surgery

Some breast reduction surgical techniques affect lactation outcomes more than others.

Breast reduction surgery, also known as ***reduction mammaplasty***, is done to decrease breast size by removing either the fat within the mammary gland via liposuction or by surgically removing mammary tissue. Unlike top surgery (see the last section), its goal is to create a smaller, female-shaped breast.

Liposuction is the breast reduction technique least likely to affect milk production, because only fatty tissue is removed and there is minimal scarring and nerve damage. However, liposuction does not usually reduce breast size by more than two cup sizes (Spear, 2006), and it is not considered the best option for younger women, because their breasts tend to contain less fatty tissue as compared with older women (Nahai & Nahai, 2008).

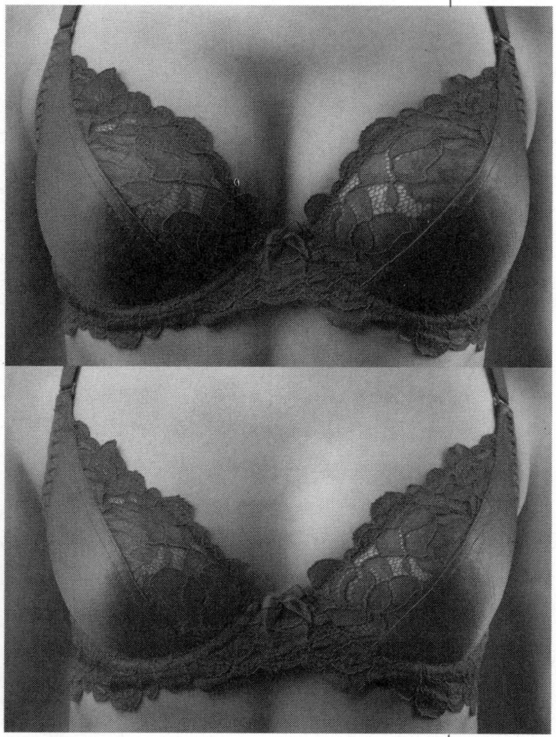

Free nipple grafts put milk production at greatest risk, because this type of breast reduction surgery involves completely detaching the nipple and areola from the mammary gland and reattaching them elsewhere for a more symmetrical appearance (Marshall, Callan, & Nicholson, 1994). This procedure, which is not as common as other techniques, severs all milk ducts, nerves, and blood vessels. Even so, due to regrowth of nerves and milk ducts, some parents who nursed after having this procedure produced milk and a few produced ample milk (West & Hirsch, 2008).

Pedicle techniques. In addition to concerns about milk ducts and nerves, there are also concerns about maintaining an adequate blood supply to the nipple and areola after surgery, as too little blood flow can cause tissue death, a very serious complication that can greatly reduce lactation potential. To protect these vital arteries while some parts of the mammary gland are being removed during surgery, a section of the gland that includes these arteries, milk ducts, and nerves can be kept completely attached down to the chest wall or partially severed. These partially or fully intact sections are called ***pedicles***, and the names of these surgical techniques (***inferior, superior, central, lateral,*** and ***medial*** pedicle techniques) refer to the specific section of the gland used to create the pedicle. Different techniques can be used with different types and shapes of incisions, which makes it impossible to tell from the shape of a scar what type of surgery was performed.

Research on lactation after pedicle techniques. Although many studies have examined the effects of different types of breast reduction techniques on nursing outcomes, unfortunately, consistent definitions of lactation success were not used. A 2017 systematic review of 51 observational studies that examined the effects on lactation of 31 distinct breast reduction techniques (Kraut et al., 2017) concluded that:

- The time elapsed between the surgery and nursing was less important to milk production than the surgical technique used.
- Fewer cases of nursing "success" occurred after free nipple grafts as compared with any other techniques.
- When pedicle techniques were used, the best nursing outcomes were among those who had the inferior or central pedicle surgeries, as compared with the superior, medial, and lateral pedicles.
- Full preservation of the attachment of the pedicle column to the chest wall resulted in better nursing outcomes as compared with surgeries in which the column was only partially preserved.

• • •

After breast reduction surgery, most parents produce some milk; the real issue is how much milk.

As described previously, the number of milk ducts cut and the number remaining will determine in part the effect of breast reduction surgery on milk production. For details on how to help families create a plan when full milk production is compromised, see p. 222-227.

Chest Masculinization or Top Surgery

Some transmasculine or gender non-conforming people have chest masculinization procedures known as top surgery, which removes much of the milk-making tissue.

Transmasculine people are those assigned as female at birth but who identify on the male end of the gender spectrum. When their physical anatomy does not match their internal sense of gender identity, they may experience a type of distress or anxiety known as ***gender dysphoria***. These negative feelings motivate some to go through the process of transitioning so their outer appearance is closer to their inner gender identity. Transitioning may involve wearing different clothes, taking testosterone, or undergoing surgeries of the chest or reproductive organs. Chest masculinization surgery, often referred to as ***top surgery*** or ***male chest contouring***, involves removing much of the mammary tissue to create a masculine-looking chest. This makes top surgery different from breast reduction surgery, which is intended to produce a smaller but definitely female-shaped breast. Unlike a mastectomy, not all of the mammary tissue is removed during top surgery, because doing so would leave a sunken-looking chest.

A 2016 qualitative study (MacDonald et al., 2016) described the experiences of pregnancy, birth, and lactation in the 22 transmasculine individuals who responded to an online survey. (Read this open-access study at **bit.ly/BA2-Transmasculine**.) Of its 22 respondents, 16 nursed their babies, which some referred to as ***chestfeeding***. Of the original 22, only 9 had the top surgery before giving birth, but others planned to have it done in the future. The techniques used to do the top surgeries varied but fell into two general categories:

- Two broad incisions under the mammary tissue, with the nipples completely removed and repositioned (much like the free nipple grafts mentioned previously)
- Removal of the mammary tissue while preserving the nipple pedicle

Of the 9 respondents who had top surgery, 5 had their nipples removed and repositioned. Some who had top surgery said it provided "immense relief" from their feelings of gender dysphoria. Some said their gender dysphoria would have been unbearable during pregnancy if they had not had the procedure.

Those who had the top surgery said that none of their surgeons discussed future infant feeding with them. The authors wrote (MacDonald et al., 2016, p. 5):

> "Participants believed that their surgeons subscribed to a binary view of gender and that pregnancy and chestfeeding would not fit with their surgeons' ideas of what a 'true' transgender man would want to do."

A "binary view of gender" means there are only two genders: male and female. With this worldview, it is inconceivable that a transgender man would decide to get pregnant and nurse his baby. But if instead gender is considered on a spectrum, with male and female at either end, the idea that an individual may be truest to their own unique gender identity by making choices from various points on this spectrum makes more sense.

During pregnancy, chest changes occurred in 6 of the 9 who previously had the top surgery. In some cases, the tissue grew back to pre-surgical size, which was a surprise After birth, 9 of the 16 who decided to nurse reported no gender dysphoria during nursing. Four reported being comfortable nursing in public. Four of the 9 who had the top surgery assumed they would be unable to nurse their babies after giving birth due to physical pain, lack of milk production, and lack of tissue for latching.

KEY CONCEPT

To provide competent lactation help to transmasculine nursing parents, start with a nuanced approach and basic knowledge about their unique needs.

Of those who had the top surgery, some reported becoming engorged from milk production in areas of their chest that did not drain due to severed milk ducts. After asking for help, one healthcare provider suggested not nursing. Another found help from a doula.

Some of those who had the top surgery nursed, and some of those who didn't have the surgery chose not to nurse because of feelings of gender dysphoria. Of the study participants who nursed, some produced ample milk. Seven of the 16 either used donor milk or said they were considering it. One used a nursing supplementer. At the end of the study, 2 of the 16 were still nursing their young babies, 3 nursed for a total of less than 6 months, and 11 nursed for more than 1 year.

The study authors noted that each transgender experience of pregnancy, birth, and nursing is unique, so healthcare providers need to take a "nuanced" approach to providing care for these families. To provide competent care, the authors recommended becoming more knowledgeable about lactation and chest care when transmasculine individuals choose to bind their mammary tissue and when they need chest care after top surgery.

Breast or Chest Injury

Ask the parent to describe the injury, and find out how long ago and at what age it occurred.

Parents with a history of breast or chest injury may worry about its effect on their milk production. The same basic considerations mentioned for breast or chest surgery apply here. Milk production should not be affected if the milk ducts and nerves were not damaged. Some examples of injuries that may affect lactation include:

- **Breast or other cancer treatments.** For example, if the mammary gland (or in a baby or child, the chest) is exposed to radiation therapy, this damages milk-making cells, which reduces milk production significantly in the exposed gland (Leal, Stuart, & Carvalho Hde, 2013)
- **Spinal cord injuries** of the T3, T4, T5, and T6 vertebrae or above could affect the sensitivity to temperature and touch in the nipple and gland. For more details, see p. 865.
- **Blunt force trauma** to the mammary gland or the chest, especially during infancy or childhood, when the gland has not yet developed
- **Severe chest burns.** See next point.

A loss of sensation on one or both glands indicates nerve damage. If so, milk ejection may be affected on that side. However, if only one side is affected, in most cases, it will be possible to establish full milk production on the unaffected side. If both mammary glands are affected, see the previous section "Initiating Nursing."

• • •

If one or both nipples were burned, scarring may affect milk flow and skin elasticity, and may cause pain during nursing and latching difficulties.

Even second- and third-degree burns do not usually extend deeply enough into the mammary tissue to affect the milk-making glands. If parents' nipples were burned and scarred, their ability to nurse would depend on how many nipple pores are blocked by scar tissue. The overall effect on nursing will depend on how many milk ducts and corresponding nipple pores that parent had before the injury. The average number of nipple pores and corresponding ducts is 9, but some parents have as few as 4 and as many as 14 (Ramsay et al., 2005). Scar tissue may also make the mammary tissue less pliable, which may make latching more challenging.

Some parents with scarred nipples report that early nursing is painful, although in some cases, the pain resolves early. In one case report (Faridi & Dewan, 2008), the pain resolved within days after birth.

• • •

The ability to express colostrum during pregnancy indicates that at least some of the nipple pores are not blocked.

Expressing colostrum during the last month of pregnancy is not a reliable gauge of how much milk parents will produce after birth. Many who are unable to express colostrum go on to produce abundant milk. However, if during pregnancy parents can express colostrum, it indicates that some nipple pores are not blocked. Suggest parents who would like to learn hand-expression during pregnancy watch the demonstration videos at **firstdroplets.com**.

RESOURCES

BFAR.org—An informational website for parents nursing after mammary reduction surgery.

bfmed.org/protocols—Free, downloadable, fully referenced clinical protocols in multiple languages are ideal for sharing with healthcare providers from the Academy of Breastfeeding Medicine:

- #4 Mastitis
- #20 Engorgement
- #26 Persistent pain with breastfeeding
- #30 Breast masses, breast complaints, and diagnostic breast imaging in the lactating woman

bit.ly/BA2-FDAImplants—A U.S. Food and Drug Administration (FDA) informational website on breast implants.

Cassar-Uhl, D. (2014). *Finding Sufficiency: Breastfeeding with Insufficient Glandular Tissue.* Amarillo, TX: Praeclarus Press.

firstdroplets.com—Videos by Dr. Jane Morton for parents of term and preterm babies show how to maximize milk production and prevent engorgement by learning hand expression before birth and using it after birth

Marasco, L. & West, D. (2020). *Making More Milk: The Breastfeeding Guide to Increasing Your Milk Production,* 2nd ed. New York, NY: McGraw Hill.

West, D. (2001). *Defining Your Own Success: Breastfeeding after Breast Reduction Surgery.* Schaumburg, IL: La Leche League International.

West, D. And Hirsch, E. (2008). Breastfeeding after breast and nipple procedures: A guide for healthcare professionals. *Clinics in Human Lactation.* Amarillo, TX: Hale Publishing.

REFERENCES

AAP. (2001). Transfer of drugs and other chemicals into human milk. *Pediatrics, 108*(3), 776-789.

ACR. (2018). *ACR Manual on Contrast Media, Version 10.3* (11th ed.). Reston, VA: American Committee on Radiology.

Ader, D. N., South-Paul, J., Adera, T., et al. (2001). Cyclical mastalgia: Prevalence and associated health and behavioral factors. *Journal of Psychosomatic Obstetrics & Gynaecology, 22*(2), 71-76.

Afshariani, R., Farhadi, P., Ghaffarpasand, F., et al. (2014). Effectiveness of topical curcumin for treatment of mastitis in breastfeeding women: A randomized, double-blind, placebo-controlled clinical trial. *Oman Medical Journal, 29*(5), 330-334.

Aksoy, H. T., Eras, Z., Erdeve, O., et al. (2013). A rare cause of hematemesis in newborn: Fibrocystic breast disease of mother. *Breastfeeding Medicine, 8*(4), 418-420.

Al Hetmi, T., Al Lahham, S., Badran, S., et al. (2019). Preserving nipple areolar complex sensitivity in augmentation mammaplasty. *Journal of General Surgery, 3*(1), 1-3.

Alekseev, N. P. (2017). Progesterone-containing gel does not eliminate postpartum breast engorgement? *Breastfeeding Medicine, 12,* 122-123.

Alekseev, N. P., Vladimir, II, & Nadezhda, T. E. (2015). Pathological postpartum breast engorgement: Prediction, prevention, and resolution. *Breastfeeding Medicine, 10*(4), 203-208.

Amir, L. H. (2003). Breast pain in lactating women--mastitis or something else? *Australian Family Physician, 32*(3), 141-145.

Amir, L. H., & Academy of Breastfeeding Medicine Protocol, C. (2014). ABM Clinical protocol #4: Mastitis, revised March 2014. *Breastfeeding Medicine, 9*(5), 239-243.

Amir, L. H., Donath, S. M., Garland, S. M., et al. (2013). Does Candida and/or Staphylococcus play a role in nipple and breast pain in lactation? A cohort study in Melbourne, Australia. *British Medical Journal Open, 3*(3).

Amir, L. H., Forster, D., McLachlan, H., et al. (2004). Incidence of breast abscess in lactating women: Report from an Australian cohort. *British Journal of Obstetrics and Gynaecology, 111*(12), 1378-1381.

Amir, L. H., Forster, D. A., Lumley, J., et al. (2007). A descriptive study of mastitis in Australian breastfeeding women: Incidence and determinants. *BMC Public Health, 7,* 62.

Amir, L. H., Griffin, L., Cullinane, M., et al. (2016). Probiotics and mastitis: Evidence-based marketing? *International Breastfeeding Journal, 11,* 19.

Amir, L. H., Trupin, S., & Kvist, L. J. (2014). Diagnosis and treatment of mastitis in breastfeeding women. *Journal of Human Lactation, 30*(1), 10-13.

Anderson, J. E., Held, N., & Wright, K. (2004). Raynaud's phenomenon of the nipple: A treatable cause of painful breastfeeding. *Pediatrics, 113*(4), e360-364.

Angelopoulou, A., Field, D., Ryan, C. A., et al. (2018). The microbiology and treatment of human mastitis. *Medical Microbiology and Immunology, 207*(2), 83-94.

Antevski, B., Jovkovski, O., Filipovski, V., et al. (2011). Extreme gigantomastia in pregnancy: Case report--My experience with two cases in last 5 years. *Archives of Gynecology and Obstetrics, 284*(3), 575-578.

Antevski, B. M., Smilevski, D. A., Stojovski, M. Z., et al. (2007). Extreme gigantomastia in pregnancy: Case report and review of literature. *Archives of Gynecology and Obstetrics, 275*(2), 149-153.

Arbour, M. W., & Kessler, J. L. (2013). Mammary hypoplasia: Not every breast can produce sufficient milk. *Journal of Midwifery & Women's Health, 58*(4), 457-461.

Arroyo, R., Martin, V., Maldonado, A., et al. (2010). Treatment of infectious mastitis during lactation: Antibiotics versus oral administration of Lactobacilli isolated from breast milk. *Clinical Infectious Diseases, 50*(12), 1551-1558.

Aryeetey, R. N., Marquis, G. S., Brakohiapa, L., et al. (2009). Subclinical mastitis may not reduce breastmilk intake during established lactation. *Breastfeeding Medicine, 4*(3), 161-166.

Aryeetey, R. N., Marquis, G. S., Timms, L., et al. (2008). Subclinical mastitis is common among Ghanaian women lactating 3 to 4 months postpartum. *Journal of Human Lactation, 24*(3), 263-267.

Auvichayapat, P., Auvichayapat, N., Tong-un, T., et al. (2003). A controlled trial of a new treatment for galactocele. *Journal of the Medical Association of Thailand, 86*(3), 257-261.

Baeza, C. (2016). Acute, subclinical, and subacute mastitis: Definitions, etiology, and clinical management. *Clinical Lactation, 7*(1), 7-10.

Balcar, V., Silinkova-Malkova, E., & Matys, Z. (1972). Soft tissue radiography of the female breast and pelvic pneumoperitoneum in the Stein-Leventhal syndrome. *Acta Radiologica: Diagnosis (Stockholm), 12*(3), 353-362.

Barco, I., Vidal, M. C., Barco, J., et al. (2014). Blood-stained colostrum and human milk during pregnancy and early lactation. *Journal of Human Lactation, 30*(4), 413-415.

Barreto, D. S., Sedgwick, E. L., Nagi, C. S., et al. (2018). Granulomatous mastitis: Etiology, imaging, pathology, treatment, and clinical findings. *Breast Cancer Research and Treatment, 171*(3), 527-534.

Benson, S. (2001). What is normal? A study of normal breastfeeding dyads during the first sixty hours of life. *Breastfeeding Review, 9*(1), 27-32.

Berens, P., & Brodribb, W. (2016). ABM Clinical Protocol #20: Engorgement, revised 2016. *Breastfeeding Medicine, 11,* 159-163.

Berens, P., Eglash, A., Malloy, M., et al. (2016). ABM Clinical Protocol #26: Persistent pain with breastfeeding. *Breastfeeding Medicine, 11*(2), 46-53.

Berens, P., Swaim, L., & Peterson, B. (2010). Incidence of methicillin-resistant Staphylococcus aureus in postpartum breast abscesses. *Breastfeeding Medicine, 5*(3), 113-115.

Berens, P. D. (2015). Breast pain: Engorgement, nipple pain, and mastitis. *Clinical Obstetrics and Gynecology, 58*(4), 902-914.

Bergmann, H., Rodriguez, J. M., Salminen, S., et al. (2014). Probiotics in human milk and probiotic supplementation in infant nutrition: A workshop report. *British Journal of Nutrition, 112*(7), 1119-1128.

Berlin, C. M., Jr. (1994). Silicone breast implants and breast-feeding. *Pediatrics, 94*(4 Pt 1), 547-549.

Bodley, V., & Powers, D. (1999). Patient with insufficient glandular tissue experiences milk supply increase attributed to progesterone treatment for luteal phase defect. *Journal of Human Lactation, 15*(4), 339-343.

Bolman, M., Saju, L., Oganesyan, K., et al. (2013). Recapturing the art of therapeutic breast massage during breastfeeding. *Journal of Human Lactation, 29*(3), 328-331.

Bompy, L., Gerenton, B., Cristofari, S., et al. (2019). Impact on breastfeeding according to implant features in breast augmentation: A multicentric retrospective study. *Annals of Plastic Surgery, 82*(1), 11-14.

Bonyata, K. (2018). Lecithin treatments for recurring plugged ducts. Retrieved from **kellymom.com/nutrition/vitamins/lecithin/**

Borucki, L. C. (2005). Breastfeeding mothers' experiences using a supplemental feeding tube device: Finding an alternative. *Journal of Human Lactation, 21*(4), 429-438.

Bowles, B. C. (2011). Breast massage: A "handy" multipurpose tool to promote breastfeeding success. *Clinical Lactation, 2*(4), 21-24.

Brown, D., & Langdon, C. (2014). Does kinesio elastic therapeutic taping decrease breast engorgement in postpartum women? *Clinical Lactation, 5*(2), 67-74.

Buck, M. L., Amir, L. H., Cullinane, M., et al. (2014). Nipple pain, damage, and vasospasm in the first 8 weeks postpartum. *Breastfeeding Medicine, 9*(2), 56-62.

Buescher, E. S., & Hair, P. S. (2001). Human milk anti-inflammatory component contents during acute mastitis. *Cellular Immunology, 210*(2), 87-95.

Bystrova, K., Widstrom, A. M., Matthiesen, A. S., et al. (2007). Early lactation performance in primiparous and multiparous women in relation to different maternity home practices. A randomised trial in St. Petersburg. *International Breastfeeding Journal, 2,* 9.

Chen, C. Y., Anderson, B. O., Lo, S. S., et al. (2010). Methicillin-resistant Staphylococcus aureus infections may not impede the success of ultrasound-guided drainage of puerperal breast abscesses. *Journal of the American College of Surgeons, 210*(2), 148-154.

Cheng, F., Dai, S., Wang, C., et al. (2018). Do breast implants influence breastfeeding? A meta-analysis of comparative studies. *Journal of Human Lactation,* 890334418776654.

Chiu, J. Y., Gau, M. L., Kuo, S. Y., et al. (2010). Effects of Gua-Sha therapy on breast engorgement: A randomized controlled trial. *Journal of Nursing Research, 18*(1), 1-10.

Christensen, A. F., Al-Suliman, N., Nielsen, K. R., et al. (2005). Ultrasound-guided drainage of breast abscesses: Results in 151 patients. *British Journal of Radiology, 78*(927), 186-188.

Cizmeci, M. N., Kanburoglu, M. K., Akelma, A. Z., et al. (2013). Rusty-pipe syndrome: A rare cause of change in the color of breastmilk. *Breastfeeding Medicine, 8*(3), 340-341.

Colin, C., Delov, A. G., Peyron-Faure, N., et al. (2019). Breast abscesses in lactating women: Evidences for ultrasound-guided percutaneous drainage to avoid surgery. *Emergency Radiology, 26*(5), 507-514.

Collado, M. C., Delgado, S., Maldonado, A., et al. (2009). Assessment of the bacterial diversity of breast milk of healthy women by quantitative real-time PCR. *Letters in Applied Microbiology, 48*(5), 523-528.

Colson, S. (2003). Biological nurturing increases duration of breastfeeding for a vulnerable cohort. *MIDRIS Midwifery Digest, 13*(1), 92-97.

Colson, S. (2019). *Biological Nurturing: Instinctual Breastfeeding* (2nd ed.). Amarillo, TX: Praeclarus Press.

Colson, S., DeRooy, L., & Hawdon, J. (2003). Biological nurturing increases duration of breastfeeding for a vulnerable cohort. *MIDIRS Midwifery Digest, 13*(1), 92-97.

Cotterman, K. J. (2004). Reverse pressure softening: a simple tool to prepare areola for easier latching during engorgement. *Journal of Human Lactation, 20*(2), 227-237. doi:10.1177/0890334404264224

Couto, L. S., Glassman, L. M., Batista Abreu, D. C., et al. (2016). Chronic galactocele. *Breast Journal, 22*(4), 471-472.

Cowley, K. C. (2014). Breastfeeding by women with tetraplegia: Some evidence for optimism. *Spinal Cord, 52*(3), 255.

Cox, D. B., Kent, J. C., Casey, T. M., et al. (1999). Breast growth and the urinary excretion of lactose during human pregnancy and early lactation: Endocrine relationships. *Experimental Physiology, 84*(2), 421-434.

Craig, H. R. (2008). *Gestational gigantomastia: Clinical and lactation management.* Paper presented at the International Lactation Consultant Association (ILCA) Conference, Las Vegas, NV, Las Vegas, NV.

Cullinane, M., Amir, L. H., Donath, S. M., et al. (2015). Determinants of mastitis in women in the CASTLE study: A cohort study. *BMC Family Practice, 16,* 181.

Dahlbeck, S. W., Donnelly, J. F., & Theriault, R. L. (1995). Differentiating inflammatory breast cancer from acute mastitis. *American Family Physician, 52*(3), 929-934.

de Paula, I. B., & Campos, A. M. (2017). Breast imaging in patients with nipple discharge. *Radiologia Brasileira, 50*(6), 383-388.

Diepeveen, L. C., Fraser, E., Croft, A. J. E., et al. (2019). Regional and facility differences in interventions for mastitis by Australian physiotherapists. *Journal of Human Lactation, 35*(4), 695-705.

DiTomasso, D., & Paiva, A. L. (2018). Neonatal weight matters: An examination of weight changes in full-term breastfeeding newborns during the first 2 weeks of life. *Journal of Human Lactation, 34*(1), 86-92.

Duran, M. S., & Spatz, D. L. (2011). A mother with glandular hypoplasia and a late preterm infant. *Journal of Human Lactation, 27*(4), 394-397.

Dutta, R., & Gowder, R. O. (2018). The prevalence and predisposing factors of mastitis in lactating mothers in puerperium. *New Indian Journal of OBGYN, 5*(1), 28-32.

Eglash, A., Simon, L., & Academy of Breastfeeding, M. (2017). ABM Clinical Protocol #8: Human milk storage information for home use for full-term infants, revised 2017. *Breastfeeding Medicine, 12*(7), 390-395.

Evans, K., Evans, R., & Simmer, K. (1995). Effect of the method of breast feeding on breast engorgement, mastitis and infantile colic. *Acta Paediatrica, 84*(8), 849-852.

Faridi, M. M., & Dewan, P. (2008). Successful breastfeeding with breast malformations. *Journal of Human Lactation, 24*(4), 446-450.

Farrokh, D., Alamdaran, A., Feyzi Laeen, A., et al. (2019). Tuberculous mastitis: A review of 32 cases. *International Journal of Infectious Diseases, 87,* 135-142.

Fernandez, L., Arroyo, R., Espinosa, I., et al. (2014). Probiotics for human lactational mastitis. *Beneficial Microbes, 5*(2), 169-183.

Fernandez, L., Delgado, S., Herrero, H., et al. (2008). The bacteriocin nisin, an effective agent for the treatment of staphylococcal mastitis during lactation. *Journal of Human Lactation, 24*(3), 311-316.

Fernandez, L., Langa, S., Martin, V., et al. (2013). The human milk microbiota: Origin and potential roles in health and disease. *Pharmacological Research, 69*(1), 1-10.

Fetherston, C. (1997). Management of lactation mastitis in a Western Australian cohort. *Breastfeeding Review, 5*(2), 13-19.

Fetherston, C. (1998). Risk factors for lactation mastitis. *Journal of Human Lactation, 14*(2), 101-109.

Fetherston, C. (2001). Mastitis in lactating women: Physiology or pathology? *Breastfeeding Review, 9*(1), 5-12.

Fetherston, C. M., Lai, C. T., & Hartmann, P. E. (2006). Relationships between symptoms and changes in breast physiology during lactation mastitis. *Breastfeeding Medicine, 1*(3), 136-145.

Fetherston, C. M., Lai, C. T., & Hartmann, P. E. (2008). Recurrent blocked duct(s) in a mother with immunoglobulin A deficiency. *Breastfeeding Medicine, 3*(4), 261-265.

Filteau, S. (2003). The influence of mastitis on antibody transfer to infants through breast milk. *Vaccine, 21*(24), 3377-3381.

Filteau, S. M., Rice, A. L., Ball, J. J., et al. (1999). Breast milk immune factors in Bangladeshi women supplemented postpartum with retinol or beta-carotene. *American Journal of Clinical Nutrition, 69*(5), 953-958.

Flores, M., & Filteau, S. (2002). Effect of lactation counselling on subclinical mastitis among Bangladeshi women. *Annals of Tropical Paediatrics, 22*(1), 85-88.

Foxman, B., D'Arcy, H., Gillespie, B., et al. (2002). Lactation mastitis: Occurrence and medical management among 946 breastfeeding women in the United States. *American Journal of Epidemiology, 155*(2), 103-114.

Galipeau, R., Dumas, L., & Lepage, M. (2017). Perception of not having enough milk and actual milk production of first-time breastfeeding mothers: Is there a difference? *Breastfeeding Medicine, 12,* 210-217.

Garbin, C. P., Deacon, J. P., Rowan, M. K., et al. (2009). Association of nipple piercing with abnormal milk production and breastfeeding. *Journal of the American Medical Assocation, 301*(24), 2550-2551.

Gastelum, D. T., Dassey, D., Mascola, L., et al. (2005). Transmission of community-associated methicillin-resistant Staphylococcus aureus from breast milk in the neonatal intensive care unit. *Pediatric Infectious Disease Journal, 24*(12), 1122-1124.

Geddes, D. T. (2007). Inside the lactating breast: The latest anatomy research. *Journal of Midwifery & Women's Health, 52*(6), 556-563.

Ghosh, K., Morton, M. J., Whaley, D. H., et al. (2004). Infected galactocele: A perplexing problem. *Breast Journal, 10*(2), 159.

Gonik, G., & Cotton, D. B. (1984). Peripartum colloid osmotic pressure changes influence of intravenous hydration. *American Journal of Obstetrics and Gynecology, 150,* 174-177.

Gonik, G., Cotton, D.B. (1984). Peripartum colloid osmotic pressure changes influence of intravenous hydration. *American Journal of Obstetrics and Gynecology, 150,* 174-177.

Goyal, A., & Mansel, R. E. (2003). Iatrogenic injury to the breast bud causing breast hypoplasia. *Postgraduate Medical Journal, 79*(930), 235-236.

Guillette, E. A., Conard, C., Lares, F., et al. (2006). Altered breast development in young girls from an agricultural environment. *Environmental Health Perspectives, 114*(3), 471-475.

Gupta, R., Gupta, A. S., & Duggal, N. (1982). Tubercular mastitis. *International Surgery, 67*(4 Suppl), 422-424.

Hagiya, H., Shiota, S., Sugiyama, W., et al. (2014). Postpartum breast abscess caused by community-acquired methicillin-resistant Staphylococcus aureus in Japan. *Breastfeeding Medicine, 9*(1), 45-46.

Haitz, K., Ly, A., & Smith, G. (2019). Idiopathic granulomatous mastitis. *Cutis, 103*(1), 38-42.

Hale, T. W. (2019). *Hale's Medications & Mothers' Milk: A Manual of Lactational Pharmacology* (18th ed.). New York, NY: Springer Publishing Company.

Hale, T. W., Bateman, T. L., Finkelman, M. A., et al. (2009). The absence of Candida albicans in milk samples of women with clinical symptoms of ductal candidiasis. *Breastfeeding Medicine, 4*(2), 57-61. doi:10.1089/bfm.2008.0144

Haliloglu, N., Ustuner, E., & Ozkavukcu, E. (2019). Breast ultrasound during lactation: Benign and malignant lesions. *Breast Care (Basel), 14*(1), 30-34.

Henriksen, T. F., Holmich, L. R., Fryzek, J. P., et al. (2003). Incidence and severity of short-term complications after breast augmentation: Results from a nationwide breast implant registry. *Annals of Plastic Surgery, 51*(6), 531-539.

Hill, P. D., Aldag, J. C., Chatterton, R. T., et al. (2005). Comparison of milk output between mothers of preterm and term infants: The first 6 weeks after birth. *Journal of Human Lactation, 21*(1), 22-30.

Hill, P. D., & Humenick, S. S. (1994). The occurrence of breast engorgement. *Journal of Human Lactation, 10*(2), 79-86.

Huggins, K. E., Petok, E. S., & Mireles, O. (2000). Markers of lactation insufficiency: A study of 34 mothers. In *Current Issues in Clinical Lactation.* Boston, MA: Jones and Bartlett.

Humenick, S. S., Hill, P. D., & Anderson, M. A. (1994). Breast engorgement: Patterns and selected outcomes. *Journal of Human Lactation, 10*(2), 87-93.

Hunt, K. M., Foster, J. A., Forney, L. J., et al. (2011). Characterization of the diversity and temporal stability of bacterial communities in human milk. *PLoS One, 6*(6), e21313.

Hurst, N. (2003). Breastfeeding after breast augmentation. *Journal of Human Lactation, 19*(1), 70-71.

Hurst, N. M. (1996). Lactation after augmentation mammoplasty. *Obstetrics & Gynecology, 87*(1), 30-34.

Hurtado, J. A., Maldonado-Lobon, J. A., Diaz-Ropero, M. P., et al. (2017). Oral administration to nursing women of Lactobacillus fermentum CECT5716 prevents lactational mastitis development: A randomized controlled trial. *Breastfeeding Medicine, 12*(4), 202-209.

Irusen, H., Rohwer, A. C., Steyn, D. W., et al. (2015). Treatments for breast abscesses in breastfeeding women. *Cochrane Database of Systematic Reviews*(8), CD010490. doi:10.1002/14651858.CD010490.pub2.

Jacobs, V. R., Golombeck, K., Jonat, W., et al. (2003). Mastitis nonpuerperalis after nipple piercing: Time to act. *International Journal of Fertility and Women's Medicine, 48*(5), 226-231.

Jahanfar, S., Ng, C. J., & Teng, C. L. (2013). Antibiotics for mastitis in breastfeeding women. *Cochrane Database of Systematic Reviews*(2), CD005458. doi:10.1002/14651858.CD005458.pub3

Jimenez, E., Arroyo, R., Cardenas, N., et al. (2017). Mammary candidiasis: A medical condition without scientific evidence? *PLoS One, 12*(7), e0181071.

Jimenez, E., de Andres, J., Manrique, M., et al. (2015). Metagenomic analysis of milk of healthy and mastitis-suffering women. *Journal of Human Lactation, 31*(3), 406-415.

Jimenez, E., Fernandez, L., Maldonado, A., et al. (2008). Oral administration of Lactobacillus strains isolated from breast milk as an alternative for the treatment of infectious mastitis during lactation. *Applied and Environmental Microbiology, 74*(15), 4650-4655.

Johansson, M., Fenwick, J., & Thies-Lagergren, L. (2019). Mothers' experiences of pain during breastfeeding in the early postnatal period: A short report in a Swedish context. *American Journal of Human Biology,* e23363.

Jonsson, S., & Pulkkinen, M. O. (1994). Mastitis today: Incidence, prevention and treatment. *Annales Chirugiae Gynaecologiae Supplementum, 208,* 84-87.

Kaski, K., & Kvist, L. J. (2018). Deep breast pain during lactation: A case-control study in Sweden investigating the role of Candida albicans. *International Breastfeeding Journal, 13,* 21.

Kasonka, L., Makasa, M., Marshall, T., et al. (2006). Risk factors for subclinical mastitis among HIV-infected and uninfected women in Lusaka, Zambia. *Paediatric and Perinatal Epidemiology, 20*(5), 379-391.

Kendall-Tackett, K. (2007). A new paradigm for depression in new mothers: The central role of inflammation and how breastfeeding and anti-inflammatory treatments protect maternal mental health. *International Breastfeeding Journal, 2,* 6.

Kent, J. C., Gardner, H., & Geddes, D. T. (2016). Breastmilk production in the first 4 weeks after birth of term infants. *Nutrients, 8*(12).

Kernerman, E., & Park, E. (2014). Severe breast pain resolved with pectoral muscle massage. *Journal of Human Lactation, 30*(3), 287-291.

Ketsuwan, S., Baiya, N., Paritakul, P., et al. (2018). Effect of herbal compresses for maternal breast engorgement at postpartum: A randomized controlled trial. *Breastfeeding Medicine, 13*(5), 361-365.

Khanal, V., Scott, J. A., Lee, A. H., et al. (2015). Incidence of mastitis in the neonatal period in a traditional breastfeeding dociety: Results of a cohort study. *Breastfeeding Medicine, 10*(10), 481-487.

Khosravan, S., Mohammadzadeh-Moghadam, H., Mohammadzadeh, F., et al. (2017). The effect of hollyhock (Althaea officinalis L) leaf compresses combined with warm and cold compress on breast engorgement in lactating women: A randomized clinical trial. *Journal of Evidence-Based Complementary and Alternative Medicine, 22*(1), 25-30.

Kinlay, J. R., O'Connell, D. L., & Kinlay, S. (1998). Incidence of mastitis in breastfeeding women during the six months after delivery: A prospective cohort study. *Medical Journal of Australia, 169*(6), 310-312.

Kinlay, J. R., O'Connell, D. L., & Kinlay, S. (2001). Risk factors for mastitis in breastfeeding women: Results of a prospective cohort study. *Australian and New Zealand Journal of Public Health, 25*(2), 115-120.

Kjoller, K., McLaughlin, J. K., Friis, S., et al. (1998). Health outcomes in offspring of mothers with breast implants. *Pediatrics, 102*(5), 1112-1115.

Kline, T. S., & Lash, S. R. (1964). The bleeding nipple of pregnancy and postpartum period; a cytologic and histologic study. *Acta Cytologica, 8,* 336-340.

Kraut, R. Y., Brown, E., Korownyk, C., et al. (2017). The impact of breast reduction surgery on breastfeeding: Systematic review of observational studies. *PLoS One, 12*(10), e0186591.

Kujawa-Myles, S., Noel-Weiss, J., Dunn, S., et al. (2015). Maternal intravenous fluids and postpartum breast changes: A pilot observational study. *International Breastfeeding Journal, 10,* 18.

Kvist, L. J. (2013). Re-examination of old truths: Replication of a study to measure the incidence of lactational mastitis in breastfeeding women. *International Breastfeeding Journal, 8*(1), 2.

Kvist, L. J. (2016). Diagnostic methods for mastitis in cows are not appropriate for use in humans: Commentary. *International Breastfeeding Journal, 11,* 2.

Kvist, L. J., Hall-Lord, M. L., & Larsson, B. W. (2007). A descriptive study of Swedish women with symptoms of breast inflammation during lactation and their perceptions of the quality of care given at a breastfeeding clinic. *International Breastfeeding Journal, 2,* 2.

Kvist, L. J., Hall-Lord, M. L., Rydhstroem, H., et al. (2007). A randomised-controlled trial in Sweden of acupuncture and care interventions for the relief of inflammatory symptoms of the breast during lactation. *Midwifery, 23*(2), 184-195.

Kvist, L. J., Larsson, B. W., Hall-Lord, M. L., et al. (2008). The role of bacteria in lactational mastitis and some considerations of the use of antibiotic treatment. *International Breastfeeding Journal, 3,* 6.

Kvist, L. J., & Rydhstroem, H. (2005). Factors related to breast abscess after delivery: A population-based study. *British Journal of Obstetrics and Gynaecology, 112*(8), 1070-1074.

Lavigne, V., & Gleberzon, B. J. (2012). Ultrasound as a treatment of mammary blocked duct among 25 postpartum lactating women: A retrospective case series. *Journal of Chiropractic Medicine, 11*(3), 170-178.

Lawrence, R. A., & Lawrence, R. M. (2016). *Breastfeeding: A Guide for the Medical Profession* (8th ed.). Philadelphia, PA: Elsevier.

Leal, S. C., Stuart, S. R., & Carvalho Hde, A. (2013). Breast irradiation and lactation: A review. *Expert Review of Anticancer Therapy, 13*(2), 159-164.

Lei, X., Chen, K., Zhu, L., et al. (2017). Treatments for idiopathic granulomatous mastitis: Systematic review and meta-analysis. *Breastfeeding Medicine, 12*(7), 415-421.

Levine, J. J., & Ilowite, N. T. (1994). Sclerodermalike esophageal disease in children breast-fed by mothers with silicone breast implants. *Journal of the American Medical Assocation, 271*(3), 213-216.

Li, C., Solomons, N. W., Scott, M. E., et al. (2018). Subclinical mastitis (SCM) and proinflammatory cytokines are associated with mineral and trace element concentrations in human breast milk. *Journal of Trace Elements in Medicine and Biology, 46,* 55-61.

Lim, A. R., Song, J. A., Hur, M. H., et al. (2015). Cabbage compression early breast care on breast engorgement in primiparous women after cesarean birth: A controlled clinical trial. *International Journal of Clinical and Experimental Medicine, 8*(11), 21335-21342.

Loukas, M., Clarke, P., & Tubbs, R. S. (2007). Accessory breasts: A historical and current perspective. *American Surgeon, 73*(5), 525-528.

Lukassek, J., Ignatov, A., Faerber, J., et al. (2019). Puerperal mastitis in the past decade: Results of a single institution analysis. *Archives of Gynecology and Obstetrics, 300*(6), 1637-1644.

MacDonald, T., Noel-Weiss, J., West, D., et al. (2016). Transmasculine individuals' experiences with lactation, chestfeeding, and gender identity: A qualitative study. *BMC Pregnancy & Childbirth, 16,* 106.

Madan, J. C., Hoen, A. G., Lundgren, S. N., et al. (2016). Association of cesarean delivery and formula supplementation with the intestinal microbiome of 6-week-old infants. *JAMA Pediatrics, 170*(3), 212-219.

Maldonado-Lobon, J. A., Diaz-Lopez, M. A., Carputo, R., et al. (2015). Lactobacillus fermentum CECT 5716 reduces staphylococcus load in the breastmilk of lactating mothers suffering breast pain: A randomized controlled trial. *Breastfeeding Medicine, 10*(9), 425-432.

Mangesi, L., & Zakarija-Grkovic, I. (2016). Treatments for breast engorgement during lactation. *Cochrane Database of Systematic Reviews*(6), CD006946. doi:10.1002/14651858.CD006946.pub3

Marasco, L., & West, D. (2020). *Making More Milk: The Breastfeeding Guide to Increasing Your Milk Production* (2nd ed.). New York, NY: McGraw Hill.

Marmet, C., & Shell, E. (2017). Therapeutic positioning for breastfeeding. In C. W. Genna (Ed.), *Supporting Sucking Skills in Breastfeeding Infants* (3rd ed., pp. 399-416). Burlington, MA: Jones & Bartlett Learning.

Marshall, D. R., Callan, P. P., & Nicholson, W. (1994). Breastfeeding after reduction mammaplasty. *British Journal of Plastic Surgery, 47*(3), 167-169.

Martin, R., Heilig, H. G., Zoetendal, E. G., et al. (2007). Cultivation-independent assessment of the bacterial diversity of breast milk among healthy women. *Research in Microbiology, 158*(1), 31-37.

Matheson, I., Aursnes, I., Horgen, M., et al. (1988). Bacteriological findings and clinical symptoms in relation to clinical outcome in puerperal mastitis. *Acta Obstetricia et Gynecologica Scandinavica, 67*(8), 723-726.

McClellan, H. L., Hepworth, A. R., Garbin, C. P., et al. (2012). Nipple pain during breastfeeding with or without visible trauma. *Journal of Human Lactation, 28*(4), 511-521.

McLachlan, Z., Milne, E. J., Lumley, J., et al. (1993). Ultrasound treatment for breast engorgement: A randomised double blind trial. *Breastfeeding Review, 2*(7), 316-320.

Meguid, M. M., Oler, A., Numann, P. J., et al. (1995). Pathogenesis-based treatment of recurring subareolar breast abscesses. *Surgery, 118*(4), 775-782.

Michaels, A. M., & Wanner, H. (2013). Breastfeeding twins after mastectomy. *Journal of Human Lactation, 29*(1), 20-22.

Michalopoulos, K. (2007). The effects of breast augmentation surgery on future ability to lactate. *Breast Journal, 13*(1), 62-67.

Michie, C., Lockie, F., & Lynn, W. (2005). The challenge of mastitis. *Breastfeeding Review, 13*(1), 13-16.

Mitchell, K. B., Eglash, A., & Bamberger, E. T. (2019). Mammary dysbiosis and nipple blebs treated with intravenous daptomycin and dalbavancin. *Journal of Human Lactation.* doi:10.1177/0890334419862214.

Mitchell, K. B., Johnson, H. M., Eglash, A., et al. (2019). ABM Clinical Protocol #30: Breast masses, breast complaints, and diagnostic breast imaging in the lactating woman. *Breastfeeding Medicine, 14*(4), 208-214.

Mizuno, K., Nishida, Y., Mizuno, N., et al. (2008). The important role of deep attachment in the uniform drainage of breast milk from mammary lobe. *Acta Paediatrica, 97*(9), 1200-1204.

Mofid, M. M., Klatsky, S. A., Singh, N. K., et al. (2006). Nipple-areola complex sensitivity after primary breast augmentation: A comparison of periareolar and inframammary incision approaches. *Plastic and Reconstructive Surgery, 117*(6), 1694-1698.

Montalto, M., & Lui, B. (2009). MRSA as a cause of postpartum breast abscess in infant and mother. *Journal of Human Lactation, 25*(4), 448-450.

Moon, J. L., & Humenick, S. S. (1989). Breast engorgement: Contributing variables and variables amenable to nursing intervention. *Journal of Obstetric, Gynecologic & Neonatal Nursing, 18*(4), 309-315.

Morton, J. (2019). Hands-on or hands-off when first milk matters most? *Breastfeeding Medicine, 14*(5), 295-297.

Morton, J. A. (1994). The clinical usefulness of breast milk sodium in the assessment of lactogenesis. *Pediatrics, 93*(5), 802-806.

Nahai, F. R., & Nahai, F. (2008). MOC-PSSM CME article: Breast reduction. *Plastic and Reconstructive Surgery, 121*(1 Supplement), 1-13.

NCI. (2020). Inflammatory breast cancer: Questions and answers. Retrieved from **cancer.gov/cancertopics/factsheet/Sites-Types/IBC**.

Neifert, M., DeMarzo, S., Seacat, J., et al. (1990). The influence of breast surgery, breast appearance, and pregnancy-induced breast changes on lactation sufficiency as measured by infant weight gain. *Birth, 17*(1), 31-38.

Neville, M. C., Keller, R., Seacat, J., et al. (1988). Studies in human lactation: Milk volumes in lactating women during the onset of lactation and full lactation. *American Journal of Clinical Nutrition, 48*(6), 1375-1386.

Noel-Weiss, J., Woodend, A. K., & Groll, D. L. (2011). Iatrogenic newborn weight loss: Knowledge translation using a study protocol for your maternity setting. *International Breastfeeding Journal, 6*(1), 10.

Nommsen-Rivers, L. A., Heinig, M. J., Cohen, R. J., et al. (2008). Newborn wet and soiled diaper counts and timing of onset of lactation as indicators of breastfeeding inadequacy. *Journal of Human Lactation, 24*(1), 27-33.

O'Callaghan, M. A. (1981). Atypical discharge from the breast during pregnancy and/or lactation. *Australian and New Zealand Journal of Obstetrics and Gynaecology, 21*(4), 214-216.

Ohene-Yeboah, M., & Amaning, E. (2008). Spectrum of complaints presented at a specialist breast clinic in kumasi, ghana. *Ghana Medical Journal, 42*(3), 110-113.

Osterman, K. L., & Rahm, V. A. (2000). Lactation mastitis: Bacterial cultivation of breast milk, symptoms, treatment, and outcome. *Journal of Human Lactation, 16*(4), 297-302.

Park, G. E., Hauch, M. A., Curlin, F., et al. (1996). The effects of varying volumes of crystalloid administration before cesarean delivery on maternal hemodynamics and colloid osmotic pressure. *Anesthesia and Analgesia, 83*(2), 299-303.

Peters, F., Diemer, P., Mecks, O., et al. (2003). Severity of mastalgia in relation to milk duct dilatation. *Obstetrics & Gynecology, 101*(1), 54-60.

Peterson, B. (2007). Incidence of MRSA in postpartum breast abscesses (abstract). *Breastfeeding Medicine, 2*(3), 190.

Pieh-Holder, K. L. (2013). Lactational ectopic breast tissue of the vulva: Case report and brief historical review. *Breastfeeding Medicine, 8,* 223-225.

Pitanguy, I., Vaena, M., Radwanski, H. N., et al. (2007). Relative implant volume and sensibility alterations after breast augmentation. *Aesthetic Plastic Surgery, 31*(3), 238-243.

Poojari, V. G., Pupadhya, R., Pai, M. V., et al. (2018). Gestational gigantomastia: Challenges in management and follow up. *Journal of Clinical and Diagnostic Research, 12*(8), 3-4.

Pringle, P. J., Stanhope, R., Hindmarsh, P., et al. (1988). Abnormal pubertal development in primary hypothyroidism. *Clinical Endocrinology, 28*(5), 479-486.

Quinn, L., Ailsworth, M., Matthews, E., et al. (2018). Serratia marcescens colonization causing pink breast milk and pink diapers: A case report and literature review. *Breastfeeding Medicine, 13*(5), 388-394.

Ramsay, D. T., Kent, J. C., Hartmann, R. A., et al. (2005). Anatomy of the lactating human breast redefined with ultrasound imaging. *Journal of Anatomy, 206*(6), 525-534.

Ramsay, D. T., Kent, J. C., Owens, R. A., et al. (2004). Ultrasound imaging of milk ejection in the breast of lactating women. *Pediatrics, 113*(2), 361-367.

Rasmussen, L. B., Hansen, D. H., Kaestel, P., et al. (2008). Milk enzyme activities and subclinical mastitis among women in Guinea-Bissau. *Breastfeeding Medicine, 3*(4), 215-219.

Rezai, S., Nakagawa, J. T., Tedesco, J., et al. (2015). Gestational gigantomastia complicating pregnancy: A case report and review of the literature. *Case Reports in Obstetrics and Gynecology, 2015,* 892369.

Rimoldi, S. G., Pileri, P., Mazzocco, M. I., et al. (2019). The role of Staphylococcus aureus in mastitis: A multidisciplinary working group experience. *Journal of Human Lactation,* 890334419876272.

Riordan, J. M., & Nichols, F. H. (1990). A descriptive study of lactation mastitis in long-term breastfeeding women. *Journal of Human Lactation, 6*(2), 53-58.

Roberts, C. L., Ampt, A. J., Algert, C. S., et al. (2015). Reduced breast milk feeding subsequent to cosmetic breast augmentation surgery. *Medical Journal of Australia, 202*(6), 324-328.

Roberts, K. L. (1995). A comparison of chilled cabbage leaves and chilled gelpaks in reducing breast engorgement. *Journal of Human Lactation, 11*(1), 17-20.

Roberts, K. L., Reiter, M., & Schuster, D. (1995). A comparison of chilled and room temperature cabbage leaves in treating breast engorgement. *Journal of Human Lactation, 11*(3), 191-194.

Roberts, K. L., Reiter, M., & Schuster, D. (1998). Effects of cabbage leaf extract on breast engorgement. *Journal of Human Lactation, 14*(3), 231-236.

Robertson, B. D. (2016). An alternative treatment: Using ultrasound for plugged ducts--An interview with Karen Lin. *Clinical Lactation, 7*(4), 148-152.

Rosenberg , C. A., Derman , G. H., Grabb , W. C., et al. (1983). Hypomastia and mitral-valve prolapse. *New England Journal of Medicine, 309*(20), 1230-1232.

Rothenberg, J. B., Jayaram, P., Naqvi, U., et al. (2017). The role of low-intensity pulsed ultrasound on cartilage healing in knee osteoarthritis: A review. *Physical Medicine & Rehabilitation, 9*(12), 1268-1277.

Sadove, A. M., & van Aalst, J. A. (2005). Congenital and acquired pediatric breast anomalies: A review of 20 years' experience. *Plastic and Reconstructive Surgery, 115*(4), 1039-1050.

Say, B., Dizdar, E. A., Degirmencioglu, H., et al. (2016). The effect of lactational mastitis on the macronutrient content of breast milk. *Early Human Development, 98,* 7-9.

Schiff, M., Algert, C. S., Ampt, A., et al. (2014). The impact of cosmetic breast implants on breastfeeding: a systematic review and meta-analysis. *International Breastfeeding Journal, 9,* 17-17.

Schlenz, I., Kuzbari, R., Gruber, H., et al. (2000). The sensitivity of the nipple-areola complex: An anatomic study. *Plastic and Reconstructive Surgery, 105*(3), 905-909.

Scott, J. A., Robertson, M., Fitzpatrick, J., et al. (2008). Occurrence of lactational mastitis and medical management: A prospective cohort study in Glasgow. *International Breastfeeding Journal, 3,* 21.

Semple, J. L., Lugowski, S. J., Baines, C. J., et al. (1998). Breast milk contamination and silicone implants: Preliminary results using silicon as a proxy measurement for silicone. *Plastic and Reconstructive Surgery, 102*(2), 528-533.

Sharma, Y., Bajpai, A., Mittal, S., et al. (2006). Ovarian cysts in young girls with hypothyroidism: Follow-up and effect of treatment. *Journal of Pediatric Endocrinology and Metabolism, 19*(7), 895-900.

Sickles, E. A., & Abele, J. S. (1981). Milk of calcium within tiny benign breast cysts. *Radiology, 141*(3), 655-658.

Silva, J. R., Carvalho, R., Maia, C., et al. (2014). Rusty pipe syndrome, a cause of bloody nipple discharge: Case report. *Breastfeeding Medicine, 9*(8), 411-412.

Skalkeas, G., Gogas, J., & Pavlatos, F. (1972). Mammary hypoplasia following irradiation to an infant breast. Case report. *Acta Chirurgiae Plasticae, 14*(4), 240-243.

Spear, S. (2006). *Surgeries of the Breast: Principles and Art.* Philadelphia, PA: Lippincott-Raven.

Stafford, I., Hernandez, J., Laibl, V., et al. (2008). Community-acquired methicillin-resistant Staphylococcus aureus among patients with puerperal mastitis requiring hospitalization. *Obstetrics & Gynecology, 112*(3), 533-537.

Stone, K., & Wheeler, A. (2015). A review of anatomy, physiology, and benign pathology of the nipple. *Annals of Surgical Oncology, 22*(10), 3236-3240.

Strom, S. S., Baldwin, B. J., Sigurdson, A. J., et al. (1997). Cosmetic saline breast implants: A survey of satisfaction, breast-feeding experience, cancer screening, and health. *Plastic and Reconstructive Surgery, 100*(6), 1553-1557.

Tang, L., Lee, A. H., Qiu, L., et al. (2014). Mastitis in Chinese breastfeeding mothers: A prospective cohort study. *Breastfeeding Medicine, 9*(1), 35-38.

Teuber, S. S., & Gershwin, M. E. (1994). Autoantibodies and clinical rheumatic complaints in two children of women with silicone gel breast implants. *International Archives of Allergy and Immunology, 103*(1), 105-108.

Thorley, V. (2005). Breast hypoplasia and breastfeeding: A case history. *Breastfeeding Review, 13*(2), 13-16.

Trupiano, J. K., Sebek, B. A., Goldfarb, J., et al. (2001). Mastitis due to mycobacterium abscessus after body piercing. *Clinical Infectious Diseases, 33*(1), 131-134.

Tsai, F. C., Hsieh, M. S., Liao, C. K., et al. (2010). Correlation between scoliosis and breast asymmetries in women undergoing augmentation mammaplasty. *Aesthetic Plastic Surgery, 34*(3), 374-380.

Tuaillon, E., Viljoen, J., Dujols, P., et al. (2017). Subclinical mastitis occurs frequently in association with dramatic changes in inflammatory/anti-inflammatory breast milk components. *Pediatric Research, 81*(4), 556-564.

Uematsu, T., Kasami, M., & Yuen, S. (2009). A cluster of microcalcifications: Women with high risk for breast cancer versus other women. *Breast Cancer, 16*(4), 307-314.

Ulitzsch, D., Nyman, M. K., & Carlson, R. A. (2004). Breast abscess in lactating women: US-guided treatment. *Radiology, 232*(3), 904-909.

Uysal, E., Soran, A., Sezgin, E., et al. (2018). Factors related to recurrence of idiopathic granulomatous mastitis: What do we learn from a multicentre study? *ANZ Journal of Surgery, 88*(6), 635-639.

von Heimburg, D., Exner, K., Kruft, S., et al. (1996). The tuberous breast deformity: Classification and treatment. *British Journal of Plastic Surgery, 49*(6), 339-345.

Walker, M. (2018). Mammary dysbiosis: An unwelcome visitor during lactation. *Clinical Lactation, 9*(3), 130-136.

Walker, M. (2019). Novel innovations and recent findings in lactation support. *Clinical Lactation, 10*(4), 175-182.

Wambach, K. (2021). Breast-related problems. In K. Wambach & B. Spencer (Eds.), *Breastfeeding and Human Lactation* (6th ed., pp. 281-312). Burlington, MA: Jones & Bartlett Learning.

Wambach, K., & Genna, C. W. (2021). Anatomy and physiology of lactation. In K. Wambach & B. Spencer (Eds.), *Breastfeeding and Human Lactation* (6th ed., pp. 49-83). Burlington, MA: Jones & Bartlett Learning.

Wambach, K. A. (2003). Lactation mastitis: A descriptive study of the experience. *Journal of Human Lactation, 19*(1), 24-34.

Wang, Z. X., Luo, D. L., Dai, X., et al. (2012). Polyacrylamide hydrogel injection for augmentation mammaplasty: Loss of ability for breastfeeding. *Annals of Plastic Surgery, 69*(2), 123-128.

Wei, J., Zhang, J., & Fu, D. (2016). Negative suction drain through a mini periareolar incision for the treatment of lactational breast abscess shortens hospital stay and increases breastfeeding rates. *Breastfeeding Medicine, 11,* 259-260.

West, D., & Hirsch, E. (2008). *Breastfeeding after Breast and Nipple Procedures.* Amarillo, TX: Hale Publishing.

Westerfield, K. L., Koenig, K., & Oh, R. (2018). Breastfeeding: Common questions and answers. *American Family Physician, 98*(6), 368-373.

WHO. (2000). Mastitis: Causes and Management. Geneva, Switzerland: World Health Organization Retrieved from **apps.who.int/iris/bitstream/handle/10665/66230/WHO_FCH_CAH_00.13_eng.pdf;jsessionid=46005F748E69A916788E58E16595E342?sequence=1**.

Wilson-Clay, B. (2008). Case report of methicillin-resistant Staphylococcus aureus (MRSA) mastitis with abscess formation in a breastfeeding woman. *Journal of Human Lactation, 24*(3), 326-329.

Wilson-Clay, B., & Hoover, K. (2017). *The Breastfeeding Atlas* (6th ed.). Manchaca, TX: LactNews Press.

Winocour, S., & Lemaine, V. (2013). Hypoplastic breast anomalies in the female adolescent breast. *Seminars in Plastic Surgery, 27*(1), 42-48.

Witt, A. M., Bolman, M., & Kredit, S. (2016). Mothers value and utilize early outpatient education on breast massage and hand expression in their self-management of engorgement. *Breastfeeding Medicine, 11,* 433-439.

Witt, A. M., Bolman, M., Kredit, S., et al. (2016). Therapeutic breast massage in lactation for the management of engorgement, plugged ducts, and mastitis. *Journal of Human Lactation, 32*(1), 123-131.

Wockel, A., Abou-Dakn, M., Beggel, A., et al. (2008). Inflammatory breast diseases during lactation: Health effects on the newborn-a literature review. *Mediators of Inflammation, 2008,* 298760.

Wolfrum, A., Kummel, S., Theuerkauf, I., et al. (2018). Granulomatous mastitis: A therapeutic and diagnostic challenge. *Breast Care (Basel), 13*(6), 413-418.

Wong, B. B., Chan, Y. H., Leow, M. Q. H., et al. (2017). Application of cabbage leaves compared to gel packs for mothers with breast engorgement: Randomised controlled trial. *International Journal of Nursing Studies, 76,* 92-99.

Wust, J., Rutsch, M., & Stocker, S. (1995). Streptococcus pneumoniae as an agent of mastitis. *European Journal of Clinical Microbiology & Infectious Diseases, 14*(2), 156-157.

Yoshida, M., Shinohara, H., Sugiyama, T., et al. (2014). Taste of milk from inflamed breasts of breastfeeding mothers with mastitis evaluated using a taste sensor. *Breastfeeding Medicine, 9*(2), 92-97.

Zelazniewicz, A., & Pawlowski, B. (2019). Maternal breast volume in pregnancy and lactation capacity. *American Journal of Physical Anthropology, 168*(1), 180-189.

Zocchi, M. L., & Zuliani, F. (2008). Bicompartmental breast lipostructuring. *Aesthetic Plastic Surgery, 32*(2), 313-328. doi:10.1007/s00266-007-9089-3.

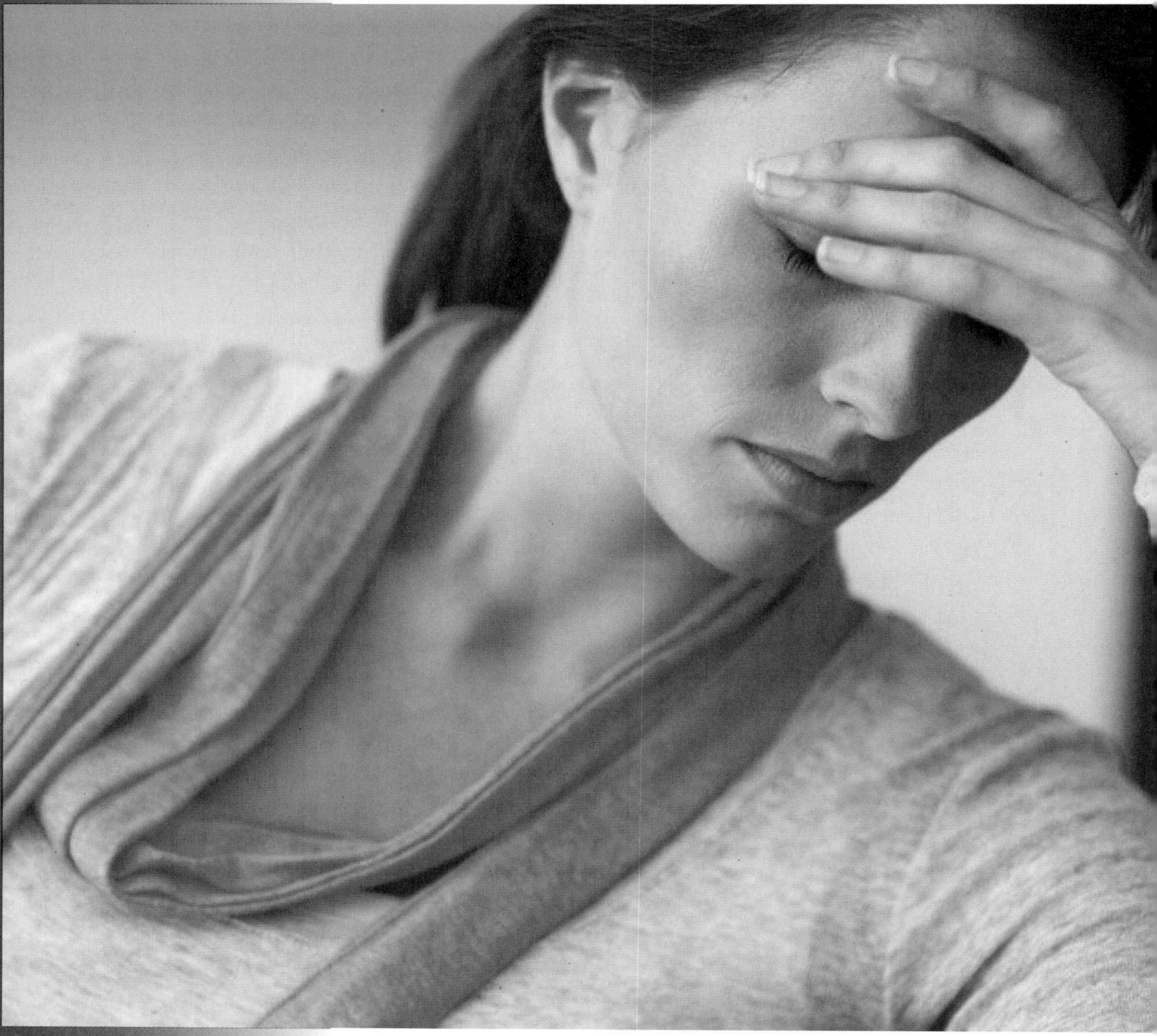

Nursing Parent's Health

19

NURSING WITH HEALTH ISSUES

When parents are ill, nursing relieves stress, enhances sleep, metabolism, and the immune system, and often provides a greater sense of control and normalcy.

When lactating parents are ill, to help speed their recovery, those supporting them may look for ways to reduce their stress and workload. Sometimes others, including healthcare providers, assume that eliminating nursing will make an ill parent's life easier. Milk-making may seem like an unnecessary physical strain on the body, and it may seem to others that the time spent nursing is extra work, an inconvenience, or an interruption of rest. But how parents feel about continuing to nurse is more important. If they want to continue, the following information may help convey to family and friends that nursing can be good for parents and aid in their recovery, as well as being good for the baby. When discussing options, follow the parent's lead.

Nursing is a stress reliever. Caring for a newborn can be intense and sometimes stressful, no matter how a baby is fed. According to research, however, when nursing is going well, not nursing is more stressful for parents than nursing. The skin-to-skin contact and oxytocin released during milk flow are no doubt factors. Swedish research (Jonas et al., 2008; Uvnas-Moberg, 1998) found that higher oxytocin blood levels decreased blood pressure and levels of cortisol, a stress hormone. In one U.S. study of 24 women who both breastfed and bottle-fed (Mezzacappa & Katlin, 2002), researchers assessed the study mothers' mood before and after breastfeeding and before and after bottle-feeding. They found that the mothers were calmer after breastfeeding than after bottle-feeding. This study was significant because it eliminated one of the major problems in comparing nursing and non-nursing parents: the often-substantial differences between parents who choose one feeding method over the other. In this study, since the same mothers were studied after both breast and bottle, this potential confounder was eliminated. The down-regulation of stress that nursing provides is one reason research linked longer nursing duration to better cardiovascular outcomes in women later in life (Peters et al., 2017; Qu, Wang, Tang, Wu, & Sun, 2018; Schwarz et al., 2009). For details, see the later section "Cardiac Issues/ Hypertension."

Nursing enhances a parent's immune system and mood. Another U.S. study of 181 mothers (Groer & Davis, 2006) measured mothers' reactions to stress, including its effect on the immune system, measured by blood cytokine balance, and their mood. The researchers found that the immune systems of non-breastfeeding mothers were more depressed by life stressors, and these mothers developed more infections than the breastfeeding mothers. The non-breastfeeding mothers also had higher levels of anxiety and fatigue. Based on their own results and German research (Dimitrov, Lange, Fehm, & Born, 2004), these authors suggested that higher levels of blood prolactin stimulated by nursing were related to more positive mood, greater immunity to infection, and decreased stress.

KEY CONCEPT

When ill, some parents want to continue nursing while others pressure them to wean. Follow parents' lead.

Nursing enhances metabolic efficiency. According to U.S. research (Hammond, 1997), nursing parents' bodies adapt to lactation by reducing the energy required to make milk, causing their metabolism to be more energy-efficient. During lactation, the intestines enlarge and change to make digestion more efficient at absorbing nutrients. After a meal, nursing mothers were found to have greater metabolic efficiency than non-nursing mothers (Illingworth, Jung, Howie, Leslie, & Isles, 1986). This greater metabolic efficiency continued long after nursing ended, improving parents' health outcomes later in life. A U.S. cross-sectional cohort analysis of 1,620 women (Ram et al., 2008) found that duration of lactation was associated with a lower incidence later in life of metabolic syndrome. (For more details, see p. 848). One of these researchers (Ram et al., 2008, p. 268) wrote: "Lactation may prime the metabolic system by making it a more energy-efficient machine...."

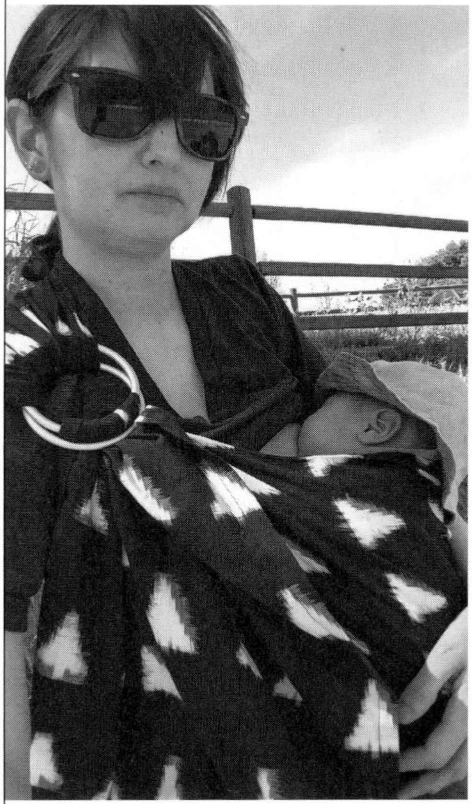

Nursing parents sleep more and spend more time in deep sleep. Some think that if someone else feeds baby at night the nursing parent will get more sleep and sleep better, but surprisingly, in families with young babies, exclusive nursing leads to more and deeper sleep in nursing parents. One U.S. study of 133 new mothers and fathers during the first 3 months post-delivery (Doan, Gardiner, Gay, & Lee, 2007) found that mothers who exclusively breastfed averaged 40 to 45 minutes more sleep at night than those who mixed fed (nursing and formula). Australian research (Blyton, Sullivan, & Edwards, 2002) found breastfeeding mothers spent more time in deep sleep than non-breastfeeding mothers. The exclusively breastfeeding mothers had "a marked alteration in their sleep architecture," giving them longer periods of slow-wave sleep (SWS), a type of deep sleep, than the formula-feeding mothers. For more details, see p. 79.

Nursing can help provide a greater sense of normalcy and control. Very ill parents may be able nurse, even when they can do little else for their baby. If appropriate, discuss ways to make continued nursing easier, such as bringing the young baby into bed during the recovery and nursing while side-lying or semi-reclining, while resting. If the baby is older and active, suggest closing the door and having toys available for him to play with while resting. A toddler may be happy spending time with others, returning to the nursing parent every now and then to nurse and "touch base." For parents with a disability or limitation, see that section (p. 862-863) for strategies for making nursing easier.

• • •

In nearly all cases, continuing to nurse will be better for the baby.

Acute illness. Even before parents exposed to an acute illness notice symptoms, they are already contagious. At this stage, one of the body's first responses is to make antibodies that pass into the milk specifically designed to protect the nursing baby from that illness. By the time parents start to feel sick, the baby is already exposed and is already receiving protection against the illness. When nursing continues, parents continue to provide their baby with protection. Because of the antibodies, if the nursing baby does become ill, he almost always gets a milder case than he would if he had weaned. In the case of a virus, most often immunity to that virus is transmitted through mother's milk.

Endocrine, metabolic, or autoimmune disorders. Some parents worry that nursing may transmit their chronic illness to their baby. Usually the opposite is true. For example, when parents with Type 2 diabetes exclusively nurse, their babies are less likely to develop this illness than formula-fed or mixed-fed babies (Horta & de Lima, 2019). The same is true for rheumatoid arthritis (Jacobsson, Jacobsson, Askling, & Knowler, 2003), and other autoimmune disorders. With a genetic disease, such as cystic fibrosis, if the baby has a genetic predisposition to it, nursing cannot prevent it, but it was found to delay the onset of its symptoms (Colombo et al., 2007).

• • •

Most medications and diagnostic tests are compatible with lactation.

If nursing parents have concerns about whether they should take a prescribed medication for a health problem, check the drug in the LactMed database (**bit.ly/BA2-LactMed**) or in the current edition of *Hale's Medications and Mothers' Milk*. (See Box 13.1 on p. 601 for a more complete listing of reliable resources.) Another book often used by healthcare providers to check a drug's compatibility with nursing is *The Physician's Desk Reference (PDR)*. However, the PDR is a compilation of package inserts from the drug manufacturers, whose main concern is avoiding lawsuits. In the PDR, weaning is recommended for many drugs research found are compatible with lactation. *Hale's Medications and Mothers' Milk*, on the other hand, provides information about the published research on each drug in nursing parents and to simplify decision-making, assigns each drug a ***Lactation Risk Category***:

- **L1** (Safest) are drugs that were taken by large numbers of nursing parents and controlled studies found no adverse effects on the baby, the possibility of risk is remote, or due to its characteristics, the drug is not orally bioavailable to the baby.
- **L2** (Safer) are drugs for which some studies exist in nursing parents without adverse effects on their baby and/or the risk during lactation is remote.
- **L3** (Moderately Safe) are newer drugs with no published research or drugs with no controlled studies in nursing parents, those with a possible risk of adverse effects on the baby, or controlled studies found minimal effects on the baby.
- **L4** (Possibly Hazardous) are drugs for which evidence exists of risk to either the nursing baby or the milk production. If there are no alternative drugs available and the parent is seriously ill, the benefit may outweigh the risk of taking these drugs while continuing to nurse.
- **L5** (Contraindicated) are drugs that should not be taken during lactation. Either studies have found a significant risk to the human-milk-fed baby or the characteristics of the drug indicate the risks to the baby would outweigh the benefits to the parent.

For important points about lactation and medications, see Box 19.1. The vast majority of medications, medical procedures, and diagnostic tests are compatible with lactation (T.W. Hale, 2019). This means that the health risks associated with feeding the baby infant formula are considered greater than the risks of continuing to nurse with a tiny amount of the drug (usually about 1%-2% of the parental dose) in the milk. However, because there are a few drugs that are not compatible with lactation, any medication should always be checked. Also, each drug needs to be evaluated by the family's healthcare providers in light of the parent's and baby's condition and health history. If an incompatible drug is recommended, there is often an alternative drug compatible with lactation that can be substituted.

• • •

If temporary or permanent weaning is necessary due to illness or treatment, help parents do so as gradually and comfortably as possible.

Continuing to nurse is nearly always the best option. But if parents must wean the baby, either temporarily or permanently, discuss how to do this with the least amount of physical and emotional stress. Sudden or abrupt weaning during an illness can cause parents intense discomfort from full mammary glands and put them at increased risk for mastitis. It can also upset the baby, making him difficult to console and increasing his odds of becoming ill.

BOX 19.1 Key Points about Medication Use during Lactation

- Most drugs are safe during lactation. The hazards of using formula are well-known and documented.
- Avoid using medications that are not necessary. Herbal preparations, high-dose vitamins, unusual supplements, etc. that are not necessary should be avoided.
- Medications used in the first 3 to 4 days are rarely of concern due to the limited volume of mother's milk the baby consumes.
- If the baby receives <10% of the parent's dose (Relative Infant Dose), the vast majority of medications are considered safe. For most drugs, the baby receives <1% of the parent's dose.
- Choose drugs for which there is published data, rather than new drugs, short-acting rather than long-acting drugs (short half-life), and drugs with high protein binding, low oral bioavailability, or high molecular weight.
- Be slightly more cautious with newborns and at-risk babies, such as those ill or preterm. Be less concerned about older, heavier babies and those no longer exclusively nursing.
- Recommend that parents with depressive symptoms or other mental disorders seek treatment. Most of the medications used to treat them are safe.
- Temporary weaning may be required for hours or days for a few drugs and nearly all radioactive compounds. Follow published guidelines.

Adapted from Hale's Medications and Mothers' Milk *(T.W. Hale, 2019, p. ix)*

If the weaning is temporary, discuss milk expression (see Chapter 11 for options). Even if the milk cannot be fed to the baby, regular milk expression will prevent pain and mastitis and maintain milk production until they are ready to resume nursing. If weaning must be permanent, discuss its timing and help families wean as slowly and gradually as possible to make it easier for both parent and baby. (For details on weaning strategies, see p. 171.)

BACTERIAL AND VIRAL ILLNESSES

When nursing parents are ill, first acknowledge their feelings and challenges, and then discuss their specific concerns.

A parent's illness can disrupt the whole household. In this situation, parents must cope with their own health issues, along with any worries they have about the effect of their illness or its treatment on the nursing baby. If they recently developed a serious or chronic illness, they may be afraid and grieving for their previous life.

Whatever the concerns and emotions, first acknowledge their feelings. Comments like "You're really having a difficult time" or "Don't worry about crying. You have so much to cope with!" can let them know they are heard and that it is okay to express strong feelings. Feeling heard first may make it possible for them to better process information and make decisions. The following sections describe nursing issues that may arise with specific illnesses.

• • •

When parents are contagious, using good hygiene, such as frequent handwashing, can reduce the baby's odds of catching the illness.

Most acute illnesses are transmitted through skin contact and nose or mouth secretions, not through nursing. When parents are ill, good personal hygiene, including regular handwashing, can decrease the baby's chances of catching the illness. Parents can also try to avoid breathing on the baby by limiting face-to-face contact. In cases of a highly contagious or serious illness, wearing a face mask whenever holding the baby can help prevent transmission through breath or nose-and-mouth secretions.

• • •

Suggest parents running a fever drink lots of fluids to stay well hydrated.

Fever can reduce the body fluids, which increases the chances of becoming constipated and dehydrated. When parents are feverish, encourage them to drink more fluids.

Common Illnesses

Cold, Virus, Mild Infection, Flu, and COVID-19

Interrupting nursing during a cold, virus, or mild infection increases the baby's chances of getting sick.

Before parents notice the symptoms of a cold, virus, or mild infection, they are already contagious (Wambach & Morrison, 2021, p. 511). At this stage, their body begins producing antibodies specific to that illness that pass into the milk to protect the baby. Continued nursing is the baby's best protection from the illness, but if he does catch it, the antibodies he receives usually make his illness less severe.

• • •

In most cases, if a lactating parent contracts seasonal influenza, nursing can continue while following recommended practices to prevent transmission to the baby.

Getting the flu is problematic for babies younger than 6 months because they are at risk for severe complications and are too young to be vaccinated. To prevent the spread of the flu, the U.S. Centers for Disease Control and Prevention (CDC, 2019a) recommends healthy pregnant and nursing parents receive the flu vaccine and follow these basic practices to avoid contracting the flu.

- Frequent handwashing
- Avoid contact with sick people
- When sneezing or coughing, use a tissue to cover their mouth, then throw it away and wash their hands
- Avoid touching their eyes, nose, and mouth
- Often clean and disinfect their living space

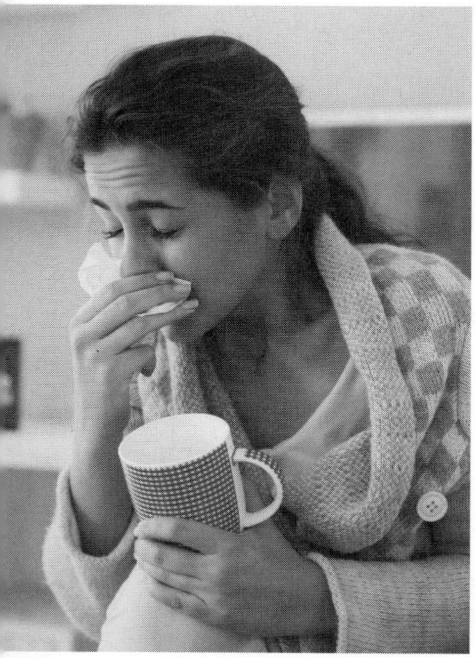

The flu and the nursing baby. According to the CDC, parents who were exposed to the seasonal flu but do not have symptoms should continue nursing. If a baby becomes ill with the flu, he should continue nursing. When a nursing parent becomes ill with the flu and the baby is healthy, the CDC (CDC, 2019a) wrote:

> "A mother's breast milk contains antibodies and other immunological factors that can help protect her infant from flu and is the recommended source of nutrition for the infant, even while the mother is ill. If a mother is too sick to feed her infant at the breast and another healthy caregiver is caring for the infant, the breastfeeding mother should be encouraged and supported to regularly express her milk so that the infant continues to receive her breast milk."

Some ways a sick nursing parent can reduce the risk of passing the flu on to the baby include:

- Wash their hands before touching the baby.
- While nursing, wear a surgical mask to protect the baby from contact with nasal secretions during coughing or sneezing.
- Use clean blankets or burp cloths at each feed.
- Be sure everyone who touches the baby follows these precautions.

An exception to these recommendations is the parent who has an active case of the flu while delivering a newborn. In this case, the CDC recommends separating the nursing couple until 24 hours after the parent's fever is gone. In this situation, the CDC suggests ill parents express their milk and have healthy caregivers feed it to the newborn.

KEY CONCEPT

The U.S. CDC encourages nursing parents with the flu to keep nursing.

Treatments for the flu and lactation. The CDC (CDC, 2019a) considers the antiviral medications used to treat nursing parents who come down with the flu to be compatible with lactation.

• • •

Nursing parents with an active case of COVID-19 can continue nursing but should take precautions to avoid transmitting it to their baby.

COVID-19 and the nursing baby. In December 2019, a novel coronavirus named COVID-19 soon spread to the entire world. Its fatality rate is 10 times higher than the seasonal flu, with elderly and compromised individuals at greatest risk.

At this writing, when nursing parents contract COVID-19, they may continue nursing. The U.S. Centers for Disease Control and Prevention (CDC) issued the following recommendation on its website (CDC, 2020):

> "A mother with confirmed COVID-19 or who is…symptomatic…should take all possible precautions to avoid spreading the virus to her infant, including washing her hands before touching the infant and wearing a face mask, if possible, while feeding at the breast."

See the previous point for other precautions to take. When recommended hygiene practices are followed, any expressed milk can be fed to the baby.

Like the seasonal flu, if a baby is born to a parent with an active case of COVID-19, separation may be recommended, with a healthy caregiver feeding the newborn the expressed milk.

Food Poisoning

Nursing does not need to be interrupted when parents contract food poisoning.

Food poisoning may occur after consuming a food or drink contaminated with specific bacteria or toxins. Bacteria that can cause food poisoning include botulism (*Clostridium botulinum*), listeriosis (*Listeria*), salmonella, *Shigella*, *E. coli*, and others.

Incubation period and symptoms. Incubation period varies by organism. Symptoms include vomiting, abdominal cramps, and diarrhea.

Food poisoning and the nursing baby. Food poisoning in the lactating parent should not affect the nursing baby.

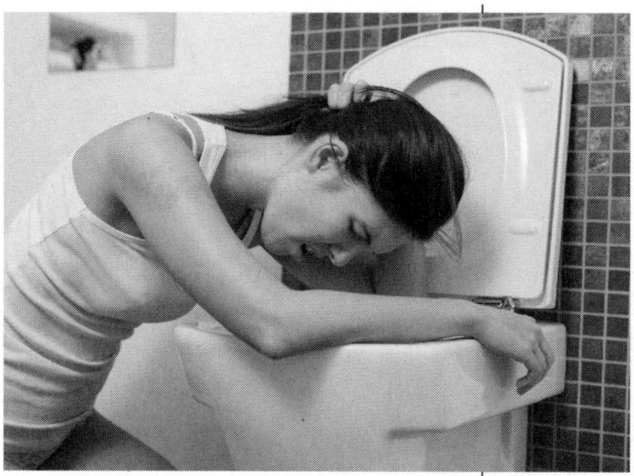

Food poisoning and the nursing parent. Parents most often recover from food poisoning within a few days without further problems. If they have diarrhea and vomiting, suggest drinking plenty of fluids to avoid dehydration.

Treatments for food poisoning and lactation. If the case of food poisoning is so severe that a parent is prescribed antibiotics, the drug's compatibility with lactation should be checked. (Most antibiotics are compatible.) In severe cases, depending on the bacteria involved, precautions may be recommended to prevent airborne or skin-contact transmission between parent and baby, such as handwashing and wearing a surgical mask while nursing.

Bacterial Infections

Group B Streptococcus

One of the most common causes of newborn infection, Group B Streptococcus, is usually transmitted before or during birth and only rarely via mother's milk.

In the U.S., Group B Strep (GBS) has been a major cause of serious infection in newborns and their parents (Puopolo et al., 2019). The GBS bacterium is part of our normal body flora, but colonization can occur if there is an overgrowth, usually in the lower reproductive organs and/or the gut. The U.S. Centers for Disease Control and Prevention (CDC, 2019d) estimates that between 15% and 40% of pregnant American women are colonized with GBS. Without treatment, about 1% to 2% of newborns become ill as a result (ACOG, 2019).

Incubation period and symptoms. The illnesses associated with GBS can be severe and even life-threatening. About 90% of newborns who become ill from GBS develop symptoms within the first 6 days after birth, which may manifest as pneumonia, meningitis, and a serious blood-borne infection known as sepsis.

Screening for GBS. In the U.K., tools to assess risk factors for GBS disease are used to screen newborns after delivery. In the U.S., universal screening for GBS by vaginal or rectal swabs is done between 35 and 37 weeks of pregnancy. If culture results are positive, IV antibiotics are given during labor. These two approaches produce similar results in decreasing newborn illness (Homer, Scarf, Catling, & Davis, 2014).

GBS and the nursing baby. One study conducted in the Czech Republic (Burianova, Paulova, Cermak, & Janota, 2013) demonstrated how rare it is for GBS to appear in mother's milk and found this unrelated to whether the nursing parent was GBS positive or negative. These researchers analyzed 243 milk samples from two groups of mothers: 1) those who cultured positive for GBS during pregnancy, and 2) those who cultured negative 1 week after delivery. Only 2 (0.8%) of the milk samples cultured positive for GBS, and both were from mothers in the GBS-negative group.

Although rare, there are case reports of GBS transmission via mother's milk to a very preterm or compromised baby (Dinger, Muller, Pargac, & Schwarze, 2002). It is also possible for the GBS organism to be passed back and forth between nursing parent and baby, especially if the baby becomes colonized (S. M. Jones & Steele, 2012; Wang, Chen, Liu, & Wang, 2007). In this case, both parent and child need treatment at the same time (Byrne, Miller, & Justus, 2006). If the milk cultures positive for GBS and the baby is ill or preterm, the milk can be pasteurized (by heating it to 63° [145° F] for 30 minutes) or discarded until the milk cultures are clear.

Treatments for GBS and lactation. In the U.S., GBS is treated during labor with IV antibiotics. The antibiotics used to treat GBS, such as penicillin, ampicillin, clindamycin, and erythromycin, are also used to treat babies and are therefore compatible with lactation (T.W. Hale, 2019).

Lyme Disease

Lyme disease is transmitted by the bite of an infected tick—not nursing—and its treatment is compatible with lactation.

Lyme disease is caused by a type of spirochete bacterium (*Borrelia burgdorferi*) that lives in rodents and other small animals. It is transmitted to humans through the bite of an infected tick. Most human cases occur in late spring and summer, when people spend more time outdoors.

Incubation period and symptoms. From the tick bite to the onset of symptoms is between 3 and 32 days, with an average of 11 days (AAP, 2018, p. 517). Symptoms usually start with a painless circular rash at the tick-bite site (usually appearing within 3 to 30 days after being bitten by an infected tick), which expands in size, reaching up to 12 inches (30 cm) in diameter. Symptoms may include fever, headache, chills, muscle and joint aches, and swollen lymph glands.

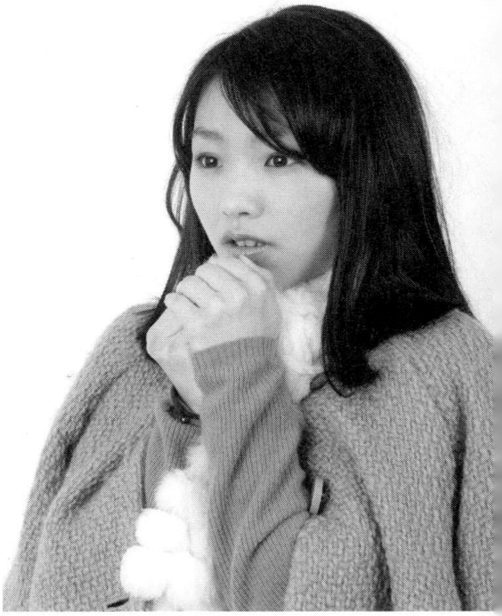

Lyme disease and the nursing baby. Although the Lyme spirochete can be transmitted to an unborn baby in utero, according to the U.S. Centers for Disease Control and Prevention (CDC, 2018c), "There are no reports of Lyme disease being spread through breast milk."

Treatments for Lyme disease and lactation. Treatment of a nursing parent with Lyme disease usually involves a several-week course of an appropriate oral antibiotic, such as doxycycline, amoxicillin, azithromycin, and cefuroxime (T.W. Hale & Berens, 2010, p. 283), which are considered compatible with lactation (T.W. Hale, 2019). Although most cases of Lyme disease treated early resolve completely, in some cases, symptoms like muscle and joint pain, sleep disturbance, and fatigue can continue long term.

Methicillin-Resistant Staphylococcus Aureus (MRSA)

When a nursing parent or baby is diagnosed with a methicillin-resistant *Staphylococcus aureus* (MRSA) infection, keep them together. Nursing can usually continue.

The *Staphylococcus aureus* bacterium (staph for short) lives on the skin of healthy people and usually causes no symptoms. Staph is so common that during the 1950s, by the fifth day after birth, 40% to 90% of newborns in hospital nurseries were colonized with it, not all of whom developed infections (Fairchild, Graber, Vogel, & Ingersoll, 1958). Over the years, with frequent use of antibiotics, strains of ***methicillin-resistant*** staph (MRSA) developed. Methicillin-resistant strains do not respond to the antibiotics often used to treat staph infections. MRSA causes more severe illness and requires different antibiotics to treat.

MRSA once existed only rarely and only then in hospitals. In some areas, it became increasingly common—about 60% of staph infections in some hospitals are now MRSA—and it spread to some communities (Salgado, Farr, & Calfee, 2003), such as in Taiwan and the U.S. One U.S. study (Stafford et al., 2008) reported that cases of community-acquired MRSA increased nine-fold in the Dallas, Texas area between 2003 and 2008 and that 63% of the breastfeeding study mothers diagnosed with breast abscesses cultured positive for MRSA. Other studies (Berens, Swaim, & Peterson, 2010; Peterson, 2007) found similar rates in Houston, Texas. Although MRSA is uncommon in other areas, it may occasionally cause mastitis and abscess. Reports in the literature identified individual cases of MRSA in:

- Japan (Hagiya, Shiota, Sugiyama, & Otsuka, 2014)
- Italy (Rimoldi et al., 2019)
- Germany (Lukassek, Ignatov, Faerber, Costa, & Eggemann, 2019)
- Australia (Montalto & Lui, 2009)

Preventing the spread of MRSA. During the hospital stay, keeping MRSA-infected parent and baby together but separate from other patients will help prevent its spread. In areas where MRSA is prevalent in the community, practicing good hygiene is especially vital. In these areas, suggest parents wash their hands often. Healthcare providers in clinics and private practices need to be vigilant about using gloves and routinely disinfecting the everyday objects they touch, such as clipboards, pens, and computer keyboards, as well as the surfaces parents and babies come in contact with, such as baby scales and breast pumps (Wilson-Clay, 2008).

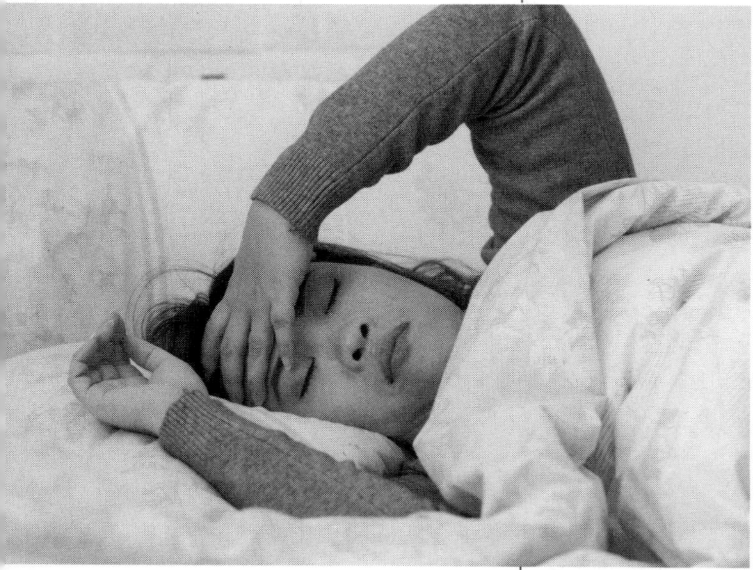

Preventing MRSA in the baby after birth. During birth, a baby is exposed to outside organisms in the birth canal. Japanese researchers (Kitajima, 2003) suggested skin-to-skin contact immediately after birth provides a defense against MRSA, colonizing newborns with their parent's normal flora, which decreases their susceptibility to MRSA colonization of their nose and throat, which can lead to infection. To lower the risk of contracting MRSA in the hospital NICU, one Japanese report (Nakamura, 2001) recommended at NICU admission to spread their mother's milk in and over the mouths of all extremely-low-birth-weight babies.

Incubation period and symptoms. MRSA may begin as a skin infection that may look like a spider bite, a boil, or an abscess. It is usually swollen, red, and painful and can progress to a fever, shortness of breath, a cough, and chills. MRSA may also be present during a bout of mastitis or in a breast abscess. The incubation period can be from 1 to 10 days, depending on its route of transmission.

MRSA and the nursing baby. When a nursing parent has MRSA, some healthcare providers question whether it is risky to continue nursing. However, ***if a parent develops a MRSA infection, the baby has already been exposed to it before the symptoms become obvious, so there is usually no reason to stop nursing if the baby is healthy*** (AAP, 2018, p. 115; CDC, 2019b). Babies can't contract MRSA from mother's milk; it is spread by contact. If the parent has an open sore that the baby might touch during nursing, it's important to completely cover it with a clean, dry bandage. If it's not possible for the baby to nurse without coming in contact with the sore, the baby can nurse on the unaffected side, and milk can be expressed from the affected side. If the baby is fragile due to illness or prematurity, the milk can be cultured to check for MRSA. If MRSA is cultured, it can be pasteurized (by heating it to 63° [145° F] for 30 minutes) before feeding (Gastelum, Dassey, Mascola, & Yasuda, 2005; Kim et al.,

2007), or if that is not an option, expressed milk may need to be discarded until it is clear of infection, usually within 24 to 48 hours of starting treatment (CDC, 2019b). Handwashing and other routine hygiene practices are important to help stop the spread of MRSA.

Treatment for MRSA and lactation. The same antibiotics used to treat babies with MRSA are also used to treat parents, making them compatible with lactation (T.W. Hale, 2019).

Tuberculosis

In cases of active tuberculosis, after parent and baby begin receiving drug therapy, nursing can continue.

Tuberculosis (TB) is an infectious disease caused by the bacterium *Mycobacterium tuberculosis,* which is usually transmitted from person-to-person via droplets in the air from coughing. TB bacteria usually attack the lungs, but can also spread to other parts of the body.

Incubation period and symptoms. The time from exposure to TB to a positive TB test is 2 to 10 weeks. Symptoms may not occur for 1 to 6 months and include weight loss, fever, cough, night sweats, and chills (AAP, 2018, p. 833).

TB and the nursing couple. Parents known to be contagious with active pulmonary TB are separated from their babies, no matter how they are fed, at least until parent and baby are started on drug therapy. Two U.S. physicians (Lawrence & Lawrence, 2016, p. 425) wrote:

> "Initiation of prophylactic isoniazid [an antimicrobial drug] in the infant has been demonstrated to be effective in preventing TB infection and disease in the infant. Therefore, continued separation of the infant and mother is unnecessary after therapy in both mother and child has begun."

This is common practice in many parts of the world.

After birth, if treatment of the nursing couple is delayed or healthcare providers recommend separation, suggest nursing parents establish their milk production using milk expression. (For details, see p. 498.) If an active case of TB develops during pregnancy and the parent receives appropriate drug therapy, separation after birth is unlikely and nursing should be encouraged (CDC, 2016).

Treatments for TB and lactation. TB requires long-term drug therapy. Many anti-tubercular drugs—such as isoniazid, rifampin, and ethambutol—are considered compatible with lactation (T.W. Hale, 2019).

Viral Infections

Hepatitis A, B, C and Others

When nursing parents contract hepatitis A, their baby can be given its immune globulin and/or vaccine, and nursing can continue.

Hepatitis means "inflammation of the liver." Hepatitis A is liver inflammation caused by the hepatitis A virus (HAV), one of the three most common hepatitis viruses. HAV can be transmitted by contact with infected blood or feces. Hepatitis B and C (see next points) are chronic diseases, but hepatitis A is not. In most people, it resolves completely without long-term damage. A case of hepatitis A also confers lifelong immunity to this illness.

Incubation period and symptoms. After exposure to HAV, it may take 15 to 50 days for symptoms to develop (AAP, 2018, p. 393). During this illness, the liver becomes tender and swollen and bilirubin accumulates in the bloodstream, causing jaundice (yellowish skin). Fever and nausea are also common.

Hepatitis A and the nursing parent. During the acute phase of hepatitis A, if parents feel too ill to nurse, they can express milk (which can be fed to the baby) or rebuild their milk production after the symptoms subside. If they decide to wean, suggest expressing at least enough milk to avoid uncomfortable mammary fullness, which can lead to mastitis, complicating their health problems.

Hepatitis A and the nursing baby. When the nursing parent of a newborn contracts hepatitis A, the American Academy of Pediatrics Committee on Infectious Diseases (AAP, 2018, p. 399) recommends treating the baby with either the hepatitis A vaccine or immune globulin or both. Hepatitis A is not a contraindication to nursing.

Hepatitis A treatments and lactation. Other than treating its symptoms with fever-reducers or pain medication, Hepatitis A has no treatment.

• • •

If parents contract hepatitis B, their baby can be given its immune globulin and vaccine, and nursing can continue.

Hepatitis B is the most common serious liver infection in the world and is caused by the hepatitis-B virus (HBV).

Incubation period and symptoms. Some carriers of HBV never become ill. Acute symptoms usually appear between 45 and 160 days after exposure (AAP, 2018, p. 401). Symptoms are similar to hepatitis A, but in about 5% to 10% of cases, hepatitis B becomes a chronic illness. It is spread whenever a body fluid (saliva, mucus, blood, etc.) containing the HBV comes in contact with broken skin. It can also be transmitted from contaminated food and sexual contact.

Hepatitis B immune globulin and lactation. When parents giving birth have hepatitis B, their newborn may be exposed to HBV through contact with body fluids during delivery. In this situation, the American Academy of Pediatrics Committee on Infectious Diseases recommends the baby of a hepatitis B positive parent be given both the first dose of the hepatitis B vaccine and the hepatitis B immune globulin within 12 hours after birth. There is no reason to delay nursing after birth. The Committee (AAP, 2018, p. 426) wrote:

> "Breastfeeding of the infant by an HBV-positive mother poses no additional risk of acquisition of HBV infection by the infant with appropriate administration of hepatitis B vaccine and HBIG."

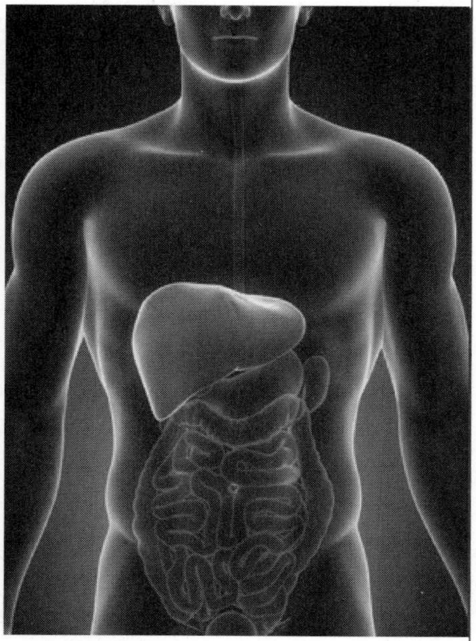

Staff training and extra lactation support are recommended when caring for these families. Despite guidelines from the World Health Association to nurse babies born to HBV-positive parents (WHO, 1996), in some parts of China, for example, nursing rates are much lower in HBV-positive families than in other families (Qiu, Binns, Zhao, Zhang, & Xie, 2010).

Hepatitis B and the nursing couple. If nursing parents contract hepatitis B after birth, the same course of action is advised. The baby (and other family members) should be vaccinated and nursing should continue (WHO, 1996).

Treatment of hepatitis B and lactation. Chronic hepatitis B may be treated with antiviral medications, such as telbivudine, which is compatible with lactation (T.W. Hale, 2019, p. 721). However, many other antiviral medications used to treat hepatitis B (for example, entecavir, tenofovir, and lamivudine.) are considered either potentially hazardous to the nursing baby (L4) or contraindicated during lactation (L5).

• • •

The hepatitis C virus (HCV) causes liver infection, which in many cases becomes chronic.

It is considered safe for asymptomatic parents with hepatitis C to nurse, but nursing with cracked or bleeding nipples is controversial.

Incubation period and symptoms. After transmission, the hepatitis C virus usually incubates for an average of 6 to 7 weeks before symptoms appear. It may start as a mild infection, or there may be no symptoms. However, 75% to 85% of those who contract HCV develop a chronic liver infection (AAP, 2018, p. 428). Hepatitis C is transmitted through sexual contact and infected blood. It occurs most often in those who received blood transfusions or had an accidental needle stick in healthcare settings, drug users who share needles, those with many sexual partners, and babies infected before or during birth (CDC, 2018a).

Hepatitis C and the nursing couple. Only about 5% to 6% of babies born to HCV-positive parents acquire the virus during pregnancy or delivery (AAP, 2018, p. 433). Studies that examined the parent-child transmission rate of hepatitis C (Resti et al., 1998) found no differences in those who nursed their babies and those who didn't, indicating that transmission takes place during pregnancy and/or birth. The U.S. Centers for Disease Control and Prevention gave the following answer to the question "Is it safe for a mother infected with hepatitis C virus (HCV) to breastfeed her infant?" (CDC, 2018a):

> "Yes. There is no documented evidence that breastfeeding spreads HCV. Therefore, having HCV-infection is not a contraindication to breastfeed."

Hepatitis C and cracked and bleeding nipples. Because HCV is transmitted via blood, controversy exists about whether HCV-infected nursing parents with cracked and bleeding nipples should interrupt nursing until their nipples are healed. The American Academy of Pediatrics Committee on Infectious Diseases (AAP, 2018, pp. 432-433) recommended a temporary weaning—discarding any expressed milk—from the affected nipple until the nipple is no longer bleeding. However, at this writing, there are no documented cases of a baby contracting hepatitis C this way. The U.S. Centers for Disease Control and Prevention (CDC, 2018a) concluded:

KEY CONCEPT

As long as the nursing parent with hepatitis C has no symptoms, nursing can continue.

> "Data are insufficient to say yes or no. However, HCV is spread by infected blood. Therefore, if the HCV-positive mother's nipples and/or surrounding areola are cracked and bleeding, she should stop nursing temporarily. To maintain her milk supply while not breastfeeding, she can express and discard her breast milk until her nipples are healed. Once her nipples are no longer cracked or bleeding, the HCV-positive mother may fully resume breastfeeding."

At this writing, the following 2002 statement from U.S. physician Lawrence Gartner, Professor Emeritus in Pediatrics at the University of Chicago (personal communication, June 21, 2002) still appears to be accurate:

> "The issue of nipple bleeding as a risk for acquisition of hepatitis C is an entirely theoretical possibility for which there is no evidence that I have ever seen. There are now more than 15 different studies comparing the

incidence of hepatitis in infants who are either breastfed or formula-fed, and none have shown any difference. I must assume that some of these hepatitis C carrier mothers had bleeding nipples. Since human milk of some carrier mothers contains hepatitis C virus, the exposure should not be different whether the virus enters in a small amount of blood or a large volume of milk. The indirect evidence is that human milk protects the infant from becoming infected when ingesting the virus through its various protective agents, which either inactivate the virus or prevent its attachment to the intestinal mucosa. The fact is that there is no evidence that breastfeeding from a mother who is infected with hepatitis C increases the risk of the infant becoming infected."

Acute hepatitis C infection after birth and the nursing parent. The rare exception is the nursing parent who becomes infected with HCV after birth and has acute symptoms while nursing but before their levels of antibodies are high enough to provide protection for the baby. In this situation, suggest parents talk to their healthcare provider about their options in light of their unique situation. One Spanish study of 63 women and 73 babies (Ruiz-Extremera et al., 2000) found the rate of transmission of HCV and the level of the virus in the milk were higher (20% versus 0%) when the HCV-positive women had active HCV symptoms as compared with being asymptomatic. Another study of 65 HCV-infected mothers conducted in the United Arab Emirates (Kumar & Shahul, 1998) found that when mothers were symptomatic, the level of virus in their milk increased along with the incidence of HCV transmission to their babies. If symptomatic HCV-positive parents and their healthcare provider decide they should wean, offer to discuss milk expression with them to either maintain their milk production until their symptoms subside or gradually decrease their milk production and wean comfortably (see Chapter 11 for milk-expression strategies).

Treatments for hepatitis C and lactation. Since this book's last edition, effective treatments that cure chronic hepatitis C were developed. These antiviral regimens usually last for 8 weeks or more and are targeted to specific genotypes of the virus. At this writing, many of these drugs are relatively new, so not much research exists on their use in lactating parents. Some drugs, such as ledipasvir, sofosbuvir, and simeprevir, are rated as L3 drugs, meaning they are considered compatible with nursing even with little research available (T.W. Hale, 2019). Others are not yet rated in reliable resources.

• • •

Not much is known about nursing with hepatitis D, E, and G.

Hepatitis D virus (delta hepatitis or HDV) may cause acute or chronic infection only in those who are already infected with hepatitis B and has an incubation period of about 2 to 8 weeks (AAP, 2018, p. 435). HDV is most common in South America, west Africa, Russia, Pacific islands, central Asia, and the Mediterranean region. Hepatitis E (HEV) is transmitted primarily via contaminated food and water, is usually short-term and self-limiting but has a high mortality rate when contracted during pregnancy. Hepatitis G (HGV) is associated mainly with blood transfusions.

Nursing and other types of hepatitis. Not much is known about the transmission of hepatitis D, E, or G through human milk. Because hepatitis D occurs only with hepatitis B infections, preventing hepatitis B by giving the baby the hepatitis-B vaccine and immune globulin also provides protection from hepatitis D, making the risk from nursing negligible (Lawrence & Lawrence, 2016, p. 439). There is no evidence of transmission of hepatitis E or G through nursing or mother's milk.

Herpes Viruses

Chickenpox

Nursing can continue when parents have chickenpox, but special precautions are needed if they become infected within days of giving birth.

Chickenpox is a common childhood illness that is highly contagious and caused by the same herpes varicella-zoster virus that causes shingles (see later section). Complications are rarely an issue if a baby catches it more than 10 days after birth. But it can cause lifelong health problems if the infection occurs in an unborn baby, a very preterm baby, and a newborn who contracted it in utero (congenital chickenpox) or right after birth. After this vulnerable period, its symptoms are usually more severe in adults than in children.

Incubation period and symptoms. Chickenpox is spread by contact with the sores (lesions) or by inhaling droplets in the air from coughing or sneezing. The incubation period of chickenpox is from 10 to 21 days, and an infected person will be contagious for about 7 days, beginning about 2 days before the lesions appear. Chickenpox is no longer contagious when there are no new eruptions for 72 hours and all lesions are crusted (AAP, 2018, p. 878).

Chickenpox and the pregnant or nursing parent. If parents exposed to chickenpox during pregnancy are unsure about whether they had it as a child (which confers lifelong immunity to the chickenpox form of the illness), a blood test can determine their immune status. When those who are not immune to chickenpox are exposed to it during pregnancy, the American Academy of Pediatrics Committee on Infectious Diseases suggests contacting their healthcare provider about getting the varicella vaccine (AAP, 2018, p. 874).

In the rare event that a parent contracts a chickenpox infection between 5 days before giving birth and 10 days after delivery and the baby is born without the disease, special precautions are needed. The risk to the uninfected newborn of catching chickenpox may be as high as 50% and in newborns who catch it during their first 10 days of life, the mortality rate is as high as 30%. After birth, to reduce the risk to the newborn, high-titer varicella immune globulin (VZIG) should be given to the newborn and the nursing couple isolated from other patients while being kept together (Schlaudecker, 2021, p. 165).

If siblings at home are infected, parents can keep them away from the baby to minimize the chances of transmission. If nursing parents have immunity to chickenpox, the baby received antibodies in utero, and the risk of the newborn catching chickenpox is greatly reduced.

Treatments for chickenpox and nursing. Other than treating the parent's symptoms, no other treatments for chickenpox are available at this writing.

Cold Sores and Genital Herpes

When nursing parents have cold sores or genital herpes, nursing is not affected as long as the newborn does not come into contact with the herpes sores.

Herpes simplex virus 1 (cold sores) and 2 (genital herpes) are two different herpes viruses spread by contact with the sores.

Incubation period and symptoms. The incubation period of these herpes simplex viruses is between 2 days and 2 weeks (AAP, 2018, p. 439). Symptoms include small, painful, fluid-filled, red-rimmed blisters that dry after a few days and form a scab. Genital herpes sores can be spread by touching the sores and then touching the mammary gland.

Herpes sores and the nursing newborn. Herpes infections can be very dangerous (even fatal) to a newborn up to 3 weeks of age (S. S. Field, 2016; Sullivan-Bolyai, Fife, Jacobs, Miller, & Corey, 1983). With quick hospitalization and care, as one case report described (D'Andrea & Spatz, 2019), it's also possible to successfully treat a newborn herpes infection, maintain lactation with milk expression, and resume nursing after discharge.

During pregnancy, if parents or their partners have recurrent herpes sores, suggest they talk to a healthcare provider knowledgeable about herpes and nursing to decide what precautions to take. If a sore on the nipple or mammary gland is suspected of being herpes, a culture can be done and the results should be available within a few days at most.

If herpes sores appear on the nipple or gland after birth, while waiting for the culture results (or after herpes is confirmed), nursing can continue if the sores can be completely covered so that the baby can't touch them. If the sores are on the nipple, areola, or anywhere else the baby might touch while nursing, express milk from that side until the sores heal, while continuing to nurse on the unaffected side. During hand expression or pumping, if the parent's hand or breast-pump parts touch the sores, the milk can become contaminated with the virus and should be discarded. If the parent's hand (if hand-expressing) or breast-pump parts do not touch the sores, the baby may be fed the milk.

Herpes sores and nursing after the newborn period. Although herpes sores can be dangerous to a baby within the first month of life, cases in the literature describe older babies touching their mother's herpes sores while breastfeeding without developing complications. There is also a documented case (Sealander & Kerr, 1989) of a breastfeeding 15-month-old with a cold sore in his mouth who passed herpes to his mother's breast. Although an older baby is not likely to develop life-threatening complications from herpes, suggest parents take steps to avoid spreading herpes to a child, as the sores can be very painful for a week or more and may make eating and drinking difficult.

Treatments for herpes sores and lactation. Antiviral drugs can be used to treat these herpes viruses in parents and children (AAP, 2018, pp. 441-444). Three oral antiviral drugs, acyclovir (L2), famciclovir (L2), and valacyclovir (L1) are compatible with lactation according to *Hale's Medications and Mothers' Milk* (T.W. Hale, 2019).

Cytomegalovirus (CMV)

When a parent is CMV-positive before pregnancy—as most adults are—nursing provides immunity to CMV infections in full-term, healthy babies.

Cytomegalovirus (CMV) is the most widespread of the herpes viruses that infect humans. By 40 years of age, between 50% and 80% of U.S. adults are infected with CMV for life.

Incubation period and symptoms. The incubation period is highly variable, from 3 to 12 weeks (AAP, 2018, p. 313). Few who become infected experience symptoms, which may include fatigue, fever, and swollen lymph glands.

CMV and the full-term nursing baby. If the initial CMV infection occurs before pregnancy, the CMV virus can be found in parents' urine, tears, saliva, and milk (Schleiss, 2006), and during pregnancy, the baby is exposed in utero to both the virus and its antibodies. In healthy term babies, mother's milk acts like a vaccine, with more than two-thirds of the full-term babies born to CMV-positive parents testing positive, despite having no symptoms (Dworsky, Yow, Stagno, Pass, & Alford, 1983). However, if the initial CMV infection occurs during pregnancy, this can result in about half of babies being born infected and about 10% of those with the symptoms of a congenital CMV infection, which can cause hearing loss, developmental delays, and a variety of health problems (CDC, 2019c).

CMV and the preterm or compromised baby. If at birth both parent and preterm baby are CMV-negative or CMV-positive, there is no concern about nursing or feeding expressed milk to the very preterm or immune-compromised baby. But when a baby born before 32 weeks and with a birth weight less than 1500 g (3 lbs. 5 oz.), is CMV-negative and his nursing parent is CMV-positive, there is a small risk the baby could become seriously ill from exposure to the CMV virus in the milk. Being born CMV-negative means the baby did not receive antibodies to the virus in utero. Plus, an immature or compromised immune system makes a baby more vulnerable to infections of all kinds (Bryant, Morley, Garland, & Curtis, 2002). For more details and ways mother's milk can be treated to decrease the risk of CMV transmission in at-risk babies, see p. 374.

Treatments for CMV and lactation. Treatments are not usually needed for lactating parents with CMV, who rarely have symptoms. Treatments for babies with congenital CMV would not affect lactation.

Shingles

When nursing parents contract shingles, the baby can be immunized and nursing can continue.

The same virus responsible for chickenpox—varicella zoster—also causes shingles. It occurs most commonly in an adult who had a mild case of chickenpox as a child and didn't become completely immune to the virus, which lays dormant until it is reactivated later in life.

Incubation period and symptoms. Because the virus that causes shingles lives dormant in the body after a previous chickenpox infection, its incubation period may be many years. Several days before the shingles rash erupts, parents may notice burning pain and sensitive skin. The rash starts as small blisters on a red base that continue to form for 3 to 5 days. They often appear in a band- or belt-like pattern on an area of skin and can be very painful. The blisters will pop, ooze, crust over, and heal. A person with shingles can give chickenpox to someone who never had it or was never vaccinated against it. It is contagious when the rash appears and until it is crusted over. The shingles episode may last 3 to 4 weeks in total.

Shingles and the nursing baby. If parents contract shingles while nursing, suggest they ask the baby's healthcare provider about administering varicella zoster immune globulin as soon as possible, as it is most effective when given soon after exposure (Isaacs, 2000). To prevent the spread of the virus to others, parents can cover their rash, avoid touching or scratching it, wash their hands often, and avoid contact with vulnerable people, including preterm babies.

Treatments for shingles and lactation. Antiviral drugs may be given. See the previous section "Cold Sores and Genital Herpes" for details on specific antiviral drugs and their compatibility with lactation.

HIV

Recommendations about nursing with HIV vary in different parts of the world.

In the 1980s and 1990s, a worldwide pandemic of human immunodeficiency virus (HIV) caused the deaths of millions from Acquired Immune Deficiency Syndrome (AIDS), which destroys parts of the immune system, leaving those affected unable to fight off illness. HIV is transmitted by the exchange of body fluids from parent to child during pregnancy and birth, from sexual contact, sharing needles, and blood transfusions. HIV can also be transmitted through nursing. Thankfully, since the late 20th century, major advances in treating HIV both improved survival rates and made nursing much safer.

Transmission of HIV through nursing was discovered in 1985. The authors of a 1992 U.K. review article (Dunn, Newell, Ades, & Peckham, 1992) estimated after 18 months of nursing, the rate of mother-to-child transmission (MTCT) of HIV was 14%. By the early 21st century, however, the combined use of antiretroviral drugs (known as antiretroviral therapy or ART) significantly reduced MTCT after 18 months of nursing to 1% or less (Lala & Merchant, 2012). As the scientific community developed effective treatments for HIV, they became widely available, and HIV was no longer a death sentence for parents and babies. This also resulted in changes in nursing recommendations for HIV-infected parents.

KEY CONCEPT

Current guidelines state that mothers with HIV in developed countries should avoid nursing.

Shifting recommendations about nursing with HIV. Shortly after the transmission of HIV via nursing was identified, the World Health Organization (WHO) issued a statement (WHO, 1987) recommending affected families nurse their babies because the risk of death from other types of infection was believed to be greater than the risk of death from the transmission of HIV via nursing. In the years since, while the American Academy of Pediatrics' recommendations have not changed (AAP, 1995, 2013), the recommendations of WHO shifted, based on new developments.

- 1987—WHO: HIV+ parents should nurse
- 1995—AAP: HIV+ parents in the U.S. should exclusively formula-feed
- 1997—WHO: In developing countries where risk of death from infection is high, HIV+ parents should nurse. In developed countries where risk of death from infection is low, HIV+ parents should formula-feed
- 2010—WHO: All HIV+ parents should receive ART for life and in high-risk areas, should nurse exclusively for 6 months
- 2013—AAP: HIV+ parents in the U.S. should exclusively formula-feed
- 2016—WHO: HIV+ parents in high-risk areas should exclusively nurse for 6 months and continue for 1 to 2 years

In 1997, as more information emerged about the risks of nursing with HIV, the original WHO recommendation for HIV-positive parents to nurse was amended to apply only to developing countries, where risk of death to babies from infection was high. Formula-feeding was recommended in developed countries, where risk of dying of infection was low. There formula was acceptable, affordable, feasible, sustainable, and less risky, in part because there was safe water and good medical care. In 2010, in light of the effectiveness of ART, WHO and UNICEF (WHO, 2010) recommended all HIV-positive parents receive ART from diagnosis throughout their lives. This kept the virus at undetectable levels in their blood and gave them a normal life span. In high-infection areas, WHO also recommended 6 months of exclusive nursing. Nursing with no other foods or drinks further reduces the risk of HIV transmission from parent to child. In 2016, the WHO guidelines for high-infection areas were expanded (WHO & UNICEF, 2016) to recommend after 6 months of exclusive nursing to continue nursing for 1 to 2 years.

Meanwhile, U.S. health organizations consistently recommended HIV-positive parents in the U.S. exclusively formula-feed. The U.S. Centers for Disease Control and Prevention (CDC), for example, (CDC, 2018b) wrote:

> "The best way to prevent transmission of HIV to an infant through breast milk is to not breastfeed. In the United States, where mothers have access to clean water and affordable replacement feeding (infant formula), CDC and the American Academy of Pediatrics recommend that HIV-infected mothers completely avoid breastfeeding their infants, regardless of ART and maternal viral load. Healthcare providers should be aware that some mothers with HIV may experience social or cultural pressure to breastfeed. These mothers may need ongoing feeding guidance and/or emotional support."

In the American Academy of Pediatrics (AAP) 2013 statement on HIV and infant feeding (AAP, 2013), it acknowledged that some U.S. HIV-positive parents on effective ART with undetectable viral loads may choose to nurse their babies. In this situation, the AAP recommended against automatically calling child protective services and instead suggested consulting a pediatric HIV specialist on how to minimize risk. In the U.K., the British HIV Association has created an information guide for HIV-positive parents at **bit.ly/BA2-BritishHIV** (BHIVA, 2018). Rather than trying to strictly prohibit nursing, encouraging honest discussion about minimizing risks enhances open communication and may ultimately produce better health outcomes.

Ways HIV-positive nursing parents can reduce risk of transmission to their baby include:

- ***Take ART medications as directed.*** Missing doses or taking breaks from ART increases health risks for both parent and baby.
- ***Nurse exclusively.*** This may be counter-intuitive for some. HIV-transmission rates are lower among exclusively nursing babies and higher among babies who are mixed-fed (nursing plus formula and other liquids or solid foods) (Becquet et al., 2008; Coutsoudis et al., 2001; Coutsoudis, Pillay, Spooner, Kuhn, & Coovadia, 1999; Kuhn et al., 2007). From birth to 3 months of age, the percentage of babies infected with HIV was higher in those mixed-fed but about the same among those exclusively nursed and those exclusively formula-fed.
- ***Follow best nursing practices.*** Risk of HIV transmission increases during bouts of mastitis and when nipples are cracked and bleeding. Knowing how to achieve a deep latch and the importance of regular nursing to reduce risk of mastitis makes transmission of HIV via nursing less likely. For many families, access to regular lactation help and support may make a major difference (Kuhn, Sinkala, Thea, Kankasa, & Aldrovandi, 2009).

Treatments for HIV and lactation. The antiretroviral drugs used to treat nursing parents are considered compatible with lactation (T.W. Hale, 2019). Many of these drugs (such as nevirapine and zidovudine) are also given directly to nursing babies and children to prevent HIV infection.

HTLV-1

HTLV-1, rare in the U.S. and Europe, can be transmitted by long-term nursing and may cause adult leukemia in a small percentage of those affected.

Discovered in 1980, human T-cell leukemia virus type 1 (HTLV-1) is spread through contact with body fluids from blood transfusions, through sexual contact, from mother to child during pregnancy and birth, and through nursing. It is rare in the U.S. and Europe, with most cases occurring in the Caribbean, Africa, South America, and southwestern Japan, where 10% of those older than 40 in one city are carriers of HTLV-1 (AAP, 2018, p. 118; Hino et al., 1997).

Incubation period and symptoms. Much later in life, 1% to 5% of those infected with HTLV-1 develop adult T-cell leukemia and lymphoma, a very malignant, usually fatal disease (Rosadas, Malik, Taylor, & Puccioni-Sohler, 2018; Tajima, 1988). Other possible illnesses associated with HTLV-1 infection include infective dermatitis of children, swelling of the eye (uveitis), and infection of the spinal cord (Manns, Hisada, & La Grenade, 1999). When HTLV-1 infection occurs during infancy, the 1% to 5% who eventually develop adult leukemia do not develop symptoms until adulthood.

HTLV-1 and the nursing baby. Lactoferrin in human milk appears to enhance transmission of this virus from parent to baby (Moriuchi & Moriuchi, 2006). In one Japanese study (Hino, 1989), about 30% of exclusively breastfed babies born to HTLV-1 positive mothers became infected, as compared with 10% of the mixed-fed babies, and none of those exclusively formula-fed. Another Japanese study (Tsuji et al., 1990) found 39% of the breastfed babies became infected as compared with none of the formula-fed babies.

Impact of nursing duration on HTLV-1 transmission. Nursing duration makes a profound difference in infection rates. A 2018 prospective Brazilian study (Paiva et al., 2018) found that nursing 12 or more months and a higher viral load in the mother increased the risk of HTLV-1 transmission. One Japanese study (Hino et al., 1997) found that children breastfed for at least 12 months had the highest infection rate (16%), while only 4% of the formula-fed children became infected during their first year. Babies breastfed for less than 6 months, however, were no more likely to develop HTLV-1 infections than those formula-fed (Takezaki et al., 1997). As an explanation, Japanese researchers suggested the antibodies to HTLV-1 in mother's milk may protect their babies from HTLV-1 infection during the first 6 months.

KEY CONCEPT

In developing countries, nursing is recommended for parents who are HTLV-1 positive.

Other Japanese retrospective and prospective studies of HTLV-1 positive women (Wiktor et al., 1993) found a significant difference between seroconversion rates of short-term (less than 7 months) and long-term (7 months or more) breastfed infants of 3.8% and 25%, respectively. Again, the short-term breastfeeding seroconversion rate was nearly equal to that of formula-fed infants. The overall prevalence of anti-HTLV-1 antibodies among children nursed more than 3 months was significantly higher (28%) than that of those nursed less than 3 months (5%) (Hirata et al., 1992). These studies found that over time 13% of formula-fed children born to carrier mothers became infected with HTLV-1, likely contracting it in utero.

Factors that increase risk of parent-to-baby transmission. Other factors that increased risk of transmission during nursing were higher blood levels of the HTLV-1 virus in the mother, older mother, and longer duration of breastfeeding (Hirata et al., 1992; Oki et al., 1992; Paiva et al., 2018; Takahashi et al., 1991;

Wiktor et al., 1993). Transmission was also more likely when infected cells appeared in the parent's blood and/or milk (Ichimaru, Ikeda, Kinoshita, Hino, & Tsuji, 1991). When no infected cells were found in the blood or milk, no babies became infected.

Nursing recommendations. Because this virus is relatively rare, most parents are not routinely tested for HTLV-1, and many healthcare providers are unfamiliar with it (Zihlmann, Mazzaia, & de Alvarenga, 2017). When parents in a developed country are diagnosed with this infection, some recommend against nursing (AAP, 2018, p. 118; Ichimaru et al., 1991). However, in areas where babies not nursed are at greater risk of life-threatening infection and disease, nursing is a better option for the HTLV-1 positive parent (van Tienen, Jakobsen, & Schim van der Loeff, 2012). In some developing countries, even shortening nursing duration to 6 months may be a greater health risk to the baby than acquiring HTLV-1 (Nyambi et al., 1996). Because the risk of adult onset leukemia from HTLV-1 infection is relatively small (1% to 5% of those infected), each carrier parent should discuss the risks with the baby's healthcare provider in light of their specific situation.

Milk treatment options to prevent HTLV-1 transmission. If HTLV-1 positive parents want to avoid any risk of transmission but want their baby to receive their milk, studies found that the HTLV-1 virus is greatly reduced when human milk is frozen to -20 degrees C (-4º F) and then thawed (Ando, Kakimoto, et al., 1989; Ando, Saito, et al., 1989). If HTLV-1 positive parents decide to exclusively express and treat their milk with this freeze-and-thaw method, offer to discuss milk-expression strategies to establish and maintain milk production (see p. 496).

Treatments for HTLV-1 and lactation. Not applicable, as symptoms appear long after lactation

Measles and Rubella

Unless the parent is contagious with measles during delivery, nursing is not usually affected.

Like chickenpox, measles is usually less severe in children than in newborns and adults. When a baby contracts measles in utero, this can be fatal (congenital measles). If the baby becomes infected with measles after birth (symptoms will not appear until the baby is at least 14 days old), his illness is likely to be mild because the baby received antibodies in utero (Lawrence & Lawrence, 2016, p. 442).

Incubation period and symptoms. Measles is spread by contact with infectious droplets or in the air. In a person infected with measles, the incubation period before symptoms appear is usually 8 to 12 days (AAP, 2018, p. 539). During the first 3 to 4 days of this illness, there is no rash, and the symptoms are similar to a bad cold: fever, watery eyes, congestion, and cough. Typically, the rash appears on about the fourth day. Measles are no longer contagious when the rash and cold symptoms are gone, about 72 hours after the rash appears. If the nursing parent catches measles after the newborn period, the baby can be given the measles immune globulin. If separation of the nursing couple is recommended, the baby can be fed the expressed milk, which contains protective antibodies.

Exposure to measles during pregnancy. If exposure to measles occurs during pregnancy and parents are unsure whether they were vaccinated or had the illness (which gives lifelong immunity), their healthcare provider can order a blood test to determine their immune status. If at delivery parent and baby have no symptoms, both can be given the measles immune globulin.

Measles in the nursing parent during birth. Because most of those currently in their childbearing years received the measles vaccine in their youth, becoming infected at birth is a rare situation. But if parents give birth with an acute case of the measles and the baby is born without the disease, the baby's healthcare provider may recommend separating the nursing couple until the parent is no longer contagious. About half of newborns in this situation will develop the disease despite the separation. If they are separated, offer to discuss milk-expression strategies to provide milk for the baby and to establish milk production (see p. 498). The antibodies in the expressed milk will help prevent the baby from becoming ill or lessen the severity of the baby's illness. When parents in this situation are no longer contagious, they can be reunited with their baby and begin nursing. If siblings at home are infected and the parent is immune, the parents can keep them away from the baby to minimize the chances of transmission. If the parent has immunity to measles, the baby will receive antibodies in utero, and the risk of the newborn catching measles from his siblings is greatly reduced.

Measles treatments and lactation. Other than treating the symptoms, there are no treatments for measles.

• • •

Neither an active case of rubella nor getting the rubella vaccine affects nursing.

Rubella, also known as German measles, is a mild infectious disease. The biggest risk of rubella is catching it during pregnancy (congenital rubella), when it can damage the unborn baby. At any other time, it is likely to be short-lived and without complications.

Incubation period and symptoms. Rubella is transmitted through contact with nose or mouth secretions, and the incubation period is 16 to 18 days (AAP, 2018, p. 706). Symptoms include a generalized rash, swollen lymph glands, and a slight fever. Between one-quarter and half of its cases have no symptoms at all. The person with rubella (other than congenital rubella) is contagious for 2 to 7 days after the rash appears.

Rubella, the rubella vaccine, and the nursing couple. The nursing baby of a parent with an active case of rubella was already exposed to it before the symptoms appeared. Nursing provides the baby with antibodies, so if he does become ill, he will likely have a milder case. If nursing parents previously had rubella or received the rubella vaccine, their milk may provide the baby a natural immunization to rubella (T.W. Hale, 2019; Losonsky, Fishaut, Strussenberg, & Ogra, 1982). According to the American Academy of Pediatrics Committee on Infectious Diseases (AAP, 2018, p. 119):

> "...[T]he presence of rubella virus in human milk has not been associated with significant disease in infants and transmission is more likely to occur via other routes. Women with rubella or women who have been immunized recently with live-attenuated rubella virus vaccine may continue to breastfeed."

Rubella treatments and lactation. Other than treating the symptoms, there are no treatments for rubella.

West Nile Virus

It is safe for nursing parents with the West Nile virus to continue nursing.

West Nile virus, which can become a serious illness, is most often transmitted by an infected mosquito, making it most common during summer and fall. But it can also be spread by blood transfusions, transplants, and from parent to child during pregnancy. It is not spread through touch or kissing.

Incubation period and symptoms. Its incubation period is usually 2 to 6 days but may extend to 14 days. Symptoms of West Nile virus include fever, headache, and neck stiffness. If severe, it can lead to disorientation, coma, tremors, vision loss, and paralysis.

West Nile virus and the nursing couple. Although West Nile virus was found in the milk of infected mothers, none of their nursing babies became ill (CDC, 2018d). In one U.S. case report, a woman received a blood transfusion later found to contain the West Nile virus. The mother developed symptoms of West Nile virus when her baby was 11 days old and breastfed him for 6 more days. Testing revealed the mother's milk and the baby's blood were both positive for the West Nile virus, but the baby stayed healthy and developed no symptoms. The CDC (CDC, 2002, p. 878) concluded: "these findings do not suggest a change in nursing recommendations." According to the American Academy of Pediatrics Committee on Infectious Diseases (AAP, 2018, p. 119): "...women who reside in areas with endemic West Nile virus infections should continue to breastfeed."

West Nile virus treatments and lactation. Other than treating the symptoms, there are no treatments for West Nile virus.

Zika

Nursing parents who contract the Zika virus can safely continue nursing.

The Zika virus is transmitted by the bite of an infected mosquito and is known to cause birth defects, such as microcephaly, if contracted during pregnancy.

Incubation period and symptoms. After being bitten by an infected mosquito, the incubation period for Zika is 3 to 14 days, and its infection is often without symptoms (AAP, 2018, p. 895). When symptoms do occur, they are often mild and include fever and rash.

Zika and the nursing couple. Much like other viruses, the Zika virus can be found in the milk of infected parents and in the blood of their nursing babies. However, this exposure does not appear to lead to infection. Two systematic reviews (Mann et al., 2018; Sampieri & Montero, 2019) agreed, supporting the position of the World Health Organization (WHO, 2016), which recommended parents with the Zika virus and who live in areas where the virus is endemic continue nursing.

Holder pasteurization of expressed milk (heating milk to 63 C [145 F] for 30 minutes) deactivates the Zika virus, as does refrigerating the expressed milk at 4 C (39 F) for 2 to 3 days, during which the antiviral properties of human milk deactivate the virus (Pfaender et al., 2017).

Zika treatments and lactation. Other than treating the symptoms, there are no treatments for Zika.

CANCER

Parents with cancer can continue to nurse through most diagnostic tests and surgeries. But some treatments require either temporary or permanent weaning.

Cancer occurs when cells in the body grow out of control. There are many kinds of cancer, but they all start with out-of-control growth of abnormal cells. Instead of eventually dying, like normal cells, cancer cells continue to grow and form new, abnormal cells. Cancer cells may invade other tissues, which normal cells cannot do. If found early and treated quickly, many types of cancer can be completely cured. As the cancerous cells spread from the original tumor through the body, the chances for a cure decrease.

Diagnostic tests, biopsy, surgery, and the nursing parent. For details on diagnostic tests and biopsy, see p. 779-780 in the previous chapter. Before having surgery, suggest discussing nursing with the surgeon and ask that medications be chosen that are most compatible with lactation. For more details, see the later section "Surgery."

Radioactive tests, treatments, and lactation. If the healthcare provider recommends the use of radioactive materials to diagnose or treat the illness (common for thyroid cancer and other thyroid problems), suggest asking what specific materials will be used. Some radioactive materials accumulate in human milk, and temporary or permanent weaning may be necessary. After some tests or treatments, nursing (or even holding the baby) may expose him to radioactivity. The specific substance, its form, and the dose will determine:

- Whether nursing can continue
- If weaning is necessary, whether the weaning will be permanent or temporary
- If temporary, its duration and when the baby can resume nursing

For example, when a radioactive iodine uptake test is performed, nursing must be interrupted for a minimum of 12 hours. Of the various radioactive substances, technetium-99m pertechnetate has the shortest half-life (6.02 hours) and requires the shortest interruption of nursing. For a listing of radioactive substances and recommended length of weaning after use in diagnosis or treatment, see Clinical Protocol #31 from the Academy of Breastfeeding Medicine, which is downloadable in multiple languages at **bfmed.org/protocols**.

Radioactive iodine ^{131}I and lactation. Although some substances can be used for diagnostic tests without interrupting nursing (see p. 779), when radioactive iodine ^{131}I is used for a thyroid scan or tumor imaging, weaning is necessary due to potentially harmful effects on both parent and baby. According to the Academy of Breastfeeding Clinical Protocol #31 on radiology and nuclear medicine (Mitchell, Fleming, Anderson, Giesbrandt, & Academy of Breastfeeding, 2019), when this substance is used, permanent weaning is necessary. At the very least, several months of weaning is required. After procedures with this substance, even holding or sleeping close to the baby is risky (T.W. Hale, 2019, p. 817) because it exposes the baby to radiation. Iodine radiation directly affects baby's thyroid gland and increases his risk of thyroid cancer later in life. Nursing parents need to completely wean at least several weeks before the treatment because about 40% of the radiation dose will be deposited in active mammary tissue, putting parents at higher risk for later breast cancer (Grunwald, Palmedo,

> **KEY CONCEPT**
>
> *Parents being treated with radioactive iodine ^{131}I must wean.*

& Biersack, 1995; Robinson et al., 1994). Weaning several weeks in advance gives parents' mammary tissue time to involute, or revert back to its prepregnancy state, so it is no longer active during the treatment. After this treatment, it may be months before the radioactivity in the milk returns to safe levels.

Questions to ask. If parents' healthcare provider recommends the use of radioactive materials and they do not want to wean, suggest telling the healthcare provider their feelings and find out if any other options are available that allow for continued nursing. Suggest they seek answers to the following questions:

- Is the radioactive procedure for diagnosis or treatment?
- What will happen if the procedure is not done or it is postponed?
- Is there an alternative that would not involve weaning?
- If the baby is younger than 12 months, can the procedure be delayed until they can express enough milk for the baby during the temporary weaning?
- Was a radioactive material chosen that will clear the milk in the shortest time possible? For example, a radioisotope in complexed form excretes less radioactivity into human milk than its uncomplexed form.
- Is there a local testing facility available to determine when the milk is clear of radioactivity? With milk testing, some parents resume nursing sooner than estimated (Saenz, 2000).
- Will the radioactive material be concentrated in one organ (i.e., the thyroid), and if so, will parents need to keep their baby away from that part of their body for a time?

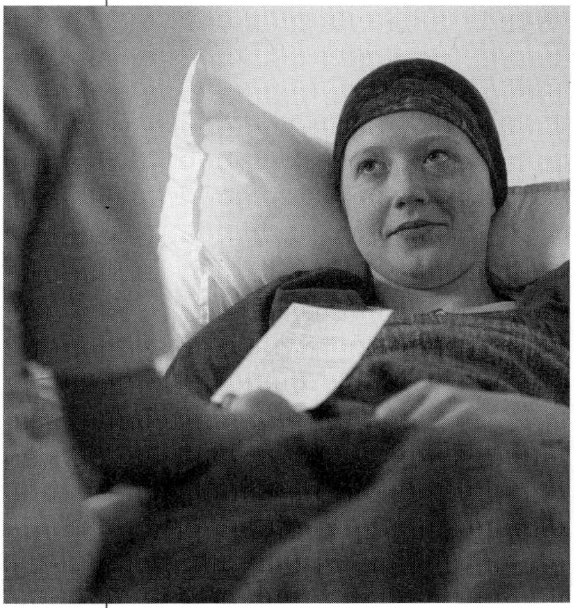

If parents are not satisfied with the healthcare provider's answers, suggest seeking a second opinion.

Milk expression after radioactive procedures. If parents undergo radioactive testing and wean temporarily, offer to discuss strategies for maintaining milk production while "pumping and dumping." Unlike medications, milk expression will help eliminate the radioactivity from the body more quickly (Rose, Prescott, & Herman, 1990).

Chemotherapy and lactation. It was once assumed that all cancer chemotherapy is incompatible with lactation. However, chemotherapy has changed, and more information is available on using these drugs during lactation (Pistilli et al., 2013). This makes a more nuanced approach possible. For example, some nursing parents receiving low-dose chemotherapy may be able to continue nursing. Or if the chemotherapy is given for short periods with longer periods in between, it may be possible for some to do a temporary weaning and go back to nursing after the drugs are eliminated from the body. Doctor of pharmacology Philip O. Anderson (Anderson, 2016, p. 165) described this option:

> "Since cancer chemotherapy is often given in cycles, highly motivated nursing mothers sometimes ask whether they can breastfeed in between cycles....Typically, a period of five half-lives would be considered a safe waiting period. If combination chemotherapy is being given, the drug with the longest half-life would usually determine the waiting period. It is important to consider any active metabolites, also, and use the longest of their half-lives."

Most drugs' half-lives can be found in the *Hale's Medications and Mothers' Milk* book and app. Anderson noted that nursing between cycles of chemotherapy would not work with the most toxic drugs that have the longest half-lives. For guidance in individual situations, suggest families and their healthcare providers contact the Infant Risk Center U.S. hotline at 1-806-352-2519 or check their online resources at **infantrisk.com**. For a more complete listing of international drug resources, see Box 13.1 on p. 601.

Radiation therapy and lactation. Like diagnostic x-rays, cancer radiation therapy does not make human milk radioactive, and nursing can continue. During treatment for breast cancer, the unradiated mammary gland will not be affected. The treated gland, however, is likely to undergo changes. Radiation therapy damages mammary tissue, which may affect its development and milk production during treatment and with subsequent pregnancies (Leal, Stuart, & Carvalho Hde, 2013; Neifert, 1992). One U.S. case report (David, 1985, p. 1425) described the effects of breast radiation as "ductal shrinkage, condensation of cytoplasm in cells lining the ducts, atrophy of the lobules, and perilobar and periductal fibrosis."

Milk production after breast cancer radiation therapy. A 2013 review article (Leal et al., 2013) noted that radiation therapy is likely to reduce milk production in the affected side. In one U.S. study of 21 women with previously irradiated breasts who later became pregnant and breastfed (Moran et al., 2005), all had little or no breast tissue growth during pregnancy. After birth 56% lactated in the irradiated breast, although 80% reported their milk production was significantly less on that side. In another U.S. study of 13 pregnancies (Higgins & Haffty, 1994), in the 10 women who breastfed, the treated breast produced milk in four cases and produced no milk in six cases. Like the previous study, all reported little or no breast changes in the irradiated breast during pregnancy. In a third U.S. study (Tralins, 1995), 18 of the 43 women (34%) reported some milk production from the irradiated breast and 13 (24.5%) breastfed, with five (9%) describing their treated breast as smaller. Two-thirds of the nine women who commented on milk production in the treated breast described it as "less but adequate." One of these babies never latched to the treated breast.

Because parents can produce enough milk to exclusively nurse twins, triplets, and quadruplets (Berlin, 2007), even if only one side is fully functional after radiation therapy, most parents will produce enough milk to exclusively nurse. One case report described the experience of a mother who exclusively nursed twins after a mastectomy (Michaels & Wanner, 2013). If parents are unable to reach full milk production or if both glands were treated, partial nursing is an option.

Recommendations to wean. An Italian study of breast cancer survivors (Azim et al., 2010) found that 50% were counseled by their healthcare providers not to nurse their babies after delivery, even though no contraindication to lactation existed. If weaning is suggested and there are no compelling medical reasons, see the first section "Nursing with Health Issues." If nursing parents diagnosed with cancer do not want to wean or feel that weaning would not make life easier, suggest talking with the healthcare provider about their feelings.

Nursing after cancer. One common worry expressed by parents who survived breast cancer is that nursing will cause a recurrence, even though there's no evidence to indicate this (Azim et al., 2010; Johnson & Mitchell, 2019). Another worry (Connell, Patterson, & Newman, 2006) is that because lactation makes mammary tissue denser, a recurrence might be more difficult to detect (see p. 780).

If surgery was performed on the mammary gland, nursing parents may have nursing issues related to decreased sensation of the areola and nipple (Leal et al., 2013), which may inhibit milk ejection (see p. 865). Low milk production from previous radiation may also affect whether baby will latch and suck well from the affected side. Parents may need extra lactation help and support as they are establishing nursing.

During pregnancy, how does cancer diagnosis and chemotherapy affect lactation outcomes? A U.S. prospective cohort study surveyed 96 women diagnosed with cancer (mostly breast cancer) during pregnancy (Stopenski, Aslam, Zhang, & Cardonick, 2017). None required chemotherapy after birth, and all nursed their babies. Of the 96 women, 74 (77%) received chemotherapy during pregnancy (which ended at least 3 weeks before delivery), and 22 (23%) didn't receive chemotherapy. The researchers did not use objective measures of milk adequacy and did not include nursing exclusivity as a measure, which are serious limitations. They found only 34% of those who received chemotherapy during pregnancy successfully nursed. Of those who received chemotherapy, 64% reported needing to supplement their babies due to low milk production, compared with only 9% of those who did not receive chemotherapy.

CARDIAC ISSUES/HYPERTENSTION

Nursing has positive effects on cardiovascular health, both in the short and long term. Many treatments for cardiac problems and hypertension are compatible with lactation.

Nursing reduces risk of cardiovascular problems later in life. Parents with a family history of cardiac issues or high blood pressure (hypertension) are likely unaware that nursing reduces risk of cardiovascular disease (K. M. Kelly, Chopra, & Dolly, 2015). According to research (Groer, Jevitt, Sahebzamani, Beckstead, & Keefe, 2013; Jonas et al., 2008), in the short term, nursing decreases heart rate and both systolic and diastolic blood pressure. During the first 6 months after birth, parents' blood pressures before nursing are lower than their prepregnancy levels. A 2018 systematic review (Bonifacino, Schwartz, Jun, Wessel, & Corbelli, 2018) identified 15 long-term studies that followed women for 2 to 3 decades, and all of the studies that evaluated for hypertension found nursing for a minimum of 1 month or more protected against high blood pressure later in life.

Nursing also reduces risk of stroke. Using data from the U.S. Women's Health Initiative study, which included nearly 100,000 women (Jacobson et al., 2018), researchers found that any nursing was associated with a lower risk of stroke after menopause, even after adjusting for multiple stroke risk factors and lifestyle variables. Nursing relatively short term, for 1 to 6 months, was found to reduce risk of stroke later in life by 19%. Longer nursing was associated with an even greater reduction of stroke risk.

Some of the first studies to evaluate the effects of nursing on cardiovascular health used data from large groups. One U.S. prospective cohort study of nearly 90,000 women (A. M. Stuebe et al., 2009) found that those with a lifetime total of 2 or more years of nursing had a 23% lower risk of coronary heart disease (the number one killer of women) as compared with those who had never nursed. A U.S. retrospective study examined data from 139,681 postmenopausal mothers (Schwarz et al., 2009). After controlling for many factors, women who breastfed for more than 12 months total (all lactations included) were less likely than women who never breastfed to develop hypertension, diabetes, and cardiovascular disease.

Nursing improves outcomes in parents with active cardiovascular disease. Preeclampsia, which includes high blood pressure, occurs in 3% to 8% of pregnancies, and it is often a precursor to other cardiovascular problems later. A 2018 Brazilian study (Strapasson, Ferreira, & Ramos, 2018) found that preeclampsia is associated with lower rates of nursing after delivery. However, a 2019 U.S. study (Burgess, McDowell, & Ebersold, 2019) found that nursing parents who had preeclampsia had healthier systolic and diastolic blood pressure levels after birth. For parents with other cardiovascular disease before and after birth, nursing leads to more positive health outcomes. A U.S. survey of 55 patients with a serious heart condition known as peripartum cardiomyopathy (PPCM) (Safirstein et al., 2012) found that nursing was significantly associated with improved heart function.

KEY CONCEPT

Nursing can lower a woman's lifetime risk of heart disease, the number one killer of women.

Treatments for cardiovascular problems and lactation. Diuretics are often used to treat hypertension by increasing the volume of urine and keeping fluid levels low. High-dose diuretics can decrease milk production, but some low-dose diuretics are compatible with lactation. Other drugs used for cardiovascular treatment, such as beta-blockers, are compatible with lactation (T.W. Hale, 2019). For an overview of the compatibility of antiarrhythmics and other cardiac agents with lactation, see (Anderson, 2019b). For an overview of treatments for hypertension, see (Anderson, 2018b).

DEPRESSION, ANXIETY, AND MENTAL HEALTH

Postpartum Depression and Psychosis

Depressive symptoms put nursing parents at risk for early weaning and if untreated may have negative physical, emotional, and social effects on their baby.

After childbirth, more than half of new parents have occasional bouts of crying, irritability, and fatigue sometimes referred to as the ***baby blues***. Postpartum depression (or depressive symptoms) refers to more consistent and severe symptoms and is also relatively common. Some estimate that during the first year of new parenthood the incidence is 12% to 25% overall and 35% to 60% among high-risk parents, including those who experience racial and economic discrimination (K. A. Kendall-Tackett, 2017; Ko, Rockhill, Tong, Morrow, & Farr, 2017).

Postpartum depressive symptoms include feelings of sadness, an absence of pleasure from activities once enjoyed (known as ***anhedonia***), sleep problems unrelated to baby care, inability to focus, feelings of hopelessness, changes in appetite, anxiety, and greater anger or hostility, including thoughts of death. Parents with these symptoms may be difficult to listen to and conversations may feel draining because their sense of hopelessness may convince them that nothing can help. Before considering treatment for depression, parents should see a healthcare provider to rule out physical causes for their symptoms, such as thyroid problems and anemia. Symptoms considered ***red flags that parents need immediate medical attention*** include (K. A. Kendall-Tackett, 2017):

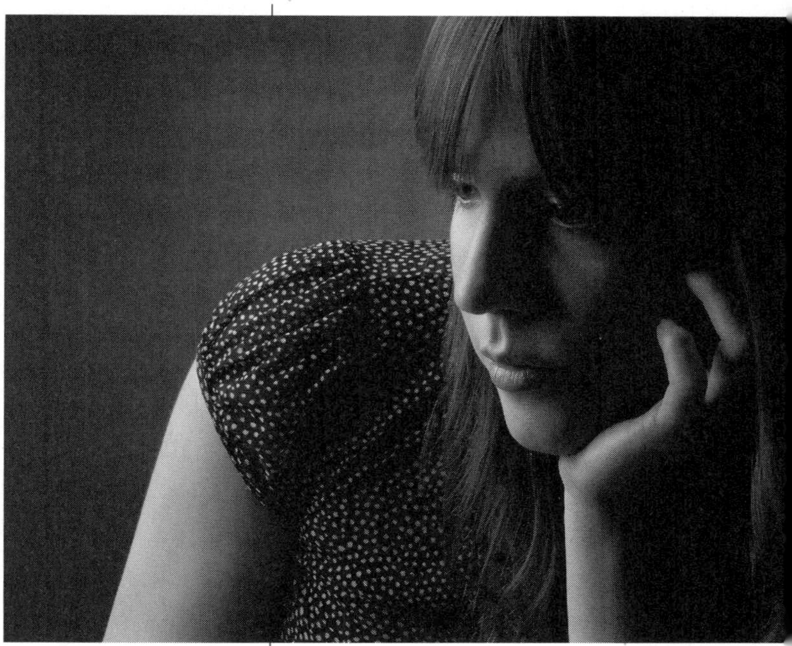

- Suicidal or bizarre statements: "My children would be better off without me," or "I'd like to give them away to strangers."
- Substance abuse
- Days without sleep
- Fast weight loss
- Lack of normal grooming
- Inability to get out of bed

See also the next point on postpartum psychosis.

Causes and risk factors for postpartum depressive symptoms. Inflammation was identified as the risk factor for depression that underlies all its other risk factors (K. Kendall-Tackett, 2007, 2015). When the other risk factors are present—sleep disturbance, stress (a fussy baby, a household move away from family and friends), physical pain, psychological trauma, or a history of abuse or trauma (including a traumatic birth)—these can cause the release of cells from the immune system (called ***proinflammatory cytokines***) that cause physical inflammation and depressive symptoms. This can go both ways. In other words, parents who have inflammation from the other risk factors are at increased risk for depression, and parents who are depressed release more of these inflammatory cells, causing more inflammation.

Nipple pain is one type of physical pain research linked to depression. An Australian study that followed 65 breastfeeding mothers (Amir, Dennerstein, Garland, Fisher, & Farish, 1997) found 38% of those with nipple pain rated as depressed compared with only 14% of those without pain. When the mothers' nipple pain resolved, the percentage of depressed mothers in the two groups became comparable. The researchers concluded that relieving nipple pain can improve mood in some cases. A U.S. retrospective chart review (Watkins, Meltzer-Brody, Zolnoun, & Stuebe, 2011) also noted this connection between nipple pain and increased risk of depressive symptoms.

The value of a listening ear. Parents with postpartum depressive symptoms may feel embarrassed, ashamed, or guilty and try to minimize their problem. This can make them feel even more isolated. They may imagine all other parents as blissfully happy and in control of their lives and believe that they are the only one with negative feelings. Offer emotional support and praise them for caring for their baby in spite of their feelings. Let them know that negative feelings are normal. Suggest taking part in peer-support groups, online and/or in person, so they can hear about other parents' down moments. Let them know about some of the factors that can influence their feelings (unusual stress, a difficult birth, little support). Offer to brainstorm about how they might get more rest or the strategies (below) that can help alleviate depressive symptoms. Encourage them to accept help and support from others.

Postpartum depressive symptoms and nursing. Nursing lowers stress and increases sleep (see the first point in this chapter), which decreases a parent's risk of depressive symptoms. When nursing is going well, it can decrease inflammation and increase parents' feelings of well-being. Overall, nursing was found to protect parents' mental health (Figueiredo, Dias, Brandao, Canario, & Nunes-Costa, 2013). Although nursing parents have a lower risk of postpartum depressive symptoms (Hatton et al., 2005; McCoy, Beal, Shipman, Payton, & Watson, 2006; Yusuff, Tang, Binns, & Lee, 2016), nursing is not a guarantee against depression. Research also found that when nursing parents become depressed, they are at increased risk of nursing less often and weaning earlier (Bascom & Napolitano, 2016; Borra, Iacovou, & Sevilla, 2015). A study using Canadian data (Adedinsewo et al., 2014) found that an increase in anxiety scores at 3 months reduced the odds of exclusive nursing by 11% at 6 months.

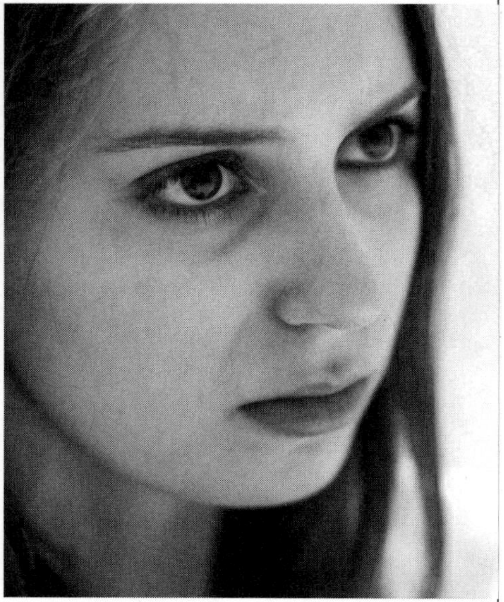

Depressed parents may describe nursing in negative terms. A Finnish study (Tamminen & Salmelin, 1991) found differences in mother-baby interactions during feeds when the mother was depressed. As compared with a group of breastfeeding mothers who were not depressed, the depressed mothers interpreted their baby's fussiness when hungry as a rejection of them or their milk rather than due to a physical cause. The depressed mothers also expressed less satisfaction in their interactions with their babies and appeared less sensitive to their babies' needs and cues (see next paragraph). Depressed parents may begin to believe that nursing is the cause of their problems. If so, let them know that caring for a newborn can be stressful, and the challenges of a fussy baby, fatigue, and feeling overwhelmed are not confined to nursing parents.

Why treatment for postpartum depressive symptoms is vital to parents and babies. Depression and anxiety negatively affect parents' health, well-being, and their relationships (Hammen & Brennan, 2002). But parents' depressive symptoms also affect their baby physically, emotionally, and socially and can impair the way they interact with their baby. Knowing this may motivate parents to seek treatment sooner. But be careful how this is shared. Never imply that their depression "damaged" their baby. Emphasize instead that when parents seek treatment, it benefits both them and their baby.

When depressed, many parents interact with their babies using one of two styles: avoidant or angry-intrusive (K. A. Kendall-Tackett, 2017). When avoidant, parents ignore many of their baby's cues. This behavior is associated with high infant blood cortisol levels (a stress hormone) and abnormal EEG patterns (T. Field, 1995). If parents' depressive symptoms are chronic, these abnormal brain patterns may extend throughout infancy (Cicchetti & Toth, 1998), and their toddlers may experience developmental delays (Cornish et al., 2005). Depressed parents who are angry-intrusive also ignore their babies' cues, but rather than being non-responsive, they take over the interactions. For example, if the baby looks or arches away because he doesn't like what his parent is doing, the parent may interpret this as a personal rejection and become hostile or abusive.

Long-term studies on children whose parents were depressed when they were infants found that by school age, they are less socially competent (Luoma et al., 2001), have lower IQs (Hay et al., 2001), and are at greater risk for depression (Murray, Woolgar, Cooper, & Hipwell, 2001). But one Dutch study (N. A. Jones, McFall, & Diego, 2004) found that if depressed mothers breastfed, their babies were protected from the harmful effects of their depression. To explain their findings, the authors noted that depressed breastfeeding mothers did not disengage from their babies. They looked at, touched, and stroked their babies more often than mothers who were depressed but bottle-feeding. This type of interaction can be taught, but it's built into the nursing relationship and is another good reason for parents with depressive symptoms to continue nursing if possible.

Non-pharmacological treatments for postpartum depressive symptoms. Many parents are reluctant to seek treatment for fear that they might have to choose between treatment and nursing (K. A. Kendall-Tackett, 2017; Spiesser-Robelet, Maurice, & Gagnayre, 2019). Fortunately, that's not usually the case. Most antidepressant medications are compatible with nursing (see next section). For parents reluctant to use medications, there are many non-medication strategies that can effectively treat depression. The most important point to emphasize is that depressive symptoms need to be treated rather than ignored. Examples of non-pharmacologic treatments include:

- **Long-chain omega-3 fatty acids.** These can be taken alone or with antidepressants. A review of the literature by a committee of the American Psychiatric Association (Freeman et al., 2006) found that DHA and EPA, which are anti-inflammatories, appear to have a protective effect on mood disorders. DHA and EPA are considered safe during pregnancy and lactation, even at high doses (K. Kendall-Tackett, 2010). **Recommendation:** For the treatment of depressive symptoms, take daily doses of 1000 mg of EPA and 200-400 mg of DHA (K. A. Kendall-Tackett, 2017).

- **Exercise** also lowers inflammation and improves mood after childbirth (Kiecolt-Glaser, Derry, & Fagundes, 2015). A review of 17 studies on exercise and postpartum depressive symptoms (Teychenne & York, 2013) found that exercise decreased these symptoms after birth. U.S. research compared the effects of a placebo, exercise, and antidepressant medication (sertraline) in 202 people with major depression (Blumenthal et al., 2007). Unlike the placebo, exercise (40 minutes three times per week) was found to be as effective at resolving depression as antidepressants. **Recommendation:** 20 to 30 minutes of exercise 2 to 3 times per week for moderate depression and 45 to 60 minutes of exercise 3 to 5 times per week for major depression (K. A. Kendall-Tackett, 2017).

- **Bright light therapy** was found to alleviate up to 75% of depressive symptoms when professionally created light boxes were used. The type of light that is therapeutic without harming users' eyes is not easily replicated by consumers. As U.S. author and researcher Kathleen Kendall-Tackett noted, just because parents can create their own light boxes doesn't mean they should (K. A. Kendall-Tackett, 2017, p. 196). What time of day light therapy is used makes a difference, too, as light therapy early in the day was found more effective than light therapy later in the day.

- **Psychotherapy** was also found to have an anti-inflammatory effect (K. A. Kendall-Tackett, 2017). Cognitive behavioral therapy (for U.S. resources, see **nacbt.org**) was found as effective as medications in treating depression, with a lower incidence of relapse (Rupke, Blecke, & Renfrow, 2006). Interpersonal therapy (see **interpersonalpsychotherapy.org**) is another type of "talk therapy" found effective in both preventing and treating postpartum depressive symptoms in high-risk groups (Weissman, 2007).

KEY CONCEPT

Effective non-drug treatments for depressive symptoms are available.

- **St. John's Wort.** The most widely used herbal antidepressant, St. John's wort (*Hypericum perforatum*) is native to the U.K. and has been used for this purpose since the Middle Ages. Several studies compared its effectiveness to the antidepressants imipramine (Philipp, Kohnen, & Hiller, 1999; Woelk, 2000), sertraline (HDTSG, 2002; van Gurp, Meterissian, Haiek, McCusker, & Bellavance, 2002), and paroxetine (Anghelescu, Kohnen, Szegedi, Klement, & Kieser, 2006; Szegedi, Kohnen, Dienel, & Kieser, 2005) and found St. John's wort as effective as prescribed antidepressants, with fewer side effects. **Recommendation:** Take 300 mg of St. John's wort 3 per day, standardized to 0.3% hypericin and/or 2% to 4% hyperforin (K. A. Kendall-Tackett, 2017).

Antidepressants and lactation. Although most antidepressant medications are considered compatible with lactation (Table 19.1), one Canadian review article (Dennis & Chung-Lee, 2006) found that even after parents were told this, they were still reluctant to take these medications due to concerns about addiction, side effects, possible harm to their nursing baby, and the perceived stigma of taking antidepressants. Suggest parents discuss their concerns with their healthcare provider, as depending on their symptoms, risk factors, and preferences, prescribed medications may or may not be the best choice. When deciding what drug to use, several factors are important (Chaudron, 2007):

- Have they used an antidepressant before that worked well for them?
- Do they find particular side effects especially concerning?
- Are they taking any other medication that might interact with the drug?

One U.S. study (Marshall et al., 2010) found an association in first-time mothers between taking serotonin-disrupting drugs, such as Prozac (fluoxetine) and other selective serotonin. reuptake inhibitors (SSRIs) listed in Table 19.1, and a delay in milk increase after birth. However, only 8 of its 431 mothers took SSRIs during this study. Other larger studies published since (Grzeskowiak, Leggett, Costi, Roberts, & Amir, 2018; K. Kendall-Tackett & T. Hale, 2009) did not find this association. Research that followed women who took antidepressants before and during pregnancy (Lewis et al., 2016; A. M. Stuebe et al., 2019) concluded that the primary cause of the reduced rates of nursing initiation and exclusivity in these families was the depressive symptoms—not the physical effects of the antidepressants.

> **KEY CONCEPT**
>
> *When nursing is going well, it reduces risk of depression and protects mental health.*

• • •

A parent with postpartum psychosis needs immediate medical attention.

Postpartum psychosis usually strikes during the first month after birth but can occur any time within the first year. It is relatively rare, occurring in only 0.1% to 0.2% of birthing parents (Hill, Law, Yelland, & Sved Williams, 2019; Rapkin, Mikacich, Moatakef-Imani, & Rasgon, 2002). But when it occurs, parents and babies need immediate help, because both parent and baby are at risk of serious harm. Parents with postpartum psychosis may have a distorted perception of reality, hallucinations, delusions, and/or suicidal or homicidal thoughts. Immediate treatment is needed.

Hospitalization. Parents with postpartum psychosis or a severe case of postpartum depressive symptoms may require hospitalization. In England and some other countries, hospitals have mother-baby units where parents can be treated while caring for their babies (Hill et al., 2019; Nicholls & Cox, 1999). This

TABLE 19.1 Antidepressants, Antipsychotics, and Their Lactation Risk Categories

Medication	Rated L2 (Safer, studies exist, risk to baby is remote)	Rated L3 (Moderately safe, no controlled studies)
SSRIs		
Citalopram (Celexa)	X	
Escitalopram (Lexapro)	X	
Fluoxetine (Prozac)	X	
Paroxetine (Paxil)	X	
Sertraline (Zoloft)	X	
Venlafaxine (Effexor)	X	
Older Antidepressants		
Buproprion (Wellbutrin)		X
Tricyclic Antidepressants		
Amitriptyline (Elavil)	X	
Imipramine (Tofranil)	X	
Nortriptyline (Pamelor)	X	
Antipsychotics		
Risperidone	X	
Clozapine		X
Olanzapine	X	

Adapted from (T.W. Hale, 2019)

allows parents to get the help they need without separation from their baby. Giving hospitalized parents the option of keeping their baby with them can boost their often-fragile self-esteem, while recognizing the baby's need for them and their adequacy as a nurturer. It also allows nursing to continue without interruption. Suggest parents and healthcare providers look into this possibility.

Medications and lactation. Many of the antipsychotic medications used to treat postpartum psychosis are compatible with lactation (Table 19.1).

If weaning is necessary. When parents are unable to care for their baby or their drug therapy is incompatible with lactation, weaning carefully should be an important part of their treatment plan. Physical, hormonal, and emotional changes take place during weaning that can affect parents' mental and emotional state. In some rare cases (Sharma, 2018), weaning may trigger a mental-health crisis. In addition to possible effects on mental health, abrupt weaning increases parents' risk for pain and mastitis, which increases inflammation. Also, weaning may be experienced as an emotional loss, because for most parents, nursing is a way of giving and receiving love and comfort, as well as a way to feed their baby. Nursing may be one of the few positive actions only parents can do for their baby during a difficult time. Losing nursing may leave them feeling useless and incompetent, interchangeable with any other caregiver. When weaning is necessary, offer to discuss ways to wean gradually (see p. 171). If the baby must stop nursing abruptly, discuss milk-expression strategies that will allow a gradual and comfortable reduction of milk production.

Past Sexual Abuse or Childhood Trauma

A history of sexual trauma and other types of child abuse are common among new parents and may or may not lead to nursing difficulties.

It's estimated that about 25% of women and 15% of men have a history of sexual abuse or assault. This may have happened within their families, or they may have been assaulted by peers. In either case, it can affect their birth, nursing, and early parenting experiences (Felitti et al., 1998; K. A. Kendall-Tackett, 2017). Childhood abuse is only rarely limited to one type. The more types of abuse and trauma children experience, the greater their long-term effects (Felitti, 2009; Felitti et al., 1998). In the Survey of Mothers' Sleep and Fatigue, which included 6,410 new mothers worldwide, the following types of childhood abuse and trauma were reported (K. Kendall-Tackett, Cong, & Hale, 2013):

- 34% were hit or slapped hard enough to leave a mark
- 32% reported parental substance abuse
- 25% experienced sexual trauma as a child, teen, or adult
- 16% reported their parent (usually their mother) was hit, bitten, or kicked
- 13% were raped as a teen or adult

Unfortunately, survivors of sexual abuse and assault have higher rates of other types of abuse or trauma, which can affect both their physical and mental health (Dong, Anda, Dube, Giles, & Felitti, 2003). For more on trauma and health, see **UppityScienceChick.com**.

Nursing with a history of sexual abuse. Although some assume that when abuse survivors become new parents, they will not want to nurse, this is not the case. Some research (Prentice, Lu, Lange, & Halfon, 2002) found significantly more abuse survivors intended to nurse and actually initiated nursing compared with their non-abused counterparts. Other studies (Coles, Anderson, & Loxton, 2016; Elfgen, Hagenbuch, Gorres, Block, & Leeners, 2017; Ukah, Adu, De Silva, & von Dadelszen, 2016) found rates of nursing initiation comparable in those with and without a history of childhood sexual abuse. Nursing duration was similar between the two groups (Coles et al., 2016). However, in one study (Elfgen et al., 2017), the incidence of nursing problems, such as pain and mastitis, was higher among abuse survivors. In other studies (Dugat, Chertok, & Haile, 2019; Ukah et al., 2016), the rates of exclusive nursing were lower among those with a history of abuse or other stressful life events.

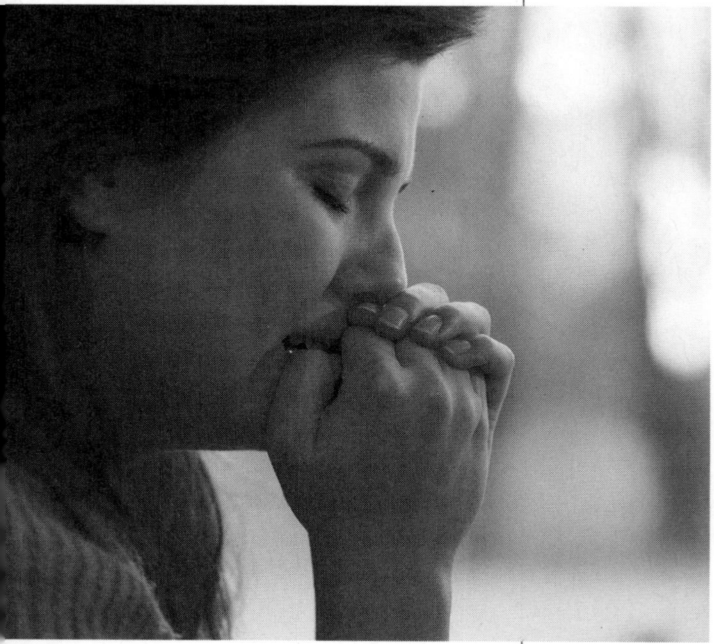

Some aspects of nursing may be challenging for abuse and trauma survivors (Klaus, 2010). For example, some find skin-to-skin contact overwhelming. Some hate the visceral sensation of their babies' mouth on their nipple. Some have post-traumatic flashbacks during birth and nursing. One of the most common challenges, however, is increased risk of depressive symptoms (see previous section), which puts nursing at risk. But this may not affect their desire to nurse. After the fact, some say they never learned to like nursing, but they learned to tolerate it, which they considered an important goal. For others, nursing was a positive and healing experience. There is a large range of possible reactions to nursing. In parents who struggle with nursing for seemingly unexplained reasons, author and researcher Phyllis Klaus described several signs of a possible history of abuse (Klaus, 2010, p. 142):

- A large file of medical or psychological complaints with no physical cause
- A history of undergoing medical procedures that did not resolve the problem

Some survivors experience very real physical pain that is an outward manifestation of the emotional pain in their psyche.

When problems occur, be flexible about nursing options. A 2013 study that included 6,410 new mothers, 994 of whom had a history of childhood sexual abuse (K. Kendall-Tackett et al., 2013), found that the abuse survivors who nursed their babies had less disrupted sleep and fewer depressive symptoms than abuse survivors who did not nurse. But in some abuse survivors, nursing triggers negative reactions. If nursing problems occur that are related to past traumatic experiences, talk about what might be triggering these negative reactions. If parents are unsure, suggest keeping a diary for a few days to try to pinpoint the problem and modify nursing to increase their comfort with it. This might include reducing the amount of skin-to-skin contact during feeds. If the problem occurs only at night, partial nursing, just during the day, may be a workable solution. To avoid the intimate contact of nursing, some parents express their milk and bottle-feed it at some feeds. Being flexible about options is vital, keeping in mind that some nursing is nearly always better than none.

Encourage parents with symptoms to seek treatment. There are several effective treatments for past trauma, most of which are compatible with nursing, (K. A. Kendall-Tackett, 2007; K. A. Kendall-Tackett & T. W. Hale, 2009) including:

- ***Education and peer counseling*** can help parents understand their experiences and their reactions to trauma. They can learn how to avoid their triggers, how to reduce their stress responses, and how to get ongoing support. By understanding that reactions after traumatic events are predictable, they are less likely to blame themselves and more likely to follow through on treatment.
- ***Trauma-focused psychotherapy.*** These types of therapy can help parents cope with past trauma.
  - *Cognitive-behavioral therapy.* Its overall focus is to help identify faulty ways of thinking that increase the risk of depressive symptoms and challenge those beliefs with more accurate interpretations. For trauma survivors, it targets distortions in their perceptions of threats and helps to desensitize them to reminders of the event.
  - *Eye movement desensitization and reprocessing (EMDR).* This highly effective therapy is approved for treating post-traumatic stress disorder by the American Psychiatric Association. Parents are asked to focus on the image, negative thought, and body sensations, while simultaneously moving their eyes back and forth, following the therapist's fingers. Sometimes sound or tactile stimulation is used instead. It allows individuals to think about their traumatic experiences without having to talk about them. For an international list of certified practitioners, see **emdr.com** or the EMDR International Association at **emdria.com**.

- ***Medications.*** Two U.S. resources (Alderman, McCarthy, & Marwood, 2009; Friedman, Davidson, & Stein, 2009) reviewed the medications recommended for trauma symptoms, including some SSRIs, SNRIs, SARIs, and atypical antipsychotics, many of which (as described in Table 19.1 on p. 839) are compatible with lactation. Other reliable resources include those listed in Box 13.1 on p. 601, which includes international resources on the safety of drugs, procedures, and treatments during lactation.

ENDOCRINE, METABOLIC, AND AUTOIMMUNE DISORDERS

Parents with a chronic illness may be advised not to nurse, in part in an effort to make their lives easier.

A chronic illness or disorder may be present at birth (congenital) or it may develop over time. Although many parents with these disorders nurse—some at about the same rate as healthy parents—they may be advised by healthcare providers or family not to nurse. Family or friends may offer to help with a new baby to ease their fatigue or stress. This type of offer is usually made out of concern for parents' well-being. But allowing others to take over the baby's care can undermine both parents' self-confidence and their relationship with their baby. For some of the ways nursing may benefit parents with a health issue, see the first point in this chapter.

Many chronically ill parents have the same questions and concerns as healthy parents. If they have questions about how their condition affects nursing, see the appropriate section. Keep in mind that most ill parents are well-educated about their health issues, so if needed, feel free to ask questions about the illness or any limitations that might affect nursing. For more details about an illness, also visit the websites of national and international organizations supporting those with chronic illnesses.

Cystic Fibrosis

Parents with cystic fibrosis can nurse while carefully monitoring their diet and weight.

Cystic fibrosis is a genetic disease which causes the secretion of a thick, gluey mucus that clogs the bronchial tubes, interfering with breathing and blocking digestive enzymes from leaving the pancreas, which causes incomplete digestion. There are more than 1,000 mutations of the gene that causes cystic fibrosis, which means parents may have a mild or severe form. Some cases of cystic fibrosis are so mild they can be detected only through laboratory tests, while some are serious enough to be life-threatening. During pregnancy, 25% of those with cystic fibrosis deliver preterm (Gilljam et al., 2000).

Nursing parents with cystic fibrosis produce normal milk. According to several studies and case reports (Kent & Farquharson, 1993; Michel & Mueller, 1994; Shiffman, Seale, Flux, Rennert, & Swender, 1989; Welch, Phelps, & Osher, 1981), mothers with cystic fibrosis who achieve full milk production make milk of normal composition, and their babies grow normally. An early case report (Alpert & Cormier, 1983) found that one mother with cystic fibrosis produced milk with high sodium levels, but this mother was not breastfeeding and had expressed her milk only for research purposes. Milk sodium levels are usually elevated as milk production declines and the breasts involute.

Parents' weight and nutrition. If parents with cystic fibrosis have issues with incomplete digestion of food (called ***pancreatic insufficiency*** or ***PI***), the nutrients in food may not be well-absorbed and parents may find it challenging to maintain a healthy weight. Parents in this situation are probably taking digestive enzymes to help break down the food more completely and may also be taking vitamin and mineral supplements. If so, they need to carefully monitor their weight and nutritional needs while pregnant and lactating (Edenborough et al., 2008). As long as parents with cystic fibrosis can maintain a healthy weight, nursing can continue (Wambach & Morrison, 2021, p. 520).

Cystic fibrosis and the nursing baby. As a genetic disease, a baby cannot "catch" cystic fibrosis by nursing. In fact, babies born with cystic fibrosis who do not nurse were found to have poorer health outcomes and earlier and more severe symptoms (Colombo et al., 2007). Also, human milk provides the baby with protection from the bacterial infections, such as Staphylococcus aureus and Pseudomonas, many parents with cystic fibrosis regularly battle. For details on nursing the baby with cystic fibrosis, see p. 314.

> **KEY CONCEPT**
>
> *Nursing parents with chronic illnesses often nurse at similar rates as healthy parents.*

Treatments for cystic fibrosis and lactation. Some parents with cystic fibrosis decide not to nurse because they are concerned their medications may negatively affect their baby, but most drugs prescribed for cystic fibrosis are compatible with lactation (Kroon et al., 2018; Panchaud et al., 2016). An Italian case report (Festini et al., 2006) documented a severe *Pseudomonas* lung infection in a breastfeeding mother with cystic fibrosis, which was treated with the IV antibiotic tobramycin. This medication was undetectable in her milk.

Diabetes Mellitus

People with diabetes produce too little insulin, or their bodies cannot use insulin normally.

Diabetes is a chronic illness that involves either inadequate production of the hormone insulin or its inefficient use. Insulin is responsible for the breakdown of carbohydrates. If diabetes is present before pregnancy, it is either Type 1 or Type 2. The most serious form of diabetes mellitus is Type 1 (see next section), which involves inadequate production of insulin. Type 2 diabetes is caused by the body's inefficient use of insulin, known as ***insulin resistance***, which may be influenced by lifestyle factors, such as weight. The third main category, gestational diabetes mellitus, occurs only during pregnancy but also indicates a higher risk of developing Type 2 diabetes later in life. Diabetes may affect lactation, because as explained in Chapter 10, "Making Milk," insulin is one of the hormones involved in milk-making. An Australian systematic review and meta-analysis (De Bortoli & Amir, 2015) examined 10 studies and concluded that diabetes of any kind during pregnancy is associated with a delay in milk increase after birth (lactogenesis II or secretory activation). Milk increase is considered delayed if it occurs more than 72 hours post-delivery.

Lactation may also affect diabetes, as lactation appears to increase insulin sensitivity, leading to better long-term health outcomes in nursing parents with gestational diabetes (Ma, Hu, Liang, Xiao, & Tan, 2019). Some researchers (Velle-Forbord et al., 2019) suggested that rather than nursing having a positive effect on metabolism, the conclusions from these long-term studies may actually be an example of "reverse causality." In other words, rather than lactation improving glucose metabolism long term, perhaps those with more severe diabetes nurse for a shorter time because diabetes negatively affects milk production and leads to more metabolic problems later in life. However, other researchers (A. Stuebe, 2019) disagree. Studies on the physiology of lactation (Diniz & Da Costa, 2004; Ozisik, Suner, & Cetinkalp, 2019; Shub, Miranda, Georgiou, McCarthy, & Lappas, 2019; Yasuhi et al., 2017) found positive metabolic changes during nursing that could explain the results of the long-term studies.

Type 1 Diabetes

In parents with Type 1 diabetes, milk increase after birth is usually delayed by about 1 day.

Type 1 diabetes is also known as insulin-dependent diabetes mellitus (or IDDM). Only 5% to 10% of diabetics have this form of the disease. It occurs when the insulin-producing beta cells in the pancreas are destroyed, leaving the body unable to produce insulin, a hormone needed to convert sugar, starches, and other foods into fuel for the body. Without insulin, blood sugar can rise to dangerous levels and cause health complications. Parents with Type 1 diabetes need to check their blood-sugar levels regularly and receive daily insulin replacement therapy via injections or subcutaneous pump, so their blood sugar doesn't become dangerously high. Some cases of Type 1 diabetes are caused by autoimmune factors (Type 1a) and others are not (Type 1b) and considered genetic. When autoimmune factors are involved, Type 1 diabetes is caused by a combination of genetics and environmental triggers, such as viral infections and obesity.

Type 1 diabetes and the nursing baby. Type 1 diabetes is not transmitted by nursing. Although some research linked early formula exposure to increased risk of Type 1 diabetes (Rosenbauer, Herzig, Kaiser, & Giani, 2007), a 2017 systematic review (Piescik-Lech, Chmielewska, Shamir, & Szajewska, 2017) found the evidence inconclusive.

Type 1 diabetes and the first hours after delivery. During pregnancy, keeping the parent's blood sugar levels within a healthy range is vital to positive birth outcomes and newborn health. In the past, babies born to parents with Type 1 diabetes were at increased risk of preterm birth, respiratory distress syndrome, heavier-than-average birth weight, exaggerated newborn jaundice, and low blood sugar (Cordero, Treuer, Landon, & Gabbe, 1998). As a result, it was common for many of these babies to spend time after birth in the special care nursery. Today, however, modern technology available in developed countries makes it possible for most parents with Type 1 diabetes to keep their blood-sugar levels within the healthy range during pregnancy, eliminating for many the need for separation after birth (Linden, Berg, Adolfsson, & Sparud-Lundin, 2018). During the first 5 to 7 hours after delivery, most parents experience low blood sugar (hypoglycemia) as their body adjusts to the rapid hormonal changes that are normal after childbirth (Wambach & Morrison, 2021, p. 516).

The same basic approach to early nursing described in Chapter 2 is vital to these families: nurse early, often, and effectively. Suggest parents plan to nurse within the first hour or two after birth and every hour or two afterward until the baby's blood sugar stabilizes. Follow nursing in the first few days by hand-expressing colostrum into a spoon and feeding it to the newborn as his "dessert." (See **firstdroplets.com** for demonstration videos and rationale.) For whatever reason, if nursing is delayed, suggest parents express their milk within the first hour or two by hand or with a breast pump to help stimulate milk production (see next paragraph). After birth, parents' blood-sugar levels need to be closely monitored to help them quickly reestablish good control.

Milk increase after birth is often delayed when early nursing is postponed or limited, but Type 1 diabetes also delays milk increase after birth by an average of about 1 day (De Bortoli & Amir, 2015; L. A. Nommsen-Rivers, Chantry, Peerson, Cohen, & Dewey, 2010). This may be in part because Type 1 diabetes lowers oxytocin levels (Kujath et al., 2015). In nursing babies, early exposure to cow-milk-based infant formula is associated with a 16-fold increased risk of sensitization to cow-milk-protein allergy (E. Kelly, DunnGalvin, Murphy, & J, 2019). So if milk production is delayed and the baby needs to be supplemented, suggest families consider these alternatives to cow-milk-based formulas.

- ***Mother's own milk hand-expressed and stored during pregnancy.*** In years past, many healthcare providers warned parents not to hand express milk during pregnancy for fear it might trigger early labor. But a 2017 Australian randomized controlled trial (Forster et al., 2017) set these fears to rest. In this study, 635 low-risk mothers with either Type 1 or Type 2 diabetes were randomly assigned to one of two groups: 1) standard care or 2) twice daily hand expression from 36 weeks of pregnancy until delivery. No adverse effects of hand expression on their pregnancies were found. See the website **firstdroplets.com** for video demos of hand expression during pregnancy.
- ***Pasteurized donor human milk.*** Many hospitals keep on hand pasteurized donor human milk from milk banks for use in the NICU (Kantorowska et al., 2016; Perrine & Scanlon, 2013). Some birthing facilities also have donor milk available for families with healthy term babies (Belfort et al., 2018; Sen et al., 2018).
- ***Elemental or amino-acid-based infant formula*** (such as Nutramigen AA or Neocate), which some research (Urashima et al., 2019) found may reduce risk of allergy sensitization.

Nursing decreases the amount of insulin parents need. Nursing has a healthy effect on a parent's insulin response (Diniz & Da Costa, 2004; Ozisik et al., 2019), increasing insulin sensitivity (Butte, Hopkinson, Mehta, Moon, & Smith, 1999; McManus, Cunningham, Watson, Harker, & Finegood, 2001). Making milk "primes" a parent's metabolism, increasing its energy efficiency. As a result, parents with Type 1 diabetes need less insulin, between 27% less (Davies, Clark, Dalton, & Edwards, 1989) and 50% less (Asselin & Lawrence, 1987). Therefore, while parents are exclusively nursing, they will likely need less insulin than before. Suggest having snacks to eat at each nursing session that includes protein and carbohydrates, as blood sugar often dips about an hour later (Walker, 2017). When the time comes for weaning, suggest doing it as gradually as possible to make maintaining blood-sugar control easier.

Type 1 diabetes and long-term nursing. When parents' blood sugar is in good control, long-term milk production does not seem to be a problem. Similar rates of long-term nursing were found in parents with and without Type 1 diabetes in studies from Australia (Webster, Moore, & McMullan, 1995), the U.S. (Ferris et al., 1993), and Denmark (Stage, Norgard, Damm, & Mathiesen, 2006). A Swedish study (Berg, Erlandsson, & Sparud-Lundin, 2012) found that during the first 6 months of nursing, mothers with Type 1 diabetes expressed more concerns about the impact of nursing on their health than the control mothers. Mothers with diabetes found the normal disruptions of daily life that occur with a baby more difficult as they tried to keep their blood-sugar levels under control. Also, since parents with Type 1 diabetes are at greater risk of developing bacterial and fungal infections of all kinds, including mastitis and candida (thrush) (Wambach & Morrison, 2021, p. 517), suggest they learn how to prevent these infections, as well as their signs and symptoms, so if needed, they can seek treatment immediately.

Treatments for Type 1 diabetes and lactation. The insulin replacement needed daily by parents with Type 1 diabetes does not affect the nursing baby. Insulin molecules are too large to pass into the milk, but even if they did, they would be broken down in the baby's gut (T.W. Hale, 2019, pp. 387-388).

Type 2 Diabetes

Nursing improves glucose metabolism, which can reduce the severity of Type 2 diabetes.

Type 2 diabetes, also known as non-insulin dependent diabetes mellitus (NIDDM), accounts for about 90% of diabetes cases. Once rare during the childbearing years, it has become more common in recent years. When parents have Type 2 diabetes, either they do not produce enough insulin or their body's insulin receptors do not respond normally to insulin, a dynamic known as insulin resistance. When sugar builds up in the blood instead of being used as fuel by cells, this causes a variety of health complications that can affect the eyes, skin, feet, heart, and other systems. Type 2 diabetes is one part of a constellation of health problems known as metabolic syndrome (including obesity, high cholesterol, and high blood pressure) that increases the risk of cardiovascular disease.

KEY CONCEPT

Lactation increases insulin sensitivity.

Type 2 diabetes and the nursing baby. Nursing babies have a reduced risk of Type 2 diabetes later in life, according to a 2019 systematic review and meta-analysis that included nearly 250,00 individuals (Horta & de Lima, 2019), with longer duration of nursing having a greater effect. A Hong Kong study that followed children for 17 years (Hui et al., 2018) found that nursing exclusively during the first 3 months was associated with less insulin resistance in adolescence.

Type 2 diabetes and early milk production. Some research (Chevalier & Fenichel, 2015; Zdrojewicz, Popowicz, Szyca, Michalik, & Smieszniak, 2017) suggests that insulin resistance—a major feature of Type 2 diabetes—may delay early milk production. As described in Chapter 10, "Making Milk," insulin is one of the hormones essential to lactation. U.S. lactation consultants Lisa Marasco and Diana West (L. Marasco & West, 2020, p. 154) wrote:

> "As milk production increases after birth, the body's metabolic needs change dramatically, and insulin requirements may also change. Depending on how quickly medication adjustments are made, this can slow the increase of milk production for up to 24 hours (Carlsen, Jacobsen, & Vanky, 2010)."

Effective treatments for insulin resistance (see last paragraph of this point) may be key to better lactation outcomes.

Type 2 diabetes and early nursing. Like babies whose parents have Type 1 diabetes, at birth these babies are at greater risk for low blood sugar (hypoglycemia). Suggest expectant parents plan to nurse within the first hour or two and at least every hour or two thereafter until the baby's blood sugar is stable. A New Zealand study (Simmons, Conroy, & Thompson, 2005) found that the main determinant of whether mothers with Type 2 diabetes were nursing at hospital discharge was whether their baby's first feed was at the breast or formula. Only 19% of those mothers whose babies received formula as their first feed were nursing at discharge compared with 78% whose first feed was nursing. During the first few days after birth, follow nursing by hand-expressing any available colostrum into a spoon and feeding it to the baby as "dessert." (See **firstdroplets.com** for demonstration videos and rationale.) This can stimulate faster milk production and prevent excess weight loss, which is associated with shorter duration of nursing (Flaherman, Beiler, Cabana, & Paul, 2016).

Type 2 diabetes and the nursing parent. Lactation improves glucose metabolism, increasing insulin sensitivity (Diniz & Da Costa, 2004; Ozisik et al., 2019), which reduces the severity of Type 2 diabetes. A 2019 South Korean nationwide population-based study (Nam et al., 2019) found that in women who gave birth to at least one previous child (multipara), breastfeeding improved their ability to control their blood-sugar levels.

Treatments for Type 2 diabetes and lactation.. During pregnancy, insulin injections are sometimes used to keep blood-sugar levels in the normal range. After birth, if needed, insulin may be continued (see the "Treatments" section in Type 1 diabetes) or hypoglycemic medications may be prescribed, along with diet and exercise (Feng, Lin, Wan, Hu, & Du, 2015; T.W. Hale, 2019). A 2018 overview article on medications commonly used to treat Type 2 diabetes in lactating parents (Anderson, 2018a, p. 239) concluded: "The most commonly used antidiabetic drugs such as insulin, metformin, and some second-generation sulfonylureas appear to be acceptable to use during breastfeeding."

Some newer, more "natural" treatments for Type 2 diabetes and insulin resistance are described in the book *Making More Milk* (L. Marasco & West, 2020, pp. 157-158). Its authors describe the use of inositol, a sugar that naturally occurs in many fruits and beans. An imbalance of myo-inositol and d-chiro-inositol is associated with insulin resistance, and new therapies are focused on correcting this imbalance with myo-inositol supplements or a specially calibrated combination of both substances (Nestler & Unfer, 2015; Unfer, Nestler, Kamenov, Prapas, & Facchinetti, 2016). Side effects are rare with these new therapies.

Gestational Diabetes

Gestational diabetes is a glucose intolerance that occurs in 7% to 9% of pregnancies (Wambach & Morrison, 2021, p. 515). About 50% of those who develop gestational diabetes will later develop Type 2 diabetes (T.W. Hale & Berens, 2010).

Parents with gestational diabetes who do not lactate after birth are more likely to develop Type 2 diabetes later in life compared with those who do lactate.

Gestational diabetes and the nursing parent. In parents who develop gestational diabetes, lactation has a long-term effect on preventing or delaying the development of Type 2 diabetes. Knowing this may motivate some parents to nurse (Wallenborn, Perera, & Masho, 2017). This beneficial effect of lactation on glucose metabolism was noted right after birth when fasting glucose levels were compared in nursing and non-nursing parents who had gestational diabetes (Shub et al., 2019). Greater nursing intensity has a more profound effect (Yasuhi et al., 2017). See the previous points about Type 1 and Type 2 diabetes for more details on the increased insulin sensitivity that occurs during lactation. A 2019 systematic review and meta-analysis that included 23 observational studies (Ma et al., 2019) found a reduced risk of progression to Type 2 diabetes with any nursing, which became stronger with longer duration and greater exclusivity of nursing. A U.S. study of 809 women with gestational diabetes (Kjos, Henry, Lee, Buchanan, & Mishell, 1993) found that those doing any amount of nursing between 4 and 12 weeks after birth had significantly better glucose metabolism than those who were not nursing. The researchers (Kjos et al., 1993, p. 454) found a "two-fold reduction in the development of diabetes mellitus in the lactating group compared to the nonlactating group…"

Another U.S. cohort study of 121,700 women (A. M. Stuebe, Rich-Edwards, Willett, Manson, & Michels, 2005) found that longer duration of nursing was associated with a reduced incidence of Type 2 diabetes. For each additional year of nursing, the study mothers had a decreased risk of contracting Type 2 diabetes over the next 15 years of 14% to 15%. A U.K. review of 23 studies (Owen, Martin, Whincup, Smith, & Cook, 2006) estimated that nursing is associated with a 15% to 56% reduction in the risk for Type 2 diabetes. A U.S. cross-sectional cohort analysis of 1,620 women (Ram et al., 2008) found that later in life duration of lactation was also associated with a lower prevalence of metabolic syndrome, of which Type 2 diabetes is a part. Nursing was associated with better measures on all aspects of metabolic syndrome, including blood pressure, abdominal obesity, fasting glucose, cholesterol, and triglycerides. Not only does lactation increase parents' insulin sensitivity while they are nursing, it appears to positively program their metabolism for years afterwards. As one U.S. researcher (Ram et al., 2008, p. 268) wrote: "Lactation may prime the metabolic system by making it a more energy-efficient machine….".

Yet even with the positive effects of lactation on metabolism, many studies found that compared with parents without gestational diabetes, those with it are:

- Less likely to start nursing after birth (Doughty, Ronnenberg, Reeves, Qian, & Sibeko, 2018),
- Less likely to be nursing at hospital discharge (Haile, Oza-Frank, Azulay Chertok, & Passen, 2016)
- Less likely to exclusively nurse, and nurse for a shorter duration (Nguyen et al., 2019)

These differences in nursing outcomes occur in studies from cultures as diverse when it comes to lactation as:

- Denmark (Fenger-Gron, et al., 2015)
- Thailand (Jirakittidul, Panichyawat, Chotrungrote, & Mala, 2019)
- United States (Glover, Berry, Schwartz, & Stuebe, 2018)
- Brazil (Reinheimer, Schmidt, Duncan, & Drehmer, 2019)

Gestational diabetes and the nursing baby. A 2018 Canadian analysis of the data from a cohort study of children exposed to gestational diabetes in utero (Dugas et al., 2018) concluded that in those exposed in the womb, more than 8 months of nursing was associated with healthier A1C test results (which tests for Type 2 diabetes) in childhood. The researchers (Dugas et al., 2018, p. 40) wrote: "Considering that these children are at high risk of developing Type 2 diabetes later in life, this suggests that the impact of in utero exposure to [gestational diabetes] can be partly attenuated by prolonged infant feeding with breast milk during early life...."

Gestational diabetes and early milk production. As previously mentioned, milk increase after birth (also known as lactogenesis II or secretory activation) is considered delayed if it occurs more than 72 hours post-delivery. A U.S. analysis of data from a prospective cohort study (Matias, Dewey, Quesenberry, & Gunderson, 2014) found that 33% of its mothers with gestational diabetes experienced delayed milk increase after birth. Treatment with insulin during pregnancy was associated with this delay, as well as obesity and suboptimal nursing in the hospital. As described in Chapter 10 (see p. 424), analysis of the milk can determine a delay, with a higher ratio of sodium to potassium indicating milk increase has not yet occurred (Morton, 1994). A Canadian study that analyzed milk samples from 252 first-time mothers at 48 hours after delivery (Galipeau, Goulet, & Chagnon, 2012) found an association between delay in milk increase and gestational diabetes. However, it also noted that nursing at least 8 to 12 times per 24 hours offset this delay.

Gestational diabetes and early nursing. As with the other types of diabetes, suggest families plan to nurse within the first hour or two after delivery and every hour or two after that until baby's blood sugar levels are stable. If early nursing is not possible, begin hand-expressing or pumping. During the first few days after birth, follow nursing by hand-expressing any available colostrum into a spoon and feeding it to the baby as "dessert." (See **firstdroplets.com** for demonstration videos and rationale.) This can stimulate faster milk production and prevent excess weight loss, which is associated with shorter duration of nursing (Flaherman et al., 2016). U.S. research (A. M. Stuebe, Bonuck, Adatorwovor, Schwartz, & Berry, 2016) found that nursing parents with gestational diabetes have better lactation outcomes when they receive targeted support.

Treatments for gestational diabetes and lactation. See "Treatments" for the previously described types of diabetes for details on common diabetic treatments.

Galactosemia and PKU

Exclusive nursing is contraindicated for babies with galactosemia and PKU, but parents with these metabolic disorders can nurse their babies.

Individuals with the metabolic disorders galactosemia and phenylketonuria (PKU) are born unable to completely metabolize specific components of human milk. In the case of galactosemia, babies with this condition cannot metabolize galactose, a milk sugar, and its accumulation in their system causes severe health problems. With PKU, the essential amino acid phenylalanine is not well metabolized, also causing severe health issues unless diet is modified. As these babies grow, no matter what their age, they must remain vigilant about diet. For their entire lives, affected individuals must monitor their diets carefully to avoid dangerously high blood levels of these substances. In those with PKU, for example, too-high levels of blood phenylalanine can lead to intellectual impairment. (See the sections on these metabolic disorders on p. 320 for details on how nursing is affected in babies with these genetic disorders.)

When people with galactosemia or PKU reach childbearing age, they can become pregnant and nurse. During a pregnancy with PKU, careful dietary control of blood levels of phenylalanine is critical, as too-high blood levels put parents at greater risk of having a baby with birth defects similar to fetal alcohol syndrome (Matalon, Michals, & Gleason, 1986). During lactation, the milk of these parents is normal (Forbes, Barton, Nicholas, & Cook, 1988; Purnell, 2001). One U.S. case report (Fox-Bacon, McCamman, Therou, Moore, & Kipp, 1997) documented identical twin mothers with PKU who breastfed their babies. After birth, the researchers found no association between the mothers' phenylalanine blood levels and their milk levels. One Swedish mother with galactosemia (Ohlsson, Nasiell, & von Dobeln, 2007) breastfed two healthy babies, one for 8 months, with measures of her disorder staying within normal treatment levels.

Gestational Ovarian Theca Lutein Cysts

After birth, parents with gestational theca lutein cysts may have inhibited milk production, but most can eventually reach full milk production.

Gestational ovarian theca lutein cysts are benign cysts that develop on the ovaries during pregnancy. They are more common among those who have undergone fertility treatments, but they can also occur during a naturally-occurring pregnancy (Montz, Schlaerth, & Morrow, 1988). These cysts produce testosterone, sometimes at levels 10 to 150 times higher than normal. When testosterone levels are very high, body or facial hair may develop and the voice may deepen. If testosterone levels are elevated to more moderate levels, there may be no obvious symptoms, and parents and their healthcare provider may be unaware they have this condition.

After birth, these cysts disappear without treatment, and within several weeks, the affected parent's testosterone levels return to normal. But during the first weeks after birth, higher-than-normal testosterone levels may inhibit milk production. If a blood test reveals high testosterone levels (a "high normal" level is 67-70 ng/dL), an ultrasound can confirm the presence of the cysts. Some parents with gestational ovarian theca lutein cysts have blood testosterone levels as high as 711 ng/dL (Hoover, Barbalinardo, & Platia, 2002).

In one U.S. article (Hoover et al., 2002), two mothers' experiences of breastfeeding with gestational ovarian theca lutein cysts were reported. After birth, despite their lack of milk, both kept stimulating their breasts 8 or more times per day either by breastfeeding (with a nursing supplementer) or with a breast pump. When these mothers' testosterone blood levels fell below 300 ng/dL, their milk finally "came in," one at 20 days after delivery and the other at 12 days post-birth. Another U.S. article (Betzold, Hoover, & Snyder, 2004) reported two other mothers' experiences. With regular breast stimulation, these mothers achieved increased milk production, one at 10 days and the other at 31 days. One of these four mothers did not achieve full milk production, but the other three did.

Multiple Sclerosis

Exclusive nursing appears to delay the post-delivery recurrence of symptoms in parents with multiple sclerosis.

Multiple sclerosis (or MS) is a chronic, often disabling disease that attacks the central nervous system. Symptoms may be mild, such as numbness in the limbs, or severe, such as paralysis or loss of vision. The development, severity, and symptoms of MS vary from person to person. Although the cause of MS is not yet known, it is thought to be a type of autoimmune disorder because the body's own defenses attack the fatty substance called myelin that surrounds and protects the nerves in the central nervous system. It may also damage the nerve fibers, which form scar tissue (***sclerosis***) that gives the disease its name. When any part of the myelin sheath or nerve fiber is damaged or destroyed, nerve impulses traveling to and from the brain and spinal cord are distorted or interrupted, producing the variety of symptoms that can occur, such as numbness, fatigue, trouble walking, vision problems, pain, vertigo, and even paralysis.

In mild cases, the affected person may completely recover after the symptoms pass and have long periods of remission. In severe cases, the symptoms may become progressively worse and not subside, or there may be repeated relapses that leave those affected permanently and increasingly disabled. It is common for MS to occur during the childbearing years.

MS and the nursing baby. Many parents with chronic illnesses worry that nursing will transmit their disorder to their baby, but in this case, the opposite appears to be true. MS cannot be transmitted by nursing, and several studies (Brenton, Engel, Sohn, & Goldman, 2017; Dalla Costa et al., 2019) found that not nursing increased baby's risk of developing pediatric MS. An Italian study (Pisacane et al., 1994) found lower rates of MS among individuals nursed for more than 6 months compared with those nursed less than 6 months or never nursed. A 2017 U.S. case-control study (Langer-Gould et al., 2017) compared nearly 400 women newly diagnosed with MS with 433 controls and concluded that those who did not nurse were at a higher risk of subsequent MS diagnosis.

KEY CONCEPT

In parents with MS, greater nursing intensity seems to be associated with a longer remission of symptoms.

MS and the nursing parent. During pregnancy, many of those with MS enjoy a remission from MS symptoms, especially during the third trimester. However, the first 3 months after birth typically bring a significant increase in symptoms (Kaplan, 2019). Some of the early research from the U.S. and Ireland (Confavreux, Hutchinson, Hours, Cortinovis-Tourniaire, & Moreau, 1998; Nelson, Franklin, & Jones, 1988) found no real difference in incidence of MS symptoms during the first months after birth in breastfeeding and non-breastfeeding mothers. But these studies did not distinguish between exclusive and partial nursing.

Studies that controlled for intensity of nursing found a significant difference. One U.S. study of 140 women with MS (Gulick & Halper, 2002) found the lower the percentage of feeds at the breast, the more likely a relapse of MS symptoms. A later U.S. prospective cohort study of 61 women (32 with MS) (Langer-Gould et al., 2009) found a five-fold increase in relapse during the first year after delivery among mothers who breastfed partially or not at all compared with those who exclusively breastfed for the first 2 months. The researchers suggested one reason may be the longer delay in the return of the menses in those exclusively nursing (see Chapter 12, "Sexuality, Fertility, and Contraception."). The difference in relapse rate was not related to the severity of illness, and the mothers' perception of their disease's severity was not related to their decision about nursing.

Controversy still exists, however, over whether nursing affects relapse rates in those with MS. Some note that the parents who nurse may have milder cases of MS, which could influence the conclusions (Portaccio & Amato, 2019). This is an important issue if treatments are recommended that are not compatible with lactation.

Treatments for MS and lactation. Many of the first-line drugs used to slow the progression of MS, known as disease-modifying treatments (or DMTs), are considered compatible with lactation (T.W. Hale, 2019). Examples include interferon beta 1a (Avonex), rated L2 (the "safer" lactation risk factor in *Hale's Medications and Mothers' Milk*), and interferon beta 1b (Betaferon), also rated L2 (safer). There are some exceptions, such as mitoxantrone (Novantrone), which is rated L5 (contraindicated). In most cases, parents with MS can take their medications and nurse. In an overview article on both old and new treatments for MS in nursing parents, doctor of pharmacology Philip O. Anderson (Anderson, 2019a, p. 358) wrote:

> "A general strategy for new mothers with MS is to encourage exclusive breastfeeding postpartum, because it might lessen relapse. Monthly IVIG or methylprednisolone injections might be adequate for many women to avoid a DMT for a few months."

Polycystic Ovary Syndrome (PCOS)

Some parents with PCOS produce overabundant milk, some have no milk production issues, and some have low milk production.

Polycystic ovary syndrome (PCOS) is not a disease but a syndrome (a constellation of symptoms) that is still poorly understood. It affects up to 15% of women and is one of the leading causes of infertility. Common symptoms of PCOS include:

- High levels of estrogen and androgens (testosterone and other male hormones), which can cause severe acne, skin discoloration, and excess hair growth
- High insulin levels, which contribute to the obesity that affects about half of those with PCOS
- Multiple ovarian cysts
- Menstrual abnormalities, which usually begin in adolescence and contribute to infertility

Many with PCOS also develop insulin resistance and Type 2 diabetes during their childbearing years. Insulin resistance (insulin receptors not responding normally to insulin in the body) appears to be a pivotal issue, as when insulin resistance is treated, it resolves many other PCOS symptoms (Sirmans & Pate, 2013). Some with PCOS experience low thyroid levels (hypothyroidism), which may contribute to infertility (Joham, Teede, Ranasinha, Zoungas, & Boyle, 2015; Wiffen & Fetherston, 2016).

PCOS and the nursing parent. Because the hormonal disruptions in those with PCOS vary in type and degree, the effect of PCOS on milk production is not consistent. Some with PCOS produce overabundant milk, others have low milk production, and still others produce milk in the normal range. One Swedish radiological study that examined breast tissue in women with PCOS (Balcar, Silinkova-Malkova, & Matys, 1972) found that some had hypoplastic breasts made mostly of fat with few milk-making glands. A Brazilian study (Fonseca, de Souza, Bagnoli, Celestino, & Salvatore, 1985) also found breast tissue abnormalities in women with PCOS. One U.S. article (L. Marasco, Marmet, & Shell, 2000) described the breastfeeding experiences of three women with PCOS, all of whom produced little milk despite expert help and the use of many usually effective strategies to increase milk production. Insulin is known to affect mammary growth and development during pregnancy and to play an important role in increasing milk production after birth (Chevalier & Fenichel, 2015; Laurie A Nommsen-Rivers, 2016). When a parent's body does not respond normally to insulin, this may potentially affect milk production.

But not all of those with PCOS have issues with mammary function and milk production. A Norwegian study of 36 women with PCOS and 99 controls (Vanky, Isaksen, Moen, & Carlsen, 2008) found that mothers with PCOS had a slightly reduced early breastfeeding rate, 75% vs. 89% among the control mothers, meaning three-quarters of the mothers with PCOS exclusively breastfed their babies. Another later Norwegian study (Carlsen et al., 2010) found an association between the high androgen levels in many women with PCOS and reduced breastfeeding duration. It is possible that higher levels of testosterone and other androgens during pregnancy may affect mammary development. When a parent with PCOS is also obese, has high blood pressure, and is insulin resistant, this increases the chances of having milk-production problems (Thatcher & Jackson, 2006). As with other lactation red flags, when a parent has PCOS, this means both parent and baby should be carefully monitored after birth without undermining their confidence in nursing.

KEY CONCEPT

The impact of PCOS on nursing varies from woman to woman.

Treatments for PCOS and lactation. A common treatment for PCOS, the hypoglycemic medication metformin, decreases the hormonal disruptions in some of those affected, even those without insulin resistance (Baillargeon, Jakubowicz, Iuorno, Jakubowicz, & Nestler, 2004; Zhao, Liu, & Zhang, 2018). This drug has helped some parents overcome infertility, and during pregnancy, metformin was found to reduce the incidence of miscarriages, gestational diabetes, hypertension, and preterm birth (Feng et al., 2015; Glueck, Wang, Goldenberg, & Sieve, 2004; Zhao et al., 2018). Metformin is rated an L1 (safest) in *Hale's Medications and Mothers' Milk*, as U.S. research (T. W. Hale, Kristensen, Hackett, Kohan, & Ilett, 2002) found that little transfers into human milk, and when taken during pregnancy and lactation, the exposed babies grew normally with no adverse effects (Glueck, Salehi, Sieve, & Wang, 2006). Some report (Gabbay & Kelly, 2003) that treatment with metformin through pregnancy and lactation helped normalize milk production in some mothers with PCOS. Doses start at about 500 mg per day and increase up to 1,000 to 2,500 mg per day (Glueck et al., 2006; L. Marasco & West, 2020). See the previous section on treatments for Type 2 diabetes (p. 847) for some newer, more natural treatments for insulin resistance that have the potential to be helpful in boosting milk production in parents with PCOS.

Rheumatoid Arthritis and Lupus

Many nursing parents with rheumatoid arthritis and lupus have physical challenges and medication concerns.

Both rheumatoid arthritis and systemic lupus erythematosus (the most common type of lupus) are autoimmune disorders caused by the immune system attacking body tissues with unusual antibodies known as "autoantibodies." Autoimmune disorders are more common in women than men, with rheumatoid arthritis occurring in 2.5 women for every one man and lupus occurring in 10 women for every one man. These disorders often occur in periods of flares and remissions. During the flares, symptoms include joint swelling, pain, fatigue, and fever. In those with lupus, neurological problems can occur and organ function may be affected. In severe cases, organ failure may occur.

Rheumatoid arthritis, lupus, and the nursing baby. The baby cannot "catch" rheumatoid arthritis or lupus by nursing. In fact, Swedish and U.S. research (Jacobsson et al., 2003; Simard et al., 2008) found nursing babies less likely to contract these autoimmune disorders than babies not nursed.

KEY CONCEPT

Nursing parents with rheumatoid arthritis or lupus may experience a relapse of their symptoms during lactation.

Rheumatoid arthritis, lupus, and the nursing parent. Nursing also appears to protect parents from developing these autoimmune disorders, with longer nursing providing greater protection than shorter nursing (Adab et al., 2014; Costenbader, Feskanich, Stampfer, & Karlson, 2007; Pikwer et al., 2009).

Many parents with rheumatoid arthritis experience a remission from their symptoms beginning in the second trimester of pregnancy and ending with their return about 3 to 4 months after delivery (Akasbi, Abourazzak, & Harzy, 2014). When a chronic illness goes into remission during pregnancy and symptoms return during nursing, parents may think nursing is the cause. If so, assure them this is not the case. In fact, for many parents, the hormonal changes of nursing actually help prolong their remission. After a long break from painful symptoms, parents may think they are worse than before. If so, gently explore the possibility that after a time of relief, they may have forgotten how severe their symptoms used to be. In parents with lupus, symptoms during pregnancy are more unpredictable, and pregnancy may be a difficult time.

A 2017 Argentinian cross-sectional study (Acevedo, Pretini, Micelli, Sequeira, & Kerzberg, 2017) examined how lupus affects nursing outcomes by comparing 31 mothers diagnosed with lupus before pregnancy with 31 healthy controls. They found the mothers with lupus less likely to initiate breastfeeding (81% versus 94%) and those with lupus weaned earlier (on average 6 months versus 12 months). The most common reason given for weaning was starting a new medication, and in half of these cases, the drug was compatible with continued nursing. A 2019 U.K. qualitative study of 128 women with autoimmune rheumatic disease (Williams et al., 2019) described why shorter nursing duration might be an issue with these parents. Its study participants described how difficult it was for them to access information about lactation with a rheumatic illness and the lack of support they felt when making decisions about nursing and treatment options. A 2016 U.K. prospective study (Noviani, Wasserman, & Clowse, 2016) found about half of its 51 study mothers breastfed after delivery, with the decision to nurse associated with plans to breastfeed and low lupus activity after a term birth.

Physical challenges and nursing. Many parents with rheumatoid arthritis and lupus struggle with pain and fatigue, especially joint pain and pain associated with Raynaud's phenomenon (see p. 710), which is more common in those with autoimmune disorders. For practical strategies for making nursing easier, see p. 862 for the section "Basic Strategies for Parents with Disabilities."

Treatments for rheumatoid arthritis and lactation. Different types of medications are used in those with rheumatoid arthritis, many of which are compatible with lactation, such as the non-steroidal anti-inflammatory drugs like ibuprofen (Advil) and aspirin. Acetaminophen (Tylenol) and meperidine are also considered compatible with lactation and may sometimes be taken for pain. The disease-modifying antirheumatic drugs (DMARDs) include steroids, antimalarial medications, and others, many of which are compatible with lactation. However, some cytotoxic drugs in this category, such as methotrexate, are questionable for lactating parents, because although only small amounts of these drugs pass into the milk, they are believed to be retained in human tissues (T.W. Hale, 2019).

Treatments for lupus and lactation. The medications used to treat lupus will depend on its severity and the organ involvement. Non-steroidal anti-inflammatories (mentioned above) may be used for inflammation and/or pain. The DMARDs mentioned may also be prescribed, many of which are compatible with lactation (T.W. Hale, 2019).

Thyroid Disease

The physical changes that occur during pregnancy and lactation can affect thyroid function, which can affect parents' health, mood, and milk production.

Located in the neck, the butterfly-shaped thyroid gland releases hormones (T_3 and T_4) that regulate much of the body's activities: metabolism, heat generation, brain and heart function, and more. When the thyroid gland becomes overactive (known as ***hyperthyroidism***), it releases too much hormone. When it becomes underactive (known as ***hypothyroidism***), it releases too little hormone. Both too much and too little thyroid hormone may affect parents' mood and energy level, as well as their health and milk production. A 2019 Turkish retrospective study of 795 women who delivered babies during a 1-year period in one hospital (Dulek, Vural, Aka, & Zengin, 2019) found that 87% had normal thyroid function, 0.5% had hypothyroidism, 9% had subclinical hypothyroidism (measurable abnormalities in lab tests without symptoms), and 3% had hyperthyroidism, Encourage parents with a history of thyroid problems to have their thyroid levels tested every few weeks during pregnancy and after birth so that their medication can be adjusted as their levels change.

Postpartum Thyroiditis

Temporary changes in parents' thyroid levels after birth are called postpartum thyroiditis.

In 5% to 10% of pregnancies, an autoimmune condition is triggered called ***postpartum thyroiditis***, which can occur even in parents without a history of thyroid problems. This condition is more common among those with autoimmune disorders, such as Type 1 diabetes, and a history of thyroid disorders (ATA, 2020).

Symptoms and diagnosis of postpartum thyroiditis. This disorder usually starts with a period of overactive thyroid (***thyrotoxicosis*** or hyperthyroidism), sometime between 1 and 4 months after birth. Symptoms may include fast heartbeat, insomnia, anxiety, weight loss, and irritability. This overactive phase may last a few weeks to a few months, and then in some, but not all, parents it is followed by a period of underactive thyroid (hypothyroidism), usually between 4 to 8 months after birth. Symptoms in this phase may include weight gain, fatigue, dry skin, constipation, depression, and decrease in milk production. Postpartum thyroiditis may be diagnosed from its symptoms alone or blood tests may detect thyroid levels that are too high or too low. Depending on its severity, treatments described in the following two sections for hypo- and hyperthyroidism may be used to bring thyroid levels back into the normal range until the thyroid function normalizes over time. In 80% of parents with this condition, its symptoms resolve within 12 to 18 months after they began. If thyroid replacement therapy is used, it is tapered off gradually as the parent's thyroid begins functioning normally.

> **KEY CONCEPT**
>
> *Postpartum hypothyroidism can mimic symptoms of postpartum depression.*

Postpartum thyroiditis may sometimes be mistaken for Graves' disease (for details, see later section "Hyperthyroidism"). But there are differences. According to U.S. physicians Ruth and Robert Lawrence (Lawrence & Lawrence, 2016, p. 586), levels of thyroid stimulation immunoglobulins are high in those with Graves' disease and normal in those with postpartum thyroiditis. Symptoms are severe with Graves' disease and more modest with postpartum thyroiditis. The thyroid gland is usually more enlarged with Graves' disease, and those with Graves' disease have blood levels of thyroid hormone that are significantly high, as opposed to the more modestly elevated levels in those with postpartum thyroiditis.

Hypothyroidism

Treatments for underactive thyroid are compatible with lactation and may boost milk production.

Causes of an underactive thyroid (hypothyroidism) include autoimmune disorders such as Hashimoto's thyroiditis, medical treatments such as surgery or radiation of the thyroid gland, medications, illness, and damage of the pituitary gland, the "master gland" that tells the thyroid how much hormone to release.

Symptoms and diagnosis of hypothyroidism. With clinical hypothyroidism, lower-than-normal levels of thyroid hormones cause symptoms that indicate the body is slowing down. Parents with low thyroid may feel cold, a lack of energy, be forgetful, and depressed. Constipation and low milk production are other possible symptoms. Because the symptoms may seem vague and start slowly, it is not unusual for hypothyroidism to be missed or misdiagnosed. This condition is usually diagnosed from a combination of symptoms, medical history, physical exam, and blood tests. If the blood TSH (***thyroid stimulating hormone***) levels are high and the T_3 (***triiodothyronine***) and T_4 (***thyroxine***) levels are low, this indicates underactive thyroid. Before any new parent is treated for depressive symptoms, first rule out hypothyroidism. Taking St. John's wort (an herbal depression treatment) can mask hypothyroidism.

Hypothyroidism and low milk production. The connection between low thyroid function and low milk production is well known. But low thyroid may also affect the release of oxytocin. In the book *Making More Milk* (L. Marasco & West, 2020, p. 162), its authors describe animal research that found impaired milk ejection in rats with hypothyroidism (Campo Verde Arbocco, Persia, Hapon, & Jahn, 2017; Hapon, Varas, Jahn, & Gimenez, 2005). Another result of hypothyroidism in the study rats was that their milk-making tissue began to shut down or involute (Campo Verde Arbocco et al., 2016). If a galactogogues is used to boost low milk production, it is important to choose wisely. In *Making More Milk*, U.S. lactation consultants Lisa Marasco and Diana West (L. Marasco & West, 2020, p. 163) wrote:

> "Parents with low milk production and low thyroid function should know that large amounts of both fenugreek and moringa [malunggay] reduced thyroid hormones in rats (Hapon, Simoncini, Via, & Jahn, 2003; Panda, Tahiliani, & Kar, 1999). While eating moringa as a vegetable or fenugreek as a spice is not a concern, it would be wise to avoid larger amounts of either; choose a thyroid-supportive or thyroid-neutral galactogogue instead."

These authors also note that the drug metformin, which is prescribed for insulin resistance (see p. 853), was found to improve low thyroid without causing problems in people with normal thyroid levels (Lupoli et al., 2014).

Subclinical hypothyroidism. When a disorder is ***subclinical***, that means lab tests show abnormal results without any obvious symptoms. As described in the first point in this section, 9% of women giving birth at one Turkish hospital had subclinical hypothyroidism (Dulek et al., 2019). The authors of *Making More Milk* (L. Marasco & West, 2020, p. 162) note that in some parents with low milk production, a "low-normal" thyroid test result may not lead to treatment. But sometimes more extensive testing may result in a diagnosis of subclinical hypothyroidism and treatment. If a parent wants information to share with a healthcare provider from the American Thyroid Association that provides treatment recommendations, suggest they share these 2017 guidelines at **bit.ly/BA2-Thyroid**. Recommendations 74 and 75 in these guidelines address treatment for hypothyroidism to address lactation-related issues.

Genetic hypothyroidism. Some genetic forms of hypothyroidism may cause low milk production, but lab tests may come back normal (Maino, Cantara, Forleo, Pilli, & Castagria, 2018). U.S. lactation consultant Elise Fulara had personal experience with this type of hypothyroidism and recommends when other causes of low milk production are ruled out and hypothyroidism is suspected to test for free/total T_3 as well as TSH and T_4 (Wiersinga, 2017), which would reveal this condition and hopefully lead to appropriate treatment (personal communication, August 22, 2019).

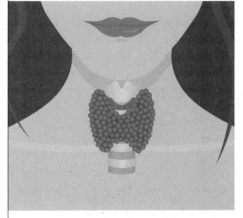

The butterfly-shaped thyroid gland is located in the neck.

Treatments for hypothyroidism and lactation. Hypothyroidism is usually treated with synthetic thyroid replacement hormones, such as levothyroxine (Synthroid), which bring parents' levels up to normal by providing the hormones that should be produced naturally. In *Hale's Medications and Mothers' Milk* (T.W. Hale, 2019), this medication is rated an L1 (safest). Many parents with hypothyroidism find that with this treatment, they not only feel better, their milk production increases, sometimes dramatically. For the normal range of thyroid hormones and the usual tests for determining if treatment is needed, see p. 443.

Hyperthyroidism

Treatments for hyperthyroidism are compatible with lactation unless radioactive iodine is used.

In more than 70% of people with overactive thyroid (hyperthyroidism), the cause is Graves' disease, an autoimmune disorder in which autoantibodies stimulate overproduction of the cells of the thyroid gland. It can also be caused by nodes or lumps in the thyroid or a temporary condition called thyroiditis, which may be triggered by a virus.

Symptoms and diagnosis of hyperthyroidism. When parents produce higher-than-normal thyroid levels, symptoms indicate the body is running faster: racing heartbeat, anxiety, insomnia, irritability, more perspiration, and weight loss. Their eyes may bulge and their thyroid gland may swell into a visible lump (goiter) on their neck. Diagnosis is usually made first with a physical exam, which reveals a swollen thyroid gland, and confirmed by a blood test. When parents' TSH (thyroid-stimulating hormone) levels are low and T_3 and T_4 levels are high, this indicates an overactive thyroid.

Hyperthyroidism and early nursing. In the book, *Making More Milk* (L. Marasco & West, 2020, pp. 163-164), its authors describe several case reports of women with severe, untreated hyperthyroidism who experienced early, rapid milk increase after delivery but were unable to remove milk by either nursing or milk expression. These cases were also noted in the 2017 guidelines of the American Thyroid Association (Alexander et al., 2017). Marasco and West suggest that parents in this situation first seek treatment for their hyperthyroidism, and if needed, consider using oxytocin nasal spray after delivery to help remove the milk.

Radioactive diagnostic tests and lactation. Once hyperthyroidism is confirmed, to determine its cause, the healthcare provider may order a scan of the thyroid to see whether lumps are present. The radioactive iodine uptake test requires an interruption of nursing until it clears the parent's system, usually at least 12 hours. If a radioactive scan is recommended, suggest parents ask if a material can be used that has the shortest half-life, which requires the shortest interruption of nursing (T.W. Hale, 2019; Mitchell et al., 2019). The Academy of Breastfeeding Medicine's Clinical Protocol #31 (downloadable at **bfmed.org/protocols**) includes this information and is suitable for sharing with healthcare providers. Hyperthyroidism can be a serious health problem that stresses the heart, muscles, and nervous system, so if a parent's condition is serious, quick treatment may be critical.

Hyperthyroidism medications and lactation. Antithyroid medications, such as propylthiouracil (PTU) and methimazole (Tapazole) and the beta-blocker propranolol (Inderal) are used to treat hyperthyroidism. All are compatible with lactation (T.W. Hale, 2019). In many cases of Graves' disease, medication alone for 12 to 18 months is enough to cause a remission of symptoms.

Radioactive iodine treatment, thyroid surgery, and lactation. Unfortunately, the above medications are not always effective for all types of hyperthyroidism and in all people. Other treatment options include surgical removal of all or part of the thyroid gland, which is compatible with continued nursing, or radioactive iodine treatment, which is not. For details on this last treatment option, see p. 830. Radioactive iodine is also used to treat thyroid cancer.

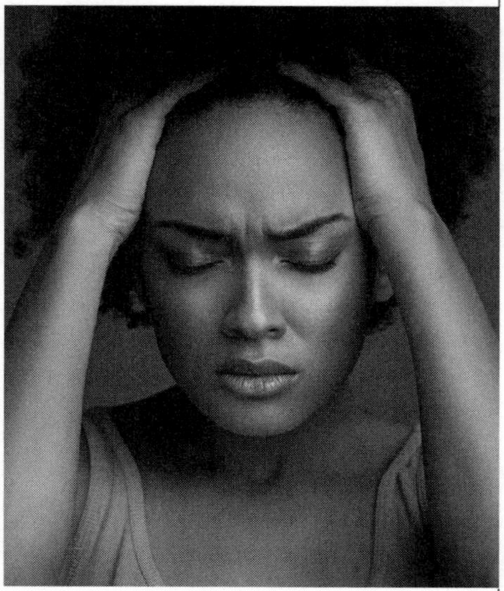

HEADACHES AND LACTATION

Rarely, headaches are associated with the hormonal changes of birth and lactation.

Some headaches, such as migraines, appear to be affected by hormonal fluctuations. For example, migraines tend to be less frequent during pregnancy and after menopause than during other times in life. In one Italian study of migraines during and after pregnancy (Sances et al., 2003), the researchers concluded that breastfeeding protected the mothers from migraine recurrence after birth. If headaches, such as a tension headaches, are not affected by hormonal fluctuations, nursing may have no effect (Marcus, Scharff, & Turk, 1999).

In rare cases, rather than preventing headaches, the hormonal changes that occur during lactation seem to trigger headaches. One U.S. article (Wall, 1992) described four cases (out of a total of about 4,500 lactation calls logged over a 6-year period) of mothers whose migraines became worse during breastfeeding. One breastfeeding mother got relief from her thrice-weekly migraines only when she weaned her 4-month-old twins. Another of these four mothers reported having migraines only during weaning, when her breasts became overly full.

An Australian case report (Thorley, 1997a) also described a mother whose headaches were related to feelings of breast fullness.

Australian author and lactation consultant Virginia Thorley wrote an overview of the cases described in the literature of mothers whose headaches appeared to be associated with breastfeeding (Thorley, 1997b). She noted two types of lactational headaches:

- Headaches that occurred during the first milk ejection, such as the Swedish mother who developed a headache within 2 minutes of every breastfeeding session (Askmark & Lundberg, 1989)
- Headaches that occurred when the mammary glands felt full, as described in the previous paragraph

For an overview on types of headaches occurring during pregnancy and lactation and treatment options, including non-drug therapies, see **bit.ly/BA2-Headaches**.

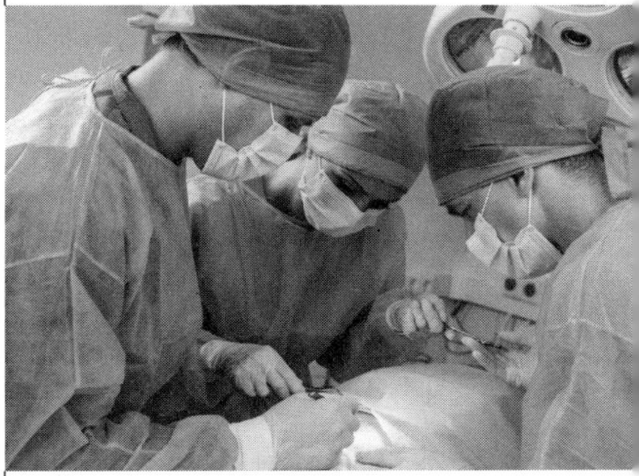

HOSPITALIZATION AND SURGERY

Hospitalization

When discussing hospitalization, talk to parents about their feelings, their situation, and their feeding goals.

Nursing parents needing hospitalization may be as worried about their baby as they are about themselves. Before discussing possible options, first ask for some basic information.

- The reason for the hospitalization and/or surgery and how long the hospital stay is estimated to be
- The ages of any nursing child and any other children
- Their long- and short-term nursing goals
- Plans for the nursing child. Will the child stay with them in the hospital (with an adult helper)? If not, can he visit, and if so, for how much of the day? (Some hospitals will make exceptions to policies if asked.) Will he be cared for elsewhere?
- Available help from family and friends while in the hospital and after
- What the healthcare provider said about nursing
- Availability of lactation consultants and breast pumps at the hospital. If parents need help expressing milk, is the nursing staff knowledgeable and willing?

> **KEY CONCEPT**
>
> *With planning and support, parents can nurse or maintain their milk production while hospitalized.*

For information about the lactation services and equipment available at the hospital, suggest contacting the lactation consultant or patient liaison. Parents—or their advocate—can explain to hospital staff that nursing or expressing milk is a vital part of the parent's medical care, as it will help avoid complications, such as pain and mastitis. If parents are told their child cannot stay with them, suggest asking if arranging for a room in another area, such as the mother-baby unit, would make a difference. If parents are discouraged from nursing or expressing milk due to health concerns, see the first point in this chapter for research on how nursing can help parents recover faster. If the healthcare providers are concerned about a young baby being exposed to organisms in the hospital, explain that a private room will decrease risk.

Feeding goals. If the family's goal is to continue nursing and parents will be separated from their baby for all or part of the hospitalization, discuss milk-expression strategies for maintaining milk production (see p. 504). If parents want to wean or slow milk production temporarily until they are feeling healthier, discuss how to use milk expression to reduce milk production gradually and avoid painful mammary fullness and mastitis (see p. 510).

• • •

Suggest parents ask for the names and spellings of all medications to check their compatibility with lactation.

Suggest making sure all healthcare providers know that parents are lactating, so the medications' compatibility with lactation can be evaluated. For the vast majority of drugs, the amount that passes into the milk is so small that the nursing child will not be affected. The older and heavier the child and the more other foods he eats, the less of a concern this is. If a drug is incompatible with lactation, suggest asking that alternatives be considered.

Suggest the resources listed in Box 13.1 on p. 601 be used to determine the medications' compatibility with lactation, as other resources, such as the *Physician's Desk Reference*, do not include the research and other specific information needed.

• • •

If nursing parents are concerned about their baby feeding well while they're separated or whether the baby will return to nursing later, discuss options and strategies.

Especially if the baby is exclusively nursing, parents may be concerned about their baby accepting a bottle or other feeding method while they're apart. If so, for strategies see p. 647 in Chapter 15, "Employment." Also see the section "Alternative Feeding Methods" on p. 894 for the range of feeding options and their advantages and disadvantages.

If parents are concerned their baby may not return to nursing when they are reunited, tell them most babies nurse after a separation, some willingly and others with coaxing. Tell them that even if the baby is reluctant to nurse at first, with patience and persistence, he will likely be persuaded to nurse again. For details on helping a non-nursing baby make the transition back to nursing, see p. 129. Also reassure parents that the loving care they provide after they are reunited will allay any unhappiness the baby felt while they were hospitalized.

Surgery

Before surgery, suggest nursing parents ask what to expect afterwards, so they can manage lactation safely and comfortably.

After surgery, the parents' condition and level of pain will determine their ability and desire to nurse and care for their child. If parents can plan ahead, are motivated, and have help, it may be possible to directly nurse soon after surgery. While some healthcare facilities put lactation programs in place for nursing parents undergoing surgery (Rieth, Barnett, & Simon, 2018), at this writing, this is the exception rather than the rule. Suggest parents ask their healthcare provider how they will feel after surgery. Depending on the procedure and the parent's condition, some will be alert and in little pain, while others will be completely incapacitated and in need of intensive medical care. Knowing what to expect will help them decide how they want to handle nursing or milk expression after surgery. Some may want to nurse as soon as possible, while others may want or need to wait several days. If there will be a wait, suggest making arrangements to have a rental-grade breast pump available, and if needed, help with expressing milk.

• • •

In most cases after surgery, when the nursing parent is alert and awake enough to hold the baby, it is safe to resume nursing.

After surgery, according to the authors of Academy for Breastfeeding Medicine's Clinical Protocol #15, "Analgesia and Anesthesia for the Breastfeeding Mother" (Reece-Stremtan, Campos, Kokajko, & Academy of Breastfeeding, 2017):

> "Mothers with healthy term or older infants can generally resume breastfeeding as soon as they are awake, stable, and alert. Resumption of normal [alertness] is a hallmark that medications have redistributed from the plasma compartment (and thus the milk compartment) and entered adipose and muscle tissue where they are slowly released."

An interruption of nursing for 6 to 12 hours after the anesthesia was administered is recommended only for parents whose babies are at risk for apnea, low blood pressure, or low muscle tone, such as some preterm babies. If healthcare providers have questions or concerns about the effects of anesthesia on the nursing baby, suggest parents share ABM Clinical Protocol #15, which is available at **bfmed.org/protocols**.

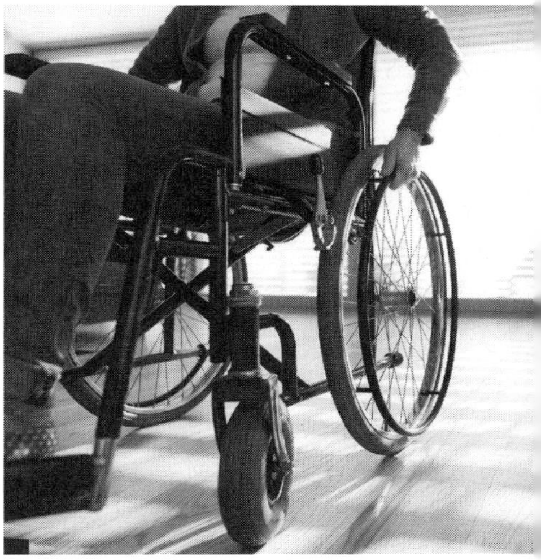

PHYSICAL IMPAIRMENT OR CHALLENGE

A parent with a physical impairment may find the act of nursing challenging, but bottle-feeding may be even more challenging.

A physical impairment may be present at birth or occur as the result of an illness or injury. Parents with physical impairments often decide to nurse their babies for the same reasons as other parents. But there may be more. For many, formula-feeding has significant drawbacks.

- Formula feeding requires buying and preparing bottles. Especially for the visually impaired, measuring and safely preparing bottles may be difficult.
- Statistically, babies who are not human-milk-fed are sick more often, requiring more visits to their healthcare provider with ear infections, digestive issues, respiratory illnesses, and allergy. Parents who do not nurse are also at greater risk of a variety of serious health problems later in life (Louis-Jacques & Stuebe, 2018).
- Bottle-feeding requires an adult to be awake, alert, and upright for feeds, whereas parents can nurse in side-lying positions and rest while baby feeds.

KEY CONCEPT

Fatigue is a common symptom for many parents with disabilities or chronic conditions.

Although many believe that nursing "takes more energy" than bottle-feeding, research found otherwise. For more details, see the first point in this chapter.

• • •

A physical limitation can be the result of a birth defect, an injury, an autoimmune disorder, or other chronic disease.

Physical limitations may be present at birth, such as a missing limb. They may occur after an accident, a spinal cord injury, or stroke. Temporary or permanent loss of function, including swelling, weakness, numbness, and fatigue can occur with autoimmune disorders, such as lupus, multiple sclerosis, myasthenia gravis (MG), and rheumatoid arthritis, as well as carpal tunnel syndrome.

• • •

Parents living with a physical limitation probably already know how to set priorities, but offer to help them brainstorm.

One of the insights described by parents with a chronic illness or physical disability is the necessity of carefully setting their priorities (see the article "The Spoon Theory" at **bit.ly/BA2-SpoonTheory**). They learn from experience ways to simplify their routine and household tasks and adjust their expectations of what really needs to be done to keep their household running. Even so, offer to brainstorm about ways others have simplified their lives after the birth of a baby.

Especially during the early post-birth period, encourage parents to accept offers of help from family and friends supportive of nursing. If no one is available to help with housework and finances allow, suggest hiring household help. What's most important during the first weeks after delivery is that any helpers focus on doing household chores, while parents nurse and establish their relationship with the new baby. Having others handle baby care can prevent them from getting in sync with their baby and gaining confidence in their baby-care skills. Having others care for the baby distances them from their baby during this vulnerable time.

Basic Strategies for Parents with Disabilities

Suggest parents create a "nursing nest" at home where everything is within easy reach and the parent can nurse comfortably.

No matter how a baby is fed and no matter how healthy or able the parent, caring for a newborn can be challenging. To make nursing easier for parents with a physical limitation or impairment, it may help to designate an area of the home a "nursing nest," where the parent can gather everything needed during feeds. Items to have on hand may include water to drink, snacks, clean diapers, a container for used diapers, cleaning supplies for diaper changes, a safe area to lay the baby, a book, phone, tablet, or television (with remote). If there are older children, toys, books, or other entertainment for them would also be a plus. Depending on their preferred nursing positions, this area may include a comfortable chair, chaise lounge, sofa, futon, or bed. Some parents find it easiest to sit or lie on the floor, where dropping the baby is not a concern.

• • •

For some parents, slings, pillows, and other tools may simplify baby care and nursing.

Many parents with physical limitations use ***adaptive equipment***, tools that allow them to more easily accomplish their goals (Powell et al., 2018). For nursing parents, this might include:

- A sling or baby carrier that supports the baby's weight during nursing
- Pillows or cushions for supporting the baby's weight in upright feeding positions or supporting parents' elbows or arms in starter positions (see p. 23-29)

- A nursing bra with velcro closures or closures in front rather than in back
- A bell to tie to the crawling baby's shoes to make his whereabouts known
- A prosthesis for missing arms and/or legs
- A stroller or pram, where they can safely strap the baby while away from home

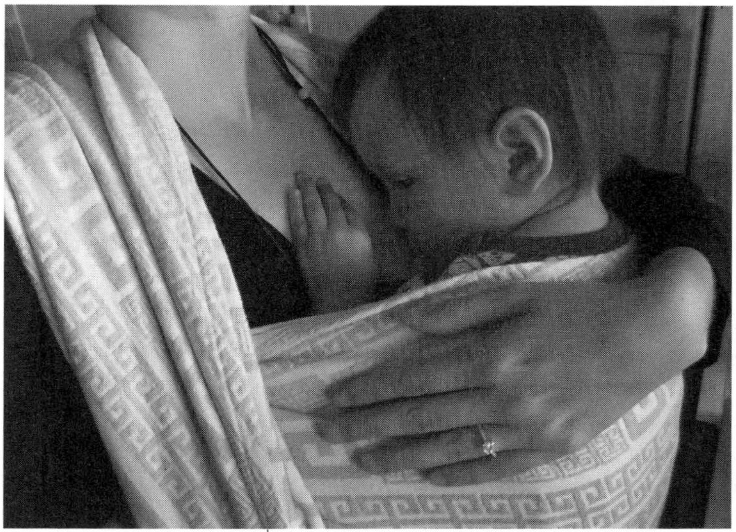

Suggest parents who have difficulty supporting the baby's weight in arms or have chronic fatigue to try nursing in the side-lying (p. 31-32) or starter positions (p. 23-29) described in Chapter 1. Some found it helpful to nurse by leaning over an elevated surface (like a crib or the drawer of a tall dresser). This positioning strategy would only work well if was possible to make it comfortable. For the parent in a wheelchair, diaper/nappy changing areas and sleep surfaces need to be made wheelchair accessible.

Pumping and bottle-feeding. U.S. researchers who conducted a 2018 semi-structured interview study (Powell et al., 2018) spoke by telephone with 25 women with disabilities who breastfed and found that some were unable to find a workable feeding position. These women reported pumping their milk and providing it by bottle instead.

Use of a mirror for pumping in parents with limited neck mobility. In one U.S. case report (Drazin, 1995), a lactation consultant discovered that a mother with limited neck movement from surgery as a child was unable to express milk using a rental breast pump because she could not see to center her nipples in the nipple tunnels. The lactation consultant suggested using a mirror, which allowed the mother to see when her nipples were centered, and she was able to pump effectively.

• • •

Parents with missing limbs have found creative ways to nurse their babies.

A U.S. case report (Dunne & Fuerst, 1995) described the experience of a mother who was a triple amputee who exclusively breastfed her baby, with her partner putting the baby to the breast. When the baby's healthcare provider suggested switching to formula, the mother explained that bottle-feeding would be more difficult for her and involve her less in her baby's care.

An Australian article (Thomson, 1995) described the breastfeeding experience of a mother who was born without part of her lower left arm. This mother breastfed two children, at first using a pillow to support her baby's weight, shaping her breast while leaning forward to put the breast in the baby's mouth. She later found another position that worked for her and her baby, with her baby straddling her thigh, while she leaned slightly forward.

Carpal Tunnel Syndrome

Conservative treatments may resolve carpal tunnel syndrome.

Carpal tunnel syndrome occurs when repetitive hand movements cause swelling in the wrist, which compresses the nerves leading to the hand. Symptoms include hand numbness, tingling, and pain that extends from wrist to shoulder.

When carpal tunnel syndrome develops during pregnancy, it usually resolves without treatment after birth, sometimes taking a month or two to resolve completely. A small number of parents develop carpal tunnel syndrome during the first month of nursing, with symptoms that only completely resolve after weaning (Snell, Coysh, & Snell, 1980; Wand, 1989, 1990).

Carpal tunnel syndrome and the nursing parent. If nursing parents find it painful to support the baby's weight with their arms, suggest as much as possible using the side-lying (p. 31-32) or starter positions (p. 23-29) described in Chapter 1. Suggest using pillows or cushions as needed in upright positions or nursing with baby in a sling or baby carrier. A 2018 Iranian study of 50 women who developed carpal tunnel syndrome during pregnancy (Yazdanpanah, Mousavizadeh, Mousavifard, & Vafaei, 2018) found that after treatment, complete recovery occurred in 11% of the breastfeeding women compared with 53% of those were not lactating. Rates of complete to partial recovery were 1.7 times higher in non-breastfeeding women. The researchers suggested that these differences may be partly due to hormonal differences and partly due to repetitive motions while nursing.

Treatments for carpal tunnel syndrome and lactation. Most parents who developed carpal tunnel syndrome while nursing reported some relief from their symptoms by wearing a splint at night, keeping the hand elevated, and taking diuretic medications. Because these parents had no symptoms later, continuing to nurse while using these conservative treatments is considered appropriate (Yagnik, 1987).

Epilepsy and Other Seizure Disorders

Nursing parents with a seizure disorder can plan ahead to ensure their baby's safety in case of a seizure during feeds.

Epilepsy is a seizure disorder that affects about 1.1 million U.S. women of childbearing age, 20,000 of whom give birth each year (Pschirrer, 2004). Medication is usually so effective at preventing seizures that they are rare, but during pregnancy, many experience more frequent seizures as their body changes and their usual dosage of medication becomes less effective (Yerby, Kaplan, & Tran, 2004).

Epilepsy and the nursing baby. A baby cannot "catch" epilepsy by nursing. In fact, one Canadian study that examined the records of all 124,207 children born between 1986 and 2000 in Nova Scotia (Whitehead et al., 2006) found that not nursing was associated with an increased incidence of epilepsy as the children grew.

Epilepsy and the nursing parent. To create a safe nursing environment in case parents have a seizure (which is important no matter how the baby is fed), suggest they choose a feeding area with padding to protect the baby, such as a bed or a chair with padded arms. If the chair doesn't have padded arms, suggest folding two towels, wrapping and securing them around the chair's arms. This creates a cushion for baby's head during a seizure. Padding and extra pillows may also help parents avoid bruising. Other strategies (Penovich, Eck, & Economou, 2004) include:

- In upright feeding positions, keep their feet elevated (i.e., use a footstool) so that if a seizure occurs the baby would roll back into their lap, not onto the floor.

- If nursing in bed, use guardrails and pillows for padding. A mattress or futon on the floor away from walls would be safer.
- Have a safe surface available on each level of the home, such as a pram, stroller, or portable crib, where parents can lay the baby if they feel a seizure coming.
- Change the baby's diaper/nappy on the floor, or if using a changing table, strap the baby securely, and bathe the baby only when another adult is present.
- When babies and toddlers are crawling and walking, use gates at staircases and doorways to prevent accidents.
- When away from home, suggest attaching a tag or sticker to the pram or stroller with information about epilepsy, the baby's name, and contact information for a friend or relative.

Treatments for epilepsy and lactation. A major concern of many parents with seizure disorders is the compatibility of their medications with lactation. However, the amount of anti-seizure medication the baby receives while nursing is much less than what he received while in utero. Although each nursing couple must be evaluated individually, most of these medications have been thoroughly studied and used in nursing parents for years (T.W. Hale & Berens, 2010, p. 438). Yet despite this, a 2013 Israeli study found that the reason nearly half of the 37 study mothers chose not to breastfeed was concerns about the possibility of their medication harming their baby. The researchers suggested epileptic specialists receive education on this so they can express their support for nursing among these parents. Some anti-epileptic medications, such as phenobarbital, have infrequently been associated with sedation in the newborn (T.W. Hale, 2019, p. 605).

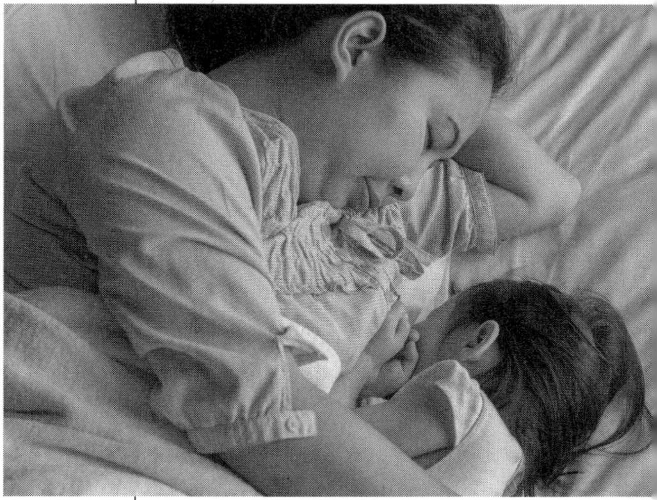

Spinal Cord Injury or Stroke

With a spinal cord injury, the degree of parents' physical limitations will be determined by the location and extent of the spinal injury. In general, the lower the spinal cord injury, the less the loss of function, and the higher and more complete the injury, the more function is lost (Cesario, 2002).

When parents with a spinal cord injury have full use of their arms, nursing is unlikely to be affected.

Lack of nipple sensation. If the spinal cord injury causes complete loss of mammary sensation, milk ejection may be inhibited because the nerve pathways between nipple and brain that trigger milk ejection are no longer functional (Craig, 1990). A 2019 Canadian case report (Lee et al., 2019) described the experience of a mother who incurred a spinal-cord injury while 6 months pregnant with her second baby. She breastfed her first child for 9 months, and despite her T6 injury, which left her without breast sensation, she successfully and exclusively breastfed her second child for nearly 3 months. Two other Canadian articles (Cowley, 2005, 2014) described the experiences of three women with damaged nerve pathways between breast and brain. Because they were unable to feel the sensations of their baby nursing, they learned to trigger milk ejections with mental imagery while their babies were at the breast. In some areas, nasal oxytocin spray is available from compounding pharmacies and can be used to help trigger milk ejection, if needed.

Nursing challenges. The 2019 Canadian case report mentioned above (Lee et al., 2019) described the experiences of a woman nursing a newborn without the full use of the hands and arms. This mother found two feeding positions worked well for her, which she accomplished only with the help of family and aides. One was side-lying, using a wedge behind her back and pillows to support her baby at nipple height. The other position involved sitting up with a nursing pillow wrapped around her waist, which kept her baby at nipple level. A 2018 retrospective survey of 52 women with a history of both spinal-cord injury and breastfeeding (Holmgren et al., 2018) described a wider range of experiences. More than half (28) had high-level injuries at or above T6. Nearly 78% of those with the high-level injuries had milk-production problems, as compared with only 35% with the low-level injuries. Those with the high-level injuries exclusively breastfed their babies for a shorter average duration (3.3 months) compared with those with low-level injuries (6.5 months).

• • •

A stroke can cause partial paralysis and affect parents' vision and judgment.

The most common type of stroke associated with childbirth is caused by a clot that blocks blood flow to the brain (referred to as an ***SSSVT*** or ***superior sagittal sinus venous thrombus***). When parents giving birth suffer a stroke, nursing is often sacrificed as the focus shifts to the parent's health and recovery (Flinn, 1995; Terhaar & Kaut, 1993). But parents who want to nurse in spite of a stroke deserve help. One U.S. article (Halbert, 1998) addressed some of the nursing issues for these parents. The physical effects of the stroke depend upon its severity and which side of the brain is affected. Suggestions for helping nursing parents include: letting them know when the baby needs to feed, providing extra pillows for support, and if paralysis is involved, helping them hold their baby. One U.S. author (Walker, 2017) suggests having parents lie on their affected side so they can use the unaffected arm and hand to help the baby latch. As with any disability, creativity and an open mind will be helpful in finding the strategies that work best.

Visual Impairment

Nursing presents challenges for some visually-impaired parents, but for many, fewer than bottle-feeding.

In parents with any type of sensory impairment, when one of the senses is unavailable, the other senses can be used to enjoy closeness with the baby. A sling or baby carrier can help parents learn to read the baby's hunger cues through movements and changes in breathing. Keeping baby close also promotes strong attachment and responsive parenting.

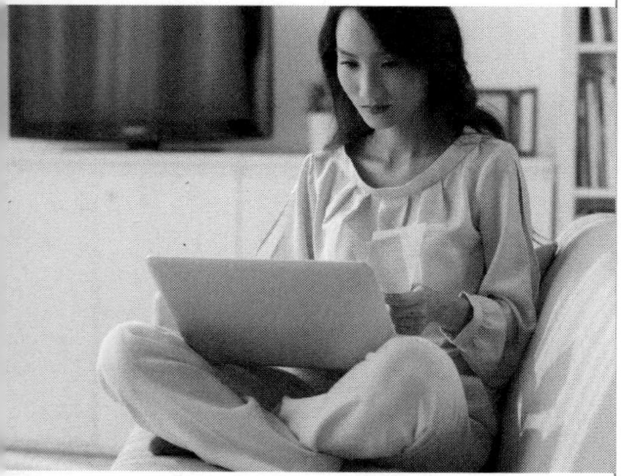

Parents who are completely blind are likely to find nursing easier to manage than formula-feeding, which involves (both at home and in unfamiliar places) measuring, preparing, pouring, and cleaning.

To better help visually impaired parents, ask about their vision limitations and how they usually access information. Some have partial vision and can read large print materials or use magnifying lenses. Others use audio materials, Braille, or computer screen reading programs with a voice synthesizer (Good-Mojab, 1999). When helping parents with latch, remember that much printed material relies on photos and drawings to convey information, which blind parents may not be able to access. Use words and ask permission before touching parent or baby.

VACCINES

Nearly all vaccines given to lactating parents are compatible with nursing.

According to the U.S. Centers for Disease Control and Prevention, with the exception of the smallpox and yellow fever vaccines (which are not recommended during lactation) (CDC, 2019e)

> "[N]either inactivated nor live-virus vaccines administered to a lactating woman affect the safety of breastfeeding for women or their infants.... Limited data (Pickering et al., 1998) indicate that breastfeeding can enhance the response to certain vaccine antigens."

See next point for details.

Timing of the rubella vaccine. The rubella vaccine is not recommended for anyone who may become pregnant within the next 28 days, as the rubella virus is associated with birth defects when contracted during pregnancy (AAP, 2018). In parents without immunity to rubella (which can be determined with a blood test), often immunization after birth is recommended.

• • •

When nursing parents are immunized, their baby also receives temporary protection from illness.

When nursing parents are exposed to an illness, as happens when they are immunized, their body produces antibodies to the illness that pass into the milk. Several studies documented this effect in nursing babies. In one U.S. study (Pickering et al., 1995), mothers were immunized with a rotavirus vaccine during the first month after birth, which provided the breastfeeding babies with passive protection from rotavirus diarrhea for their first 4 months. A U.K. study (Shahid et al., 1995) found that vaccinating pregnant mothers against pneumococci (the leading cause of severe bacterial disease in children worldwide) resulted in passive immunization for their breastfed babies for up to 5 months. These effects are temporary and do not take the place of immunizations for babies. (See p. 293 for details on how nursing enhances a baby's response to infant immunizations.)

• • •

Nursing is not affected when an Rh negative parent receives the Rh immune globulin (RhoGAM) after birth.

When an Rh-negative parent gives birth to an Rh-positive baby, an injection of Rh immune globulin (RhoGAM) is recommended to prevent complications in future pregnancies. Any Rh antibodies in the mother's milk are inactivated in the baby's stomach, so parents should be encouraged to nurse, even when high doses are given (Lawrence & Lawrence, 2016, p. 402).

RESOURCES

bfmed.org/protocols—Free, downloadable, fully referenced clinical protocols in multiple languages are ideal for sharing with healthcare providers from the Academy of Breastfeeding Medicine:

- #15: Analgesia and anesthesia for the breastfeeding mother
- #18: Use of antidepressants in nursing mothers
- #30: Breast masses, breast complaints, and diagnostic breast imaging in the lactating woman
- #31: Radiology and nuclear medicine studies in lactating women

Hale, T. W. (2019). *Hale's Medications & Mothers' Milk: A Manual of Lactational Pharmacology* (18th ed.). New York, NY: Springer Publishing Company.

Kendall-Tackett, K.A. (2017). *Depression in New Mothers: Causes, Consequences and Treatment Alternatives.* New York and London: Routledge.

Lawrence, R. A., & Lawrence, R. M. (2016). *Breastfeeding: A Guide for the Medical Profession* (8th ed.). Philadelphia, PA: Elsevier.

REFERENCES

AAP. (1995). Human milk, breastfeeding, and transmission of human immunodeficiency virus in the United States. *Pediatrics, 96*(5), 977-979.

AAP. (2013). Infant feeding and transmission of human immunodeficiency virus in the United States. *Pediatrics, 131*(2), 391-396.

AAP. (2018). *Red Book: 2018-2021 Report of the Committee on Infectious Diseases* (31st ed.). Elk Grove Village, IL: American Academy of Pediatrics.

Acevedo, M., Pretini, J., Micelli, M., et al. (2017). Breastfeeding initiation, duration, and reasons for weaning in patients with systemic lupus erythematosus. *Rheumatology International, 37*(7), 1183-1186.

ACOG. (2019). Prevention of Group B Streptococcal Early-Onset Disease in Newborns: ACOG Committee Opinion, Number 782. *Obstetrics & Gynecology, 134*(1), e19-e40.

Adab, P., Jiang, C. Q., Rankin, E., et al. (2014). Breastfeeding practice, oral contraceptive use and risk of rheumatoid arthritis among Chinese women: The Guangzhou Biobank Cohort Study. *Rheumatology (Oxford), 53*(5), 860-866.

Adedinsewo, D. A., Fleming, A. S., Steiner, M., et al. (2014). Maternal anxiety and breastfeeding: Findings from the MAVAN (Maternal Adversity, Vulnerability and Neurodevelopment) Study. *Journal of Human Lactation, 30*(1), 102-109.

Akasbi, N., Abourazzak, F. E., & Harzy, T. (2014). Management of pregnancy in patients with rheumatoid arthritis. *OA Musculoskelatal Medicine, 2*(1), 3.

Alderman, C. P., McCarthy, L. C., & Marwood, A. C. (2009). Pharmacotherapy for posttraumatic stress disorder. *Expert Review in Clinical Pharmacology, 2,* 77-86.

Alexander, E. K., Pearce, E. N., Brent, G. A., et al. (2017). 2017 guidelines of the American Thyroid Association for the diagnosis and management of thyroid disease during pregnancy and the postpartum. *Thyroid, 27*(3), 315-389.

Alpert, S. E., & Cormier, A. D. (1983). Normal electrolyte and protein content in milk from mothers with cystic fibrosis: An explanation for the initial report of elevated milk sodium concentration. *Journal of Pediatrics, 102*(1), 77-80.

Amir, L. H., Dennerstein, L., Garland, S. M., et al. (1997). Psychological aspects of nipple pain in lactating women. *Breastfeeding Review, 5,* 29-32.

Anderson, P. O. (2016). Cancer chemotherapy. *Breastfeeding Medicine, 11,* 164-165.

Anderson, P. O. (2018a). Treating diabetes during breastfeeding. *Breastfeeding Medicine, 13*(4), 237-239.

Anderson, P. O. (2018b). Treating hypertension during breastfeeding. *Breastfeeding Medicine, 13*(2), 95-96.

Anderson, P. O. (2019a). Breastfeeding in the multiple sclerosis patient. *Breastfeeding Medicine, 14*(6), 356-358.

Anderson, P. O. (2019b). When the heart is not in it: Breastfeeding with cardiovascular disease. *Breastfeeding Medicine, 14*(2), 80-82.

Ando, Y., Kakimoto, K., Tanigawa, T., et al. (1989). Effect of freeze-thawing breast milk on vertical HTLV-I transmission from seropositive mothers to children. *Japanese Journal of Cancer Research, 80*(5), 405-407.

Ando, Y., Saito, K., Nakano, S., et al. (1989). Bottle-feeding can prevent transmission of HTLV-I from mothers to their babies. *Journal of Infection, 19*(1), 25-29.

Anghelescu, I. G., Kohnen, R., Szegedi, A., et al. (2006). Comparison of Hypericum extract WS 5570 and paroxetine in ongoing treatment after recovery from an episode of moderate to severe depression: Results from a randomized multicenter study. *Pharmacopsychiatry, 39*(6), 213-219.

Askmark, H., & Lundberg, P. O. (1989). Lactation headache—A new form of headache? *Cephalalgia, 9*(2), 119-122.

Asselin, B. L., & Lawrence, R. A. (1987). Maternal disease as a consideration in lactation management. *Clinical Perinatology, 14*(1), 71-87.

ATA. (2020). Postpartum thyroiditis. Retrieved from **thyroid.org/wp-content/uploads/patients/brochures/Postpartum_Thyroiditis_brochure.pdf**.

Azim, H. A., Jr., Bellettini, G., Liptrott, S. J., et al. (2010). Breastfeeding in breast cancer survivors: Pattern, behaviour and effect on breast cancer outcome. *Breast, 19*(6), 527-531.

Baillargeon, J. P., Jakubowicz, D. J., Iuorno, M. J., et al. (2004). Effects of metformin and rosiglitazone, alone and in combination, in nonobese women with polycystic ovary syndrome and normal indices of insulin sensitivity. *Fertility and Sterility, 82*(4), 893-902.

Balcar, V., Silinkova-Malkova, E., & Matys, Z. (1972). Soft tissue radiography of the female breast and pelvic pneumoperitoneum in the Stein-Leventhal syndrome. *Acta Radiologica: Diagnosis, 12*(3), 353-362.

Bascom, E. M., & Napolitano, M. A. (2016). Breastfeeding duration and primary reasons for breastfeeding cessation among women with postpartum depressive symptoms. *Journal of Human Lactation, 32*(2), 282-291.

Becquet, R., Ekouevi, D. K., Menan, H., et al. (2008). Early mixed feeding and breastfeeding beyond 6 months increase the risk of postnatal HIV transmission: ANRS 1201/1202 Ditrame Plus, Abidjan, Cote d'Ivoire. *Preventive Medicine, 47*(1), 27-33.

Belfort, M. B., Drouin, K., Riley, J. F., et al. (2018). Prevalence and trends in donor milk use in the well-baby nursery: A survey of northeast United States birth hospitals. *Breastfeeding Medicine, 13*(1), 34-41.

Berens, P., Swaim, L., & Peterson, B. (2010). Incidence of methicillin-resistant Staphylococcus aureus in postpartum breast abscesses. *Breastfeeding Medicine, 5*(3), 113-115.

Berg, M., Erlandsson, L. K., & Sparud-Lundin, C. (2012). Breastfeeding and its impact on daily life in women with type 1 diabetes during the first six months after childbirth: A prospective cohort study. *International Breastfeeding Journal, 7*(1), 20.

Berlin, C. M. (2007). "Exclusive" breastfeeding of quadruplets. *Breastfeeding Medicine, 2*(2), 125-126. doi:10.1089/bfm.2007.0001

Betzold, C. M., Hoover, K. L., & Snyder, C. L. (2004). Delayed lactogenesis II: A comparison of four cases. *Journal of Midwifery & Women's Health, 49*(2), 132-137.

BHIVA. (2018). General information on infant feeding for women living with HIV. Hertfordshire, UK: British HIV Association.

Blumenthal, J. A., Babyak, M. A., Doraiswamy, P. M., et al. (2007). Exercise and pharmacotherapy in the treatment of major depressive disorder. *Psychosomatic Medicine, 69*(7), 587-596.

Blyton, D. M., Sullivan, C. E., & Edwards, N. (2002). Lactation is associated with an increase in slow-wave sleep in women. *Journal of Sleep Research, 11*(4), 297-303.

Bonifacino, E., Schwartz, E. B., Jun, H., et al. (2018). Effect of lactation on maternal hypertension: A systematic review. *Breastfeeding Medicine, 13*(9), 578-588.

Borra, C., Iacovou, M., & Sevilla, A. (2015). New evidence on breastfeeding and postpartum depression: The importance of understanding women's intentions. *Maternal and Child Health Journal, 19*(4), 897-907.

Brenton, J. N., Engel, C. E., Sohn, M. W., et al. (2017). Breastfeeding during infancy is associated with a lower future risk of pediatric multiple sclerosis. *Pediatric Neurology, 77,* 67-72.

Bryant, P., Morley, C., Garland, S., et al. (2002). Cytomegalovirus transmission from breast milk in premature babies: Does it matter? *Archives of Disease in Childhood. Fetal and Neonatal Edition, 87*(2), F75-77.

Burgess, A., McDowell, W., & Ebersold, S. (2019). Association between lactation and postpartum blood pressure in women with preeclampsia. *MCN: American Journal of Maternal/Child Nursing, 44*(2), 86-93.

Burianova, I., Paulova, M., Cermak, P., et al. (2013). Group B streptococcus colonization of breast milk of group B streptococcus positive mothers. *Journal of Human Lactation, 29*(4), 586-590.

Butte, N. F., Hopkinson, J. M., Mehta, N., et al. (1999). Adjustments in energy expenditure and substrate utilization during late pregnancy and lactation. *American Journal of Clinical Nutrition, 69*(2), 299-307.

Byrne, P. A., Miller, C., & Justus, K. (2006). Neonatal group B streptococcal infection related to breast milk. *Breastfeeding Medicine, 1*(4), 263-270. doi:10.1089/bfm.2006.1.263.

Campo Verde Arbocco, F., Persia, F. A., Hapon, M. B., et al. (2017). Hypothyroidism decreases JAK/STAT signaling pathway in lactating rat mammary gland. *Molecular and Cellular Endocrinology, 450,* 14-23.

Campo Verde Arbocco, F., Sasso, C. V., Actis, E. A., et al. (2016). Hypothyroidism advances mammary involution in lactating rats through inhibition of PRL signaling and induction of LIF/STAT3 mRNAs. *Molecular and Cellular Endocrinology, 419,* 18-28.

Carlsen, S. M., Jacobsen, G., & Vanky, E. (2010). Mid-pregnancy androgen levels are negatively associated with breastfeeding. *Acta Obstetricia et Gynecologica Scandinavica, 89*(1), 87-94.

CDC. (2002). Possible West Nile virus transmission to an infant through breast-feeding--Michigan, 2002. MMWR. *Morbidity and Mortality Weekly Report, 51*(39), 877-878.

CDC. (2016, April 5, 2016). Tuberculosis: TB treatment & pregnancy. Retrieved from **cdc.gov/tb/topic/treatment/pregnancy.htm**.

CDC. (2018a, January 24, 2018). Breastfeeding: Hepatitis B or C infections. Retrieved from **cdc.gov/tb/topic/treatment/pregnancy.html**.

CDC. (2018b, 24 January 2018). Breastfeeding: HIV. Retrieved from **cdc.gov/breastfeeding/breastfeeding-special-circumstances/maternal-or-infant-illnesses/hiv.html**.

CDC. (2018c, 24 May 2018). Breastfeeding: Lyme Disease. Retrieved from **cdc.gov/breastfeeding/breastfeeding-special-circumstances/maternal-or-infant-illnesses/lyme.html**.

CDC. (2018d, 24 January 2018). Breastfeeding: West Nile Virus. Retrieved from **cdc.gov/breastfeeding/breastfeeding-special-circumstances/maternal-or-infant-illnesses/west-nile-virus.html**.

CDC. (2019a, November 2019). Breastfeeding: Influenza. Retrieved from **cdc.gov/breastfeeding/breastfeeding-special-circumstances/maternal-or-infant-illnesses/influenza.html**.

CDC. (2019b, June 2019). Breastfeeding: Methicillin-resistant Staphylococcus aureus (MRSA). Retrieved from **cdc.gov/breastfeeding/breastfeeding-special-circumstances/maternal-or-infant-illnesses/mrsa.html**.

CDC. (2019c, 31 May 2019). Congenital CMV infection. Retrieved from **cdc.gov/cmv/clinical/congenital-cmv.html**.

CDC. (2019d, June 2019). Group B Strep (GBS). Retrieved from **cdc.gov/groupbstrep/**.

CDC. (2019e, 15 November 2019). Vaccine recommendations and guidelines of the ACIP: Special situations. Retrieved from **cdc.gov/vaccines/hcp/acip-recs/general-recs/special-situations.html#breastfeeding**.

CDC. (2020, 17 March 2020). Pregnancy & Breastfeeding: Information about Coronavirus Disease 2019. Retrieved from **cdc.gov/coronavirus/2019-ncov/prepare/pregnancy-breastfeeding.html#anchor_1584169714**.

Cesario, S. K. (2002). Spinal cord injuries. Nurses can help affected women & their families achieve pregnancy birth. *AWHONN Lifelines, 6*(3), 224-232.

Chaudron, L. H. (2007). Treating pregnant women with antidepressants: The gray zone. *Journal of Women's Health (Larchmont), 16*(4), 551-553.

Chevalier, N., & Fenichel, P. (2015). Endocrine disruptors: New players in the pathophysiology of type 2 diabetes? *Diabetes & Metabolism, 41*(2), 107-115.

Cicchetti, D., & Toth, S. L. (1998). The development of depression in children and adolescents. *American Psychologist, 53*(2), 221-241.

Coles, J., Anderson, A., & Loxton, D. (2016). Breastfeeding duration after childhood sexual abuse: An Australian cohort study. *Journal of Human Lactation, 32*(3), NP28-35.

Colombo, C., Costantini, D., Zazzeron, L., et al. (2007). Benefits of breastfeeding in cystic fibrosis: A single-centre follow-up survey. *Acta Paediatrica, 96*(8), 1228-1232.

Confavreux, C., Hutchinson, M., Hours, M. M., et al. (1998). Rate of pregnancy-related relapse in multiple sclerosis. Pregnancy in Multiple Sclerosis Group. *New England Journal of Medicine, 339*(5), 285-291.

Connell, S., Patterson, C., & Newman, B. (2006). A qualitative analysis of reproductive issues raised by young Australian women with breast cancer. *Health Care for Women International, 27*(1), 94-110.

Cordero, L., Treuer, S. H., Landon, M. B., et al. (1998). Management of infants of diabetic mothers. *Archives of Pediatrics and Adolescent Medicine, 152*(3), 249-254.

Cornish, A. M., McMahon, C. A., Ungerer, J. A., et al. (2005). Postnatal depression and infant cognitive and motor development in the second postnatal year: The impact of depression chronicity and infant gender. *Infant Behavior and Development, 28,* 407-417.

Costenbader, K. H., Feskanich, D., Stampfer, M. J., et al. (2007). Reproductive and menopausal factors and risk of systemic lupus erythematosus in women. *Arthritis & Rheumatology, 56*(4), 1251-1262.

Coutsoudis, A., Pillay, K., Kuhn, L., et al. (2001). Method of feeding and transmission of HIV-1 from mothers to children by 15 months of age: Prospective cohort study from Durban, South Africa. *AIDS, 15*(3), 379-387.

Coutsoudis, A., Pillay, K., Spooner, E., et al. (1999). Influence of infant-feeding patterns on early mother-to-child transmission of HIV-1 in Durban, South Africa: A prospective cohort study. South African Vitamin A Study Group. *Lancet, 354*(9177), 471-476.

Cowley, K. C. (2005). Psychogenic and pharmacologic induction of the let-down reflex can facilitate breastfeeding by tetraplegic women: A report of 3 cases. *Archives of Physical Medicine and Rehabilitation, 86*(6), 1261-1264.

Cowley, K. C. (2014). Breastfeeding by women with tetraplegia: Some evidence for optimism. *Spinal Cord, 52*(3), 255.

Craig, D. I. (1990). The adaptation to pregnancy of spinal cord injured women. *Rehabilitation Nursing, 15*(1), 6-9.

D'Andrea, M. A., & Spatz, D. L. (2019). Maintaining breastfeeding during severe infant and maternal HSV-1 infection: A case report. *Journal of Human Lactation, 35*(4), 737-741.

Dalla Costa, G., Romeo, M., Esposito, F., et al. (2019). Caesarean section and infant formula feeding are associated with an earlier age of onset of multiple sclerosis. *Multiple Sclerosis and Related Disorders, 33,* 75-77.

David, F. C. (1985). Lactation following primary radiation therapy for carcinoma of the breast. *International Journal of Radiation Oncology, Biology, Physics, 11*(7), 1425.

Davies, H. A., Clark, J. D., Dalton, K. J., et al. (1989). Insulin requirements of diabetic women who breast feed. *British Medical Journal, 298*(6684), 1357-1358.

De Bortoli, J., & Amir, L. H. (2015). Is onset of lactation delayed in women with diabetes in pregnancy? A systematic review. *Diabetic Medicine, 33*(1), 17-24.

Dennis, C. L., & Chung-Lee, L. (2006). Postpartum depression help-seeking barriers and maternal treatment preferences: A qualitative systematic review. *Birth, 33*(4), 323-331.

Dimitrov, S., Lange, T., Fehm, H. L., et al. (2004). A regulatory role of prolactin, growth hormone, and corticosteroids for human T-cell production of cytokines. *Brain, Behavior, and Immunity, 18*(4), 368-374.

Dinger, J., Muller, D., Pargac, N., et al. (2002). Breast milk transmission of group B streptococcal infection. *Pediatric Infectious Disease Journal, 21*(6), 567-568.

Diniz, J. M., & Da Costa, T. H. (2004). Independent of body adiposity, breast-feeding has a protective effect on glucose metabolism in young adult women. *British Journal of Nutrition, 92*(6), 905-912.

Doan, T., Gardiner, A., Gay, C. L., et al. (2007). Breast-feeding increases sleep duration of new parents. *Journal of Perinatal & Neonatal Nursing, 21*(3), 200-206.

Dong, M., Anda, R. F., Dube, S. R., et al. (2003). The relationship of exposure to childhood sexual abuse to other forms of abuse, neglect, and household dysfunction during childhood. *Child Abuse & Neglect, 27*(6), 625-639.

Doughty, K. N., Ronnenberg, A. G., Reeves, K. W., et al. (2018). Barriers to exclusive breastfeeding among women with gestational diabetes mellitus in the United States. *Journal of Obstetric, Gynecologic & Neonatal Nursing, 47*(3), 301-315.

Drazin, P. B. (1995). Use of a mirror to assist breast pumping. *Journal of Human Lactation, 11*(3), 219.

Dugas, C., Kearney, M., Mercier, R., et al. (2018). Early life nutrition, glycemic and anthropometric profiles of children exposed to gestational diabetes mellitus in utero. *Early Human Development, 118,* 37-41.

Dugat, V. M., Chertok, I. R. A., & Haile, Z. T. (2019). Association between stressful life events and exclusive breastfeeding among mothers in the United States. *Breastfeeding Medicine, 14*(7), 475-481.

Dulek, H., Vural, F., Aka, N., et al. (2019). The prevalence of thyroid dysfunction and its relationship with perinatal outcomes in pregnant women in the third trimester. *Northern Clinics of Istanbul, 6*(3), 267-272.

Dunn, D. T., Newell, M. L., Ades, A. E., et al. (1992). Risk of human immunodeficiency virus type 1 transmission through breastfeeding. *Lancet, 340*(8819), 585-588.

Dunne, G., & Fuerst, K. (1995). Breastfeeding by a mother who is a triple amputee: A case report. *Journal of Human Lactation, 11*(3), 217-218.

Dworsky, M., Yow, M., Stagno, S., et al. (1983). Cytomegalovirus infection of breast milk and transmission in infancy. *Pediatrics, 72*(3), 295-299.

Edenborough, F. P., Borgo, G., Knoop, C., et al. (2008). Guidelines for the management of pregnancy in women with cystic fibrosis. *Journal of Cystic Fibrosis, 7 Supplement 1,* S2-32.

Elfgen, C., Hagenbuch, N., Gorres, G., et al. (2017). Breastfeeding in women having experienced childhood sexual abuse. *Journal of Human Lactation, 33*(1), 119-127.

Fairchild, J. P., Graber, C. D., Vogel, E. H., Jr., et al. (1958). Flora of the umbilical stump; 2,479 cultures. *Journal of Pediatrics, 53*(5), 538-546.

Felitti, V. J. (2009). Adverse childhood experiences and adult health. *Academic Pediatrics, 9*(3), 131-132.

Felitti, V. J., Anda, R. F., Nordenberg, D., et al. (1998). Relationship of childhood abuse and household dysfunction to many of the leading causes of death in adults. The Adverse Childhood Experiences (ACE) Study. *American Journal of Preventive Medicine, 14*(4), 245-258.

Feng, L., Lin, X. F., Wan, Z. H., et al. (2015). Efficacy of metformin on pregnancy complications in women with polycystic ovary syndrome: A meta-analysis. *Gynecological Endocrinology, 31*(11), 833-839.

Fenger-Gron, J., Fenger-Gron, M., Blunck, C. H., et al. (2015). Low breastfeeding rates and body mass index in Danish children of women with gestational diabetes mellitus. *International Breastfeeding Journal, 10,* 26.

Ferris, A. M., Neubauer, S. H., Bendel, R. B., et al. (1993). Perinatal lactation protocol and outcome in mothers with and without insulin-dependent diabetes mellitus. *American Journal of Clinical Nutrition, 58*(1), 43-48.

Festini, F., Ciuti, R., Taccetti, G., et al. (2006). Breast-feeding in a woman with cystic fibrosis undergoing antibiotic intravenous treatment. *Journal of Maternal and Fetal Neonatal Medicine, 19*(6), 375-376.

Field, S. S. (2016). Fatal neonatal herpes simplex infection likely from unrecognized breast lesions. *Journal of Human Lactation, 32*(1), 86-88.

Field, T. (1995). Infants of depressed mothers. *Infant Behavior and Development, 18,* 1-13.

Figueiredo, B., Dias, C. C., Brandao, S., et al. (2013). Breastfeeding and postpartum depression: State of the art review. *Jornal de Pediatria (Rio J), 89*(4), 332-338.

Flaherman, V. J., Beiler, J. S., Cabana, M. D., et al. (2016). Relationship of newborn weight loss to milk supply concern and anxiety: The impact on breastfeeding duration. *Maternal and Child Nutrition, 12*(3), 463-472.

Flinn, N. (1995). A task-oriented approach to the treatment of a client with hemiplegia. *American Journal of Occupational Therapy, 49*(6), 560-569.

Fonseca, A. M., de Souza, A. Z., Bagnoli, V. R., et al. (1985). Histologic and histometric aspects of the breast in polycystic ovary syndrome. *Archives of Gynecology, 237,* 380-381.

Forbes, G. B., Barton, L. D., Nicholas, D. L., et al. (1988). Composition of milk produced by a mother with galactosemia. *Journal of Pediatrics, 113*(1 Pt 1), 90-91.

Forster, D. A., Moorhead, A. M., Jacobs, S. E., et al. (2017). Advising women with diabetes in pregnancy to express breastmilk in late pregnancy (Diabetes and Antenatal Milk Expressing [DAME]): A multicentre, unblinded, randomised controlled trial. *Lancet, 389*(10085), 2204-2213.

Fox-Bacon, C., McCamman, S., Therou, L., et al. (1997). Maternal PKU and breastfeeding: Case report of identical twin mothers. *Clinical Pediatrics (Philadelphia), 36*(9), 539-542.

Freeman, M. P., Hibbeln, J. R., Wisner, K. L., et al. (2006). Omega-3 fatty acids: Evidence basis for treatment and future research in psychiatry. *Journal of Clinical Psychiatry, 67*(12), 1954-1967.

Friedman, M. J., Davidson, J. R. T., & Stein, D. J. (2009). Psychopharmacotherapy for adults. In E. B. Foa, T. M. Keane, M. J. Friedman, & J. A. Cohen (Eds.), *Practice Guidelines from the International Society for Traumatic Stress Studies* (pp. 245-268). New York: Guilford.

Gabbay, M., & Kelly, H. (2003). Use of metformin to increase breast milk production in women with insulin resistance: Case series. *ABM News and Views, 9,* 20.

Galipeau, R., Goulet, C., & Chagnon, M. (2012). Infant and maternal factors influencing breastmilk sodium among primiparous mothers. *Breastfeeding Medicine, 7,* 290-294.

Gastelum, D. T., Dassey, D., Mascola, L., et al. (2005). Transmission of community-associated methicillin-resistant Staphylococcus aureus from breast milk in the neonatal intensive care unit. *Pediatric Infectious Disease Journal, 24*(12), 1122-1124.

Gilljam, M., Antoniou, M., Shin, J., et al. (2000). Pregnancy in cystic fibrosis. Fetal and maternal outcome. *Chest, 118*(1), 85-91.

Glover, A. V., Berry, D. C., Schwartz, T. A., et al. (2018). The association of metabolic dysfunction with breastfeeding outcomes in gestational diabetes. *American Journal of Perinatology, 35*(14), 1339-1345.

Glueck, C. J., Salehi, M., Sieve, L., et al. (2006). Growth, motor, and social development in breast- and formula-fed infants of metformin-treated women with polycystic ovary syndrome. *Journal of Pediatrics, 148*(5), 628-632.

Glueck, C. J., Wang, P., Goldenberg, N., et al. (2004). Pregnancy loss, polycystic ovary syndrome, thrombophilia, hypofibrinolysis, enoxaparin, metformin. *Clinical and Applied Thrombosis/Hemostasis, 10*(4), 323-334.

Good-Mojab, C. (1999). Helping the visually impaired or blind mother breastfeed. *Leaven, 35*(3), 51-56.

Groer, M. W., & Davis, M. W. (2006). Cytokines, infections, stress, and dysphoric moods in breastfeeders and formula feeders. *Journal of Obstetric, Gynecologic & Neonatal Nursing, 35*(5), 599-607.

Groer, M. W., Jevitt, C. M., Sahebzamani, F., et al. (2013). Breastfeeding status and maternal cardiovascular variables across the postpartum. *Journal of Women's Health (Larchmont), 22*(5), 453-459.

Grunwald, F., Palmedo, H., & Biersack, H. J. (1995). Unilateral iodine-131 uptake in the lactating breast. *Journal of Nuclear Medicine, 36*(9), 1724-1725.

Grzeskowiak, L. E., Leggett, C., Costi, L., et al. (2018). Impact of serotonin reuptake inhibitor use on breast milk supply in mothers of preterm infants: A retrospective cohort study. *British Journal of Clinical Pharmacology, 84*(6), 1373-1379.

Gulick, E. E., & Halper, J. (2002). Influence of infant feeding method on postpartum relapse of mothers with MS. *International Journal of MS Care, 4*(4), 4-12.

Hagiya, H., Shiota, S., Sugiyama, W., et al. (2014). Postpartum breast abscess caused by community-acquired methicillin-resistant Staphylococcus aureus in Japan. *Breastfeeding Medicine, 9*(1), 45-46.

Haile, Z. T., Oza-Frank, R., Azulay Chertok, I. R., et al. (2016). Association between history of gestational diabetes and exclusive breastfeeding at hospital discharge. *Journal of Human Lactation, 32*(3), NP36-43.

Halbert, L. A. (1998). Breastfeeding in the woman with a compromised nervous system. *Journal of Human Lactation, 14*(4), 327-331.

Hale, T. W. (2019). *Hale's Medications & Mothers' Milk: A Manual of Lactational Pharmacology* (18th ed.). New York, NY: Springer Publishing Company.

Hale, T. W., & Berens, P. D. (2010). *Clinical Therapy in Breastfeeding Patients.* Amarillo, TX: Hale Publishing.

Hale, T. W., Kristensen, J. H., Hackett, L. P., et al. (2002). Transfer of metformin into human milk. *Diabetologia, 45*(11), 1509-1514.

Hammen, C., & Brennan, P. A. (2002). Interpersonal dysfunction in depressed women: Impairments independent of depressive symptoms. *Journal of Affective Disorders, 72*(2), 145-156.

Hammond, K. A. (1997). Adaptation of the maternal intestine during lactation. *Journal of Mammary Gland Biology and Neoplasia, 2*(3), 243-252.

Hapon, M. B., Simoncini, M., Via, G., et al. (2003). Effect of hypothyroidism on hormone profiles in virgin, pregnant and lactating rats, and on lactation. *Reproduction, 126*(3), 371-382.

Hapon, M. B., Varas, S. M., Jahn, G. A., et al. (2005). Effects of hypothyroidism on mammary and liver lipid metabolism in virgin and late-pregnant rats. *Journal of Lipid Resesarch, 46*(6), 1320-1330.

Hatton, D. C., Harrison-Hohner, J., Coste, S., et al. (2005). Symptoms of postpartum depression and breastfeeding. *Journal of Human Lactation, 21*(4), 444-449; quiz 450-444.

Hay, D. F., Pawlby, S., Sharp, D., et al. (2001). Intellectual problems shown by 11-year-old children whose mothers had postnatal depression. *Journal of Child Psychology and Psychiatry and Allied Disciplines, 42*(7), 871-889.

HDTSG. (2002). Effect of Hypericum perforatum (St John's wort) in major depressive disorder: A randomized controlled trial. *Journal of the American Medical Association, 287*(14), 1807-1814.

Higgins, S., & Haffty, B. G. (1994). Pregnancy and lactation after breast-conserving therapy for early stage breast cancer. *Cancer, 73*(8), 2175-2180.

Hill, R., Law, D., Yelland, C., et al. (2019). Treatment of postpartum psychosis in a mother-baby unit: Do both mother and baby benefit? *Australasian Psychiatry, 27*(2), 121-124.

Hino, S. (1989). Milk-borne transmission of HTLV-I as a major route in the endemic cycle. *Acta Paediatrica Japonica, 31*(4), 428-435.

Hino, S., Katamine, S., Miyata, H., et al. (1997). Primary prevention of HTLV-1 in Japan. *Leukemia, 11 Supplement 3,* 57-59.

Hirata, M., Hayashi, J., Noguchi, A., et al. (1992). The effects of breastfeeding and presence of antibody to p40tax protein of human T cell lymphotropic virus type-I on mother to child transmission. *International Journal of Epidemiology, 21*(5), 989-994.

Holmgren, T., Lee, A. H. X., Hocaloski, S., et al. (2018). The influence of spinal cord injury on breastfeeding ability and behavior. *Journal of Human Lactation, 34*(3), 556-565.

Homer, C. S., Scarf, V., Catling, C., et al. (2014). Culture-based versus risk-based screening for the prevention of group B streptococcal disease in newborns: A review of national guidelines. *Women and Birth, 27*(1), 46-51.

Hoover, K. L., Barbalinardo, L. H., & Platia, M. P. (2002). Delayed lactogenesis II secondary to gestational ovarian theca lutein cysts in two normal singleton pregnancies. *Journal of Human Lactation, 18*(3), 264-268.

Horta, B. L., & de Lima, N. P. (2019). Breastfeeding and type 2 diabetes: Systematic review and meta-analysis. *Current Diabetes Reports, 19*(1), 1.

Hui, L. L., Kwok, M. K., Nelson, E. A. S., et al. (2018). The association of breastfeeding with insulin resistance at 17 years: Prospective observations from Hong Kong's "Children of 1997" birth cohort. *Maternal and Child Nutrition, 14*(1).

Ichimaru, M., Ikeda, S., Kinoshita, K., et al. (1991). Mother-to-child transmission of HTLV-1. *Cancer Detection and Prevention, 15*(3), 177-181.

Illingworth, P. J., Jung, R. T., Howie, P. W., et al. (1986). Diminution in energy expenditure during lactation. *British Medical Journal (Clinical Research Edition), 292*(6518), 437-441.

Isaacs, D. (2000). Neonatal chickenpox. *Journal of Paediatrics and Child Health, 36,* 76-77.

Jacobson, L. T., Hade, E. M., Collins, T. C., et al. (2018). Breastfeeding history and risk of stroke among parous postmenopausal women in the Women's health Initiative. *Journal of the American Heart Association, 7*(17), e008739.

Jacobsson, L. T., Jacobsson, M. E., Askling, J., et al. (2003). Perinatal characteristics and risk of rheumatoid arthritis. *British Medical Journal, 326*(7398), 1068-1069.

Jirakittidul, P., Panichyawat, N., Chotrungrote, B., et al. (2019). Prevalence and associated factors of breastfeeding in women with gestational diabetes in a University Hospital in Thailand. *International Breastfeeding Journal, 14,* 34.

Joham, A. E., Teede, H. J., Ranasinha, S., et al. (2015). Prevalence of infertility and use of fertility treatment in women with polycystic ovary syndrome: Data from a large community-based cohort study. *Journal of Women's Health (Larchmont), 24*(4), 299-307.

Johnson, H. M., & Mitchell, K. B. (2019). Breastfeeding and breast cancer: Managing lactation in survivors and women with a new diagnosis. *Annals of Surgical Oncology, 26*(10), 3032-3039.

Jonas, W., Nissen, E., Ransjo-Arvidson, A. B., et al. (2008). Short- and long-term decrease of blood pressure in women during breastfeeding. *Breastfeeding Medicine, 3*(2), 103-109.

Jones, N. A., McFall, B. A., & Diego, M. A. (2004). Patterns of brain electrical activity in infants of depressed mothers who breastfeed and bottle feed: The mediating role of infant temperament. *Biological Psychology, 67*(1-2), 103-124.

Jones, S. M., & Steele, R. W. (2012). Recurrent group B streptococcal bacteremia. *Clinical Pediatrics (Philadelphia), 51*(9), 884-887.

Kantorowska, A., Wei, J. C., Cohen, R. S., et al. (2016). Impact of donor milk availability on breast milk use and necrotizing enterocolitis rates. *Pediatrics, 137*(3), e20153123.

Kaplan, T. B. (2019). Management of demyelinating disorders in pregnancy. *Neurologic Clinics, 37*(1), 17-30.

Kelly, E., DunnGalvin, G., Murphy, B. P., et al. (2019). Formula supplementation remains a risk for cow's milk allergy in breast-fed infants. *Pediatric Allergy and Immunology.* doi:10.1111/pai.13108.

Kelly, K. M., Chopra, I., & Dolly, B. (2015). Breastfeeding: An unknown factor to reduce heart disease risk among breastfeeding women. *Breastfeeding Medicine, 10*(9), 442-447.

Kendall-Tackett, K. (2007). A new paradigm for depression in new mothers: The central role of inflammation and how breastfeeding and anti-inflammatory treatments protect maternal mental health. *International Breastfeeding Journal, 2,* 6.

Kendall-Tackett, K. (2010). Long-chain omega-3 fatty acids and women's mental health in the perinatal period and beyond. *Journal of Midwifery & Women's Health, 55*(6), 561-567.

Kendall-Tackett, K. (2015). The new paradigm for depression in new mothers: Current findings on maternal depression, breastfeeding and resiliency across the lifespan. *Breastfeeding Review, 23*(1), 7-10.

Kendall-Tackett, K., Cong, Z., & Hale, T. W. (2013). Depression, sleep quality, and maternal well-being in postpartum women with a history of sexual assault: A comparison of breastfeeding, mixed-feeding, and formula-feeding mothers. *Breastfeeding Medicine, 8*(1), 16-22.

Kendall-Tackett, K., & Hale, T. (2009). The use of antidepressants in pregnant and breastfeeding women: A review of recent studies. *Journal of Human Lactation.*

Kendall-Tackett, K. A. (2007). Diagnosis and treatment of posttraumatic stress disorder (PTSD): Compatibility of treatment choices with breastfeeding. *Medications & More, 23* ((October)), 1-3.

Kendall-Tackett, K. A. (2017). *Depression in New Mothers: Causes, Consequences and Treatment Alternatives.* London and New York: Routledge.

Kendall-Tackett, K. A., & Hale, T. W. (2009). Medication use for trauma symptoms and PTSD in pregnant and breastfeeding women. *Trauma Psychology, 4*(2), 12-15.

Kent, N. E., & Farquharson, D. F. (1993). Cystic fibrosis in pregnancy. *Canadian Medical Association Journal, 149*(6), 809-813.

Kiecolt-Glaser, J. K., Derry, H. M., & Fagundes, C. P. (2015). Inflammation: Depression fans the flames and feasts on the heat. *American Journal of Psychiatry, 172*(11), 1075-1091.

Kim, Y. H., Chang, S. S., Kim, Y. S., et al. (2007). Clinical outcomes in methicillin-resistant Staphylococcus aureus-colonized neonates in the neonatal intensive care unit. *Neonatology, 91*(4), 241-247.

Kitajima, H. (2003). Prevention of methicillin-resistant Staphylococcus aureus infections in neonates. *Pediatrics International, 45*(2), 238-245. doi:1719 [pii]

Kjos, S. L., Henry, O., Lee, R. M., et al. (1993). The effect of lactation on glucose and lipid metabolism in women with recent gestational diabetes. *Obstetrics & Gynecology, 82*(3), 451-455.

Klaus, P. (2010). The impact of childhood sexual abuse on childbearing and breastfeeding: The role of maternity caregivers. *Breastfeeding Medicine, 5*(4), 141-145.

Ko, J. Y., Rockhill, K. M., Tong, V. T., et al. (2017). Trends in postpartum depressive symptoms - 27 states, 2004, 2008, and 2012. *MMWR Morbidity and Mortality Weekly Report, 66*(6), 153-158.

Kroon, M., Akkerman-Nijland, A. M., Rottier, B. L., et al. (2018). Drugs during pregnancy and breast feeding in women diagnosed with cystic fibrosis—An update. *Journal of Cystic Fibrosis, 17*(1), 17-25.

Kuhn, L., Sinkala, M., Kankasa, C., et al. (2007). High uptake of exclusive breastfeeding and reduced early post-natal HIV transmission. *PLoS One, 2*(12), e1363.

Kuhn, L., Sinkala, M., Thea, D. M., et al. (2009). HIV prevention is not enough: Child survival in the context of prevention of mother to child HIV transmission. *Journal of the International AIDS Society, 12*(1), 36.

Kujath, A. S., Quinn, L., Elliott, M. E., et al. (2015). Oxytocin levels are lower in premenopausal women with type 1 diabetes mellitus compared with matched controls. *Diabetes/Metabolism Research and Review, 31*(1), 102-112.

Kumar, R. M., & Shahul, S. (1998). Role of breast-feeding in transmission of hepatitis C virus to infants of HCV-infected mothers. *Journal of Hepatology, 29*(2), 191-197. doi:S0168-8278(98)80003-2 [pii].

Lala, M. M., & Merchant, R. H. (2012). Prevention of parent to child transmission of HIV - What is new? *Indian Journal of Pediatrics, 79*(11), 1491-1500.

Langer-Gould, A., Huang, S. M., Gupta, R., et al. (2009). Exclusive breastfeeding and the risk of postpartum relapses in women with multiple sclerosis. *Archives of Neurology, 66*(8), 958-963.

Langer-Gould, A., Smith, J. B., Hellwig, K., et al. (2017). Breastfeeding, ovulatory years, and risk of multiple sclerosis. *Neurology, 89*(6), 563-569.

Lawrence, R. A., & Lawrence, R. M. (2016). *Breastfeeding: A Guide for the Medical Profession* (8th ed.). Philadelphia, PA: Elsevier.

Leal, S. C., Stuart, S. R., & Carvalho Hde, A. (2013). Breast irradiation and lactation: A review. *Expert Review of Anticancer Therapy, 13*(2), 159-164.

Lee, A. H. X., Wen, B., Hocaloski, S., et al. (2019). Breastfeeding before and after spinal cord injury: A case report of a mother with C6 tetraplegia. *Journal of Human Lactation, 35*(4), 742-747.

Lewis, B. A., Schuver, K., Gjerdingen, D., et al. (2016). The relationship between prenatal antidepressant use and the decision to breastfeed among women enrolled in a randomized exercise intervention trial. *Journal of Human Lactation, 32*(3), 67-72.

Linden, K., Berg, M., Adolfsson, A., et al. (2018). Well-being, diabetes management and breastfeeding in mothers with type 1 diabetes—An explorative analysis. *Sexual & Reproductive Healthcare, 15,* 77-82.

Losonsky, G. A., Fishaut, J. M., Strussenberg, J., et al. (1982). Effect of immunization against rubella on lactation products. II. Maternal-neonatal interactions. *Journal of Infectious Diseases, 145*(5), 661-666.

Louis-Jacques, A., & Stuebe, A. M. (2018). Long-term maternal benefits of breastfeeding. *Contemporary OB-GYN, 64*(7).

Lukassek, J., Ignatov, A., Faerber, J., et al. (2019). Puerperal mastitis in the past decade: Results of a single institution analysis. *Archives of Gynecology and Obstetrics, 300*(6), 1637-1644.

Luoma, I., Tamminen, T., Kaukonen, P., et al. (2001). Longitudinal study of maternal depressive symptoms and child well-being. *Journal of the American Academy of Child and Adolescent Psychiatry, 40*(12), 1367-1374.

Lupoli, R., Di Minno, A., Tortora, A., et al. (2014). Effects of treatment with metformin on TSH levels: A meta-analysis of literature studies. *Journal of Clinical Endocrinology and Metabolism, 99*(1), E143-148.

Ma, S., Hu, S., Liang, H., et al. (2019). Metabolic effects of breastfeed in women with prior gestational diabetes mellitus: A systematic review and meta-analysis. *Diabetes/Metabolism Research and Review, 35*(3), e3108.

Maino, F., Cantara, S., Forleo, R., et al. (2018). Clinical significance of type 2 iodothyronine deiodinase polymorphism. *Expert Review of Endocrinology & Metabolism, 13*(5), 273-277.

Mann, T. Z., Haddad, L. B., Williams, T. R., et al. (2018). Breast milk transmission of flaviviruses in the context of Zika virus: A systematic review. *Paediatric and Perinatal Epidemiology, 32*(4), 358-368.

Manns, A., Hisada, M., & La Grenade, L. (1999). Human T-lymphotropic virus type I infection. *Lancet, 353*(9168), 1951-1958.

Marasco, L., Marmet, C., & Shell, E. (2000). Polycystic ovary syndrome: A connection to insufficient milk supply? *Journal of Human Lactation, 16*(2), 143-148.

Marasco, L., & West, D. (2020). *Making More Milk: The Breastfeeding Guide to Increasing Your Milk Production* (2nd ed.). New York, NY: McGraw Hill.

Marcus, D. A., Scharff, L., & Turk, D. (1999). Longitudinal prospective study of headache during pregnancy and postpartum. *Headache, 39*(9), 625-632.

Marshall, A. M., Nommsen-Rivers, L. A., Hernandez, L. L., et al. (2010). Serotonin transport and metabolism in the mammary gland modulates secretory activation and involution. *Journal of Clinical Endocrinology & Metabolism, 95*(2), 837-846.

Matalon, R., Michals, K., & Gleason, L. (1986). Maternal PKU: Strategies for dietary treatment and monitoring compliance. *Annals of the New York Academy of Sciences, 477,* 223-230.

Matias, S. L., Dewey, K. G., Quesenberry, C. P., Jr., et al. (2014). Maternal prepregnancy obesity and insulin treatment during pregnancy are independently associated with delayed lactogenesis in women with recent gestational diabetes mellitus. *American Journal of Clinical Nutrition, 99*(1), 115-121.

McCoy, S. J., Beal, J. M., Shipman, S. B., et al. (2006). Risk factors for postpartum depression: A retrospective investigation at 4-weeks postnatal and a review of the literature. *Journal of the American Osteopathic Association, 106*(4), 193-198.

McManus, R. M., Cunningham, I., Watson, A., et al. (2001). Beta-cell function and visceral fat in lactating women with a history of gestational diabetes. *Metabolism, 50*(6), 715-719.

Mezzacappa, E. S., & Katlin, E. S. (2002). Breast-feeding is associated with reduced perceived stress and negative mood in mothers. *Health Psychology, 21*(2), 187-193.

Michaels, A. M., & Wanner, H. (2013). Breastfeeding twins after mastectomy. *Journal of Human Lactation, 29*(1), 20-22.

Michel, S. H., & Mueller, D. H. (1994). Impact of lactation on women with cystic fibrosis and their infants: A review of five cases. *Journal of the American Dietetic Association, 94*(2), 159-165.

Mitchell, K. B., Fleming, M. M., Anderson, P. O., et al. (2019). ABM Clinical Protocol #31: Radiology and nuclear medicine studies in lactating women. *Breastfeeding Medicine, 14*(5), 290-294.

Montalto, M., & Lui, B. (2009). MRSA as a cause of postpartum breast abscess in infant and mother. *Journal of Human Lactation, 25*(4), 448-450.

Montz, F. J., Schlaerth, J. B., & Morrow, C. P. (1988). The natural history of theca lutein cysts. *Obstetrics & Gynecology*(2), 247-251.

Moran, M. S., Colasanto, J. M., Haffty, B. G., et al. (2005). Effects of breast-conserving therapy on lactation after pregnancy. *Cancer Journal, 11*(5), 399-403.

Moriuchi, M., & Moriuchi, H. (2006). Induction of lactoferrin gene expression in myeloid or mammary gland cells by human T-cell leukemia virus type 1 (HTLV-1) tax: Implications for milk-borne transmission of HTLV-1. *Journal of Virology, 80*(14), 7118-7126.

Morton, J. A. (1994). The clinical usefulness of breast milk sodium in the assessment of lactogenesis. *Pediatrics, 93*(5), 802-806.

Murray, L., Woolgar, M., Cooper, P., et al. (2001). Cognitive vulnerability to depression in 5-year-old children of depressed mothers. *Journal of Child Psychology and Psychiatry and Allied Disciplines, 42*(7), 891-899.

Nakamura, T. (2001). Studies of colonization of MRSA and normal bacterial flora in the upper airway of extremely low birth weight infants. In *Annual Report: Risk Assessments and Preventive Measure for Nosocomial Infections Including MRSA One in Newborns and Infants* (pp. 27-30).

Nam, G. E., Han, K., Kim, D. H., et al. (2019). Associations between breastfeeding and type 2 diabetes mellitus and glycemic control in parous women: A nationwide, population-based study. *Diabetes & Metabolism Journal, 43*(2), 236-241.

Neifert, M. (1992). Breastfeeding after breast surgical procedure or breast cancer. *NAACOGS Clinical Issues in Perinatal Women's Health Nursing, 3*(4), 673-682.

Nelson, L. M., Franklin, G. M., & Jones, M. C. (1988). Risk of multiple sclerosis exacerbation during pregnancy and breast-feeding. *Journal of the American Medical Association, 259*(23), 3441-3443.

Nestler, J. E., & Unfer, V. (2015). Reflections on inositol(s) for PCOS therapy: Steps toward success. *Gynecological Endocrinology, 31*(7), 501-505.

Nguyen, P. T. H., Binns, C. W., Nguyen, C. L., et al. (2019). Gestational diabetes mellitus reduces breastfeeding duration: A prospective cohort study. *Breastfeeding Medicine, 14*(1), 39-45.

Nicholls, K. R., & Cox, J. L. (1999). The provision of care for women with postnatal mental disorder in the United Kingdom: An overview. *Hong Kong Medical Journal, 5*(1), 43-47.

Nommsen-Rivers, L. A. (2016). Does insulin explain the relation between maternal obesity and poor lactation outcomes? An overview of the literature. *Advances in Nutrition, 7*(2), 407-414.

Nommsen-Rivers, L. A., Chantry, C. J., Peerson, J. M., et al. (2010). Delayed onset of lactogenesis among first-time mothers is related to maternal obesity and factors associated with ineffective breastfeeding. *American Journal of Clinical Nutrition, 92*(3), 574-584.

Noviani, M., Wasserman, S., & Clowse, M. E. (2016). Breastfeeding in mothers with systemic lupus erythematosus. *Lupus, 25*(9), 973-979.

Nyambi, P. N., Ville, Y., Louwagie, J., et al. (1996). Mother-to-child transmission of human T-cell lymphotropic virus types I and II (HTLV-I/II) in Gabon: A prospective follow-up of 4 years. *Journal of Acquired Immune Deficiency Syndromes and Human Retrovirology, 12*(2), 187-192.

Ohlsson, A., Nasiell, J., & von Dobeln, U. (2007). Pregnancy and lactation in a woman with classical galactosaemia heterozygous for p.Q188R and p.R333W. *Journal of Inherited Metabolic Disease, 30*(1), 105. doi:10.1007/s10545-006-0383-z.

Oki, T., Yoshinaga, M., Otsuka, H., et al. (1992). A sero-epidemiological study on mother-to-child transmission of HTLV-I in southern Kyushu, Japan. *Asia-Oceania Journal of Obstetrics and Gynaecology, 18*(4), 371-377.

Owen, C. G., Martin, R. M., Whincup, P. H., et al. (2006). Does breastfeeding influence risk of type 2 diabetes in later life? A quantitative analysis of published evidence. *American Journal of Clinical Nutrition, 84*(5), 1043-1054. doi:84/5/1043 [pii].

Ozisik, H., Suner, A., & Cetinkalp, S. (2019). Prolactin effect on blood glucose and insulin in breastfeeding women. *Diabetes & Metabolic Syndrome: Clinical Research & Review, 13*(3), 1765-1767.

Paiva, A. M., Assone, T., Haziot, M. E. J., et al. (2018). Risk factors associated with HTLV-1 vertical transmission in Brazil: Longer breastfeeding, higher maternal proviral load and previous HTLV-1-infected offspring. *Scientific Reports, 8*(1), 7742.

Panchaud, A., Di Paolo, E. R., Koutsokera, A., et al. (2016). Safety of drugs during pregnancy and breastfeeding in cystic fibrosis patients. *Respiration, 91*(4), 333-348.

Panda, S., Tahiliani, P., & Kar, A. (1999). Inhibition of triiodothyronine production by fenugreek seed extract in mice and rats. *Pharmacological Research, 40*(5), 405-409.

Penovich, P. E., Eck, K. E., & Economou, V. V. (2004). Recommendations for the care of women with epilepsy. *Cleveland Clinic Journal of Medicine, 71 Suppl 2,* S49-57.

Perrine, C. G., & Scanlon, K. S. (2013). Prevalence of use of human milk in US advanced care neonatal units. *Pediatrics, 131*(6), 1066-1071.

Peters, S. A. E., Yang, L., Guo, Y., et al. (2017). Breastfeeding and the risk of maternal cardiovascular disease: A prospective study of 300 000 Chinese women. *Journal of the American Heart Association, 6*(6).

Peterson, B. (2007). Incidence of MRSA in postpartum breast abscesses [abstract]. *Breastfeeding Medicine, 2*(3), 190.

Pfaender, S., Vielle, N. J., Ebert, N., et al. (2017). Inactivation of Zika virus in human breast milk by prolonged storage or pasteurization. *Virus Research, 228,* 58-60.

Philipp, M., Kohnen, R., & Hiller, K. O. (1999). Hypericum extract versus imipramine or placebo in patients with moderate depression: Randomised multicentre study of treatment for eight weeks. *British Medical Journal, 319*(7224), 1534-1538.

Pickering, L. K., Granoff, D. M., Erickson, J. R., et al. (1998). Modulation of the immune system by human milk and infant formula containing nucleotides. *Pediatrics, 101*(2), 242-249.

Pickering, L. K., Morrow, A. L., Herrera, I., et al. (1995). Effect of maternal rotavirus immunization on milk and serum antibody titers. *Journal of Infectious Diseases, 172*(3), 723-728.

Piescik-Lech, M., Chmielewska, A., Shamir, R., et al. (2017). Systematic review: Early infant feeding and the risk of type 1 diabetes. *Journal of Pediatric Gastroenterology and Nutrition, 64*(3), 454-459.

Pikwer, M., Bergstrom, U., Nilsson, J. A., et al. (2009). Breast feeding, but not use of oral contraceptives, is associated with a reduced risk of rheumatoid arthritis. *Annals of the Rheumatic Diseases, 68*(4), 526-530.

Pisacane, A., Impagliazzo, N., Russo, M., et al. (1994). Breast feeding and multiple sclerosis. *British Medical Journal, 308*(6941), 1411-1412.

Pistilli, B., Bellettini, G., Giovannetti, E., et al. (2013). Chemotherapy, targeted agents, antiemetics and growth-factors in human milk: How should we counsel cancer patients about breastfeeding? *Cancer Treatment Reviews, 39*(3), 207-211.

Portaccio, E., & Amato, M. P. (2019). Breastfeeding and post-partum relapses in multiple sclerosis patients. *Multiple Sclerosis, 25*(9), 1211-1216.

Powell, R. M., Mitra, M., Smeltzer, S. C., et al. (2018). Breastfeeding among women with physical disabilities in the United States. *Journal of Human Lactation, 34*(2), 253-261.

Prentice, J. C., Lu, M. C., Lange, L., et al. (2002). The association between reported childhood sexual abuse and breastfeeding initiation. *Journal of Human Lactation, 18*(3), 219-226.

Pschirrer, E. R. (2004). Seizure disorders in pregnancy. *Obstetrics and Gynecology Clinics of North America, 31*(2), 373-384, vii.

Puopolo, K. M., Lynfield, R., Cummings, J. J., et al. (2019). Management of infants at risk for Group B Streptococcal disease. *Pediatrics, 144*(2).

Purnell, H. (2001). Phenylketonuria and maternal phenylketonuria. *Breastfeeding Review, 9*(2), 19-21.

Qiu, L., Binns, C. W., Zhao, Y., et al. (2010). Hepatitis B and breastfeeding in Hangzhou, Zhejiang Province, People's Republic of China. *Breastfeeding Medicine, 5*(3), 109-112.

Qu, G., Wang, L., Tang, X., et al. (2018). Association between duration of breastfeeding and maternal hypertension: A systematic review and meta-analysis. *Breastfeeding Medicine, 13*(5), 318-326.

Ram, K. T., Bobby, P., Hailpern, S. M., et al. (2008). Duration of lactation is associated with lower prevalence of the metabolic syndrome in midlife--SWAN, the study of women's health across the nation. *American Journal of Obstetrics & Gynecology, 198*(3), 268 e261-266.

Rapkin, A. J., Mikacich, J. A., Moatakef-Imani, B., et al. (2002). The clinical nature and formal diagnosis of premenstrual, postpartum, and perimenopausal affective disorders: *Current Psychiatry Reports, 4*(6), 419-428.

Reece-Stremtan, S., Campos, M., Kokajko, L., et al. (2017). ABM Clinical Protocol #15: Analgesia and anesthesia for the breastfeeding mother, revised 2017. *Breastfeeding Medicine, 12*(9), 500-506.

Reinheimer, S. M., Schmidt, M. I., Duncan, B. B., et al. (2019). Factors associated with breastfeeding among women with gestational diabetes. *Journal of Human Lactation.* doi:10.1177/0890334419845871.

Resti, M., Azzari, C., Mannelli, F., et al. (1998). Mother to child transmission of hepatitis C virus: Prospective study of risk factors and timing of infection in children born to women seronegative for HIV-1. Tuscany Study Group on Hepatitis C Virus Infection. *British Medical Journal, 317*(7156), 437-441.

Rieth, E. F., Barnett, K. M., & Simon, J. A. (2018). Implementation and organization of a perioperative lactation program: A descriptive study. *Breastfeeding Medicine, 13*(2), 97-105.

Rimoldi, S. G., Pileri, P., Mazzocco, M. I., et al. (2019). The role of Staphylococcus aureus in mastitis: A multidisciplinary working group experience. *Journal of Human Lactation,* 890334419876272.

Robinson, P. S., Barker, P., Campbell, A., et al. (1994). Iodine-131 in breast milk following therapy for thyroid carcinoma. *Journal of Nuclear Medicine, 35*(11), 1797-1801.

Rosadas, C., Malik, B., Taylor, G. P., et al. (2018). Estimation of HTLV-1 vertical transmission cases in Brazil per annum. *PLoS Neglected Tropical Diseases, 12*(11), e0006913.

Rose, M. R., Prescott, M. C., & Herman, K. J. (1990). Excretion of iodine-123-hippuran, technetium-99m-red blood cells, and technetium-99m-macroaggregated albumin into breast milk. *Journal of Nuclear Medicine, 31*(6), 978-984.

Rosenbauer, J., Herzig, P., Kaiser, P., et al. (2007). Early nutrition and risk of type 1 diabetes mellitus--A nationwide case-control study in preschool children. *Experimental and Clinical Endocrinology & Diabetes, 115*(8), 502-508.

Ruiz-Extremera, A., Salmeron, J., Torres, C., et al. (2000). Follow-up of transmission of hepatitis C to babies of human immunodeficiency virus-negative women: The role of breast-feeding in transmission. *Pediatric Infectious Disease Journal, 19*(6), 511-516.

Rupke, S. J., Blecke, D., & Renfrow, M. (2006). Cognitive therapy for depression. *American Family Physician, 73*(1), 83-86.

Saenz, R. B. (2000). Iodine-131 elimination from breast milk: A case report. *Journal of Human Lactation, 16*(1), 44-46.

Safirstein, J. G., Ro, A. S., Grandhi, S., et al. (2012). Predictors of left ventricular recovery in a cohort of peripartum cardiomyopathy patients recruited via the internet. *International Journal of Cardiology, 154*(1), 27-31.

Salgado, C. D., Farr, B. M., & Calfee, D. P. (2003). Community-acquired methicillin-resistant Staphylococcus aureus: A meta-analysis of prevalence and risk factors. *Clinical Infectious Diseases, 36*(2), 131-139.

Sampieri, C. L., & Montero, H. (2019). Breastfeeding in the time of Zika: A systematic literature review. *PeerJ, 7,* e6452.

Sances, G., Granella, F., Nappi, R. E., et al. (2003). Course of migraine during pregnancy and postpartum: A prospective study. *Cephalalgia, 23*(3), 197-205.

Schlaudecker, E. R. (2021). Viral infections and breastfeeding. In K. Wambach & B. Spencer (Eds.), *Breastfeeding and Human Lactation* (6th ed., pp. 159-174). Burlington, MA: Jones & Bartlett Learning.

Schleiss, M. R. (2006). Acquisition of human cytomegalovirus infection in infants via breast milk: Natural immunization or cause for concern? *Reviews in Medical Virology, 16*(2), 73-82.

Schwarz, E. B., Ray, R. M., Stuebe, A. M., et al. (2009). Duration of lactation and risk factors for maternal cardiovascular disease. *Obstetrics & Gynecology, 113*(5), 974-982.

Sealander, J. Y., & Kerr, C. P. (1989). Herpes simplex of the nipple: Infant-to-mother transmission. *American Family Physician, 39*(3), 111-113.

Sen, S., Benjamin, C., Riley, J., et al. (2018). Donor milk utilization for healthy infants: Experience at a single academic center. *Breastfeeding Medicine, 13*(1), 28-33.

Shahid, N. S., Steinhoff, M. C., Hoque, S. S., et al. (1995). Serum, breast milk, and infant antibody after maternal immunisation with pneumococcal vaccine. *Lancet, 346*(8985), 1252-1257.

Sharma, V. (2018). Weaning and mixed mania-A case report. *Journal of Human Lactation, 34*(4), 745-748.

Shiffman, M. L., Seale, T. W., Flux, M., et al. (1989). Breast-milk composition in women with cystic fibrosis: Report of two cases and a review of the literature. *American Journal of Clinical Nutrition, 49*(4), 612-617.

Shub, A., Miranda, M., Georgiou, H. M., et al. (2019). The effect of breastfeeding on postpartum glucose tolerance and lipid profiles in women with gestational diabetes mellitus. *International Breastfeeding Journal, 14,* 46.

Simard, J. F., Karlson, E. W., Costenbader, K. H., et al. (2008). Perinatal factors and adult-onset lupus. *Arthritis & Rheumatology, 59*(8), 1155-1161.

Simmons, D., Conroy, C., & Thompson, C. F. (2005). In-hospital breast feeding rates among women with gestational diabetes and pregestational type 2 diabetes in South Auckland. *Diabetes Medicine, 22*(2), 177-181.

Sirmans, S. M., & Pate, K. A. (2013). Epidemiology, diagnosis, and management of polycystic ovary syndrome. *Clinical Epidemiology, 6,* 1-13.

Snell, N. J., Coysh, H. L., & Snell, B. J. (1980). Carpal tunnel syndrome presenting in the puerperium. *Practitioner, 224*(1340), 191-193.

Spiesser-Robelet, L., Maurice, A., & Gagnayre, R. (2019). Understanding breastfeeding women's behaviors toward medication: Healthcare professionals' viewpoint. *Journal of Human Lactation, 35*(1), 137-153.

Stafford, I., Hernandez, J., Laibl, V., et al. (2008). Community-acquired methicillin-resistant Staphylococcus aureus among patients with puerperal mastitis requiring hospitalization. *Obstetrics & Gynecology, 112*(3), 533-537.

Stage, E., Norgard, H., Damm, P., et al. (2006). Long-term breast-feeding in women with type 1 diabetes. *Diabetes Care, 29*(4), 771-774.

Stopenski, S., Aslam, A., Zhang, X., et al. (2017). After chemotherapy treatment for maternal cancer during pregnancy, is breastfeeding possible? *Breastfeeding Medicine, 12,* 91-97.

Strapasson, M. R., Ferreira, C. F., & Ramos, J. G. L. (2018). Feeding practices in the first 6 months after delivery: Effects of gestational hypertension. *Pregnancy Hypertension, 13,* 254-259.

Stuebe, A. (2019). Does breastfeeding prevent metabolic disease or does metabolic disease prevent breastfeeding? *British Journal of Obstetrics and Gynaecology, 126*(4), 535.

Stuebe, A. M., Bonuck, K., Adatorwovor, R., et al. (2016). A cluster randomized trial of tailored breastfeeding support for women with gestational diabetes. *Breastfeeding Medicine, 11,* 504-513.

Stuebe, A. M., Meltzer-Brody, S., Propper, C., et al. (2019). The Mood, Mother, and Infant study: Associations between maternal mood in pregnancy and breastfeeding outcome. *Breastfeeding Medicine, 14*(8), 551-559.

Stuebe, A. M., Michels, K. B., Willett, W. C., et al. (2009). Duration of lactation and incidence of myocardial infarction in middle to late adulthood. *American Journal of Obstetrics & Gynecology, 200*(2), 138 e131-138.

Stuebe, A. M., Rich-Edwards, J. W., Willett, W. C., et al. (2005). Duration of lactation and incidence of type 2 diabetes. *Journal of the American Medical Association, 294*(20), 2601-2610.

Sullivan-Bolyai, J. Z., Fife, K. H., Jacobs, R. F., et al. (1983). Disseminated neonatal herpes simplex virus type 1 from a maternal breast lesion. *Pediatrics, 71*(3), 455-457.

Szegedi, A., Kohnen, R., Dienel, A., et al. (2005). Acute treatment of moderate to severe depression with hypericum extract WS 5570 (St John's wort): Randomised controlled double blind non-inferiority trial versus paroxetine. *British Medical Journal, 330*(7490), 503.

Tajima, K. (1988). Malignant lymphomas in Japan: Epidemiological analysis of adult T-cell leukemia/lymphoma (ATL). *Cancer Metastasis Reviews, 7*(3), 223-241.

Takahashi, K., Takezaki, T., Oki, T., et al. (1991). Inhibitory effect of maternal antibody on mother-to-child transmission of human T-lymphotropic virus type I. The Mother-to-Child Transmission Study Group. *International Journal of Cancer, 49*(5), 673-677.

Takezaki, T., Tajima, K., Ito, M., et al. (1997). Short-term breast-feeding may reduce the risk of vertical transmission of HTLV-I. The Tsushima ATL Study Group. *Leukemia, 11 Supplement 3,* 60-62.

Tamminen, T. M., & Salmelin, R. K. (1991). Psychosomatic interaction between mother and infant during breast feeding. *Psychotherapy and Psychosomatics, 56*(1-2), 78-84.

Terhaar, M. F., & Kaut, K. (1993). Perinatal superior sagittal sinus venous thrombosis. *Journal of Perinatal and Neonatal Nursing, 7*(1), 35-48.

Teychenne, M., & York, R. (2013). Physical activity, sedentary behavior, and postnatal depressive symptoms: A review. *American Journal of Preventive Medicine, 45*(2), 217-227.

Thatcher, S. S., & Jackson, E. M. (2006). Pregnancy outcome in infertile patients with polycystic ovary syndrome who were treated with metformin. *Fertility and Sterility, 85*(4), 1002-1009.

Thomson, V. M. (1995). Breastfeeding and mothering one-handed. *Journal of Human Lactation, 11*(3), 211-215.

Thorley, V. (1997a). Lactational headache: A lactation consultant's diary. *Journal of Human Lactation, 13*(1), 51-53.

Thorley, V. (1997b). Lactational headaches. *Breastfeeding Review, 5*(1), 23-25.

Tralins, A. H. (1995). Lactation after conservative breast surgery combined with radiation therapy. *American Journal of Clinical Oncology, 18*(1), 40-43.

Tsuji, Y., Doi, H., Yamabe, T., et al. (1990). Prevention of mother-to-child transmission of human T-lymphotropic virus type-I. *Pediatrics, 86*(1), 11-17.

Ukah, U. V., Adu, P. A., De Silva, D. A., et al. (2016). The impact of a history of adverse childhood experiences on breastfeeding initiation and exclusivity: Findings from a national population health survey. *Breastfeeding Medicine, 11,* 544-550.

Unfer, V., Nestler, J. E., Kamenov, Z. A., et al. (2016). Effects of inositol(s) in women with PCOS: A systematic review of randomized controlled trials. *International Journal of Endocrinology, 2016,* 1849162.

Urashima, M., Mezawa, H., Okuyama, M., et al. (2019). Primary prevention of cow's milk sensitization and food allergy by avoiding supplementation with cow's milk formula at birth: A randomized clinical trial. *JAMA Pediatrics.* doi:10.1001/jamapediatrics.2019.3544.

Uvnas-Moberg, K. (1998). Antistress pattern induced by oxytocin. *News in Physiological Sciences, 13,* 22-25.

van Gurp, G., Meterissian, G. B., Haiek, L. N., et al. (2002). St John's wort or sertraline? Randomized controlled trial in primary care. *Canadian Family Physician, 48,* 905-912.

van Tienen, C., Jakobsen, M., & Schim van der Loeff, M. (2012). Stopping breastfeeding to prevent vertical transmission of HTLV-1 in resource-poor settings: Beneficial or harmful? *Archives of Gynecology and Obstetrics, 286*(1), 255-256.

Vanky, E., Isaksen, H., Moen, M. H., et al. (2008). Breastfeeding in polycystic ovary syndrome. *Acta Obstetricia et Gynecologica Scandinavica, 87*(5), 531-535.

Velle-Forbord, V., Skrastad, R. B., Salvesen, O., et al. (2019). Breastfeeding and long-term maternal metabolic health in the HUNT Study: A longitudinal population-based cohort study. *British Journal of Obstetrics and Gynaecology, 126*(4), 526-534.

Walker, M. (2017). *Breastfeeding Management for the Clinician: Using the Evidence* (4th ed.). Burlington, MA: Jones & Bartlett Learning.

Wall, V. R. (1992). Breastfeeding and migraine headaches. *Journal of Human Lactation, 8*(4), 209-212.

Wallenborn, J. T., Perera, R. A., & Masho, S. W. (2017). Breastfeeding after gestational diabetes: Does perceived benefits mediate the relationship? *Journal of Pregnancy, 2017,* 9581796.

Wambach, K., & Morrison, B. (2021). Women's health and breastfeeding. In K. Wambach & B. Spencer (Eds.), *Breastfeeding and Human Lactation* (6th ed., pp. 481-547). Burlington, MA: Jones & bartlett Learning.

Wand, J. S. (1989). The natural history of carpal tunnel syndrome in lactation. *Journal of the Royal Society of Medicine, 82*(6), 349-350.

Wand, J. S. (1990). Carpal tunnel syndrome in pregnancy and lactation. *Journal of Hand Surgery. British Volume, 15*(1), 93-95.

Wang, L. Y., Chen, C. T., Liu, W. H., et al. (2007). Recurrent neonatal group B streptococcal disease associated with infected breast milk. *Clinical Pediatrics (Philadelphia), 46*(6), 547-549.

Watkins, S., Meltzer-Brody, S., Zolnoun, D., et al. (2011). Early breastfeeding experiences and postpartum depression. *Obstetrics & Gynecology, 118*(2 Pt 1), 214-221.

Webster, J., Moore, K., & McMullan, A. (1995). Breastfeeding outcomes for women with insulin dependent diabetes. *Journal of Human Lactation, 11*(3), 195-200.

Weissman, M. M. (2007). Recent non-medication trials of interpersonal psychotherapy for depression. *International Journal of Neuropsychopharmacology, 10*(1), 117-122.

Welch, M. J., Phelps, D. L., & Osher, A. B. (1981). Breast-feeding by a mother with cystic fibrosis. *Pediatrics, 67*(5), 664-666.

Whitehead, E., Dodds, L., Joseph, K. S., et al. (2006). Relation of pregnancy and neonatal factors to subsequent development of childhood epilepsy: A population-based cohort study. *Pediatrics, 117*(4), 1298-1306.

WHO. (1987). *Special Programme on AIDS Statement: Breast-feeding/Breast Milk and Human Immunodeficiency Virus (HIV).* In. Geneva, Switzerland: World Health Organization.

WHO. (1996). *Hepatitis B and Breastfeeding.* Geneva, Switzerland: World Health Organization.

WHO. (2010). *Guidelines on HIV and Infant Feeding.* Geneva, Switzerland: World Health Organization.

WHO. (2016). Infant feeding in areas of Zika virus transmission: Summary of rapid advice guideline 29 June 2016. Retrieved from **apps.who.int/iris/bitstream/handle/10665/204473/WHO_ZIKV_MOC_16.5_eng.pdf?sequence=1**.

WHO, & UNICEF. (2016). *Guideline Updates on HIV and Infant Feeding.* Geneva, Switzerland: World Health Organization.

Wiersinga, W.M. (2017). Therapy of endocrinology disease: T4 + T3 combination therapy: Is there a true effect? *European Journal of Endocrinology, 177*(6), R287-R296.

Wiffen, J., & Fetherston, C. (2016). Relationships between assisted reproductive technologies and initiation of lactation: Preliminary observations. *Breastfeeding Review, 24*(1), 21-27.

Wiktor, S. Z., Pate, E. J., Murphy, E. L., et al. (1993). Mother-to-child transmission of human T-cell lymphotropic virus type I (HTLV-I) in Jamaica: Association with antibodies to envelope glycoprotein (gp46) epitopes. *Journal of Acquired Immune Deficiency Syndome, 6*(10), 1162-1167.

Williams, D., Webber, J., Pell, B., et al. (2019). "Nobody knows, or seems to know how rheumatology and breastfeeding works": Women's experiences of breastfeeding whilst managing a long-term limiting condition—A qualitative visual methods study. *Midwifery, 78,* 91-96.

Wilson-Clay, B. (2008). Case report of methicillin-resistant Staphylococcus aureus (MRSA) mastitis with abscess formation in a breastfeeding woman. *Journal of Human Lactation, 24*(3), 326-329.

Woelk, H. (2000). Comparison of St John's wort and imipramine for treating depression: Randomised controlled trial. *British Medical Journal, 321*(7260), 536-539.

Yagnik, P. M. (1987). Carpal tunnel syndrome in nursing mothers. *Southern Medical Journal, 80*(11), 1468.

Yasuhi, I., Soda, T., Yamashita, H., et al. (2017). The effect of high-intensity breastfeeding on postpartum glucose tolerance in women with recent gestational diabetes. *International Breastfeeding Journal, 12,* 32.

Yazdanpanah, P., Mousavizadeh, A., Mousavifard, P., et al. (2018). Comparison course of pregnancy related carpal tunnel syndrome in breastfeeding and non-breastfeeding women during the first 6 months after delivery [abstract]. *Annals of Physical Rehabilitation Medicine, 61S,* e116.

Yerby, M. S., Kaplan, P., & Tran, T. (2004). Risks and management of pregnancy in women with epilepsy. *Cleveland Clinic Journal of Medicine, 71 Supplement 2,* S25-37.

Yusuff, A. S., Tang, L., Binns, C. W., et al. (2016). Breastfeeding and postnatal depression: A prospective cohort study in Sabah, Malaysia. *Journal of Human Lactation, 32*(2), 277-281.

Zdrojewicz, Z., Popowicz, E., Szyca, M., et al. (2017). TOFI phenotype—Its effect on the occurrence of diabetes. *Pediatric Endocrinology, Diabetes and Metabolism, 23*(2), 96-100.

Zhao, J., Liu, X., & Zhang, W. (2018). The effect of metformin therapy for preventing gestational diabetes mellitus in women with polycystic ovary syndrome: A meta-analysis. *Experimental and Clinical Endocrinology & Diabetes.*

Zihlmann, K. F., Mazzaia, M. C., & de Alvarenga, A. T. (2017). Meaning of breastfeeding interruption due to infection by human T cell lymphotrophic virus type 1 (HTLV-1). *Acta Paulista de Enfermagem, 30*(1), 80-88.

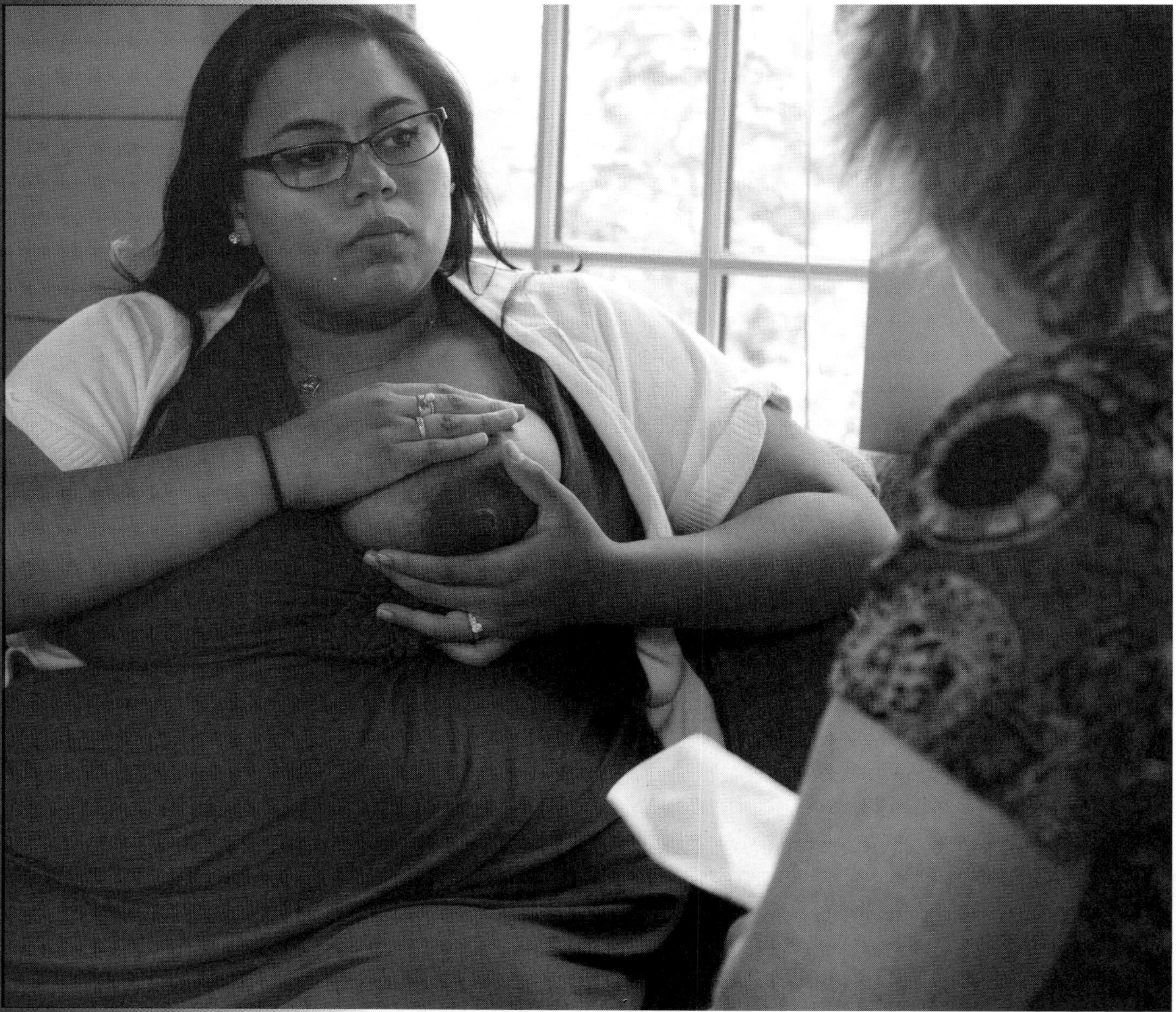

Techniques

A

ASYMMETRICAL LATCH

When a baby is latched deeply and nursing actively, on average, the nipple extends to within about 5 mm of the junction on the roof of baby's mouth where her hard and soft palates meet (Elad et al., 2014; Jacobs, Dickinson, Hart, Doherty, & Faulkner, 2007). Some call this area in the baby's mouth the "comfort zone," because in most cases, when the nipple reaches this area, nursing is comfortable and effective (Mohrbacher & Kendall-Tackett, 2010).

When upright and side-lying feeding positions are used, the ***asymmetrical latch*** can help some nursing couples achieve deep latch. An asymmetrical latch is different from a "centered" or "bull's-eye" latch, which was once taught in the U.S. and Canada. The asymmetrical latch was popularized in North America and the U.K. by British midwife Chloe Fisher and Canadian pediatrician Jack Newman.

The baby's working jaw. During an asymmetrical latch, the baby latches off-center, with her lower jaw further from the nipple than her upper jaw (Figure A.1). This allows the nipple to extend deeper into the baby's mouth, which makes nursing more comfortable and effective. A Japanese study (Mizuno et al., 2008) found that when babies latched shallowly, they drained the mammary gland unevenly, with some lobes left fuller, while others were well-drained. A deep latch, on the other hand, drained the gland evenly.

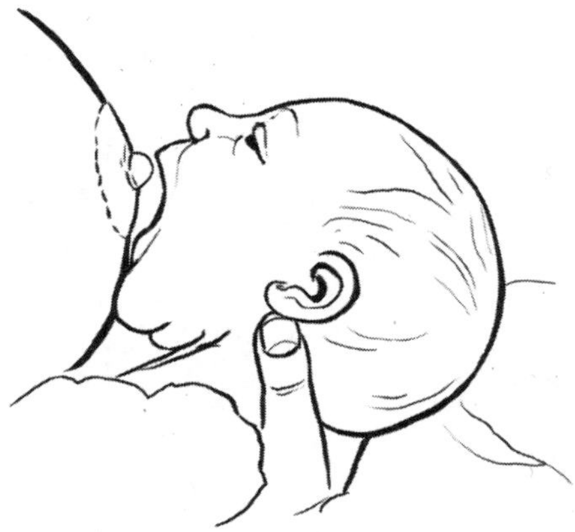

Figure A.1 During an asymmetrical latch, baby's lower jaw lands further from the nipple than her upper jaw, allowing the nipple to extend deeper in baby's mouth. ©2020, Nancy Mohrbacher Solutions, Inc.

To understand this better, when eating or talking, notice how only the lower jaw moves. The same is true during nursing, which is why some refer to the lower jaw as the "working jaw" (Wiessinger, 1998). The lower jaw does all the work of feeding, while the upper jaw simply helps keeps the mammary tissue in place. The further away from the nipple the lower jaw lands during latch, the further back in her mouth the nipple can extend.

The effects of early positioning. As described in Chapter 1, feeding position can make achieving a deep latch easier or more difficult, especially during the early weeks, when the newborn lacks much head-and-neck control. The feeding position determines whether the baby or the parent has primary responsibility for the depth of latch. When a baby is resting tummy down on the parent's semi-reclined body (***starter positions***, p. 23-29), the baby can self-attach. Self-attaching during latch makes several aspects of a deep latch automatic: a wide-open mouth, a relaxed jaw, and the tongue forward. In these starter positions, thanks to baby's inborn feeding behaviors, the baby can readjust the latch as needed until the nipple reaches the area that triggers active and effective nursing. With the baby in control of the latch, there is no need for the parent to manipulate its angle.

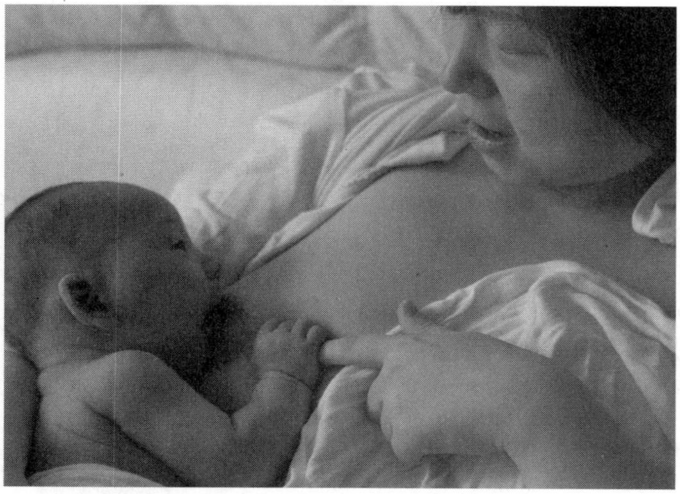

Figure A.2 Newborns can self-attach in starter positions like this one, which simplifies early nursing. ©2020 Melanie Ham, used with permission.

During the early weeks, however, if upright or side-lying positions are used, the newborn cannot self-attach as easily. In these positions (which work well when baby is a little older, stronger, and more coordinated), gravity pulls the baby's body away from the nipple, so the parent needs to provide much more help. Latching in an upright or side-lying position can be trickier during the early learning period. Parents need to support the baby's body, either in arms or with pillows. They need to make sure the baby's body is in good alignment with the nipple (see below). They need to keep baby's body pressed against theirs to help her orient and trigger her inborn feeding behaviors. When she opens wide, they need to provide a gentle push at just the right moment to help baby well onto the mammary gland so the nipple reaches the comfort zone. This involves normal dexterity, practice, and requires the parent remember many steps in the right order at a time when—due to the brain changes that occur during pregnancy and after birth—most new parents have difficulty following instructions (Kim, 2016; Zheng et al., 2018).

To achieve a deep latch in an upright position, suggest parents:

1. Start by aligning the baby's body with the nipple so that the baby is "nose to nipple" (Figure A.3), supporting the baby's shoulders and neck, so her head can tilt back slightly (the ***instinctive feeding position***, see p. 8).

2. Make sure the baby's chin, torso, hips, legs, and feet are pulled in close with the baby's whole body touching the parent (no gaps between them).

3. Wait until the stimulation of the baby's chin and torso against the mammary gland triggers a wide-open mouth (Figure A.4).

4. As the baby moves toward the nipple, apply gentle pressure on the baby's back and shoulders (avoid pushing on baby's head) to help her get onto the gland deeply, so the nipple extends back to the comfort zone (Figure A.5).

5. Positioning baby nose to nipple makes it possible for her to take enough of the areola below the nipple (3 to 4 cm) into her mouth so that the nipple can extend back into the comfort zone (Glover & Wiessinger, 2017).

During latch, if baby's lower jaw lands at the base of the nipple, a shallow latch is the result. Even when the nipple is centered in the baby's mouth, it is more difficult for it to stretch back far enough to reach the comfort zone. The baby who latches with her head tilted forward instead of slightly back is at the same disadvantage. When baby's head tilts forward, it also tilts the lower jaw (the working jaw) away from the mammary gland, resulting in a shallow latch.

BREAST MASSAGE AND MANUAL THERAPY

Research and Practice of Breast Massage

Many cultures use breast massage to prevent and treat a variety of lactation issues. Touch has a profound effect on the release of hormones in our bodies (Uvnas-Moberg, 2014). For example, a newborn's touch after birth raises a birthing parent's oxytocin levels (Matthiesen, Ransjo-Arvidson, Nissen, & Uvnas-Moberg, 2001). Knowing this, it's not surprising that breast massage is practiced in various forms around the world. But just as post-birth beliefs and practices vary internationally (Wambach & Spencer, 2021), beliefs about breast massage techniques and the importance of breast massage to lactation vary greatly from place to place. In some cultures, very little emphasis is put on breast massage during the early weeks after birth, while in others, it is considered essential to successful lactation.

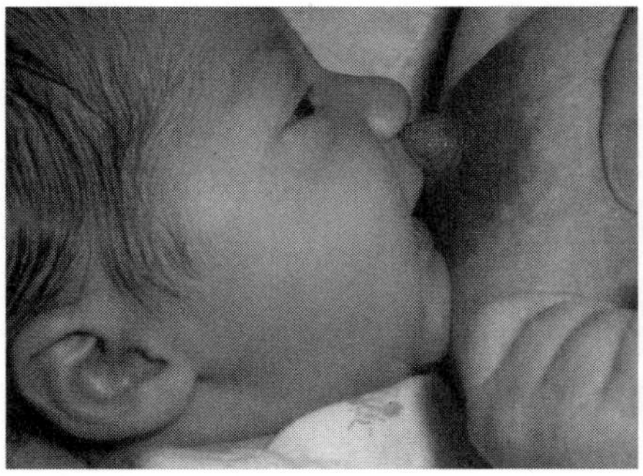

Figure A.3 Nose to nipple. ©2020 Catherine Watson Genna, used with permission.

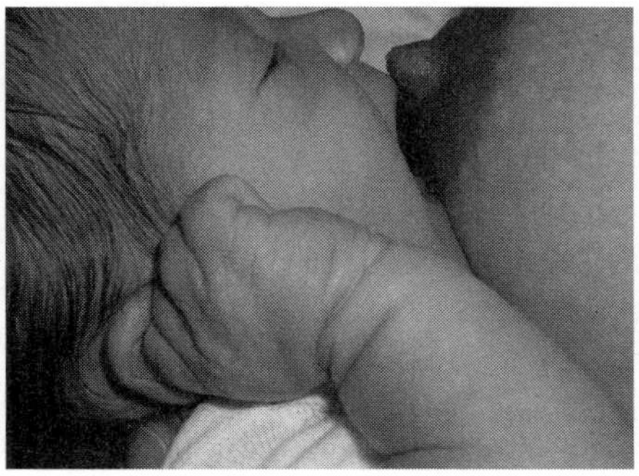

Figure A.4 Baby's lower jaw lands on the gland off-center, well away from the nipple. ©2020 Catherine Watson Genna, used with permission.

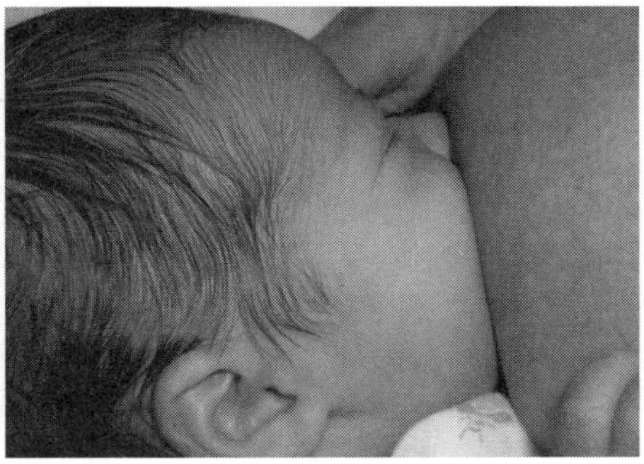

Figure A.5 Baby takes a big mouthful. ©2020 Catherine Watson Genna, used with permission.

At least 10 different breast massage techniques. A 2015 systematic review attempted to categorize breast massage techniques by the specific lactation problem they are intended to solve (Sadovnikova, 2015). After searching YouTube videos and the databases of Pub Med and Google Scholar, its authors found 10 different breast massage techniques. They noted that research articles rarely describe in detail the specific techniques used and suggested that studies are needed to determine which breast massage techniques are most suited for specific issues.

Lactation issues treated with breast massage. The 2015 systematic review described above noted the lactation issues treated with breast massage:

- Engorgement
- Plugged ducts/mastitis
- Mammary tenderness and pain
- Concerns about milk volume or milk-fat content
- Milk ejection

A 2019 systematic review of the literature on breast massage (Anderson, Kynoch, Kildea, & Lee, 2019) concluded that despite the differences in the studies it included (3 randomized controlled trials and 3 quasi-experimental studies), all found reduction in pain and other symptoms, regardless of the specific massage technique used.

Research on breast massage and pumping milk yields. A small U.S. study (Stutte, 1988) found that in the 18 mothers who double-pumped while massaging one breast, the massaged side had both greater milk yield, and higher fat content. A 2018 Indian study with a similar design (Kraleti, Lingaldinna, Kalvala, Anjum, & Singh, 2018) also found greater milk yield when one breast was massaged 10 minutes before pumping. In 2001, U.K. researchers (Jones, Dimmock, & Spencer, 2001) noted that when its study mothers used breast massage immediately before pumping for their preterm babies, their milk yields increased by about 40%. In 2009, U.S. pediatrician Jane Morton published her study on hands-on pumping (Morton et al., 2009), which used massage and compression during pumping in mothers pumping exclusively for their preterm babies in the NICU. The researchers found that the study mothers in the hands-on group pumped on average nearly 50% more milk than those who used the pump alone. Hands-on pumping was also found to double milk-fat content (Morton et al., 2012). See p. 492 for instructions on hands-on pumping, and see it in action at **bit.ly/BA2-HandsOnPumpingDemo**.

Research on Russian breast massage, engorgement, and plugged ducts. Maya Bolman, RN, IBCLC came to the U.S. from Russia and brought with her knowledge about traditional Russian breast massage techniques. In her work at a U.S. practice, Bolman used these techniques, which she called therapeutic breast massage during lactation (or TBML). She participated in studies that tested the effectiveness of TBML in solving lactation problems such as engorgement and plugged ducts (Bolman, Saju, Oganesyan, Kondrashova, & Witt, 2013). Two 2016 U.S. studies (Witt, Bolman, & Kredit, 2016; Witt, Bolman, Kredit, et al., 2016) found that TBML effectively decreased pain and resolved engorgement more quickly than usual care. The study mothers found TBML a useful skill that helped them effectively solve lactation problems. See Box 18.1 on p. 752 for TBML massage techniques recommended for engorgement and a video demonstrating TBML at **bit.ly/BA2-BolmanMassage**.

Research on Japanese (Oketani) breast massage. The Oketani method of breast massage was developed in Japan and named for its founder (Kabir & Tasnim, 2009). A 2012 study done in Korea using this technique (Cho, Ahn, Ahn, Lee, & Hur, 2012) found that it significantly reduced breast pain among new mothers. Researchers analyzed milk samples immediately before and after Oketani massage was performed by professionals (Foda, Kawashima, Nakamura, Kobayashi, & Oku, 2004). The researchers found increased fat content in the milk in later lactation (more than 11 months after birth) but not in early lactation. From birth to 11 months, the milk samples expressed after Oketani massage were higher in milk solids and casein.

Breast massage in China. When a baby is born in China, many families believe that breast massage is necessary to reach full milk production. In China, an entire profession exists consisting of hundreds of thousands of women who were trained to provide breast massage to new families. To Westerners, this practice may seem unnecessary (Eidelman, 2016), but in China, breast massage is considered by many to be a requirement for successful nursing. This cultural belief motivated Chinese researchers to study the effects of breast massage on lactation. A 2017 Chinese study randomized 80 women after a cesarean delivery into 4 groups (Chu et al., 2017). In 3 groups, breast massage began after birth at 2, 12, or 24 hours respectively and continued 3 times per day for 3 days. The fourth group (the controls) received no massage. The group that started earliest had the highest blood prolactin levels and reached what the researchers defined as "adequate lactation" the fastest. The blood prolactin levels were higher in all of the three massage groups as compared with the control group, and these differences were statistically significant.

International research on breast massage found that these practices may give early milk production a boost, as well as increasing nursing parents' comfort. A U.S. overview article on breast massage (Bowles, 2011) summarized some of the reasons families should consider using these techniques.

- To enhance normal nursing for all lactating families
- To maximize colostrum intake during early nursing in order to prevent exaggerated jaundice
- To enhance effective milk removal during nursing and pumping
- To boost milk production and transfer

In addition to the breast-massage practices mentioned here, other highly effective techniques that originiated in China can be used to help lactating families. Some techniques are intended to solve one specific lactation problem, such as plugged ducts (Zhao et al., 2014). But others are intended more holistically, such as the approach to manual therapy developed by author, lactation specialist, and certified practitioner of traditional Chinese medicine, Huimin (Daphne) Di, who incorporated ancient Chinese principles into effective modern strategies for solving a wide variety of lactation problems. After years of practice and training students in China, Di's U.S. workshops offer skills-training for lactation supporters outside of China, so they can incorporate this manual therapy into their own practices. The next section is an excerpt from Di's popular book, which was written in Chinese and describes an approach she calls ***Both Hands 10 Fingers and Love (BHTFL)***. At this writing, Di's book is being translated into English. For information on manual-therapy workshops, email Di at **554816924@qq.com**.

Manual Therapy and Traditional Chinese Medicine

From Di, Huimin (Daphne). (2012). *New Therapies for the Breastfeeding Mother: Using Traditional Chinese Medicine with Manual Therapy to Support Lactation.* China Labor & Social Security Press.

Theory and Overview

Traditional Chinese medicine (TCM) is a unique health science that gradually took shape over 3,500-years of continuous medical practice and observation, influenced by the ancient Chinese schools of thinking known as materialism and dialectic thought. Its evolution occurred while the Chinese people struggled against disease, and today it is a highly valued part of Chinese traditional culture and is used in many forms worldwide.

Breastfeeding is as old as humankind, so of course, in China, nursing is the traditional way to feed a baby. Like other aspects of TCM, the manual therapies described here were developed over thousands of years and employ a holistic approach to supporting lactation and maternal health. These techniques are intended to be used with parents and babies along with conventional medicine and other alternative and complementary treatments.

One of the most famous TCM references is the 2,500-year-old treatise on medicine and disease, *Huangdi Neijing (The Yellow Emperor's Classic of Medicine)*. This book explains the theoretical principles of TCM, which can be applied to the mammary gland and the physiology of nursing and lactation. Its principles can also be used to address pathologies, as it provides guidance on diagnosing, treating, and preventing problems. The theoretical system described in this ancient text is the basis for how TCM is used when practicing manual therapy in lactating parents.

TCM envisions the human body as a unified whole with connections between all parts of the body and the ***Viscera*** (capitalized to distinguish them from the anatomical organs they are named for), the main organs in the torso. The heart, liver, spleen, lung, and kidney are the center of the five Viscera along with the six Fu: the gallbladder, stomach, small intestine, large intestine, bladder and three Jiao. The three Jiao are also known as the Triple Burner, which does not have a counterpart in Western medicine. This consists of the upper burner, consisting of the organs in the chest and the breathing process; the middle burner, consisting of the abdominal organs related to digestion and the digestive process; and the lower burner, involving the lower abdominal organs and their urogenital functions. If the Triple burner functions well, then the organs are said to be in synergy. In TCM, the three burners transport fluids throughout the body, treating all conditions. All of the organs consist of ***Qi*** (the vital life force that underlies everything), blood, essence, and other body fluids. The

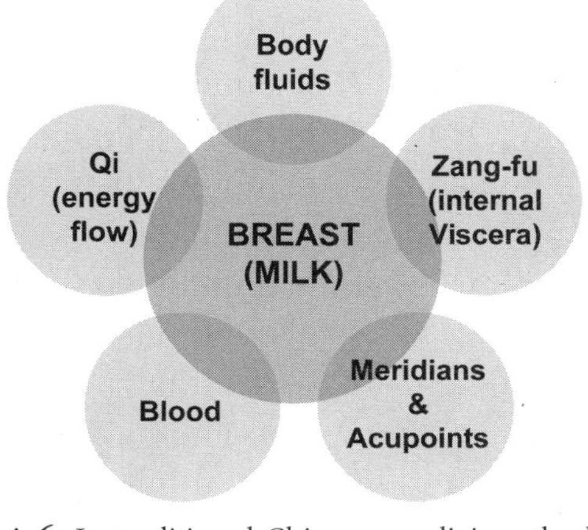

Figure A.6 In traditional Chinese medicine, the body is seen as a unified whole, with lactation influenced by other aspects of the body to which it is connected.

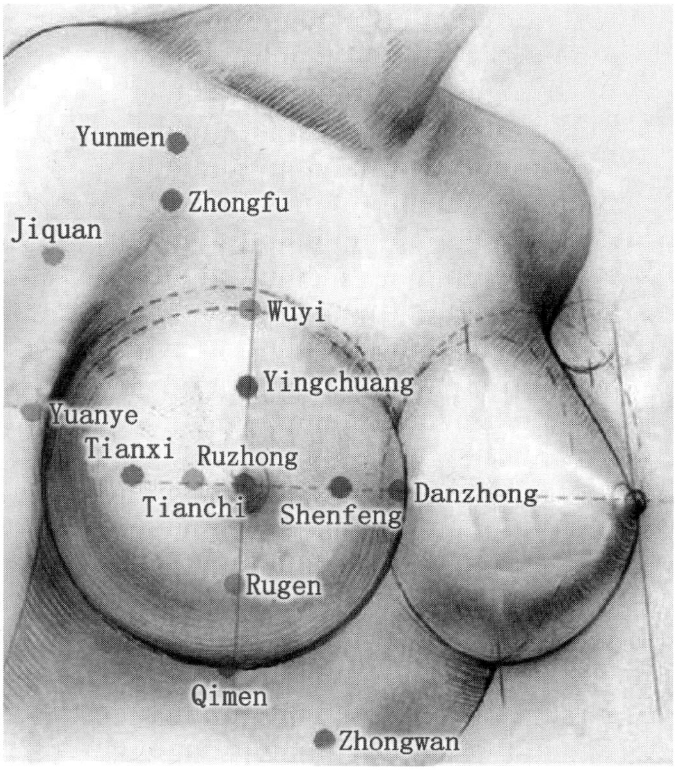

Figure A.7 Location of acupoints on the chest and mammary glands.

meridians, the channels in the body through which the Qi flows, transport fluids which connect the internal Viscera with the external features of the body (including the mammary glands) at the ***acupoints***. These body parts along with the nine orifices, limbs, and bones, constitute an organic whole that is unified with the external environment.

The ancient TCM text takes a holistic view of the human body, which considers milk secretion by the normal mammary gland closely related to the physiological function of the Viscera, meridians, Qi, blood, essence, and other body fluids. The focus in TCM is on treating the whole person. This involves using the meridians and acupoints that connect with the breast to solve lactation problems, such as plugged ducts, mastitis, low milk production, nipple pain, and breast lumps.

Emotional care is a vital part of TCM, so it uses meridians and acupoints to make sure parents' bodies (including their mammary glands) are relaxed. With relaxation comes the

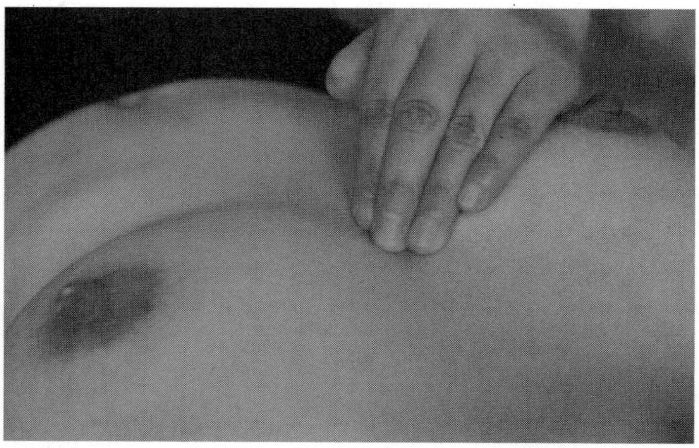

Figure A.8a Acupoint Danzhong. Indication: Lack of milk, mastitis.

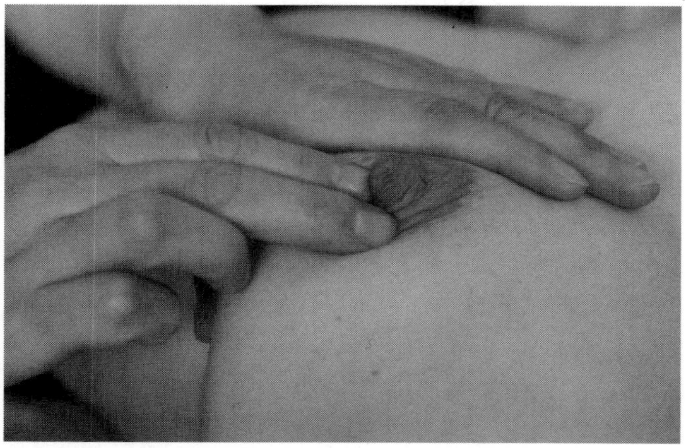

Figure A.8b Acupoint Ruzhong. Indication: Mammary swelling and pain, mastitis.

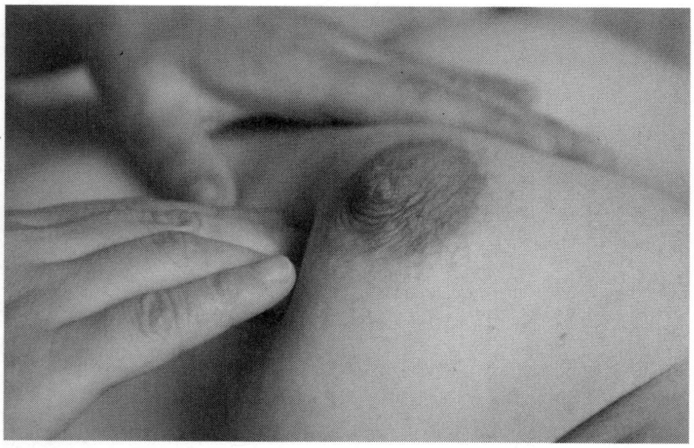

Figure A.8c Acupoint Rugen. Indication: Mammary swelling and pain, mastitis, lack of milk.

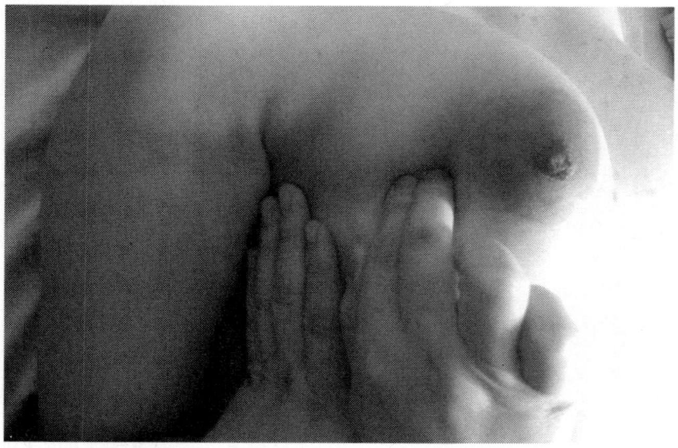

Figure A.8d Acupoint Tianchi. Indication: Axillary swelling, headache, mastitis.

release of oxytocin, and milk ejection occurs easily. A relaxed and positive mood enhances milk production. Otherwise, post-birth feelings of injury, (suppressed anger, worry, stress) will harm the Qi (energy flow), which causes obstruction and stagnation through the body's meridians, resulting in obstructed milk flow, aggravating any existing plugged ducts.

Meridians and Acupoints

According to TCM, there are 14 meridians, which act like a network on the surface of the body. These meridians are the main channels for transmitting and regulating the flow of information, blood, and energy within the entire body. The mammary glands are part of an organic whole. The body as a whole maintains with its local parts (like the breasts) a relationship of mutual restriction and coordination. To treat a lactation problem, therefore, the focus is on the whole, paying attention to the overall regulation within the body. This is why TCM uses the meridians and acupoints to solve nursing problems.

Regarding the acupoints, there are:

- 2 on the head: Baihui, Shenting
- 5 on the upper arm: Shaoze, Qiangu, Hegu, Quchi, Jiquan
- 5 on the back: Geshu, Ganshu, Pishu, Weishu, Shenshu
- 2 on the neck and shoulders: Fengchi, Jianjing
- 12 on the chest: Yunmen, Zhongfu, Wuyi, Yingchuang, Danzhong, Shenfeng, Ruzhong, Rugen, Qimen, Tianchi, Tianxi, Yuanye
- 2 on the belly: Zhongwan, Shenque
- 4 on the leg: Liang Qiu, Xuehai, Zusanlia, Sanyinjiao
- 2 on the foot: Taichong, Zulinqi

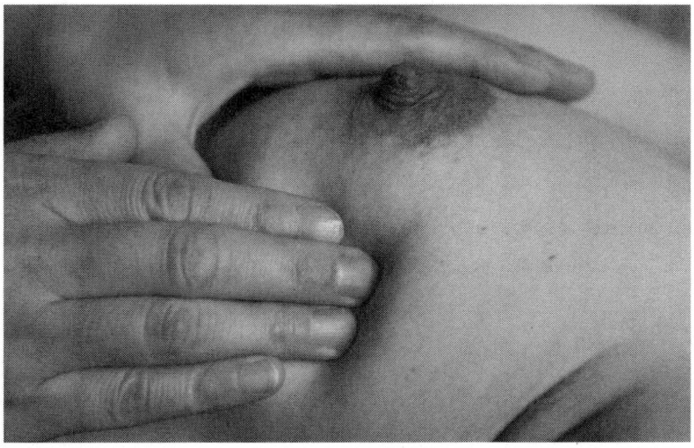

Figure A.8e Acupoint Tianxi. Indication: Mammary swelling and pain, mastitis, lack of milk.

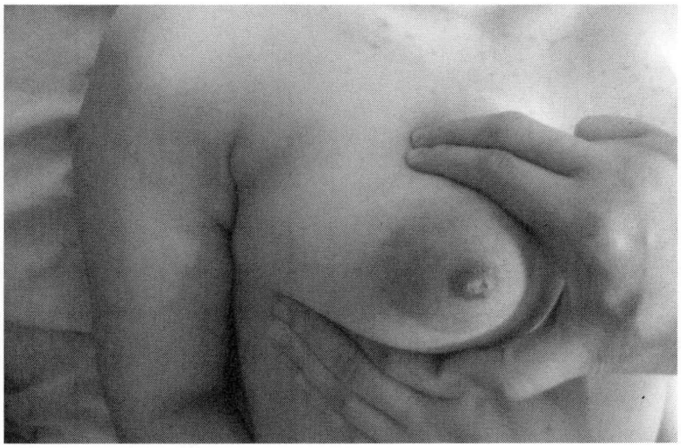

Figure A.8f Acupoint Wuyi. Indication: Mammary swelling and pain, mastitis.

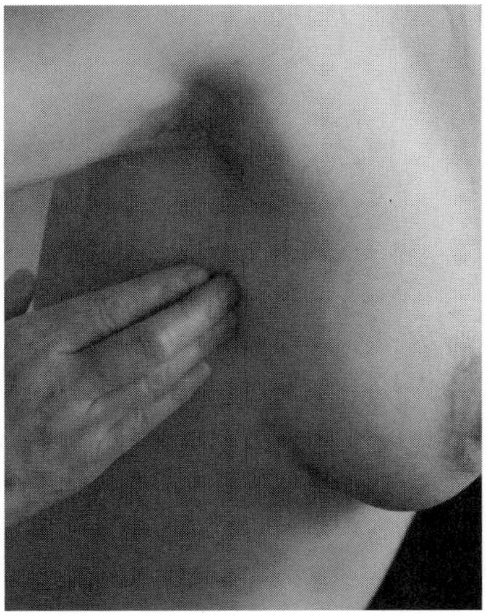

Figure A.8g Acupoint Yuanye. Indication: Reduced swelling and mammary pain relief.

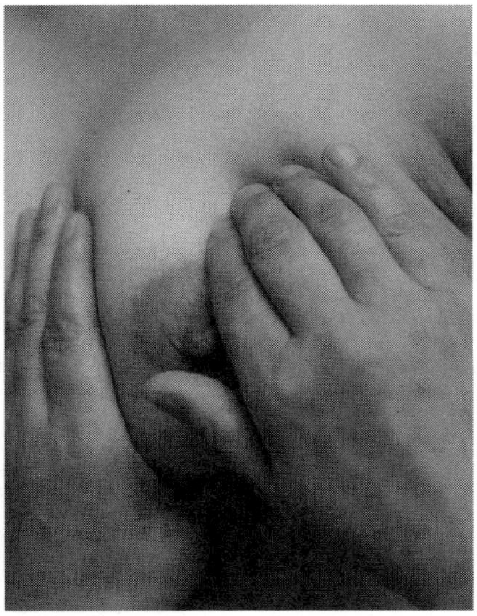

Figure A.8h Acupoint Yingchuang. Indication: mastitis, cough, chest pain.

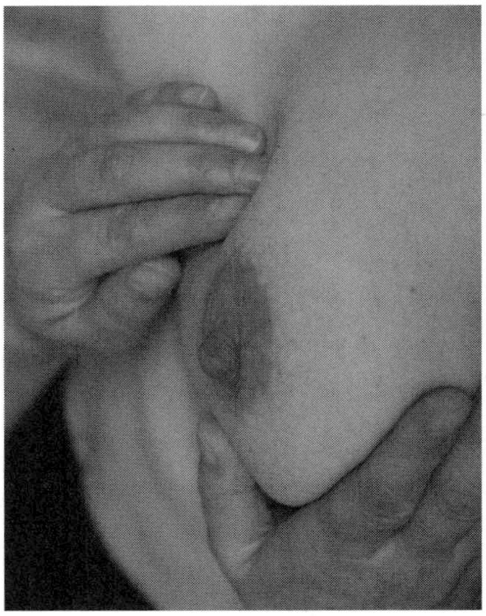

Figure A.8i Acupoint Shenfeng. Indication: mastitis, mammary swelling and pain, vomiting.

Acupoints act as the resources for energy and blood. There are 34 acupoints in total that are widely used in clinical practice, healthcare, and disease treatment. Although the breast is a local organ, 14 meridians connect the mammary glands to the internal Zang-fu organs. Through the flow of Qi, blood, essence, and other body fluids, these meridians fulfill their functional activities. Acupoints belong to different meridians, and meridians belong to different Zang-fu Viscera. Acupoints used for treatment are healing to the corresponding organs, so different acupoints have different indications. Some acupoints are used primarily for emotional care. Some acupoints are used to resolve fever. Some acupoints are used to treat plugged ducts and mastitis.

Manual Therapy

When manual therapy is used in lactating parents, we use both hands, 10 fingers, and love (BHTFL). Therapeutic treatments use different acupoints for different conditions, finding the right location of the acupoints, pressing on particular points on a parent's body with the fingertips or thumbs.

Begin by having parents lie down. Start with the hand, shoulder, back, chest, belly, legs, and feet. After that, use both hands on the breasts to resolve lactation problems, such as plugged ducts. Finish the manual therapy with the acupoints on the back. After the manual therapy, milk ejection usually occurs, increasing parents' confidence in their milk production.

TCM-based manual therapy—which is ideally practiced with patience and love—is natural and safe. It promotes relaxation, relieves pain, increases energy, enhances mammary blood circulation, encourages the body to heal itself, and can help resolve disease. New parents treated with manual therapy consider it to be like magic. Some specialized study is required to master this method, but it can be learned quickly. These skills provide lactation supporters with new, more effective treatment options.

MAMMARY SHAPING

When a baby has trouble latching deeply, tissue-shaping techniques can sometimes make a deep latch easier. Breast sandwich and nipple tilting are two mammary-shaping techniques that can help some babies more easily take a larger mouthful of mammary tissue, which can make a huge difference, especially during the early learning period.

Breast Sandwich

Using this technique, the parent gently squeezes the mammary tissue near the areola (fingers on one side and thumb on the other) to narrow its shape and make it easier for the baby's lower jaw to land further onto the areola so the nipple extends deeper in her mouth (Wilson-Clay & Hoover, 2017, p. 43). This technique can be especially helpful for parents with firm mammary tissue, either naturally occurring or from engorgement or tissue swelling from excess IV fluids during labor. It can also be helpful during the newborn period for any nursing couple who is struggling with latch.

For the breast sandwich technique to help, the oval of the compressed tissue must match the oval of the baby's mouth—wider at the corners and narrower between upper and lower lips. If the directions of these two ovals do not match, mammary shaping can make latching more difficult rather than less.

Two approaches can make this concept easier to understand.

- **Hamburger, not taco.** Imagine taking a bite out of a sandwich. First we line it up horizontally with our mouth to make it easier to take a big bite (Wiessinger, 1998). Think about how much harder it would be to take a bite if we rotated the sandwich 90º, so it was vertical rather than horizontal. Suggest when shaping the mammary tissue, as the baby approaches the gland, parents think "hamburger," not "taco."
- **Finger moustache.** Whether parents' thumb or fingers are closest to baby's upper lip, think of them as the baby's "mustache." For the tissue and mouth ovals to align, the parents' thumb and fingers run parallel to the baby's lips (Figure A.9).

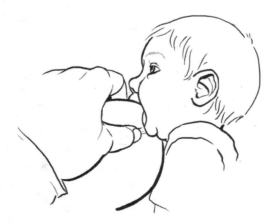

Figure A.9 The breast sandwich can help baby get a bigger mouthful and a deeper latch. ©2020 Nancy Mohrbacher Solutions, Inc.

When forming a breast sandwich, it's also important for parents to keep their fingers far enough back on the mammary tissue, so they don't get in baby's way as she latches.

Nipple Tilting

Nipple tilting (sometimes called ***The Flipple***) is a shaping strategy developed by Australian midwife and lactation consultant Rebecca Glover, which can sometimes make it easier for the baby's lower working jaw to land further back on the areola for a deeper latch (Glover & Wiessinger, 2017). Here's how this technique works.

- With the baby's body pulled in close to the parent and her chin touching the gland, parents press on the gland just above the nipple with a thumb or finger running parallel to the baby's upper lip. This action causes the nipple to point up and away from the baby (Figure A.10).
- The touch of the gland on the baby's chin triggers a wide-open mouth (gape).
- Parents then use this top thumb or finger to press into the gland and roll the underside of the areola into baby's wide-open mouth.
- As the areola enters the baby's mouth, parents can use the top finger or thumb to gently push the nipple inside the baby's upper gum before removing their finger.

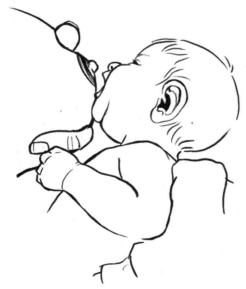

Figure A.10 Nipple tilting. ©2020 Nancy Mohrbacher Solutions, Inc.

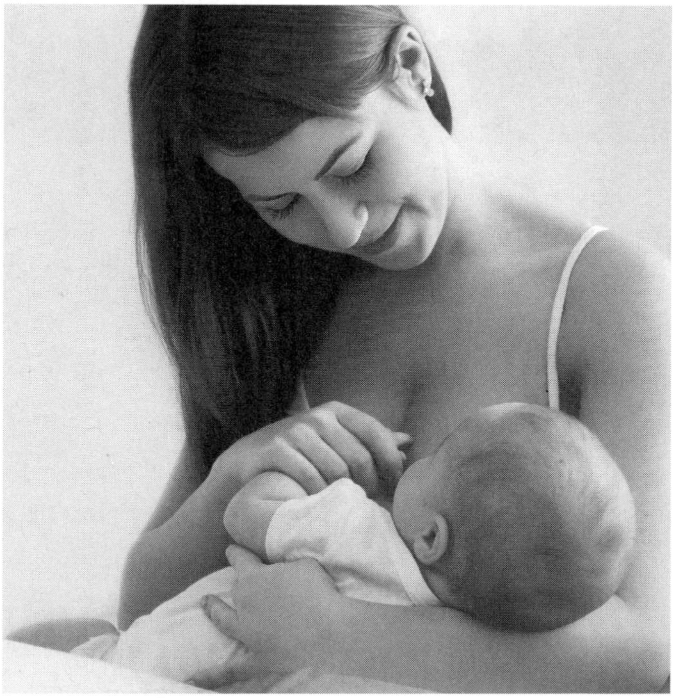

REVERSE PRESSURE SOFTENING (RPS)

Developed by U.S. lactation consultant and nurse Jean Cotterman, ***reverse pressure softening*** (or RPS) can be helpful any time a nursing parent's areola is so firm that latching or milk expression is challenging (Cotterman, 2004). This technique is used most often during the first week or two after birth when the mammary glands become swollen from excess IV fluids given during labor or when a nursing parent becomes engorged (see p. 748). RPS can also be used at any stage of lactation to trigger milk ejection before expressing milk or whenever the glands are so full that the areola needs to be softened.

Reverse pressure softening involves applying gentle pressure to the areola to soften it by moving the swelling (edema) farther back into the mammary tissue. With the areola soft and the swelling out of the way, the baby can latch deeper and nursing parents have easier access to their milk during milk expression.

Refer to the handout on the following three pages for more details. These handouts may be photocopied and distributed with no further permission required.

Reverse Pressure Softening for Helpers

Illustrations by Kyle Cotterman, Reverse Pressure Softening by K. Jean Cotterman © 2008

Try this if pain, swelling, or fullness creates problems during the early weeks of learning to nurse. The key is making the areola **very soft** right around the base of the nipple for better latching.

- A softer areola protects the nipple deep in baby's mouth, helping his tongue remove milk better.
- Parents say curved fingers work best (Figure 1 or 2).
- Press inward toward the chest wall and **count slowly to 50**.
- Pressure should be **steady and firm**, and **gentle enough to avoid pain**.
- If desired, someone other than the nursing parent may help, using thumbs (Figure 5).
- (For long fingernails, try another way shown below.)
- If glands are quite large or **very** swollen, count **very** slowly, with parents **lying down on their back**.
- This delays return of swelling to the areola, giving more time to latch.
- Soften the areola **right before each feeding** (or pumping) till swelling goes away.
- For some, this takes 2-4 days.
- Make any pumping sessions short, with pauses to re-soften the areola if needed.
- Use medium or low vacuum, to reduce the return of swelling into the areola.

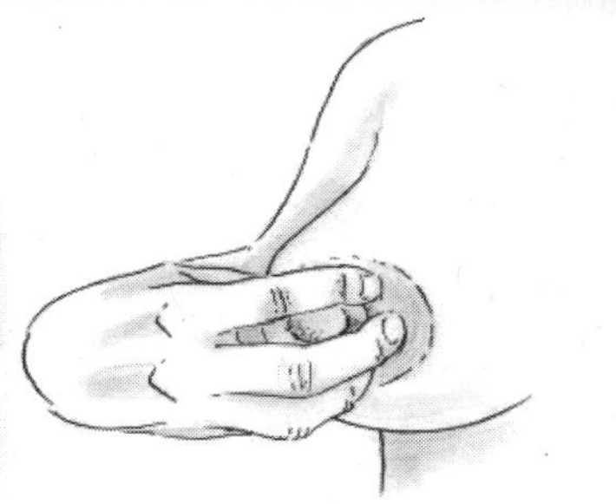

Figure 1 One handed "flower hold": Fingernails short, Fingertips curved, placed where baby's tongue will go.

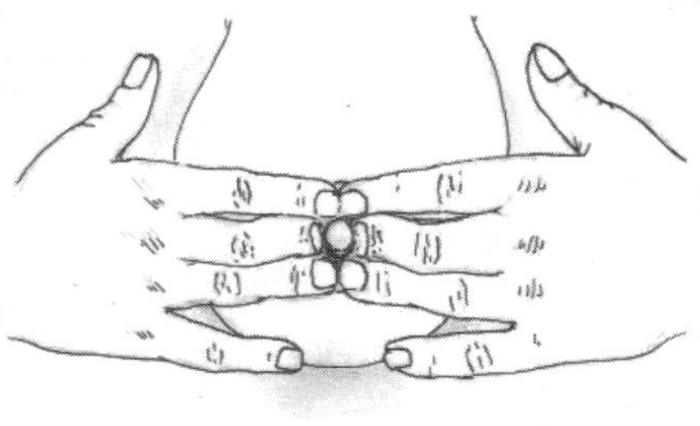

Figure 2 Two handed, one-step method: Fingernails short, Fingertips curved, each one touching the side of the nipple.

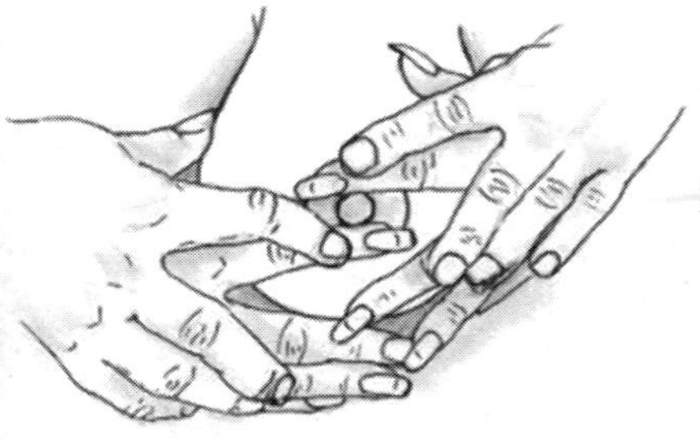

Figure 3 You may ask someone to help press by placing fingers or thumbs on top of yours.

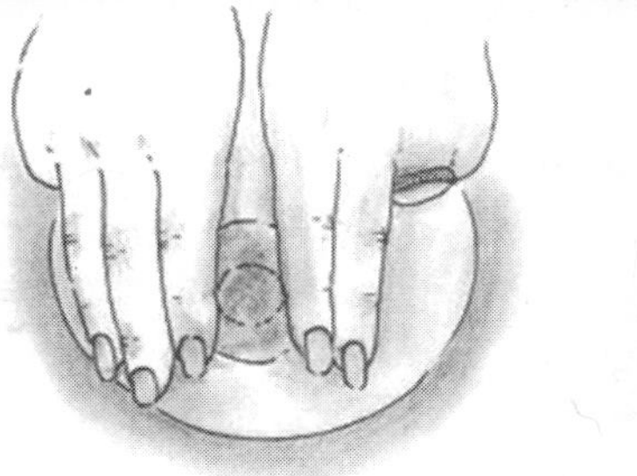

Figure 4 Two step method, two hands: using 2 or 3 straight fingers each side, first knuckles touching nipple. Move ¼ turn, repeat above and below nipple.

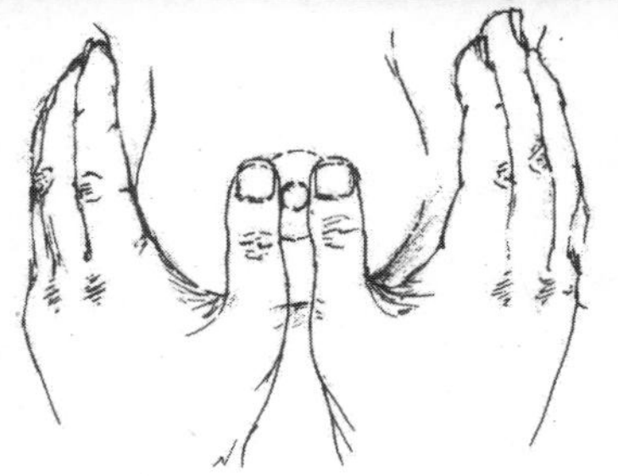

Figure 5 Two step method, two hands: using straight thumbs, base of thumbnail at side of nipple. Move ¼ turn, repeat, thumbs above and below nipple.

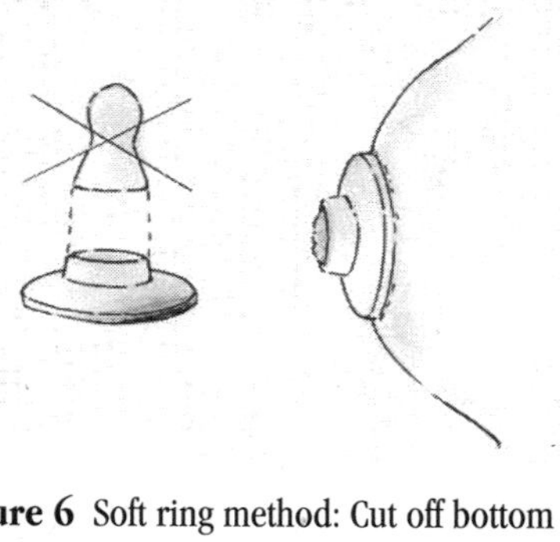

Figure 6 Soft ring method: Cut off bottom half of an artificial nipple to place on areola to press with fingers.

Reverse Pressure Softening for Parents

Developed by K. Jean Cotterman RNC, IBCLC

What is it?

REVERSE PRESSURE SOFTENING is a way to soften the **circle around your nipple (the a-re-o-la)** to make latching and getting your milk out easy while your baby and you are learning. **LATCHING SHOULDN'T BE PAINFUL**. If your **areola** is soft enough to **change shape** while feeding, it helps your baby **gently extend your nipple deep inside his mouth**, so his tongue and jaws can press on milk ducts under the **areola**.

(These motions differ from those that artificial nipples force a baby to use.)

This new method is **NOT THE SAME** as removing milk with your fingers. **DON'T EXPECT MILK TO COME FROM YOUR NIPPLE** while you soften your **areola** this way. (But it's OK if some milk does come out.)

When is it helpful?

Try **REVERSE PRESSURE SOFTENING** in the early days after birth if you begin to notice firmness of the **areola**, latch pain, or breast fullness. (This full feeling is **only partly due to milk**. Delayed or skipped feedings may also cause **the tissue around your milk ducts** to hold extra fluid much like a sponge does. **This fluid never goes to your baby.)** **Intravenous (IV) fluids**, or drugs such as **pitocin** may cause even more retained tissue fluid, which often takes **7-14 days** to go away. **Avoid long pumping sessions and high vacuum settings on breast pumps to prevent extra swelling of the areola itself.**

Feel your **areola and the tissue deeper inside it**. Is it soft and easy to squeeze, like **your earlobe or your lip**? Or does it feel **FIRMER and harder to compress, like your chin**? If so, it's time to try **REVERSE PRESSURE SOFTENING** just before each time you offer your baby your breast. (Some mothers soften their **areola** before feeding, for a week or longer, till swelling goes down, baby can be heard swallowing milk regularly, and latching is always pain-free without softening first.)

Why does it work?

REVERSE PRESSURE SOFTENING briefly moves some swelling **backward and upward into your breast** to soften your **areola** so it can change shape and extend your nipple. It sends a **special signal to the back of your breasts to start moving milk forward (let-down reflex)** where your baby's tongue can reach it. It also makes it easy to remove milk with your fingertips or with **SHORT PERIODS OF SLOW GENTLE PUMPING**, combined with gentle forward massage of the upper breast, if you need to remove milk for your baby.

Where should I press?

It is most important to soften the **areola** in the whole **one-inch area all around where it joins your nipple**. Soften even more of the **areola** if you wish. You may also want to soften a place where your baby's chin will be able to move easily against the breast. **REVERSE PRESSURE SOFTENING** should cause **NO DISCOMFORT**.

Reverse Pressure Softening for Parents

How do I do Reverse Pressure Softening?

- You (or your helper, from in front, or behind you) choose one of the patterns pictured.
- Place the fingers/thumbs on the circle **touching the nipple**.
- (If swelling is very firm, lie down on your back, and/or ask someone to help by pressing his or her fingers on top of your fingers.)
- Push **gently but firmly** straight inward toward your ribs.
- Hold the pressure **steady** for a period of **1 to 3 full minutes**.
- Relax, breathe easy, sing a lullaby, listen to a favorite song or have someone else watch a clock or set a timer. To see your **areola** better, try using a hand mirror.
- It's OK to repeat the inward pressure again as often as you need. Deep "dimples" may form, lasting long enough for easy latching. Keep testing how soft your **areola** feels.
- You may also press with a soft ring made by cutting off half of an artificial nipple.
- Offer your baby your breast promptly while the circle is soft.

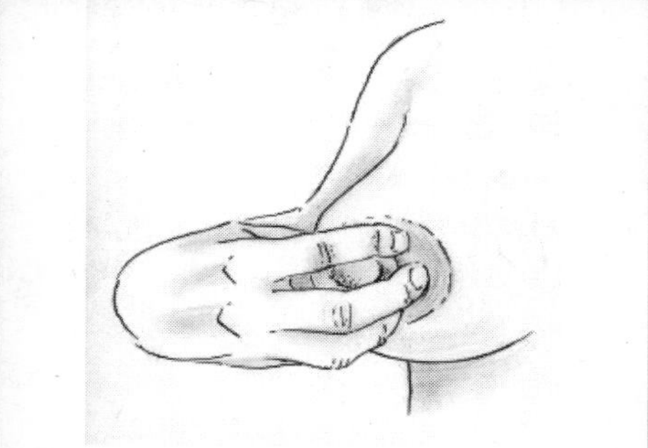

Figure 1 One handed "flower hold": Fingernails short, Fingertips curved, placed where baby's tongue will go.

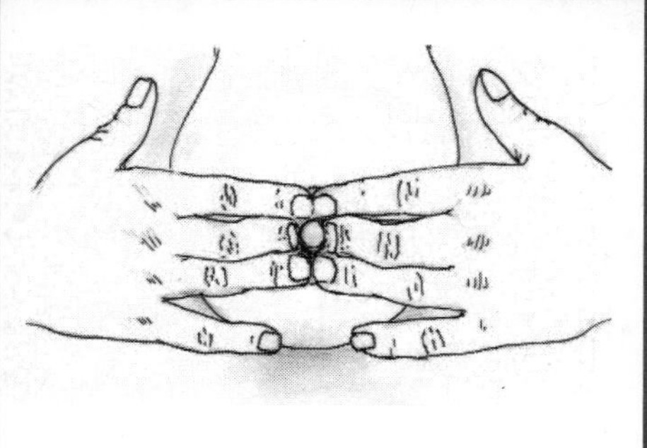

Figure 2 Two handed, one-step method: Fingernails short, Fingertips curved, each one touching the side of the nipple.

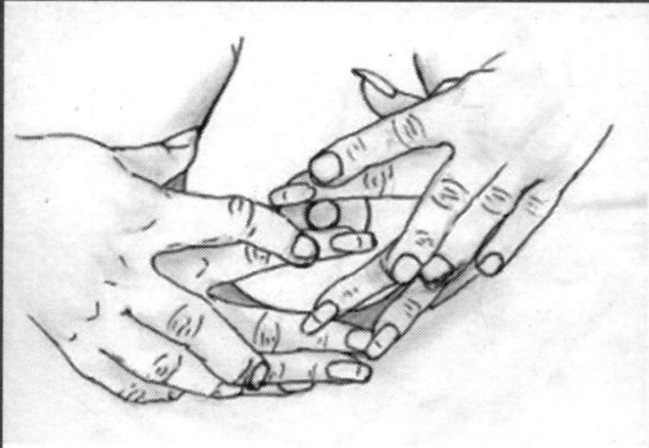

Figure 3 You may ask someone to help press by placing fingers or thumbs on top of yours.

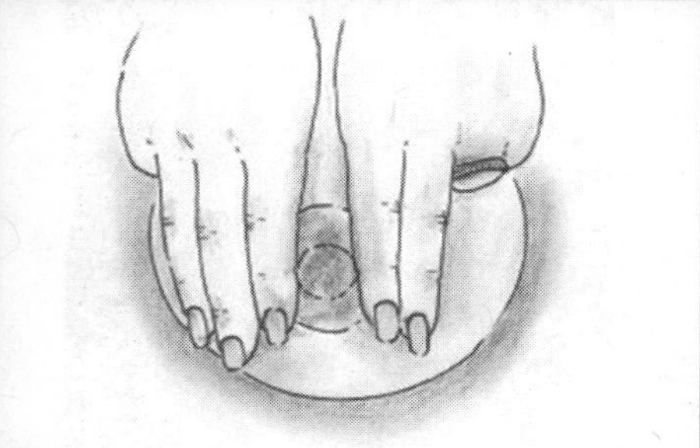

Figure 4 Two step method, two hands: using 2 or 3 straight fingers each side, first knuckles touching nipple. Move ¼ turn, repeat above and below nipple.

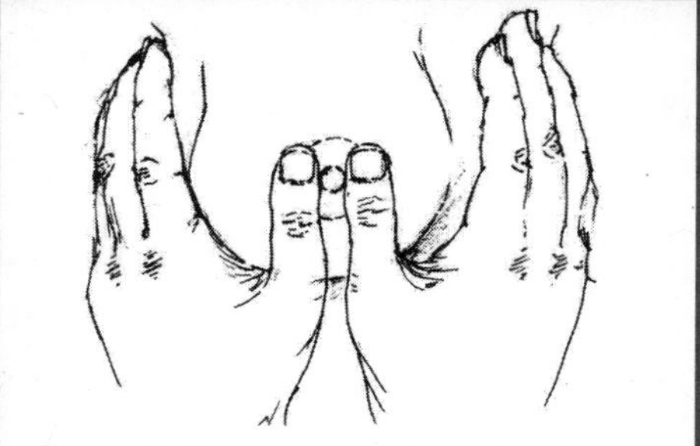

Figure 5 Two step method, two hands: using straight thumbs, base of thumbnail at side of nipple. Move ¼ turn, repeat, thumbs above and below nipple.

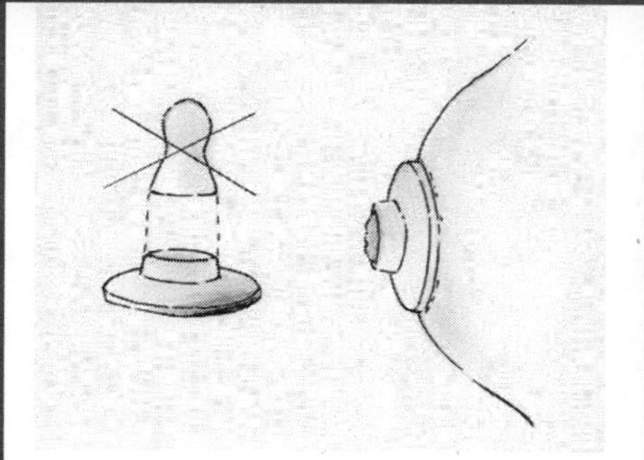

Figure 6 Soft ring method: Cut off bottom half of an artificial nipple to place on areola to press with fingers.

BREAST COMPRESSION

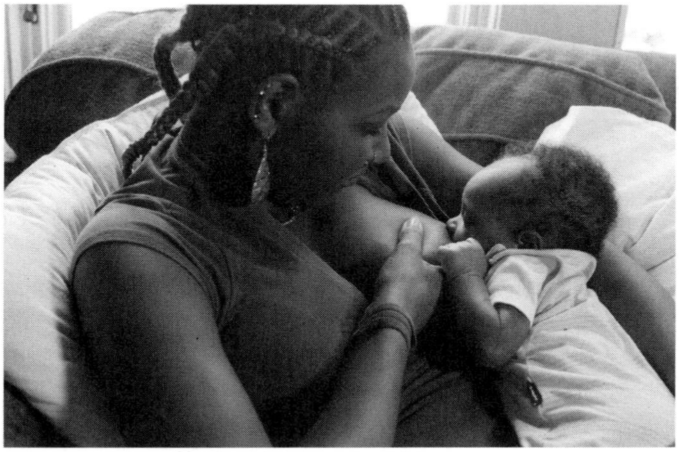

Breast compression keeps many babies actively sucking for a longer time.

Breast compression is a simple technique parents can use to help keep their nursing baby actively sucking longer to increase milk intake, which also increases the milk's fat content. (Morton et al., 2012; Stutte, 1988). This technique can be useful for:

- Healthy babies who are gaining weight slowly
- Newborns with hypoglycemia or exaggerated jaundice
- Babies with cardiac problems or any other health or neurological problems that compromise baby's weight gain or growth
- Parents trying to increase milk production

This technique was popularized by Canadian pediatrician Jack Newman. Here's how he described the technique (Newman, 2017).

How to Do Breast Compression

1. Parents need to know when the baby is getting milk (open mouth wide—pause—close mouth type of sucking.
2. When the baby is drinking milk actively, parents do not need to do any compression.
3. Once the baby is sucking, but no longer drinking, just nibbling, parents should start with the compression.
4. The baby should be sucking but not actually drinking (open mouth wide—pause—close type of sucking). As the baby sucks, the parents holding their gland with one hand, the thumb on one side and the other fingers on the other side of the gland, with a good amount of gland in their hand, should just bring their thumb and fingers together, compressing the tissue. This should be done firmly but not so hard it hurts.
5. The baby may start to drink again (open mouth wide—pause—close mouth type of sucking). If so, parents should keep up the pressure until the baby is back to nibbling. Once the baby is nibbling only, parents should release the pressure on the gland so their hand does not get tired, and allow milk to start flowing again.
6. When parents release the pressure, a young baby, say under 2 or 3 weeks of age, will stop sucking. She will restart sucking when she tastes milk again. An older baby may continue to suck. If the baby drinks, fine. If she sucks but does not drink, parents should restart the compression.
7. If the compression has no effect at a particular moment, this does not mean parents must immediately switch sides. Sometimes compression will work, other times not. But as the baby has nursed longer and longer, it will work less and less, as the flow of milk slows. This means not that the gland is "empty," but that the baby is getting less and less. Babies respond to flow of milk.
8. If the compression is no longer having an effect and the baby is getting sleepy, or starting to fuss because flow is slow, parents should unlatch the baby and offer the other side. Parents should then repeat the process.
9. Parents should experiment....do whatever works best for them. As long as it does not hurt to compress, and the baby gets milk, the technique is working.

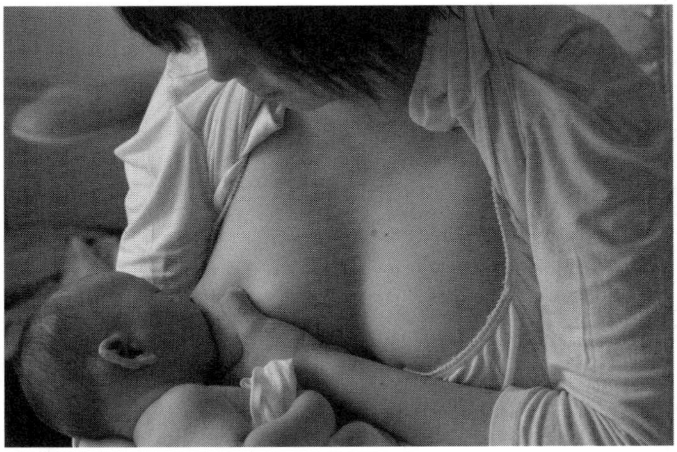

It's time to either compress or relax when baby stops sucking actively and is just nibbling.

DANCER HAND POSITION

The Dancer hand position was named after U.S. midwife Sarah DANner and physician Edward CERutti (Danner & Cerutti, 1984). It provides jaw support and reduces the space inside baby's mouth during nursing, which increases the vacuum a special-needs baby can generate. Enough (but not too much) vacuum is vital to milk transfer during nursing (Elad et al., 2014; Geddes et al., 2017; Geddes, Kent, Mitoulas, & Hartmann, 2008). The Dancer hand position may help the preterm baby, the baby with a cleft palate, or the baby with high or low tone who (Marmet & Shell, 2017):

- Has trouble maintaining an air seal during nursing
- Sucks weakly (may have unusually wide jaw movements)
- Has difficulty staying latched

To use the Dancer Hand Position, suggest parents (Figure A.11):

1. Support their mammary tissue with their hand, thumb on one side, and four fingers on the other.
2. Slide this hand forward, supporting the tissue with their palm and middle, ring, and little fingers. Their index finger and thumb should now be free in front of the nipple.
3. Bend their index finger slightly as the baby latches, so their finger gently presses the baby's cheek on one side, while the thumb presses the other cheek. The baby's chin rests on the bottom of the "U."
4. Maintain this hand position during nursing, using this position with the other hand when the baby changes sides.

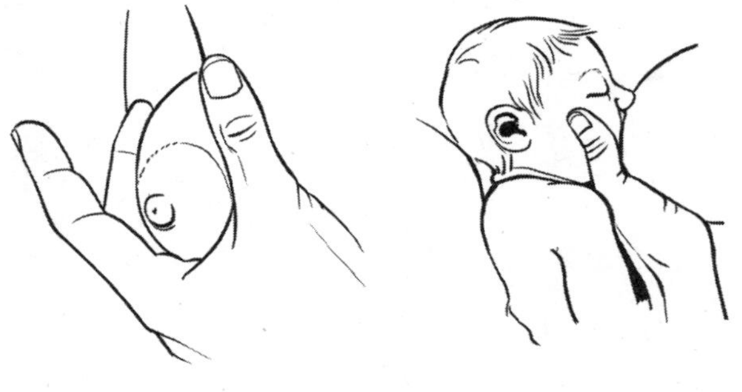

Figure A.11 Dancer Hand Position. ©2020 Nancy Mohrbacher Solutions, Inc.

TONGUE EXERCISES

When a baby has difficulty nursing due to high or low muscle tone (or due to a neurological impairment), mouth and tongue exercises may help. But to be effective, they should be tailored to the baby's specific issues. Some babies having nursing problems become more organized when oral exercises are used and some become less organized. There is a wide range of possible tongue and mouth exercises, but choosing an oral exercise should be done by someone familiar with the underlying cause of the baby's problem and the techniques that best address it (Genna, 2017). Unless the person providing skilled lactation help is trained in oral-motor evaluation and therapy, she/he should consider referring the nursing couple to someone with this training, especially if the baby has difficulty both nursing and bottle-feeding. The following U.S. websites list local people trained in oral-motor evaluation and therapy. Because many in these fields were trained using bottle-feeding norms, ask if they are familiar with the nursing baby.

asha.org—American Speech and Hearing Association, where parents can find a speech pathologist trained in assessing and treating feeding problems.

ndta.org—Neuro-Developmental Treatment Association, where parents can find a therapist who uses a neuro-developmental (whole child) approach.

Mouth and tongue exercises should always be enjoyable for everyone. The baby should be actively involved, and because her mouth is a private space, the baby should be the one to decide if others can enter it and for how long (Genna, 2017). When showing parents how to do the exercises below, it is important to model sensitivity to the baby's responses. To avoid overstimulation, in some cases, these exercises may be best timed before the baby shows feeding cues or when switching sides during a nursing session.

Walking Back on the Tongue

- Wash hands well with soap and water. Trim the fingernail of the index finger to be used.
- Touch baby's cheek lightly with the index finger and move it against the baby's skin to her lips, brushing her lips several times to trigger an open mouth.
- When she opens, massage the outside of her gums with the index finger, starting at the middle of the upper or low gum, moving toward either side.

- As she opens wide, use the fingertip to press down firmly near the tip of the baby's tongue and count slowly to three before releasing the pressure, keeping the finger in the baby's mouth.
- Move this finger a little farther back on her tongue, pressing again to a count of three.
- Move farther back on the baby's tongue once or twice more.
- Avoid making the baby gag. If she gags, avoid going that far back on the tongue the next time.
- If the baby enjoys this exercise, repeat it three or four times. If not, stop.

Pushing the Tongue Down and Out

- Wash and rinse hands well and trim the index finger to be used.
- Insert an index finger, pad side up, gently into the baby's mouth, pressing gently on her tongue.
- Leave the finger in that position for about 30 seconds while the baby sucks on it.
- Turn the finger over, so it is pad side down on the baby's tongue, and push down gently, while gradually pulling the finger out of her mouth.
- Repeat several times, then nurse the baby.

REFERENCES

Anderson, L., Kynoch, K., Kildea, S., et al. (2019). Effectiveness of breast massage for the treatment of women with breastfeeding problems: A systematic review. *JBI Database of Systematic Reviews and Implementation Reports, 17*(8), 1668-1694.

Bowles, B. C. (2011). Breast massage: A "handy" multipurpose tool to promote breastfeeding success. *Clinical Lactation, 2*(4), 21-24.

Cho, J., Ahn, H. Y., Ahn, S., et al. (2012). Effects of Oketani breast massage on breast pain, the breast milk pH of mothers, and the sucking speed of neonates. *Korean Journal of Women Health Nursing, 18*(2), 149-158.

Cotterman, K. J. (2004). Reverse pressure softening: A simple tool to prepare areola for easier latching during engorgement. *Journal of Human Lactation, 20*(2), 227-237.

Danner, S., & Cerutti, E. (1984). *Nursing Your Neurologically Impaired Baby.* Rochester, NY: Childbirth Graphics.

Eidelman, A. I. (2016). The appropriate use of breast massage. *Breastfeeding Medicine, 11,* 423.

Elad, D., Kozlovsky, P., Blum, O., et al. (2014). Biomechanics of milk extraction during breast-feeding. *Proceedings of the National Academy of Sciences of the USA, 111*(14), 5230-5235.

Foda, M. I., Kawashima, T., Nakamura, S., et al. (2004). Composition of milk obtained from unmassaged versus massaged breasts of lactating mothers. *Journal of Pediatric Gastroenterology and Nutrition, 38*(5), 484-487.

Geddes, D. T., Chooi, K., Nancarrow, K., et al. (2017). Characterisation of sucking dynamics of breastfeeding preterm infants: A cross sectional study. *BMC Pregnancy and Childbirth, 17*(1), 386.

Geddes, D. T., Kent, J. C., Mitoulas, L. R., et al. (2008). Tongue movement and intra-oral vacuum in breastfeeding infants. *Early Human Development, 84*(7), 471-477.

Genna, C. W. (2017). The influence of anatomic and structural issues on sucking skills. In C. W. Genna (Ed.), *Supporting Sucking Skills in Breastfeeding Infants* (3rd ed., pp. 209-267). Burlington, MA: Jones & Bartlett Learning.

Glover, R., & Wiessinger, D. (2017). They can do it, you can help: Building breastfeeding skill and confidence in mother and helper. In C. W. Genna (Ed.), *Supporting Sucking Skills in Breastfeeding Infants* (3rd ed., pp. 113-155). Burlington, MA: Jones & Bartlett Learning.

Jacobs, L. A., Dickinson, J. E., Hart, P. D., et al. (2007). Normal nipple position in term infants measured on breastfeeding ultrasound. *Journal of Human Lactation, 23*(1), 52-59.

Jones, E., Dimmock, P. W., & Spencer, S. A. (2001). A randomised controlled trial to compare methods of milk expression after preterm delivery. *Archives of Disease in Childhood. Fetal and Neonatal Edition, 85*(2), F91-95.

Kim, P. (2016). Human maternal brain plasticity: Adaptation to parenting. *New Directions for Child and Adolescent Development*(153), 47-58.

Kraleti, S. K., Lingaldjnna, S., Kalvala, S., et al. (2018). To study the impact of unilateral breast massage on milk volume among postnatal mothers—A quasi-experimental study. *Indian Journal of Child Health, 5*(12), 731-734.

Marmet, C., & Shell, E. (2017). Therapeutic positioning for breastfeeding. In C. W. Genna (Ed.), *Supporting Sucking Skills in Breastfeeding Infants* (3rd ed., pp. 399-416). Burlington, MA: Jones & Bartlett Learning.

Matthiesen, A. S., Ransjo-Arvidson, A. B., Nissen, E., et al. (2001). Postpartum maternal oxytocin release by newborns: Effects of infant hand massage and sucking. *Birth, 28*(1), 13-19.

Mizuno, K., Nishida, Y., Mizuno, N., et al. (2008). The important role of deep attachment in the uniform drainage of breast milk from mammary lobe. *Acta Paediatrica, 97*(9), 1200-1204.

Mohrbacher, N., & Kendall-Tackett, K. (2010). *Breastfeeding Made Simple: Seven Natural Laws for Nursing Mothers* (2nd ed.). Oakland, CA: New Harbinger Publications.

Morton, J., Hall, J. Y., Wong, R. J., et al. (2009). Combining hand techniques with electric pumping increases milk production in mothers of preterm infants. *Journal of Perinatology, 29*(11), 757-764.

Morton, J., Wong, R. J., Hall, J. Y., et al. (2012). Combining hand techniques with electric pumping increases the caloric content of milk in mothers of preterm infants. *Journal of Perinatology, 32*(10), 791-796.

Newman, J. (2017). Breast compression. Retrieved from **ibconline.ca/information-sheets/breast-compression/**.

Sadovnikova, A., Sanders, I., Koehler, S., et al. (2015). Systematic review of breast massage techniques around the world in databases and on YouTube [abstract]. *Breastfeeding Medicine, 10*(S1)(S1), S17.

Stutte, P. (1988). The effects of breast massage on volume and fat content of human milk. *Genesis, 10*(2), 22-25.

Uvnas-Moberg, K. (2014). *Oxytocin: The Biological Guide to Motherhood.* Amarillo, TX: Praeclarus Press.

Wambach, K., & Spencer, B. (2021). The cultural context of breastfeeding. In K. Wambach & B. Spencer (Eds.), *Breastfeeding and Human Lactation* (6th ed., pp. 739-758). Burlington, MA: Jones & Bartlett Learning.

Wiessinger, D. (1998). A breastfeeding teaching tool using a sandwich analogy for latch-on. *Journal of Human Lactation, 14*(1), 51-56.

Wilson-Clay, B., & Hoover, K. (2017). *The Breastfeeding Atlas* (6th ed.). Manchaca, TX: LactNews Press.

Zhao, C., Tang, R., Wang, J., et al. (2014). Six-step recanalization manual therapy: A novel method for treating plugged ducts in lactating women. *Journal of Human Lactation, 30*(3), 324-330.

Zheng, J. X., Chen, Y. C., Chen, H., et al. (2018). Disrupted spontaneous neural activity related to cognitive impairment in postpartum women. *Frontiers in Psychology, 9,* 624.

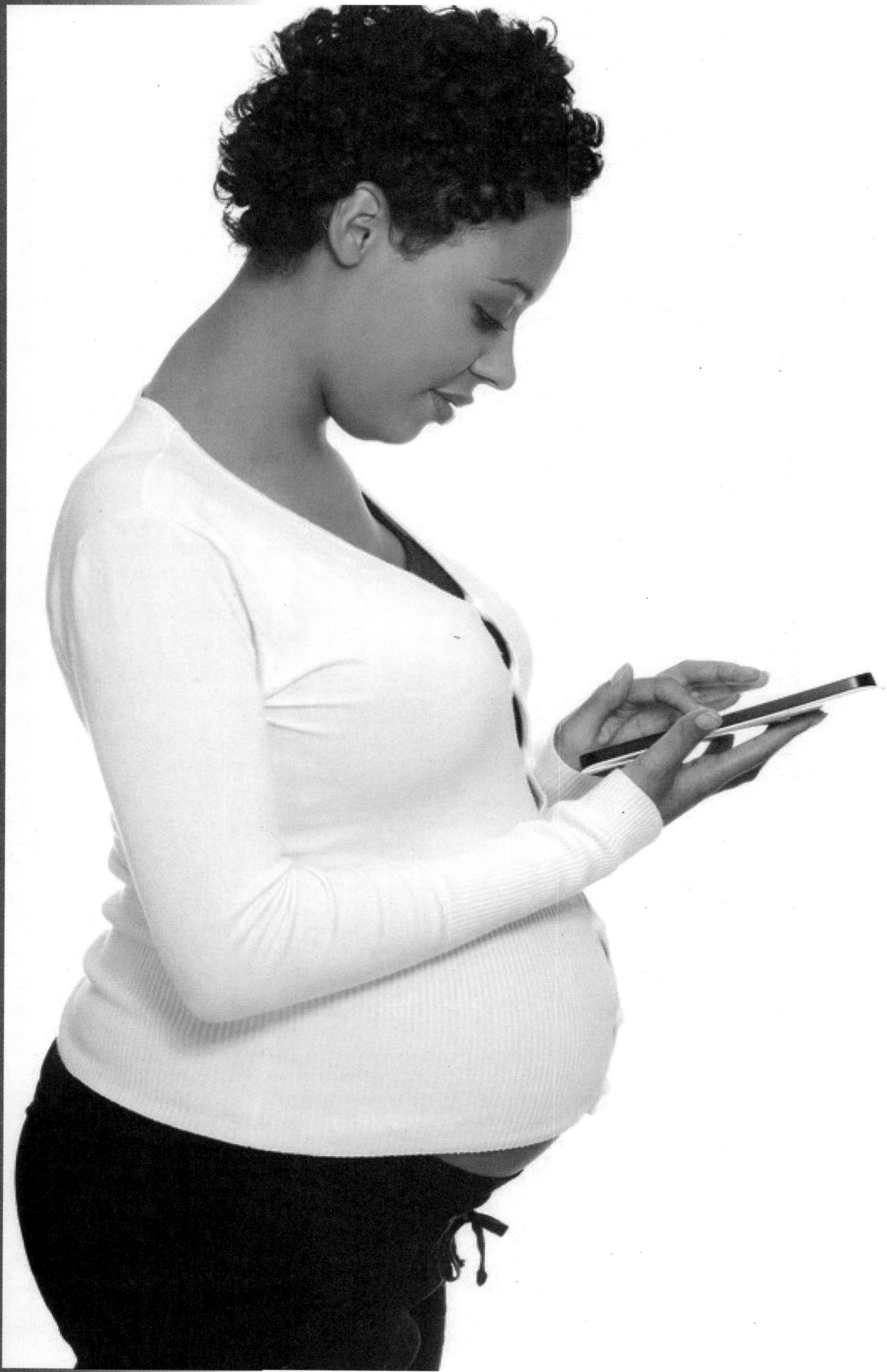

Tools and Products

B

ALTERNATIVE FEEDING METHODS

Indications for Use

An alternative to nursing is needed when the nursing couple is separated at feeding times, the baby can't directly nurse or nurse effectively, or the family decides to feed the nursing baby in other ways.

Choosing a Method

Nursing parents and their partners should be the final decision-makers on feeding method, ideally after reviewing each possibility's pros and cons, which are listed in Table B.1. U.S. lactation consultants Barbara Wilson-Clay and Kay Hoover (Wilson-Clay & Hoover, 2017, p. 115) explain that any eligible feeding method should have the following characteristics:

- It cannot harm the baby.
- It is a good match for the baby's size and condition.
- It is accessible and affordable.
- It is easy to use and clean.
- It is suitable for the length of time needed.
- It promotes the transition to direct nursing.

Also, it is important that the parents and others feeding the baby are comfortable with the feeding method. All the methods described in this section require instruction and practice. But most can be mastered quickly and get easier over time.

Cultural differences and the decision-maker. Alternatives to nursing vary by culture. A 2012 roundtable discussion (Bandara, Nyqvist, Musmar, Procaccini, & Wang, 2012) summarized alternative feeding methods commonly used in hospitals in Sri Lanka, the U.S., Palestine, Sweden, and Taiwan:

- Sri Lanka: cups, syringes, spoons, tube (no bottles)
- U.S.: bottles, but other methods are available if requested: cups, periodontal syringes, oral syringes, feeding-tube devices, and spoons
- Palestine: spoons syringes, or NG tube, and bottles if all other methods fail
- Sweden: cups, bottles are used only in non-nursing families and those who do not want to use cups for supplementing
- Taiwan: About 20%-30% of babies in the NICU use methods other than bottles, usually cups

A 2019 exploratory descriptive cross-sectional survey of 2,308 IBCLCs (Penny, Judge, Brownell, & McGrath, 2019) found that most IBCLCs believed that nursing supplementers (feeding-tube devices) were the best method for preserving the nursing relationship and was their preferred method. But only 18% thought the IBCLC had input on the method chosen. Feeding bottles were ranked as the most used method in the U.S., Australia, and Canada.

Early use of alternative feeding methods and breast-feeding self-efficacy. Research (Hussien, Refaat, & Arafa, 2019; Keemer, 2013) examined the use of alternative feeding methods with nursing babies soon after hospital discharge and found an association between their use and lower breastfeeding self-efficacy (BSE), or parents' confidence in their ability to nurse their baby. But what is the cause and what is the effect? Did parents use these methods because they doubted their ability to nurse, or did lactation problems, such as pain or latching struggles require them to use these methods, causing them to doubt their ability to nurse? An Australian study (Keemer, 2013) found that by the time a newborn was 7 days old, 48% of its 128 study mothers had used an alternative feeding method or a nipple shield, with 77% using feeding bottles with regular teats, 44% using syringes, and 34% using feeding bottles with wide-based teats.

Comparative Research

Much of the research comparing feeding methods is focused on preterm babies. Some study results may not apply to healthy term babies.

NG tube versus feeding bottles in preterm babies. In many hospitals, small preterm babies receive their first oral feeds by tube. One type of tube-feeding is done by nasogastric tube, NG tube for short. Using this method, the milk flows through a thin tube inserted through the baby's nose directly into his stomach. An advantage of supplementing a baby this way is there is no exposure to artificial nipples/teats. Some babies transition from NG-tube feedings to direct nursing without the use of feeding bottles. One U.S. randomized controlled trial (Kliethermes, Cross, Lanese, Johnson, & Simon, 1999) found that preterm babies supplemented only by NG tube were 4.5 times more likely to be directly nursing at hospital discharge and more than 9.0 times more likely to be exclusively nursing than the babies who were supplemented by bottle. At 3 months, the babies supplemented by NG tube were 3 times more likely to be nursing and 3 times more likely to be fully nursing than the preemies who were supplemented by bottle.

Syringe feeding versus feeding bottles in preterm babies. A 2019 Turkish prospective experimental study followed 103 preterm babies who were being transitioned from NG tube to full oral feeds (Say et al., 2019). These babies, who ranged in gestational age from 26 to 32 weeks, were randomized into one of two groups whose supplementary feeds were given: 1) by syringe or 2) by feeding bottle. The syringe was placed in the middle of baby's tongue, gently touching the baby's palate to promote sucking of the syringe. The feeder applied gentle pressure to the syringe plunger to provide 3 to 5 mL of milk, and baby was given time to swallow before more milk was given. The researchers found that compared with the babies fed by bottle, the babies in the syringe group reached full oral feeds sooner (40 days versus 54 days) and they transitioned to nursing sooner (43 days versus 54 days). The researchers recommended syringe feeding as a transitional method for preterm babies.

Cups versus feeding bottles in term and preterm babies. The results of any study on feeding methods depend in part on whether those using the method or teaching parents are skilled in its use. Every method takes practice to master. With cup-feeding, some early U.S. studies found that cup-feedings took more time than bottle-feeding, resulted in more milk spillage, and delayed hospital discharge for up to 10 days (Collins et al., 2004; Dowling, Meier, DiFiore, Blatz, & Martin, 2002; Marinelli, Burke, & Dodd, 2001), but this was not the case in research conducted in areas where cup-feeding is the norm.

Preterm babies have a much more difficult time safely bottle-feeding compared with term newborns, in part because preterm babies find it more challenging to coordinate sucking, swallowing, and breathing with a fast and consistent milk flow. A 2018 integrative review, which examined in depth 14 studies on cup-feeding preterm babies (Penny, Judge, Brownell, & McGrath, 2018a), concluded that use of cup-feeding resulted in more stable heart rate and oxygen saturation than bottle-feeding with a similar weight gain. Also, nursing rates were higher at discharge with continued higher rates of nursing among cup-fed infants at both 3 and 6 months post-discharge. A Cochrane Review that examined the safety of feeding methods for preterm babies (Collins, Gillis, McPhee, Suganuma, & Makrides, 2016) recommended against bottle-feeding preterm babies. Cup-feeding is common in many developing countries for health and sanitation reasons. Because cup-feeding produces better health and nursing outcomes, it is also used routinely in some developed countries (Bandara et al., 2012). Another Cochrane Review that focused on cup-feeding in both term and preterm babies (Flint, New, & Davies, 2016) concluded that supplementing late preterm babies with cups rather than bottles improves nursing outcomes for up to 6 months of age.

Physiology of cup-feeding. Why does cup-feeding lead to better nursing outcomes? Brazilian research (Franca, Sousa, Aragao, & Costa, 2014; Gomes, Trezza, Murade, & Padovani, 2006) found that during cup-feeding, the feeding behaviors and muscles used were closer to nursing than other feeding methods.

Full-term babies may react differently than preterm babies to cup- and bottle-feeding. A Taiwanese study of 138 full-term babies found that although nursing outcomes were virtually the same between the groups supplemented by cup and bottle, in the early days, those supplemented by bottle were more fretful while nursing than those supplemented by cup (Huang, Gau, Huang, & Lee, 2009). The researchers also noted that the mothers who supplemented by bottle were more likely to believe they had insufficient milk compared with those who supplemented by cup. A U.S. study (Howard et al., 1999) found no difference in milk intake and feeding time among full-term babies supplemented by cup or bottle, and later nursing rates later were the same in both groups. Another U.S. study (Howard et al., 2003) found that cup-feeding improved nursing outcomes only among parents who gave birth by cesarean section and babies who received more than two supplemental feeds in the hospital.

The paladai, a type of feeding cup used traditionally in India, is a low bowl with a small spout that is shaped like Aladdin's lamp. During feeds, the milk is poured from its spout into the baby's mouth. In a study done in India of 100 babies, which included full-term, growth retarded, and preterm babies (Malhotra, Vishwambaran, Sundaram, & Narayanan, 1999b), those fed by paladai had the greatest milk intake in the shortest time and were quiet longer after feeds than babies fed by regular cup or bottle. This study found higher rates of milk spillage with a straight-sided cup compared to a paladai or a bottle. As with any type of cup, technique is obviously important when feeding with a paladai. A study of preterm babies in the U.K.—where the paladai is not traditionally used—found longer feeding times, more milk spillage, and more stress cues among the babies fed by a paladai (Aloysius & Hickson, 2007).

Cup-feeding versus nursing supplementer. A Thai randomized controlled trial (Puapornpong, Raungrongmorakot, Hemachandra, Ketsuwan, & Wongin, 2015) included 120 nursing couples who delivered without complications but whose babies needed to be fed a supplement at 48 hours post-delivery. These nursing couples were randomized into two group 1) supplemented by cup and 2) supplemented by a nursing supplementer consisting of a syringe and attached tube. About 72 hours after birth (24 hours after the supplements began), all 120 babies received a latch score. Those supplemented by nursing supplementer scored significantly higher than those supplemented by cup.

Finger-feeding versus cup. A 2017 Brazilian prospective longitudinal randomized experimental study (Moreira, Cavalcante-Silva, Fujinaga, & Marson, 2017) followed 53 preterm babies who were born at less than 37 weeks gestation and were transitioning from NG tube to nursing. The researchers divided the supplemented babies into two groups: 1) those supplemented by cup and 2) those supplemented via finger-feeding. Finger-feeding was done by taping a feeding tube along the inside of a gloved little finger of the feeder with the finger pad side up. The milk was inside a syringe with plunger removed positioned horizontally at the level of the baby's head. The baby's sucking drew out the milk rather than gravity. The researchers found the finger-feeding group had less milk loss, longer feeding times, and lower frequency of complications, such as gagging, respiratory problems, and reduced oxygen levels. They concluded finger-feeding was a better transitional feeding method than cup-feeding.

TABLE B.1 Advantages and Disadvantages of Alternative Feeding Methods

Feeding Method	Advantages	Disadvantages
Nursing Supplementer	• Reinforces direct nursing • Reduces or eliminates the need to feed baby again after nursing • Babies latch easier when using this method • Can improve sucking skills in some babies • If latched deeply, sucking stimulates milk production during supplementation	• Unfamiliar to many • Equipment care may be stressful and time consuming • Some babies suck on tubing like a straw, which reduces stimulation • If latching with tubing in place, may add stress • If tape is used often, it may cause skin damage • Some commercial devices are expensive
Feeding Bottles	• Culturally acceptable and readily avaiable in the West • Familiar to many parents • Some babies consume more milk in a shorter time • Relatively inexpensive	• Can replace nursing • Fast flow causes more heart-rate and breathing problems in preemies • May complicate transition to nursing if used for >2 feedings or after a c-section • Baby uses different mouth muscles; so long-term regular use increases risk of oral malformations • Fast flow may cause overfeeding; so long-term, regular use increases risk of obesity
Finger-Feeding	• May make transition to nursing easier • Can be used to improve sucking in some babies • Viewed as temporary	• Unfamiliar to many parents • Finger-feeding equipment may not be easily available to parents • Little research
Sipping/Lapping Methods (cup, bowl, spoon, eyedropper, syringe)	• Easy to clean • Readily available • Inexpensive • In preemies, fewer heart-rate and breathing problems than bottles • More direct nursing at discharge • May make transition to nursing easier • Muscles used similar to nursing	• If hospital staff or parents are not well trained, can lead to feeding problems • Feeding may take longer • May be some milk loss from spillage

For research citations, see earlier and later sections.

Nursing Supplementers

Sometimes called ***feeding-tube devices, tube-feeding devices, at-breast supplementers,*** or ***nursing supplementers***, these devices deliver extra milk to the baby during nursing through a thin tube. The baby's natural response to a swallow is to suck. Some babies learn to suck more effectively when the steady milk flow from the tube stimulates more active and consistent sucking and swallowing. When a baby latches deeply and sucks longer or more vigorously, he also takes more milk directly from the mammary gland and stimulates faster milk production. A nursing supplementer can allow parents with low milk production to feed their baby exclusively during nursing, eliminating the need to feed him again afterwards. Unlike other feeding methods, supplementing while baby nurses provides positive reinforcement for direct nursing.

Commercially manufactured nursing supplementers can be purchased or parents can create their own. One easy-to-make ***lactation aid*** functions as a siphon and consists of a bottle with a hole cut in the nipple/teat to insert one end of a feeding tube into the milk and the other end into the nursing baby's mouth (Newman, 2016). To learn more about how to make, use, and clean a homemade lactation aid, go to **bit.ly/BA2-LactationAid**. These devices can be used alone or—if latching is a problem—with a nipple shield. U.S. lactation consultant Catherine Watson Genna suggested in her book about lactation tools (Genna, 2016) that if a nursing supplementer is used with a nipple shield, choose a device with softer tubing, so during nursing, positioning the tubing inside the shield is less likely to disrupt the shield from the mammary gland.

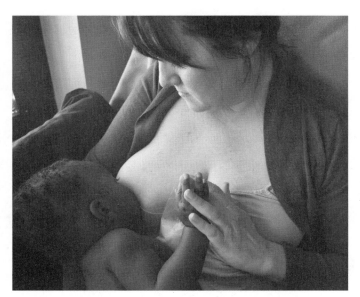

The milk container can hang around the parent's neck, be clipped to clothing, set nearby, or held.

Indications for Use

Nursing supplementers may be a good choice if milk production is low or baby is gaining weight slowly. It can provide a faster, more consistent milk flow during relactation or induced lactation. This immediate milk flow may help some babies more easily transition to nursing from other feeding methods. It can provide extra milk for babies with special needs, such as those with cardiac issues, neurological impairment, cleft palate, Down syndrome, and prematurity, which—depending on the issue—can sometimes help a baby with challenges learn to nurse more effectively.

Two Types of Nursing Supplementers

Nursing supplementers fall into two general categories:

- **Suction required.** These devices can be makeshift or manufactured. They include a container to hold the supplement, which hangs around the user's neck, clips to clothing, or is held or set/hung from a nearby surface. When the baby latches, in addition to the nipple and areola, he also takes its thin tubing. As he sucks, milk flows through the tubing. When used effectively, the nursing baby receives both the supplement through the tubing and milk directly from the mammary gland.
- **Suction not required.** These makeshift devices (at this writing, no manufactured versions are commercially available) consist of either a periodontal syringe or a syringe with needle removed attached by port to a thin feeding tube. With these supplementers, the feeder controls milk flow, and the baby does not need to generate suction.

The suction-required nursing supplementers are only a useful tool if the baby can generate enough suction to draw the supplement through the tubing. The suction-not-required supplementers can be used with babies who can't generate suction, such as those with a cleft palate or those weakened from underfeeding. The suction-not-required devices should be used with caution with babies who have cardiac defects and airway abnormalities. These babies must breathe more times per minute to maintain adequate oxygen levels. If a faster milk flow generated by the feeder forces these babies swallow more often, this may compromise their oxygen levels (Genna, LeVan Fram, & Sandora, 2017).

Research on Nursing Supplementers

A 2018 review of the evidence on nursing supplementers (Penny, Judge, Brownell, & McGrath, 2018b) concluded that these devices could be useful tools when nursing babies need extra milk and that all healthcare providers who help lactating families should be familiar with them and trained in their use. One U.S. survey of 22 mothers who used a suction-required nursing supplementer (Borucki, 2005) reported very mixed feelings about their experiences. Some considered the device a "necessary evil" that allowed them to maintain the nursing relationship. Some described it as "cumbersome, time-consuming, compromising, artificial, complicated, and messy" (Borucki, 2005, p. 435). One mother used the device twice for a short-term issue; another mother used it continuously for 13 months. Five of the 22 mothers stopped nursing within a week due to struggles with the device. Sixteen of the 22 mothers breastfed longer than 6 months and one nursed for 4.5 years. Parent-related reasons for using this device included insufficient milk production, delay in milk increase after birth, nipple pain and trauma, history of breast-reduction surgery, and adoption. Baby-related reasons for its use included shallow latch, weak suck, slow weight gain, and prematurity-related feeding problems. As described on p. 684, according to U.S. lactation consultant Alyssa Schnell, author of *Breastfeeding Without Birthing*, families who intend to use these devices may find them more manageable and less intimidating if after they buy them, they practice assembling, using, and cleaning them before using them with the baby. One way to practice is to set them up as directed with water instead of milk in the container and have the partner suck the water out. For podcasts and articles that feature tips and tricks for using these devices, go to **bit.ly/BA2-TipsTricks**.

Using a Nursing Supplementer

Knowing something about the following practical details of using a nursing supplementer may make it a much more effective tool.

Milk type, volume, and tubing care. If the parent is using infant formula as a supplement, suggest using either the concentrate or ready-to-feed form, as powdered formula can clump and clog the thin tubing. To make sure the baby gets the milk he needs, suggest adding enough milk to the container so that about a half-ounce (15 mL) is left after every feed. If baby takes it all, add more at that feed and start the next feed with 1 ounce (30 mL) more. If more than a half-ounce (15 mL) is left consistently, decrease the volume of milk in the supplementer at the next feed. See Table 6.4 on p. 226 for milk-volume suggestions as a starting point. Unless the parent is using disposable tubing, suggest either washing the tubing immediately after feeds or immersing it in a container of cool or warm water (not hot, which can cook the milk), so the milk doesn't dry. Tubing with dried milk inside needs to be replaced.

Latching with tubing in place. One of the challenges parents report when using a nursing supplementer is achieving a deep latch while the tubing is positioned on the nipple. Some devices include surgical tape to keep the tubing in place while baby latches. Usually the tubing is taped just behind the areola to keep it out of baby's way, with the tape running lengthwise on the tubing and the tubing tip extending about a quarter-inch (6 mm) past the nipple tip. Finding a good spot to tape the tubing so it doesn't get in the baby's way can be a challenge.

An alternative to tape is for the parent to place a self-adhesive bandage on the appropriate place on the

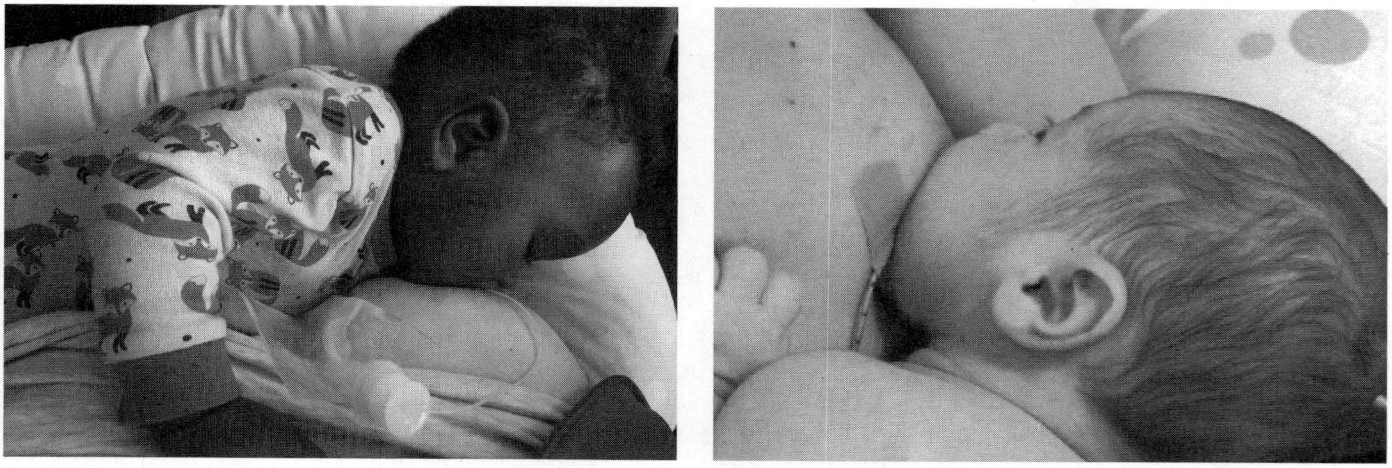

Figure B.1 Feeds with a nursing supplementer go more smoothly for some nursing couples when the tubing is positioned under baby's top lip (left), but others prefer a lower-lip position (right). Note on the right the bandage holding the tubing under the areola. ©2020 Catherine Watson Genna, BS, IBCLC, used with permission.

mammary gland after bathing and leave it there until the next bath or shower. At each feed, the bandage can be pinched to allow the tubing to thread through it underneath its pad. Although some devices recommend positioning the tubing on top of the nipple when baby latches (Figure B.1 left), some suggest instead positioning it on the underside of the nipple so that it rests against baby's tongue during feeds (Figure B.1 right). Some babies find it irritating when the tubing rubs against their palate during nursing (Genna, 2016).

Latching first and then inserting the tubing. To make it easier to get a deep latch to both mammary gland and tubing, if the nursing supplementer tubing is firm enough, such as the tubing used with the lactation aid, it may be possible for baby to latch first without the tubing and then push the firmer tubing into the corner of the baby's mouth until milk starts to flow (Newman, 2016).

Sucking the tubing like a straw. Another challenge when using this device is that some babies learn to latch shallowly and suck the tubing like a straw without stimulating the mammary gland. If this happens, the baby will not have wide jaw movements when nursing, which are needed to stimulate faster milk production. If latching deeper doesn't correct this, this device may not be helpful.

Adjusting milk flow of a nursing supplementer. To provide enough mammary stimulation with this feeding method, the goal is for feeds to last 20 to 40 minutes, or 10 to 20 minutes per side. To achieve this, suggest the user adjust the device's milk flow so that at each nursing, the baby sucks actively for about 10 to 20 minutes per side, switching sides about halfway through. If the milk flow is too fast, the baby may finish before 20 minutes total. If the milk flow is too slow, feeds may take more than 45 minutes, which may cause the baby to quickly lose interest in feeding or make it difficult to fit in enough feeds per day. Milk flow can be adjusted in suction-required nursing supplementers in the following ways.

- **Raise or lower the container.** These devices work like a siphon, with a higher container providing faster flow and a lower container providing slower flow.
- **Increase or decrease tubing diameter.** Some nursing supplementers include different size tubing (small, medium, large). Larger diameter tubing provides faster flow; smaller diameter tubing provides slower flow.
- **Open or clamp one tubing.** Nursing supplementers with a closed container and two tubes can be set up with either both tubes open or one or both clamped closed. Both tubes open provides faster milk flow; one tube closed provides slower milk flow.
- **Position one or two tubes at the nipple.** When the device includes two tubes, they can either be positioned with one at each nipple to make switching sides easier, or for faster flow, both can be positioned at one nipple.

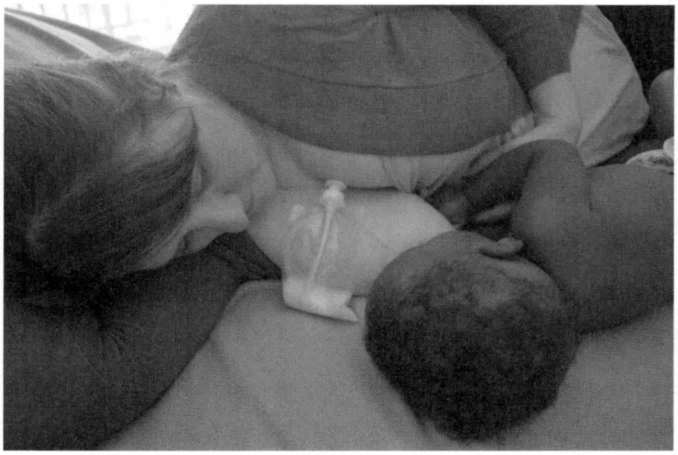

With some types of nursing supplementers, it's possible to nurse in a side-lying position.

If the baby begins to nurse more effectively and/or the milk production increases, adjust the supplementer in the above ways to slow milk flow as needed to maintain ideal feeding times.

Determining volume of supplement needed. Encourage the baby who was underfed to take as much milk as possible to increase his energy for more effective nursing. But when a baby's weight gain is just a little slow, a balance needs to be found between providing him with the milk he needs to gain weight normally and not giving him so much supplement that he takes less milk from the nursing parent. For the baby younger than 4 months, see Table 6.4 on p. 226 for the average recommended volume of supplement to increase weight gain to the average weight gain of 7 ounces (198 g.) per week as described by the World Health Organization's Growth Standards for nursing babies at **bit.ly/BA2-WHOweight**.

Weaning from a nursing supplementer. During the baby's first 6 months, if a nursing parent's milk production cannot be increased enough to fully meet the baby's needs for milk, such as parents with inadequate glandular tissue or a history of breast reduction or top surgery, the supplementer may be needed until solid foods eventually reduce baby's need for milk to match the parent's production. In most cases, though, this device will be needed short-term until the baby's nursing effectiveness improves and/or the milk production increases.

If the baby begins feeding more effectively, he may start taking all of the supplement in a shorter time. If the baby finishes feeding in less than 20 minutes, and the nursing supplementer has multiple tubing sizes, suggest switching to a smaller size tubing to slow the flow and increase feeding time for better stimulation.

If parents want to know how much milk the baby is taking directly from them, they can do a test-weight (see last section) and subtract the amount the baby took from the supplementer from his total milk intake at the feed. As the baby takes more milk from the parent, the following strategies can be used to gradually wean from the device:

- Lower the height of the container to slow milk flow.
- Clamp the tubing shut before baby latches and wait to unclamp it until the sound of baby's swallowing stops.
- Try nursing without the supplementer at the first morning feed, which is usually when the most milk is available.
- Use the supplementer at gradually fewer feeds each day.

As parents wean the baby from the supplement, they should expect the baby will want to nurse more often. Some use their baby's behavior as a guide. As one U.S. mother (Borucki, 2005, p. 433) said, "When I really felt like he didn't have a good feeding, and he really seemed like he was hungry, I would put it on." Suggest having the baby weighed regularly while weaning from the supplementer to ensure he gets enough milk.

Some parents have a difficult time emotionally weaning from the supplementer, considering it a kind of "security blanket." As one U.S. mother (Borucki, 2005, pp. 433-434) said:

> "I think that, towards the end, I might have tried to do plain breastfeeding without the system, but he never wanted to do that. I wasn't too supportive of that anyway, because I had lost confidence in my ability to do it on my own."

Support, encouragement, and the use of test-weighing to provide objective reassurance of baby's milk intake may be helpful in convincing parents that the nursing supplementer is no longer needed.

Feeding Bottles

Research on Feeding Bottles

Nursing and bottle-feeding differ. Some—but not all—newborns have difficulty transitioning from bottle-feeding to nursing, especially during the early weeks. This may be in part because of the differences between these feeding methods. Research on 12 healthy term babies who acted as their own controls during nursing and bottle-feeding (Aizawa, Mizuno, & Tamura, 2010) found significant differences in the movements of their mouth, throat, and jaws, depending on the method used. A Japanese study that examined the sucking patterns in breastfed and bottle-fed babies (Taki et al., 2010) found a different sucking pattern in the two groups, with bottle-fed babies having longer sucking bursts and more sucks per burst. A Brazilian retrospective study of 25 newborns undergoing swallow studies, some of whom were nursing and some of whom were bottle-feeding (Hernandez & Bianchini, 2019), found significant differences in how the two groups swallowed.

Does bottle-feeding affect nursing? Do these differences in how babies suck and swallow affect how babies nurse after being bottle-fed? A 2019 Brazilian prospective cross-sectional study of 427 mothers and babies (Batista, Rodrigues, Ribeiro, & Nascimento, 2019) tried to answer this question. The researchers found there were greater changes in the babies' nutritive sucking patterns (when they sucked for milk) over time in the group fed by bottle as compared with those who exclusively nursed. In another study using data from this same group (Batista, Ribeiro, Nascimento, & Rodrigues, 2018), the Brazilian researchers concluded that more of the babies who received bottles were rated as "poor" or "fair" in their nursing behaviors, as compared with the babies who exclusively nursed. The researchers concluded that bottle-feeding may be associated with unfavorable nursing behaviors.

In *The Breastfeeding Atlas*, its authors suggest that the nursing parent's anatomy may play a role in a baby's response to a bottle teat. They wrote: "If women have erectile nipples with good elasticity, their babies may not be vulnerable…." (Wilson-Clay & Hoover, 2017, p. 46). In other words, bottles may pose a greater risk of feeding problems in babies whose nursing parents have flat or inverted nipples. They suggest the fast flow of the bottle and the firm teat provide a "supernormal stimulus" in the baby's mouth, which may lead to feeding problems for parents with non-protruding nipples.

Drawbacks of bottle-feeding with preterm babies. As described in the earlier section, "Comparative Research," bottle-feeding preterm babies has significant health drawbacks. After examining seven trials that included 1,152 preemies, the authors of a 2016 Cochrane Review (Collins et al., 2016) concluded that due to the heart-rate and breathing irregularities common among preemies during bottle-feeding, when supplementing preterm babies, bottle-feeding should be avoided and cups should be used instead. Bottle-feeding preterm babies was also associated with lower nursing rates at hospital discharge, at 3 months, and at 6 months.

Long-term drawbacks of regular bottle-feeding. The baby's oral cavity develops differently when exposed to different feeding methods. Bottle-feeding, for example, is associated with a greater likelihood of oral malformations. A 2017 systematic review and meta-analysis examined 31 observational studies of moderate to high quality (Boronat-Catala, Montiel-Company, Bellot-Arcis, Almerich-Silla, & Catala-Pizarro, 2017). Its authors concluded that risk of posterior crossbite was nearly 4 times higher in children who never breastfed compared with those who breastfed for more than 6 months. The risk of this condition was 8 times higher when the never-breastfed babies were compared with those who breastfed for 12 months or longer. Odds of class II malocclusion and irregularly-spaced teeth were also higher in children who never nursed.

Another long-term drawback associated with bottle-feeding is a higher risk of overweight and obesity in children. See p. 192-194 for an overview of the research and a summary of how both bottle-feeding (even bottle-feeding expressed human milk) and exposure to formula affects the risk of childhood overweight and obesity.

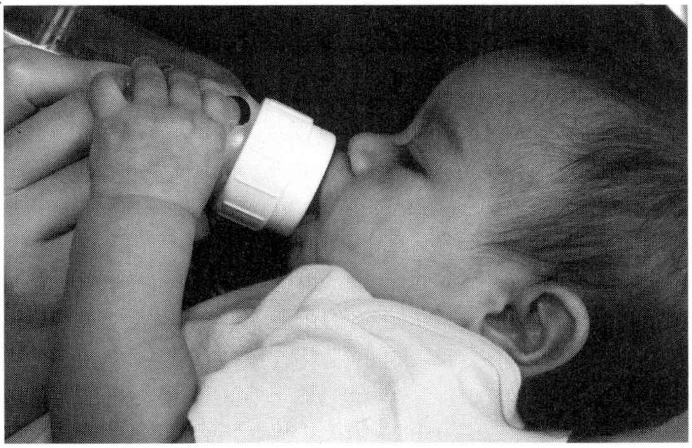

Figure B.2 This baby's lips are closed on the bottle collar rather than the base of the teat, a sign the teat may be too short.

Feeding-Bottle Options

Two basic aspects of bottle-feeding may affect how easily a nursing baby transitions between nursing and the bottle. One is the shape and flow of the bottle nipple, also known as its ***teat***. The other is feeding technique. Research found that using a larger bottle, as compared with a smaller bottle, is more likely to lead to greater weight gain in formula-fed babies (Wood et al., 2016), but for the most part the milk container is not going to have a significant effect on nursing. Regarding type of bottle to use, parents need to decide whether they want to use a standard size bottle and teat or the brands (such as Avent and Dr. Brown's) whose parts are not interchangeable with other brands. Also, keep in mind that despite the reassuring volume markers on the sides of most bottles, amazingly, research found many to be significantly inaccurate (Gribble, Berry, Kerac, & Challinor, 2017).

Teat characteristics. What should nursing parents who are planning to use bottles look for in a bottle teat? There are many choices and many brands. First, make sure they know that despite marketing claims, none are like the real thing! An excellent general resource is the book *Balancing Breast and Bottle* by Amy Peterson and Mindy Harmer (Peterson & Harmer, 2010). Here are some teat characteristics to consider.

- ***Teat material.*** Nearly all bottle teats are made of either silicone or latex. Silicone is firmer and more durable. Latex is softer, less durable, and causes allergic reactions in some parents and babies.
- ***Teat length.*** Mouth shape varies from baby to baby, which is why one teat length does not fit all! To quantify one difference among babies, U.S. lactation consultant Barbara Wilson-Clay measured the ***oral reach*** of 98 babies in her practice (Wilson-Clay & Hoover, 2017) by allowing the babies to suck on her gloved finger and then marking the distance between the area in the babies' mouth that triggered active sucking and their closed lips. She found their oral reach ranged from 1.9 cm to 3.2 cm. To find their baby's best teat length, parents can experiment with different teats. If baby gags, the teat is too long. If baby's lips close on the bottle collar rather than the teat base (Figure B.2), it is probably too short.
- ***Teat shape.*** At this writing, expert opinion is the best evidence we have on what teat shape to choose. U.S. co-authors Amy Peterson, an IBCLC, and Mindy Harmer, a speech-and-language pathologist (Peterson & Harmer, 2010), suggest starting with teats—independent of their style—

that widen gradually rather than teats that widen abruptly, which they found in their practice were more difficult for many nursing babies to master. See Figure B.3 for an illustration of what these differences look like with different style teats.

- ***Teat flow rate.*** Suggest parents use feeding bottles that provide the slowest flow rate the baby will accept. Slow-flow teats are less likely to cause overfeeding. With a slower flow, baby is satisfied with less milk, reducing risk of overweight and minimizing the volume of expressed milk needed. A slower flow also makes it easier for a compromised baby to coordinate sucking, swallowing, and breathing. Shouldn't this be easy for parents to find since manufacturers label their teats as slow flow, medium flow, and fast flow? Actually not, because there is little relation between the package labels and the teats' actual flow rates. U.S. researchers (Pados, Park, & Dodrill, 2019) examined the milk-flow rates of 25 different slow-flow and standard teats. Even among those labeled "slow flow," the flow rates differed by more than 20 times. For example, the slowest milk-flow rate was the Avent Natural First Flow teat at 0.86 mL/min. while the Medela Wide-Base Slow Flow teat was the fastest at 22.03 mL/min. The milk-flow rate of the Medela Calma teat was the fastest, at 37.61 mL/min. A chart showing the milk-flow rates is available to use as a reference in this Pados study. A teat's milk-flow rate may be too slow for a baby if he starts biting the teat or seems frustrated.
- ***Teat style.*** Should parents choose a wide-based or narrow-based teat? Experimenting can help determine the answer. How the baby latches to the teat makes a difference, too. When a baby takes a wide-based nipple into his mouth by opening wide and closing his lips on its wide base rather than the nipple shaft, this mimics the wider gape of a baby nursing. However, one size does not fit all. As two U.S. IBCLCs (Wilson-Clay & Hoover, 2017, pp. 123-124) wrote: "Some infants require a narrow based teat owing to poor lip tone and inability to seal to a wider base. Some infants will gag if the teat is too long. Other infants seem not to respond if the teat is too short…"
- ***Specialty feeding bottles.*** Most feeding bottles flow freely. Some specialty feeding bottles give a baby who is physically compromised more control over milk flow during bottle-feeds. One example is the Haberman Feeder (Figure B.4.) This bottle does not rely on suction. It flows only when the baby compresses the teat. Babies who benefit from these devices include babies with an airway abnormality or those with a cleft palate, who can easily become overwhelmed when milk flows through the opening in their palate into their nasal cavity and ear tubes.

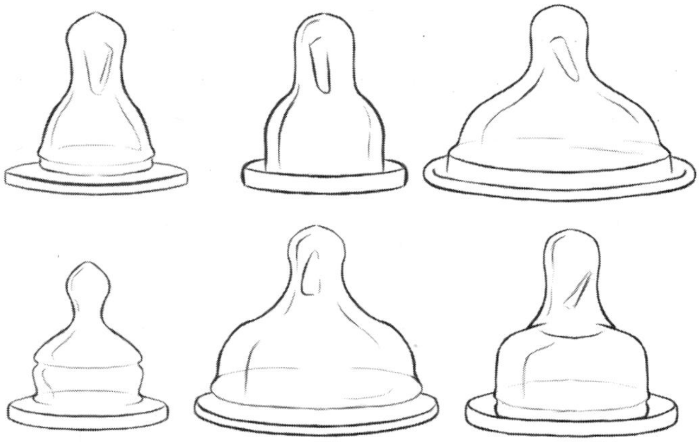

Figure B.3 Experts recommend nursing babies start with teats shaped like those pictured in the top row, which widen gradually, rather than those in the bottom row, which widen abruptly. ©2020 Nancy Mohrbacher Soltions, Inc.

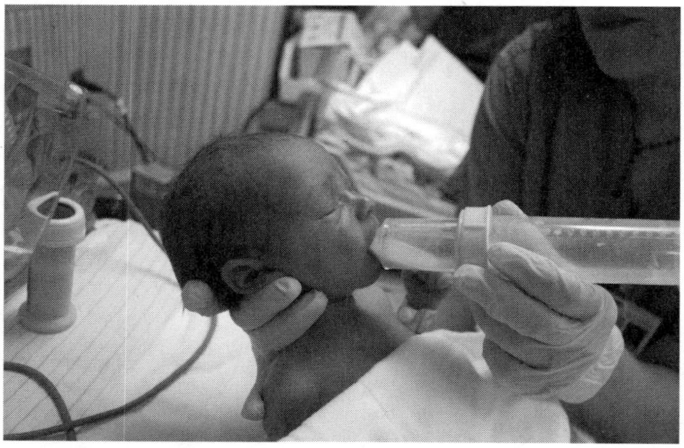

Figure B.4 This compromised baby is being bottle-fed in the hospital with a specialty feeding bottle in which milk flows only when baby compresses its teat.

Pacing and Other Bottle-Feeding Techniques

Make bottle-feeding more like nursing. When nursing parents or other caregivers bottle-feed, encourage them to use feeding techniques that reinforce nursing behaviors. U.S. lactation consultant Dee Kassing described how bottle-feeding techniques can mimic nursing to make the transition back to nursing easier (Kassing, 2002). For example, rather than inserting the bottle teat into the baby's mouth, hold the baby on the feeder's lap in a semi-upright position with the bottle held horizontally and brush the bottle teat lightly against the baby's lips, waiting for a wide gape before allowing the baby to draw it in.

Pacing bottle-feeds. Pacing also mimics nursing. Unlike the fast, consistent milk flow that occurs when babies are bottle-fed in the usual way, pacing provides the fast-then slow-then fast milk flow that occurs with milk ejections during nursing sessions. This technique was originally used for preterm or compromised babies who struggled during bottle feeds with fast milk flow. But many parents and lactation specialists found that it can help all bottle-feeding babies avoid overfeeding and give them more control over milk flow. Here's how paced bottle-feeding works:

- Position baby semi-upright or upright (Figure B.4).
- Touch baby's lips with the bottle teat and wait until he opens wide (Figure B.5).
- Allow baby to draw in the teat so that his lips close on the teat base, not its shaft or bottle collar, with top and bottom lips flanged out.
- Hold the bottle nearly horizontal (Figure B.6). As baby starts to suck and swallow, build in pauses every few minutes by lowering the end of the bottle so milk runs out of the teat, giving baby a breathing break.
- When the baby begins sucking again, lift the end of the bottle so milk flows back into the teat.
- Repeat until baby is finished.

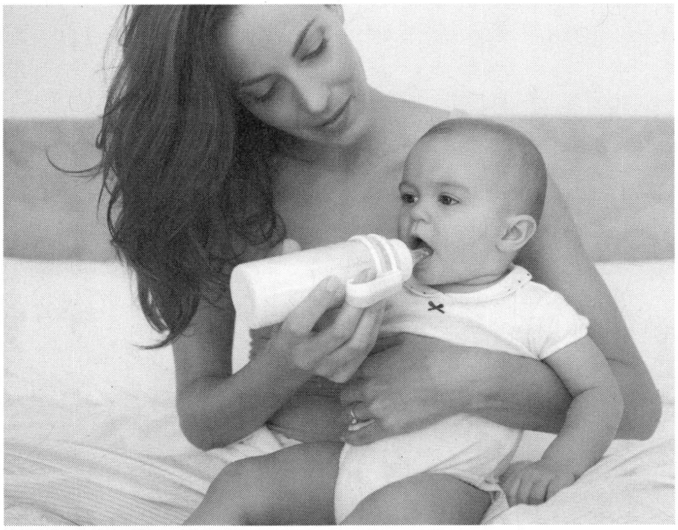

Figure B.5 Rather than pushing the bottle teat into baby's mouth, tap his lips until he opens wide. Then let him draw it in far enough so his lips close on the teat base, not its shaft or the bottle collar.

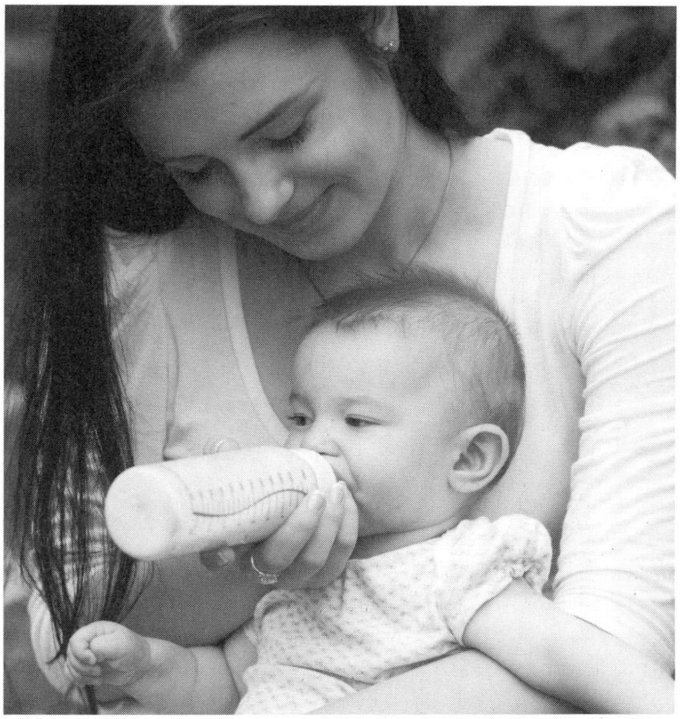

Figure B.6 During paced bottle-feeds, every few minutes tilt the end of the bottle down to give baby a breathing break.

Bottle-feeds should ideally take between 15 to 30 minutes. An average feeding volume for a nursing baby 1 month or older is about 3 to 4 oz. (89-113 mL) (Kent et al., 2013). One common concern about paced bottle-feeds is whether allowing the milk to drain out of the teat means that baby swallows air. Assure families that we all swallow air while we eat, and it is easy for baby to burp up any air after feeds. A too-fast milk flow, however, can lead to aspirating (breathing in) milk, which is a much more serious concern. Some employed nursing parents report that when their baby's caregiver uses paced bottle-feeding, this sometimes decreases milk volumes needed during the workday by as much as 50%.

Finger-Feeding

Finger-feeding involves feeding milk to a baby while he's sucking on the feeder's finger.

Indications for Use

Finger-feeding can be used with any baby to provide extra milk and can be used therapeutically to teach more normal sucking to babies with poor oral-motor skills by rewarding them with milk when they make correct feeding movements (Genna, 2016).

Research on Finger-Feeding

See the previous section "Comparative Research" (starting on p. 894) for a description of a study of preterm babies that compared finger-feeding to cup-feeding.

Tools and Strategies for Finger-Feeding

Whichever tool is used to finger-feed, tell the feeders the first step is to wash their hands well and make sure the finger used to feed the baby has a closely-trimmed nail:

- Any nursing supplementer can be used to finger-feed by placing its tubing along an adult's finger, pad side up, and extending it about a quarter-inch (6 mm) past the fingertip. If desired, the tubing can be taped to the finger, ideally lengthwise, so the baby can't suck the tape into his mouth. Tap baby's lips with the finger and wait until he opens. Allow baby to draw the finger into his mouth to the area where active sucking is triggered.
- Periodontal syringes, which typically hold 10 to 20 mL of milk each, can be used by pulling back on the plunger to draw milk into the syringe and resting the curved tip against the feeder's finger just inside the corner of the baby's mouth (about one-sixteenth of an inch or 2 mm). The plunger should be depressed slowly, only while the baby is sucking. When the baby pauses, the feeder pauses to avoid overwhelming the baby with milk.

Sipping and Lapping Methods

Feeding methods that require the baby to sip or lap the milk (as opposed to sucking) include cup, bowl, spoon, eyedropper, and syringe.

Research on Sipping/Lapping Methods

As one Swedish researcher (Nyqvist & Ewald, 2006, p. 85) wrote, "Cup-feeding has been used for feeding infants and young children as far back in history as we have any insight." In many parts of the developing world, cups and spoons are considered the only safe alternatives to nursing, because clean water for washing feeding utensils is not always available and dangerous bacteria can grow in the cracks and crevices of feeding bottles, spreading illness (Bergman & Jurisoo, 1994). In the 1980s, journal articles described cup-feeding of low birthweight babies in Kenya (Armstrong, 1987) and a UNICEF video was widely distributed, increasing interest in cup-feeding in the U.K., spurring research.

Studies in both India and the U.K. found that very preterm babies as young as 30 weeks gestation could effectively cup-feed even before they could bottle-feed (Gupta, Khanna, & Chattree, 1999; Lang, Lawrence, & Orme, 1994; Malhotra, Vishwambaran, Sundaram, & Narayanan, 1999a). In some developed countries, cups are recommended over bottles for hospitalized babies (Nyqvist, 2017). Research found that unlike bottle-feeding, the muscles and feeding behaviors babies use while cup-feeding are similar to nursing (Franca, Sousa, Aragao, & Costa, 2014). See the earlier section "Comparative Research" (p. 895) for the effects of cup-feeding on infant stability and nursing outcomes compared with other feeding methods.

Feeding with a Cup, Bowl, Spoon, Eyedropper, or Syringe

Technique is key when feeding a baby with a sipping or lapping method. When cup-feeding, any small cup can be used, such as a shot glass or the plastic cup included with children's liquid medicines. Commercial baby feeding cups are also available, some with snap-on lids and some with valves that regulate the baby's access to milk. If a bowl is used for feeding, a small, flexible bowl may be easier to manage than a rigid one. But any clean cup, glass, or bowl can be used, even those that are adult-sized. Spoon-feeding (Figure B.7) can also be used when supplements are needed after birth. In some hospitals, parents routinely express colostrum into a spoon after nursing and feed babies this "dessert." See **firstdroplets.com** for videos demonstrating this practice and its rationale. Any spoon can be used. Other sipping/lapping tools include an eyedropper or a syringe (with needle removed) for dripping milk into baby's mouth.

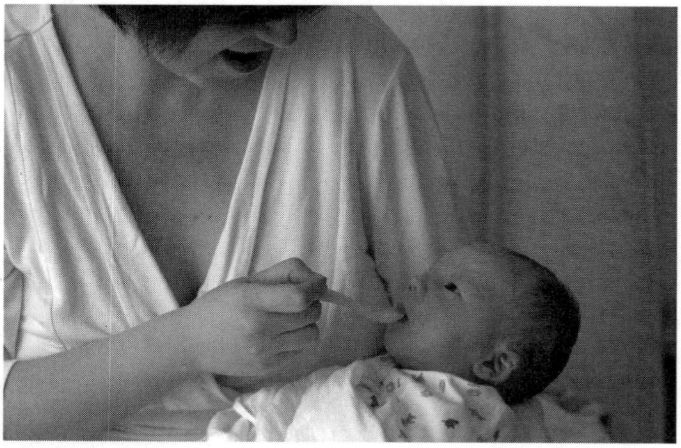

Figure B.7 Spoon-feeding is not intimidating to most parents, because it is low-tech and familiar. ©2020 Melanie Ham, used with permission.

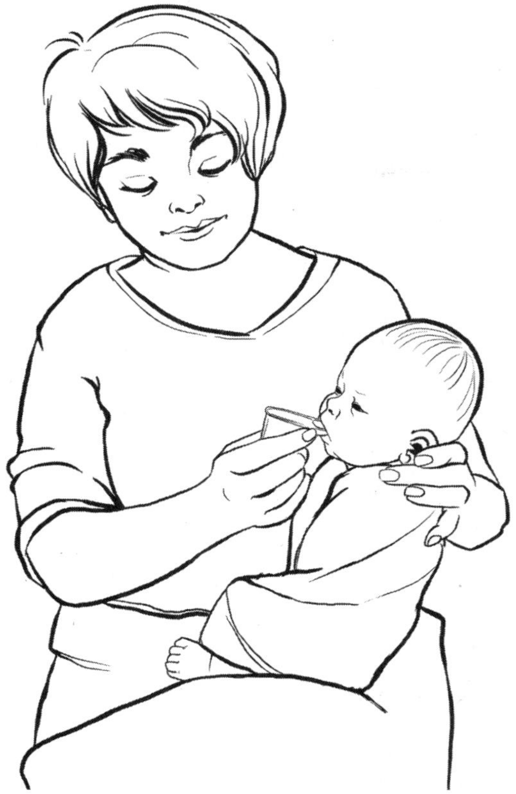

Figure B.8 Sit a baby upright when using a sipping/lapping feeding method, such as cup-feeding. ©2020 Nancy Mohrbacher Solutions, Inc.

While parent and baby are learning, it is best to go slowly. As both have more practice, feeds are often quick. No matter what container is used, when starting:

- Make sure baby is awake and alert before feeding.
- Wrap the baby's hands securely to prevent them from bumping the feeding container, and use a bib or cloth to protect baby's clothes from spills.
- Hold the baby in a sitting position (Figure B.8).

When cup-feeding:

- Raise the cup and rest its rim lightly on baby's lower lip.
- Tip the cup so the milk just touches his lips and he can sip or lap it in, but not so much that it pours into his mouth.
- Let the baby set his own sipping or lapping rhythm, pausing when needed, until he finishes. Some babies prefer the cup be tilted away between swallows, others prefer to feed continuously. Some use their tongue to lap the milk, others sip it in.

A variation of the cup is a feeding device used traditionally in India, called the paladai, which is shaped like Aladdin's lamp. When feeding with the paladai, milk is poured from its small spout into the baby's mouth. See the earlier section "Comparative Research" (p. 894) for studies comparing the paladai with a regular cup and feeding bottle.

When spoon-feeding:

- Fill the spoon with a mouthful of milk.
- Rest the spoon lightly on baby's lower lip and tilt it so the milk touches his lips.
- Either pour the milk into baby's mouth or allow him to sip or lap it, whichever he prefers.
- Give the baby time to swallow, refill the spoon, and repeat until baby is done.

When feeding with an eyedropper or syringe:

- Fill the eyedropper or syringe with a mouthful of milk.
- Raise it and drip the milk into baby's mouth at a slow enough pace so that he can swallow it before more is given.

BREAST PUMPS

Indications for Use

See p. 474 for the many reasons parents express milk. Although hand expression is an option for most parents and is used exclusively for milk expression in some parts of the world, there are some situations, such as establishing milk production after birth when baby is not yet nursing, in which a breast pump along with hand expression may produce better results than either method alone. Work settings where parents have limited milk-expression time may be another situation in which a breast pump might be helpful, as double-pumping can cut milk expression time in half (Becker, Smith, & Cooney, 2016). In some cultures, parents prefer breast pumps to hand expression, and in some cultures, it is common to use both. For details on choosing a breast pump, see Table 11.3 on p. 487 and p. 488-489.

Research on Breast Pumps

One of the first breast pump studies was done by Swedish civil engineer Einar Egnell and published in 1956 in the journal of the Swedish medical association (Egnell, 1956). In the early 1940s, Egnell spent 3 years developing a better breast pump, because the U.S. pumps available at the time caused skin rupture in one-third of the mothers who used them. In his landmark article, Egnell described the science behind the suction and cycling parameters he developed, which are still used today to gauge breast-pump safety and efficacy. By decreasing pump vacuum to 250 mmHg and increasing the number of suction-and-release cycles per minute to around 50, Egnell created a breast pump that was both comfortable and effective. Since then, many breast pump studies have been published. Although significant improvements have been made in pump fit and portability, as yet no one has improved upon Egnell's basic pump design, which is still used by the vast majority of pumps currently sold and rented.

That said, however, parents vary in their response to pump stimulation, and subtle differences between brands and models may produce different results. For this reason, those who work with lactating parents should be familiar with locally available equipment and their differences. For example, some pumps offer lower vacuum levels, which may make them a better choice for parents who are in pain or engorged. It is also important to be aware of available fit options (see later section) for situations in which a pump's nipple tunnel is too large or too small. As one U.S. lactation consultant (Genna, 2016, p. 124) wrote:

> "The take-home message here is that mothers differ...and so far no one pump has been developed that works optimally for absolutely all mothers."

Pump Suction, Speed, and Fit

If parents have never used a breast pump, they may be confused about how to set the pump suction and speed to their best advantage. They may, for example, think that setting suction and speed on the highest setting will produce the best milk yields. Some guidance can shorten their learning curve for better milk yields more quickly.

Setting breast pump suction (vacuum). Many think "more is better" when it comes to pump suction. But expressing milk with a pump is not like sucking a drink through a straw. For the highest milk yields, milk ejections (ideally more than one) need to occur. When suction levels are high enough to become uncomfortable, this may actually inhibit milk ejection, resulting in less milk expressed. Suggest when parents begin pumping, they set their pump suction to the highest level that is truly comfortable, both during and after pumping. Unlike many other medical devices, this setting will vary from person to person. For some, it may be at the pump's highest suction setting and for others, it may be at the pump's lowest suction setting, or anywhere in between.

To find the highest comfortable pump suction level, suggest parents:

- Turn up the pump suction until they feel a slight discomfort.
- Turn it down slowly, just until it feels completely comfortable.

Some lactation specialists recommend starting a pump session at a low suction and gradually increasing it over time. But that recommendation produces lower milk yields. According to Australian research (Ramsay et al., 2006), the most effective strategy for pump suction is to set it at the highest comfortable setting by the time the first milk ejection occurs. Milk yields averaged 33% higher with that strategy as compared to being at a lower suction setting during the first milk ejection.

Setting breast pump speed (cycles). The unit ***cycles per minute*** (or ***cpm***) refers to the number of times each minute the pump suction builds, peaks, and releases. This is one variable that distinguishes more-effective from less-effective breast pumps. Pump comfort and effectiveness depends on a speed of at least 40 to 60 cpm. As Einar Egnell found, slower speed can cause greater discomfort and even skin damage.

Many pump brands and models now use what some call ***2-phase*** cycling. This means the pumps are set to automatically start at the high-cycle setting of 120 cpm. After a specific time, usually 2 minutes, they automatically shift to a slower speed. According to pump marketing, this is meant to mimic a nursing baby, who sucks faster at first to trigger a milk ejection and then sucks slower to drain the milk faster. If parents use a pump with this feature, encourage them to press its "let-down" button as soon as their milk flow begins. If the first milk ejection occurs before 2 minutes, staying for a longer time at the fast 120 cycles per minute may lower their milk yield. Australian research (Ramsay et al., 2006) found that 86% of its study mothers expressed no milk at all during this very fast first phase, and other research (Ramsay et al., 2006) found that taking maximum advantage of that first milk ejection is key to better milk yields.

Research comparing time to milk ejection did not find that 2-phase pumping resulted in more milk expressed as compared with pumps that run at a single speed. In fact, one small Australian study of 28 mothers (Kent, Ramsay, Doherty, Larsson, & Hartmann, 2003) found that mothers experienced milk ejection about 30 seconds faster with a

2-phase pump but expressed slightly less milk overall than a pump cycling at a set 50 cpm. One larger U.S. study of 100 mothers of preterm babies who initiated lactation after birth with a breast pump set at 50 cpm (P. P. Meier et al., 2008) reported that when the mothers were switched to a 2-phase pump, their milk ejection was delayed by an average of nearly a minute compared with the single-phase pump. Milk ejection is a conditioned response, and these mothers had become conditioned to the feel of the single-phase pump.

If parents are using a pump with separate suction and speed controls, suggest they:

- Start pumping at the fastest speed
- When milk flow starts, turn it down to a slow speed.
- As milk flow slows, return to a fast speed to trigger the next milk ejection faster.
- Repeat, alternating between fast and slow speeds (like a nursing baby) for the fastest and highest milk yields

That said, encourage parents to experiment and use whatever settings produce the best results.

Getting a good pump fit is vital, especially for parents who pump often and who use a pump with a nipple tunnel made of rigid plastic. Pump fit affects both nipple comfort and milk flow. A poor fit can lead to pain, skin trauma, and reduced milk flow, putting milk production at risk in pump-dependent families.

Pump fit is about nipple diameter. Pump fit is based on how well parents' nipples fit into the pump's ***nipple tunnel*** (Figure B.9), the opening the mammary gland is drawn into during pumping. Pump manufacturers call this pump part by different names (flange, breastshield). Parents often refer to it as the "horn" or "funnel."

Nipple tunnel diameter varies slightly by brand, with 24 or 25 mm the standard size of most pumps. One sign a different size nipple tunnel is needed is pain or discomfort during pumping, even near the lowest suction setting. Because nipple sizes can vary, some parents may need one size on one side and another size on the other side.

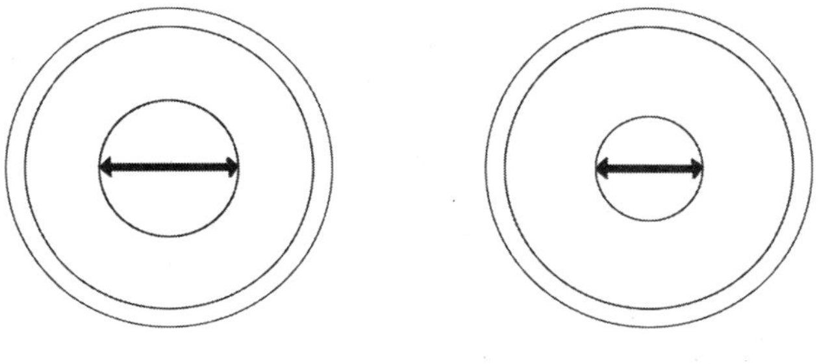

Figure B.9 Pump nipple tunnels come in different diameters, and getting a good fit is vital to comfort and milk flow. ©2020 Nancy Mohrbacher Solutions, Inc.

If pumping is comfortable with good milk flow, parents probably have a good fit. If there is discomfort, even on low suction settings, suggest parents watch their nipples during a pump session and report on what they see. Suggest they look online at the following link and compare the line drawings (below) to what they see while pumping: **bit.ly/BA2-PumpFit**.

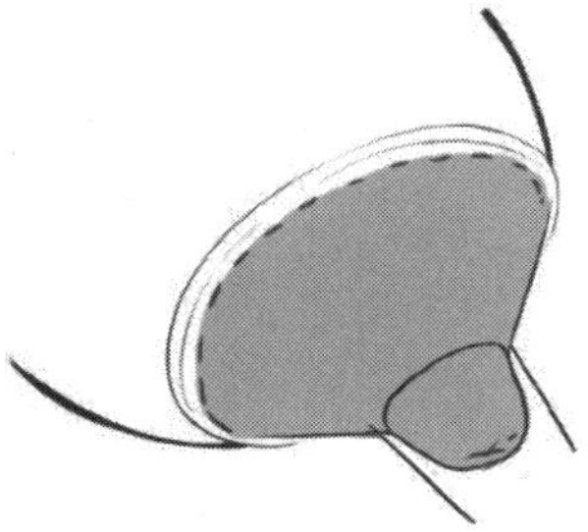

Figure B.10a ***Good fit:*** Can see some, but not too much, space around the nipple as it moves freely in the pump's nipple tunnel. ©2020 Nancy Mohrbacher Solutions, Inc.

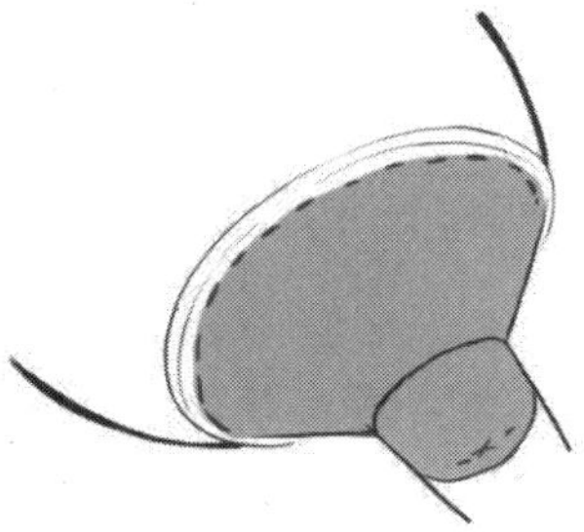

Figure B.10b ***Too small:*** The nipple rubs along the sides of the nipple tunnel, even when centered. Rubbing may cause blanching, pain, or skin damage, limit the movement of the nipple, and squeeze the nipple, slowing milk flow. ©2020 Nancy Mohrbacher Solutions, Inc.

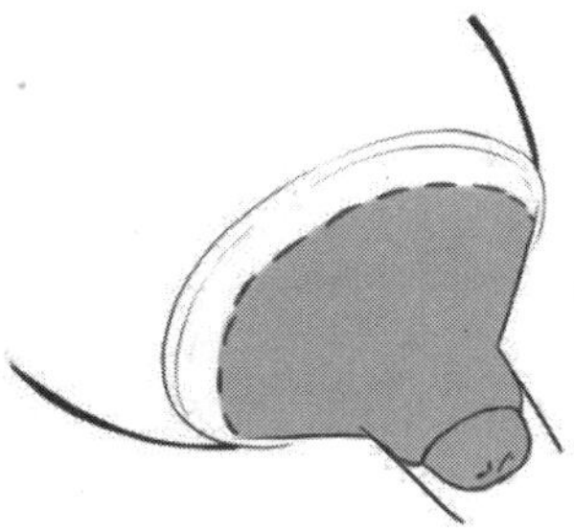

Figure B.10c ***Too large:*** Too much areola is pulled in, which can cause rubbing and soreness. The nipple may bounce in and out of the tunnel during pumping or there may be difficulty maintaining an air seal. ©2020 Nancy Mohrbacher Solutions, Inc.

Depending on the pump brand, larger or smaller nipple tunnels may be available to purchase separately.

How common is the need for larger or smaller nipple tunnels? In one U.K. study, 36 mothers with babies in the NICU pumped with a standard 25 mm nipple tunnel, and the researchers noted that the opening was too small for 28%. The authors (Jones, Dimmock, & Spencer, 2001, p. F94) wrote: "If the [opening] is too small, pressure is highest on the nipple tissue, which can cause sore nipples and ineffective drainage." In a U.S. NICU study, a different brand of pump with a 24 mm standard nipple tunnel was used. When both milk flow and comfort were assessed, a much higher percentage of mothers had better results with a larger nipple tunnel (P. Meier, 2004, p. 8):

> [W]e found that 51.4%—or about half—of the 35 mothers who served as subjects in the research initially required either the 27 or 30 mm shield in order to achieve optimal, pain-free nipple and areolar movement during milk expression. As lactation progressed, 77.1%—or slightly more than three quarters—of the mothers eventually found they needed these larger shields."

Pump fit can change with regular pumping. A 2019 U.S. randomized crossover study compared the effects of nursing, hand expression and pumping on the nipple sizes of 46 lactating women (Francis & Dickton, 2019). The researchers found that unlike direct nursing and hand expression, with pumping, nipple length and diameter increased in size. Two U.S. lactation consultants used an engineer's template to measure mothers' nipples before and after pumping and also found that pumping causes nipples to increase in size. They (Wilson-Clay & Hoover, 2017, pp. 80-81) wrote: "Pre- and post-pumping measurements taken with a circle template reveal that nipple size can increase 3 to 4 millimeters." So even if parents are fitted well when they start pumping, it makes sense for them to check their pump fit over time to see if it has changed and whether they need a larger diameter nipple tunnel. See Box B.1 for signs that a new nipple-tunnel size may be needed.

BOX B.1 Signs Parents May Need a Larger or Smaller Nipple Tunnel

Suggest a larger nipple tunnel if parents report:

- Discomfort, even on low suction settings
- Nipple rubs along the tunnel, despite efforts to center it
- Nipple blanches, or turns white
- Nipple does not move freely in the nipple tunnel
- Slow milk flow or less milk expressed than expected

Suggest a smaller nipple tunnel if parents report:

- Discomfort, even on low suction settings.
- More than about 1/8 inch (3 mm) of the areola is pulled into the nipple tunnel
- Nipple bounces in and out of the tunnel
- Difficulty maintaining an air seal

BREAST SHELLS AND NIPPLE EVERTERS

Breast shells are hard-plastic cups worn over the nipples (usually in a bra) during pregnancy or between nursing sessions. Their intended purpose is to either protect painful nipples from pressure and clothing friction or to draw out flat or inverted nipples. Most versions include a dome (usually with holes for air circulation) and a backing (either hard plastic or silicone) that rests against the skin (Figure B.11). In some versions, only one type of backing (one size opening) is included. In other versions, two different backings are included and either size can be snapped onto the dome. The backing with the smaller opening is designed to apply pressure to the areola and draw out non-protruding nipples. The backing with the larger opening is designed to protect painful nipples from pressure and clothing friction.

Indications for Use

Breast shells. When used to draw out flat or inverted nipples, breast shells may be worn during the last trimester of pregnancy for increasing lengths of time each day or in the early post-birth period for about 30 minutes before feeds. If they are used after the milk increased and they are worn inside a bra, suggest parents be sure the bra cups are large enough to accommodate them without putting too much pressure on the mammary gland. If the bra cup is too small, consistent pressure on the gland increases the risk of mastitis.

Nipple everters. The purpose of these devices is to physically pull out flat or inverted nipples to make them easier for the baby to latch and nurse. This device may be helpful for parents with flat or inverted nipples that are not caused by shortened milk ducts (tethered) and whose baby is having difficulty latching (Genna, 2016).

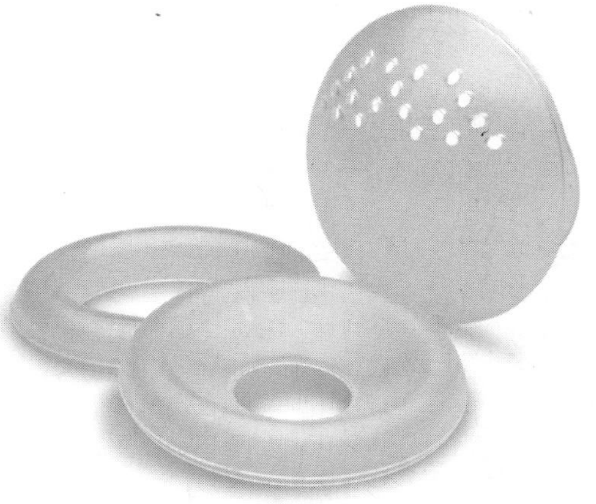

Figure B.11 This package of breast shells includes two sets of backings that snap onto the dome: one set with a small hole for inverted nipples and the other with a large hole to protect sore nipples. ©2020 Ameda, Inc., used with permission.

Research on Breast Shells and Nipple Everters

Breast shells. Although these devices were commonly recommended for decades to draw out flat or inverted nipples, research found they may cause more nursing problems than they solve. Two U.K. studies (Alexander, Grant, & Campbell, 1992; MAIN, 1994) found that identifying flat or inverted nipples during pregnancy and "treating" them with either breast shells or the Hoffman technique (using the fingers to pull back on the areolae to draw out the nipples) resulted in fewer women breastfeeding. The first of these two studies, which followed 96 first-time mothers with flat or inverted nipples, found that more of those in the treatment group either decided ***not*** to breastfeed or stopped breastfeeding earlier than those whose nipples were not identified and treated. The researchers expressed concern that telling a pregnant woman her nipples could be problematic may act as a disincentive to successful nursing, because it calls into question her ability to breastfeed. They concluded that during pregnancy recommending breast shells may reduce the chances of successful breastfeeding (Alexander et al., 1992).

The second study, which followed 463 mothers with flat or inverted nipples, found that babies whose mothers did ***not*** receive treatment during pregnancy had fewer latching problems than babies whose mothers received treatments. They therefore recommended that healthcare professionals stop screening mothers during pregnancy for flat or inverted nipples. Due to these research findings, the U.K. Royal College of Midwives warned against focusing on "inadequate nipples," encouraging a focus instead on basic nursing dynamics that make early latching easier.

A 2013 Thai study followed 90 women who were judged to have "short nipples," half of whom wore breast shells during pregnancy and half who didn't (Chanprapaph, Luttarapakul, Siribariruck, & Boonyawanichkul, 2013). The researchers found that although there appeared to be an increase in the length of the treated nipples, on Day 3 after delivery, the group who wore the breast shells had significantly lower rates of breastfeeding compared with those who did not wear the breast shells.

Nipple everters. Several commercially manufactured products and two makeshift devices can be used to draw out flat, retracted, or inverted nipples. If an inverted nipple is tethered so it cannot be pulled out manually or during nursing (Grade 3 inverted nipple, see p. 736), these products may make nursing possible (Genna, 2016, p. 35).

Supple Cups. A 2011 U.S. case series (Boucher-Horwitz, 2011) described the use of Supple Cups™ with 12 women, some of who began using them in the 37th week of pregnancy and some of whom used them after delivery. This all-silicone product is worn over the nipple, which it draws out with gentle, continuous suction. According to the author, this product is inexpensive and easy to use. During pregnancy, when the mothers began wearing them inside their bra, they started with 15 minutes per day and gradually lengthened their wear time to 4 hours per day. In these two cases, by birth, the adhesions that tethered the nipples were painlessly broken and these two mothers exclusively breastfed. When started after delivery, the Supple Cups were worn under breast shells to prevent them from falling off. These women used this product (along with some lanolin to increase comfort) for between 2 days and 2 weeks. Among the 12 women followed in this case series, 83% of their babies were able to consistently latch and 67% exclusively breastfed.

Rubber bands. A 2011 Indian study (Chakrabarti & Basu, 2011) described the use of rubber bands to evert the nipples of 19 women with flat or inverted nipples whose babies were between 9 and 38 days old. This makeshift solution was created by using a condom rim, which was applied with a syringe to tie it to the base of the nipple, drawing it out. Of the 19 study mothers, 63% were able to successfully latch and nurse their babies with the help of this device, and there were no reports of pain or the band slipping during feeds.

Disposable syringe. In a 1992 Indian study, researchers followed eight mothers with flat or inverted nipples whose babies were unable to latch and used a makeshift nipple everter created from a disposable syringe. (Kesaree, Banapurmath, Banapurmath, & Shamanur, 1993). When the study started, the mothers had bottle-fed for 28 to 103 days. To create this device, the researchers transformed a 10 or 20 mL syringe (depending on nipple size) into a small suction device. After receiving positioning help and using the modified syringe before feeds, seven of eight babies latched. Within 4 to 6 weeks of breastfeeding often, six of the eight women were exclusively breastfeeding.

To transform a 10 or 20 mL syringe into a nipple suction device:

1. Remove the piston from the syringe and cut off the nozzle with a sharp blade.
2. Reinsert the piston through the cut end of the syringe so that the piston is pulled away from the smooth end of the syringe.
3. Put the smooth end of the syringe over the nipple and onto the areola.
4. Gently pull the piston to maintain steady but gentle pressure for 30 to 60 seconds, adjusting the pressure to comfort.

Commercial nipple everters. Along with the makeshift devices described above, commercial products are available in some areas that are specifically designed to draw out non-protractile nipples. Examples other than the Supple Cups include Evert-It™, Niplette™ (McGeorge, 1994). and LatchAssist™.

DIGITAL AND ONLINE LACTATION TOOLS

Not so long ago, nursing parents relied on books, magazines, in-person consults, and telephone conversations to get the lactation information and help they needed. At this writing, many new families look first to online and digital platforms for lactation information, support, and help.

Lactation Support in the Digital Age

Although families giving birth and raising babies in the digital age are not all alike, they have some qualities in common. Two U.S. authors (McCulloch & McCann, 2017) note that today's parents value their online communities.

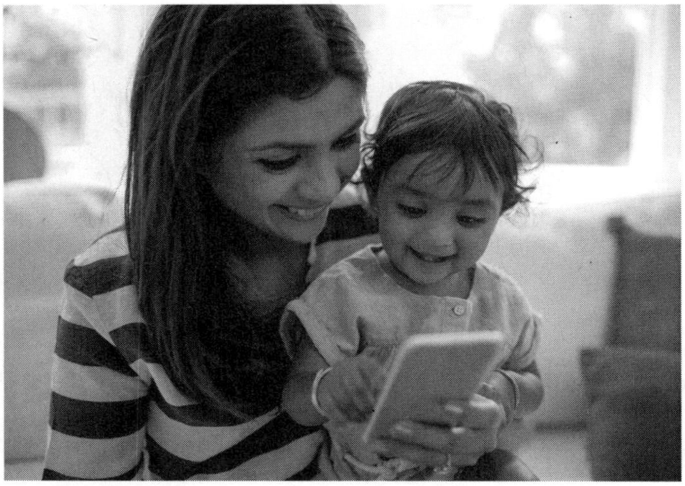

A 2019 New Zealand qualitative study of 30 mothers (Alianmoghaddam, Phibbs, & Benn, 2019) concluded that to achieve 6 months of exclusive breastfeed, these parents:

- Accessed factual lactation information online
- Relied on the "strength of weak ties" through social-media groups consisting of other nursing parents
- Contacted family members who were geographically distant with Skype and other videoconferencing software to get the emotional support they needed
- Found smartphone apps helpful in meeting their goals

An Australian longitudinal prospective cohort study (Wheaton, Lenehan, & Amir, 2018) examined the impact of this author's Breastfeeding Solutions app on 29 mothers living in rural Australia without access to in-person lactation help. It found that nearly 80% of those who used the app and completed the study surveys at 3 and 6 months were breastfeeding at 6 months. The local average of any breastfeeding at this stage was 50%. For the study mothers, having a reliable lactation resource on their phone reduced their confusion about breastfeeding. As one participant noted (Wheaton et al., 2018, p. 718):

> "Searching the web comes up with all sorts of contradictions; books become outdated. I think the app…feels much more trustworthy."

Closed social-media groups on platforms like Facebook, WeChat, WhatsApp, and others were found to provide both answers to specific lactation questions and emotional support by volunteers working with organizations such as La Leche League's local and national entities and the Australian Breastfeeding Association (Bridges, Howell, & Schmied, 2018). In her book, *The Virtual Breastfeeding*

Culture, author Lara Audelo (Audelo, 2013) describes the experiences of many parents who found lactation support from other parents who were living through unusual situations, such as induced lactation, nursing a chronically ill or hospitalized child, exclusive pumping, parenting the nursing child with allergies, and many more.

Digital Forms of Lactation Education and Help

Nursing parents in the digital age do not confine themselves to the lactation informational options of the past. Today's parents want to access information and help in the formats they are most comfortable using (Mohrbacher, 2015). This includes smartphone apps and social media groups, but it also includes online videos, texting, lactation consults on Skype and Facetime, and on-demand digital learning.

What does research tell us about the use of hi-tech lactation tools? For one, modern families value on-demand and self-directed learning (McCulloch & McCann, 2017). A 2015 U.S. study evaluated the efficacy of tablet-based lactation education during pregnancy (Pitts, Faucher, & Spencer, 2015) and found that 95% of the women who took this lactation course on tablets at their obstetrician's office during their prenatal appointments preferred it over group education. The study also confirmed that the information in the course was effectively retained. A 2019 U.S. study that evaluated the effectiveness of online video instruction on hand expression during pregnancy (O'Sullivan, Cooke, McCafferty, & Giglia, 2019) found that its 95 mothers felt more confident in their ability to hand express after watching the video, and 98% said they would recommend it to a friend. A 2018 survey of 101 U.S. mothers about teleconferencing for lactation consultations (Habibi, Springer, Spence, Hansen-Petrik, & Kavanagh, 2018) found general acceptance of this alternative to a home or office visit with greater acceptance among younger parents and those who wanted more control over their privacy.

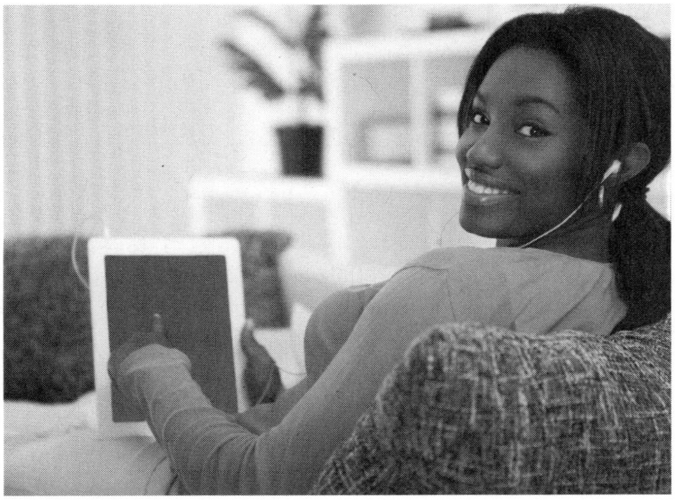

NIPPLE CREAMS, OINTMENTS, AND PADS

Indications for Use

Nipple creams, ointments, and hydrogel pads are commonly used by nursing parents. One 2015 Australian prospective cohort study of 360 first-time mothers (Buck, Amir, & Donath, 2015) found that 91% used some type of topical treatment on their nipples. Parents often use these treatments in the hope they will speed the healing of painful or traumatized nipples and reduce nipple pain. Research, however, casts doubt on their effectiveness.

Research on Topical Nipple Treatments

Over the years, an incredible number of studies compared various treatment options for early nipple pain and trauma. Some found their participants expressed greater satisfaction when their painful nipples were treated with something rather than nothing (Cadwell, Turner-Maffei, Blair, Brimdyr, & Maja McInerney, 2004). However, as a 2014 Cochrane Review (Dennis, Jackson, & Watson, 2014) found, the quality of the vast majority of these studies was so low that only four met their criteria for review. After close examination of these four studies, its authors concluded that there is not enough evidence to recommend any specific type of treatment for painful or damaged nipples in nursing parents. This Cochrane Review also noted that—whether or not a topical nipple treatment is used—within 7 to 10 days after birth, nipple pain is reduced to mild in most nursing parents.

Although many lactation specialists recommend all-purpose nipple ointment (APNO) (a combination of antibiotic, anti-inflammatory, and antifungal mixed by the pharmacist), a randomized controlled trial (Dennis, Schottle, Hodnett, & McQueen, 2012) found that APNO was no more effective than lanolin. This same research team (Jackson & Dennis, 2017) also found that lanolin was no more effective than applying warm compresses. For more details about the research on these treatments and others, such as silver cups, laser, and LED light phototherapy, see the section starting on p. 719.

For traumatized nipples with broken skin, some recommend applying an antibiotic ointment after nursing to help prevent infection (Witt, Burgess, Hawn, & Zyzanski, 2014). For more details and a summary of the research, see p. 724.

NIPPLE SHIELDS

Unlike hard plastic breast shells, flexible nipple shields are worn over the nipple during nursing, with the baby getting milk through the holes in their tip. Most are made of silicone and consist of a thin ***brim*** that covers all or part of the areola and a firmer, protruding ***tip*** that fits over the nipple (Figure B.12). Over time, the pendulum has swung to both extremes regarding nipple shield use. After a time of being used often during the post-delivery hospital stay in the late 1980s and early 1990s, their use was strongly discouraged. Like any tool, nipple shields can be used appropriately or misused. In some situations, nipple shields can support and preserve direct nursing.

Indications for Use

A 2010 review of the literature on nipple shields (McKechnie & Eglash, 2010, p. 313) concluded:

> "The current literature does not support many of the current practices regarding [nipple shield] use. The available evidence does not demonstrate that [nipple shields] are safe in the long term for milk supply, infant weight gain, or duration of breastfeeding. Rather than assuming that [nipple shields] are safe until proven otherwise, healthcare providers should consider [nipple shields] an unknown risk and limit their duration of use whenever possible, until further evidence demonstrates their long-term safety."

Nipple shields have other downsides in addition to concerns about possible impact on long-term milk production and infant weight gain. Their use complicates direct nursing, and they are often difficult to wean from (Flacking & Dykes, 2017). In light of this, it's best to proceed with the understanding that nipple shields are almost never a good first strategy. Yet their use is common. An anonymous online survey of 490 healthcare providers (Eglash, Ziemer, & Chevalier, 2010) found that 95% of lactation consultants and 80% of other healthcare professionals use nipple shields with the families they serve.

The most common reasons nipple shields are used (Kronborg, Foverskov, Nilsson, & Maastrup, 2017) are:

- Painful nursing
- Latching struggles

Despite the potential downsides of nipple shield use, some studies also found positives. A 2015 review of the literature (Chow et al., 2015) noted that in some situations, a nipple shield makes latching less stressful, which may boost parents' feeling of accomplishment, reduce their frustration, and keep them nursing longer. Shield use may also eliminate the need to supplement and shorten the time to exclusive nursing. If a nipple shield helps increase milk intake during nursing and time spent nursing directly, encourage parents to use it as needed. Box B.2 lists a variety of situations in which nipples shields might be used.

BOX B.2 Situations in Which a Nipple Shield Might Be Used After Other Strategies Failed

Latching difficulties due to:

- Flat or inverted nipples
- Poor fit (large nipple, small infant mouth)
- Infant alertness issues from labor medications
- Birth trauma
- Oral aversion after vigorous suctioning
- Preference for artificial teats

An ineffective infant suck due to:

- Tongue-tie
- Small or receding jaw
- Cleft palate
- Unusually shaped palate (high, bubble, channel)
- Painful cephalohematoma
- Prematurity
- Airway abnormality (tracheomalacia, laryngomalacia)

Nipple pain so severe that the nursing parent dreads every feed

Overabundant milk production

History of sexual abuse in the nursing parent

Adapted from (D. C. Powers & Tapia, 2012; Walker, 2016)

A U.S. lactation consultant described some specific ways nipple shields may help babies latch and nurse (Walker, 2016, p. 100). Nipple shields may:

- Moderate a fast milk flow for a struggling baby.
- Supply greater oral stimulation due to their firm feel
- Help compensate for a weak suck.
- Remain in place during pauses and continue to protrude throughout feed (for parents with inverted or retractable nipples).
- Extend back far enough in baby's mouth to trigger active sucking.

Regarding this last point, for the baby with high muscle tone or tongue-tie, the firm shield may help push the nipple past a retracted or humped tongue to trigger active sucking (Genna, 2017). When parents have traumatized nipples, another way temporary use of a nipple shield may help is by providing just enough pain relief to avoid interrupting direct nursing. For some preterm babies, use of a nipple shield may improve milk intake during nursing just enough to avoid the need for supplementation (Clum & Primomo, 1996; P. P. Meier et al., 2000).

But Walker also noted what nipple shields ***cannot*** do:

- Improve milk intake if the problem is low milk production
- Improve damaged nipples if the root cause is not identified and corrected
- Take the place of skilled lactation help and close follow-up

One Australian case report (Perrella & Geddes, 2016) described the experience of a breastfeeding mother with painful nipples whose 3-month-old baby generated very high suction levels (intraoral pressures) in his mouth. She experienced an unusual downside of nipple-shield use when she tried one in an attempt to moderate the pain of nursing. As a result, she developed blisters at the sites of each of the holes in the nipple shield tip. Her son's suction was so high, it damaged her nipple tissue by pulling in and trapping her nipple skin in the holes of the nipple shield.

Although nipple shields may help preserve nursing in some situations, whenever possible, it is always better to solve a nursing problem by improving feeding dynamics rather than by using a nipple shield. The authors of a large Danish study described in the next section noted the dependence on the shield that occurred in many families (Kronborg et al., 2017, p. 2) and wrote:

> "Health professionals should be aware that the use of nipple shields may be an easy but not necessarily supportive solution to the inexperienced mother who needs extra support in the early process of breastfeeding."

Examples of misuse of nipple shields include offering it as the first solution to a problem or giving it to parents as an alternative to spending time improving nursing dynamics.

Follow-up is vital. Sending nursing parents home from the hospital with a nipple shield without a scheduled follow-up appointment is a recipe for failure. When nipple shields are used, the nursing couple needs to be seen regularly to make sure the baby is feeding effectively and the family has the support they need to meet their nursing goals. If a hospital does not offer outpatient help for nursing families, the alternative is to provide referrals to local lactation specialists who can see families shortly after discharge, after milk production increases, so they can be evaluated and assisted in weaning from the shield at the appropriate time.

Research on Nipple Shields

A 2017 Danish observational cross-sectional study that included 4,815 mothers (Kronborg et al., 2017) found that 22% (1 in 5) used a nipple shield at the beginning of nursing and 7% used a shield the entire time they nursed. The most common reasons the shield was used were painful nursing and difficulty latching. Lower gestational age was associated with a higher likelihood of shield use. Among those who gave birth to very or moderately preterm babies, 32% used a shield. Shield use was 3 times more likely to lead to shorter duration (≤17 weeks) of exclusive nursing among first-time mothers who used the shield in the beginning. Other research found, too, that nipple-shield use leads to shorter duration of nursing (Maastrup et al., 2014; Pincombe et al., 2008).

Preterm babies and nipple shields. One 2000 U.S. study (P. P. Meier et al., 2000) found the use of a nipple shield increased milk intake during nursing in some preterm babies. In this study, nipple shields were used with 34 preemies who were slipping off the nipple during pauses or falling asleep early in nursing sessions. Milk transfer was greater for all 34 babies, with a mean increase of 14.4 mL or about a half-ounce. With the shield, the babies sucked for longer bursts and stayed awake nursing longer. These preterm babies used the shield for a mean of 32.5 days out of a mean nursing duration of 169 days. Overall the parents used the shield for about 24% of their time nursing. The babies who were previously unable to transfer milk without the shield used it longer than the babies who took some milk without the shield. There was no association between the length of time the shield was used and duration of nursing.

Why did the nipple shields increase milk intake in some preterm babies? A 2017 Australian prospective cross-sectional crossover study (Geddes et al., 2017) measured suction levels (intraoral pressures) while preterm babies nursed with and without a nipple shield and found that the babies generated weaker suction levels with the nipple shield but they nursed actively for longer. The researchers noted that suction is generated when babies lower the back of their tongue during nursing but that suction levels are not related to milk volumes consumed. What matters to milk intake is the length of time babies actively nurse. It is likely that the firmer tip of the nipple shield (as compared with the parents' softer nipples) provides extra stimulation and may also push deeper into baby's mouth triggering more active sucking. The 2000 U.S. study (P. P. Meier et al., 2000) found that the preterm babies who consumed more milk with the nipple shield continued to take more milk with the shield until they reached their term-corrected age of about 40 weeks.

Is it necessary to pump after feeds? More research is needed, but there is cause for concern about the effect of nipple-shield use on milk production. Several studies examined their impact on milk intake. One early U.K. study (Woolridge, Baum, & Drewett, 1980) found that thick nipple shields altered babies' sucking patterns and the babies took less milk during nursing. The babies using the thick rubber "Mexican hat" nipple shields took 58% less milk than they did without the shield, and those using the thinner latex nipple shields took 22% less milk. A Swedish study (Amatayakul et al., 1987) found no difference in the blood prolactin and cortisol levels when its study mothers breastfed with or without a thin latex nipple shield. But like the previous U.K. study, it also found a significant decrease in milk transfer during nursing. In this case, 42% less milk was transferred during shield use. A U.S. study (Auerbach, 1990) used a breast pump with a nipple shield and also found a significant difference in milk transfer. The women pumping without the nipple shield had milk yields 4 times higher than when they used the nipple shield during pumping.

A U.S. descriptive longitudinal study examined weight gain in 54 breastfeeding babies using a nipple shield whose mothers were not expressing milk after feeds and found no statistically significant difference in weight gain at 2 weeks, 1 month, and 2 months between babies using a nipple shield and babies who were not (Chertok, 2009). The problem with this study is that 41% of the study babies were fed formula supplements by 2 weeks and 59% by 2 months, and the researcher did not include the volume of formula given in relation to the duration of nipple-shield use. It's possible that the weight gain of the two groups were so similar because the babies using the nipple shields were receiving formula.

So where do we stand? It's important that recommendations be tailored to individual circumstances. As U.S. lactation consultant Catherine Watson Genna (Genna, 2016, p. 57) wrote:

> "Many LCs encourage mothers using a nipple shield to pump. I originally followed the 'party line' and encouraged mothers to express milk while using a nipple shield, but soon found that some mothers were developing uncomfortable hyperlactation and recurrent plugged ducts. Now instructions are individualized. If the infant feeds efficiently and effectively with the nipple shield, the mother is encouraged to watch the baby for normal energy, copious stools, and sated behaviors. If the infant is sleepier than usual, has fewer than four or five stools per day in the early weeks, or is unsettled, she is encouraged to express and feed sufficient milk to the infant to resolve these concerns."

In some situations, expressing after feeding with a shield makes sense, such as right after birth, when it's vital to support early milk increase. Another situation is when milk production is low, or if parents are unsure about whether milk transfer during nursing is effective or ineffective with the shield. Regular weight checks are recommended until it is clear regular milk expression is not needed. Other signs parents can look for between weight checks include visible milk in the tip of the shield after feeds and a decrease in mammary fullness after feeds.

Nipple Shield Styles, Shapes, and Sizes

If a nipple shield is not the right size or shape for a nursing couple, it may not be an effective tool. But it's always helpful to know the options.

Nipple shield styles: regular and contact. The two basic nipple shield styles have much in common. Both are made of ultra-thin silicone and have a firm, protruding tip surrounded by a soft brim that lays flat on the areola. One, referred to as a ***regular*** nipple shield, has a completely circular brim and is preferred by some lactation helpers because in some cases, it stays in place more securely during feeds. One U.S. lactation consultant (Genna, 2016) suggested that the more spherical the mammary gland, the better the regular style seems to fit.

The other style, referred to as a ***contact*** nipple shield, has a cutout area on its brim that can be positioned for skin-to-skin contact with the baby's nose or chin. Some prefer this second style because of this increased skin-to-skin contact and because aligning the cutout with the baby's nose prevents the shield brim from bending back into the baby's face during nursing. It also allows the baby to smell the parent's skin during feeds instead of the shield. Because parents' anatomy and helpers' preferences vary, it may be wise to suggest parents start with one of each style and see which works better.

Nipple shield shapes. Nipple shields come in two basic shapes: conical and cherry-shaped (Figure B,12) (Walker, 2016). As with the other nipple-shield variations, some babies may respond better to one shape than another.

Nipple shield sizes. A nipple shield will only be an effective tool if is a good fit for both parent and baby. If the shield is too large for the baby, it can cause gagging (which can lead to feeding aversion), and if his jaws close on its tip rather than its soft brim, it can prevent effective milk transfer. A too-small shield may fail to stimulate baby to suck actively because it doesn't extend deep enough into the baby's mouth.

Most nipple shields tips are close to the same length. The measurement often listed on the package (Table B.2) that varies most is the diameter of the tip opening. To fit the parent's nipple, the tip opening must be wide enough to comfortably accommodate it.

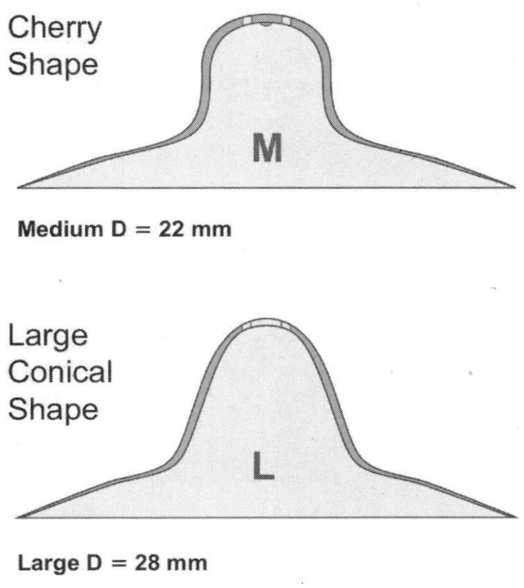

Figure B.12 The two basic nipple-shield shapes are cherry-shaped (top) and conical (bottom). ©2020 Mamivac®, used with permission.

TABLE B.2 Some Nipple Shield Brands and Sizes

Brand/Style/Shape	Sizes (mm)
Ameda regular style	24
Ameda contact style	24, 20, 16
Ardo regular style	24, 20
Avent contact style	21
Mamivac (all regular style)	
• conical shape	28, 20, 18
• cherry shape	22, 18
Medela regular style	24, 20, 16
Medela contact style	24, 20, 16

Adapted from (D. C. Powers & Tapia, 2012; Walker, 2016)

Some lactation specialists fit nipple shields primarily to the parent (D. C. Powers & Tapia, 2012). Others fit nipple shields primarily to the baby or a mix of both. When fitting a shield to the baby, many recommend the narrower tip openings (16 mm and 20 mm) for preterm babies and newborns. Those with wider tip openings (24 mm) are most often chosen for term or older or larger babies. But the size of the baby is unrelated to the width of his parent's nipple, which means the nipple shield that is a good fit for a baby may not be a good fit for the parent, and vice versa. The parent's nipples may not fit comfortably into the shield tip (which can slow milk flow like a too-small pump nipple tunnel) and the shield that fits the parent may not fit comfortably in the baby's mouth. In this case, a nipple shield would not be a helpful tool.

Nipple Shield Application and Latch Dynamics

Several different strategies can be used to apply a nipple shield. Some simply center the nipple inside the tip and place the shield on the mammary gland. If this method is used, to keep the shield in place during nursing, the parent places a thumb on one side of the brim's border and fingers on the other side.

Figure B.13 illustrates another method of applying a shield that draws the nipple farther in to the tip, reducing the suction needed by the baby and keeping the shield in place more easily:

1. Turn half of the shield tip inside out (Figure B.13a).

2. Place the shield over the nipple (Figure B.13b).

3. When the shield is slowly turned right side out and smoothed into place, the nipple is drawn into the tip (Figure B.13c).

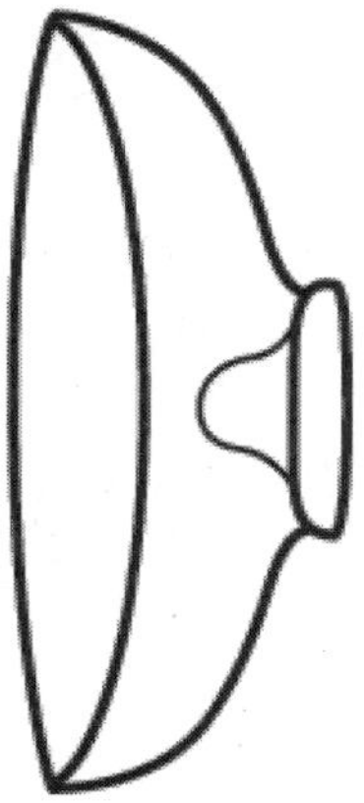

Figure B.13a To apply a nipple shield, first turn its tip halfway inside out.

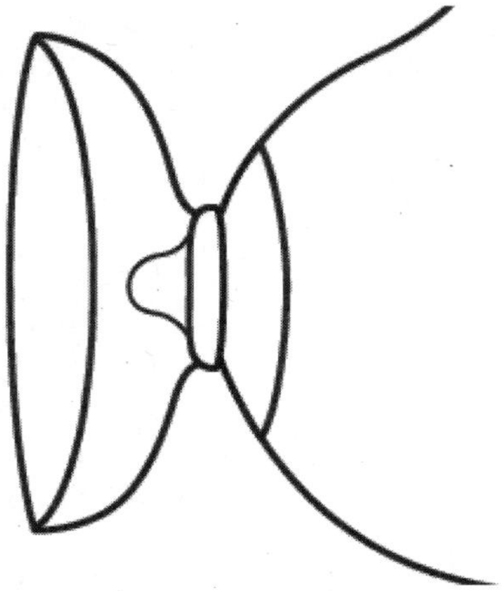

Figure B.13b Place the shield over the nipple.

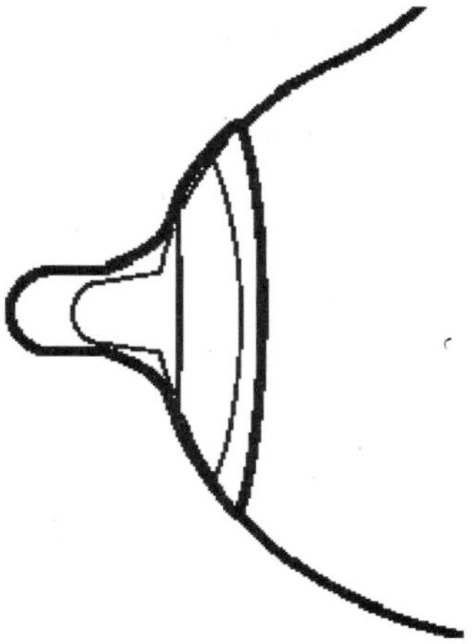

Figure B.13c Smooth the shield onto the mammary gland, which draws the nipple into its tip.

Other ways to help keep the shield in place during nursing include running hot or warm water over it before applying it (Walker, 2016) or applying a small amount of USP-modified lanolin to the inside borders of the brim to help it stick to the skin.

Latching to a nipple shield. In addition to a well-fitted shield and its effective application, parents need to be sure the baby latches deeply to the shield for effective nursing (Figure B.14a left). If the baby's jaws close on the shield's tip instead of its brim (Figure B.14b right), the shield is less likely to trigger active sucking. As when nursing without the shield, the baby needs to open wide and latch deeply.

If parents can see any part of the firmer tip of the shield while the baby nurses, suggest unlatching the baby by breaking the suction and trying again, making sure his mouth is open very wide as he latches. One U.S. lactation consultant (Genna, 2016, p. 55) wrote:

> "Infants who are repeatedly allowed to slide down the teat with pursed lips are being set up for failure once the shield is removed. Sliding pursed lips along the soft human nipple pushes it out of the mouth. LCs always want to consider that any movement provides for future normal function of the infant and promote as close to normal as the infant can perform."

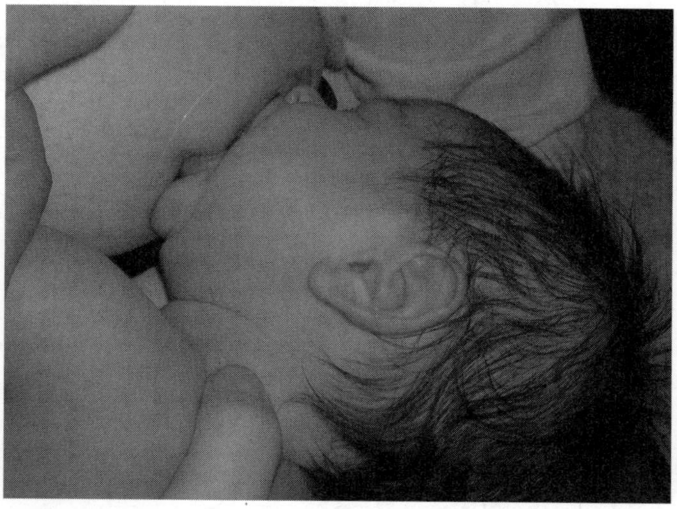

Figure B.14a Baby latched deeply with a nipple shield (wide gape, no tip showing). ©2020 Catherine Watson Genna, used with permission.

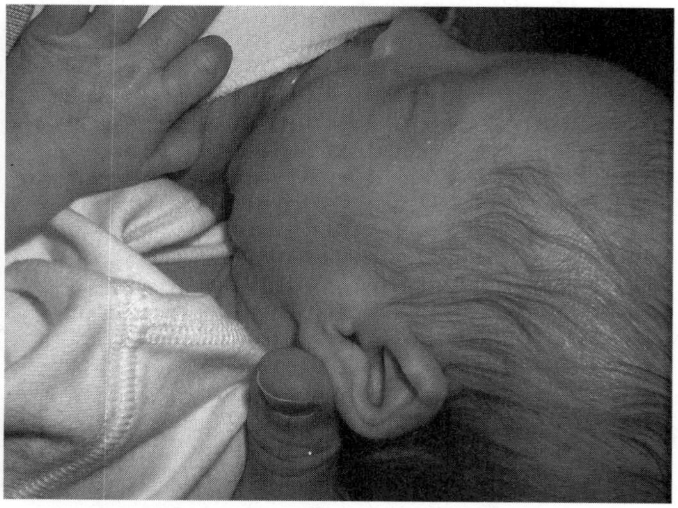

Figure B.14b Baby latched shallowly with a nipple shield (narrower gape, tip showing). Needs to be unlatched and latched deeper for effective feeding. ©2020 Catherine Watson Genna, used with permission.

Genna suggests starting baby in a "nose-to-nipple" position (see p. 879) with both lips on the underside of the shield to help mimic what he will do later on the bare gland.

Assessing feeding effectiveness with the nipple shield. After each feed, suggest looking for signs of effective feeding, such as milk in the tip of the shield and a decrease in mammary fullness. The baby's behavior can also provide clues. A satisfied baby will release the nipple when he's full. He may rest his head on the gland or be quietly alert, hands will be relaxed, and he will not begin to fuss right away if laid down. As a precaution, it is wise to have the baby's weight checked after a day or two on the shield and weekly after that to be sure he is getting enough milk and is stimulating adequate milk production.

Weaning from a Nipple Shield

The right time to wean from the shield will depend in large part on the reason it was used. For example, if it is used to help a baby who was bottle-feeding recognize the mammary gland as a source of milk, it may only be useful at one feed. But if the nursing couple was struggling with nursing for some time and the baby associates the parent's chest with frustration, a longer time of easier nursing to build positive associations may be better. The preterm baby using the nipple shield to improve milk intake may need to grow and mature for several weeks before he can feed well without the shield (P. P. Meier et al., 2000).

In one U.S. retrospective telephone survey of 202 mothers who used a nipple shield, 67% eventually weaned from the shield and breastfed without it, with the length of shield use ranging from 1 day to 5 months and the median duration 2 weeks (D. Powers & Tapia, 2004). Of the 33% who used the shield for the duration of nursing, 11% said the baby would have nursed without it at any time, but they continued using it because nursing was more comfortable with it. One mother used the nipple shield for the entire 15 months she and her baby nursed.

Strategy for weaning from the shield. When a shield is used for latching struggles, suggest starting nursing with the shield on. After milk ejection occurs and audible swallowing is heard, try removing the shield quickly, allowing baby to latch immediately. If the baby latches, use this strategy whenever needed to move from shield to bare nipple. Usually, as the baby becomes more coordinated and has more practice, the shield will be needed at fewer and fewer feeds.

If this strategy doesn't work, suggest parents continue using the shield throughout the feed and try again a few days later when parent and baby are feeling relaxed, perhaps at a time when the baby is not too hungry. Suggest keeping the parent's chest a pleasant place for the baby and avoid the stress of trying to nurse without the shield at every feed.

Encourage parents to use the shield as long as it helps the baby nurse more effectively. In general, as the baby matures, his coordination will increase. As he has more practice and develops more positive associations during nursing sessions, the easier it will be to wean him off the shield. A baby may need the shield for one feed, a few feeds, a few days, a few weeks, or very rarely, a few months. If the baby is unable or unwilling to nurse without the shield, chances are the problem that caused the baby to need the nipple shield is not yet completely resolved. Encourage parents to follow their baby's cues, but keep trying to nurse without the shield every few days.

Although it was once recommended to wean a baby from a nipple shield by gradually cutting off more of the tip of the shield until it is gone, this strategy is not recommended for the ultra-thin silicone shields used today. When cut, silicone has rough edges that can irritate the baby's mouth.

SCALES FOR WEIGHING BABIES

Scales can serve multiple purposes for nursing families. Regular pediatric scales can be used to monitor babies' weight gain. More accurate scales (to 2 g) can be used to measure babies' milk intake during nursing, known as test-weighing, which can be a vital part of pinpointing the cause of a lactation problem and finding an effective solution.

Indications for Use

Weight checks and test-weighing of nursing babies. Regular weight checks are a vital part of routine monitoring of healthy growth and development for all nursing babies. Test-weighing, on the other hand, may be helpful in some situations by allowing parents to monitor milk intake while a baby transitions from other feeding methods to exclusive nursing. Knowing baby's milk intake at each feed can prevent unnecessary supplementation or over-supplementation as baby weans off of other forms of nourishment. When dealing with lactation problems, test-weighing can also be useful to gauge a baby's milk intake during nursing. Even if there are no nursing problems, if parents are very anxious about their baby's milk intake, test-weighing can provide reassurance. It can also reveal when a baby is nursing ineffectively so that supplements can be started before the baby becomes severely underfed.

Test-weighing preterm babies. When a preterm baby begins nursing, test-weighing can be a helpful tool to determine milk intake. It can also prevent delays in initiating direct nursing, as some healthcare providers are reluctant to allow early nursing when a preterm baby's milk intake cannot be accurately measured. Knowing how much milk a preterm baby takes during nursing can prevent over-supplementation, which can delay the transition to full nursing (Hurst, Meier, Engstrom, & Myatt, 2004). In some countries, knowing how effectively a preterm baby nurses can also affect discharge plans, as feeding competence is usually one of the determining criteria (Nye, 2008).

Research on Weighing Babies

Parents' reactions to weighing babies. Some assume that regular weight checks and test-weighing increases parents' anxiety. A 2019 Irish mixed-methods study that interviewed 75 individuals, both public health nurses and new mothers (Hanafin, 2019) found these two groups had very different views about weighing babies at nursing support group meetings. The public health nurses, in keeping with their national policy, believed that mothers should be confident in their ability to breastfeed without relying on weighing their babies at these meetings. The mothers, on the other hand, viewed their infants' weight as an important and objective measure of their breastfeeding success and felt that having their baby's weight information could counter some of the negative attitudes they encountered.

Having a scale at home for daily weight checks. Is it anxiety producing for parents to do daily weight checks at home? Not for most, according to 2018 U.S. research. One cross-sectional sub-study within a larger prospective study examined responses from 69 mothers of term babies to its online survey about their experiences of doing daily weight checks at home with a pediatric baby scale for the first 2 weeks after hospital discharge (DiTomasso, Roberts, & Parker Cotton, 2018). Ninety percent of these mothers reported increased confidence in breastfeeding, although daily weight checks were most helpful to first-time mothers. In some cases, knowing their baby's weight convinced them to increase feeding frequency during this critical period. In another 2018 article that used data from this same survey (DiTomasso & Ferszt, 2018), researchers found that 81% felt positively about the use of the scale at home, 67% said it provided valuable knowledge, and 32% said it provided reassurance. The authors concluded that nursing parents may benefit from the use of a scale at home, which not only increases confidence, but can alert them early to problems that need attention. A 2014 Canadian qualitative interview study of eight mothers who participated in a larger study on infant weight loss after birth did daily weight checks at home during the first 14 days with a pediatric scale. The researchers (Noel-Weiss & Lada, 2014, p. 157) concluded:

> "The overall theme to emerge from the data was 'the baby scale as a tool' and five subthemes emerged: builds confidence, fosters reassurance, offers convenience, provides information, and satisfies curiosity....weighing babies did not cause mothers distress and worry; it usually provided reassurance."

Research on the accuracy of test-weighing. Dutch research (Savenije & Brand, 2006) found that the baby scales typically found in healthcare offices are not accurate enough to assess milk intake during nursing. U.S. research (P. P. Meier, Engstrom, Fleming, Streeter, & Lawrence, 1996) found that neither parents nor lactation consultants could accurately estimate preterm babies' milk intake during nursing by observing behaviors, such as audible swallowing and wide jaw movements. But doing pre- and post-feed weights with a scale accurate to 2 g was found reliable for measuring milk intake during nursing (P. P. Meier & Engstrom, 2007; Rankin et al., 2016). Even when hospitalized babies have leads (wires) attached that connect them to medical equipment, test-weighing was found to be reliable in measuring milk intake during nursing (Haase, Barreira, Murphy, Mueller, & Rhodes, 2009).

Test-weighing term babies. A 2015 study surveyed 120 mothers who participated in a previous study in which they did 24-hour test-weights with their nursing baby sometime between 2 and 14 weeks after birth. The survey measured their confidence in breastfeeding after undergoing the 24-hour test weights. The authors concluded that 66% of the mothers who were initially confident in nursing maintained their confidence after the test weights. Eleven percent of the mothers who were not confident originally became more confident after having an objective measure

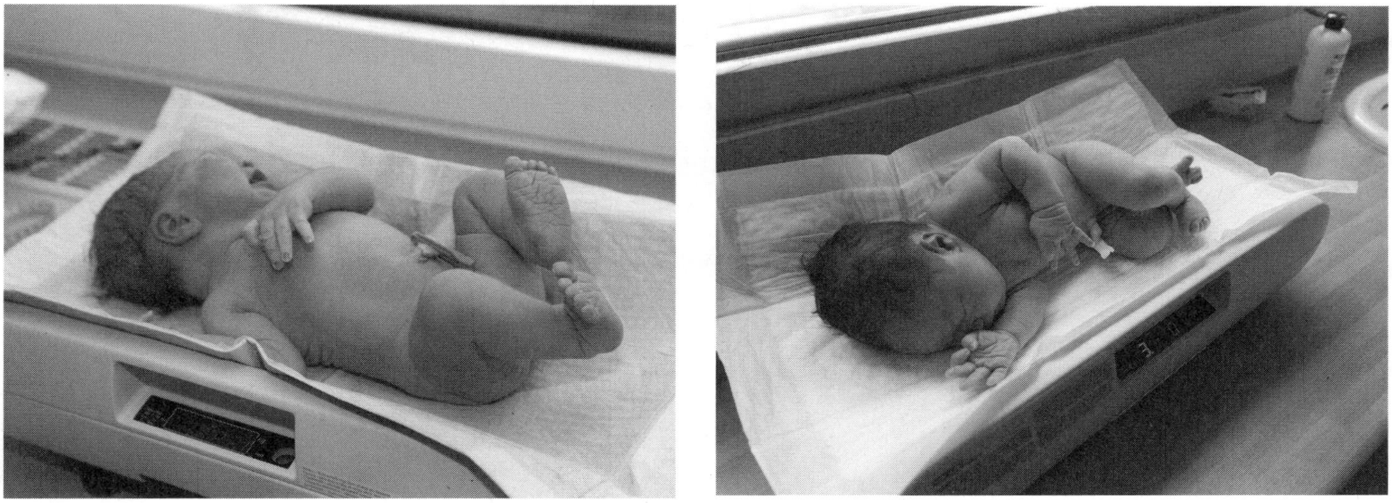

Figure B.15 The baby on the left is crying, which is not only upsetting, it takes longer to get a final weight. The baby on the right is calm. Either side-lying or tummy down positions make weights faster and more pleasant for everyone.

of their baby's milk intake. The authors concluded that this objective measure can be helpful to maintaining and improving confidence in nursing.

Test-weighing preterm babies. A U.S. study (Hurst et al., 2004) examined mothers' reactions to either using or not using a scale as they transitioned their preterm baby to breastfeeding. All the mothers who used the scale found it either very or extremely helpful, and 75% of the mothers who didn't use the scale reported it would have been somewhat to extremely helpful to them to know exactly how much milk their baby was taking at the breast. If parents find test-weighing stressful or low milk intake leaves them feeling discouraged, as an alternative, one strategy used in Sweden (Flacking, Nyqvist, Ewald, & Wallin, 2003) is to reduce the baby's supplement gradually, while carefully monitoring his weight and growth at regular check-ups.

Avoiding Test-Weighing Errors

Although the scales suitable for test-weighing are accurate to 2 g, common mistakes sometimes affect results.

- Don't weigh naked babies. If they urinate or defecate during the feed, the measure of milk intake will be inaccurate. At minimum baby should be in a diaper.
- Keep the same diaper on until the "after" weight is taken.
- Keep any clothing exactly the same. If a sock falls off or the baby's diaper is changed, the measure of milk intake will not be accurate.
- Milk dripped onto the baby's clothes either from dribbling during feeding or milk leaked onto the baby from the other side will also throw off the calculation.
- The extension of a blanket or baby's arm or leg over the side of the scale basket can affect the weight. Make sure baby and blanket stay inside the basket for both the before and after weights.

Weigh small babies either side-lying or tummy down. Newborns laid on their backs on a hard surface usually get upset and cry, which prolongs an electronic weighing process and may make it difficult or impossible for an electronic scale to lock in a weight. Most small babies find being weighed much less stressful if they are placed on their sides or on their tummies (Figure B.15).

Where to find scales for test-weighing. These very accurate scales are available in many hospitals, clinics, and lactation practices. In some areas, they can be rented for home use, usually from medical supply companies, lactation clinics, or breast-pump rental businesses. The scales that feature buttons to automatically calculate the difference between the before and after weights are made by the Japanese company Tanita. These scales are also rebranded through other companies, but they are available more economically from the manufacturer.

RESOURCES

Audelo, L. (2013). *The Virtual Breastfeeding Culture: Seeking Mother-to-Mother Support in the Digital Age.* Amarillo, TX: Praeclarus Press.

Breastfeeding Solutions app—Available from the App Store and Google Play for families and lactation specialists. When this app was provided to isolated breastfeeding mothers in rural Australia, exclusive nursing rates at 6 months were 80% compared with a local rate of 50%. (Wheaton et al., 2018).

Genna, C.W. (2016). *Selecting and Using Breastfeeding Tools: Improving Care and Outcomes.* Amarillo, TX: Praeclarus Press.

NaturalBreastfeeding.com/Professional—Annual subscription to the Professional Package offers licensing rights for the educational use of video clips, images, staff-training videos, and a digital lactation course that can be shared with an unlimited number of families.

Peterson, A. and M. Harmer. *Balancing Breast & Bottle: Reaching Your Breastfeeding Goals.* Amarillo, TX: Hale Publishing, 2010.

Wilson-Clay, B. & Hoover, K. (2017). *The Breastfeeding Atlas,* 6th ed. Manchaca, TX: LactNews Press.

REFERENCES

Aizawa, M., Mizuno, K., & Tamura, M. (2010). Neonatal sucking behavior: Comparison of perioral movement during breast-feeding and bottle feeding. *Pediatrics International, 52*(1), 104-108.

Alexander, J. M., Grant, A. M., & Campbell, M. J. (1992). Randomised controlled trial of breast shells and Hoffman's exercises for inverted and non-protractile nipples. *British Medical Journal, 304*(6833), 1030-1032.

Alianmoghaddam, N., Phibbs, S., & Benn, C. (2019). "I did a lot of Googling": A qualitative study of exclusive breastfeeding support through social media. *Women and Birth, 32*(2), 147-156.

Aloysius, A., & Hickson, M. (2007). Evaluation of paladai cup feeding in breast-fed preterm infants compared with bottle feeding. *Early Human Development, 83*(9), 619-621.

Amatayakul, K., Vutyavanich, T., Tanthayaphinant, O., et al. (1987). Serum prolactin and cortisol levels after suckling for varying periods of time and the effect of a nipple shield. *Acta Obstetricia et Gynecologica Scandinavica, 66*(1), 47-51.

Armstrong, H. C. (1987). Breastfeeding low birthweight babies: Advances in Kenya. *Journal of Human Lactation, 3*(2), 34-37.

Audelo, L. (2013). *The Virtual Breastfeeding Culture: Seeking Mother-to-Mother Support in the Digital Age.* Amarillo, TX: Praeclarus Press.

Auerbach, K. G. (1990). The effect of nipple shields on maternal milk volume. *Journal of Obstetric, Gynecologic & Neonatal Nursing, 19*(5), 419-427.

Bandara, S., Nyqvist, K. H., Musmar, S. M., et al. (2012). RoundTable discussion: Use of alternative feeding methods in the hospital. *Journal of Human Lactation, 28*(2), 122-124.

Batista, C. L. C., Ribeiro, V. S., Nascimento, M., et al. (2018). Association between pacifier use and bottle-feeding and unfavorable behaviors during breastfeeding. *Jornal de Pediatria* (Rio J), 94(6), 596-601.

Batista, C. L. C., Rodrigues, V. P., Ribeiro, V. S., et al. (2019). Nutritive and non-nutritive sucking patterns associated with pacifier use and bottle-feeding in full-term infants. *Early Human Development, 132,* 18-23.

Becker, G. E., Smith, H. A., & Cooney, F. (2016). Methods of milk expression for lactating women. *Cochrane Database of Systematic Reviews, 9,* CD006170. doi:10.1002/14651858.CD006170.pub5

Bergman, N. J., & Jurisoo, L. A. (1994). The 'kangaroo-method' for treating low birth weight babies in a developing country. *Tropical Doctor, 24*(2), 57-60.

Boronat-Catala, M., Montiel-Company, J. M., Bellot-Arcis, C., et al. (2017). Association between duration of breastfeeding and malocclusions in primary and mixed dentition: A systematic review and meta-analysis. *Scientific Reports, 7*(1), 5048.

Borucki, L. C. (2005). Breastfeeding mothers' experiences using a supplemental feeding tube device: Finding an alternative. *Journal of Human Lactation, 21*(4), 429-438.

Boucher-Horwitz, J. (2011). The use of supple cups for flat, retracting, and inverted nipples. *Clinical Lactation, 2*(3), 30-33.

Bridges, N., Howell, G., & Schmied, V. (2018). Exploring breastfeeding support on social media. *International Breastfeeding Journal, 13,* 22.

Buck, M. L., Amir, L. H., & Donath, S. M. (2015). Topical treatments used by breastfeeding women to treat sore and damaged nipples. *Clinical Lactation, 6*(1), 16-23.

Cadwell, K., Turner-Maffei, C., Blair, A., et al. (2004). Pain reduction and treatment of sore nipples in nursing mothers. *Journal of Perinatal Education, 13*(1), 29-35.

Chakrabarti, K., & Basu, S. (2011). Management of flat or inverted nipples with simple rubber bands. *Breastfeeding Medicine, 6*(4), 215-219.

Chanprapaph, P., Luttarapakul, J., Siribariruck, S., et al. (2013). Outcome of non-protractile nipple correction with breast cups in pregnant women: A randomized controlled trial. *Breastfeeding Medicine, 8*(4), 408-412.

Chertok, I. R. (2009). Reexamination of ultra-thin nipple shield use, infant growth and maternal satisfaction. *Journal of Clinical Nursing, 18*(21), 2949-2955.

Chow, S., Chow, R., Popovic, M., et al. (2015). The use of nipple shields: A review. *Front Public Health, 3,* 236.

Clum, D., & Primomo, J. (1996). Use of a silicone nipple shield with premature infants. *Journal of Human Lactation, 12*(4), 287-290.

Collins, C. T., Gillis, J., McPhee, A. J., et al. (2016). Avoidance of bottles during the establishment of breast feeds in preterm infants. *Cochrane Database of Systematic Reviews, 10,* CD005252. doi:10.1002/14651858.CD005252.pub4

Collins, C. T., Ryan, P., Crowther, C. A., et al. (2004). Effect of bottles, cups, and dummies on breast feeding in preterm infants: A randomised controlled trial. *British Medical Journal, 329*(7459), 193-198.

Dennis, C. L., Jackson, K., & Watson, J. (2014). Interventions for treating painful nipples among breastfeeding women. *Cochrane Database of Systematic Reviews, 12,* Cd007366. doi:10.1002/14651858.CD007366.pub2

Dennis, C. L., Schottle, N., Hodnett, E., et al. (2012). An all-purpose nipple ointment versus lanolin in treating painful damaged nipples in breastfeeding women: A randomized controlled trial. *Breastfeeding Medicine, 7*(6), 473-479.

DiTomasso, D., & Ferszt, G. (2018). Mothers' thoughts and feelings about using a pediatric scale in the home to monitor weight changes in breastfed newborns. *Nursing for Women's Health, 22*(6), 463-470.

DiTomasso, D., Roberts, M., & Parker Cotton, B. (2018). Postpartum mothers' experiences with newborn weight checks in the home. *Journal of Perinatal & Neonatal Nursing, 32*(4), 333-340.

Dowling, D. A., Meier, P. P., DiFiore, J. M., et al. (2002). Cup-feeding for preterm infants: Mechanics and safety. *Journal of Human Lactation, 18*(1), 13-20; quiz 46-19, 72.

Eglash, A., Ziemer, A. L., & Chevalier, A. (2010). Health professionals' attitudes and use of nipple shields for breastfeeding women. *Breastfeeding Medicine, 5*(4), 147-151.

Egnell, E. (1956). The mechanics of different methods of emptying the female breast. *Svenska Lakartidningen*(40), 1-7.

Flacking, R., & Dykes, F. (2017). Perceptions and experiences of using a nipple shield among parents and staff - An ethnographic study in neonatal units. *BMC Pregnancy and Childbirth, 17*(1), 1.

Flacking, R., Nyqvist, K. H., Ewald, U., et al. (2003). Long-term duration of breastfeeding in Swedish low birth weight infants. *Journal of Human Lactation, 19*(2), 157-165.

Flint, A., New, K., & Davies, M. W. (2016). Cup feeding versus other forms of supplemental enteral feeding for newborn infants unable to fully breastfeed. *Cochrane Database of Systematic Reviews*(8), CD005092. doi:10.1002/14651858.CD005092.pub3

Franca, E. C., Sousa, C. B., Aragao, L. C., et al. (2014). Electromyographic analysis of masseter muscle in newborns during suction in breast, bottle or cup feeding. *BMC Pregnancy and Childbirth, 14,* 154.

Francis, J., & Dickton, D. (2019). Physical analysis of the breast after direct breastfeeding compared with hand or pump expression: A randomized clinical trial. *Breastfeeding Medicine, 14*(10), 705-711.

Geddes, D. T., Chooi, K., Nancarrow, K., et al. (2017). Characterisation of sucking dynamics of breastfeeding preterm infants: A cross sectional study. *BMC Pregnancy and Childbirth, 17*(1), 386.

Genna, C. W. (2016). *Selecting and Using Breastfeeding Tools: Improving Care and Outcomes.* Amarillo, TX: Praeclarus Press.

Genna, C. W. (2017). The influence of anatomic and structural issues on sucking skills. In C. W. Genna (Ed.), *Supporting Sucking Skills in Breastfeeding Infants* (3rd ed., pp. 209-267). Burlington, MA: Jones & Bartlett Learning.

Genna, C. W., LeVan Fram, J., & Sandora, L. (2017). Neurological issues and breastfeeding. In C. W. Genna (Ed.), *Supporting Sucking Skills in Breastfeeding Infants* (3rd ed., pp. 335-397). Burlington, MA: Jones & Bartlett Learning.

Gribble, K., Berry, N., Kerac, M., et al. (2017). Volume marker inaccuracies: A cross-sectional survey of infant feeding bottles. *Maternal and Child Nutrition, 13*(3).

Gupta, A., Khanna, K., & Chattree, S. (1999). Cup feeding: An alternative to bottle feeding in a neonatal intensive care unit. *Journal of Tropical Pediatrics, 45*(2), 108-110.

Haase, B., Barreira, J., Murphy, P. K., et al. (2009). The development of an accurate test weighing technique for preterm and high-risk hospitalized infants. *Breastfeeding Medicine, 4*(3), 151-156.

Habibi, M. F., Springer, C. M., Spence, M. L., et al. (2018). Use of videoconferencing for lactation consultation: An online cross-sectional survey of mothers' acceptance in the United States. *Journal of Human Lactation, 34*(2), 313-321.

Hanafin, S. (2019). Views of public health nurses and mothers on weighing infants at breastfeeding support groups. *Journal of Health Visiting, 7*(2), 85-91.

Hernandez, A. M., & Bianchini, E. M. G. (2019). Swallowing analyses of neonates and infants in breastfeeding and bottle-feeding: Impact on videofluoroscopy swallow studies. *International Archives of Otorhinolaryngology, 23*(3), e343-e353.

Howard, C. R., de Blieck, E. A., ten Hoopen, C. B., et al. (1999). Physiologic stability of newborns during cup- and bottle-feeding. *Pediatrics, 104*(5 Pt 2), 1204-1207.

Howard, C. R., Howard, F. M., Lanphear, B., et al. (2003). Randomized clinical trial of pacifier use and bottle-feeding or cupfeeding and their effect on breastfeeding. *Pediatrics, 111*(3), 511-518.

Huang, Y. Y., Gau, M. L., Huang, C. M., et al. (2009). Supplementation with cup-feeding as a substitute for bottle-feeding to promote breastfeeding. *Chang Gung Medical Journal, 32*(4), 423-431.

Hurst, N. M., Meier, P. P., Engstrom, J. L., et al. (2004). Mothers performing in-home measurement of milk intake during breastfeeding of their preterm infants: Maternal reactions and feeding outcomes. *Journal of Human Lactation, 20*(2), 178-187.

Hussien, N. N., Refaat, D. O., & Arafa, N. E. (2019). Alternative feeding techniques and its effect on breastfeeding self-efficacy. *Journal of Family Medicine and Health Care, 5*(2), 22-27.

Jackson, K. T., & Dennis, C. L. (2017). Lanolin for the treatment of nipple pain in breastfeeding women: A randomized controlled trial. *Maternal & Child Nutrition, 13*(3).

Jones, E., Dimmock, P. W., & Spencer, S. A. (2001). A randomised controlled trial to compare methods of milk expression after preterm delivery. *Archives of Disease in Childhood. Fetal and Neonatal Edition, 85*(2), F91-95.

Kassing, D. (2002). Bottle-feeding as a tool to reinforce breastfeeding. *Journal of Human Lactation, 18*(1), 56-60.

Keemer, F. (2013). Breastfeeding self-efficacy of women using second-line strategies for healthy term infants in the first week postpartum: An Australian observational study. *International Breastfeeding Journal, 8*(1), 18.

Kent, J. C., Hepworth, A. R., Sherriff, J. L., et al. (2013). Longitudinal changes in breastfeeding patterns from 1 to 6 months of lactation. *Breastfeeding Medicine, 8,* 401-407.

Kent, J. C., Ramsay, D. T., Doherty, D., et al. (2003). Response of breasts to different stimulation patterns of an electric breast pump. *Journal of Human Lactation, 19*(2), 179-186; quiz 187-178, 218.

Kesaree, N., Banapurmath, C. R., Banapurmath, S., et al. (1993). Treatment of inverted nipples using a disposable syringe. *Journal of Human Lactation, 9*(1), 27-29.

Kliethermes, P. A., Cross, M. L., Lanese, M. G., et al. (1999). Transitioning preterm infants with nasogastric tube supplementation: Increased likelihood of breastfeeding. *Journal of Obstetric, Gynecologic & Neonatal Nursing, 28*(3), 264-273.

Kronborg, H., Foverskov, E., Nilsson, I., et al. (2017). Why do mothers use nipple shields and how does this influence duration of exclusive breastfeeding? *Maternal and Child Nutrition, 13*(1).

Lang, S., Lawrence, C. J., & Orme, R. L. (1994). Cup feeding: An alternative method of infant feeding. *Archives of Disease in Childhood, 71*(4), 365-369.

Maastrup, R., Hansen, B. M., Kronborg, H., et al. (2014). Factors associated with exclusive breastfeeding of preterm infants. Results from a prospective national cohort study. *PLoS One, 9*(2), e89077.

MAIN. (1994). Preparing for breast feeding: Treatment of inverted and non-protractile nipples in pregnancy. The MAIN Trial Collaborative Group. *Midwifery, 10*(4), 200-214.

Malhotra, N., Vishwambaran, L., Sundaram, K. R., et al. (1999a). A controlled trial of alternative methods of oral feeding in neonates. *Early Human Development, 54*(1), 29-38.

Malhotra, N., Vishwambaran, L., Sundaram, K. R., et al. (1999b). A controlled trial of alternative methods of oral feeding in neonates. *Early Human Development, 54*(1), 29-38. doi:S0378378298000826 [pii]

Marinelli, K. A., Burke, G. S., & Dodd, V. L. (2001). A comparison of the safety of cupfeedings and bottlefeedings in premature infants whose mothers intend to breastfeed. *Journal of Perinatology, 21*(6), 350-355.

McCulloch, J., & McCann, A. (2017). Communicating to connect-Reaching today's new families. *Journal of Human Lactation, 33*(3), 570-572.

McGeorge, D. D. (1994). The "Niplette": An instrument for the non-surgical correction of inverted nipples. *British Journal of Plastic Surgery, 47*(1), 46-49.

McKechnie, A. C., & Eglash, A. (2010). Nipple shields: A review of the literature. *Breastfeeding Medicine, 5*(6), 309-314. doi:10.1089/bfm.2010.0003

Meier, P. (2004). Choosing a correctly-fitted breastshield. *Medela Messenger, 21,* 8-9.

Meier, P. P., Brown, L. P., Hurst, N. M., et al. (2000). Nipple shields for preterm infants: Effect on milk transfer and duration of breastfeeding. *Journal of Human Lactation, 16*(2), 106-114; quiz 129-131.

Meier, P. P., & Engstrom, J. L. (2007). Test weighing for term and premature infants is an accurate procedure. *Archives of Disease in Childhood. Fetal and Neonatal Edition, 92*(2), F155-156.

Meier, P. P., Engstrom, J. L., Fleming, B. A., et al. (1996). Estimating milk intake of hospitalized preterm infants who breastfeed. *Journal of Human Lactation, 12*(1), 21-26.

Meier, P. P., Engstrom, J. L., Hurst, N. M., et al. (2008). A comparison of the efficiency, efficacy, comfort, and convenience of two hospital-grade electric breast pumps for mothers of very low birthweight infants. *Breastfeeding Medicine, 3*(3), 141-150.

Mohrbacher, N. (2015). Hi-Tech breastfeeding tools: Meeting the needs of today's parents. *International Journal of Childbirth Education, 30*(4), 1-4.

Moreira, C. M. D., Cavalcante-Silva, R., Fujinaga, C. I., et al. (2017). Comparison of the finger-feeding versus cup feeding methods in the transition from gastric to oral feeding in preterm infants. *Jornal de Pediatria (Rio de Janeiro), 93*(6), 585-591.

Newman, J. (2016). Lactation aid. Retrieved from **ibconline.ca/information-sheets/lactation-aid/**.

Noel-Weiss, J., & Lada, N. S. (2014). Mothers' experiences with baby scales in the first two weeks post birth: A qualitative study. *Journal of Women's Health Care, 3*(3), 157.

Nye, C. (2008). Transitioning premature infants from gavage to breast. *Neonatal Network, 27*(1), 7-13.

Nyqvist, K. H. (2017). Breastfeeding preterm infants. In C. W. Genna (Ed.), *Supporting Sucking Skills in Breastfeeding Infants* (3rd ed., pp. 181-208). Burlington, MA: Jones & Bartlett Learning.

Nyqvist, K. H., & Ewald, U. (2006). Surface electromyography of facial muscles during natural and artificial feeding of infants: Identification of differences between breast-, cup- and bottle-feeding. *Jornal de Pediatria (Rio de Janeiro), 82*(2), 85-86.

O'Sullivan, T. A., Cooke, J., McCafferty, C., et al. (2019). Online video instruction on hand expression of colostrum in pregnancy is an effective educational tool. *Nutrients, 11*(4).

Pados, B. F., Park, J., & Dodrill, P. (2019). Know the flow: Milk flow rates from bottle nipples used in the hospital and after discharge. *Advances in Neonatal Care, 19*(1), 32-41.

Penny, F., Judge, M., Brownell, E., et al. (2018a). Cup feeding as a supplemental, alternative feeding method for preterm breastfed infants: An integrative review. *Maternal and Child Health Journal, 22*(11), 1568-1579.

Penny, F., Judge, M., Brownell, E., et al. (2018b). What is the evidence for use of a supplemental feeding tube device as an alternative supplemental feeding method for breastfed infants? *Advances in Neonatal Care, 18*(1), 31-37.

Penny, F., Judge, M., Brownell, E. A., et al. (2019). International board certified lactation consultants' practices regarding supplemental feeding methods for breastfed infants. *Journal of Human Lactation, 35*(4), 683-694.

Perrella, S. L., & Geddes, D. T. (2016). A case report of a breastfed infant's excessive weight gains over 14 months. *Journal of Human Lactation, 32*(2), 364-368.

Peterson, A., & Harmer, M. (2010). *Balancing Breast and Bottle: Reaching Your Breastfeeding Goals.* Amarillo, TX: Hale Publishing.

Pincombe, J., Baghurst, P., Antoniou, G., et al. (2008). Baby Friendly Hospital Initiative practices and breast feeding duration in a cohort of first-time mothers in Adelaide, Australia. *Midwifery, 24*(1), 55-61.

Pitts, A., Faucher, M. A., & Spencer, R. (2015). Incorporating breastfeeding education into prenatal care. *Breastfeeding Medicine, 10*(2), 118-123.

Powers, D., & Tapia, V. B. (2004). Women's experiences using a nipple shield. *Journal of Human Lactation, 20*(3), 327-334.

Powers, D. C., & Tapia, V. B. (2012). Clinical decision making when to consider using a nipple shield. *Clinical Lactation, 3*(1), 26-29.

Puapornpong, P., Raungrongmorakot, K., Hemachandra, A., et al. (2015). Comparisons of latching on between newborns fed with feeding tubes and cup feedings. *Journal of the Medical Association of Thailand, 98 Suppl 9,* S61-65.

Ramsay, D. T., Mitoulas, L. R., Kent, J. C., et al. (2006). Milk flow rates can be used to identify and investigate milk ejection in women expressing breast milk using an electric breast pump. *Breastfeeding Medicine, 1*(1), 14-23.

Rankin, M. W., Jimenez, E. Y., Caraco, M., et al. (2016). Validation of test weighing protocol to estimate enteral feeding volumes in preterm infants. *Journal of Pediatrics, 178,* 108-112.

Savenije, O. E., & Brand, P. L. (2006). Accuracy and precision of test weighing to assess milk intake in newborn infants. *Archives of Disease in Childhood. Fetal and Neonatal Edition, 91*(5), F330-332.

Say, B., Buyuktiruaki, M., Okur, N., et al. (2019). Evaluation of syringe feeding compared to botle feeding for the transition from gavage feding to oral feeding in preterm infants. *Journal of Pediatric Research, 6*(2), 94-98.

Taki, M., Mizuno, K., Murase, M., et al. (2010). Maturational changes in the feeding behaviour of infants - A comparison between breast-feeding and bottle-feeding. *Acta Paediatrica, 99*(1), 61-67.

Walker, M. (2016). Nipple shields: What we know, what we wish we knew, and how best to use them. *Clinical Lactation, 7*(3), 100-107.

Wheaton, N., Lenehan, J., & Amir, L. H. (2018). Evaluation of a breastfeeding app in rural Australia: Prospective cohort study. *Journal of Human Lactation, 34*(4), 711-720.

Wilson-Clay, B., & Hoover, K. (2017). *The Breastfeeding Atlas* (6th ed.). Manchaca, TX: LactNews Press.

Witt, A. M., Burgess, K., Hawn, T. R., et al. (2014). Role of oral antibiotics in treatment of breastfeeding women with chronic breast pain who fail conservative therapy. *Breastfeeding Medicine, 9*(2), 63-72.

Wood, C. T., Skinner, A. C., Yin, H. S., et al. (2016). Bottle size and weight gain in formula-fed infants. *Pediatrics, 138*(1).

Woolridge, M. W., Baum, J. D., & Drewett, R. F. (1980). Effect of a traditional and of a new nipple shield on sucking patterns and milk flow. *Early Human Development, 4*(4), 357-364.

Index

A

B

D

G

H

I

J

K

L

M

N

O

P

Q

R

S

T

U

V

W

X

Y

Z